Target Organ Toxicology Series

Immunotoxicology and Immunopharmacology

Second Edition

Target Organ Toxicology Series

Series Editors

A. Wallace Hayes, John A. Thomas, and Donald E. Gardner

Immunotoxicology and Immunopharmacology, Second Edition
Jack H. Dean, Michael I. Luster, Albert E. Munson, and Ian Kimber, editors, 784 pp., 1994

Nutrition Toxicology
Frank N. Kotsonis, Maureen Mackey, and Jerry J. Hjelle, editors, 336 pp., 1994

Carcinogenesis
Michael P. Waalkes and Jerrold M. Ward, editors, 496 pp., 1994

Toxicology of the Lung, Second Edition
Donald E. Gardner, James D. Crapo, and Roger O. McClellan, editors, 688 pp., 1993

Cardiovascular Toxicology, Second Edition
Daniel Acosta, Jr., editor, 576 pp., 1992

Ophthalmic Toxicology
George C. Y. Chiou, editor, 352 pp., 1992

Neurotoxicology
Hugh A. Tilson and Clifford L. Mitchell, editors, 416 pp., 1992

Toxicology of the Lung
Donald E. Gardner, James D. Crapo, and Edward J. Massaro, editors, 540 pp., 1988

Endocrine Toxicology
John A. Thomas, Kenneth S. Korach, and John A. McLachlan, editors, 414 pp., 1985

Immunotoxicology and Immunopharmacology
Jack H. Dean, Michael I. Luster, Albert E. Munson, and Harry Amos, editors, 528 pp., 1985

***Reproductive Toxicology**
Robert L. Dixon, editor, 368 pp., 1985

Toxicology of the Blood and Bone Marrow
Richard D. Irons, editor, 192 pp., 1985

Toxicology of the Eye, Ear, and Other Special Senses
A. Wallace Hayes, editor, 264 pp., 1985

***Toxicology of the Immune System**
Jack H. Dean and Albert E. Munson, editors, 528 pp., 1985

Cutaneous Toxicity
Victor A. Drill and Paul Lazar, editors, 288 pp., 1984

Intestinal Toxicology
Carol M. Schiller, editor, 252 pp., 1984

---

*Out of print.

Target Organ Toxicology Series

Immunotoxicology and Immunopharmacology

Second Edition

Editors

Jack H. Dean, Ph.D., Diplomate A.B.T.

Executive Vice President
Drug Development
Sterling Winthrop Pharmaceuticals Research Division
Sterling Winthrop Inc.
Collegeville, Pennsylvania

Michael I. Luster, Ph.D.

Section Head, Department of Environmental
Immunology and Neurobiology
Laboratory of Biochemical Risk Analysis
Division of Intramural Research
National Institute of Environmental Health Sciences
Research Triangle Park, North Carolina

Albert E. Munson, Ph.D.

Professor, Department of Pharmacology and Toxicology
Medical College of Virginia
Virginia Commonwealth University
Richmond, Virginia

Ian Kimber, Ph.D.

Head, Research Toxicology Section
ZENECA Central Toxicology Laboratory
Macclesfield, Cheshire, United Kingdom

Raven Press New York

Raven Press, Ltd., 1185 Avenue of the Americas, New York, New York 10036

Made in the United States of America

Library of Congress Cataloging-in-Publication Data

Immunotoxicology and immunopharmacology / editors, Jack H. Dean . . .
[et al.]. — 2nd ed.
p. cm.
Includes bibliographical references and index.
ISBN 0-7817-0219-4
1. Immunotoxicology. 2. Immunopharmacology. I. Dean, Jack H.
[DNLM: 1. Immunotoxins—pharmacology. 2. Immune System—drug effects. 3. Immunity—drug effects. 4. Immune System—immunology.
QW 630 I325 1994]
RC582.17.I46 1994
616.97—dc20
DNLM/DLC
for Library of Congress 94-11198
CIP

---

9 8 7 6 5 4 3 2 1

Contents

Immunotoxicity and the Skin

Selective Immunotoxicity

Autoimmunity

Clinical Aspects of Hypersensitivity

Contributing Authors

Steven G. Armstrong, Ph.D.
Department of Pharmacology
Dalhousie University
Sir Charles Tupper Medical Building
Halifax, Nova Scotia, B3H 4H7, Canada

John B. Barnett, Ph.D.
Professor of Microbiology and Immunology
Departments of Microbiology and Immunology
West Virginia University School of Medicine
2095 Health Sciences North, P.O. Box 9177
Morgantown, West Virginia 26506

David A. Basketter, B.Sc.
Immunology Group Manager
Department of Biology
Unilever Environmental Safety Laboratory
Colworth House
Sharnbrook, MK44 1LQ United Kingdom

Blanche Bellon, Ph.D.
INSERM U28
Hospital Broussais
96 rue Didot
75674 Paris Cedex, France

I. Leonard Bernstein, M.D.
Department of Internal Medicine
Division of Immunology and Allergy
University of Cincinnati Medical Center
231 Bethesda Avenue
Cincinnati, Ohio 45267

Jonathan A. Bernstein, M.D.
Assistant Professor of Clinical Medicine
Department of Internal Medicine
Division of Immunology and Allergy
University of Cincinnati Medical Center
231 Bethesda Avenue, ML-563
Cincinnati, Ohio 45267

Raymond E. Biagini, Ph.D.
Research Toxicologist
Applied Biology Branch
Immunochemistry Research Section
Division of Biomedical and Behavioral Sciences
Centers for Disease Control and Prevention
National Institute for Occupational Safety and Health
4676 Columbia Parkway
Cincinnati, Ohio 45226

Nanne Bloksma, Ph.D.
Associate Professor of Immunotoxicology
Research Institute of Toxicology
Section of Immunotoxicology
Utrect University
Yalellan 2, P.O. Box 80.176
NL 3508 TD Utrect, The Netherlands

Genevieve S. Bondy, Ph.D.
Research Scientist
Toxicology Research Division
Food Directorate
Health Protection Branch
Health Canada
Ottawa, Ontario, K1A OL2, Canada

Philip A. Botham, Ph.D.
ZENECA Central Toxicology Laboratory
Alderley Park
Macclesfield, Cheshire, SK10 4TJ United Kingdom

Florence G. Burleson, Ph.D.
Environmental Immunology and Neurobiology Section
National Institute of Environmental Health Sciences
Research Triangle Park, North Carolina 27709

Gary R. Burleson, Ph.D.
Miami Valley Laboratory
Procter & Gamble
P.O. Box 398707
Cincinnati, Ohio 45239

Leigh Ann Burns, Ph.D.
Department of Immunology
Mayo Clinic and Foundation
Guggenheim, Room 338
Rochester, Minnesota 55905

Bruce D. Car, Ph.D.
Professor
Institute of Toxicology
University of Zürich
Schorenstrasse 16
CH-8603 Schwerzenbach ZH, Switzerland

Maria Castedo, Ph.D.
INSERM U28
Hospital Broussais
96 rue Didot
75674 Paris Cedex, France

John W. Coleman, Ph.D.
Senior Lecturer
Department of Pharmacology and Therapeutics
University of Liverpool
P.O. Box 147
Liverpool, L69 3BX, United Kingdom

Christine E. Comment, ASCP
Department of Occupational and Environmental Medicine
National Jewish Center for Immunology and Respiratory Medicine
1400 Jackson Street, Room D311
Denver, Colorado 80206

Jack H. Dean, Ph.D., Diplomate A.B.T.
Executive Vice President
Drug Development
Sterling Winthrop Pharmaceuticals Research Division
Sterling Winthrop Inc.
P.O. Box 5000
Collegeville, Pennsylvania 19426

Rebecca J. Dearman, Ph.D.
Immunology Group
Research Toxicology Section
ZENECA Central Toxicology Laboratory
Alderley Park
Macclesfield, Cheshire, SK10 4TJ United Kingdom

Jacques G. Descotes, M.D., Ph.D., Pharm.D.
Professor of Medical Pharmacology
Laboratory of Fundamental and Clinical Immunotoxicology
INSERM 80
Alexis Carrel Faculty of Medicine
69008 Lyon, France

Philippe Druet, M.D.
Professor of Medicine
Department of Nephrology
INSERM U28
Hospital Broussais
University of Paris
96 rue Didot
75674 Paris Cedex, France

Craig A. Elmets, M.D.
Professor of Dermatology and Environmental Health Sciences
Director of Skin Diseases Research Center
Department of Dermatology
Case Western Reserve University
University Hospital of Cleveland
11100 Euclid Avenue
Cleveland, Ohio 44106

Hans-Pietro Eugster, M.D.
Professor
Institute of Toxicology
University of Zürich
Schorenstrasse 16
CH-8603 Schwerzenbach ZH, Switzerland

Herman Friedman, Ph.D.
Professor and Chairman of Medical Microbiology and Immunology
Department of Medical Microbiology and Immunology
University of South Florida College of Medicine
12901 Bruce B. Downs Boulevard
Tampa, Florida 33612

Peter S. Friedmann, M.D., F.R.C.P.
Professor of Dermatology
Department of Medicine
University of Liverpool
Royal Liverpool University Hospital
P.O. Box 147
Liverpool, L69 3BX, United Kingdom

G. Frank Gerberick, Ph.D.
Section Head
Human Safety Division
Procter & Gamble
P.O. Box 398707
Cincinnati, Ohio 45239

Dori R. Germolec, M.A.
Biologist
Environmental Immunology and Neurobiology Section
National Institute of Environmental Health Sciences
111 TW Alexander Drive
Research Triangle Park, North Carolina 27709

Matthew I. Gilmour, Ph.D.
Research Associate
Center for Environmental Medicine and Lung Biology
University of North Carolina
Medical Research Building C, CB 7310
Chapel Hill, North Carolina 27599

Niranjan S. Goud, Ph.D.
Assistant Professor
Department of Microbiology and Immunology
University of Kentucky College of Medicine
800 Rose Street
Lexington, Kentucky 40536

Lesley Helyar, Ph.D.
Research Associate
Department of Pharmacology and Toxicology
Rutgers University
681 Frelinghuysen Road
Piscataway, New Jersey 08855

Gerry M. Henningsen, D.V.M., Ph.D.
Regional Senior Toxicologist
United States Public Health Service
United States Environmental Protection Agency
999 18th Street, Region 8, Suite 500
Denver, Colorado 80202

Thomas W. Hesterberg, Ph.D.
Senior Toxicologist
Department of Health, Safety, and Environment
Schuller International, Inc.
P.O. Box 625005
Littleton, Colorado 80162

Thomas R. Jerrells, Ph.D.
Professor of Cellular Biology
Department of Cellular Biology and Anatomy
Louisiana State University Medical Center
1501 Kings Highway
Shreveport, Louisiana 71130

Mikael B. Jondal, M.D., Ph.D.
Professor of Immunology
Departments of Microbiology and Tumor Biology
Karolinska Institute
S-171 77 Stockholm, Sweden

Norbert E. Kaminski, Ph.D.
Assistant Professor
Departments of Pharmacology and Toxicology
Michigan State University
Life Sciences Building
East Lansing, Michigan 48824

Michael E. Kammüller, Ph.D.
Department of Drug Safety and Toxicology
Sandoz Pharma, Ltd.
CH-4002 Basel, Switzerland

Alan M. Kaplan, Ph.D.
Professor of Microbiology and Immunology
Department of Microbiology and Immunology
University of Kentucky College of Medicine
800 Rose Street
Lexington, Kentucky 40536

Meryl H. Karol, Ph.D.
Professor of Environmental and Occupational Health
Department of Environmental and Occupational Health
University of Pittsburgh
260 Kappa Drive
Pittsburgh, Pennsylvania 15238

Thomas T. Kawabata, Ph.D.
Research Scientist
Procter & Gamble
P.O. Box 398707
Cincinnati, Ohio 45239

Fujio Kayama, M.D., Ph.D.
Instructor
Department of Environmental Health
University of Occupational and Environmental Health
P.O. Orio
Kitakyushu 807, Japan

Nancy I. Kerkvliet, Ph.D.
Department of Agriculture Chemistry and Environmental Health Sciences
Oregon State University
Agricultural and Life Sciences 1007
Corvallis, Oregon 97331

Kaye H. Kilburn, M.D.
Professor of Medicine
Department of Medicine
Division of Pulmonary
University of Southern California School of Medicine
2025 Zonal Avenue, CSC 201
Los Angeles, California 90033

Ian Kimber, Ph.D.
Head, Research Toxicology Section
ZENECA Central Toxicology Laboratory
Alderley Park
Macclesfield, Cheshire, SK10 4TJ United Kingdom

Thomas W. Klein, Ph.D.
Professor of Immunology
Department of Medical Microbiology and Immunology
University of South Florida College of Medicine
12901 Bruce B. Downs Boulevard
Tampa, Florida 33612

Michael Kowolenko, Ph.D.
Senior Scientist
Department of Pre-Clinical Biology
Miles Pharmaceutical Company
400 Morgan Lane
West Haven, Connecticut 06516

Gregory S. Ladics, Ph.D.
Research Toxicologist
Department of Central Research and Development
DuPont Company
Haskell Laboratory
P.O. Box 50
Newark, Delaware 19714

Debra L. Laskin, Ph.D.
Professor
Department of Pharmacology and Toxicology
Rutgers University
681 Frelinghuysen Road
Piscataway, New Jersey 08855

David G. LeVier, Ph.D.
Department of Pharmacology and Toxicology
Medical College of Virginia
Virginia Commonwealth University
P.O. Box 98063
Richmond, Virginia 23298

Michael I. Luster, Ph.D.
Head, Environmental Immunology and Neurobiology Section
Laboratory of Biochemical Risk Analysis
Division of Intramural Research
National Institute of Environmental Health Sciences
P.O. Box 12233
Research Triangle Park, North Carolina 27709

Michael J. McCabe, Jr., Ph.D.
Assistant Professor
Institute of Chemical Toxicology
Wayne State University
2727 Second Avenue
Detroit, Michigan 48201

David J. McConkey, Ph.D.
Assistant Professor of Cell Biology
Department of Cell Biology
University of Texas
M.D. Anderson Cancer Center
1515 Holcombe Boulevard, Box 173
Houston, Texas 77030

Hasan Mukhtar, Ph.D.
Professor, Director of Research
Department of Dermatology
Case Western Reserve University
2074 Abington Road
Cleveland, Ohio 44106

Albert E. Munson, Ph.D.
Professor
Department of Pharmacology and Toxicology
Medical College of Virginia
Virginia Commonwealth University
527 North 12th Street, Box 98063
Richmond, Virginia 23298

Lee S. Newman, M.D.
Associate Professor of Medicine and Preventive Medicine
Department of Medicine
Occupational and Environmental Medicine Division
Pulmonary Division
National Jewish Center for Immunology and Respiratory Medicine
University of Colorado School of Medicine
1400 Jackson Street, Room D-104
Denver, Colorado 80206

Sten G. Orrenius, M.D.
Professor
Institute of Environmental Medicine
Karolinska Institute
Tomtebodavagen 30, Box 210
S-171 77 Stockholm, Sweden

Gabriel S. Panayi, M.D., F.R.C.P.
Professor of Rheumatology
Rheumatology Unit
Guy's Hospital
London SE1 9RT, United Kingdom

Lucette Pelletier, M.D., Ph.D.
INSERM U28
Hospital Broussais
96 rue Didot
75674 Paris Cedex, France

James J. Pestka, Ph.D.
Professor
Department of Food Science and Human Nutrition
Michigan State University
234A Trout Food Science and Human Nutrition Building
East Lansing, Michigan 48824

Stephen B. Pruett, Ph.D.
Associate Professor of Immunology
Department of Biological Sciences
Mississippi State University
Harned Biology Building, Room 130
P.O. Drawer GY
Mississippi State, Mississippi 39762

Kenneth W. Renton, Ph.D.
Professor and Head of Pharmacology
Department of Pharmacology
Dalhousie University
Sir Charles Tupper Medical Building
Halifax, Nova Scotia, B3H 4H7, Canada

Jorge M. Rivas, Ph.D.
Department of Immunology
University of Texas
M.D. Anderson Cancer Center
1515 Holcombe Boulevard
Houston, Texas 77030

Kathleen E. Rodgers, Ph.D.
Research Associate Professor
Department of Obstetrics and Gynecology
University of Southern California
Livingston Research Center
1321 North Mission Road
Los Angeles, California 90033

Noel R. Rose, M.D., Ph.D.
Professor of Immunology and Infectious Diseases, Medicine, and Environmental Health Sciences
Department of Immunology and Infectious Diseases
Johns Hopkins University School of Hygiene and Public Health
615 North Wolfe Street
Baltimore, Maryland 21205

Gary J. Rosenthal, Ph.D.
Director of Pharmacology and Toxicology
Department of Drug Development
Somatogen Inc.
2545 Central Avenue
Boulder, Colorado 80301

Bernhard Ryffel, M.D., Ph.D.
Professor
Institute of Toxicology
University of Zürich
Schorenstrasse 16
CH-8603 Schwerzenbach ZH, Switzerland

Katherine Sarlo, Ph.D.
Senior Research Scientist
Procter & Gamble
P.O. Box 398707
Cincinnati, Ohio 45239

MaryJane K. Selgrade, Ph.D.
Chief, Immunotoxicology Branch
Health Effects Research Laboratory
United States Environmental Protection Agency, MD-92
Research Triangle Park, North Carolina 27711

Steven C. Shivers, Ph.D.
Bone Marrow Transplant Program
H. Lee Moffitt Cancer Center and Research Institute
12902 Magnolia Drive
Tampa, Florida 33612

Edith Sim, D.Phil.
Welcome Senior Lecturer
Department of Pharmacology
Oxford University
Mansfield Road
Oxford OX1 3QT United Kingdom

Ralph J. Smialowicz, Ph.D.
Health Effects Research Laboratory
United States Environmental Protection Agency
Research Triangle Park, North Carolina 27711

Mohan L. Sopori, Ph.D.
Senior Scientist
Department of Immunotoxicology
The Lovelace Institutes
2425 Ridgecrest Road, South East
Albuquerque, New Mexico 87108

Carroll A. Snyder, Ph.D.
Research Professor
Department of Environmental Medicine
New York University Medical Center
Long Meadow Road
Tuxedo, New York 10987

James E. Talmadge, Ph.D.
Professor of Pathology and Microbiology
Departments of Pathology and Microbiology
University of Nebraska Medical Center
600 South 42nd Street, Box 985660
Omaha, Nebraska 68198

Eric L. Teasdale, F.R.C.G.P.
Group Chief Medical Officer
Department of Safety, Health, and Environment
ZENECA Pharmaceuticals
Alderley House
Alderley Park
Macclesfield, Cheshire, SK10 4TF, United Kingdom

Uwe Trefzer, M.D.
Senior Research Fellow
Department of Dermatology
Case Western Reserve University
11100 Euclid Avenue
Cleveland, Ohio 44106

Ernest S. Tucker III, M.D.
Chairman
Department of Pathology
Scripps Clinic and Research Foundation
10666 North Torrey Pines Road
La Jolla, California 92037

Stephen E. Ullrich, Ph.D.
Associate Professor of Immunology
Department of Immunology
University of Texas
M.D. Anderson Cancer Center
1515 Holcombe Boulevard
Houston, Texas 77030

Henk van Loveren, Ph.D.
Head, Section of Immunotoxicology
Laboratory of Pathology
National Institute of Public Health and Environmental Protection
P.O. Box 1
3720 BA Bilthoven, The Netherlands

Johanna J. Verwilghen, M.D., Ph.D., M.R.C.P.
Fellow in Rheumatology
Department of Rheumatology
Northwestern Memorial Hospital
303 East Chicago, W3-315
Chicago, Illinois 60611

Thierry Vial, M.D.
Assistant Professor of Medical Pharmacology
Laboratory of Clinical and Fundamental Immunotoxicology
Faculte Alexis Carrel
Rue Guillanme Parradin
69008 Lyon, France

Robert Vogt, Ph.D.
Clinical Biochemistry Branch
Centers for Disease Control and Prevention
1600 Clifton Road
Atlanta, Georgia 30333

Joseph G. Vos, D.V.M., Ph.D.
Laboratory of Pathology
National Institute of Public Health and Environmental Protection
P.O. Box 1
3720 BA Bilthoven, The Netherlands

Elizabeth M. Ward, Ph.D.
Assistant Chief, Industrywide Studies Branch
Division of Surveillance, Hazard Evaluation, and Field Studies
National Institute for Occupational Safety and Health
4676 Columbia Parkway
Cincinnati, Ohio 45226

David B. Warheit, Ph.D.
Senior Research Toxicologist
DuPont Haskell Laboratory for Toxicology and Industrial Medicine
Eckton Road, P.O. Box 50
Newark, Delaware 19714

Raphael H. Warshaw, B.A.
Associate
Department of Medicine
University of Southern California School of Medicine
2025 Zonal Avenue, CSC 201
Los Angeles, California 90033; and
Working Diseases Detection Services Inc.
112 North Harvard Avenue
Suite 258
Claremont, California 91711

Kimber L. White, Jr., Ph.D.
Departments of Biomedical Engineering, Pharmacology, and Toxicology
Medical College of Virginia
Virginia Commonwealth University
Richmond, Virginia 23298

James L. Wilmer, Ph.D.
Environmental Immunology and Neurobiology Section
National Institute of Environmental Health Sciences
Research Triangle Park, North Carolina 27709

Gaetane Woerly, Ph.D.
Professor
Institute of Toxicology
University of Zürich
Schorenstrasse 16
CH-8603 Schwerzenbach ZH, Switzerland

Judith T. Zelikoff, Ph.D.
Assistant Professor
Department of Environmental Medicine
Institute of Environmental Medicine
New York University Medical Center
Long Meadow Road
Tuxedo, New York 10987

Preface to the First Edition

Traditional methods for toxicological assessment have implicated the immune system as a frequent target organ of toxic insult following chronic or subchronic exposure to certain chemicals or therapeutic drugs (e.g., xenobiotics). Interaction of the immune system with these xenobiotics may result in three principal undesirable effects: (1) those determined by immune suppression; (2) those determined by immune dysregulation (e.g., autoimmunity); and (3) those determined by the response of immunologic defense mechanisms to the xenobiotic (e.g., hypersensitivity). The first section of this volume reviews the basic organization of the immune system and describes the cellular and humoral elements involved, the interactions and regulation of lymphoid cells, and their dysregulations that result in disease.

Toxicological manifestations in the immune system following xenobiotic exposure in experimental animals appear as alterations in lymphoid organ weights or histology: quantitative or qualitative changes in cellularity of lymphoid tissue, peripheral leukocytes, or bone marrow; impairment of cell functions; and increased susceptibility to infectious agents or tumors. Allergy, and to a lesser extent autoimmunity, have also been associated with exposure to xenobiotics in animals and man. Chapters are included in the second section which describe approaches and methodology for assessing chemical- or drug-induced immunosuppression or hypersensitivity.

Awareness of immunotoxicology was stimulated by a comprehensive review by Vos in 1977, in which he provided evidence that a broad spectrum of xenobiotics alter immune responses in laboratory animals and subsequently may affect the health of exposed individuals. Several additional reviews, as well as national and international scientific meetings, have reinforced these early observations. In several studies, alteration of immune function was accompanied by increased susceptibility to challenge with infectious agents or transplantable tumor cells, indicating that the resulting immune dysfunction in altered host resistance. Clinical studies in humans exposed to xenobiotics have confirmed the parallelism with immune dysfunction observed in rodents. The latter sections in this volume describe studies with xenobiotics that resulted in immune modulation in rodents and man.

The sensitivity or utility of the immune system for detecting subclinical toxic injury has likewise been demonstrated. This may occur for one of several reasons: functionally immunocompetent cells are required for host resistance to opportunistic infectious agents or neoplasia; immunocompetent cells require continued proliferation and differentiation for self-renewal and are thus sensitive to agents which affect cell proliferation or differentiation; and finally, the immune system is a tightly regulated organization of lymphoid cells which are interdependent in function. These cells communicate through soluble mediators and cell-to-cell interactions. Any agent that alters this delicate regulatory balance, that functionally affects a particular cell type, or alters proliferation or differentiation can lead to an immune alteration. One section of this volume is devoted to possible mechanisms by which xenobiotics may perturb lymphoid cells.

This volume should be of interest to toxicologists, immunologists, cell biologists, and clinicians who are studying mechanisms of xenobiotic-induced diseases. It should also be of interest to scientists faced with the challenge of the safety assessment of immunotherapeutics, biological responses modifiers, recombinant DNA products, drugs under development, and other consumer products. This volume should better prepare toxicologists for the challenges of the 21st century.

Jack H. Dean

Preface

Although the philosophy and design of the second edition is consistent with the first, many changes have been made to reflect the metamorphosis of this area from a subdiscipline of toxicology to an independent area of research that can best be described as "Environmental Immunology." For example, chapters have been added that describe the role of immune mediators in liver, lung, and skin toxicity, in regulating drug- and chemical-metabolizing enzymes and in the immunosuppression produced by ultraviolet light, as well as immunotoxicology studies of nonmammalian systems. More emphasis has been placed upon the clinical consequences of immunotoxicity as well as on the interpretation of experimental data for predicting human health risk. A number of chapters from the first edition have been deleted, particularly those that provided descriptive overviews of the immune system, in order to limit the size of this edition while increasing the scope of immunotoxicology subjects.

Unlike the first edition, this book is divided into three major subsections, comprising immunosuppression, autoimmunity, and hypersensitivity. This division allows for a more comprehensive treatment of these important subjects with greater attention to test methods, theoretical considerations, and clinical significance. The section on immunosuppression begins with introductory chapters discussing consequences of immunodeficiency, human and animal test systems, and risk assessment. This is followed by chapters discussing various environmental agents, therapeutic drugs, biological agents, and drugs of abuse as well as immune-mediated toxicity that occur in specific organ systems. The second section is devoted to autoimmunity and includes discussions on the immunopathogenesis of autoimmunity as well as examples of chemical- and drug-induced autoimmune disease. The last section, which is devoted to hypersensitivity, has been greatly expanded from the first edition. This section begins with discussions on the clinical aspects of allergic contact dermatitis and respiratory hypersensitivity. This is followed by chapters describing mechanistic aspects of sensitization and the methods available for the toxicologic evaluation of chemical allergens.

This volume will be of interest to toxicologists, immunologists, clinicians, and scientists working in the area of environmental health. It should also be of interest to individuals involved in occupational health, safety assessment, and regulatory decisions. Although we assume that most readers have at least some understanding of immunology, we have attempted to prepare this book so that any individual interested in environmental sciences could follow it.

Michael I. Luster

Acknowledgments

Again, the volume editors would like to thank the series editors for their vision and wisdom in recognizing the importance of such a volume in this series. We are also grateful to our colleagues who contributed to the volume and whose combined expertise made possible the breadth of coverage of this multifaceted discipline. Finally, appreciation goes to our families who tolerated our usual lack of attention during the editing of this edition.

Immunotoxicology and Immunopharmacology, Second Edition, edited by J. H. Dean, M. I. Luster, A. E. Munson, and I. Kimber.
Raven Press, Ltd., New York © 1994.

1

Consequences of Immunodeficiency

Ernest S. Tucker III

Department of Pathology, Scripps Clinic and Research Foundation, La Jolla, California 92037

ESSENTIALS OF IMMUNOLOGIC COMPETENCE/RESPONSIVENESS

Significance of an Immune Response

The ability of humans and other vertebrates to develop an immune response is the essential characteristic of immunologic competence. An immune response is usually directed against hazardous molecules and biologic factors that are foreign to the host. Three "end products" may develop from an immune response: notably, the production of antibody, the proliferation of specific effector killer cells, or clonal expansion of memory cells that increases the number of specific reactive cells in the lymphocytic repertoire (1–3). Any one or all of these responses may be an important component of an immune response; however, usually one of the three predominates (4–7). In some instances, antibody production may be the principal response (8,9). In others, increased numbers of specific effector killer cells may be most prominent (10,11). An immune response tends to be protective and results in the inactivation or destruction of potentially injurious toxic chemical factors and infectious agents (12–17). Because of its protective effect, the immune response has important survival value.

Development and Maturation of the Immune System

Normal development and maturation of the immune system continue throughout life beginning *in utero* until senescence and death in old age. The most significant development and maturation of the immune systems begin in the third trimester of pregnancy in humans and progresses to full maturation by the time of late puberty and early adulthood, around the age of 19 to 24 years. Thereafter, there is a slow decline into the fifth and sixth decades of life (18–23).

The lymphocytic tissues are the principle component of the immune system. The cells originate from stem cells in the bone marrow (24) followed by selective differentiation in the thymus (25–27) (T cells) and in specific loci in the bone marrow (B cells) (19,28). The bone marrow and thymus are regarded as central lymphatic tissues. Peripheral lymphatic tissues are lymph nodes that are distributed through the body, the spleen, and mucosa-associated lymphoid tissue (MALT) that is prominent in the respiratory and gastrointestinal tracts (29,30). As the T and B cells differentiate, they acquire specific identity due to the appearance of specific antigen receptors on their cell membranes (31–33). The antigen receptors are genetically determined and determine the phenotype of the individual (32,34,35). They are coded in the immune response (IR) genes located in the major histocompatibility complex (MHC) (34–37).

With development of specific antigen receptors, the T and B cells are capable of binding the specific molecular configurations that are called immunogens, or more commonly designated as antigens (38–40). In humans, abundant lymphocytes populate the peripheral lymphatic tissues by late childhood. Approximately 80% are T cell types and 20% are B cells (19). B cells differentiate into antibody-secreting cells following antigen receptor binding (41–46). Antigen-activated T cells may differentiate into specific effector cells but also proliferate as memory cells or as regulatory T cells called helper and suppressor cells (47–49). The cell membrane receptors for binding a specific antigen on a lymphocyte are genetically determined and each receptor is unique to each cell and specific for a particular antigen (50). Only a few of the lymphocytes within the entire repertoire of lymphocytic tissues will have receptors for the same antigen (51,52). This restriction of specific antigen receptors to a few lymphocytes limits the extent of the initial immune response following antigen exposure and explains the great diversity of reactivity of the immune system (31,53–57).

CRITICAL STEPS IN AN IMMUNE RESPONSE

Antigen Presentation and Lymphocyte Activation

Specific antigen binding to the receptor on the lymphocyte membrane sets in motion a series of complex cellular and biochemical events that must occur sequentially and within a close spatial setting in order for an effective response to develop (3,58–60). Figure 1 provides a diagram that shows a model of the immune system as a self-regulating interaction of the major components. The model identifies each component by analogy with a computer-controlled servo-regulated system. Immunogen or antigen is the initial input signal, the lymphocytic tissues are the central processor, and the output products are antibodies and effector T cells. Downregulation occurs by negative feedback that results from immunogen (antigen) inactivation by products of the immune response (61–63). Secondary activation of ancillary factors such as complement may occur to augment antigen inactivation and removal (64). Antigen or immunogen usually enters the tissues by absorption, contact, injec-

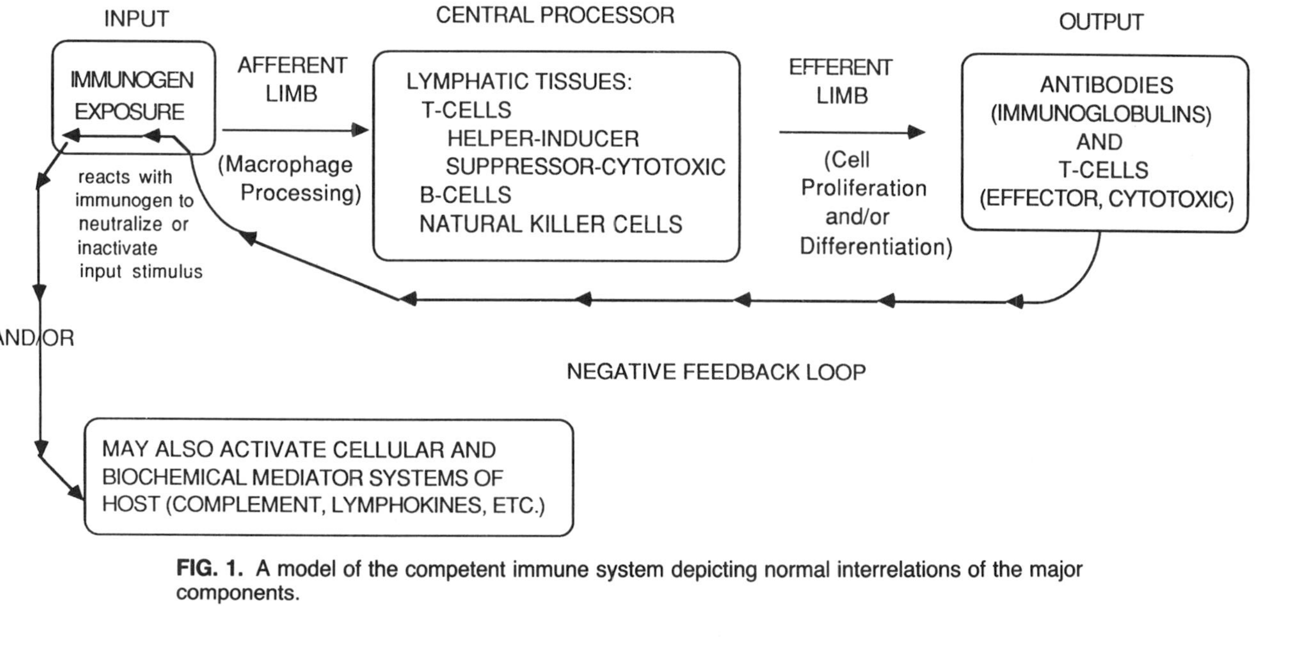

FIG. 1. A model of the competent immune system depicting normal interrelations of the major components.

tion, or ingestion or indirectly as a result of infection or secondary contamination. The antigen is initially phagocytosed by cell types such as those of the reticuloendothelial system, tissue macrophages, or macrophage–monocytes that are recruited from peripheral blood by cytokines. Phagocytic cells subserve the important function in the immune response of degrading the complex chemical structure of an antigen to simplified chemical fragments that possess individual antigenic determinants. Phagocytes also are the cells that present antigen to the specific receptor on the lymphocyte membrane (65). This antigen presentation occurs by linkage of antigen to the specific receptor along with secondary coreceptor linkage through a MHC class II molecule on the lymphocyte and a MHC class II receptor on the phagocyte (58,66,67). Figure 2 shows a diagram of the sequence of cellular and biochemical factors (cytokines) that participate in immunogen (antigen) processing, recognition, and presentation to specific lymphocytes that become activated to differentiate and/or proliferate (53,68–71). Proper presentation of antigen does not occur without the concurrent linkage with the MHC class II molecule and its receptor (72–74). This accounts for unique individual phenotypic restriction of the immune response that only occurs between cells of identical MHC class II type (75). This MHC restriction, in addition to the antigen receptor restriction, are two important factors that limit development of a specific immune response.

Cellular Proliferation and Differentiation

Antigen presentation by the phagocytic cell occurs as a primary interaction with specialized T cells known as T helper (T_H) cells (48,65,76). T_H cells then in turn distribute antigen to other specific T and B cells (see Fig. 2) (77). The T_H cell acts as a secondary presenting cell. Beginning with the time of contact with other T and B cells, the T_H cell secretes lymphokines that stimulate differentiation and proliferation of the recipient B and T cells (78–81). Antigen presented to B cells via receptors leads to activation and differentiation of B cells into plasma cells that secrete antibody specific for the particular antigenic determinant (77). In a similar manner, T cell antigen receptors are activated on antigen presentation and are stimulated to proliferate by clonal expansion either as memory T cells, regulator T cells, or effector T cells (killer T cells) (82). These specific products of the immune response, antibody and effector T cells, mediate the immune activities of neutralization, inactivation, or destruction of the target antigens in tissue fluids or on cell membranes (13,15,83,84).

Regulatory Factors

In addition to effector molecules and cells, there are other T cells that proliferate in an immune response that exert important regulatory effects on the immune system. Some of the regulatory factors such as MHC molecules and antigen receptors that restrict an immune response have been discussed; however, the regulatory T

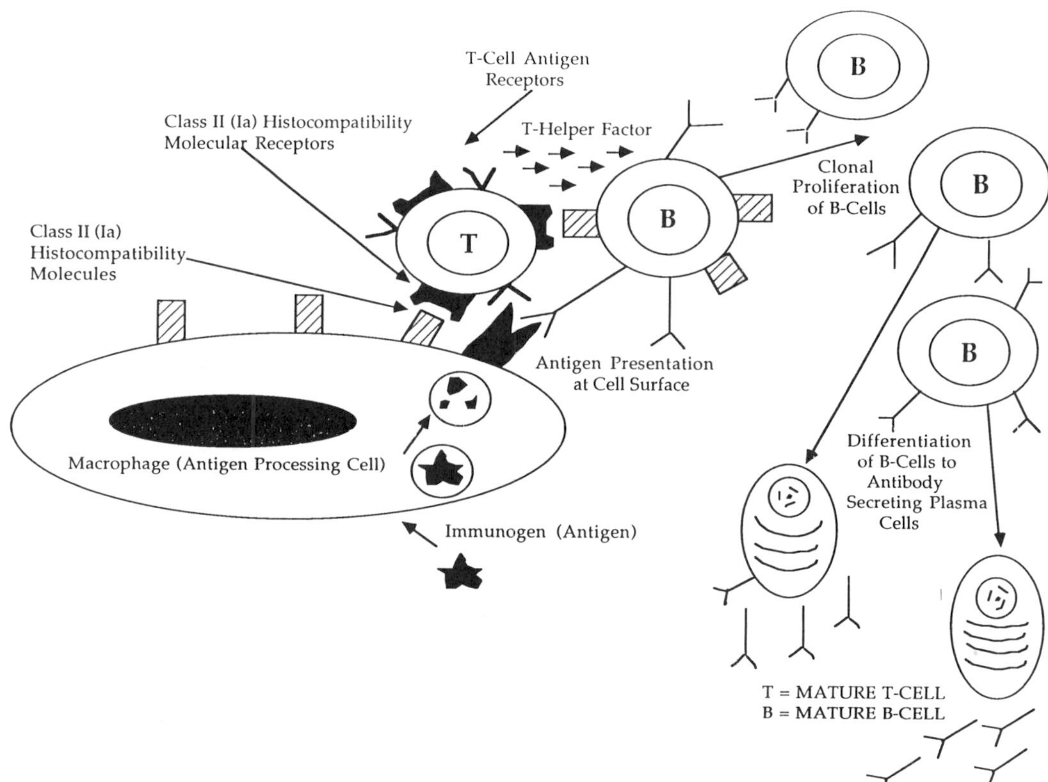

FIG. 2. Cellular events in the course of B cell immune response.

cells and biochemical factors (cytokines) are of key importance in either upregulation or downregulation of the immune response (7,85–88). Other regulatory factors are genetic determinants and variables such as the age and sex of the host as well as nutritional state (19,20,22,23). The physical form of the antigen, the amount of antigen, and the route of exposure are variables that often determine whether an immune response yields antibody or leads to proliferation of specific effector cells (43,70,89). The factors that influence the isotype of immunoglobulin, the avidity of the antibody, and the time course of an immune response are not yet understood (90–92).

Effect on Target Antigens

The impact of antibody or effector T cells on target antigen is the inactivation, degradation, or destruction of the target that results in a negative feedback effect. The immune response is downregulated as the antigenic stimulus is destroyed or inactivated (see Fig. 1). Antibody and cytotoxic or T killer cell activity on target antigens or cells is frequently augmented by secretion of biochemical mediators known as cytokines (78). These factors include the interleukins (ILs), interferon (IFN), tumor necrosis factor (TNF), and lymphotoxin (LT), as well as activation of plasma factors such as the complement and kinin systems (64,71,78,93–95). These mediators cause important secondary biologic effects such as increased phagocytic activity, granule release by specific cells such as basophils, eosinophils, and neutrophils, and rupture of cell membranes.

Homeostatic System

An immune response in the fully mature, immunologically competent individual provides critical protection against a myriad of environmental hazards that include chemicals, infectious agents, and biomolecular toxins. The immune system acts as a self-restoring homeostatic system that returns to normal levels of function after periods of marked stimulation and response (7,19,96). The immune system is comparable in intricacy and complexity to the nervous system. The self-restoring immune system can usually recover and bypass or circumvent the effects of many potentially damaging environmental hazards such as injurious chemicals and drugs when the offending agent is removed.

DEFECTIVE/DEFICIENT IMMUNOLOGIC RESPONSIVENESS

Concept of Immunosuppression/Immunodeficiency

In the foregoing section, it is apparent that a degree of deficiency in immune function persists to the time of young adulthood in humans until maturation and development are complete and reactivity is at maximum. The state of maturity of the immune system varies with different individuals, often reaching the peak of immune function at different ages but always at puberty or early adulthood. There are many well-known clinical conditions of inherited deficiencies in immunologic function (97,98). Some exhibit specific defects in antibody formation while others show T cell and/or metabolic defects, while others show combined impairment of both B and T cell function. These disorders are known as primary immunodeficiencies due to definable genetic defects with specific faulty genes identified on specific chromosomes. The importance of the immune system to individual survival has been shown by the information gathered from clinical studies of these disorders. Studies have shown that individuals with partial or absolute defects in T cell function rarely survive beyond infancy or early childhood. In contrast, individuals with defects in B cell function that exhibit deficiency of antibody formation may suffer from a variety of chronic recurrent infectious diseases and diminished health but they do survive with appropriate therapy when the underlying disorder is recognized. Study of these genetic immunodeficiency states has also provided considerable information about functions of human B and T cells that could not otherwise be determined. T cells have been found to have key roles in the normal development and functioning of the human immune system. They function as regulator and effector cells. T cell defects are clearly shown by the types of immunodeficiency in those disorders.

Acquired Immunodeficiency

Figure 3 is a diagram of the interacting components of the immune system from Fig. 1 which also shows potential target sites that may be affected by xenobiotics or other toxic factors. Impairment of function of a key component at any of these sites could result in a diminished response (immunosuppression) or immunodeficiency.

The occurrence of acquired immunodeficiency states was recognized sporadically in scattered individuals during the 1960s and 1970s. In the late 1970s and early 1980s, a syndrome appeared that spread quite rapidly through certain groups of individuals and was identified as a generalized type of acquired immunodeficiency syndrome (AIDS). This disorder was found to be due to a specific retrovirus that infects and destroys T_H cells in humans (99). These helper lymphocytes have been identified in experimental studies as the key cells in the recognition and secondary processing of antigen. Decrease in numbers of T_H cells leads to impaired immune responses to a variety of infectious agents as well as the occurrence of certain types of neoplasms. AIDS appears to result from declining numbers of T_H cells (CD4+ lymphocytes) with persistence of residual populations of T suppressor cells (CD8+ lymphocytes). Progression of AIDS is associated with progressive loss of the T_H (CD4+) cells and an increased frequency of infections by bacterial, fungal, viral, and parasitic agents.

Other types of acquired immunodeficiency conditions have been recognized and

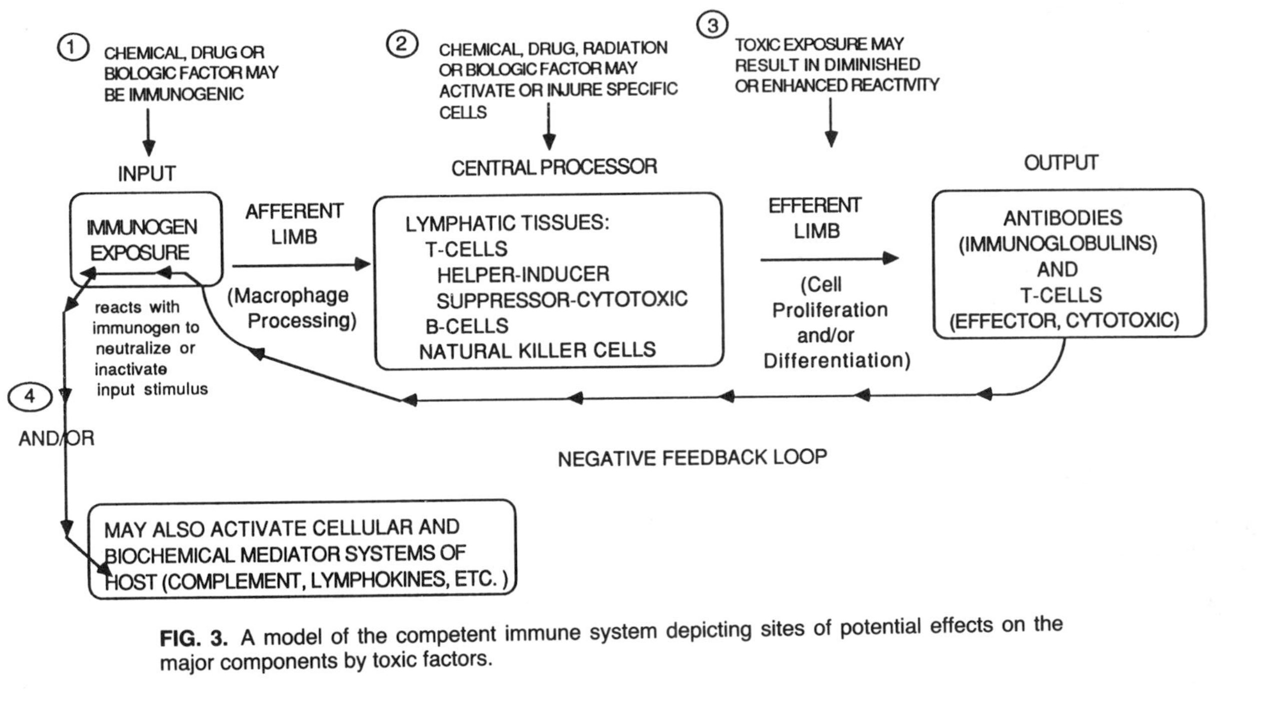

FIG. 3. A model of the competent immune system depicting sites of potential effects on the major components by toxic factors.

more clearly defined in the past two decades. Many have been related to specific immunosuppressive drugs, chemotherapeutic agents, and certain chemicals (100–103). Cyclosporin A (CsA) is a cyclic decapeptide derived from a fungus that exhibits a notable effect on lymphocyte function, which significantly reduces allograft rejection and prolongs graft survival in both humans and experimental animals (100,104–108). There have also been sporadic reports of depressed immune function associated with exposure to certain xenobiotics in some humans environmentally exposed to toxicants, but most data come from studies in experimental animals. Some of the animal studies have used exposures to xenobiotics at high levels, well above those that would mimic low-level ambient exposure in the environment to humans. In addition, the animal studies have been short-term and immune effects were determined by quantitative counts of lymphocyte and other cell populations, gross changes induced in lymphoid organs, and quantitative measures of immunoglobulin levels or assessment of immune function. Most of the immunologic data collected in human studies after accidental xenobiotic exposure have been the determination of immunoglobulin levels and counts of specific populations of blood lymphocytes (109–111). These studies have often lacked clear documentation and confirmation of the amount of individual exposure to the xenobiotic by measurements of blood or tissue levels (112,113) and have not included adequate functional assessment of immune responsiveness (114). The immunosuppressive effects of xenobiotics in humans due to environmental exposure when compared to genetically determined immunodeficiency defects do not reveal the same degree of severity and persistence in the xenobiotic-related immune defects as seen in the genetic disorders.

Based on our current knowledge of components of the immune system and their functional interactions as discussed earlier, it is apparent that there are a number of potential sites where an acquired defect could lead to failure of immune responsiveness (115) (Fig. 3). Defective phagocytic function could result in impaired antigen recognition and processing with failure of antigen presentation to the receptors on lymphocytes (116). Such a defect would lead to a complete lack of an immune response that would appear as a clinical problem of immunosuppression (117). Studies are needed to determine whether such a mechanism is important in acquired immune suppression following drug or xenobiotic exposure.

Another potential site of immune suppression would be at the level of lymphocyte antigen recognition and cell activation. This could occur due to impaired expression of antigen receptor and/or failure of biochemical mechanisms that would cause failure of activation and subsequent failure of proliferation or differentiation of the recognition lymphocyte (118). This would result in immunosuppression because of failure to form specific antibody (119) or specific effector cells (120). Experimental studies are needed to confirm the occurrence of this mechanism.

Impaired immune responsiveness could also be due to specific inhibitors of cell activation or the inhibition of biochemical mediators. This could prevent cell proliferation and differentiation resulting in immunosuppression. Study of this possibility is also needed.

An absolute or relative decrease in numbers of lymphocytes and quantity of immunoglobulins has been used as a measure of immunosuppression in a number of sporadic studies in humans who have been exposed to various xenobiotics such as asbestos, silica, polychlorinated biphenyls (PCBs), dibenzofurans, lead, pesticides, dioxin, and benzene (100,103,105,106,109,121–125). However, the findings in these studies have been quite variable and generally inconclusive in defining specific immunosuppressive effects related to a particular xenobiotic or in elaborating a specific mechanism of immunosuppression. Many animal studies have reported immunosuppressive effects of xenobiotics and some have provided more conclusive data than others (126–129). These studies have included xenobiotics such as dioxin, pesticides, PCBs and other halogenated aromatic hydrocarbons, polycyclic aromatic hydrocarbons (PAHs), as well as a variety of heavy metals (130,131). In these animal studies, the mechanisms of action of particular xenobiotics appear to vary widely and there is no evidence of a common pathway or a uniform injurious effect on the target cells. The types of immunosuppressive effects found in animals have included bone marrow suppression, atrophy of the thymus and spleen, inhibition of complement component activation, suppression of lymphocyte response to mitogens and antigens along with termination of suppressed cytotoxic and regulatory T cell activity, inhibition of stem cell proliferation, decrease in natural killer cell activity, impairment of phagocytic activity, and defective host resistance (118,132–136).

In human studies, there are considerable difficulties in comparing data from one study to another because of lack of uniformity in protocol development and study design as well as considerable variation in technical procedures and methods. In many instances the studies lack appropriate and proper controls, along with lack of standardized quantitative data analysis and unclear time course and exposure variables. Often, these variations are substantial and make it difficult to draw meaningful conclusions from some of the studies reported in the literature (137). It is clear from some animal studies that immunosuppressive effects do occur, but the severity, duration, and mechanisms are yet to be clearly understood. There is a significant need for more rigorous scientific animal studies as well as a more rigorous approach to evaluate human cohort studies of xenobiotic exposure to properly assess their immunosuppressive potential.

Consequences of Immunodeficiency/Immunosuppression

The major consequence of immunodeficiency or impaired immune responsiveness is failure of protection of the host by antibody or effector cells directed against specific target antigens. Antibody and effector cells are essential for a protective effect against infectious and toxic agents that can cause destructive tissue injury and disseminated infections (97). An impaired immune response also limits the response to protective vaccines that normally build adequate levels of cellular and antibody protection against infectious agents (61). Selective impairment of immune responsiveness in some instances may also lead to hypersensitivity states due to dysregulation. This effect could also result in autoimmune disease by promoting recognition of self-antigens and hyperresponsiveness with increased antibody and effector cell production (138–141). Increased potential development of neoplasia and disseminated malignancies, especially those of the lymphocytic tissues, may occur with impaired immune surveillance (122,142,143).

The duration of immunodeficiency states might be transient or long-lasting depending on the severity and site of the specific xenobiotic effect (100,106,140,144–146). However, as noted earlier, there are no reported, long-lasting immunodeficiency syndromes due to xenobiotics in humans (115,147–151). The immune impairment that results from continued specific drug therapy with immunosuppressive agents or human immunodeficiency virus (HIV) infection are the only examples of long-lasting acquired immunodeficiency in humans (99,152,153). Indeed, studies that have reported acquired deficiency of immune function as a result of xenobiotics or radiation have shown the marked capacity for self-restoring activity of the immune system so that once an offending agent has been cleared from the body, the various cellular components return to a normal state (19,57,154).

HORIZONS IN RESEARCH

Currently, the lack of clear, convincing evidence that humans suffer significant immunosuppression or defective immune responsiveness from xenobiotics indicates a need for well-designed cohort studies to effectively evaluate their effects on immune function in humans (106,142,155–157). Because immune systems in vertebrates are generally similar to humans, animal studies can be effective in defining potential harmful effects of xenobiotics (107,145,158). Such studies are needed to clarify mechanisms and assess functional impairment in order to define the risks of xenobiotic exposure (159,160). The endpoint in those studies should be determination of the biochemical defects in the animal's ability to develop an antibody and/or cellular immune response to specific antigens under standardized exposure and time-course parameters (107,161,162). The capacity for self-restoration of the immune system needs additional study. It appears that, in most animals, transient effects of various xenobiotics are readily corrected by the homeostatic biochemical and cellular mechanisms in the immune system (34,35,48,54,163). In addition, the importance of genetic determinants that underlie immune function and susceptibility to environmental factors needs more study and definition. Finally, there is a need to understand the factors and mechanisms that can be protective and shield the immune system from the effects of hazardous agents. Such knowledge could be used to obviate potential injury of the immune system. In addition to knowledge of protective mechanisms, information about specific regulator factors and/or cytokines (86,164) that augment or restore immune function is also lacking in our current understanding (23,165,166).

Finally, there is a need to develop a national information resource or database to track the effects of xenobiotic exposure on immune function (167). Such a database could be established as a registry by a consensus of knowledgeable experts using rigorous standards for valid data collection from animal and human studies. A mechanism to provide for longevity and continued support of such a resource should be sought within a government agency, major research institute, or university. Such a registry would accumulate and focus data from a wide range of studies and be the key to a coherent approach in determining whether there is a significant risk to human immune function due to xenobiotics.

REFERENCES

1. Paul WE. *Fundamental immunology*, 2nd ed. New York: Raven Press; 1989.
2. Roitt I, Brostoff J, Male D. *Immunology*, 2nd ed. London: Gower Medical Publishing; 1989.
3. Terhorst C, Alarcon B, de Vries J, Spits H. T lymphocyte recognition and activation. In: Hames BD, Glover DM, eds. *Molecular immunology*. Oxford: IRL Press; 1988.
4. Aloisi RM. *Principles of immunology and immunodiagnostics*. Philadelphia: Lea & Febiger; 1988.
5. Andersson J, Möller G, Sjöberg O. Selective induction of DNA synthesis in T and B lymphocytes. *Cell Immunol* 1972;4:381–393.
6. Bick PH. The immune system: organization and function. In: Dean J, Luster MI, Munson AE, Amos H, eds. *Immunotoxicology and immunopharmacology*. New York: Raven Press; 1985:1–10.
7. Claman HN. The biology of the immune response. *JAMA* 1987;258:2834–2840.
8. Katz DH. Genetic controls and cellular interactions in antibody formation. *Hosp Pract* 1977;12:85–99.
9. *Clinical aspects of immunology*, vols 1 and 2, 4th ed. St Louis: Blackwell–Mosby; 1982.
10. Raidt DJ, Mishell RI, Dutton RW. Cellular events in the immune response. Analysis of *in vitro* response of mouse spleen cell populations separated by differential flotation in albumin gradients. *J Exp Med* 1968;128:681–698.
11. Redelman D, Scott CB, Sheppard HW Jr, Sell S. *In vitro* studies of the rabbit immune system. V. Suppressor T cells activated by concanavalin A block the proliferation, not the induction of anti-erythrocyte plaque-forming cells. *J Exp Med* 1976;143:919–936.
12. Schrier RD, Gnann JW, Landes R, et al. T cell recognition of HIV synthetic peptides in a natural infection. *J Immunol* 1989;142:1166.
13. Townsend J, Bastin J, Bodmer H, et al. Recognition of influenza virus proteins by cytotoxic T cells. *Philos Trans R Soc Lond [Biol]* 1989;323:527.
14. Palker TJ, Matthews TJ, Langlois A, et al. Polyvalent HIV synthetic immunogen compromised of envelope gp120, T helper cell sites and B cell neutralisation epitopes. *J Immunol* 1989;142:3612.
15. Romero P, Marvanski JL, Corradin G, Nussenzweig RS, Nussenzweig V, Zavala F. Cloned cytotoxic T cells recognize an epitope in the circumsporozoite protein and protect against malaria. *Nature* 1989;341:323.
16. Müller-Eberhard HJ. The molecular basis of target cell killing by human lymphocytes and of killer self-protection. *Immunol Rev* 1988;103:87.
17. Bradley SG. Immunologic mechanisms of host resistance to bacteria and parasites. In: Dean JH, Luster MI, Munson AE, Amos H, eds. *Immunotoxicology and immunopharmacology*. New York: Raven Press; 1985:45–54.
18. Gell PGH, Coombs RRA, Lachman PJ. *Clinical aspects of immunology*. Oxford: Blackwell Scientific Publications; 1975.
19. Golub ES. *Immunology: a synthesis*. Sunderland, MA: Sinauer Associates; 1987.
20. Hausman PB, Weksler ME. Changes in the immune response with age. In: Finch CE, Schneider EL, eds. *Handbook of the biology of aging*. New York: Van Nostrand Reinhold; 1985:414–432.
21. Katz S, Branch LG, Branson MH, Papsidero JA, Beck JC, Greer DS. Active life expectancy. *N Engl J Med* 1983;309:1218–1224.
22. Lewis VM, Twomey JJ, Bealmear P, Goldstein G, Good RA. Age, thymic involution and circulating thymic hormone activity. *J Clin Endocrinol* 1978;47:145–150.
23. Makinodan T, Kay MM. Age influence on the immune system. *Adv Immunol* 1980;29:287–330.
24. Dorshkind K. Regulation of haemopoiesis by bone marrow stromal cells and their products. *Annu Rev Immunol* 1990;8:137.

25. Blackman M, Kappler JW, Marrack P. The role of the T-cell receptor in positive and negative selection of developing T-cells. *Science* 1990;248:1335.
26. Marrack P, Lo D, Brinster R, Palmiter R, Burkly L, Flavell RA, Kappler J. The effect of thymus environment on T cell development and tolerance. *Cell* 1988;53:627.
27. Von Boehmer H, Kisielow P. Self–non-self discrimination by T cells. *Science* 1990;248:1369.
28. Twomey JJ. *The pathophysiology of human immunologic disorders*. Baltimore: Urban & Schwarzenberg; 1982.
29. Bonneville M, Janeway CA Jr, Ito K, Haser W, Ishida I, Nakanishi N, Tonegawa S. Intestinal intraepithelial lymphocytes are a distinct set of τδ T-cells. *Nature* 1988;336:479.
30. Takagaki Y, DeCloux A, Bonneville M, Tonegawa S. Diversity of τδ T-cell receptors on murine intestinal intra-epithelial lymphocytes. *Nature* 1989;339:712.
31. Owen MJ, Lamb JR. *Immune recognition in focus*. Oxford: IRL Press at Oxford University Press; 1988.
32. Toyonaga B, Mak TW. Genes of the T-cell antigen receptor in normal and malignant T cells. *Annu Rev Immunol* 1987;5:585.
33. Fink PJ, Matis LA, McElligott DL, Bookman M, Hendrick SM. Correlations between T-cell specificity and the structure of the antigen receptor. *Nature* 1986;321:219.
34. Davis MM, Bjorkman PJ. T-cell antigen receptor genes and T-cell recognition. *Nature* 1988; 334:395.
35. Kronenberg M, Siu G, Hood L, Shastri N. The molecular genetics of the T-cell antigen receptor and T-cell antigen recognition. *Annu Rev Immunol* 1986;4:529.
36. Bjorkman PJ, Saper MA, Samraoui B, Bennett WS, Strominger JL, Wiley DC. The foreign antigen binding site and T cell recognition regions of class I histocompatibility antigens. *Nature* 1987; 329:512.
37. Spies T, Bresnahan M, Strominger JL. Human major histocompatibility complex contains a minimum of 19 genes between the complement cluster and HLA-B. *Proc Natl Acad Sci USA* 1989;86:8955.
38. Minami Y, Samelson LE, Klausner RD. Internalisation and cycling of the T cell antigen receptor. *J Biol Chem* 1987;262:13342.
39. Goldsmith MA, Weiss A. New clues about T-cell antigen receptor complex function. *Immunol Today* 1988;9:220.
40. Williams AF, Barclay AN. The immunoglobulin superfamily—domains for cell surface recognition. *Annu Rev Immunol* 1988;6:381.
41. Cambier JC, Ransom JT. Molecular mechanisms of transmembrane signalling in B lymphocytes. *Annu Rev Immunol* 1987;5:175.
42. Klaus GGB, Bijsterbosch MK, O'Garra A, Harnett M, Rigley KP. Receptor signalling and cross-talk in B lymphocytes. *Immunol Rev* 1987;99:19.
43. Hayakawa K, Hardy RR. Characterization of the secondary antibody response using purified memory B and T cells. In: Melchers F, ed. *Progress in immunology VII*. Berlin: Springer-Verlag; 1989:439.
44. Berek C, Milstein C. The dynamic nature of the antibody repertoire. *Immunol Rev* 1988;105:5.
45. Manser T. Evolution of antibody structure during the immune response. The differentiative potential of a single B lymphocyte. *J Exp Med* 1989;170:1211.
46. van Rooijen N. Direct intrafollicular differentiation of memory B cells into plasma cells. *Immunol Today* 1990;11:154.
47. Cerottini J-C, MacDonald HR. The cellular basis of T-cell memory. *Annu Rev Immunol* 1989;7:77.
48. Powrie F, Mason D. Phenotypic and functional heterogeneity of $CD4^+$ T cells. *Immunol Today* 1988;9:274.
49. Liu Y-J, Joshua DE, Williams GT, Smith CA, Gordon J, MacLennan ICM. Mechanism of antigen-driven selection in germinal centres. *Nature* 1989;342:929.
50. Happ MP, Kubo RT, Palmer E, Born WK, O'Brien RL. Limited receptor repertoire in a mycobacteria-reactive subset of τδ T lymphocytes. *Nature* 1989;342:696.
51. Hata S, Clabby M, Devlin P, Spits H, de Vries J, Krangel MS. Diversity and organisation of human T cell receptor δ variable gene segments. *J Exp Med* 1989;169:41.
52. French DL, Laskov R, Scharff MD. The role of somatic hypermutation in the generation of antibody diversity. *Science* 1989;244:1152.
53. Terhorst C. Alarcon B, de Vries J, Spits H. T lymphocyte recognition and activation. In: Hames BD, Glover DM, eds. *Molecular immunology*. Oxford: IRL Press; 1988:145.
54. Hunkapiller T, Hood L. Diversity of the immunoglobulin gene superfamily. *Adv Immunol* 1989; 44:1–63.

55. Ohashi PS, Pircher H, Mak TW, Buerki K, Zinkernagel RM, Hengartner H. Ontogeny and selection of the T-cell repertoire in transgenic mice. *Semin Immunol* 1989;1:95.
56. Rothbard JB, Pemberton RM, Bodmer HC, Askonas BA, Taylor WR. Identification of residues necessary for clonally specific recognition of a cytotoxic T cell determinant. *EMBO J* 1989;8:2321.
57. Hay FC. The generation of diversity. In: Roitt IM, Brostoff J, Male DK, eds. *Immunology*, 2nd ed. London: Gower Medical Publishing; 1989.
58. Weaver CT, Unanue ER. The costimulatory function of antigen presenting cells. *Immunol Today* 1990;11:49.
59. Adams DO, Hamilton DA. The cell biology of activation. *Annu Rev Immunol* 1984;2:283.
60. Pingel JT, Thomas ML. Evidence that the leukocyte-common antigen is required for antigen-induced T lymphocyte proliferation. *Cell* 1989;58:1055.
61. Lehner P, Hutchings P, Lydyard PM, Cooke A. Regulation of immune responses by antibody. II. IgM-mediated enhancement: dependency on antigen dose, T cell requirement and lack of evidence for an idiotype related mechanism. *Immunology* 1983;50:503.
62. Muller I, Pedrazzini T, Farrell JP, Louis J. T cell responses and immunity to experimental infection with *Leishmania major*. *Annu Rev Immunol* 1989;7:561.
63. Wakelin D, Blackwell JK. Genetic variations in immunity to parasite infection. In: Warren KS, ed. *Immunology and molecular biology of parasitic infections*. Oxford: Blackwell Scientific Publications; 1992.
64. Reid KBM. Structure function relationships of the complement components. *Immunol Today* 1989;10:177.
65. Shevach EM, Rosenthal AS. Function of macrophages in antigen recognition by guinea pig T lymphocytes. II. Role of the macrophage in the regulation of genetic control of the immune response. *J Exp Med* 1973;138:1213.
66. Koch N, Lipp J, Pessara U, Schenck K, Wraight C, Dobberstein B. MHC class II invariant chains in antigen processing and presentation. *Trends Biochem Sci* 1989;14:232.
67. van Rooijen N. Antigen processing and presentation *in vivo*: the microenvironment as a crucial factor. *Immunol Today* 1990;11:436.
68. Long EO. Intracellular traffic and antigen processing. *Immunol Today* 1989;10:232.
69. Bierer BE, Sleckman BP, Ratnofsky SE, Burakoff SJ. The biologic roles of CD2, CD4 and CD8 in T cell activation. *Annu Rev Immunol* 1989;7:579.
70. Yokoyama WM, Maxfield SR, Shevach EM. Very early (VEA) and very late (VLA) activation antigens have distinct functions in T lymphocyte activation. *Immunol Rev* 1989;109:153.
71. Hamblin AS. *Lymphokines: in focus*. Oxford: IRL Press; 1988.
72. Kozbor D, Trinchieri G, Monos DS, et al. Human TRC-τ^+/δ^+, $CD8^+$ T lymphocytes recognize tetanus toxoid in an MHC-restricted fashion. *J Exp Med* 1989;169:1847.
73. Altmann DM, Trowsdale J. Major histocompatibility complex structure and function. *Curr Opin Immunol* 1989;2:93.
74. Brown JH, Jardetzky T, Saper MA, Samraoui B, Bjorkman PJ, Wiley DC. A hypothetical model of the foreign antigen binding site of class II histocompatibility molecules. *Nature* 1988;332:845.
75. Demotz S, Grey HM, Appella E, Sette A. Characterization of a naturally processed MHC class II-restricted T-cell determinant of hen egg lysozome. *Nature* 1989;342:682.
76. Anderson P, Blue M-L, Morimoto C, Schlossman SF. Cross-linking of T3 (CD3) with T4 (CD4) enhances the proliferation of resting T lymphocytes. *J Immunol* 1987;139:678.
77. Cambier J. Transmembrane signalling in T lymphocyte-dependent B lymphocyte activation. *Semin Immunol* 1989;1:43.
78. Balkwill FR, Burke F. The cytokine network. *Immunol Today* 1989;10:299.
79. Mizel SB. The interleukins. *FASEB J* 1989;3:2379.
80. Yoshimoto T, Nakanishi K, Kiyoshi M, et al. IL-5 upregulates but IL-4 downregulates IL-2R expression on a cloned B lymphoma line. *J Immunol* 1990;144:183.
81. Bottomly K. Subsets of $CD4^+$ T cells and B cell activation. *Semin Immunol* 1989;1:21.
82. Weiss A, Imboden JB. Cell surface molecules and early events in human T lymphocyte activation. *Adv Immunol* 1987;41:1–38.
83. Makela MJ. Antibody responses to different antigenic sites on measles virus surface polypeptides in patients with multiple sclerosis. *J Neurol Sci* 1989;90:239.
84. Berke G. The cytolytic T lymphocyte and its mode of action. *Immunol Lett* 1989;20:169.
85. Jung TM, Gallatin WM, Weissmann IL, Dailey MO. Down regulation of homing receptors after T cell activation. *J Immunol* 1988;141:4110.

86. Arai K, Lee F, Miyajima A, et al. Cytokines: coordinators of immune and inflammatory responses. *Annu Rev Biochem* 1990;59:783–836.
87. Cantrell DA, Collins MKL, Crumpton MJ. Autocrine regulation of T-lymphocyte proliferation: differential induction of IL-2 and IL-2 receptor. *Immunology* 1988;65:343–349.
88. Fibbe WE, Schaafsma MR, Falkenburg JH, Willemze R. The biological activities of interleukin-1. *Blut* 1989;59:147–156.
89. Daynes RA, Araneo BA, Dowell TA, Huang K, Dudley D. Regulation of murine lymphokine production *in vivo*. III. The lymphoid microenvironment exerts regulatory influences over T helper cell function. *J Exp Med* 1990;171:979.
90. Esser C, Radbruch A. Immunoglobulin class switching: molecular and cellular analysis. *Annu Rev Immunol* 1990;8:717.
91. Petrini J, Dunnick WA. Products and implied mechanism of H chain switch recombination. *J Immunol* 1989;142:2932.
92. Coffman RL, Savelkoul HE, Lebman DA. Cytokine regulation of immunoglobulin isotype switching and expression. *Semin Immunol* 1989;1:55.
93. Beutler B, Cerami A. The biology of cachectin/TNF. *Annu Rev Immunol* 1989;7:625.
94. Frank MD. Complement in the pathophysiology of human disease. *N Engl J Med* 1987;316:1525.
95. Proud D, Kaplan AP. Kinin formation: mechanisms and role in inflammatory disorders. *Annu Rev Immunol* 1988;6:49.
96. Burnet M. *The clonal selection theory of acquired immunity*. Nashville: Vanderbilt University Press; 1959.
97. Buckley RH. Primary immunodeficiency diseases. In: Wyngaarden J, Smith L, eds. *Cecil textbook of medicine*. Philadelphia: Saunders; 1992:1446–1453.
98. Waldmann TA, Wedgwood RJ, Cooper MD, et al. Primary immunodeficiency diseases: report of a WHO-scientific group. *Immunodefic Rev* 1992;3:195–236.
99. Fauci A, Schnittman SM, Poli G. Immunopathologenic mechanisms in human immunodeficiency virus (HIV) infection. *Ann Intern Med* 1991;114:678–693.
100. Bekesi JG, Roboz JP, Fischbein A, Mason P. Immunotoxicology: environmental contamination by polybrominated biphenyls and immune dysfunction among residents of the State of Michigan. *Cancer Detect Prev Suppl* 1987;1:29–37.
101. Borel JF, Feurer C, Gubler HU, Stahelin H. Biological effects of cyclosporin A: a new antilymphocytic agent. *Agents Actions* 1976;6:468–475.
102. Faith RE, Luster MI, Kimmel CA. Effect of chronic developmental lead exposure on cell-mediated immune functions. *Clin Exp Immunol* 1979;35:413–420.
103. Fiore MC, Anderson HA, Hong R, et al. Chronic exposure to aldicarb-contaminated groundwater and human immune function. *Environ Res* 1986;41:633–645.
104. Barnett JB, Barfield R, Walls R, Joyner R, Ownes R, Soderberg LSF. The effect of *in utero* exposure to hexachlorobenzene on the developing immune response of BALB/c mice. *Toxicol Lett* 1987;39:263–274.
105. Bekesi JG, Holland JF, Anderson HA, Fischbein AS, Rom W, Wolff MS, Selikoff IJ. Lymphocyte function of Michigan dairy farmers exposed to polybrominated biphenyls. *Science* 1978;199:1207–1209.
106. Bick PH, Holsapple MP, White KL. Assessment of the effects of chemicals on the immune system. In: Li AP, Blank TL, Flaherty DK, Ribelin WE, Wilson AGE, eds. *Toxicity testing: new approaches and applications in human risk assessment*. New York: Raven Press; 1985:165–178.
107. Dean JH, Cornacoff JB, Luster MI. Toxicity to the immune system. In: Hadden JW, Szentivanyi A, eds. *Immunopharmacology reviews*, vol. 1. New York: Plenum Press; 1990:377–408.
108. Germolec DR, Yang RSH, Ackermann MF, Rosenthal GJ, Boorman GA, Blair P, Luster MI. Toxicology studies of a chemical mixture of 25 groundwater contaminants. II. Immunosuppression in $B6C3F_1$ mice. *Fundam Appl Toxicol* 1989;13:377–387.
109. Hoffman RE, Stehr-Green PA, Webb KB, et al. Health effects of long-term exposure to 2,3,7,8-tetrachloro-dibenzo-*p*-dioxin. *JAMA* 1986;255:2031–2038.
110. Knutsen AP, Roodman ST, Evans RG, et al. Immune studies in dioxin-exposed Missouri residents: Quail Run. *Bull Environ Contam Toxicol* 1987;39:481–489.
111. Lotzová E, Savary CA, Hersh EM, Khan AA, Rosenblum M. Depression of murine natural killer cell cytotoxicity by isobutyl nitrate. *Cancer Immunol Immunother* 1984;17:130–134.
112. Patterson DG Jr, Fingerhut MA, Roberts DW, et al. Levels of polychlorinated dibenzo-*p*-dioxins and dibenzofurans in workers exposed to 2,3,7,8-tetrachlor-dibenzo-*p*-dioxin. *Am J Ind Med* 1989; 16:135–146.

113. Pirkle JL, Wolfe WH, Patterson DG, et al. Estimates of the half-life of 2,3,7,8-tetrachloro-dibenzo-*p*-dioxin in Vietnam veterans of Operation Ranch Hand. *J Toxicol Environ Health* 1989;27:165–171.
114. Reggiani G. Acute human exposure to TCDD in Saveso, Italy. *J Toxicol Environ Health* 1980; 6:27–43.
115. Speirs RS, Speirs EE. An *in vivo* model for assessing effects of drugs and toxicants on immunocompetence. *Drug Chem Toxicol* 1979;2:19–23.
116. Suzuki T, Ikeda S, Kanoh T, Mizoguchi I. Decreased phagocytosis and superoxide anion production in alveolar macrophages of rats exposed to nitrogen dioxide. *Arch Environ Contam Toxicol* 1986;15:733–739.
117. Vos JG. Immune suppression as related to toxicology. *CRC Crit Rev Toxicol* 1977;5:67–101.
118. Seinen W, Penninks A. Immune suppression as a consequence of a selective cytotoxic activity of certain organo metallic compounds on thymus and thymus-dependent lymphocytes. *Ann NY Acad Sci* 1979;320:499–517.
119. Ward EC, Murray MJ, Lauer LD, House RV, Irons R, Dean JH. Immunosuppression following 7,12-dimethylbenz[*a*]anthracene exposure in B6C3F1 mice. I. Effects on humoral immunity and host resistance. *Toxicol Appl Pharmacol* 1984;75:299–308.
120. Wojdani A, Alfred LJ. Alterations in cell-mediated immune functions induced in mouse splenic lymphocytes by polycyclic aromatic hydrocarbons. *Cancer Res* 1984;44:942–945.
121. Bice DE, Hahn FF, Benson J, Carpenter RL, Hobbs CH. Comparative lung immunotoxicity of inhaled quartz and coal combustion fly ash. *Environ Res* 1987;43:374–389.
122. Denkhaus W, von Steldern D, Botzenhardt U, Konietzko H. Lymphocyte subpopulations in solvent-exposed workers. *Int Arch Occup Environ Health* 1986;57:109–115.
123. Evans RG, Webb KB, Knutsen AP, et al. A medical follow-up of the health effects of long-term exposure to 2,3,7,8-tetrachlorodibenzo-*p*-dioxin. *Arch Environ Health* 1988;43:273–278.
124. Kimber I, Stonard MD, Gidlow DA, Niewola Z. Influence of chronic low-level exposure to lead on plasma immunoglobulin concentration and cellular immune function in man. *Int Arch Occup Environ Health* 1986;57:117–125.
125. Lew F, Tsang P, Holland JF, Warner N, Selifoff IJ, Bekesi JG. High frequency of immune dysfunctions in asbestos workers and in patients with malignant mesothelioma. *J Clin Immunol* 1986; 6:225–233.
126. Koller LD, Exon JH, Norbury KC. Induction of humoral immunity to protein antigen without adjuvant in rats exposed to immunosuppressive chemicals. *J Toxicol Environ Health* 1983;12:173–181.
127. Luster MI, Tucker AN, Hayes HT, Pung OJ, Burka T, McMillan R, Eling T. Immunosuppressive effects of benzidine in mice: evidence of alterations in arachidonic acid metabolism. *J Immunol* 1985;135:2754–2761.
128. Lynch DW, Moorman WJ, Burg JR, et al. Subchronic inhalation toxicity of isobutyl nitrite in BALB/c mice. I. Systemic toxicity. *J Toxicol Environ Health* 1985;15:823–833.
129. Lyte M, Bick PH. Modulation of interleukin-1 production by macrophages following benzo-[*a*]pyrene exposure. *Int J Immunopharmacol* 1986;8:377–381.
130. Shopp GM Jr, Sanders VM, White KL Jr, Munson AE. Humoral and cell-mediated immune status of mice exposed to *trans*-1,2-dichloroethylene. *Drug Chem Toxicol* 1985;8:393–407.
131. Talcott PA, Koller LD, Exon JH. The effect of lead and polychlorinated biphenyl exposure on rat natural killer cell cytotoxicity. *Int J Immunopharmacol* 1985;7:255–261.
132. Selgrade MJ, Daniels MJ, Burleson GR, Lauer LD, Dean JH. Effects of 7,12-dimethylbenz-[*a*]anthracene, benzo[*a*]pyrene and cyclosporin A on murine cytomegalovirus infection: studies of resistance mechanisms. *Int J Immunopharmacol* 1989;10:811–818.
133. Silkworth JB, Antrim L, Grabstein EM. Correlations between polychlorinated biphenyl immunotoxicity, the aromatic hydrocarbon locus and liver microsomal enzyme induction in C57BL/6 and DBA/2 mice. *Toxicol Appl Pharmacol* 1984;75:156–165.
134. Thomas PT, Faith RE. Adult and perinatal immunotoxicity induced by halogenated aromatic hydrocarbons. In: Dean JA, Luster MI, Munson AE, Amos H, eds. *Immunotoxicology and immunopharmacology*. New York: Raven Press; 1985:305–313.
135. Vos JG, Brouwer GMJ, van Leeuwen FXR, Wagenaar SJ. Toxicity of hexachlorobenzene in the rat following combined pre- and postnatal exposure: comparison of effects on immune system, liver, and lung. In: Gibson GG, Hubbard R, Parke DV, eds. *Immunotoxicology*. New York: Academic Press; 1983:219–235.
136. Vos JG, Moore JA. Suppression of cellular immunity in rats and mice by maternal treatment with 2,3,7,8-tetrachlorodibenzo-*p*-dioxin. *Int Arch Allergy Appl Immunol* 1974;47:777–794.

137. Yoshida S, Golub MS, Gershwin ME. Immunological aspects of toxicology: premises, not promises. *Regul Toxicol Pharmacol* 1989;9:56–80.
138. Davidson A, Shefner R, Livneh A, Diamond B. The role of somatic mutation in immunoglobulin genes in autoimmunity. *Annu Rev Immunol* 1987;5:85.
139. Bigazzi PE. Autoimmunity induced by chemicals. *J Toxicol Clin Toxicol* 1988;26:125–156.
140. Broughton A, Thrasher JD. Antibodies and altered cell-mediated immunity in formaldehyde-exposed humans. *Comments Toxicol* 1988;2:155–174.
141. Chandor SB. Autoimmune phenomena in lymphoid malignancies. *Clin Lab Med* 1988;8:373–384.
142. Byers VS, Levin AS, Ozonoff DM, Baldwin RW. Association between clinical symptoms and lymphocyte abnormalities in a population with chronic domestic exposure to industrial solvent-contaminated domestic water supply and a high incidence of leukaemia. *Cancer Immunol Immunother* 1988;27:77–81.
143. Radl J, Valentijn RM, Haaijman JJ, Paul LC. Monoclonal gamma-pathies in patients undergoing immuno-suppressive treatment after renal transplantation. *Clin Immunol Immunopathol* 1985;37:98–102.
144. Coleman RM, Lombard MF, Sicard RE, Rencricca NJ. Immune deficiency. In: Coleman RM, ed. *Fundamental immunology*. Debuque, IA: William C Brown; 1989:379–401.
145. Dean JH, Thurmond LM. Immunotoxicology: an overview. *Toxicol Pathol* 1987;15:265–271.
146. Gardner DE, Coffin DL, Pinigin MA, Sidorenko GI. Role of time as a factor in the toxicity of chemical compounds in intermittent and continuous exposures. Part I. Effects of continuous exposure. *J Toxicol Environ Health* 1977;3:811–820.
147. Riegart JR, Graber CD. Evaluation of the humoral immune response of children with low level lead exposure. *Bull Environ Contam Toxicol* 1976;16:112–117.
148. Rosen FS, Wedgwood RF, Eibl M, et al. Primary immunodeficiency diseases: report of a WHO scientific group. *Clin Immunol Immunopathol* 1986;40:166–196.
149. Shopp GM, Edwards BS, Coons TA, et al. Laboratory assessment of the immune system in individuals occupationally exposed to 2,3,7,8-tetrachlorodibenzo-*p*-dioxin (2,3,7,8-TCDD): quality control in a cross-sectional epidemiologic study. *Chemosphere* 1989;18:867–874.
150. Stehr-Green PA, Andrews JS Jr, Hoffman RE, Webb KB, Schramm WF. An overview of the Missouri dioxin studies. *Arch Environ Health* 1988;43:174–177.
151. Trizio D, Basketter DA, Botham PA, et al. Identification of immunotoxic effects of chemicals and assessment of their relevance to man. *Food Chem Toxicol* 1988;26:527–539.
152. Jenkins MK, Schwartz RH, Pardoll DM. Effects of cyclosporine A on T-cell development and clonal deletion. *Science* 1988;248:1655.
153. Talal N. Cyclosporine as an immunosuppressive agent for autoimmune disease: theoretical concepts and therapeutic strategies: *Transplant Proc* 1988;20:11–15.
154. Kishimoto T, Hirano T. β-Lymphocyte activation, proliferation, and immunoglobulin secretion. In: Paul WE, ed. *Fundamental immunology*, 2nd ed. New York: Raven; 1984.
155. Bentwich Z, Beverley PCL, Hammarstrom L, Kalden JR, Lambert PH, Rose NR, Thompson RA. Laboratory investigations in clinical immunology: methods, pitfalls, and clinical considerations. A second IUIS/WHO working report. *Clin Immunol Immunopathol* 1988;49:478–497.
156. Burleson GR. Alteration of cellular interactions in the immune system: natural killer activity and N lymphocytes. In: Milman HA, Elmore E, eds. *Biochemical mechanisms and regulation of intercellular communication*, vol 14. Princeton, NJ: Princeton Scientific; 1987:51–96.
157. Capurro PU. The effects of solvents and pesticides on health. *Clin Toxicol* 1980;16:549–553.
158. Descotes J. *Immunotoxicology of drugs and chemicals*, 2nd ed. Amsterdam: Elsevier; 1988.
159. Dean JH, Luster MI, Boorman GA, Lauer LD. Procedures available to examine the immunotoxicity of chemistry and drugs. *Pharmacol Rev* 1982;34:137–148.
160. Dean JH, Luster MI, Munson AE, Amos H, eds. *Immunotoxicology and immunopharmacology*. New York: Raven; 1985.
161. Dean JH, Murray MJ, Ward EC. Toxic responses of the immune system. In: Klaassen CD, Amdur MO, Doull J, eds. *Casarett and Doull's toxicology: the basic science of poisons*, 3rd ed. New York: Macmillan; 1986:248–285.
162. Exon JH, Koller LD, Talcott PA, O'Reilly CA. Henningsen GM. Immunotoxicity testing: an economical multiple-assay approach. *Fundam Appl Toxicol* 1986;7:387–397.
163. Nepom GT. Determinants of genetic susceptibility in HLA-associated autoimmune disease. *Clin Immunol Immunopathol* 1989;53(Pt 2):S53–S62.
164. Lindsten T, June CH, Ledbetter JA, Stella G, Thompson CB. Regulation of lymphokine messenger RNA stability by a surface-mediated T cell activation pathway. *Science* 1989;244:339–343.

165. Luster MI, Blank JA, Dean JH. Molecular and cellular basis of chemically induced immunotoxicity. *Annu Rev Pharmacol Toxicol* 1987;27:23–49.
166. Neckers LM, Cossman J. Transferrin receptor induction in mitogen-stimulated human T lymphocytes is required for DNA synthesis and cell division and is regulated by interleukin-2. *Proc Natl Acad Sci USA* 1983;80:3494–3498.
167. Burg JAR. The National Exposure Registry: a community's reaction. In: *Superfund '90. Proceedings of the 11th National Conference of the Hazardous Materials Control Research Institute*. Silver Spring, MD: Hazardous Materials Control Research Institute; 1990:161–163.

Immunotoxicology and Immunopharmacology, Second Edition, edited by J. H. Dean, M. I. Luster, A. E. Munson, and I. Kimber.
Raven Press, Ltd., New York, 1994.

2

Animal Models for Assessment

Joseph G. Vos, *Ralph J. Smialowicz, and Henk van Loveren

*Laboratory of Pathology, National Institute of Public Health and Environmental Protection, 3720 BA Bilthoven, The Netherlands; and *Health Effects Research Laboratory, United States Environmental Protection Agency, Research Triangle Park, North Carolina 27711*

A major focus of immunotoxicology is the detection and evaluation of undesired effects of chemicals and drugs by way of toxicity tests using rodent species. Toxic responses may occur when the immune system acts as a passive target of chemical insult. This can result in decreased resistance to infectious diseases, certain tumor diseases, immune dysregulation, stimulation promoting allergy or autoimmunity.

Mouse and rat species have enjoyed the most popularity in immunotoxicity testing. This is due to a variety of factors: mice are well-defined immunologically; a variety of cytokines, antibodies, and reagents are commercially available for the mouse; and mice are less expensive to purchase and maintain than larger animals. These benefits are counterbalanced by the fact that the rat is the most commonly employed species in routine toxicity testing. Consequently, a great deal of data exist for many xenobiotics in regard to their toxicity, metabolism and pharmacokinetics in rats. This information on a particular xenobiotic can provide important insights into the relationship(s) between these endpoints and the effects that the agent may have on the immune system. Furthermore, the rat as a model in immunotoxicity testing has become more attractive in recent years because of our increasing knowledge of the immune system of this species, the commercial availability of rat-specific cytokines and antibodies, and the availability of strains associated with immunogenetics.

In this chapter emphasis is placed on the tier test system in rat and mouse. Moreover, special models are discussed that can be of value in mechanism studies and in studies aimed at risk assessment. Promising models include the so-called severe combined immunodeficient (SCID) mouse and transgenic animals.

ANIMAL MODELS

Several laboratories have developed and validated a variety of methods to determine the effects of xenobiotics on the immune system of rats and mice (Table 1).

TABLE 1. *Immunotoxicology approaches in rodents*

Model	Species	Reference
Tier system developed at RIVM (extension of OECD guideline #407 for testing repeated dose oral toxicity)	Rat	1,2
Tier system adopted by NIEHS-NTP	Mouse	3,4
Tier system of the U.S. Environmental Protection Agency (evaluation of biochemical pest control agents)	Rat or mouse	5
Tier system of the U.S. Food and Drug Agency (evaluation of food additives)	Rat	6
Multiple testing in a single animal	Rat	7,8

Most employ a tier testing approach, while some investigators have advocated multiple testing in a single animal. The tier testing approaches are similar in design in that the first tier is a screen for immunotoxicity with the second tier consisting of more specific or confirmatory studies, host resistance studies, or in-depth mechanistic studies. At present, most information regarding these models comes from the U.S. National Institute of Environmental Health Sciences National Toxicology Program (NIEHS-NTP) followed by the model developed at the National Institute of Public Health and Environmental Protection (RIVM) in Bilthoven, The Netherlands. These models are described in more detail.

Dutch National Institute of Public Health and Environmental Protection Model in the Rat

Shown in Table 2 is the tier approach for immunotoxicologic evaluation followed at RIVM in The Netherlands (1,2). The first-tier screening consists of a set of tests for general parameters of specific and nonspecific immunity. No functional parameters are included in this screening tier for concern that this may compromise these routine toxicity studies (e.g., immunization). In this screening battery, histopathology of lymphoid organs is pivotal. Routine histopathology of lymphoid organs has been shown to be useful in assessing the potential immunotoxicity of a chemical, in particular when these results are combined with the effects observed on the weight of the lymphoid organs (9,10). If the results in tier I suggest immunotoxicity, tier II function studies can be performed to confirm and further investigate the nature of the immunotoxic effect. Information on structure–activity relationships of immunotoxic chemicals can also lead to the decision to initiate function testing. The choice for further studies depends on the type of immune abnormality observed. The second tier consists of a panel of *in vivo,* and *ex vivo/in vitro* assays including cell-mediated immunity, humoral immunity, macrophage and natural killer (NK) cell function, as well as host resistance assays.

Recently, it was suggested that the NK cell assay be added to RIVM's tier 1 (11).

TABLE 2. *Panel of the RIVM for detecting immunotoxic alterations in the rat*

Parameters	Procedures
Tier 1	
Nonfunctional	Routine hematology, including differential cell counting
	Serum IgM, IgG, IgA, and IgE determination
	Lymphoid organ weights (spleen, thymus, local and distant lymph nodes)
	Histopathology of thymus, spleen, lymph nodes and mucosa-associated lymphoid tissue
	Bone marrow cellularity
	Analysis of lymphocyte subpopulations in spleen by flow cytometry
Tier 2	
Cell-mediated immunity	Sensitization to T-cell-dependent antigens (e.g., ovalbumin, tuberculin, and *Listeria*) and skin test challenge
	Lymphoproliferative responses to specific antigens (*Listeria*) and mitogen responses (Con-A, PHA)
Humoral immunity	Serum titration of IgM, IgG, IgA, IgE responses to T-cell-dependent antigens (ovalbumin, tetanus toxoid, *Trichinella spiralis*, SRBCs) with ELISA
	Serum titration of T-cell-independent IgM response to LPS with ELISA
	Mitogen response to LPS
Macrophage function	*In vitro* phagocytosis and killing of *Listeia monocytogenes* by adherent spleen and peritoneal cells
	Cytolysis of YAC-1 lymphoma cells by adherent spleen and peritoneal cells
NK cell function	Cytolysis of YAC-1 lymphoma cells by nonadherent spleen and peritoneal cells
Host resistance	*Trichinella spiralis* challenge (muscle larvae counts and worm expulsion)
	Listeria monocytogenes challenge (spleen and lung clearance)
	Rat cytomegalovirus challenge (clearance from salivary gland)
	Endotoxin hypersensitivity
	Autoimmune models (adjuvant arthritis, experimental allergic encephalomyelitis)

The NK cell assay does not require that animals are sensitized or challenged and thus the assay can be performed with the same animals without affecting other toxicologic parameters.

The RIVM approach is based on the Organization for Economic Cooperation and Development (OECD) guideline for testing of chemicals—#407, Repeated Dose Oral Toxicity—Rodent: 28-day or 14-day Study—which suggests the maximum tolerated dose (MTD), to be used as the high dose level for studies. The standard exposure period is 28 days and the animal species routinely used is the rat. These tests can be performed in the context of studies aimed at determining the toxicologic profile of the compound. Testing is conducted on at least three dose levels, the highest dose being the MTD and the lowest producing no evidence of toxicity.

U.S. National Toxicology Program (NTP) Model in the Mouse

A tier testing approach for screening drugs and chemicals for their potential to alter immune function in the mouse was developed and validated by the National Toxicology Program at the U.S. National Institute of Environmental Health Sciences (3,4,12). This effort involved the participation of four separate laboratories. The panel is divided into two tiers (Table 3). Tier I tests include the following: immunopathology (i.e., complete blood counts and differentials; body, spleen, thymus, liver, and kidney weights; spleen cellularity; and spleen, thymus, and lymph node histology); humoral immunity [i.e., primary response to sheep red blood cells (SRBCs) and lipopolysaccharide (LPS) mitogen response]; cell-mediated immunity [i.e., lymphoproliferation to allogeneic leukocytes in the mixed leukocyte reaction (MLR) and to T cell mitogens]; and nonspecific immunity (i.e., NK cell activity). Tier II tests include the following: immunopathology (i.e., quantitation of T and B cells); humoral immunity (i.e., secondary response to SRBCs); cell-mediated immunity [i.e., cytotoxic T lymphocyte (CTL) cytotoxicity and delayed-type hypersensitivity (DTH) response]; and host resistance challenge models (i.e., syngeneic tumor models and bacterial, viral, and parasitic infectivity models).

In this approach, animals are usually only evaluated at one time point; thus the possibility for recovery or reversibility of immunologic changes are not evaluated. In conducting the studies, routinely a 14-day exposure period is employed. However, 30- and 90-day exposure periods have been used based on the pharmacokinetic properties of the chemical being tested. The selection of the dose to be used in this tier system tends to be lower than the MTD. In the NTP approach, a dose-ranging study is usually performed initially to determine the toxic dose and then immune endpoints are performed in a second study at subtoxic dose levels.

Several laboratories have used this panel of tests or modifications of it to evaluate the potential immunotoxicity of a variety of xenobiotics in mice. The sensitivity and predictability of the murine immune function test panel outlined above were reported in recent publications by Luster et al. (4,12). Analysis of the results, from studies in which over 50 selected compounds were evaluated, indicated that the tests or test combinations from the panel varied in their ability to identify immunotoxic compounds. Furthermore, the analysis revealed a concordance of more than 90% for the prediction of immunotoxic compounds in mice when certain groups of immune tests were performed. The two immune function tests that displayed the greatest association with immunotoxicity of the compounds studied were lymphocyte phenotype analysis (83%) and the antibody plaque-forming cell (PFC) response to SRBCs (78%). The combination of either of these two tests with almost any other parameter markedly increased the ability to predict immunotoxicity. On the other hand, several other tests were found to be rather poor predictors of immunotoxicity. These included leukocyte counts (43%), lymphoproliferative responses to LPS (50%), and spleen cellularity (56%). Luster et al. (4) concluded that their results indicated that many of the tests described in the screening panel did not improve the ability of the

TABLE 3. *Panel of the NIEHS-NTP for detecting immune alterations following chemical or drug exposure in rodents*[a]

Parameter	Procedures
Screen (tier I)	
Immunopathology	Hematology—complete blood count and differential
	Weights—body, spleen, thymus, kidney, liver
	Cellularity—spleen, bone marrow
	Histology—spleen, thymus, lymph nodes
Humoral immunity	IgM antibody PFCs to T-cell-dependent antigen (SRBCs)
	LPS mitogen response
Cell-mediated immunity	Lymphocyte blastogenesis (Con A) and MLR against allogeneic leukocytes
Nonspecific immunity	NK cell activity
Comprehensive (tier II)	
FACS analysis	Quantitation of splenic B and T cell numbers
Humoral immunity	IgG antibody response to SRBCs (PFCs)
Cell-mediated immunity	CTL cytolysis or DTH response
Host resistance challenge models (*end points*)[b]	Syngeneic tumor cells—PYB6 sarcoma (tumor incidence), B16F10 melanoma (lung burden)
	Bacterial models—*Listeria monocytogenes* (mortality), *Streptococcus* species (mortality)
	Viral models—influenza (mortality)
	Parasite models—*Plasmodium yoelli* (parasitemia)

[a]The testing panel was developed using B6C3F1 female mice.

[b]For any particular chemical tested only two or three host resistance models are selected for examination.

panel to discriminate a potential immunotoxicant. In other words, they now suggest that the PFC assay, in conjunction with fluorescence-activated cell sorter (FACS) analysis and perhaps measuring NK cell activity, would provide as high an ability to detect immunotoxicants as all the combined tests in tier I. Likewise, they suggest that similar results should be obtained with rats, although this remains to be confirmed.

In comparing the RIVM and NIEHS-NTP approaches, one striking difference concerns the dose levels that are used. The RIVM approach differs from the NIEHS-NTP model in mice, in which the highest dose level to which the mice are exposed is chosen, so that no overt toxicity (i.e., body weight changes and gross pathologic effects) is observed. It is clear that the choice of the dose regimen avoiding overt toxicity at the top dose requires a fair sensitivity of the immunotoxicity tests, in order to preclude false negatives. For this reason, the NIEHS-NTP's tier I includes functional assays. With the broader dose range, that includes overt toxicity, it is rather likely that potential immunotoxicity is observed, using the panel that does not include functional tests. Including functional assays in the first tier, especially those tests that require sensitization of the animals, would require satellite groups to be tested. It should be borne in mind that in the OECD guideline #407 for testing toxicants, none of the other systems are evaluated functionally.

While studies at RIVM have indicated that measurement of basal immunoglobulin (Ig) levels are useful in predicting immunotoxic effects of compounds in the rat (11,13,14,15), studies conducted in mice by the NIEHS-NTP did not (4). Accordingly, the measurement of basal Igs has not been included in either tier of the testing panel used by the NIEHS-NTP. There are several possible reasons for the discrepancy in the usefulness of basal Ig levels in rats versus mice. First, in the rat studies cited above, the exposure period was routinely longer than the 14-day studies conducted by the NIEHS-NTP. Since the ability to detect changes in antibody level is a function of the antibody's half-life, the longer the study the more likely an effect will be observed. Furthermore, the dose levels used by the NIEHS-NTP were often lower, by design, than those used in the rat studies.

It is clear that the current OECD guideline #407 is not suited to adequately assess potential adverse effects of exposure to the test chemical on the immune system, since, with respect to immunologic parameters, it is restricted to total and differential leukocyte counting and histopathology of the spleen. An evaluation of this test scheme (11) indicated that in a series of almost 20 chemicals over 50% of the immunotoxic chemicals would not have been identified as such if the tests would have strictly adhered to the guideline. In fact, it is even doubtful if those chemicals that were indicated to be immunotoxic only on the basis of guideline #407 would have been identified as such. For example, in a toxicologic experiment a small, but significant, change in the percentage of basophilic leukocytes, without any other parameter to suggest that an effect on the immune system might have been present, would of itself probably not be considered biologically relevant.

With the increased application of the tier testing approach in rats, information has become available for comparing the effects of certain chemicals on the immune system between rats and mice. Not surprisingly, there have been instances where the responses to certain agents have not correlated between species. For example, hexachlorobenzene effects on the immune system are highly species dependent. In mice, reduced levels of serum Ig and secondary antibody responses have been reported. However, in rats an increase in weight of lymphoid organs and enhancement of serum antibody levels occurred (16). It has recently been shown that while the immune system of mice is not affected by exposure to the glycol ether 2-methoxyethanol or its principal oxidative metabolite 2-methoxyacetic acid (17,18), these compounds are immunosuppressive in rats (18–20). In contrast, while exposure of mice to carbon tetrachloride results in immunosuppression (21), rats exposed to carbon tetrachloride at levels that induced hepatotoxicity fail to demonstrate altered immune function (22). More recently, a species comparison of the effect that 2,3,7,8-tetrachlorodibenzo-*p*-dioxin (TCDD) has on the primary antibody response to SRBCs revealed that this response was suppressed in mice but enhanced in rats following exposure to TCDD (23). While it should be emphasized that there is no evidence to suggest that any particular animal model, perhaps with the exception of the nonhuman primate, is more predictive of xenobiotic-induced immunotoxicity in humans, immunotoxicity testing should continue to be performed in a variety of species.

Nonhuman Primate Models

Various nonhuman primates including the *Macaca mulatta* (rhesus macaques), *Macaca nemestrina* (pig-tailed macaques), *Cerocebus atys* (sooty mangabeys), *Macaca fascicularis* (cynomolgus monkeys), and the marmoset have been used in immunotoxicologic studies. Virtually all the immunotoxicology assays that are carried out in the mouse or rat can be and have been adapted for use with the nonhuman primates. While most of the assays conducted in nonhuman primates have utilized serum or peripheral blood, some assays such as those used to measure DTH have been holistic in nature in that the animals were sensitized *in vivo* and then evaluated *in vivo* at the challenge site (24,25).

Assays utilized in the rhesus monkey to investigate the effects of chronic exposure to polychlorinated biphenyl (PCB) (Aroclor 1254) on the immune response are lymphocyte transformation to concanavalin A (Con A) and phytohemagglutinin (PHA), total serum Ig levels, antibodies to SRBCs, and the enumeration of T and B cells in the peripheral blood (26). Later studies by this group (27) also evaluated NK cell activity, complement activity, and production of thymosins, interferon (IFN), and tumor necrosis factor (TNF) from PCB-exposed animals.

Studies by Ahmed-Ansari et al. (28) evaluated phenotypic markers and functional assays in three different species of nonhuman primates. Functional assays included NK cell activity, lymphocyte transformation, and antigen presentation. The extensive phenotypic marker studies included the evaluation of over 20 markers or combination of markers for each of the three monkey species. The use of nonhuman primates as a test species for immunotoxicity assessment will continue to increase with the greater commercial availability of biotechnology products.

Models to Investigate Local Immunity

While the preceding discussion has dealt with the evaluation of xenobiotic-induced alterations in systemic immune responses, it is important to consider models for the evaluation of alterations in immune responses that may be confined within specific anatomic compartments of the body. There are three such compartmentalized immune systems in mammals: bronchus-associated lymphoid tissue (BALT), gut-associated lymphoid tissue (GALT), and skin immune system (SIS). Animal models of hypersensitivity responses in the respiratory tract (e.g., pulmonary hypersensitivity), skin (e.g., contact dermatitis), and gut (e.g., food allergies) will be discussed in subsequent chapters. The brief discussion that follows deals only with a consideration of immune alterations in localized lymphoid tissues, which results from either inhalation or dermal exposure.

Inhalation of chemical pollutants by rodents has been shown to result in decreased resistance to a variety of infectious agents, which have been shown to be associated with impaired pulmonary immune function. For example, mice and rats exposed to ozone have increased susceptibility to infection with bacteria and viruses

(29–31). Decreased resistance to streptococcal infection in ozone-exposed mice was found to be associated with reduced alveolar macrophage phagocytic ability (29). Murine alveolar macrophage phagocytic activity has also been shown to be suppressed following inhalation exposure to nitrogen dioxide with resultant increased susceptibility to bacterial and viral infections (32,33). Besides macrophage activity, oxidant gases also affect lung NK cell activity (34). Inhalation exposure of mice to phosgene resulted in increased mortality from streptococcal infection and increased B16 syngeneic lung tumor burdens, while virus titers in the lung were only minimally affected (35). The observed effects of phosgene on lung tumor burdens may result from alterations in pulmonary NK cell activity as has been demonstrated in rats (36). While xenobiotic-induced humoral immunocompetence, following intratracheal installation of SRBCs, has been evaluated successfully in rat models (37,38), there are no reports in which mice have been used. This is likely due to the technical difficulties associated with performing this type of immunization in the smaller mice. The examples presented here indicate that alterations in natural, cell-mediated, and/or humoral pulmonary immune defense mechanisms, resulting from exposure to inhaled xenobiotics, can be identified.

Dermal exposure of mice to certain environmental agents has been shown to result in immunosuppression through alterations in the SIS. Perhaps the best example is exposure to ultraviolet (UV) radiation in the UVB range (280 to 320 nm), which produces local as well as systemic immune alterations in mice (39). Local effects, which are responsible for initiating the systemic effects of UVB exposure, include alterations in the number and function of epidermal Langerhans cells and keratinocytes, alterations in antigen-presenting cells, and the induction of anti-UV tumor-specific suppressor T cells (39). The systemic effects of UVB irradiation include depression of the contact hypersensitivity reaction and the reduced ability to reject highly immunogenic syngeneic tumors. The tests used to delineate UVB-induced immunosuppression should be applicable to immunotoxicity testing of other dermally applied xenobiotics.

SPECIAL MODELS

The progress that has occurred in immunotoxicology research and testing is a direct result of the application of the advances that have been made in basic immunology and molecular biology. Immunotoxicology research has employed a variety of immunologic and molecular biologic models, which have resulted in the refinement of immune function assays, the characterization of the mechanism(s) of toxicant-induced immune alterations, and the identification of genetic elements that play a role in the predisposition to xenobiotic-induced immunotoxicity. For example, athymic (nude) mice and rats (40) have been used to investigate effects of immunotoxic agents on B lymphocytes without interference by T lymphocytes. Interesting new models for studying effects on specific arms of the immune system are transgenic animals and mice with the SCID mutation, which show severe combined immunodeficiency.

Transgenic Mice

One model of great utility in providing insights into a variety of immunologic phenomena is the transgenic mouse. Transgenic mice, in which genetically different deoxyribonucleic acid (DNA) is permanently introduced into the germ line, have served to elucidate, among other things, the mechanisms of gene regulation, biologic development, and pathogenesis (41). In immunology, our understanding of T lymphocyte differentiation in the thymus, B lymphocyte differentiation, and self-tolerance has greatly been advanced by transgenic mice models (42,43). For example, transgenic models that may be of value in immunotoxicology are animals transgenic with respect to certain specificities of the T cell receptor. If a gene that encodes for a certain antigen specificity is introduced in the genome, this specificity may be the only one that is expressed by the T cells. Effects of immunotoxicants that alter the process of selection (positive and/or negative) that takes place in the thymus could be studied using such models, where either undesired specificities (that should be negatively selected) or desired specificities (that should be positively selected) are introduced. The application of these transgenic mice models could provide important information that will help to elucidate the mechanism(s) of xenobiotic-induced immunosuppression, which in turn may help to reduce the uncertainty associated with human risk assessments based on results from animal testing.

SCID Mice

Another approach that may warrant further exploration is the use of SCID mice, C.B-17 *scid/scid*, engrafted with human immune cells. The lack of immunocompetent T and B cells in this mutant is related to a defective recombinase function. SCID mice have been engrafted with human fetal lymphoid tissue to study human hematopoiesis (44) or engrafted with human peripheral blood lymphocytes that are capable of producing human immunoglobulins as a result of primary and secondary antibody responses (45). Furthermore, the SCID mouse coimplanted with human fetal thymus and liver tissue fragments (SCID/hu mouse) offers the possibility of studying the human thymus *in vivo* in an isolated xenogeneic environment (44,46), as well as determining the effects that immunotoxicants may have on these grafts. This is particularly interesting for thymotoxic agents. In these types of studies, when experimental animal data have to be extrapolated to humans, a "control" model between the SCID/hu mouse model and the intact laboratory animal (rat) is desirable. This control model can provide important information about the possible differences in "thymic behavior" because of the placement of the engrafted thymus beneath the kidney capsule. For this reason, a SCID/ra mouse model was developed by implanting rat fetal thymus and liver tissue fragments under the SCID mouse renal capsule (47).

CONCLUSIONS

The goal of animal models for immunotoxicity testing is to provide sensitive predictors of xenobiotic-induced immune dysfunction in humans. Such models should be capable of identifying the target(s) (i.e., tissue, cell, and/or molecule) within the immune system that is affected by the xenobiotic and defining the resultant immune dysfunction (i.e., immunosuppression, autoimmunity, or hypersensitivity). The models discussed in this chapter have been used successfully to identify and characterize a variety of different immunotoxicants in animals leading predominantly to immune suppression. A large amount of data have been generated by the application of these animal models, which demonstrate that xenobiotics alter the immune system of animals. This database is being used increasingly for toxicologic assessment of chemicals and drugs for human health hazard evaluation.

It is now recognized that cytokines are important mediator molecules that are crucial for the physiologic function of the immune system as well as being involved in pathologic conditions. Subsequently, qualitative or quantitative cytokine measurement is increasingly being incorporated in immunotoxicity investigations. Cytokines can be measured at various levels [i.e., at the level of function using biologic assays; at the level of production using enzyme-linked immunoadsorbent assay (ELISA); and at the level of transcription using messenger ribonucleic acid (mRNA) assays]. However, validation of cytokine measurement in the context of immunotoxicity testing has yet to be performed.

In general terms, extrapolations between alterations in a specific immune function in animals to that of humans is often very difficult. This process is also hindered by the limited database for xenobiotic-induced human immunotoxicity. Consequently, efforts should be made to identify and clinically evaluate human populations who have experienced industrial or accidental high level exposures to known animal immunotoxicants. These evaluations should employ endpoints that can easily be done in both humans and animals such as hematology, FACS analysis, functionality of lymphocyte subpopulations, examining biopsies, and perhaps cytokine profiles. The information gained from such clinical studies would not only broaden the human database but also afford direct comparisons with the animal data.

REFERENCES

1. Vos JG. Immunotoxicity assessment screening and function studies. *Arch Toxicol* 1980;4:95–108.
2. Van Loveren H, Vos JG. Immunotoxicological considerations: a practical approach to immunotoxicity testing in the rat. In: Dayan AD, Paine AJ, eds. *Advances in applied toxicology*. New York: Taylor & Francis; 1989:143–164.

3. Luster MI, Munson AE, Thomas PT, et al. Development of a testing battery to assess chemical-induced immunotoxicity: National Toxicology Program's guidelines for immunotoxicity evaluation in mice. *Fundam Appl Toxicol* 1988;10:2–19.
4. Luster MI, Portier C, Pait DG. Risk assessment in immunotoxicology. I. Sensitivity and predictability of immune tests. *Fundam Appl Toxicol* 1992;18:200–210.
5. Sjoblad RD. Potential future requirements for immunotoxicology testing of pesticides. *Toxicol Ind Health* 1989;4:391–395.
6. Hinton DM. Testing guidelines for evaluation of the immunotoxic potential of direct food additives. *Crit Rev Food Sci Nutr* 1992;32:173–190.
7. Exon JH, Koller LD, Henningsen GM, Osborne CA. Multiple immunoassays in a single animal: practical approach to immunotoxicologic testing. *Fundam Appl Toxicol* 1984;4:278–283.
8. Exon JH, Bussiere JL, Mather GC. Immunotoxicity testing in the rat: an improved multiple assay model. *Int J Immunopharmacol* 1990;12;699–701.
9. Vos, JG, Krajnc-Franken MAM. Toxic effects on the immune system, rat. In: Jones TC, Ward JM, Mohr U, Hunt RD, eds. *Hemopoietic system*. New York: Springer Verlag; 1990:168–181.
10. Schuurman HJ, Krajnc-Franken MAM, Kuper CF, Van Loveren H, Vos JG. Immune system. In: Haschek-Hock WM, Rousseaux CG, eds. *Handbook of toxicologic pathology*. Orlando, FL: Academic Press; 1991:421–487.
11. Van Loveren H, Vos JG. Evaluation of OECD guideline #407 for assessment of toxicity of chemicals with respect to potential adverse effects to the immune system. *Report of the National Institute of Public Health and Environmental Protection*. Bilthoven: The Netherlands; 1992.
12. Luster MI, Portier C, Pait DG, et al. Risk assessment in immunotoxicology. II. Relationships between immune and host resistance tests. *Fundam Appl Toxicol* 1993;21:71–82.
13. Vos JG, Krajnc EI, Beekhof P. Use of the enzyme-linked immunosorbent assay (ELISA) in immunotoxicity testing. *Environ Health Perspect* 1982;43:115–121.
14. Vos JG, de Klerk A, Krajnc EI, Kruizinga W, Van Ommen B, Rozing J. Toxicity of bis(tri-*n*-butyltin)oxide in the rat. II. Suppression of thymus-dependent immune responses and of parameters of nonspecific resistance after short-term exposure. *Toxicol Appl Pharmacol* 1984;75:387–408.
15. Vos JG, de Klerk A, Krajnc EI, Van Loveren H, Rozing J. Immunotoxicity of bis(tri-*n*-butyltin)oxide in the rat: effects on thymus-dependent-immunity and non-specific resistance following long-term exposure in young versus aged rats. *Toxicol Appl Pharmacol* 1990;105:144–155.
16. Vos JG. Immunotoxicity of hexachlorobenzene. In: Morris CR, Cabral JRP, eds. *Hexachlorobenzene*. Lyon: International Agency for Research on Cancer; 1986:347–356
17. House RV, Lauer LD, Murray MJ, Ward EC, Dean JH. Immunological studies in B6C3F1 mice following exposure to ethylene glycol monomethyl ether and its principal metabolite methoxyacetic acid. *Toxicol Appl Pharmacol* 1985;776:358–362.
18. Smialowicz RJ, Riddle MM, Williams WC, Copeland CB, Luebke RW, Andrews DL. Differences between rats and mice in the immunosuppressive activity of 2-methoxyethanol and 2-methoxyacetic acid. *Toxicology* 1992;74:57–67.
19. Smialowicz RJ, Riddle MM, Luebke RW, et al. Immunotoxicity of 2-methoxyethanol following oral administration in Fischer 344 rats. *Toxicol Appl Pharmacol* 1991;109:494–506.
20. Smialowicz RJ, Riddle MM, Rogers RR, Copeland CB, Luebke RW, Andrews DL. Evaluation of the immunotoxicity of orally administered 2-methoxyacetic acid in Fischer 344 rats. *Fundam Appl Toxicol* 1991;17:771–781.
21. Kaminski NE, Jordan SD, Holsapple MP. Suppression of humoral and cell-mediated immune responses by carbon tetrachloride. *Fundam Appl Toxicol* 1989;12:117–128.
22. Smialowicz RJ, Simmons JE, Luebke RW, Allis JW. Immunotoxicologic assessment of the subacute exposure of rats to carbon tetrachloride with comparison to hepatotoxicity and nephrotoxicity. *Fundam Appl Toxicol* 1991;17:186–196.
23. Smialowicz RJ, Riddle MM, Williams WC, Diliberto JJ. Effects of 2,3,7,8-tetrachlorodibenzo-*p*-dioxin (TCDD) on humoral immunity and lymphocyte subpopulations: differences between mice and rats. *Toxicol Appl Pharmacol* 1994;124:248–256.
24. Bugelski PJ, Thiem PA, Solleveld HA, Morgan DG. Effects of sensitization to dinitrochlorobenzene (DNCB) on clinical pathology parameters and mitogen-mediated blastogenesis in cynomolgus monkeys (*Macaca fascicularis*). *Toxicol Pathol* 1990;18:643–650.
25. Bleavins MR, Alvey JD. Immunotoxicologic evaluation of a purine nucleoside phosphorylase inhibitor in the cynomolgus monkey. *Toxicologist* 1991;11:205.

26. Tryphonas H, Hayward S, O'Grady L, Loo JCK, Arnold DL, Bryce F, Zawidzka ZZ. Immunotoxicity studies of PCB (Aroclor 1254) in the adult rhesus (*Macaca mulatta*) monkey—preliminary report. *Int J Immunopharmacol* 1989;11:199–206.
27. Tryphonas H, Luster MI, White KL, et al. Effects of PCB (Aroclor 1254) on non-specific immune parameters in rhesus (*Macaca mulatta*) monkeys. *Int J Immunopharmacol* 1991;13:639–648.
28. Ahmed-Ansari A, Brodie AR, Fultz PN, Anderson DC, Sell KW, McClure HM. Flow microfluorometric analysis of peripheral blood mononuclear cells from nonhuman primates: correlation of phenotype with immune function. *Am J Prim* 1989;17:107–131.
29. Gilmour MI, Park P, Selgrade MJK. Ozone-enhanced pulmonary infection with *Streptococcus zooepidemicus* in mice: the role of alveolar macrophage function and capsular virulence factors. *Am Rev Respir Dis* 1993;147:753–760.
30. Selgrade MJK, Illing JW, Starnes DM, Stead AG, Menache MG, Stevens MA. Evaluation of effects of ozone on influenza infection in mice using several indicators of susceptibility. *Fundam Appl Toxicol* 1988;11:169–180.
31. Van Loveren H, Rombout PJA, Wagenaar SJSC, Walvoort HC, Vos JG. Effects of ozone on the defense to a respiratory *Listeria monocytogenes* infection in the rat. Suppression of macrophage function and cellular immunity and aggravation of histopathology in lung and liver during infection. *Toxicol Appl Pharmacol* 1988;94:374–393.
32. Gardner DE, Coffin DL, Pinigin MA, Sidorenko GI. Role of time as a factor in the toxicity of chemical compounds in intermittent and continuous exposure. Part I. Effects of continuous exposure. *J Toxicol Environ Health* 1977;3:811–820.
33. Rose RM, Fuglestad JM, Skornik WA, et al. The pathophysiology of enhanced susceptibility to murine cytomegalovirus respiratory infection during short-term exposure to 5 ppm nitrogen dioxide. *Am Rev Respir Dis* 1988;137:912–917.
34. Van Loveren H, Krajnc EI, Rombout PJA, Blommaert FA, Vos JG. Effect of ozone, hexachlorobenzene, and bis(tri-*n*-butyltin)oxide on natural killer activity in the rat lung. *Toxicol Appl Pharmacol* 1990;102:21–33.
35. Selgrade MJK, Starnes DM, Illing JW, Daniels MJ, Graham JA. Effects of phosgene exposure on bacterial, viral and neoplastic lung disease susceptibility in mice. *Inhal Toxicol* 1989;1:243–259.
36. Burleson GR, Keyes LL. Natural killer activity in Fischer-344 rat lungs as a method to assess pulmonary immunocompetence: immunosuppression by phosgene inhalation. *Immunopharmacol Immunotoxicol* 1989;11:421–443.
37. Bice DE, Hahn FF, Benson J, Carpenter RL, Hobbs CH. Comparative lung immunotoxicity of inhaled quartz and coal combustion fly ash. *Environ Res* 1987;43:374–389.
38. Sopori ML, Cherian S, Chilukuri R, Shopp GM. Cigarette smoke causes inhibition of the immune response to intratracheally administered antigens. *Toxicol Appl Pharmacol* 1989;97:489–499.
39. Daynes RA, Samlowski WE, Burnham DK, Gahring LC, Roberts LK. Immunobiological consequences of acute and chronic UV exposure. *Curr Probl Dermatol* 1986;15:176–194.
40. Van Loveren H, Schuurman HJ, Vos JG. Immune deficiency syndrome in rodents: the nude rat. In: Beynen AC, Solleveld HA, eds. *New developments in biosciences: their implications for laboratory animal science*. Dordrecht: Martinus Nijhoff; 1989:17–28.
41. Merlino GT. Transgenic animals in biomedical research. *FASEB J* 1991;5:2996–3001.
42. Morahan G. Transgenic mice as immune system models. *Curr Opin Immunol* 1991;3:219–223.
43. Goodnow CC. Transgenic mice and analysis of B-cell tolerance. *Annu Rev Immunol* 1992;10:489–518.
44. McCune JM, Namikawa R, Kaneshima H, Shultz LD, Lieberman M, Weissman IL. The SCID-hu mouse: murine model for the analysis of human hematolymphoid differentiation and function. *Science* 1988;241:1632–1639.
45. Mosier DE. Immunodeficient mice xenografted with human lymphoid cells: new models for in vivo studies of human immunobiology and infectious diseases. *J Clin Immunol* 1990;10:185–191.
46. Namikawa R, Weilbaecher KN, Kaneshima H, Yee EJ, McCune JM. Long-term human hematopoiesis in the SCID-hu mouse. *J Exp Med* 1990;172:1055–1063.
47. De Heer C, Verlaan APJ, Penninks AH, Schuurman HJ, Van Loveren H. The SCID-RA mouse: rat T cell differentiation in the severe combined immunodeficient mouse. *Arch Pathol Microbiol Immunol Scand* 1993;101:467–479.

Immunotoxicology and Immunopharmacology, Second Edition, edited by J. H. Dean, M. I. Luster, A. E. Munson, and I. Kimber.
Raven Press, Ltd., New York, 1994.

3

Targeted Epidemiology and Clinical Assessment Studies of the Immune System in Humans

Raymond E. Biagini, *Elizabeth M. Ward, **Robert Vogt, and †Gerry M. Henningsen

*Applied Biology Branch, Immunochemistry Research Section, Division of Biomedical and Behavioral Sciences, Centers for Disease Control and Prevention, National Institute for Occupational Safety and Health, Cincinnati, Ohio 45226; *Division of Surveillance, Hazard Evaluation, and Field Studies, National Institute for Occupational Safety and Health, Cincinnati, Ohio 45226; **Clinical Biochemistry Branch, Centers for Disease Control, Atlanta, Georgia 30333; and †United States Public Health Service, United States Environmental Protection Agency, Denver, Colorado 80202*

Field studies in humans designed to detect immunomodulation from exposure to xenobiotics present some of the most challenging problems to epidemiologists and immunotoxicologists. Investigators must choose exposed populations with adequate dose to detect an effect if one is present, quantitate exposure on an individual basis if possible, and rule out concurrent exposure of the population to other potential immunotoxicants. A control group must be identified that is similar to the exposed group in all characteristics except for exposure to the xenobiotic under study. Many exposures and circumstances can affect immune function in an individual, including sunlight, stress, medication use, and illness; some of these factors may produce immune alterations as great or greater than those predicted from occupational or environmental exposure to xenobiotics (1–5). Such exposures can be evaluated by administering questionnaires to subjects, which must necessarily include sensitive topics such as recreational drug use and human immunodeficiency virus (HIV) infection. Sample acquisition (usually of peripheral blood and/or saliva) is performed at sites geographically and temporally distant from the controlled environment of an investigator's laboratory, yielding an assortment of new problems that would not occur in a clinical or hospital situation. Some assays, such as lymphocyte transformation tests, which require almost immediate processing of blood samples, may not be possible in field studies where blood samples must be transported to the laboratory over large distances or from remote locales. Some immunologic and clinical tests that might yield important data in some studies (e.g., vaccination of study subjects to measure primary antibody responses and bronchial provocation testing with workplace antigens) are rarely used in immunotoxicity studies because of unfounded concerns about the risk to study subjects. Subjects involved in immunotoxicity field studies must be briefed about the nature and purpose of the study, must provide informed consent, and must be notified of their individual test results and their possible clinical significance as soon as feasible after testing is complete. Since the application of immunotoxicologic techniques to populations exposed to xenobiotics is relatively new, there are difficulties in the interpretation of statistically positive results and their potential health significance.

REVIEW OF THE HUMAN IMMUNE SYSTEM

Effect of Xenobiotics

The mammalian host defense system consists of an integrated network of cells and mediators with recognition and response functions throughout most tissues. Primary functions of the host defense system include tissue repair, the identification and removal of foreign substances, destruction or containment of infectious agents, and the removal of neoplastic cells. These functions are performed both through nonspecific mechanisms (innate or natural immunity) and through specific mechanisms (acquired immunity).

Much current literature on immune assessment concerns severe immunodeficiency, the first clinical evidence of which is usually frequent or prolonged infections. Such deficiencies can be acquired or congenital, and excellent reviews of the assessment of each type are available (6–10). Current efforts in the area of immunotoxicology concern the possibility of subtle xenobiotic-induced defects that may exert their adverse effects over a long period of time, such as in the development of cancer, hypersensitivity reactions, or clinically relevant autoimmunities. There are excellent reviews available on immune biomarkers and clinical immunotoxicology (1,11,12).

Table 1 presents a summary of the major molecular and cellular constituents of the host defense system. Many of the defense and regulatory functions of the immune system are carried out by peptide and nonpeptide chemical mediators released from cells. Antibodies (which constitute the humoral branch of the immune response) are antigen specific. They are secreted by stimulated B lymphocytes and are comprised of several major classes with different functional capacities. Immunoglobulin M (IgM) and immunoglobulin G (IgG) antibodies facilitate phagocytosis, antigen clearance, and the destruction of parasites. IgA antibodies are secreted at mucous membranes, where they help to prevent attachment and invasion by microbes and parasites that come in contact with the surface tissues. IgE antibodies, bound to the outer membrane of mast cells and basophils, help initiate immune responses and are involved with immunity against worms and mites and are also responsible for classic allergic reactions such as hay fever and asthma.

TABLE 1. *Major components of the host defense system*

Component	Function
Molecular mediators	
Proteins	Viral inactivation, antigen clearance, complement activation, opsonization
Immunoglobulins (antibodies)	
Cytokines	Intercellular signaling
Interferons	
Interleukins	
Growth factors	
Complement (interacting with the kinin, fibrin, and plasmin systems)	Parasite destruction, chemotactic stimulation, acute inflammatory reactions
Heat shock	Protein binding and preservation, cross-reactive antigenicity
Lipid-derived	
Prostaglandins	
Leukotrienes	Intercellular signaling
Molecular cell surface receptors	
Immunoglobulins; T cell antigen receptor	Specific antigen recognition on lymphocytes
Immunoglobulin E	Specific antigen recognition on mast cells and basophils
Class I histocompatibility proteins	
Class II histocompatibility proteins	Cell–cell interactions
Immunoglobulin-related proteins (CD4, CD8, β_2-microglobulin)	
Cytokine receptor proteins	Receptors for the various cytokines
Cell adhesion molecules	Cell traffic and migration control
Cell lineages and subsets	
Granulocytes	
Neutrophils	Phagocytosis and antigen destruction
Eosinophils	Parasite destruction, regulation
Basophils	Parasite destruction, regulation
Monocytes/macrophages	Phagocytosis and antigen destruction, antigen processing and presentation, regulation
T lymphocytes	
Helper (CD4) cells	Activation of antigen-specific responses
Suppressor (CD8) cells	Suppression of antigen-specific responses
Cytotoxic (CD8) cells	Destruction of virus-infected and neoplastic cells
B lymphocytes	Antibody production, regulation
Plasma cells	
NK cells	Destruction of virus-infected and certain neoplastic cells
Dendritic cells	Antigen presentation
Platelets	Blood clotting, activation

Adapted from ref. 8.

Cytokines are extremely potent peptide molecules that activate or suppress target cell populations supporting appropriate receptors. More than a dozen immune cytokines (many called interleukins, ILs) have been identified as participants in the complicated network of immune regulation. Complement is one of several plasma proteins involved in acute nonspecific responses to tissue injury and invasion. Complement is actually a cascading system of different protein molecules that can be activated by a variety of stimuli, including antigen–antibody complexes, blood clotting proteins, and other mediators. Complement activation products have a number of activities, including chemotaxis, clearance, and destruction of cells. Other such "acute phase" serum proteins include transferrin and plasmin. Several nonpeptide molecules are also important immune mediators. They include different lipid-derived chemicals (such as prostaglandins) that have a wide variety of effects on many different tissues, including the activation or suppression of immune cells and the dilation or constriction of blood vessels and airways. Histamine, which is stored in the granules of mast cells and basophils, causes dilation and leakage in small blood vessels and has effects on immune cells and other tissues; it is responsible for many of the symptoms of allergy. Several other chemical mediators impact the activity of cells in the immune system, although they are not central to its function. Such include catecholamines (such as epinephrine), endorphins, and insulin. Most of the several different types of cells that constitute the cellular branch of the immune response spend at least part of their lifetime in the peripheral blood, where they constitute the white blood cells or leukocytes. The major types of leukocytes are lymphocytes, monocytes, and granulocytes. Lymphocytes (B cells and T cells) are the specific recognition cells of the immune system. Each family (clone) of lymphocytes has unique recognition molecules on its surface. If the lymphocyte is activated by recognizing a foreign protein (antigen), a specific immune response is initiated. Activated lymphocytes proliferate and engage in a variety of host defense functions, such as producing antibodies (B cells), killing virus-infected cells, or regulating immune activities (T cells). Monocytes are immature cells that differentiate into macrophages after emigration from the blood. Macrophages are distributed throughout many tissues including the lung, liver, skin, brain, and bone marrow. Their innate activities of phagocytosis and digestion are nonspecific, but they become part of the specific immune response when they "present" processed fragments of foreign protein to lymphocytes. Granulocytes are important auxiliary cells with activities that are critical to host defense but also may contribute to disease processes. Neutrophils, like macrophages, are avid phagocytes but are short-lived and less versatile. Mast cells, basophils, and eosinophils are involved in immunity to larger parasites, such as worms, and are also primary participants in the allergic responses to pollens, foods, and other substances. In addition, they appear to be involved in inflammatory reactions to certain toxic and sensitizing chemical exposures (12,13).

Immunotoxic agents can affect either the cellular, the humoral, or both branches of the immune response. Classes and examples of chemicals causing immunologic changes are shown in Table 2. Coincident hematologic changes (deficiencies involving erythrocytes, platelets, or leukocytes) give evidence for toxic effects at the level of the stem cell. Chronic benzene exposure may induce pancytopenia by a direct effect on bone marrow (14). Reduction in the immune response may result in decreased host resistance to infection and malignancy. If the deficiency occurs in the T cell lineage, it characteristically presents clinically as repeated infections by intracellular pathogens (including some protozoan parasites, pathogenic fungi, viruses, and certain bacteria). Because the T cell also seems to play a role in re-

TABLE 2. *Classes and examples of chemicals causing immunologic changes*

Class	Examples
Polyhalogenated aromatic hydrocarbons	TCDD, PBBs, PCDF, PCBs, hexachlorobenzene
Metals	Lead, calcium, arsenic, methyl mercury
Aromatic hydrocarbons (solvents)	Benzene, toluene
Polycyclic aromatic hydrocarbons	DMBA, BaP, MCA
Pesticides	Trimethyl phosphorothioate, carbofuran, chlordane, malathion
Organotins	TBTO
Aromatic amines	Benzidene, acetyl aminofluorene
Oxidant gases	Nitrogen dioxide, ozone, sulfur dioxide
Particles	Silica, asbestos
Natural products	Selected vitamins, antibiotics, vinca alkaloids, estrogen, plant alkaloids, mycotoxins
Drugs of abuse	Ethanol, cannabinoids, cocaine, opioids
Therapeutic drugs	Diphenylhydantoin, lithium
Others	Nitrosamine, BHA

Adapted from ref. 6.

TCDD, 2,3,7,8-tetrachlorodlbenzo-*p*-dioxin; PBBs, polybrominated biphenyls; PCDF, polychlorinated dibenzofuran; PCBs, polychlorinated biphenyls; DMBA, dimethylbenzanthracene; BaP, benzo[*a*]pyrene; MCA, methylcholanthrene; TBTO, bis(tris-*n*-butylin)oxide: BHA, butylated hydroxyanisole.

sistance to certain malignancies, either directly through the action of cytotoxic T cells or indirectly through the production of lymphokines, an increased incidence of malignancy may also be a manifestation of cellular immunodeficiency. However, it should be noted that only a few environmental exposures have been shown to have caused a cellular immunodeficiency that can be correlated to increased opportunistic infections or neoplasms. In addition, the neoplasms that occur with increased frequency in immunocompromised individuals, such as non-Hodgkin's lymphoma, are derived from cells of the immune system, making it difficult to determine if the immune defect is responsible for the neoplasms or whether some other factor causes both the neoplasms and the immunodeficiency. B cell deficiency produces a distinct clinical syndrome characterized by increased susceptibility to acute infections with pyogenic bacteria, such as recurrent pneumonia, meningitis, or abscesses, against which antibody is the main protective mechanism. Complement deficiencies show many similarities with B cell deficiencies. Complement deficiencies involving C6 and C8 characteristically predispose to infections with gram-negative cocci. The manifestations of defects in phagocytes also can mimic B cell deficiency because of the role of opsonins in facilitating phagocytosis. However, neutrophils from persons with chronic granulomatous disease phagocytose normally but are incapable of producing an oxidative burst in metabolism following phagocytosis. These individuals are prone to chronic infections because the phagocytes can ingest the common organisms but cannot digest and kill them. Although the importance of natural killer (NK) cells for human health is not as well established as that of B cells and T cells, they are believed to be important in host defense against viruses and tumors (15). A recent case report describes a patient with recurrent herpesvirus infections who was shown to have a selective absence of NK cells (16).

Autoimmune diseases are immune reactive disorders in which the immune system reacts against the host's tissues. Autoimmune reactions often are associated with antibodies that react to self-proteins, in particular, tissues or cell components. Autoimmune reactions can damage the skin, liver, kidneys, various glands, joints, and other tissues, leading to diseases such as rheumatoid arthritis, ankylosing spondylitis, systemic lupus erythematosis (SLE), thyroiditis, multiple sclerosis, myasthenia gravis, and some types of diabetes (12). SLE (evaluated by titer of antinuclear autoantibodies) has been shown to be associated with exposure to trichloroethylene and other chemicals in contaminated well water (17) and by occupational exposure to hydralazine (18).

Consequences of Immunosuppression

The study of human immunodeficiency disease syndromes reveals a clear association between the suppression or absence of an immunologic function and an increased incidence of infectious or neoplastic disease. Numerous examples of such deficiency diseases have been reported and are well characterized in humans (Table 3). A deficiency in one or more immunologic functions can lead to severe, recurrent infections throughout life. These infections can be bacterial, viral, fungal, or protozoan, and the predominant type of infection depends on the associated immunologic lesion. Some infections can be treated with antibiotics or gamma globulin, and in some cases the immunologic defect can be restored by bone marrow transplantation. However, other immunodeficiency diseases are much more severe. For example, children born with reticular dysgenesis have no white blood cells and usually die from infectious disease in the first year of life; children born with ataxia-telangiectasia rarely survive past puberty. These diseases of genetic deficiency are more severe than those caused by environmental toxicants, because they are the result of the absence of part of the immune system. They demonstrate well-characterized consequences of immunosuppression. These same diseases would be expected to be associated with specific immunosuppression, whether the cause were genetic or environmental (1).

Nonxenobiotic Immunomodulators

Stress (from psychosocial or occupational stressors) may result in immune suppression, which may, in turn, lead to reduced disease resistance (19). In animal models, lowered disease resistance has resulted in infections, cancer, or autoimmunity, while clinical case studies have shown severe stress (i.e., bereavement) to be associated with increased mortality, altered immunity including suppression of lymphocyte responses to mitogens, reduced NK cell activity, and changes in T cell

TABLE 3. *Consequences of immunosuppression: primary deficiencies and diseases*

Syndrome	Cell type affected	Result
DiGeorge's syndrome	T cell	Increased bacterial, viral, and yeast infections
Nezelof's syndrome	T cell	Increased bacterial, viral, and protozoan infections
Common variable immunodeficiency (CVD)	B cell (T cell)	Increased bacterial infections
Bruton's disease X-linked infantile hypogammaglobulinemia	B cell	Increased bacterial infections
Selective IgA deficiency	B cell	Increased bacterial infections
Wiskott–Aldrich syndrome	B and T cells, monocytes	Increased bacterial and viral infections
Ataxia-telangiectasia (A-T)	B and T cells	Increased bacterial and viral infections
Severe combined immunodeficiency disease (SCID)	B and T cells	Increased bacterial and viral infections
Reticular dysgenesis	Leukocytes	Increased bacterial and viral infections
Adenosine deaminase (ADA) deficiency	T_H cells (direct), B cells (indirect)	Increased bacterial and viral infections
Chédiak–Higashi syndrome	Phagocytes, NK cells, and T_c cells	Increased bacterial infections
Chronic granulomatous disease	Phagocytes (primarily neutrophils)	Increased bacterial infections
Complement deficiency C1–C8	—	Increased bacterial infections

Adapted from ref. 6.

subpopulations (2). Stress also can affect the normal homeostatic relationships between the immune, nervous, and endocrine systems (20,21).

Psychometric instruments (questionnaires) for measuring job stress have been developed and applied to the workplace; however, biologic indicators of stress (biomarkers) would be a valuable objective measure to complement these questionnaires (22). Validated biomarkers could be used to measure a worker's exposure, susceptibility for developing an occupational disease, or early (preclinical/reversible) health effects resulting from occupational exposures.

Several biologic indices have been studied in the past to ascertain their value in detecting physiologic and health effects of various types of stress. Levels of cortisol in saliva, urine, and serum have been studied most often (23), while other endpoints examined include blood pressure, heart rate, visual accommodation, adrenocorticotropic hormone (ACTH), catecholamines, blood counts, immunoglobulins, cytokines, and immunocompetency (2,24). Due to problems with methods/design, these studies have had varying degrees of success. Changes in cortisol, catecholamines, and other hormones are usually only transient responses to acute stressors and have not proved to be appropriate measures of chronic stress. Many of the transient responses have relatively large natural fluctuations due to biologic rhythms (24) and are also quite variable in heterogeneous human populations and environments.

Salivary IgA (sIgA) is another potential biomarker for stress-induced immunologic effects in workers (25,26). sIgA has particular appeal as a potential biomarker because (a) it can be obtained noninvasively, easily, and frequently compared to blood; (b) it is biologically relevant as a functional immune endpoint; (c) it can be quantitated; and (d) it is more stable with a longer biologic half-life than cortisol and catecholamine. Controversy remains concerning the best methodology to measure sIgA (24,27,28); therefore total IgA levels, specific IgA titers, or both, and total salivary protein concentration and/or salivary flow rates have been measured in previous studies (29). Procedural variations occur in collection methods (stimulated versus nonstimulated salivation), in sampling times (biorhythms, frequency, storage), in sources (whole saliva versus parotid), in immunoassays [enzyme-linked immunoadsorbent assay (ELISA) versus radioimmunodiffusion, standards, antibody specificity], in IgA endpoints (monomeric versus polymeric, secretory component, J chain, subclass A1 or A2, specific antigen tested), and in designs (population size, replicates). Some important confounding factors that may affect sIgA levels include disease, nutrition, age, hormonal activity, certain medications, trauma or exertion, and biorhythms (12).

It is well known that exposure to ionizing radiation damages the immune, hematopoietic, and gastrointestinal components of the host defense system. This may lead to serious endogenous or exogenous infections. When radiation injury is combined with other physical trauma (e.g., burns or wounds), the resulting damage to these systems is synergistic (30).

Exposure to nonionizing ultraviolet (UV) radiation (sunlight) is the most common nonchemical exposure that affects the immune system. UV exposure can lead to suppression of the normal immune response, which may play an important part in the development of skin cancers, infectious diseases, and autoimmune responses (3). NK cell activity has been shown to be suppressed in volunteer subjects exposed to UV radiation from solarium lamps (4). In studies using xenon arc lamp sources, it also appears that UVA may have equivalent or greater direct immunosuppressive effects than UVB (4). Epidermal cells from UV-exposed skin, in contrast to epidermal cells from normal skin, potently activate autologous CD4+ T cells and, in particular, the CD45RA+ (2H4+) (suppressor-inducer) subset, suggesting that UV exposure in humans leads to a T cell response in which suppression dominates (5).

DESIGN OF FIELD STUDIES

Clinical assessment of individuals usually starts with evidence of an immunologic alteration that may lead to clinical diseases. This immunologic change is then investigated in order to associate the effect of exposure to a particular drug, toxic agent, or exposure. This chapter focuses on studies of groups of individuals with occupational or environmental exposure and methods to detect subclinical changes in immune function. General issues in epidemiologic study design and analysis are discussed in several texts (31,32). The most common epidemiologic study design used in immunotoxicity research is the cross-sectional study. In such a study, exposure status and disease status (in this case, changes in immunologic function) are measured at one point in time or over a short period in study subjects (33). The immune function of "exposed" subjects is compared to the immune function of a comparable group of "nonexposed" individuals.

The first challenge in conducting an immune assessment study is to identify the exposed group. In studies designed to evaluate the immunotoxicity of a chemical (as opposed to studies where immune function evaluation is prompted by a public health concern), the study should include populations at the upper end of human exposure unless previous studies have already established an immunotoxic effect in that range. Where possible, the study should incorporate individual estimates or measurement of dose and utilize biologic monitoring to estimate internal dose. Once the exposed group has been identified, a clear definition is needed of who is eligible to participate in the study. For example, in an occupational study, all individuals who have worked in a particular department might be considered eligible exposed subjects; in an environmental study, eligible persons might include all residents of a community or a sample of households in a community. It is important to enumerate the number of potentially eligible subjects, as well as the number who eventually participated, in order to assess the likelihood that selection bias has influenced the study findings. Selection bias may occur when an individual's willingness to participate varies with characteristics related to exposure status or health status of the individual. Although it is difficult to avoid or detect selection bias in a voluntary study, a high degree of participation makes it less likely that selection bias has influenced the results.

In many field situations, the potential immune effects of other chemicals present in the industrial or residential environment need to be considered. The investigator should assess all chemicals present in the exposed and control environments and whether any of these other chemicals has either known or suspected effects on the immune system. Exposures of individual study subjects to chemicals outside the study environment should also be evaluated. For example, in an occupationally based study, subjects could be questioned about chemical exposures in hobbies or second jobs. In a study of community residents exposed to an immunotoxin as a result of environmental contamination from a nearby factory, an assessment should by made of other contaminants in the local environment, as well as potential occupational chemical exposures.

Known risk factors that might influence the outcome of immune function tests, such as age, gender, cigarette smoking, sunlight exposure, stress, and use of certain medications and recreational drugs, should be matched into the design of the study or controlled for in the analysis. However, there is limited qualitative or quantitative data on the influence of these factors on immune function in the general population, and it is impossible for an epidemiologic study to match for or analyze all potential factors. For example, differences in dietary habits, exercise levels, or community-specific exposures to particular viruses might conceivably influence comparisons between an exposed and nonexposed population. Yet it is often not practical to collect information on all such factors. It is therefore desirable to select the comparison group to be as similar as possible to the exposed group in order to hopefully match factors that cannot be measured. For example, in an occupationally based study, the comparison group should be selected so that the community of residence, socioeconomic status, and ethnicity are similar to the exposed group. In an environmental study, the comparison group should be selected from a geographic area whose residents have a similar ethnic distributionl socioeconomic status, and employment pattern as residents in the exposed area.

The study should account for medical factors that might have a major impact on immune function. For example, individuals who are immunosuppressed as a result of chemotherapy or steroid treatment should be excluded from the study. Other medications and medical exposures (immunizations, medications, radiation) in the recent time period should be inquired about and evaluated in the statistical analyses.

Because many of the immune function tests have potential variability between laboratories or within a laboratory over time, it is desirable to have each test run by the same laboratory for all exposed and nonexposed subjects in a particular study (or if that is not possible, to at least ensure that equal proportions of exposed and nonexposed subjects are tested by each laboratory). The laboratory conducting the tests should validate each test procedure to assess technical and subject variability before the analysis of study samples begins. It is desirable to recruit exposed and unexposed subjects into the study during the same time period, so that the samples analyzed on a particular day include both types of subjects. This will minimize the effect on the study findings of any undetected changes in laboratory conditions that shift test results upward or downward on a particular day.

In addition to the characteristics that should be considered in evaluating the methodology of study, there are some issues that are particularly important in the interpretation of positive studies, and others that are particularly important in the interpretation of negative studies. In interpreting studies that show significant differences between the exposed and nonexposed populations, it is important to recognize that large cross-sectional studies (i.e., studies with 100 to 200 exposed and control subjects will have adequate statistical power to detect relatively small differences, on the order of 10%) in immunologic endpoints such as proportion of CD4+ and CD8+ cells. Although such studies might be interpreted as positive, particularly if there is evidence of a dose–response relationship, there will be considerable overlap between the values of nonexposed and exposed individuals, and it is possible that none of the individual values will fall outside the clinically normal range. Interpretation of such findings is complicated because there is little quantitative data on the degree to which such parameters need to be modified in a population before the population experiences an increased risk of disease (34).

In addition, because statistically significant differences measured between the two populations may be small in magnitude, and of unknown clinical significance, the possibility that they reflect methodologic errors rather than a true biologic effect is of concern. Methodologic problems that might spuriously produce such a finding might include selection bias, laboratory variability, or lack of control for confounding variables. Careful design and analysis of studies examining changes in immune function tests as the primary outcome are therefore of critical importance.

Evidence of a dose–response relationship is usually an important criterion in the assessment of a toxic exposure. However, both biologic and methodologic factors complicate the assessment of dose–response relationships in human immunotoxicity studies. Traditional dose–response relationships may not always be present for immunologically mediated effects. For example, experimental models suggest that higher doses might be tolerogenic, while moderate doses might be immunogenic (35). For some hypersensitivity phenomena, the question of individual susceptibility may complicate the assessment of "dose–response" in the population.

In evaluating a positive study that does not demonstrate a dose–response relationship, a general issue is whether the dose estimate employed takes into account data on the absorption, metabolism, and distribution of the chemical. Frequently, epidemiologic studies assume that the quantitative dose measurements available (i.e., concentration of the chemical in air, blood, or urine) are proportional to potential dose at the target organ of concern (i.e., bone marrow, primary or secondary lymphatic organs). This is not always the case. For example, air concentration may be a poor surrogate for internal dose if the compound can be absorbed through the skin as well as inhaled, or if respiratory protection has been used by some workers and not others. For chemicals with a long half-life, such as lead, an identical urinary lead concentration may reflect substantially different tissue-specific concentrations in long- versus short-term workers. In addition to inferring dose level estimates for individual subjects from quantitative measurements taken at the time of the study (or from using available historical measurements), the dose estimate used in the model should be restricted to what is considered the most biologically relevant time period. For example, in a cross-sectional immunotoxicity study, the relevant time period may be the previous 6 months rather than the cumulative lifetime exposure. Because the biologically relevant time interval is not known and may differ for different immunologic outcomes, the assessment of dose response is even more complex than in epidemiologic studies of other outcomes.

In evaluating a negative study, one important issue is whether the study size is adequate to detect a difference of a specified size in the immune function parameters of interest, which is called statistical power. The statistical power of a study to detect a difference between two populations in the mean of a continuous variable (such as serum IgG level or proportion of CD4+ lymphocytes) depends on the size of the study groups, the mean and variance of the outcome in the study groups, the specified type I difference, and the size of the difference to be detected (33). Power calculations are usually *a priori* in planning an epidemiologic study. However, there are occasions when they may be useful in interpreting a negative study result. In comparing the results of contradictory studies, one issue that can be considered is the precision of the point estimate (i.e., the confidence interval for the estimated difference between the two groups). Of equal importance in evaluating a negative study is whether there is evidence that the "exposed population" actually had substantial exposure to the xenobiotic of interest.

Other types of data on the immunotoxic effects of chemicals in humans are potentially useful. Case reports may arise from clinical identification of individuals with a particular exposure who have immune function changes or immune-mediated diseases. Such reports are particularly valuable in generating hypotheses for well-designed epidemiologic studies and may provide support for other toxicologic or epidemiologic data.

Aside from the cross-sectional study design, two alternative epidemiologic study designs may be utilized in immunotoxicity studies. In longitudinal studies, one or more groups of people who are free of disease and who differ according to extent of exposure are compared with respect to incidence of the disease after exposure (31). A variant of this design that might be utilized in immunotoxicity studies would compare immune function tests results within individuals before and after a defined exposure. Another variant would define "exposed" and "nonexposed" groups cross sectionally, administer immune function tests, and follow the subjects prospectively to assess relationships between immune function test results and development of clinical disease.

In case–control studies, individuals with a given disease and appropriate controls are selected: the proportion of cases and controls who have certain background characteristics or have been exposed to possible risk factors are compared (32). Case–control studies of the etiology of immunologically mediated diseases might 28identify increased risk of previous exposure to particular chemicals among the cases; such a finding would be particularly relevant if supported by toxicologic studies or evidence of immune function changes among humans exposed to the chemical.

Similar methodologic considerations apply to the evaluation of findings from cohort studies and case–control studies as were discussed for cross-sectional studies. These are discussed in textbooks of epidemiology (31,32).

Logistics of Sample Acquisition and Analysis

Presample acquisition planning is the hallmark of a successful and safe field study designed to investigate immunologic endpoints. Human field studies often are limited to sampling peripheral blood, which provides a convenient source of cells and mediators. However, it should be kept in mind that peripheral blood by no means represents the entire immune system. Host defense activities take place primarily in the lymphoid tissues (spleen, lymph nodes, epithelial-associated lymphoid tissues) and in interstitial tissue at local sites of injury and infection. Cell traffic and recirculation through the blood are controlled carefully and activated cells and molecules are removed quickly. In contrast, some cells and mediators persist within or outside the bloodstream for days and even years (12).

Before the actual acquisition of the first sample, numerous technical and safety details must be accounted. The recognition of the possibility of transmission of the human immunodeficiency virus (HIV) and with it the acquired immunodeficiency syndrome (AIDS) to health-care workers is a contemporary reality (36). Other infectious agents such as hepatitis B virus (HBV) and tuberculosis (37) pose a risk to health-care workers (38). A thorough understanding of the appropriate procedures, responsibilities, and risks inherent in the collection and handling of patient specimens should be acquired by everyone with potential exposure. Methods for decontaminating surfaces, disposal of broken glass, contaminated equipment, and so on, in the event of a spill or accident at the field site, also need to be planned in advance of a study. The Agent Summary Statement for Human Immunodeficiency Virus (HIVs) (39) is a valuable resource document. The Occupational Safety and Health Administration (OSHA) has promulgated "Enforcement Procedures for Occupational Exposure to Hepatitis B Virus and HIV" (40). Universal Precautions as appropriate practices for laboratory personnel exposed to human samples have been addressed by the National Committee for Clinical Laboratory Standards (NCCLS) (41). Glove use by health-care workers is a major aspect of Universal Precautions.

The collection of blood in a field situation requires planning for emergencies such as cardiovascular responses to phlebotomy in middle-aged and elderly subjects (42). Phlebotomy technicians should have recent certification in cardiopulmonary resuscitation (CPR) techniques. The location of the nearest hospital with emergency services, and the telephone number to summon emergency medical assistance should be immediately available. A private site without through traffic, with appropriate chairs and space for phlebotomy, should be utilized.

Additional planning is needed to ensure that samples collected in the field are accurately labeled and transported to the laboratory quickly and safely. A labeling scheme and system that are designed to unequivocally identify samples and withstand the rigors of transport have to be designed. All state and federal regulations concerning the transport of blood or blood products should be adhered to (43,44). Cardboard boxes with styrofoam liners are the transport system of choice for blood samples. Whole blood for immunologic analyses is best transported and maintained at room temperature (18 to 22° C). Temperatures below 10° C and above 37° C should be avoided (45,46). This can be accomplished (depending on the season or the expected temperatures to which the shipment may be subjected) by adding a cooling pack and/or insulation to the transport box with the addition of an insulating material (such as newspaper). A maximum–minimum recording thermometer should also be added to the shipment container to document temperature transients experienced.

The time between phlebotomy and sample preparation/measurement at the investigator's laboratory should be kept to a minimum. The choice of anticoagulants is also important. No change in complete blood counts (CBCs) with "five-part" differentials have been reported using automated blood analyzers and blood samples stored at 20° C for 18 to 24 hr using ethylenediamine tetraacetic acid (EDTA) (47). For immunophenotyping, acid, citrate, dextrose (ACD), or heparin are the anticoagulants of choice, and samples may be processed for up to 30 hr postdraw (48). Sera for biochemical and immunologic analyses can be separated, frozen on-site, and shipped frozen or transported in serum-separator tubes. As a design control for transport, blood from exposed subjects should be included in the same shipment as blood from nonexposed individuals to control for significant shipment effects.

Choice of Tests

Tests for immune markers used in field studies should be selected to provide the most cost-effective information relevant to the focus of investigation. Infectious or constitutive diseases that involve any organ tissues are likely to cause changes in the host defense system. In fact, many of the symptoms associated with infections are caused not by the infectious agents themselves but by cellular and molecular processes from the host. Some solid tumors that release tumor-specific antigens may elicit autoimmune responses that could serve as markers of the malignancy (49). Malnutrition, stress, pregnancy, and a variety of other factors all can influence the immune system (13). Immune markers and clinical chemical markers can be used as indicators of such health effects; conversely, these effects can be confounding variables when immune markers are used in attempts to characterize the host defense system itself. An approach to categorizing and selecting immune markers was developed by a subcommittee of the Centers for Disease Control and Prevention (CDC) and the Agency for Toxic Substances and Disease Registry (ATSDR), convened to develop guidelines for the use of biomarker tests in health assessment studies conducted at Superfund sites (50). The subcommittee identified three general categories of tests: (a) basic tests that provide a general evaluation of immune status; (b) focused/reflex tests that address particular aspects of immune function as indicated by clinical findings, suspected exposures, or results of prior tests; and (c) research tests that require evaluation in well-defined control populations (Table 4).

Tests in both the basic group and the focused/reflex group should have clinical interpretations for disease endpoints when values lie outside established reference ranges. Tests from the basic group should be included in most studies, since they provide the minimal "core" assessment of immune status. Although they may be omitted in studies addressing very specific concerns, the interpretation of other tests may suffer without the supporting data. Tests from the focused/reflex panel are suggested by particular clinical symptoms, prior laboratory findings, or specific exposures; they may be used individually or augmented by tests from the basic group. Research tests should be used under the auspices of an investigative protocol with control populations that have known exposure or disease endpoints. Before a test is considered to have completed the investigative phases, the biochemical or physical abnormalities associated with changes in the marker should be identified, and the nature of any disease associations should be determined. Because of the intrinsic variability of the immune system within and between individuals, longitudinal studies are essential in evaluating research tests for immune markers. In addition to test selection, the overall study design must be orchestrated carefully to ensure interpretability of results. The basic goal should be to identify all sources of variability in the tests: analytic (laboratory error), within individuals (over time), among individuals within each group, and among study groups. Analytic variability can be assessed by including a subset of duplicate (split) samples. Variability within individuals can be assessed only by longitudinal studies. Variability among individuals within a study group may be quite high and may require a large number of

TABLE 4. *Classification of tests for immune markers*

Test category	Characteristics	Specific tests
Basic—general Should be included with general panels	Indicators of general health and organ system status	BUN, blood glucose, SALT, etc.
Basic—immune Should be included with general panels	General indicators of immune status Relatively low cost Assay methods are standardized among laboratories Results outside reference ranges are clinically interpretable	Complete blood counts Serum IgG, IgA, IgM levels Surface marker phenotypes for major lymphocyte subsets
Focused/reflex Should be included when indicated by clinical findings, suspected exposures, or prior test results	Indicators of specific immune functions/events Cost varies Assay methods are standardized among laboratories Results outside reference ranges are clinically interpretable	Histocompatibility genotype Antibodies to infectious agents Total serum IgE Allergen-specific IgE Autoantibodies Skin tests for hypersensitivity Granulocyte oxidative burst Histopathology (tissue biopsy)
Research Should be included only with control populations and careful study design	Indicators of general or specific immune functions/events Cost varies; often expensive Assay methods are usually not standardized among laboratories Results outside reference ranges are often not clinically interpretable	*In vitro* stimulation assays Cell activation surface markers Cytokine serum concentrations Clonality assays (antibody, cellular, genetic) Cytotoxicity tests

Adapted from ref. 8.
BUN, blood urea nitrogen; SALT, skin-associated lymphoid tissue.

subjects per group to assess properly. Identification of biologically significant variability among groups, the general goal of controlled studies, is possible only with careful selection of the populations to control for the many differences in susceptibility and the confounding variables that influence the immune system.

Other Immunologic and Clinical Tests of Potential Usefulness in Field Studies

Many xenobiotics produce sensitization reactions in a proportion of subjects. For example, in study of opiate production workers, National Institutes for Occupational Safety and Health (NIOSH) investigators found both evidence of immunosuppression [significantly decreased percentages of T helper-inducer (CD4+) cells]

(51) and evidence of sensitization (lowered epicutaneous thresholds to dihydrocodeine, hydrocodone, codeine, and morphine) (52), elevated serum anti-morphine IgG antibodies (53), and an elevated prevalence of asthma (52). In designing studies of immunomodulation by exposure to mycotoxins, potential immunologic outcomes include sensitization by fungi or their products (leading to clinical disorders such as asthma and hypersensitivity pneumonitis) as well as direct toxicity of the mycotoxin leading to immunosuppression. Frequently, some clinical assessment must be incorporated into the field study. Techniques readily incorporated into field studies include assessment of respiratory tract symptoms by questionnaire, pre- and postshift, and waking hour peak flow testing (54,55). Tests that are valuable in clinical assessment but are less readily administered in field situations include skin testing (56,57) and bronchial provocation testing (58). Such tests require greater medical expertise on the part of the field team and in some tests (i.e., bronchial provocation testing) require transportation of the study subjects to a clinical facility. Although skin testing to detect sensitization to specific allergens is a well-accepted clinical procedure when Food and Drug Administration (FDA)-approved test batteries are used (59), antigens of concern in the occupational or environmental setting may not be available in FDA-approved form.

Limitations exist in the immunotoxicity test battery in which components of the immune system are quantitated (i.e., serum immunoglobulin levels and lymphocyte subset analysis) or specific functional activities measured (i.e., NK cell activity) in peripheral blood samples. For example, the battery does not measure the ability of the immune system to respond in an integrated fashion to an antigenic challenge. For many immunotoxicants a decreased primary antibody response is one of the most sensitive indicators observed in animals (60). In theory, the primary antibody response could be measured in pediatric populations who receive many routine immunizations, although the difficulties of venipuncture in young children is an important consideration. In adults, the primary antibody response can be measured by administering vaccines that have a low frequency of side effects and some potential benefits to the general population (61). For example, although public health guidelines limit hepatitis B vaccination in the adult population to certain risk groups, including workers at risk of occupational contact with blood, approximately 30% of cases occur in individuals with no known risk factors (61). It could be argued that studies utilizing hepatitis B vaccination as an investigational tool to measure the primary antibody response would be of minimal risk, and some potential benefit, to study participants who receive the vaccine. However, to our knowledge, administration of vaccines to measure primary antibody response has not been performed in field studies to assess the immunotoxicity of occupational or environmental exposures.

Clinical Laboratory Improvement Amendments (CLIA '88)

The Clinical Laboratory Improvement Amendments (CLIA '88) legislation grew out of a series of media reports of patient harm and missed diagnoses arising from poor clinical laboratory performance. Congress responded to these reports by passing the CLIA '88 law. CLIA '88 is actually an amendment and technical revision to the Clinical Laboratory Improvement Act of 1967, which was intended to update laboratory requirements and impose new quality assurance standards applicable to laboratories participating in Medicare and Medicaid programs (62). In 1990, the Department of Health and Human Services issued a set of their own regulations implementing the legislation (63). The new law and the regulations that support it expand the application of laboratory registration as well as personnel and performance requirements. In 1991, rules were published that set forth sanctions that could be imposed on laboratories that do not meet federal requirements (64). Most evaluations of immunologic endpoints used in immunotoxicology studies would fall under either the moderately or highly complex test categories of CLIA. Specific requirements for proficiency testing, subject test management, quality assurance, personnel, and inspections are outlined in the amendments. A valuable resource document for implementing the CLIA amendments is available (65).

Human Subjects Issues

The immune function tests routinely used in immunotoxicity studies by the CDC and NIOSH currently require only 40 to 50 ml of blood and 1 to 5 ml of saliva, which presents minimal risk to study subjects (66). Immunotoxicity protocols, informed consent documents, and letters notifying subjects of their individual test results are reviewed by each agency's Institutional Review Board. This ensures that subjects are being adequately informed of the nature and purpose of the study, their rights as study subjects, circumstances under which federal regulations allow release of individual identifying data, that adequate emergency plans, including the availability of NIOSH staff trained in cardiopulmonary resuscitation, are present, and that subjects will be informed of their own test results and the overall results of the study. One difficulty in immunotoxicity studies, and other studies where a large number of tests are conducted, is to explain the results in a succinct but understandable way to the study participants. Since occasionally the results of a clinical or immunologic test may suggest a serious clinical abnormality, it is important that test results outside the reference range be flagged by the laboratory and reviewed by a qualified physician so that the participant may be informed promptly that he or she should seek medical attention. The use of computerized data acquisition and analyses and relational databasing of individual results with an embedded link to an "expert system" or "neural network" to help flag individuals with potentially severe clinical immune abnormalities are future goals of NIOSH studies designed to evaluate the effect of workplace chemicals on the immune system.

CONCLUSION

Field studies in humans designed to detect immunomodulation from exposure to xenobiotics present challenging problems to epidemiologists, immunotoxicologists, and occupational physicians. Exposed and control groups should be selected carefully, exposure to the xenobiotic must be sufficiently high and well documented, and the control population should be as similar as possible to the exposed. Immune biomarkers/function tests in an individual may be influenced by stress, sunlight exposure, medication, illness, and use of recreational drugs—all of which must be taken into account. Sample acquisition usually is performed at sites geographically distant from the controlled environment of an investigator's laboratory, yielding an assortment of new problems that would not occur in clinical or hospital situations. Regulations and guidelines concerning the transport of biologic samples and potential HIV and HBV exposure to personnel must be adapted to field conditions. Since the application of immunotoxicologic techniques to populations exposed to xenobiotics is relatively new, and the ability to measure an increasing number of immune biomarkers of activation, suppression, autoimmunity, or hypersensitivity is rapidly expanding, there are difficulties in the interpretation of statistically positive results (sometimes within the "normal range") and their potential health significance. Finally, both biologic and methodologic factors complicate the assessment of dose–response/concentration–effect relationships in human immunotoxicity studies, and traditional dose–response relationships may not always be present.

ACKNOWLEDGMENTS

The authors would like to thank Eric Baumgardner of Xavier University, Cincinnati, Ohio, for careful editing of the final draft of the manuscript for this chapter.

REFERENCES

1. National Research Council. *Biologic markers in immunotoxicology*. Washington, DC: National Academy Press; 1992. 206 pp.
2. Plotnikoff NP, Faith RE, Murgo AJ, Wybran J, eds. *Stress and immunity*. Boca Raton, FL: CRC Press; 1991.
3. Clement-Lacroix P, Dubertret L. Ultraviolent rays and the skin. Modulation of immune functions. *Pathol Biol (Paris)* 1992;40:178–183.
4. Hersey P, Magrath H, Wilkinson F. Development of an in vitro system for the analysis of ultraviolet radiation-induced suppression of natural killer cell activity. *Photochem Photobiol* 1993;57:279–284.
5. Baadsgaard O, Salvo B, Mannie A, Dass B, Fox DA, Cooper KD. In vivo ultraviolet-exposed human epidermal cells activate T suppressor cell pathways that involve CD4+CD45RA+ suppressor-inducer T cells. *J Immunol* 1990;145:2854–2861.
6. Stiehm ER. *Immunologic disorders in infants and children*. Philadelphia: Saunders; 1989.
7. Samter M. *Immunological disease*. Boston: Little, Brown; 1988.
8. Hood LE, Weissman L, Wood WB. *Immunology*. Menlo Park, CA: Benjamin/Cummings; 1978.
9. Paul W. *Fundamental immunology*, 2d ed. New York: Raven Press; 1989.
10. Roitt IM, Brostoff J, Male DK. *Immunology*. St Louis: Mosby; 1987.
11. Rose NR, Margolick JB. *The immunological assessment of immunotoxic effects in man in clinical immunotoxicology*. New York: Raven Press; 1992. 449 pp.
12. Vogt RF, Schulte PA. Molecular epidemiology. In: Schulte PA, Perrera FA, eds. *Immune markers in epidemiologic field studies*. San Diego, CA: Academic Press; 1993. 588 pp.
13. Vogt RF, Dannenberg AM, Papirmeister B, Scofield B. Pathogenesis of skin lesions caused by sulfur mustard. *Fundam Appl Toxicol* 1984;4:S71–S78.

14. Snyder R. The benzene problem in historical perspectivc. *Appl Toxicol* 1984;4:692–699.
15. Penn I. Depressed immunity and the development of cancer. *Clin Exp Immunol* 1981;46:459–474.
16. Biron CA, Byron KS, Sullivan JL. Severe herpesvirus infections in an adolescent without natural killer cells. *N Engl J Med* 1990;320:1731–1735.
17. Kilburn KH, Warshaw RH. Prevalence of symptoms of systemic lupus erythematosus (SLE) and of fluorescent antinuclear antibodies associated with chronic exposure to trichloroethylene and other chemicals in well water. *Environ Res* 1992;57:1–9.
18. Reidenberg MM, Durant PJ, Harris RA, De Boccardo G, Lahita R, Stenzel KH. et al. Lupus erythematosus-like disease due to hydrazine. *Am J Med* 1983;75:365–370.
19. Cohen S, Williamson GM. Stress and infectious disease in humans. *Psychol Bull* 1991;109:5–24.
20. Institute of Medicine. *Behavioral influences on the endocrine and immune systems*. Research Briefing, NRC. Washington, DC: National Academy Press; 1989:1–9.
21. Jankovic BD, Markovic BM, Spector NH, eds. *Neuroimmune interactions: Proceedings of the 2nd International Workshop on Neuroimmunomodulation*. New York: New York Academy of Science; 1987. 496 pp.
22. Hurrell JJ Jr, McLaney MA. Exposure to job stress—a new psychometric instrument. *Scand J Work Environ Health* 1988;14(Suppl 1):27–28.
23. Fibiger W, Singer G, Kaufman H. Diurnal changes of cortisol and IgA in saliva and life events. *J Occup Health Safety Aust/NZ* 1985;1:21–25.
24. Jemmott JB, McClelland DC. Secretory IgA as a measure of resistance to infectious disease: comments on Stone et al. *Behav Med* 1989;15:63–71.
25. Kugler J. Emotional status and immunoglobulin A in saliva—review of the literature. *Psychother Psychosom Med Psychol* 1991;41:232–242.
26. Henningsen GM, Hurrell JJ Jr, Baker F, Douglas C, MacKenzie BA, Robertson SK, Phipps FC. Measurement of salivary immunoglobulin A as an immunologic biomarker of job stress. *Scand J Work Environ Health* 1992;18(2):133–136.
27. Mouton C, Fillion L, Tawadros E, Tessier R. SIgA is a weak stress marker. *Behav Med* 1989;15: 179–186.
28. Stone AA, Cox DS, Valdimarsdottir H, Neale JM. Secretory IgA as a measure of immunocompetence. *J Hum Stress* 1987;13:136–140.
29. O'Reilly CA. *Effects of psychological stress and stress reduction on salivary IgA levels* [Dissertation]. Pullman, WA: Washington State University, 1989.
30. Ledney GD, Madonna GS, DeBell RM, Walker RI. Therapies for radiation injuries: research perspectives. *Mil Med* 1992;157:130–136.
31. Rothman KJ. *Modern epidemiology*. Boston: Little, Brown; 1986.
32. Kelsey JL, Thompson WD, Evans AS. *Methods in observational epidemiology*. New York: Oxford University Press; 1986.
33. Colton T. *Statistics in medicine*. Boston: Little, Brown; 1974.
34. Trizio D, Basketter DA, Botham PA, et al. Identification of immunotoxic effects of chemicals and their relevance to man. *Food Chem Toxicol* 1988;26:527–539.
35. Biagini RE, Moorman WJ, Smith RJ, Lewis TR, Bernstein IL. Pulmonary hyperreactivity in cynomolgus monkeys (*Macaca fasicularis*) from nose-only inhalation exposure to disodium hexachloroplatinate, Na_2PtCl_6. *Toxicol Appl Pharmacol* 1983;69:377–384.
36. Wicher CP. AIDS and HIV: the dilemma of the health care worker. *Todays OR Nurse* 1993;15:14–22.
37. Hellman SL, Gram MC. The resurgence of tuberculosis: risk in health care settings. *AAOHN J* 1993;41:66–72.
38. Jackson MM, Pugliese G. The OSHA bloodborne pathogens standard. *Todays OR Nurse* 1992;14: 11–16.
39. Agent Summary Statement for Human Immunodeficiency Virus (HIVs) including HTLV-III, LAV, HIV-1, and HIV-2. *MMWR Morb Mortal Wkly Rep* 1988;37:1–17.
40. Enforcement procedures for occupational exposure to hepatitis B virus and human immunodeficiency virus (HIV). OSHA Instruction CPL-2-2-44A, August 15, 1988, Office of Health Compliance Assistance.
41. NCCLS. Protection of laboratory workers from infectious diseases transmitted by blood, body fluids and tissue. Document M29-T, 1989.
42. Kuchel GA, Avorn J, Reed MJ, Fields D. Cardiovascular responses to phlebotomy and sitting in middle-aged and elderly subjects. *Arch Intern Med* 1992;152:366–370.
43. Interstate shipment of etiologic agents. *Fed Regul* 1987;Pt72:59–63.

44. NCCLS, Document H5-A2. Procedures for the domestic handling and transport of diagnostic specimens and etiologic agents-second edition. *Fed Regul* 1985;Pt 49372.
45. Shield CF, Manlett P, Smith A, Gunter L, Goldstein G. Stability of human leukocyte differentiation antigens when stored at room temperature. *J Immunol Methods* 1983;62:347–352.
46. McCoy JP Jr, Carey JL, Krause JR. Quality control in flow cytometry for diagnostic pathology: 1. Cell surface phenotyping and general laboratory procedures. *Am J Clin Pathol* 1990;93:S27–S37.
47. Warner BA, Reardon DM. A field evaluation of the Coulter STKS. *Am J Clin Pathol* 1991;95:207–217.
48. Guidelines for the performance of CD4+ T-cell determinations in persons with human immunodeficiency virus infection. *MMWR Morb Mortal Wkly Rep* 1992;41:1–17.
49. Mavligit GM, Stuckey S. Colorectal carcinoma. Evidence for circulating CEA–anti-CEA complexes. *Cancer* 1983;52(1):146–149.
50. Centers for Disease Control and Prevention. Internal report on biomarkers of organ damage and dysfunction for the renal, hepatobiliary, and immune systems. Subcommittee on Biomarkers of Organ Damage and Dysfunction of the Centers for Disease Control and Prevention and Agency for Toxic Substances and Disease Registry, Atlanta, Georgia. [Available from Clinical Biochemistry Branch, Mailstop F-19, CDC, Atlanta, GA 30333.]
51. Henningsen GM, Biagini RE, Klincewicz SL, et al. Flow cytometric analyses of peripheral leucocytes from workers exposed occupationally to opiates. *Toxicologist* 1990;10:135.
52. Biagini RE, Bernstein DM, Klincewicz SL, Mittman R, Bernstein IL, Henningsen GM. Evaluation of cutaneous responses and lung function from exposure to opiate compounds among ethical narcotics-manufacturing workers. *J Allergy Clin Immunol* 1992;89:108–118.
53. Biagini RE, Klincewicz SL, Henningsen GM, MacKenzie BA, Gallagher JS, Bernstein DI, Bernstein IL. Antibodies to morphine in workers occupationally exposed to opiates at a narcotics manufacturing facility and evidence for similar antibodies in heroin abusers. *Life Sci* 1990;47:897–908.
54. Cote J, Kennedy S, Chan-Yeung MQ. Quantitative versus qualitative analysis of peak expiratory flow in occupational asthma. *Thorax* 1993;48(1):48–51.
55. Neukirch F, Liard R, Segala C, Korobaeff M, Henry C, Cooreman J. Peak expiratory flow variability and bronchial responsiveness to methacholine. *Am Rev Respir Dis* 1992;146:71–75.
56. Van-Metre TE Jr, Adkinson NF Jr, Kagey-Sobotka A, Marsh DG, Normal PS, Rosenberg GL. How should we use skin testing to quantify IgE sensitivity? *J Allergy Clin Immunol* 1990;86(4 Pt 1):583–586.
57. Brand PLP, Kerstjens HIM, Jansen HM, Kauffman HF, de Monchy JGR, Dutch CNSLD Study Group. Interpretation of skin tests to house dust mite and relationship to other allergy parameters in patients with asthma and chronic obstructive pulmonary disease. *J Allergy Clin Immunol* 1991;91:560–570.
58. Irwin RS, Pratter MR. The clinical value of pharmacologic bronchoprovocation challenge. *Med Clin North Am* 1990;74(3):767–778.
59. Adinoff AD, Rosloniec DM, McCall LL, Nelson HS. Immediate skin test reactivity to Food and Drug Administration-approved standardized extracts. *J Allergy Clin Immunol* 1990;86(5):766–774.
60. Descotes J. *Immunotoxicology of drugs and chemicals*. Amsterdam: Elsevier; 1988.
61. Gardner P, Schaffner W. Immunization of adults. *N Engl J Med* 1993;328:1252–1258.
62. *Federal Register* 1988;53:29590.
63. *Federal Register* 1990;55:9536.
64. *Federal Register* 1991;56:13430.
65. Regulations for implementing the clinical laboratory improvement amendments of 1988: a summary. *MMWR Morb Mortal Wkly Rep* 1992;41:1–17.
66. Turkeltaub PC, Gergen PJ. The risk of adverse reactions from percutaneous prick-puncture allergen skin testing, venipuncture, and body measurements: data from the second National Health and Nutrition Examination Survey 1976-80 (NHANES II). *J Allergy Clin Immunol* 1989;84(6 Pt 1):886–890.

Immunotoxicology and Immunopharmacology, Second Edition, edited by J. H. Dean, M. I. Luster, A. E. Munson, and I. Kimber.
Raven Press, Ltd., New York, 1994.

4

Experimental Studies on Immunosuppression

Approaches and Application in Risk Assessment

Michael I. Luster, *MaryJane K. Selgrade, Dori R. Germolec, Florence G. Burleson, †Fujio Kayama, **Christine E. Comment, and James L. Wilmer

*Environmental Immunology and Neurobiology Section, Laboratory of Biochemical Risk Analysis, Division of Intramural Research, National Institute of Environmental Health Sciences, Research Triangle Park, North Carolina 27709; *Immunotoxicology Branch, Health Effects Research Laboratory, United States Environmental Protection Agency, Research Triangle Park, North Carolina 27711; †Department of Environmental Health, University of Occupational and Environmental Health, Kitakyushu 807, Japan; **Department of Occupational and Environmental Medicine, National Jewish Center for Immunology and Respiratory Medicine, Denver, Colorado 80206*

As evidenced by documents prepared by the Commission of European Communities/International Program on Chemical Safety (1), Office of Technology Assessment (2), and the National Research Council (3) focusing on immunotoxicology, there has been growing interest and concern within the scientific and public communities on the capacity of environmental agents to perturb normal immune processes. Subsequently, incorporating experimental data on toxicant-induced alterations in the immune system as part of evaluation of drugs, chemicals, and biologicals for human risk assessment has become increasingly common. For example, in addition to previously established test guidelines developed by the Environmental Protection Agency (EPA) for hypersensitivity testing, the EPA (4) and Food and Drug Administration (FDA) (5,6) have recently discussed the benefits of testing the immunosuppressive potential of biochemical pest control agents, antiviral drugs, and food additives. Furthermore, the EPA has established reference doses [Rf or no observed

This chapter has been reviewed by the Health Effects Research Laboratory, U.S. Environmental Protection Agency, and approved for publication. Approval does not signify that the contents necessarily reflect the views and policies of the agency, nor does mention of trade names or commercial products constitute endorsement or recommendation for use.

adverse effect level (NOAEL)/Safety Factor] using immunotoxicity data for several compounds including 1,1,2-trichloroethane, 2,4–dichlorophenol, and dibutyltin oxide, while the Agency for Toxic Substances and Disease Registry has derived *minimum risk levels* for arsenic, dieldrin, nickel, 1,2–dichloroethane, and 2,4–dichlorophenol from immune endpoints.

Two critical questions in immunotoxicology are: (a) under certain conditions can chemical agents suppress the immune response within the general population and (b) if so, what are the quantitative relationships of immunosuppression to clinical diseases (i.e., is there a hazard)? Such diseases would most likely be manifested as increases in the frequency, duration, or severity of infections and increased incidences of certain cancers such as Kaposi's sarcoma or non-Hodgkin's lymphoma, malignancies often observed in immunosuppressed individuals. The basis for these concerns has been provided by a number of clinical and experimental observations. First, the association between primary immunodeficiency diseases and the incidence of recurrent infections and neoplastic diseases is well documented; a similar association with these diseases has been recognized with the chronic low-level use of immunosuppressive agents (7). For example, in one study 30% of cardiac transplant patients treated with cyclosporin developed pulmonary infections within the first year after surgery (8), while in another study 50% of renal transplant patients on immunosuppressive therapy were found to develop cancer within 10 years following surgery (9). Second, there are an increasing number of reports describing various immune changes in individuals who have been inadvertently or occupationally exposed to chemical agents. These range from unconfirmed reports on compounds such as trichloroethylene and methyl isocyanate to confirmed studies with polychlorinated biphenyls (PCBs) and asbestos (3). As may be expected, it is considerably more difficult to identify subtle immune changes in humans that may occur following inadvertent or occupational exposure as compared to severe immune dysfunction such as that observed in individuals with human immunodeficiency virus (HIV) infection or primary immunodeficiency disease. This is due to the lack of highly sensitive immune assays that normally accompany routine clinical assessment in humans, an inability to identify recently exposed, well-defined (e.g., exposure level) cohorts, and immunologic variability within the general population. The third observation, which has fueled interest in chemical-induced immunosuppression, stems from *in vitro* and *in vivo* experimental studies, suggesting that many environmental chemicals can inhibit the immune system and alter host resistance to infectious agents or tumor cells (10,11). Additional credence is ascribed to such studies since the immune system of laboratory animals, including rodents, is remarkably similar to that in humans with respect to organization, cell function, and responsiveness. However, at present, animal data serve best as "warning flags," since the doses used in laboratory studies are usually much higher than estimated in human exposures and difficulties remain in accurately extrapolating animal studies to humans. This chapter focuses on approaches, assessment, and interpretation of animal studies dealing with the ability of environmental agents to suppress local and/or systemic immune functions.

CONSIDERATIONS IN EXPERIMENTAL STUDIES

Systemic Immunity

The sensitivity of the immune system to suppression by exogenous agents is due as much to the general properties of the agent as to the complex nature of the immune system. Because of this complexity, the initial strategies devised by immunologists working in toxicology and safety assessment have been to select and apply a tiered panel of assays to identify immunosuppressive or, in rare instances, immunostimulatory agents in laboratory animals. Although the configurations of these testing panels vary depending on the laboratory conducting the test and the animal species employed, they include measures for one or more of the following: (a) altered lymphoid organ weights and histology; (b) quantitative changes in cellularity of lymphoid tissue, peripheral blood leukocytes, and/or bone marrow; (c) impairment of cell function at the effector or regulatory level; and/or (d) increased susceptibility to infectious agents or transplantable tumors. Some of the tests that have commonly been used for evaluating the immune system in experimental animals and humans are listed in Table 1. There are, of course, a number of limitations in using such test panels. For example, highly specific effects would likely be missed. Furthermore, such test panels seldom examine the effects of chronic exposure, or whether tolerance or reversibility can result from the treatment. In humans, assays that involve *in vivo* antigenic challenge, which are usually accepted as the most sensitive and informative of immune tests, are considered "invasive" procedures since they involve immunization and, as such, are not usually feasible or practical for inclusion in human studies.

A variety of factors need to be considered when evaluating the potential of an environmental agent or drug to adversely influence the immune system of experi-

TABLE 1. *Assays commonly employed to assess immune function in experimental animals and humans*

Assay/endpoint	Species		
	Rodent	Nonhuman primate	Human
Surface markers	+	+	+
NK cell activity	+	+	+
Primary antibody response	+	−	−
Hematology	+	+	+
Lymphoid organ weight	+	−	−
Serum Ig levels	−	+	+
Delayed hypersensitivity	+	−	+
Cytotoxic T lymphocyte	+	−	−
Mixed lymphocyte reactions and mitogen assays	+	+	+
Host resistance	+	−	−

+, Routinely performed; −, not routinely performed.

mental animals. These include appropriate selection of animal models and exposure variables, inclusion of general toxicologic parameters, and an understanding of the biologic relevance of the endpoints to be measured. Treatment conditions should take into account the potential route and level of human exposure, biophysical properties of the agent such as half-life, and any available information on the mechanism of action. Doses and adequate sample sizes should be selected, which attempt to establish clear dose–response curves as well as NOAELs or no observed effect levels (NOELs). Although in some instances it is beneficial to include a dose level that induces clear evidence of toxicity, any immune change observed at such a dose should not be considered biologically significant since severe stress and malnutrition are known to impair immune responsiveness. Although our laboratory routinely uses three dose levels, we normally conduct dose-range-finding studies prior to full-scale immunotoxicologic evaluation. If studies are being designed specifically to establish reference doses for toxic chemicals, additional exposure levels are advisable. In addition, the inclusion of a positive control agent that shares characteristics of the test compound may be advantageous under certain circumstances when experimental and fiscal constraints permit.

The selection of the exposure route should parallel the most probable route of human exposure, which is most frequently oral, respiratory, or dermal. A requirement for an accurate delivered dose may be the use of a parenteral exposure route. However, this may significantly alter the metabolism or distribution of the agent from that which would occur following natural exposure and prevents any evaluation of effects on local immune responses at the site of entry.

The selection of the most appropriate animal model for immunotoxicology studies has been a matter of great concern. Ideally, toxicity testing should be performed with species that will respond to a test chemical in a pharmacologic and toxicologic manner similar to that anticipated in humans (i.e., the test animals and humans metabolize the chemical similarly and will have identical target organ responses and toxicity). Toxicologic studies are often conducted in several animal species, since it is assumed that the more species showing a specific toxic response, the more likely that the response will occur in humans. For most immunosuppressive therapeutics, rodent data on target organ toxicities and the comparability of immunosuppressive doses have generally been predictive of later observations in the clinic. Exceptions to the predictive value of rodent toxicologic data are infrequent but have occurred, such as in studies of glucocorticoids, which are lympholytic in rodents but not in primates (12). Although certain compounds may exhibit different pharmacokinetic properties in rodents from that in humans, rodents still appear to be the most appropriate animal model for examining the immunotoxicity of non-species-specific compounds, based on established similarities of toxicologic profiles as well as the relative ease of generating host resistance and immune function data. Comparative toxicologic studies should be continued and expanded, particularly for novel recombinant biologic materials and natural products, since their safety assessment will likely present species-specific host interactions and unique toxicologic profiles.

The quantitative and possibly qualitative susceptibility of an individual animal to immunotoxicity by an agent can be influenced by its genetic characteristics, indicating not only a need to consider species but also strain. Rao et al. (13) described two approaches for selecting appropriate genotypes for toxicity studies. The first approach is to select genotypes that are representative of an animal species, which by virtue of similar metabolic profiles may also exhibit sensitivities similar to humans, such as the use of random bred mice. A second approach attempts to identify genotypes that are uniquely suitable for evaluation of a specific class of chemicals, such as the use of *Ah* responsive rodent strains in studies with polyhalogenated aromatic hydrocarbons. In many cases, however, this requires considerable knowledge of the mechanisms for toxicity for the particular compound. One compromise has been the use of F1 hybrids, which contain the stability, phenotypic uniformity, and genetic information of an inbred animal and yet have the vigor associated with heterozygosity. The genetic relationships between inbred mouse strains based on the distribution of allelles at 16 loci have been described (14) and have allowed for the rational selection of appropriate F1 hybrids such as the B6C3F1 mouse. Other approaches, of course, have been to employ nonrodent species, including primates, as additional test species.

Lung Immunity

It is important to consider the effects of inhaled compounds on local lung responses because the lung is the portal of entry for many infectious agents, and immune cells in the lung represent the first line of defense against these organisms. Environmental agents can alter pulmonary immune function in humans and experimental animals. Compounds implicated in the induction of immune-mediated lung pathogenesis include oxidant gases, such as ozone and nitrogen oxides, and particulates such as asbestos, silica, coal dust, and diesel exhaust. Clinical and epidemiologic studies have demonstrated associations between a number of inhaled pollutants and chronic lung diseases including fibrosis, granulomas, and asthma. Recent studies have provided an understanding of the immune-mediated mechanism(s) associated with the development of certain occupational pneumoconioses (disorders caused by inhalation of particulates or aerosols) such as beryliosis (beryllium), byssinosis (cotton dust), and occupational asthmas (red cedar). While these will be discussed in detail in later chapters, assessment of general lung immunity requires unique considerations.

Cellular and biochemical profiles of bronchoalveolar lavage (BAL) constituents following inhalation exposure in experimental animals and humans have been an increasingly used tool for screening immune-mediated lung injury. The secretion of bioactive products from pulmonary epithelial cells and alveolar macrophages is a key event in lung diseases following inhalation of certain environmental agents and a number of studies have implicated the progression of lung disease with postactivational release of cytokines, such as interleukin-1 (IL-1), tumor necrosis factor-α

(TNF-α) (15,16), platelet-derived growth factor (PDGF) (17), and transforming growth factor-β (TGF-β) (18). In addition to the release of cytokines, alveolar macrophages secrete a variety of short-lived products that may contribute to altering resistance to pulmonary infections and inflammation. Among these are the reactive oxygen species such as superoxide anions and hydrogen peroxide as well as arachidonic acid metabolites (19). Analyses of soluble enzymatic and nonenzymatic products in the BAL, such as immunoglobulins, elastase, and lactate dehydrogenase (LDH), may also be useful indices to detect acute immune-mediated damage as well as chronic lung disease (20).

Other immunologic defenses operating in the lung include humoral and cell-mediated immunity derived from bronchus-associated lymphoid tissue (BALT) as well as interstitial lymphocytes. The lung also possesses a significant number of natural killer (NK) cells, possibly an evolutionary development to combat lung neoplasia induced by inhaled carcinogens. Functional tests for these cell types are similar to those used for examining systemic immunosuppression but require more elaborate cell isolation procedures.

Skin Immunity

Mammalian skin is a complex organ that contains many immune components. The term skin-associated lymphoid tissue (SALT) was coined to include the Langerhans cells with their antigen-presenting properties, the cytokine-producing keratinocytes, homing T lymphocytes, vascular endothelial cells, and the draining lymph nodes (21). The cells of the skin can respond to environmental agents by the induction of allergic contact dermatitis (to be discussed in subsequent chapters) or with a nonspecific inflammatory response resulting in irritant contact dermatitis. In irritant contact dermatitis, a common dermatologic condition that occurs when an agent, such as phenol, acts directly to damage the skin, mediators are released that induce an inflammatory response manifested by vascular dilation, edema, and cellular infiltration (22,23). Although the primary function of keratinocytes is to provide structural integrity and barrier function of the epidermis, recent studies have demonstrated the importance of keratinocytes in the initiation and perpetuation of cutaneous inflammation. For example, various environmental stimuli can induce epidermal keratinocytes to release immunomodulating cytokines [IL-1, IL-3, IL-6, IL-8, IL-10, granulocyte–macrophage colony-stimulating factor (GM-CSF), granulocyte colony-stimulating factor (G-CSF), macrophage colony-stimulating factor (M-CSF), TGF-α and TGF-β, and TNF-α], and to express MHC class II antigens and adhesion molecules (24–26).

Since a broad spectrum of topical agents exists, considerable efforts have been made to develop predictive tests that assess their potential dermatotoxicity and, more recently, immunotoxicity. Many laboratory animal species have been used in skin irritancy testing but the most common has been the rabbit, where the skin test developed by Draize et al. (27) has received considerable attention. Another *in vivo* method used to assess irritancy is the mouse ear swelling test, where dermal irritation is correlated to an increase in ear thickness (28). Considerable efforts to develop *in vitro* tests are underway. Several *in vitro* model systems are commercially available and include the neutral red dye assay, Testskin, the chorioallantoic membrane (CAM) system, and Skintex. In the former, uptake of dye by viable human keratinocytes is measured spectrophotometrically. The Testskin utilizes a multilayer epidermal system of keratinocytes, dermal fibroblasts, and a collagen matrix. Cytotoxicity is assessed histologically and by measuring the release of inflammatory mediators. Although not strictly *in vitro*, the CAM of embryonated chicken eggs is used as an indication of vascular response by observing the appearance of hemorrhaging blood vessels in response to a test substance. The Skintex system is a membrane barrier/protein matrix system that detects changes in the intact barrier matrix via the release of an indicator dye and the use of reagents that increase turbidity (29). *In vitro* tests are often used as "prescreens," which, if positive, may preclude the need for animal tests.

Another model system employs human peripheral blood mononuclear cells and rabbit splenocytes as cellular test substrates where viability, growth characteristics, and metabolic and functional activities are measured (30). The amount of cell products, such as cytokines and prostaglandins, produced as a result of irritant exposure is yet another potential means of quantitating inflammation. The presence of certain cytokines can be measured in supernatants from skin cell cultures by bioassay or enzyme-linked immunoadsorbent assay (ELISA) or in tissue by immunohistochemical techniques. The presence of cytokine messenger ribonucleic acid (mRNA) can be determined by polymerase chain reaction (PCR) (31) or *in situ* hybridization.

Considerable effort continues to improve assays for the detection and characterization of skin irritants and immunotoxicity. As we achieve a better understanding of the mechanisms involved in chemically induced cutaneous irritancy, molecular methods of analysis may be developed that will provide a more objective, quantifiable, and simpler means of measuring the irritative potential of a test substance.

INTERPRETATION OF IMMUNE FUNCTION TESTS

Primary Antibody Response as a Measure of Humoral Immunity

Quantitating primary antibody responses following antigen challenge, such as in the plaque-forming cell (PFC) assay or ELISA, provides information on multiple components in the immune system (i.e., antigen-presenting cells, helper T lymphocytes and B lymphocytes) working in concert. Defects in any of the cellular pathways contributing to this response may lead to measurable decreases in antibody-forming cells. Both *in vivo* and *in vitro* ELISA and PFC assays have been used to assess antibody responses in experimental animals. In immunotoxicology studies in humans, assessment of antibody responses has been limited to *in vitro* tests (32). Clinically, suppression of antibody production may impair the host's ability to combat a wide variety of pathogens as well as the effectiveness of certain vaccinations. In the human population, these alterations may be manifested as increased susceptibility and frequent recurrences of bacterial infections such as pneumonia and meningitis and/or blood-borne parasitic infections such as malaria (*Plasmodium* species) or sleeping sickness (*Trypanosoma* species).

Cytotoxic T Lymphocyte as a Measure of Cellular Immunity

While alterations in the function of CD4+ T lymphocytes may influence antibody responses, suppression of CD8+ T lymphocytes, as measured in both humans and rodents in the cytotoxic T lymphocyte (CTL) assay, leads to an inability to kill cells expressing specific antigens in conjunction with self major histocompatibility complex (MHC) class I molecules. Host cells infected with virus and expressing viral antigens, or tumor cells bearing altered self-antigens, may be destroyed by previously sensitized CTLs in the absence of both antibody and complement. Clinically, abnormalities of CD8+ cell function result in persistent systemic infections with deoxyribonucleic acid (DNA) viruses [cytomegalovirus (CMV) or herpes simplex] or opportunistic pathogens such as *Candida albicans*. Suppression of CTLs also results in an increased susceptibility to the intracellular stages of numerous parasites and probably to virally induced cancers.

Natural Killer Cells

Similar to antibody and CTL responses, NK cell-mediated responses are believed to play a role in defense against viruses, many types of tumor cells, and, in some cases, bacterial infections. In experimental animals, suppression of NK cell activity has been shown to lead to increased numbers of lung tumors following intravenous inoculation of syngeneic tumor cells and increased susceptibility to CMV infection (33,34). Enhanced susceptibility to herpesvirus infections including CMV was reported in a patient who had a complete and specific lack of NK cell and inducible NK cell activity (35). In another study, three bone marrow transplant patients lacking NK cell activity developed fatal CMV pneumonia, while those patients with NK cell activity intact experienced nonfatal CMV infections (36). There is also evidence from longitudinal epidemiologic studies using large populations that asymptomatic individuals with low NK cell responses may be at some risk for developing upper respiratory infections and increased morbidity (37).

Flow Cytometry and Surface Markers

The enumeration of lymphocyte subsets is commonly used to help assess immunocompetence. The increased availability of monoclonal antibodies against specific leukocyte proteins and the use of flow cytometry can allow relatively accurate and reproducible analysis of lymphocyte populations, although, as with most immune tests, considerable variability exists within the human population (38). The assessment of certain cell surface antigens has been successfully used in the clinic to detect and monitor the progression or regression of leukemias, lymphomas, and HIV infection. However, the clinical significance of slight-to-moderate quantitative changes in the numbers of immune cell populations has not been established.

Surface marker analysis has been used extensively in studies of AIDS and has provided some quantitative information on several cell populations. For example, the depletion of CD4+ cells following HIV-1 infection has been a clinical hallmark of acquired immunodeficiency syndrome (AIDS) patients. The normal human range for CD4+ cells is 800 to 1200 cells/μl. This generally declines to less than 500 cells/μl within 3 to 4 years after HIV-1 infection and to a level of 200 cells/μl before overt pathogenesis of opportunistic infections is seen (39,40). However, it has been shown that a drop by 7% or more in a year increases the relative hazard to 35% of developing AIDS (41). Interestingly, *in vitro* lymphocyte proliferation to anti-CD3 monoclonal antibodies may even be a better prognostic marker for AIDS, where CD3 reactivity has been shown to be severely decreased already up to 4 years before development of symptoms (42).

In immunotoxicology, splenocytes, thymocytes, and bone marrow are most frequently evaluated in rodent studies, while peripheral blood is typically assessed in humans. Tissues such as bone marrow and lymph nodes as well as various body fluids (e.g., bronchial lavage fluid) are not routinely examined. Procedures for cell isolation, staining cells with monoclonal antibodies, and flow cytometric analyses have been detailed extensively elsewhere (43). Some commonly used cell surface antigens that enumerate immunocytes in humans and mice are listed in Table 2. In addition, the fluorescent intensity of cell populations may be used to monitor changes in antigen density occurring with cellular activation, such as upregulation of IL-2 receptors or expression of MHC class II molecules.

Host Resistance

There is continued interest in developing sensitive and reproducible experimental host resistance models to define altered immune function following exposure to

TABLE 2. *Cell surface antigens commonly used as leukocyte markers*

Cell description	Human	Mouse
Pan T cell	CD3, CD2	CD3, Thy 1
Pan B cell	CD19, CD20	B220, anti-Ig
NK cell	CD56, CD16	NK-1.1
T helper/inducer	CD4	CD4
T suppressor/cytotoxic	CD8	CD8
Monocytes	CD14, CD11b,c	Mac-1, F4-80
L-2 receptor	CD25	CD25 (7D4)
MHC class II	HLA-DR	Ia

environmental agents. For the most part, these models have been developed in the mouse and to a lesser extent in the rat and include bacterial, viral, protozoan, fungal, and syngeneic or semisyngeneic transplantable tumor cell models. Although the target organs and general host defense activities have been defined for most of these models, multiple immune mechanisms are normally involved in resistance, making it difficult to determine the exact immunologic defect without assessing immune function responses to the challenge agent. For example, defense against extracellular organisms involves the interactions of T lymphocytes, B lymphocytes, macrophages, and polymorphonuclear neutrophils (PMNs) in addition to a variety of cell-secreted products, whereas resistance to generalized infection from intracellular pathogens and neoplastic diseases is likely to involve NK and T cell-mediated immune processes.

Although many host resistance assays are relatively simple to perform, they normally require large numbers of animals and appear less sensitive than immune function tests (44,45). The dose of challenge agent used in experimental studies is important in any potential outcome since too low or too high a dose will fail to detect changes in immunocompromised groups when compared to controls (33,45). The sensitivity of a host resistance assay also depends on the measured endpoint. For example, tests that employ survival or tumor-takes (i.e., dichotomous) are by nature less sensitive than those utilizing endpoints that provide continuous data such as enumeration of tumors, bacteria, or soluble immune activation markers. This can partly be attributed to the differences in the types of statistical analyses applied to establish group differences. With dichotomous data, such as survival, two approaches can be taken. Our laboratory has historically used a challenge dose that produces a response in 10% to 30% of the animals within the control group. An alternative method has been to use a dose slightly below that which would induce the desired response in any of the animals from the control group. This latter design provides for a more liberal analysis of the data, but, in most cases, extreme accuracy must be achieved in the delivery of the agent to ensure that the administered dose of agent is only slightly below that which will give the response. In either approach, the ability to obtain statistical significance is highly dependent on the dose of challenge agent and number of animals in each treatment group and are hypothetically shown in Table 3.

COMPLEMENTS TO EXTRAPOLATING EXPERIMENTAL DATA

In Vitro Approaches

The complexities of the immune system, combined with the need for metabolism and distribution to ultimately produce an immunotoxic response by many agents, have resulted in the almost exclusive use of *in vivo* animal models for immunotoxicity assessment. However, *in vitro* culture systems have been used extensively to study the mechanisms by which agents produce immunosuppression. Predictive *in vitro* test systems using immune cells of human origin are particularly attractive

TABLE 3. *Chi-square values (hypothetical)*

	p-value		*p*-value		*p*-value	
Treatment group	Number effected/ number tested	One tailed	Number effected/ number tested	One tailed	Number effected/ number tested	One tailed
Control	3/15	—	6/30	—	0/15	—
Dose 1	4/15	0.532	8/30	0.428	1/15	0.516
2	5/15	0.411	10/30	0.273	2/15	0.274
3	6/15	0.312	12/30	0.165	3/15	0.150
4	7/15	0.233	14/30	0.096	4/15	0.084
5	8/15	0.173	16/30	0.055	5/15	0.048[a]
6	9/15	0.128	18/30	0.031[a]	6/15	0.028[a]
7	10/15	0.094	20/30	0.017[a]	7/15	0.017[a]
8	11/15	0.069	22/30	0.009[a]	8/15	0.010[a]
9	12/15	0.051	24/30	0.005[a]	9/15	0.006[a]
10	13/15	0.038[a]	26/30	0.003[a]	10/15	0.004[a]
11	14/15	0.028[a]	28/30	0.002[a]	11/15	0.002[a]
12	15/15	0.021[a]	30/30	0.001[a]	12/15	0.002[a]

These hypothetical values demonstrate the relative differences in obtaining statistically significant changes in susceptibility assays by modifying the experimental design. In the first design, an effective dose (ED_{30}) in the control group (i.e., a concentration of agent that produces a response in 30% of normal animals) with 15 animals per treatment group is shown. In the second design, increasing the group size to 30 allows for greater statistical significance. In the third design, a challenge inoculation is given, which produces no effect in the control group (ED_0) and which allows for greater statistical significance.

[a]Significant at $p < 0.05$.

given the uncertainties in extrapolating animal studies to humans and the accessibility of human peripheral blood cells. Although many of the immune cells obtained from human blood represent immature cell forms, the large numbers and diverse populations (i.e., PMNs, monocytes, NK cells, T cells, and B cells) that may be obtained provide an attractive alternative or adjunct to more conventional animal studies. Surprisingly, few laboratories have conducted studies comparing *in vitro* functional responses between human and rodent lymphocytes to immunosuppressive agents (32,46–48). Although these *in vitro* studies have been hampered by the lack of assays to assess primary antigen-specific immune responses with human lymphocytes, a relatively good interspecies correlation has been observed with the limited responses examined. Furthermore, some of these assays (49) have been modified successfully to include metabolic fractions of liver homogenates (50) or coculture with primary hepatocytes (51) to allow for chemical metabolism.

Parallelogram

Interpretation of animal or *in vitro* studies may be improved in cases where even limited human *in vivo* exposure data are available using a *parallelogram* approach. In general, if a parallelogram can be constructed in which data are available for three of the four corners, it may be easier to predict the outcome at the fourth corner, at least in a qualitative fashion, particularly if there are examples with other agents for which data can be obtained at all four corners. For example, data on cytokine and phagocytic responses following *in vitro* exposure of alveolar macrophages or pulmonary epithelial cells to ozone can be compared to similar responses following *in vivo* exposures in both humans and animals (Fig. 1). If the *in vitro* data prove to be predictive indicators of the *in vivo* effects in humans, increased weight can be given to *in vitro* studies with other agents, such as phosgene, or similar compounds that are too toxic to be assessed in human clinical studies but for which *in vivo* animal data as well as animal and human *in vitro* data are available. A similar approach can also be used to establish the relationships between acute and subchronic effects in animals, as a means of extrapolating from acute effects in humans to chronic effects, for which little data are usually available. Another example where this approach may be applicable is in extrapolating deficits in immune function to increased susceptibility to disease in animal models as a means of interpreting the risk of disease in humans for which immune function data, but not infectious disease data, may be available.

Severe Combined Immunodeficient (SCID) Mice

Another approach, which warrants further exploration, is the use of SCID mice engrafted with human immune cells. SCID mice have been engrafted successfully with human fetal lymphoid tissue to study human hematopoiesis (52) or with human peripheral blood lymphocytes, which allow production of human immunoglobulins and secondary antibody responses (53). Reconstituted mice have been used to study autoimmunity as well as the efficacy of antiviral therapeutics against HIV. Limitations presently exist in the use of these animals for immunotoxicity studies (54).

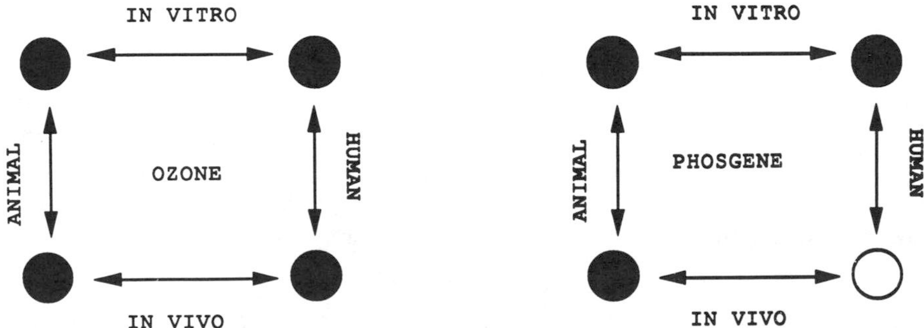

FIG. 1. Use of a parallelogram in immunotoxicology studies. Added weight may be given to agents, like phosgene, where three of the four corners are known when similar studies have been conducted on another agent (ozone) where a more complete data set is available. It follows that structure–activity relationships are important. ●, Known; ○, unknown.

MOLECULAR APPROACHES IN IMMUNOTOXICOLOGY

Appropriate assessment of immunotoxicity may also include understanding the molecular mechanisms by which an agent exerts its toxicity. This may require assessing the effects of the agent on gene expression and protein translation. One of the more promising methods in molecular biology adaptable for routine assessment in immunotoxicology is the quantitative analysis of RNA for specific proteins including cytokines and second messengers. Such analysis may be accomplished through quantitative PCR with an internal standard, which has become a powerful technique to elucidate early kinetic changes of cytokine expression prior to translation and secretion (55–57). In addition, since immunosuppressive agents can enhance or inhibit the ultimate production and secretion of cytokines at various stages such as transcription, the splicing of mRNA, the translation of mRNA to polypeptides on ribosomes, post-translational processing, and secretion, it is possible to dissect potential molecular targets using such techniques.

In addition to PCR, several other molecular approaches can be utilized for immunotoxicology studies including Northern blotting, *in situ* hybridization, and antisense oligonucleotides for inhibiting the translation of specific mRNAs, as well as the use of genetically altered mice. Northern blotting is probably the most accepted approach for quantitating gene products among the various techniques, but it lacks sensitivity, and relatively large amounts of RNA are often required to conduct the assay. *In situ* hybridization is used to show the precise location of specific mRNA within single cells or tissue sections. When combined with immunohistochemistry and PCR, *in situ* hybridization can be a powerful method to identify the source of a cytokine in a tissue, as well as to assay the extent of cytokine expression in a semiquantitative manner by counting silver grains in the specimen. *In situ* hybridization is a technically difficult approach for analyzing cytokine mRNA due to the potentially high levels of nonspecific binding and lack of sensitivity. Antisense oligodeoxynucleotides are sequences that are synthesized to be complementary to a specific gene or mRNA of interest (58,59). Transcription of the gene or translation of its mRNA is selectively blocked through the binding of the oligomers to actively transcribing regions of chromosomal DNA or mRNA. Oligomers targeted upstream of the AUG initiation codon can block the initiation step. Antisense oligonucleotides have been directed successfully against a number of cytokines and growth factors. However, if the intracellular reservoir of the mRNA is abundant, it may be difficult to suppress the production of cytokines.

The development of molecular genetic techniques has allowed not only the isolation and analysis of specific genes but also the manipulation of embryonic genes. The application of transgenic technology in immunology can be used to generate mice that lack virtually any genetic control mechanism or specific cell subpopulations. As a consequence, complex systemic responses can be dissected into individual components and the mechanism by which immunosuppressive agents exert their effects can be better understood. There are two strategies used to induce genetic aberrations in transgenic mice (60). One strategy involves the introduction of genes that code for toxins, such as diphtheria toxin or the A subunit of ricin, in targeted cell subpopulations. The second strategy uses the thymidine kinase (*tk*) gene from herpes simplex virus (HSV). When certain nucleotide analogs are administered and metabolized exclusively by the viral thymidine kinase, the metabolites are lethal only to cell subpopulations expressing the HSV *tk* gene. Both approaches serve as an inducible system for killing cells *in vivo*. Although gene ablation techniques can be used to generate mutant animals that lack specific cells *in vivo*, a small proportion of cells appear to escape from targeted cell death in virtually every study utilizing bacterial toxins or the viral *tk* genes. While this may present difficulties in addressing the qualitative roles of ablated cell populations, such techniques certainly hold promise.

APPROACHES FOR RISK ASSESSMENT IN IMMUNOTOXICOLOGY

Risk assessment is a process whereby relevant biologic, dose–response, and exposure data for a particular agent are analyzed in an attempt to establish qualitative and quantitative estimates of adverse outcomes. Such data are sometimes used in the development of standards for regulating the manufacture, use, and release of chemicals into the environment. For the most part, risk assessment for chemical agents has focused on estimating the incidence of cancer from lifetime exposures to a chemical agent at some unit dose; however, the use of noncancer endpoints, including disorders of the immune system, has received increasing attention. Although threshold rather than linear models are more applicable, establishing risk estimates using noncancer endpoints is to some degree similar to the process used for cancer, in that the estimates involve calculations that include both assumptions and uncertainties. For example, considerations in conducting risk assessments include the following: (a) ranking the value of epidemiologic versus experimental data; (b) extrapolations from high to low dose, from subchronic to chronic exposure, and from animals to humans; and (c) the appropriate use of mechanistic and pharmacokinetic data.

As defined by the often cited National Academy of Science Report (61), risk assessment comprises four steps: hazard identification, dose–response assessment, exposure assessment, and risk characterization. As indicated earlier, while experimental data have been used in risk assessment in several instances, the majority of data from immunotoxicity studies have not progressed beyond hazard identification. Although comparisons of clinical and animal studies are limited, other factors may also be responsible for the minimal use of these data in risk assessment including the concern that immunotoxicity testing has often been conducted without full knowledge of its predictive value in humans or its quantitative relationship to immune-mediated diseases. We have previously reported on the design and content of a screening battery involving a "tier" approach for detecting potential immunosuppressive compounds in mice (62). This battery has been used to examine a variety of compounds, and the database generated from these studies, which consists of over

50 compounds, has been collected and analyzed in an attempt to improve the accuracy and efficiency of screening chemicals for immunosuppression and to identify better those tests that predict experimentally induced, immune-mediated diseases (45,63).

Specifically, these analyses attempted to develop an improved testing configuration for the accurate prediction of immunotoxic agents and to provide insight into the qualitative and quantitative relationships between a number of immune and host resistance assays commonly employed to examine potential immunotoxic chemicals in experimental animals. While a number of limitations existed in the analyses, several conclusions could be drawn from the results: (a) With the testing configuration, examination of only two or three immune parameters was needed to successfully identify immunotoxicants. In particular, lymphocyte subpopulation enumeration and quantitation of the T-cell-dependent antibody response appeared particularly beneficial. Furthermore, some commonly employed measures (e.g., leukocyte counts and lymphoid organ weights) were fairly insensitive. (b) A good correlation existed between changes observed in the immune tests and altered host resistance in that there were no instances when host resistance was altered without significant changes in the immune test(s). However, in many instances immune changes were observed in the absence of detectable changes in host resistance (Table 4). This can be interpreted to reflect that immune tests are generally more sensitive than the host resistance assays. (c) We could not identify any single immune test that could be considered highly predictive for altered host resistance. However, many assays were good indicators while others, such as leukocyte counts and proliferative response to lipopolysaccharide (LPS), were relatively poor indicators for host resistance changes. Combining two immune tests increased the ability to predict host resistance deficits to about 80% in some cases. Some of the tests that gave

TABLE 4. *Association of each of the host resistance models with the immune tests*

Challenge agent	Number of tests	Frequency[a] Specificity −/−	Sensitivity +/+	Concordance total
Listeria monocytogenes	34	100	52	65[b]
PYB6 tumor	24	100	39	54
Streptococcus pneumoniae	19	100	38	58
B16F10 melanoma	19	100	40	68
Plasmodium yoelii	11	100	38	55
Influenza	9	100	17	44
Any of the above[c]	46	100	68	78[b]

Reproduced from ref. 43, with permission.

[a]Frequencies are defined as: specificity—the percentage of nonimmunotoxic chemicals yielding no effect on the host resistance models; sensitivity—the percentage of potential immunotoxic chemicals yielding a change in a host resistance model; concordance—percentage of qualitative agreement.

[b]Agreement statistically significant at $p < 0.05$.

[c]Frequency calculated on all host resistance models used to study an agent.

the highest association with host resistance were those that we described previously to be the best indicators for immunotoxicity, such as the PFC assay and surface markers, but also included tests such as delayed hypersensitivity reaction (DHR) and thymic weights. (d) Considering that there is a "background" level of infectious diseases in the population, it is possible that moderate changes in immune function would translate to a clinically significant change in host resistance given that the population exposed is large enough. While we were able to show this experimentally in an animal model, it would be difficult to demonstrate in a human population where "infectivity" (i.e., virulence or dose of infectious agent) cannot be controlled. (e) Regression modeling, using a large data set collected from one chemical agent, indicated that most, but not all, of the immune function–host resistance relationships follow a linear model. However, it was not possible to establish linear or threshold models for most of the chemicals studied when the data from all 50 chemicals were combined, and thus a more mechanistically based mathematical model will have to be developed. (f) Finally, using one data set, we developed methods for modeling quantitative relationships between changes in selected immune assays and host resistance tests. It is impossible, at present, to determine how applicable these analyses will be for immunotoxic compounds with different immune profiles. However, as more analyses become available, our ability to accurately estimate potential clinical effects from immunologic tests should increase.

SUMMARY

In the past decade we have observed increased efforts to assess the potential of environmental, therapeutic, and biologic agents to suppress the immune system and its consequences, which include increased susceptibility to infectious and neoplastic diseases. As a result, a variety of testing strategies have been developed in rodents, primates, and humans, which attempt to provide a balance between sensitivity, predictability, and simplicity associated with examining a complex system with multiple interacting and overlapping components (3,62). Efforts to improve these strategies are continuing and are focusing on the development of more predictive tests that quantifiably relate to clinical disease. In addition, efforts continue in the development of techniques that involve *in vitro* methodology, examination of local immune responses, such as in the skin and lung, and the implementation of molecular immunology techniques. Whether these efforts become an integral component of routine toxicity assessment and risk evaluation is uncertain at this time and will depend on a number of factors. Most notable will be the ability to accurately extrapolate alterations observed in experimental animals to potential human disease.

REFERENCES

1. Berlin A, Dean J, Draper MH, Smith EMB, Spreafico F, eds. *Immunotoxicology*. Hingham, MA:Martinus Nijhoff; 1987.

2. Office of Technology Assessment. *Identifying and controlling immunotoxic substances*, OTA-BP-BA-75, 1991.
3. National Research Council. *Biologic markers in immunotoxicology*. Washington, DC: National Academy Press; 1992.
4. Sjoblad RD. Potential future requirements for immunotoxicology testing of pesticides. *Toxicol Ind Health* 1988;4:391–395.
5. Hoyle PC, Cooper EC. Nonclinical toxicity studies of antiviral drugs indicated for the treatment of non-life-threatening diseases: evaluation of drug toxicity prior to phase I clinical studies. *Regul Toxicol Pharmacol* 1990;11:81–89.
6. Hinton DM. Testing guidelines for evaluation of the immunotoxic potential of direct food additives. *Crit Rev Food Sci Nutr* 1992;32:173–190.
7. Ehrke MJ, Mihich E. Effects of anticancer agents on immune responses. *Trends Pharmacol Sci* 1985;6:412–417.
8. Austin JH, Schulman LC, Mastrobattista JD. Pulmonary infection after cardiac transplantation: clinical and radiologic correlations. *Radiology* 1989; 172:259–265.
9. Penn I. Neoplastic consequences of immunosuppression. In: Dean JD, Luster MI, Munson AE, Amos H, eds. *Immunotoxicology and immunopharmacology*. New York: Raven Press; 1985:79–90.
10. Luster MI, Wierda D, Rosenthal GJ. Environmentally related disorders of the hematologic and immune systems. *Med Clin North Am* 1990;74:425–440.
11. Dean JH, Murray MJ. Toxic responses of the immune system. In: Amdur MO, Doull J, Klaassen CD, eds. *Casarett and Doull's toxicology*. New York: Pergamon Press; 1991:283–333.
12. Haynes RC, Murad F. Adrenocortical steroids and their synthetic analogs: inhibitors of adrenocortical steroid biosynthesis. In: Gilman AG, Goodman LS, Rall TW, Murad F, eds. *Goodman and Gilman's pharmacological basis of therapeutics*. New York: Macmillan; 1985:1459–1489.
13. Rao GN, Birnbaum LS, Collins JJ, Tennant RW, Skow LC. Mouse strains for chemical carcinogenicity studies: overview of workshop. *Fundam Appl Toxicol* 1988;10:385–394.
14. Taylor BA. Genetic relationships between inbred strains of mice. *J Hered* 1972;63:83–86.
15. Driscoll K, Linderschmidt R, Maurer J, Higgens J, Ridder G. Pulmonary response to silica or titanium dioxide: inflammatory cells, alveolar macrophage derived cytokines and histopathology. *Am J Respir Cell Mol Biol* 1990;2:381–390.
16. Ryan L, Karol M. Release of TNF in guinea pigs upon acute inhalation of cotton dusts. *Am J Respir Cell Mol Biol* 1991;5:93–98.
17. Brody AR, Overby LH, Badgett A, Kalter V, Kumas RK, Bennett RA. Interstitial pulmonary macrophages produce platelet-derived growth factor which stimulates rat lung fibroblast proliferation in vitro. *J Leukoc Biol* 1992;57:640–648.
18. Khalil N, Bereznay O, Sporn M, Greenberg A. Macrophage production of TGFB and fibroblast collagen synthesis in chronic pulmonary inflammation. *J Exp Med* 1989;170:727–737.
19. Koren HS, Devlin RB, Graham DE, et al. Ozone-induced inflammation in the lower airway of human subjects. *Am Rev Respir Dis* 1989;139:407–415.
20. Khan MF, Gupta GSD. Cellular and biochemical indices of bronchoalveolar lavage for detection of lung injury following insult by airborne toxicants. *Toxicol Lett* 1991;58:239–255.
21. Streilein JW. Skin-associated lymphoid tissues (SALT): origins and functions. *J Invest Dermatol* 1983;80:12s–16s.
22. Andersen KE, Benezra C, Burrows D, et al. Contact dermatitis: a review. *Contact Dermatitis* 1987;16:55–78.
23. DeLeo VA. Cutaneous irritancy. In: Frazier JM, ed. *In vitro toxicity testing—applications to safety evaluation*. New York: Marcel Dekker; 1992:191–203.
24. Kupper TS. Role of epidermal cytokines. In: Oppenheim JJ, Shevach EM, eds. *Immunophysiology: the role of cytokines in immunity and inflammation*. New York: Oxford University Press; 1990:285–305.
25. Barker JNWN, Mitra RS, Griffiths CEM, Dixit VM, Nickoloff BJ. Keratinocytes as initiators of inflammation. *Lancet* 1991;337:211–214.
26. Enk AH, Katz SI. Identification and induction of keratinocyte-derived IL-10. *J Immunol* 1992; 149:92–95.
27. Draize J, Woodward G, Calvery HO. Methods for the study of irritation and toxicity of substances applied topically to the skin and mucous membranes. *J Pharmacol Exp Ther* 1944;83:377–390.
28. Patrick E, Maiback HI, Burkhalter A. Mechanisms of chemically-induced skin irritation. I. Studies of time course, dose response, and components of inflammation in the laboratory mouse. *Toxicol Appl Pharmacol* 1985;81:476–490.

29. Harvell J, Bason MM, Maibach HI. In vitro skin irritation assays—relevance to human skin. *J Toxicol Clin Toxicol* 1992;30:359–369.
30. Jirova D, Nikolova Z, Fiker S, Janci H. Some new and alternative approaches to skin irritation testing. In: Marks R, Plowig G, eds. *The environmental threat to the skin*. London: Martin Dunitz Ltd; 1992:239–245.
31. Wilmer JL, Burleson FG, Kayama F, Kanno J, Luster MI. Chemically-induced inflammation in mouse skin and its relationship to patterns of cytokine production in human epidermal keratinocytes exposed to skin toxicants. *Invest Dermatol [in press]*.
32. Wood SC, Karras JG, Holsapple MP. Integration of the human lymphocyte into immunotoxicological investigations. *Fundam Appl Toxicol* 1992;18:450–459.
33. Selgrade MJK, Daniels MJ, Hu PC, Miller FJ, Graham JA. Effects of immunosuppression with cyclophosphamide on acute murine cytomegalovirus infection and virus-augmented natural killer cell activity. *Infect Immun* 1982;38:1046–1055.
34. Selgrade MJK, Daniels MJ, Dean JH. Correlation between chemical suppression of natural killer cell activity in mice and susceptibility to cytomegalovirus: rationale for applying murine cytomegalovirus as a host resistance model and for interpreting immunotoxicity testing in terms of risk of disease. *J Toxicol Environ Health* 1992;37:123–137.
35. Biron CA, Byron KS, Sullivan JL. Severe herpesvirus infections in an adolescent without natural killer cells. *N Engl J Med* 1989;320:1731–1735.
36. Quinnan GV, Kirmani N, Esber E, et al. HLA-restricted cytotoxic T lymphocyte and nonthymic cytotoxic lymphocyte responses to cytomegalovirus infection of bone marrow transplant recipients. *J Immunol* 1981;126:2036–2041.
37. Levy SM, Herberman RB, Lee J, Whiteside T, Beadle M, Heiden L, Simons A. Persistently low natural killer cell activity, age, and environmental stress as predictors of infectious morbidity. *Nat Immun Cell Growth Regul* 1991;10:289–307.
38. Vogt RF Jr, Henderson LO, Straight JM, Orti DL. Immune biomarkers demonstration project: standardized data acquisition and analysis for flow cytometric assessment of immune status in toxicant-exposed persons. *Cytometry Suppl* 1990; 4:103.
39. Masur H, Ognibene FP, Yarchoan R, et al. CD4 counts as predictors of opportunistic pneumonias in human immunodeficiency virus (HIV) infection. *Ann Intern Med* 1989;111:223–231.
40. Phair J, Munoz A, Detels RI, Kaslow R, Rinaldo C, Saah A, Multicenter AIDS Cohort Study Group. The risk of *Pneumocystis carinii* pneumonia among men infected with human immunodeficiency virus type 1. *N Engl J Med* 1990;322:1607–1608.
41. Gruters RA, Terpstra FG, Lange JMA, et al. Differences in clinical course in zidovudine-treated asymptomatic HIV-infected men associated with T-cell function at intake. *AIDS* 1991;5:43–47.
42. Miedema F, Roos MThL, Schellekens P. Low T-cell reactivity by CD3 monoclonal antibody is prognostic marker for AIDS. *J NIH Res* 1993;5:99–100.
43. Parks DR, Herzenberg LA. Flow cytometry and fluorescence activated cell sorting. In: Paul WE, ed. *Fundamental immunology*. New York: Raven Press; 1989:781–802.
44. Burcham J, Marmor M, Dubin N, Tindall B, Cooper DA, Berry G, Penny R. $CD4^+$ is the best predictor of development of AIDS in a cohort of HIV-infected homosexual men. *AIDS* 1991;5:365–372.
45. Luster MI, Portier C, Pait DG, et al. Risk assessment in immunotoxicology. II. Relationship between immune and host resistance tests. *Fundam Appl Toxicol* 1993;21:71–82.
46. Luo YD, Patel MK, Wiederholt MD, Ou DW. Effects of cannabinoids and cocaine on the mitogen-induced transformations of lymphocytes of human and mouse origins. *Int J Immunopharmacol* 1992;14:49–56.
47. Lang D, Luster MI. Comparative effects of immunotoxic chemicals on changes in the *in vitro* proliferative response in human and rodent lymphocytes. *Fundam Appl Toxicol* 1993;21:535–545.
48. Cornacoff JB, Tucker AN, Dean JH. Development of a human peripheral blood mononuclear leukocyte cell model for immunotoxicity evaluation. *In Vitro Toxicol* 1989;2:81–90.
49. Mishell RI, Dutton RW. Immunization of dissociated spleen cell cultures from normal mice. *J Exp Med* 1967;126:423–442.
50. Shand FL. The capacity of microsomally-activated cyclophosphamide to induce immunosuppression in vitro. *Immunology* 1978;35:1017–1025.
51. Kim DH, Yang KH, Johnson KW, Holsapple MP. Suppression of in vitro antibody production by dimethylnitrosamine in mixed cultures of mouse primary hepatocytes and mouse splenocytes. *Toxicol Appl Pharmacol* 1987;87:32–42.
52. McCune JM, Namikawa R, Kaneshima H, Shultz LD, Lieberman M, Weissman IC. The SCID-hu

mouse: murine model for the analysis of human hematolymphoid differentiation and function. *Nature* 1988;241:1632–1639.
53. Mosier DE. Immunodeficient mice xenografted with human lymphoid cells: new models for in vivo studies of human immunobiology and infectious diseases. *J Clin Immunol* 1990;10:185–191.
54. Pollock PL, Germolec DR, Comment CE, Rosenthal GJ, Luster MI. Human lymphocyte engrafted SCID mice as a model for immunotoxicity assessment: studies with cyclosporine A and TCDD. *Fundam Appl Toxicol* 1994;22:130–138.
55. Saiki RK, Scharf SJ, Faloona FA, Mullis KB, Horn GT, Erlich HA, Arnheim N. Enzymatic amplification of β-globulin genomic sequences and restriction site analysis for diagnosis of sickle cell anemia. *Science* 1985;230:1350–1354.
56. Gilliland G, Perrin S, Blanchard K, Bunn HF. Analysis of cytokine mRNA and DNA: detection and quantitation by competitive polymerase chain reaction. *Proc Natl Acad Sci USA* 1990;87:2725–2729.
57. Platzner C, Richter G, Uberla K, Muller W, Blocker H, Diamantstein T, Blankenstein T. Analysis of cytokine mRNA levels in interleukin-4–transgenic mice by quantitative polymerase chain reaction. *Eur J Immunol* 1992;22:1179–1184.
58. Toulme JJ, Verspieren P, Boiziau C, Loreau N, Cazanave C, Thuong NT. Les oligonucleotides antisens: outils de genetique moleculaire et agents therapeutiques. *Ann Parasitol Hum Comp* 1990; 65:11–14.
59. Rothenberg M, Johnson G, Laughlin C, Green I, Cradock J, Sarver N, Cohen JS. Oligonucleotides as anti-sense inhibitors of gene expression: therapeutic implications. *J Natl Cancer Inst* 1989;81: 1539–1544.
60. Bernstein A, Breitman M. Genetic ablation in transgenic mice. *Mol Biol Med* 1989;6:523–530.
61. National Academy of Science Report. *Risk assessment in the federal govemment: managing the process*. Washington, DC: National Academy Press; 1983.
62. Luster MI, Munson AE, Thomas PT, et al. Development of a testing battery to assess chemical-induced immunotoxicity. National Toxicology Program's criteria for immunotoxicity evaluation in mice. *Fundam Appl Toxicol* 1988;10:2–19.
63. Luster MI, Portier C, Pait DG, White KL, Gennings C, Munson AE, Rosenthal GJ. Risk assessment in immunotoxicology. I. Sensitivity and predictability of immune tests. *Fundam Appl Toxicol* 1992; 18:200–210.

Immunotoxicology and Immunopharmacology, Second Edition, edited by J. H. Dean, M. I. Luster, A. E. Munson, and I. Kimber.
Raven Press, Ltd., New York © 1994.

5

Fish Immunotoxicology

Judith T. Zelikoff

Department of Environmental Medicine, Institute of Environmental Medicine, New York University Medical Center, Tuxedo, New York 10987

Immune defense mechanisms of fish have not been studied as extensively as those of mammals, but they share a number of structural and functional characteristics important to the humoral, cell-mediated, and nonspecific aspects of the immune response (1,2). Because of this, there is increasing interest in the immune responses of fish as models for higher vertebrates in immunotoxicologic studies and as indicators of the effects of environmental pollutants.

Fish offer a number of advantages over the current immunotoxicologic mammalian models (i.e., the mouse and rat): (a) larger species are available, which can easily be maintained and can provide large numbers of immune cells for study; (b) fish are amenable to laboratory and field studies and thus can be exposed to toxicants in well-defined laboratory situations and under more "natural conditions"; (c) fish are less expensive to buy and maintain than their mammalian counterparts; (d) fish are more diverse morphologically than mammals, thus providing more alternative animal models for study; and (e) results can provide evolutionary reference points for other vertebrate studies.

Fish are exposed to toxic chemicals mainly from discharges to rivers, lakes, and oceans; marine dumping; and atmospheric fallout. In the North Atlantic ecosystem alone, hundreds of pollutant chemicals have been identified and quantified (3–6). These chemicals include metals and metalloids, synthetic and chlorinated organics, and polycyclic aromatic hydrocarbons (PAHs). For example, more than 300 aromatic hydrocarbons have been detected in Chesapeake Bay, and polychlorinated biphenyls (PCBs) are found in high concentrations in the sediments of New Bedford Harbor. In addition, the growing environmental pollution by potentially toxic metals gives rise to particular problems in the aquatic environment. Both the close contact and reactivity of these metal pollutants on aquatic organisms can result in bioaccumulation, which is dangerous not only for their survival but also for humans, with unpredictable consequences.

The biologic effects of toxic contaminants in aquatic environments are significant. Documented effects include alterations in hematologic parameters, homeostasis, carbohydrate metabolism, embryonic and/or ova development, and immunologic competence (7–9). Effects on aquatic life may be surmised from these biologic responses as well as from the incidence of pollution-related disease in these exposed organisms.

While effects of toxicants on the immune defense mechanisms of mammals are well known, toxicant-induced effects on fish immunity are not well characterized and are often scattered throughout ichthyology and toxicology literature. This lack of focus is unfortunate, since fish are frequently the organisms directly exposed environmentally to a wide variety of potentially toxic agents and are capable of accumulating high levels of many of these chemicals, which may then enter the food chain.

FISH IMMUNE SYSTEMS

Only in the last two decades has interest in, and information on, fish immune systems been the primary subject of review articles and books (10–12). Some of the generalizations about fish may, however, prove premature, since so few of the more than 20,000 known fish species have been examined for their immune structures and/or functions.

Fish are the oldest and most diverse of the vertebrate groups; their immune systems are quite varied and appear to be associated with fish phylogeny (13). Although even the most advanced teleost species do not have bone marrow or lymph nodes, fish possess functionally equivalent hematopoietic tissues primarily in areas of the spleen, head, kidney, and thymus (1,2,10), as well as circulating white blood cells functionally and morphologically similar to mammalian lymphocytes, granulocytes, and monocytes (1,2).

Fish and mammalian species share a number of structural and functional characteristics important in the humoral, cell-mediated, and nonspecific aspects of the immune response (1,2). For example, fish can reject allografts (14), exhibit hypersensitivity responses (15,16), and synthesize specific antibodies following antigenic stimulation (1,14,17). In addition, immune cells from fish can respond to mitogens and elicit a mixed lymphocyte response (18,19), release biologic response modifiers [including interleukins, arachidonic acid metabolites, and cytokines (20–22)], process and present antigen to T lymphocytes (23), effectively kill tumor cells (24), and phagocytose and kill foreign pathogens (25,26) by mechanisms that are accompanied by the release of reactive oxygen intermediates (27).

Since the purpose of this chapter is to gain a working knowledge of the fish immune response so as to more fully understand how toxicants act to bring about alterations in host defense, a brief discussion of fish immunity follows. For more detailed information on the fish immune system, a number of excellent review papers are available to the reader (1,10,11,28).

Nonspecific Immunity

Nonspecific immune reactions in fish are general responses to injury and/or invasion by foreign organisms. Phagocytosis and inflammation are two nonspecific responses that appear to be universal in fish (10). In these reactions, white blood cell responses are assisted and/or heightened by a variety of nonspecific factors found in fish serum, consisting primarily of complement, lysozyme, interferon, transferrin, C-reactive protein, and various natural hemolysins and hemagglutinins (1,10,29).

It has been demonstrated from early studies that fish produce an inflammatory reaction in response to a number of different agents (30). It was concluded that this process was basically similar to that observed in mammals, except that the response in fish was less intense and slower to appear and to resolve. It has also been observed that morphologically, at least, nonspecific immunity in fish is mediated largely by blood and tissue phagocytic cells (i.e., granulocytes and mononuclear phagocytes), which participate in acute and chronic inflammatory responses (31).

Specific Immunity

The specific immune defense mechanisms of fish are the same as those for mammals and include cell- and humoral-mediated responses (1,10). As observed in mammalian systems, each of these specific sets of immune responses shows negative memory (tolerance) as well as positive anamnestic (memory) characteristics of quicker, and more prolonged, immune responses after a second contact with foreign antigens.

Humoral-Mediated Immunity

Cells producing antibodies, thought to be analogous to mammalian B lymphocytes and plasma cells, are located primarily in the spleen and/or kidney of fish. Like mammalian cells, fish B lymphocytes are stimulated to proliferate by the B cell mitogen lipopolysaccharide (LPS) and carry immunoglobulin (Ig) on their surface membranes. The latter, in turn, can be induced to form "caps," which may constitute a triggering mechanism whereby lymphocytes are induced to transform into antibody-producing cells (APCs) or their precursors (17,32). It is known that lymphocytes in higher vertebrates are capable of secreting antibody before differentiating into plasma cells (or APCs), and it is possible that much of the Ig in fish is produced by stimulated lymphocytes that do not undergo full differentiation into APCs (1,10,32).

The antibodies produced by fish appear to be restricted to one major class of Ig, most resembling (in terms of heavy chain mass, interchain disulfide bonding, amino acid and carbohydrate content, and solution conformation) mammalian IgM (31,33).

Cell-Mediated Immunity

Cell-mediated immunity in teleosts is comparable to that found in higher vertebrates both in the diversity of cell types present and effector cell activities. While some investigators are reluctant to accept the presence of individual populations of lymphocytes in fish, several lines of evidence strongly suggest that fish do possess at least two groups of lymphocytes functioning in a fashion similar to the T lymphocytes and aforementioned B lymphocytes of higher vertebrates (10,32,34).

T lymphocytes are the primary cell type responsible for cell-mediated immunity in mammals and most likely in fish. Peripheral blood lymphocytes of mammals can be stimulated to undergo blast transformation by nonspecific stimulants. Fish T cells are also responsive to mitogens such as phytohemagglutinin (PHA) and concanavalin A (Con A) (18). These cells participate in other cell-mediated immune activities such as rejection of foreign tissue grafts (35), hypersensitivity responses (15,16), and mixed-leukocyte reactions (MLRs) (19).

Macrophage-Mediated Immune Functions

In addition to their importance for nonspecific immunity, fish macrophages play a key role in cell-mediated immunity as accessory, secretory, and effector cells. These cells (a) can be stimulated to a higher state of activation *in vitro* and *in vivo* by a variety of chemical agents (36), (b) can act as antigen-processing and -presenting cells (23), (c) can be mobile and respond to a variety of chemical stimulants (36), and (d) can be highly phagocytic (1,10,31,36). In fish, as in mammalian species, phagocytosis appears to be receptor mediated (26,31) and enhanced by opsonization.

Fish macrophages also act as secretory and effector cells and possess bactericidal, larvacidal, and cytotoxic activities (26,37). The microbicidal activity of fish macrophages is mediated by both aerobic and anaerobic defense mechanisms (26,27). The role of macrophages as secretory cells in immune responses is well known in higher vertebrates. Some of the same mediators released by mammalian macrophages, including arachidonic acid metabolites (38,39), interleukins, and cytokines (40,41), have recently been characterized in fish as well.

Nonspecific Cytotoxic Cells (NCCs)

Cells possessing nonspecific cytotoxic effector activity, equivalent to mammalian natural killer (NK) cells, have been characterized in channel catfish (42) and other fish species (43). The NCCs consist of a highly active effector population found in fish anterior kidney, spleen, and peripheral blood (42–44). The NCCs lyse a wide variety of transformed target cells and their cytotoxicity can be enhanced by immunoregulatory substances including retinolacetate (44). In addition to a probable role in tumor surveillance, mammalian NK cells function in antimicrobial and antiparasitic immunity (45); studies with channel catfish demonstrated that fish NCCs also possess antiparasitic activity (46).

IMMUNOMODULATION BY CHEMICALS

While a wide variety of toxic agents have been tested for acute and chronic lethal effects in fish, far fewer studies have examined the effects of chemical toxicants on fish immune systems, and thus relatively little is known concerning the toxic effects of xenobiotics on fish immune defense mechanisms.

Some of the same criteria used to determine the immunotoxic potential of xenobiotics in mammalian systems are also used to assess immunotoxicity in fish. These include immunopathology (i.e., thymic atrophy), alterations in nonspecific and specific immune functions, and changes in immune-system-regulated functions (i.e., host resistance challenge models).

Environmental Toxicants

A large number of environmental pollutants are capable of suppressing avian and mammalian immune responses, which may then lead to increased host susceptibility to infectious diseases or possibly cancer. Some of these same pollutants also act to alter immune responses of fish. Stresses imposed on the immune system of fish by environmental pollutants may not be overtly apparent. Stressors may act directly to kill the fish or indirectly to exacerbate disease states by lowering resistance and allowing the invasion of environmental pathogens. Although the relationship between environmental pollution and diseases in aquatic organisms has not been clearly defined, a large amount of circumstantial evidence exists linking various diseases in feral fish with pollutant discharges (47,48). A widely accepted mechanism by which aquatic pollutants are thought to increase disease incidence in fish is via suppression of immune responses (49).

Metals

Municipal wastes, industrial discharges, surface runoff, damage to and weathering of vessel protective paints, ocean dumping, and aerial inputs account for most ocean metal pollution. Some of the routes of entry for metals into the oceans have been slowed or stopped in recent years, but too little regulation has been implemented too late.

The effects of metal pollution are measurable on both ecologic and economic scales. Ecosystem impacts include contamination of sediments and the water column, accumulation of pollutants in biota over a wide area, and apparent increases in pollutant-related anomalies in the species that reside there.

Although the number of studies evaluating the effects of metals on fish is extensive, relatively little is known concerning effects of metals on fish immunocompetence. This chapter presents an overview of metal-induced immunotoxicity in fish, but for a more comprehensive review of the effects of metals on fish immune systems, the reader is referred to a recent paper by Zelikoff (49).

Oral exposures to cadmium (Cd^{2+}) and lead (Pb^{2+}) have been shown to reduce antibody responses in rabbits and other mammalian species (50,51). Similar to the effects observed for mammals, O'Neill (52) demonstrated that a single intraperitoneal (ip) injection of Pb^{2+} and Cd^{2+} (at 0.01 to 0.3 mg/100 g and 0.05 to 0.1 mg/100 g, respectively) resulted in a pronounced reduction of antibody titer to *MS2* bacteriophage in brown trout. Viale and Calamari (53) also reported a reduction in antibody production in response to human red blood cells (RBCs) following Cd^{2+} exposure of trout. The suppressive effect observed on antibody response in these studies has been speculated to be due to changes in lymphocyte numbers (54), the same mechanism by which Pb^{2+} and Cd^{2+} are thought to reduce antibody responses in mammalian species (50,51). Conversely, Thuvander (55) demonstrated that water bath exposure to low levels of Cd^{2+} for 12 weeks enhanced humoral antibody response to *Vibrio anguillarum* O-antigen. Such differences in metal-induced effects on immunocompetence are not that surprising, since the immunotoxic effects of metals in mammals have been shown to be dependent on a number of variables including animal species, dose, and both route and duration of metal exposure (56). For example, a stimulatory effect of Cd^{2+} on IgM production (as measured by the number of plaque-forming cells) in mice has been reported (57), while a suppression of the primary antibody response was observed by changing either the route of exposure or the timing of Cd^{2+} exposure relative to the presentation of the antigen. In support of this hypothesis, it appears from the literature (49) that *in vitro* exposure of fish immune cells to Cd^{2+} enhances immunocompetence, while *in vivo* exposure depresses host immunoregulatory mechanisms.

Cd^{2+}-induced modulation of cellular immunity has also been observed in mammalian species. For example, Bozelka and Burkholder (58) reported an inhibition of T lymphocyte reactivity in mice (as measured by the MLRs of splenocytes), although the mitogenic response to Con A was not affected. Müller et al. (59) also reported a suppression of T-cell-mediated responses in mice exposed to relatively low doses of Cd^{2+}. In agreement with these mammalian studies, Thuvander (55) demonstrated that, in the absence of any clinical or histologic changes, cells recovered from Cd^{2+}-exposed trout had a suppressed lymphoproliferative response to mitogens as well as to an extract of *V. anguillarum* antigen.

Macrophage functions in fish are also disrupted by exposure to Cd^{2+}. Zelikoff (49) has shown that *Aeromonas salmonicida*-injected rainbow trout exposed to Cd^{2+}-contaminated water at 2 ppb for either 8, 17, or 30 days showed depressed phorbol myristate acetate (PMA)-stimulated production of superoxide and hydrogen peroxide and enhanced phagocytic competence by activated trout macrophages. Similarly, in rodents, low dose *in vivo* exposure to Cd^{2+} also enhanced the phagocytic activity of rat pulmonary macrophages (60) as well as depressing the respiratory burst by mouse pulmonary and peritoneal macrophages (61). The reduction in respiratory burst observed in fish was most likely due to the inhibitory effects of Cd^{2+} on cellular respiration (62).

In mammals, Pb^{2+}-induced effects on APCs is thought to be due to a suppression of the clonal expansion of B lymphocytes (51). A reduction in the number of B-like cells, as well as the loss of helper and memory cell activity, could be responsible for the reduction in antibody titer observed by O'Neill (52) in Pb^{2+}-exposed brown trout. In support of this hypothesis, Dawson (63) found that brown bullheads exposed to 50 ppm of lead acetate in the water for up to 183 days had reduced spleen size and depressed hematopoietic activity. In addition, Crandall and Goodnight (64) found similar results with guppies following 60 days of exposure to lead nitrate.

Manganese (Mn^{2+}), at low levels, is a necessary constituent for life in both fish and mammalian species. However, when released at high concentrations into freshwater ecosystems by neighboring steel, mining, paint, and pesticide industries, Mn^{2+} can induce symptoms in fish of slow suffocation, paralysis, mucous cell depletion, and gill damage. *In vitro* studies by Ghanmi et al. (65,66) demonstrated an increase in both mitogen-induced lymphocyte proliferation and NCC activity in fish in response to Mn^{2+}. These results were in agreement with those observed in some mammalian studies. *In vivo* exposure of rodents to Mn^{2+} enhanced NK cell activity (67), lymphocyte proliferation in response to allogeneic cells (68), and some macrophage functions (68). It has been suggested by Smialowicz et al. (69) that the stimulation of NK cell activity might be due to increased production of interferon. The enhancing effects of Mn^{2+} on mammalian and fish NK cell activity may actually play a beneficial role in immunosurveillance against tumors. It has been speculated that the anticarcinogenic properties of Mn^{2+} in rodents, as well as its antagonist properties against the toxic and carcinogenic effects of nickel (Ni^{2+}) (70), may be due to the ability of Mn^{2+} to enhance NK cell activity. More studies, however, need to be performed before a clear association between waterborne Mn^{2+} and the incidence of tumors in fish can be assessed.

Although nickel (Ni^{2+}) is found as a contaminant in aquatic environments due to industrial discharges and other anthropogenic sources (71) and is a potent immunotoxicant in mammalian systems (72), the effects of Ni^{2+} on the immune responses of aquatic organisms are not well known. Studies by Bowser et al. (73) and O'Neill (74) indicated that Ni^{2+} acts as an immunosuppressant (with the exception of effects on macrophage migration) in fish affecting both macrophage- and humoral-mediated immunity. Similar effects of Ni^{2+} have also been observed for mammalian species. For example, Waters and Gardner (75) reported that *in vitro* exposure of rabbit alveolar macrophages to soluble nickel at millimolar concentrations induced severe functional deficits (i.e., inability to phagocytose latex beads and diminished release of lysozyme) but had no effects on macrophage viability (as measured by trypan blue exclusion). Gardner (76) showed that inhalation of atmospheric nickel chloride (0.4 mg Ni/m^3 for 2 hr) drastically reduced the phagocytic and bactericidal capabilities of mouse alveolar macrophages, but neither the yield nor the viability of those cells. The lack of effects on macrophage viability reported in these mammalian studies is in agreement with the observations by Bowser et al.

(73) following *in vitro* exposure of trout peritoneal macrophages to Ni^{2+} at concentrations between 10 and 1000 μM.

Ni^{2+} also acts to compromise humoral immunity in mammalian species. For example, Ni^{2+} depresses circulating antibody titers to *T-1* bacteriophage in rats following antigen injection (77). The suppressive effects on humoral immunity observed for rodents are similar to those observed by O'Neill (74) following waterborne exposure of carp and rainbow trout to Ni^{2+} at 7.5 mg/liter for 38 weeks.

Chromium (Cr) is a highly toxic metal often found as an aquatic pollutant as the result of spills and other anthropogenic sources. It is a suspected carcinogen (78) and potent immunomodulator that poses a substantial health risk to directly exposed organisms. The study by O'Neill (74) indicated that Cr^{6+} acted to suppress fish humoral immune responses. In addition, brown trout and carp exposed *in vivo* to Cr^{6+} at 1 mg/liter for 38 weeks had reduced primary and secondary humoral antibody responses to viral challenge (*MS2* bacteriophage). Figoni and Treagen (77) demonstrated similar Cr^{6+}-induced effects in rodents. In this latter study, injection of rats with nontoxic doses of disodium chromate depressed circulating antibody titers to injected viral antigen (*T-1* phage) (77). The authors speculated that the reduced antibody titers were due, in part, to effects on antigen-processing cells of the reticuloendothelial system.

It can be concluded that exposure to many heavy metals alters the immunologic competence of fish. Metals active in this capacity include Al^{2+}, Cd^{2+}, Cr^{6+}, Cu^{2+}, Pb^{2+}, Mn^{2+}, Ni^{2+}, Sn^{2+}, and Zn^{2+}. Metal-induced immune alterations may occur either directly by binding to, or readjusting, the tertiary structures of biologically active molecules, or indirectly by acting as "stressors" to modify corticosteroid levels in fish. Regardless of the mechanism(s) by which these effects occur, a depression of macrophage-, cell-, or humoral-mediated immunity by metal pollutants may act to alter host immunocompetence, leading ultimately to increased susceptibility of the fish to infectious diseases or possibly cancer.

Pesticides

Pesticides represent a diverse group of poisonous chemicals that are primarily used to control pest species of insects, weeds, or fungi. Many of the more persistent pesticides, especially the chlorinated hydrocarbons, are common pollutants of aquatic ecosystems. Pesticides enter the aquatic environment and become rapidly distributed through intentional application, aerial drift or runoff following application, or accidental release. Fish residing in contaminated areas frequently encounter and accumulate sublethal levels of pesticides from their surrounding water and/or food, which may then enter the food chain.

In addition to the carcinogenic potential of some pesticides and their toxicity to the nervous and reproductive systems (79), pesticides represent a possible immunotoxic threat to all directly exposed organisms. Yet despite this, relatively few studies have been performed examining the toxicity of pesticides on the immune responses of fish.

Organochlorine Insecticides

Studies (80,81) have demonstrated that carp fed a diet containing lindane at 0.1, 1, and 10 mg/kg fish/day for 2.5 months demonstrated no change in antibody production against *Yersinia ruckeri*, even though the lymphoid organs were highly contaminated; exposure to an even higher concentration of lindane (1000 mg/kg food) had no effect on graft rejection time or on *in vitro* uptake of *Y. ruckeri* and zymosan by macrophages. In addition, Saxena et al. (82) demonstrated that catfish exposed to 1.3 mg/liter lindane as hexachlorocyclohexane, alone or in combination with Cd^{2+} (0.2 mg/liter), also had no effect on humoral immunity. In contrast to the lack of effects observed on humoral responses in fish, studies in rabbits demonstrated that lindane depressed antibody responses to *Salmonella typhimurium* antigen (83).

While lindane appears to have no effects on fish humoral immunity, other organochlorines have been shown to be potent immunomodulators. Fish and some lower aquatic organisms appear to be extremely sensitive to the acute toxicity of the chlorinated ethane derivative, dichlorodiphenyltrichloroethane (DDT). Zeeman and Brindley (84) have shown that DDT significantly decreased antibody titers to bovine serum albumin in exposed goldfish; effects were persistent for at least 2 weeks following the second immunization of albumin. The persistence of effects was most likely due to residual DDT in the tissues (85). Although the immunotoxic effects of DDT in mammalian systems are ambiguous, in general, DDT appears to suppress humoral immune functions. For example, oral exposure of rats to DDT at 200 ppm (86) depresses serum antibody titers against ovalbumin, while, in chickens, exposure to DDT or Mirex significantly reduced total antibody production and serum IgG levels, although serum IgM levels were elevated (86).

DDT has also been implicated in affecting the incidence of fish diseases. Research by Schoenthal (87) demonstrated that several different species of fish exposed to DDT in the laboratory for 2 days had an increased incidence of protozoan and fungal diseases as compared with unexposed fish. The association between DDT exposure and disease incidence in fish has also been observed in feral populations collected from heavily contaminated sites off the Palos Verdes peninsula of southern California (88). In this field study, almost 40% of all fish collected from the area showed fish erosion disease. Since very few mammalian studies have examined the effects of DDT on cell-mediated immunity and/or on host resistance, interspecies comparisons are difficult to assess.

Although there is little direct evidence in humans, DDT is considered an epigenetic carcinogen in laboratory animals (89). In fish, exposure to DDT is also associated with an increased incidence of tumor formation. Trout exposed to DDT in their food for up to 20 months demonstrate an elevated number (compared to unexposed control fish) of hepatomas (90). The question then arises whether DDT acts directly as a tumor-causing agent in fish, or whether it is the result of compromised immunologic responses that act to increase host susceptibility to other tumorigens.

Regarding other chlorinated insecticides, Rogillio (91) demonstrated that large doses of Mirex fed to channel catfish for up to 4 weeks changed the differential counts of leukocytes in the peripheral blood. These alterations included a nonsignificant increase in lymphocytes, significantly decreased numbers of thrombocytes, and altered monocyte numbers.

Organophosphate Insecticides

In general, the evidence is strong that organophosphate insecticides are immunosuppressive in mammals (86,92). For example, Street and Sharma (92) observed that a 28-day oral exposure of rabbits to methylparathion (1.5 mg/kg/day) produced a marked reduction in splenic germinal centers following antigenic stimulation, as well as thymus cortical atrophy, and a reduced delayed-type hypersensitivity response to tuberculin. Studies by Desi et al. (83) demonstrated that exposure of rodents to malathion depressed antibody responses to *Salmonella typhimurium*. Malathion also suppresses humoral immune responses in fish. For example, exposure to malathion at 1.75 and 0.5 mg/liter depressed agglutinating antibody titers against *Edwardsiella ictaluri* in channel catfish following a 30-day water bath exposure (93).

The immunosuppressive effects of another organophosphorus insecticide, trichlorphon, has also been demonstrated in fish. Siwicki et al. (94) has shown that high doses of trichlorphon produced leukopenia and compromised neutrophil phagocytic ability, lysozyme levels in serum (compared to that of control), and the percentage of nitroblue tetrazolium (NBT)-positive neutrophils. Depressive effects of trichlorphon on the nonspecific immune functions of mammalian species have also been observed (86).

Organophosphate insecticides have been shown to alter circulating white blood cell numbers in exposed fish. For example, fish exposed to malathion for 24 and 48 hr demonstrate initial increased white blood cell counts, with the numbers returning to control levels after 72 hr (95). Phasolone has also been reported to produce similar stimulatory effects on white blood cell numbers (96). At fourfold higher malathion concentrations, channel catfish fingerlings exposed for 12, 24, 48, 72, and 96 hr demonstrate leukopenia at 48, 72, and 96 hr after exposure; differential leukocyte counts were unchanged by insecticide exposure. The latter findings are supported by early studies, which demonstrated that malathion reduced the numbers of splenic lymphocytes in exposed fish (97).

Carbamates

Aldicarb, a highly toxic oxime carbamate insecticide used against a variety of insects and nematodes, is distributed in groundwater resources throughout the world. Since aldicarb and its metabolites are relatively water soluble, aquatic organisms are at a high risk for exposure to these chemicals via agricultural runoff. Although the toxicity of aldicarb associated with inactivation of acetylcholinesterase is well studied, little is known concerning its effects on host resistance and immune function in fish inhabiting polluted environments. In one study (98), fish exposed to sublethal concentrations of aldicarb (0.86 mg/liter) over a 4-week exposure period demonstrated pronounced lymphocytosis that was caused by a statistically significant increase in large lymphocyte populations; small lymphocyte counts were also found to be raised with the peak occurring 2 weeks after exposure. The aberrant lymphocyte counts returned to baseline values following a week in clean water. The authors suggested that aldicarb-induced lymphocytosis was not due to the transformation of small lymphocytes into large ones but may have been due to an accelerated production of lymphocytes and/or to the early release into circulating blood of already differentiated lymphocytes from hematopoietic tissue. Chronic aldicarb poisoning also elicited marked thrombocytosis (which persisted even after recovery in clean water), neutropenia, and a marked monocytosis and basophilia. The authors suggested that a sustained stimulation of the granulopoietic precursors to meet increased demand for circulating neutrophils during aldicarb intoxication may lead to exhaustion and eventually a reduction in the circulating numbers of cells. Although most laboratory studies suggest that the carbamate class of insecticides is fairly nonimmunotoxic for laboratory animals (86), women chronically exposed to aldicarb at levels ranging from 1 to 61 μg/liter in the drinking water (99) demonstrated an association between aldicarb ingestion and increased IgG levels, the numbers and percentages of CD8+ T lymphocytes, and decreased ratios of CD4+/CD8+ cells.

Other carbamate pesticides have also been reported to produce immunotoxic effects in fish. Carbaryl has been shown to suppress humoral, cell-mediated, and nonspecific immunity in rodents as well as to compromise host resistance to infectious agents (89). Studies in fish demonstrate that lake trout and coho salmon kept for up to 100 days in waters containing various concentrations of carbaryl had significantly reduced spleen weights and depressed numbers of splenic lymphocytes (97). It appears from the limited number of studies that carbamate insecticides may be immunotoxic to fish via their effects on leukopoiesis.

Herbicides

Atrazine, a triazine herbicide commonly employed for agricultural purposes, is often implicated in acute aquatic environmental pollution. Although very few studies have been performed examining the immunotoxic effects of atrazine on fish, Walsh and Ribelin (97) and Cossarini-Dunier (80) reported no effects of atrazine on cell- and/or macrophage-mediated immunity in some fish species. In contrast to the lack of effects observed on immune functions, water bath exposure of tilapia to sublethal concentrations of atrazine produced a substantial decrease in red and white blood cell counts and in hemoglobin content (100). Other than the studies performed by Vos et al. (101), which demonstrate a "marked" effect of atrazine on the immune system of rats, limited evidence exists demonstrating the immunotoxicity of atrazine for mammalian systems.

Fungicides

Pentachlorophenol (PCP) and other chlorinated phenols are ubiquitous and persistent environmental contaminants that are highly toxic to aquatic organisms. PCP, a well-known uncoupler of mitochondrial oxidative phosphorylation and a modulator of cytochrome P 450 (102), produced numerous physiologic effects including immunotoxicity in both fish and mammalian species. In fish, kidney phagocytic cells exposed *in vitro* to analytic or technical grade PCP at concentrations ranging from 5 to 75 ppm demonstrated a dose–response reduction in chemiluminescence (CL) (103). Technical grade PCP (T-PCP), containing dioxin contaminants, elicited a slightly greater suppression of CL in medaka than did pure PCP (P-PCP). Differences in immunotoxic activity between P-TCP and T-PCP were similar to those reported in mammalian studies. While P-PCP appears to have little immunotoxicity, T-PCP produces substantial immunosuppressive activity in rodents (104). These latter authors suggested that the differences observed between the compounds are due to the presence of contaminants such as 1,2,3,6,7-8-hexachlorodibenzo-*p*-dioxin.

The immunosuppressive effects of PCP in fish appear similar to those observed in birds and mammals. For example, chickens fed a diet of P-PCP at 2500 ppm demonstrated suppressed lectin-induced lymphoproliferation, reduced white blood cell counts, and decreased humoral response to bovine serum albumin (105). In addition, other studies have demonstrated P-PCP-induced suppression of tumor surveillance mechanisms (i.e., cytotoxic T cell activity) and increased susceptibility of rodents to virus-induced tumor formation (106). In contrast, however, to the relative sensitivity of fish macrophages, mammalian macrophages were relatively resistant to the immunotoxicity of PCP. Discrepancies between the studies may be due to differences in the route of PCP exposure. The effects on fish macrophages are produced *in vitro*, while those effects observed in mammalian studies appeared following *in vivo* exposures.

Halogenated Aromatic Hydrocarbons (HAHs)

Environmental HAH congeners that resist metabolic detoxification accumulate in body fat and remain there as a residue with a long biologic half-life (79). Such body burdens are found in humans, in wildlife, and in commercially important species. In nature, marine and freshwater fish tend to bioaccumulate high levels of HAHs from the aquatic environment. For example, HAH levels in Lake Ontario coho salmon have been found to be 1.5 million times that measured in Lake Ontario water (107).

There is substantial evidence that a number of isomers of halogenated aromatics are carcinogenic, teratogenic, neurotoxic, and immunotoxic in mammalian systems. Although not to the same extent in fish, the immunotoxicity of mixtures and individual isomers of HAHs, particularly the more common chemicals such as polychlorinated biphenyls and 2,3,7,8-tetrachlorodibenzo-*p*-dioxin (TCDD), have been relatively well studied.

Polychlorinated Biphenyls (PCBs)

Because of their persistence in the environment (3,5), PCBs, ubiquitous contaminants of soil and water, represent a serious environmental threat (108). Although a number of studies investigating the immunotoxicity of PCBs in mammalian systems have been performed (108), investigations concerning the immunomodulating potential of PCBs in fish are extremely limited.

While humoral immunity appears to be particularly sensitive to the immunotoxic effects of PCBs in mammalian systems (109), the same does not appear true for fish. In one study (110), juvenile rainbow trout were fed diets containing Aroclor 1254 (a commercial mixture of a number of PCB congeners containing 54% chlorine) alone and as a mixture with Mirex (5 ppm) for 12 months. Dietary exposure to 300 ppm Aroclor 1254 did not significantly alter the humoral immune plaque-forming center response of rainbow trout, even at concentrations that produced severe generalized toxicity (i.e., body wasting and hepatomegaly). These findings appear contrary to those observed on humoral-mediated immune functions in exposed mammals. For example, exposure to PCB mixtures lowered circulating immunoglobulin levels, decreased anamnestic responses (IgG and IgM) to a T-cell-dependent antigen, and decreased specific antibody responses following immunization with antigens (109). Discrepancies between the species are not surprising, since the immunotoxic effects of HAHs depend, at least in part, on the Ah receptor (111). Thus immunotoxicity depends greatly on the species of animals used as well as the particular congener/isomer studied. Whether the effect of PCBs on cell-mediated immune functions in fish will be similar to the immunosuppression produced in mammalian species (including humans) is difficult to assess due to the lack of fish data.

PCBs cause dramatic changes in the lymphoid organs of both mammals and fish. In mammalian studies, PCB toxicosis is usually accompanied by atrophy of primary and secondary lymphoid organs (101,108,109). Early reports with chickens indicated that exposure to commercial PCBs resulted in decreased spleen and bursa weights. In fish, Nestel and Budd (112) observed that 80% of the rainbow trout fed diets containing Aroclor 1254 had reduced amounts of splenic white pulp.

PCB exposure also appears to compromise host susceptibility (113). For example, field studies have demonstrated that, at concentrations producing a low rate of mortality, long-term exposure of fish to Aroclor 1254 increases host susceptibility to fin-rot disease (114). While PCB-induced alteration in tumor resistance remains unclear for both species, resistance to bacterial and/or viral challenge is compromised in fish by PCB exposure (114).

Dioxins

Polychlorinated dibenzo-*p*-dioxins, as exemplified by the most potent isomer, TCDD, are the focus of great concern because of the extreme toxicity of some congeners and their ubiquity in food and the aquatic environment. One major point of concern involves the accumulation of dioxins in the food chain and the potential for human exposure from ingesting contaminated food items.

In addition to their carcinogenicity (115), chlorinated dioxins are immunosuppressive for many species including some nonhuman primates (116). Because TCDD is the most biologically active chemical in the family of isosteric HAHs, its effects on immunocompetence have been studied extensively in a variety of mammalian species (116). Far less, however, is known concerning their effects on fish. While it seems certain that exposure to TCDD produces thymic involution in fish, TCDD-induced effects on fish humoral- and cell-mediated immune functions are dubious (117). In studies by Spitsbergen (117), the immunotoxic effects of TCDD on yearling rainbow trout injected intraperitoneally with TCDD was evaluated. Trout receiving the highest dose of TCDD (10 μg/kg) were hypophagic and exhibited fin necrosis, ascites, thymic atrophy, and suppression of hematopoiesis, but no alterations in humoral- or macrophage-mediated immune functions [except for pokeweed mitogen (PWM)-induced lymphoproliferation] were observed. Spitsbergen et al. (118) also demonstrated that TCDD, at levels below those that caused clinical toxicology (1 μg/kg and <500 ppm, respectively), had no effects on host resistance to challenge with infectious hematopoietic necrosis virus in trout fingerlings. These results are contrary to an earlier report by Anderson et al. (119), who demonstrated that the primary immune response of rainbow trout to sheep red blood cells (sRBCs), as measured by the Jerne plaque assay, was dramatically lower following TCDD exposure.

The general failure of TCDD to suppress immune responses of rainbow trout at doses below those producing clinical toxicity parallels the finding regarding effects of a number of other pharmacologic immunomodulators in trout. For example, cyclophosphamide suppresses humoral immune responses of trout only at doses approaching those causing lethality. Of the drugs successful in suppressing immune responses in mammals, only corticosteroids suppressed humoral immune responses in trout at doses below those causing clinical toxicity (120). While the trout is among the more sensitive of species with regard to lethal effects of TCDD (117), rainbow trout are relatively resistant to the immunosuppressive effects of this toxicant. As is true for other HAHs, these discrepancies may be due to interspecies differences in Ah receptors. It is interesting, however, that humans, like fish, also appear to be relatively resistant to the immunotoxic effects of TCDD (121).

Polycyclic Aromatic Hydrocarbons (PAHs)

PAHs, well-known toxicants and carcinogens resulting from the combustion of some fossil fuels, wood, and tobacco, have made their way into the major waterways. Data from field and laboratory studies have linked PAH contamination to high frequencies of neoplasms in several of the fish species that reside there (122). Although the exact mechanism(s) of PAH-related tumor formation is not clearly defined, it is of interest that those PAHs that are carcinogenic also possess potent immunosuppressive properties (123). A number of field studies performed by investigators from the Virginia Institute of Marine Science have demonstrated that feral fish collected from the PAH-contaminated Elizabeth River (in Virginia) have altered immunologic responses. Faisal et al. (124) have demonstrated that lymphoproliferation by cells from the marine fish spot (collected from the Elizabeth River) were depressed in response to the T cell mitogens, Con A, and PHA and augmented by the B cell mitogen LPS, as well as to PWM and peanut agglutinin. Immune alterations were strongly correlated with sediment PAH levels from the sampling site. In additional studies by these same investigators (125), NCC cytotoxic activity was also found to be depressed in feral fish populations exposed to PAH-contaminated sediments. Analysis of leukocyte–tumor cell conjugates indicated that the NCCs from Elizabeth River fish were unable to recognize and subsequently bind to the tumor target cells. The authors suggested that this may be due to alterations in NCC surface receptors. Macrophage activity in the same feral fish population was also found to be suppressed by PAH-contaminated sediments (126) as well as in fish exposed to PAH-contaminated sediments in the laboratory.

In mammals, most PAHs also act to suppress cell-mediated immune responses. For example, benzo[*a*]pyrene (BaP)-exposed mice have depressed responses to T and B cell mitogens, but not to allogeneic cell stimulation (127). Stimulatory effects of PAHs observed on fish B cells appear to be contradictory to those observed for rodents. Interspecies differences may be due to differences in the cytosolic surface receptor on B cells that bind PAHs, the nature of the specific chemicals used in the studies, or the fact that, although the sediments contained primarily PAHs (4), other contaminants may act with these chemicals to produce synergistic or antagonistic effects.

While field studies such as these have their limitations and suffer in their lack of knowledge about fish history and the length of pollutant exposure, as well as to unknown differences in diet, which may influence immunoresponsiveness and disease susceptibility, results of these studies strongly suggest that PAHs found in the aquatic environment act to suppress fish immunocompetence in ways similar to that observed for mammalian species.

Drugs

Except for extensive testing of certain drugs (i.e., antimetabolites, hormones, and antibiotics) on fish scale allograft rejection rate, few drugs have been tested for their effects on other fish immune responses. Hormonal preparations are the most broadly tested drugs, with the majority of these being the corticosteroids. Unfortunately, doses of corticosteroids needed to produce quantifiable effects are often near or at lethal levels.

Antibiotics

One of the major problems of large-scale fish culture is the outbreak of epizotic diseases. As in animal husbandry, antibiotics are commonly used in a prophylactic and therapeutic way. However, the use of these drugs has some major drawbacks, including the risk of raising resistant pathogens, production of toxic effects on liver cells and/or hypersensitivity responses, and adverse effects on the immune system. It has been demonstrated that antibiotics can induce immunosuppression in avian and mammalian species (128,129), including humans (130). Effects of antibiotics in fish are similar to those observed for the other vertebrate species. While early fish studies focused primarily on antibiotic-induced changes in allograft rejection time, more recent studies were concerned with effects on humoral immunity and other aspects of cell-mediated responses. Wishkovsky et al. (131) demonstrated that *in vitro* exposure of trout kidney phagocytes to tetracycline (TC) and oxytetracycline (OTC) at concentrations between 0.1 and 50 μg/ml produced a dose-dependent suppression of CL in response to zymosan or latex particles. These findings were in agreement with previous reports of the suppressive effects of tetracyclines on other components of the fish immune system. Rijkers et al. (132) demonstrated a suppression of serum Ig levels and plaque-forming cells in response to sRBCs in carp exposed to OTC either in the food or by ip injections. Grondel et al. (133) examined the immunomodulating effects of two tetracycline analogs, OTC and doxycycline (DC), on mitogenic and allogeneic cell stimulation of carp lymphocytes *in vitro*. At concentrations of 4 to 6 μg OTC and 1 to 2.5 μg DC, mitogen-induced lymphoproliferative responses were reduced to about 50% of control values; at higher OTC (10 μg/ml) and DC (5 μg/ml) concentrations, MLR was also markedly reduced. Lymphoproliferative responses of human T and B lymphocytes have also been shown to be suppressed by exposure to tetracycline analogs.

Hormones

Recent evidence reveals that a number of hormones act as immunomodulators in mammalian species. For example, the propiomelanocortin gene products β-endorphin and adrenocorticotropic hormone (ACTH) modulate cytotoxic and proliferative immune responses (134). Animals of different phylogenetic groups exhibited neuroendocrine responses to a variety of stressful stimuli; some of these stressors induced production and secretion of endogenous opioids, which in turn produced analgesia and cross-tolerance to morphine and other opiates. Studies in fish demonstrated that "stressed" tilapia were more susceptible to experimental infection with *Aeromonas hydrophila* (135); fish also showed a decrease in nonspecific cytotoxicity (136). Faisal et al. (137) have suggested that the immunosuppression observed in these studies was due to the release of endogenous opioids.

In mammalian systems, corticosteroids and their synthetic analogs can suppress both inflammatory and immune responses. Although the precise basis for their immunologic effects is unknown, corticosteroids cause a transient lymphopenia, alter macrophage phagocytosis, and depress T and B lymphocyte function (138). Similar immunosuppressive effects are also observed in fish. Immature rainbow trout implanted with hydrocortisone pellets (10 mg) had reduced numbers of splenic and thymic lymphocytes in the absence of degenerative changes (139). At higher concentrations (40 to 50 mg), fish showed thymic involutions and appeared to be more susceptible to fungal and protozoan skin diseases (139). As with mammals, cortisone also reduced inflammation and retarded normal wound healing in fish (140). In a study by Bisset (141), perch injected with either a 0.1- or 0.2-ml dose of an adrenal cortical extract demonstrated increased serum bacteria agglutinin titers after injections. However, since corticosteroids are suspected of causing lymphocyte lysis, it was possible that these results may have reflected lysis and subsequent antibody release.

Alkylating Agents

Alkylating agents, chemicals that form covalent linkages (alkylation) with biologically important molecules, including DNA, are particularly toxic to rapidly proliferating cells including precursor bone marrow cells and those of lymphoid origin (79). Unlike the abundant information available in mammalian systems concerning the immunosuppressive effects of alkylating agents, particularly cyclophosphamide (CP), far fewer studies have been performed using fish. Of those few studies reported, immunosuppression was either not produced or effects were observed only at very high CP concentrations. While antibacterial agglutinating antibody titers to *A. salmonicida* were unchanged in adult trout injected with CP at 50 mg/kg, studies by Sakai (142) demonstrated a markedly immunosuppressive effect against the antibody response of trout, but only at 400 to 500 mg CP/kg. Other alkylating agents such as mustargens prolonged scale graft survival times in mummichogs from three to five extra days, suggesting that some alkylating agents were effective in suppressing cell-mediated responses in fish.

Natural Products

The necessity of certain vitamins in the diet for disease resistance has been implicated in fish as well as for mammals. Dietary levels of vitamin E (α-tocopherol), a component of subcellular membranes and an antioxidant controlling peroxidation of unsaturated lipids, appears important for maintaining immunoresponsiveness in fish. Blazer and Wolke (143) demonstrated a depression of cell-mediated immunity, macrophage phagocytosis, release of macrophage inhibitory factor, plaque-forming cell (PFC) numbers, and serum antibody titers in rainbow trout fed vitamin E-depleted diets. In contrast, however, Hardie et al. (144) showed that vitamin E deficiency had no effects on leukocyte numbers, respiratory burst activity by macrophages, antibody production, or lymphokine secretion by lymphocytes. However, vitamin E-deprived fish did show impaired serum complement function with respect to total hemolytic activity and the ability of serum to opsonize bacteria, compared with fish fed graded amounts of vitamin E. α-Tocopherol-deprived fish also demonstrated a significantly increased mortality rate following exposure to a virulent strain of *A. salmonicida*. In mammalian systems, vitamin E enhanced both humoral and cellular defenses (145). Mice and chicks fed vitamin E-supplemented diets exhibited enhanced PFC responses to sRBCs, while in guinea pigs, serum antibody levels to viral antigens were elevated. Macrophage phagocytosis was also enhanced in mice fed vitamin E-supplemented diets. Alternatively, vitamin E-deficient diets have been related to reduced proliferative responses in dog and rodent lymphocytes (146).

Beneficial effects of elevated levels of vitamin C (ascorbate) on resistance to infection have been reported for humans and guinea pigs. Leukocyte responses in humans (147) increased in a dose–response fashion when up to ten times the normal dietary requirement of vitamin C was given prior to challenge with various antigens. In studies using fish, Durve and Lovell (148) have observed similar results in channel catfish fingerlings fed vitamin C-enriched diets. Catfish fed vitamin C at 150 mg/kg for 14 weeks and then infected with *Edwardsiella tarda* had enhanced resistance against the bacterial challenge. These results indicated that levels of vitamin C, fivefold higher than the minimum dietary requirement for normal growth and bone development (30 mg/kg), provided increased resistance to bacterial infection in certain species of fish. Since supplemented vitamin C has also been shown to increase macrophage phagocytosis and migration in guinea pigs and to increase antibody production in chickens fed vitamin C prior to infection with Newcastle vaccine, it is possible that increased resistance observed in ascorbate-supplemented fish was due to effects on macrophage and/or humoral-mediated immunity.

Radiation

Radiation has been, and will continue to be, of concern to aquatic organisms because of contributions from nuclear power plant effluents and other sources. Fish exposed to radiation demonstrate severe immunosuppression, lymphoid tissue and hematopoietic cell atrophy (149), and severe depletions of circulating white blood cells (150). Of the circulating population, lymphocytes appeared to be the most sensitive white blood cells affected; doses of x-rays greater than 200 rads resulted in almost complete elimination of these cells from the circulation.

In addition, exposure to x-rays suppressed nonspecific immune responses, bacterial agglutination titers, susceptibility to bacterial and trematode infection, and scale allograft rejection times in a variety of fish species (151). Radiation-induced effects in fish are almost identical to those observed in mammalian species. As early as 1903, Heineke noted that all lymphoid organs of mammals were extremely sensitive to radiation (152). Even moderate levels of ionizing radiation (500 to 1000 rads) damaged hematopoietic tissues, destroyed circulating white blood cells (particularly lymphocytes), and increased host susceptibility to diseases and cancer. The effects of radiation are thought to be due, at least in part, to the reduction in normal immune capacities resulting from depletion of leukocytes in the lymphoid organs and circulation.

CONCLUSION

In mammalian systems, the integrity of disease resistance and the immune responses are very sensitive parameters altered by low levels of toxicant exposure (109,113). Interestingly, many of the same chemicals that alter immune responses of mammals (including humans) also act as immunotoxicants for fish and in many cases bring about similar effects and appear to act by similar mechanisms. These similarities suggest the applicability of the fish immune response as an alternative model for the immune responses of higher vertebrates in immunotoxicologic studies.

In addition to their potential as alternative models and their use as biomarkers of pollutant exposure, an important practical reason for investigating the effects of toxicants on fish immune responses is that fish culture is a major industry. In the United States, state fish hatcheries spend an estimated $100 million annually to produce the one-half billion fish grown for anglers to catch. In such cases, the control of fish disease is a major concern. It is also beginning to be appreciated that fish can serve as vectors of human diseases. The role that fish immunology can play in the control of fish diseases has just begun to be appreciated.

REFERENCES

1. Ellis AE. The leukocytes of fish: a review. *J Fish Biol* 1977;1:453–491.
2. Caspi RR, Shahrabani R, Avtalion RR. The cells involved in the immune response of fish: I. The separation and study of lymphocyte subpopulations in carp—a new approach. In: Manning MJ, ed. *Phylogeny of immunological memory*. Amsterdam: Elsevier/North-Holland Biomedical Press; 1980:83–92.
3. O'Connor JM, Huggett RJ. Aquatic pollution problems, North Atlantic coast, including Chesapeake Bay. *Aquatic Toxicol* 1987;318:28–53.
4. Bieri R, Hein C, Huggett R, Sou P, Slone H, Smith C, Su C. *Toxic organic compounds in surface sediment from the Elizabeth and Patapsco rivers and estuaries*. Presented at VA Institute of Marine Science, Goucester Point, VA, 1982. 135 p.
5. O'Connor JM, Stanford H. *Chemical pollutants of the New York Bight: priorities for research*. Boulder, CO: US Department of Commerce, NOAA-ERL; 1979:217–240.
6. Meyerson AL, Luther GW, Krajewski J, Hires RI. Heavy metal distribution in Newark Bay sediments. *Mar Pollut Bull* 1981;12:244–250.
7. Johannson-Sjobeck M-L, Larsson A. Effects of inorganic lead on delta-aminolevulinic acid dehydratase activity and hematological variables in the rainbow trout, *Salmo gairdneri*. *Arch Environ Contam Toxicol* 1979;8:419–431.
8. Bengtsson B-E, Bengtsson A, Himberg M. Fish deformities and pollution in some Swedish waters. *Ambio* 1985;14:32–35.
9. Larsson A, Bengtsson B-E, Haux C. Disturbed ion balance in flounder, *Platichthys flesus L.* exposed to sublethal levels of cadmium. *Aquatic Toxicol* 1981;1:19–35.
10. Corbel MJ. The immune response in fish: a review. *J Fish Biol* 1975;7:539–563.
11. Faisel M, Hetrick F. *Ann Rev Fish Dis* 1992;2:1–403.
12. Stolen JS, Fletcher TC, Anderson DP, Kaattari SL, Rowley AF, eds. *Techniques in fish immunology*. Fair Haven, NJ:SOS Publications; 1992;107–124.
13. Borysenko M. Phylogeny of immunity: an overview. *Immunogenetics* 1976;3:305–321.
14. Botham JW, Grace MF, Manning MJ. Ontogeny of first and second set alloimmune reactivity in fish. In: Manning MJ, ed. *Phylogeny of immunological memory*. Amsterdam: Elsevier/North-Holland Biomedical Press; 1980:83–92.

15. Baldo BA, Fletcher TC. Phylogenetic aspects of hypersensitivity: immediate hypersensitivity reactions in flatfish. *Adv Exp Med Biol* 1975;64:365–372.
16. Fletcher TC, Baldo BA. Immediate hypersensitivity responses in flatfish. *Science* 1974;185:360–364.
17. Lobb CJ, Clem LW. Phylogeny of immunoglobulin structure and function—XII. Secretory immunoglobulins in the bile of the marine teleost. *Arch Prob Mol Immunol* 1981;18:615–619.
18. Yui MA, Kaattari SL. *Vibrio-anguillarum* antigen stimulates mitogenesis and polyclonal activation of salmonid lymphocytes. *Dev Comp Immunol* 1987;11:539–549.
19. Miller NW, Deuter A, Clem LW. Phylogeny of lymphocyte heterogeneity: the cellular requirements for the mixed leukocyte reaction in channel catfish. *Immunology* 1986;59:123–128.
20. Grondel JL, Harmsen EGM. Do fish have interleukins? In: Manning MJ, Tatner MF, eds. *Fish immunology*. London: Academic Press; 1985:123–130.
21. Pettitt TR, Barrow SE, Rowley AF. Thromboxane, prostaglandin, and leukotriene generation by rainbow trout blood. *Fish Shellfish Immmunol* 1991;1:71–73.
22. Tocher DR, Sargent JR. The effect of calcium ionophore A23187 on the metabolism of arachidonic and eicosapentaenoic acids in neutrophils from a marine teleost fish rich in (n-3) polyunsaturated fatty acids. *Comp Biochem Physiol* 1987;87B:733–739.
23. Vallejo AN, Miller NW, Clem W. Antigen processing and presentation in teleost immune responses. *Annu Rev Fish Dis* 1992;2:167–183.
24. Hinuma S, Abo T, Kumagai K, Hata M. The potent activity of fresh water fish kidney cells in cell-killing. I. Characterization and species-distribution of cytotoxicity. *Dev Comp Immunol* 1980; 4:653–666.
25. Graham D, Jeffries AH, Secombes CJ. A novel assay to detect macrophage bactericidal activity in fish: factors influencing the killing of *Aeromonas salmonicida*. *J Fish Dis* 1988;11:389–396.
26. Avtalion RR, Shahrabani R. Studies on phagocytosis in fish. I. *In vitro* uptake and killing of living *Staphylococcus aureus* by peripheral leukocytes of carp *(Cyprinus carpio)*. *Immunology* 1975; 29:1181–1187.
27. Nagelkerke LAJ, Pannevis MC, Houlihan DF, Secombes CJ. Oxygen uptake by rainbow trout *Oncorhynchus mykiss* phagocytes following stimulation of the respiratory burst. *J Exp Biol* 1990; 154:339–353.
28. Van Muiswinkel WB, Anderson DP, Lamers CHJ, Egberts E, Van Loon JJA, Ijssel JP. Fish immunology and fish health. In: Manning MJ, Tatner MF, eds. *Fish immunology*. London: Academic Press; 1985:316–333.
29. Fletcher TC, White A, Baldo BA. C-reactive protein-like precipitin and lysozyme in the lumpsucker *Cyclopterus lumpus* during the breeding season. *Comp Biochem Physiol* 1977;57B:353.
30. Finn JP. The protective mechanisms in diseases of fish. *Vet Bull* 1970;40:873.
31. MacArthur JI, Fletcher TC. Phagocytosis in fish. In: Manning MJ, Tatner MF, eds. *Fish immunology*. London: Academic Press; 1985:29–46.
32. Etlinger HM, Hodgins HO, Chiller JM. Characterization of lymphocytes in a primitive teleost *Salmo gairdneri*. In: Wright RK, Cooper EL, eds. *Phylogeny of thymus and bone marrow-bursa cells*. Amsterdam: Elsevier/North Holland Biomedical Press; 1976:83–91.
33. Fiebig H, Gruhn R, Ambrosius H. Studies on the control of IgM functional affinity in the course of the immune response in carp. *Immunochemistry* 1977;14:721–726.
34. Miller NW, Bly JE, van Ginkel FW, Ellsaesser CF, Clem LW. Phylogeny of lymphocyte heterogeneity: identification and separation of functionally distinct subpopulation of channel catfish lymphocytes. *Dev Comp Immunol* 1987;11:739–747.
35. McKinney EC, McLeod TF, Sigel MM. Allograft rejection in a holostean fish, *Lepisosteus platyrhincus*. *Dev Comp Immunol* 1981;10:497–508.
36. Zelikoff JT, Enane NA, Bowser D, Squibb KS, Frenkel K. Development of fish peritoneal macrophages as a model for higher vertebrates in immunotoxicological studies. I. Characterization of macrophage morphological, functional, and biochemical properties. *Fundam Appl Toxicol* 1991; 16:576–589.
37. Whyte SK, Chappell LH, Secombes CJ. Cytotoxic reactions of rainbow trout, *Salmo gairdneri* Richardson, macrophages for larvae of the eye fluke *Diplostomum spathaceum* (Digenea). *J Fish Biol* 1989;35:333–345.
38. Pettitt TR, Rowley AF, Secombes CJ. Lipoxins are major lipoxygenase products of rainbow trout macrophages. *FEBS Let* 1989;259:168–170.
39. Rowley AF, Barrow SE, Hunt TC. Preliminary studies on eicosanoid production by fish leucocytes, using GC-mass spectrometry. *J Fish Biol* 1987;31A:107–111.

40. Graham S, Secombes CJ. The production of a macrophage-activating factor from rainbow trout *Salmo gairdneri* leucocytes. *Immunology* 1988;65:293–297.
41. Graham S, Secombes CJ. Do fish lymphocytes secrete interferon-γ? *J Fish Biol* 1990;36:563–573.
42. Evans DL, Carlson RL, Graves SS, Hogan KT. Nonspecific cytotoxic cells in fish (*Ictalurus punctatus*). II. Parameters of target cell lysis and specificity. *Dev Comp Immunol* 1984;8:303–312.
43. Faisal M, Ahmed II, Peters G, Cooper EL. Natural cytotoxicity of tilapia leucocytes. *Dis Aquatic Org* 1989;7:17–22.
44. Greenley AR, Brown RA, Ristow SS. Nonspecific cytotoxic cell of rainbow trout *(Oncorhynchus mykiss)* kill YAC-1 targets by both necrotic and apoptic mechanisms. *Dev Comp Immunol* 1991;29:1181–1187.
45. Hatcher FM, Kuhn RE. Destruction of *Trypanosoma cruzi* by natural killer cells. *Science* 1982; 218:295–301.
46. Graves SS, Evans DL, Dawe DL. Mobilization and activation of nonspecific cytotoxic cells (NCC) in the channel catfish *(Ictalurus punctatus)* infected with *Ichthyophthirius multifiliis*. *Comp Immunol Microbiol Infect Dis* 1985;8:43–51.
47. Waterman B, Kranz H. Pollution and fish diseases in the North Sea. Some historical aspects. *Mar Pollut Bull* 1992;24:131–137.
48. Mearns AJ, Sherwood MJ. Ocean wastewater discharge and tumors in a southern California flatfish. *Prog Exp Tumor Res* 1976;20:75–85.
49. Zelikoff JT. Metal pollution-induced immunomodulation in fish. *Annu Rev Fish Dis* 1993;2:305–325.
50. Koller LD. Immunosuppression produced by lead, cadmium and mercury. *Am J Vet Res* 1973; 34:1456–1459.
51. Koller LD, Kovaic S. Decreased antibody formation in mice exposed to lead. *Nature* 1974;250: 148–152.
52. O'Neill JG. Effects of intraperitoneal lead and cadmium on the humoral immune response of *Salmo trutta*. *Bull Environ Contam Toxicol* 1981;27:42–48.
53. Viale G, Calamari D. Immune response in rainbow trout *Salmo gairdneri* after long-term treatment with low levels of Cr, Cd and Cu. *Environ Pollut* 1984;35:247–257.
54. Sjobeck ML, Haux C, Larsson A, Lithner G. Biochemical and hematological studies on perch, *Perca fluviatilis*, from the cadmium-contaminated river Emän. *Ecotoxicol Environ Safety* 1984; 8:303–312.
55. Thuvander A. Cadmium exposure of rainbow trout, *Salmo gairdneri* Richardson: effects on immune functions. *J Fish Biol* 1989;35:521–529.
56. Treagan L. A survey of the effect of metals on the immune response. *Biol Trace Element Res* 1979;1:141–148.
57. Kawamura R, Shimizu F, Fujimaki H, Kubota K. Effects of single exposure to cadmium on the primary humoral antibody response. *Arch Toxicol* 1983;54:289–296.
58. Bozelka BE, Burkholder PM. Inhibition of mixed leukocyte culture responses in cadmium-treated mice. *Environ Res* 1982;27:421–432.
59. Müller S, Gillert K-E, Krause C, Jautzke G, Gross U, Diamanstein T. Effects of cadmium on the immune system of mice. *Experimentia* 1979;35:909–910.
60. Greenspan BJ, Morrow PE. The effects of *in vitro* and aerosol exposures to cadmium on phagocytosis by rat pulmonary macrophages. *Fundam Appl Toxicol* 1984;4:48–57.
61. Loose LD, Silkworth JB, Warrington D. Cadmium-induced depression of the respiratory burst in mouse pulmonary alveolar macrophages, peritoneal macrophages and polymorphonuclear neutrophils. *Biochem Biophys Res Commun* 1977;79:326–332.
62. Mustafa MG, Cross CE. Pulmonary alveolar macrophage. Oxidative metabolism of isolated cells and mitochondria and effect of cadmium ion on electron- and energy-transfer reactions. *Biochemistry* 1971;10:4176–4185.
63. Dawson AB. The hemopoietic response in the catfish, *Ameiurus nebulosus*, to chronic lead poisoning. *Biol Bull* 1935;68:335–342.
64. Crandall CA, Goodnight GJ. The effects of sublethal concentrations of several toxicants to the common guppy, *Lebistes reticularus*. *Trans Am Microsc Soc* 1963;82:59–64.
65. Ghanmi Z, Rouabhia M, Alifuddin M, Troutaud D, Deschaux P. Modulatory effects of metal ions on the immune response of fish: *in vivo* and *in vitro* influence of $MnCl_2$ on NK activity of carp pronephros cells. *Ecotoxicol Environ Safety* 1990;20:241–245.
66. Ghanmi Z, Rouabhia M, Othmane O, Deschaux PA. Effects of metal ions on cyprinid fish immune

response: *in vitro* effects of Zn^{2+} and Mn^{2+} on the mitogenic response of carp pronephros lymphocytes. *Ecotoxicol Environ Safety* 1989;17:183–189.
67. Rogers RR, Gardner RJ, Riddle MM, Luebke RW, Smialowicz RJ. Augmentation of murine natural killer cell activity by manganese chloride. *Toxicol Appl Pharmacol* 1983;70:7–14.
68. Smialowicz RJ, Luebke RW, Rogers RR, Riddle MM, Rowe DG. Manganese chloride enhances natural cell-mediated immune effector cell function: effects on macrophages. *Immunopharmacology* 1985,9:1–9.
69. Smialowicz RJ, Riddle MM, Rogers RR, Leubke RW, Burleson GR. Enhancement of natural killer cell activity and interferon production by manganese in young mice. *Immunopharmacol Immunotoxicol* 1988;10:93–102.
70. Costa M, Abbracchio MP, Simmons-Hausen J. Factors influencing the phagocytosis, neoplastic transformation and cytotoxicity of particulate nickel compounds in tissue culture systems. *Toxicol Appl Pharmacol* 1981;60:313–326.
71. US Department of Health and Human Services (USDHHS). *Toxicological profile for nickel*. Syracuse, NY: Syracuse Research Corp; 1991.
72. Sunderman FW, Hopfer SM, Lin S-M, et al. Toxicity to alveolar macrophages in rats following parenteral injection of nickel chloride. *Toxicol Appl Pharmacol* 1989;100:107–118.
73. Bowser D, Frenkel K, Zelikoff JT. Effects of *in vitro* nickel exposure on macrophage functions in rainbow trout (*Oncorhynchus mykiss*). *Bull Environ Contam Toxicol* 1994;52:367–373.
74. O'Neill JG. The humoral immune response of *Salmo trutta L.* and *Cyprinus carpio L.* exposed to heavy metals. *J Fish Biol* 1981;19:297–306.
75. Waters MD, Gardner DE. Metal toxicity for rabbit alveolar macrophages *in vitro*. *Environ Res* 1975;9:32–47.
76. Gardner DE. Dysfunction of host defenses following nickel inhalation. In: Brown SS, Sunderman FW Jr, eds. *Nickel toxicology*. New York: Academic Press; 1980:121–124.
77. Figoni RA, Treagan L. Inhibitory effect of nickel and chromium upon antibody response of rats to immunization with *T-1* phage. *Res Commun Chem Pathol Pharmacol* 1975;11:335–338.
78. IARC. Monograph on the evaluation of the carcinogenic risk of chemicals to humans. *IARC Lyon* 1980;23:1–210.
79. Klaassen CD, Amdur MO, Doull J, eds. *Toxicology*, 3rd ed. New York: Macmillan; 1986.
80. Cossarini-Dunier M. Effects of the pesticides atrazine and lindane and of manganese ions on cellular immunity of carp, *Cyprinus carpio*. *J Fish Biol* 1987;31:67–73.
81. Cossarini-Dunier M, Monod G, Demael A, Lepot D. Effects of gamma hexachlorocyclohexane (lindane) on carp (*Cyrinus carpis*). I. Effect of chronic intoxication on humoral immunity in relation with tissue pollutant levels. *Ecotoxicol Environ Safety* 1987;13:339–345.
82. Saxena MP, Gopal K, Jones W, Ray PK. Immune responses to *Aeromonas hydrophila* in catfish (*Heteropneustis fossilis*) exposed to cadmium and hexachlorocyclohexane. *Bull Environ Contam Toxicol* 1992;48:194–201.
83. Desi I, Varga L, Farkas I. Studies on the immunosuppressive effect of organochlorine and organophosphoric pesticides in subacute experiments. *J Hyg Epidemiol Microbiol Immunol* 1978; 22:115–122.
84. Zeeman MG, Brindley WA. DDT-induced antibody immunosuppression in goldfish. *Proc Utah Acad Sci Arts Lett* 1982;52:46.
85. Zavon MR, Tye R, Latorre, L. Chlorinated hydrocarbon insecticide content of the neonate. *Ann NY Acad Sci* 1969;160:196–200.
86. Street JC. Pesticides and the immune system. In: Sharma RP, ed. *Immunologic consideration in toxicology*. Boca Raton, FL: CRC Press; 1981:46–66.
87. Schoenthal ND. Some effects of DDT on cold water fish and fish-food organisms. *Proc Montana Acad Sci* 1963;23:63–70.
88. McDermott-Ehrlich DJ, Sherwood MJ, Heesen TC, Young DR, Mearns AJ. Chlorinated hydrocarbons in Dover sole, *Microstomus pacificus*: local migrations and fin erosion. *Fish Bull* 1977;75: 513–530.
89. Exon JH, Kerkvliet NI, Talcott PA. Immunotoxicity of carcinogenic pesticides and related chemicals. *Environ Carcinog Rev (J Environ Sci Health)* 1987;C5(1):73–120.
90. Halver JE. Crystalline aflatoxin and other vectors for trout hepatoma. In: Halver JE, Mitchell IA, eds. *Trout hepatoma research conference papers*, Rep 70. Washington, DC: Bureau of Sport Fisheries and Wildlife Research; 1967;78–85.
91. Rogillio GJ. *Effects of Mirex on selected organs of the channel catfish (Ictalurus punctatus): a light*

and electromicroscopic study [Ph.D. Dissertation]. Mississippi State: Mississippi State University, 1974.

92. Street JC, Sharma RP. Quantitative aspects of immunosuppression by selected pesticides. *Toxicol Appl Pharmacol* 1974;29:135–136.
93. Plumb JA, Areechon N. Effect of malathion on humoral immune response of channel catfish. *Dev Comp Immunol* 1990;14:355–358.
94. Siwicki AK, Cossarin-Dunier M, Studnicka M, Demael A. *In vivo* effect of the organophosphorus insecticide trichlorphon on immune response of carp (*Cyprinus carpio*). *Ecotoxicol Environ Safety* 1990;19:99–105.
95. Areechon N, Plumb JA. Sublethal effects of malathion on channel catfish, *Ictalurus punctatus*. *Bull Environ Contam Toxicol* 1990;44:435–442.
96. Reddy SJ, Reddy BV, Ramamurthi R. Impact of chronic phosalone toxicity on erythropoietic activity of fish, *Oreochromis mossambicus*. *Biochem Int* 1991;25:547–552.
97. Walsh AH, Ribelin WE. The pathology of pesticide poisoning. In: Ribelin WE, Migaki G, eds. *The pathology of fishes*. Madison: University of Wisconsin Press; 1975.
98. Gill TS, Pande J, Tewari H. Hemopathological changes associated with experimental aldicarb poisoning in fish (*Puntius conchonius Hamilton*). *Bull Environ Contam Toxicol* 1991;47:628–633.
99. Fiore MC, Anderson HA, Hong R, et al. Chronic exposure to aldicarb-containing groundwater and human immune function. *Environ Res* 1986;41:633–645.
100. Prasad TAV, Srinivas T, Rafi G, Reddy DC. Effect *in vivo* of atrazine on haematology and O_2 consumption in fish, *Tilapia mossambica*. *Biochem Int* 1991;23:157–161.
101. Vos JG, Faith RE, Luster MI. *Immune alterations*. New York: Elsevier/North-Holland Biomedical Press; 1980:241–266.
102. Arrhenius E, Renberg L, Johansson L, Zetterqvist M-A. Disturbance of microsomal detoxication mechanisms in liver by chlorophenol pesticides. *Chem Biol Interact* 1977;18:35–47.
103. Anderson RS. *In vitro* inhibition of medaka phagocyte chemiluminescence by pentachlorophenol. *Fish Shellfish Immunol* 1992;2:299–310.
104. Kerkvliet NI, Brauner JA, Matlock JP. Humoral immunotoxicity of polychlorinated diphenyl ethers, phenoxyphenols, dioxins and furans present as contaminants of technical grade pentachlorphenol. *Toxicology* 1985;36:307–324.
105. Prescott CA, Wilkie BN, Hunter B, Julian RJ. Influence of a purified grade of pentachlorophenol on the immune response of chickens. *Am J Vet Res* 1982;43:481–487.
106. Kerkvliet NI, Baecher-Steppan L, Shmitz J. Immunotoxicity of pentachlorophenol (PCP): increased susceptibility to tumor growth in adult mice fed technical PCP-contaminated diets. *Toxicol Appl Pharmacol* 1982;62:55–64.
107. Norstrom RJ, Hallett D, Sonstegard RA. Coho salmon (*Oncorhynchus kisutch*) and herring gulls (*Larus argentatus*) as indicators of organochlorine contamination in Lake Ontario. *J Fish Res Board Can* 1978;35:1401–1409.
108. Safe S. Polychlorinated biphenyls (PCBs) and polybrominated biphenyls (PBBs): biochemistry, toxicology, and mechanism of action. *CRC Crit Rev Toxicol* 1985;13:319–381.
109. Thomas PT, Faith RE. Adult and perinatal immunotoxicity induced by halogenated aromatic hydrocarbons. In: Dean JH, Luster MI, Munson AE, Amos H, eds. *Immunotoxicolgy and immunopharmacology*. New York: Raven Press; 1985:305–313.
110. Cleland GB, McElroy PJ, Sonstegard RA. The effect of dietary exposure to Aroclor 1254 and/or Mirex on humoral immune expression of rainbow trout (*Salmo gairdneri*). *Aquatic Toxicol* 1988; 2:141–146
111. Kerkvliet NI, Baecher-Steppan L, Smith BB. Role of the *Ah* locus in suppression of cytotoxic T lymphocyte activity in halogenated aromatic hydrocarbons (PCBs and TCDD): structure–activity relationships and effects in C57B1/6 mice congenic at the *Ah* locus. *Fundam Appl Toxicol* 1990;62:55–64.
112. Nestel H, Budd J. Chronic oral exposure of rainbow trout (*Salmo gairdneri*) to a polychlorinated biphenyl (Aroclor 1254): pathological effects. *Can J Comp Med* 1975;39:208–213.
113. Dean JH, Luster MI, Boorman GA, Leubke RW, Lauer LD. Application of tumor, bacterial, and parasite susceptibility assays to study immune alterations induced by environmental chemicals. *Environ Health Perspect* 1982;43:81–88.
114. Hensen DJ, Parrish PR, Lowe JI, Wilson AJ, Wilson PD. Chronic toxicity, uptake and retention of Aroclor 1254 in two estuarine fishes. *Bull Environ Contam Toxicol* 1971;6:113–125.
115. Johnson ES. Human exposure to 2,3,7,8-TCDD and risk of cancer. *Crit Rev Toxicol* 1991;21: 451–463.

116. Vos JG, Kreeftenberg JG, Engel HW, Minderhoud A, van Noorlejansen LM. Studies on 2,3,7,8-tetrachlorodibenzo-*p*-dioxin-induced immune suppression and decreased resistance to infection: endotoxin hypersensitivity, serum zinc concentrations and effect of thymosin treatment. *Toxicology* 1978;9:75–86.
117. Spitsbergen JM, Schat KA, Kleeman JM, Peterson RE. Interactions of 2,3,7,8-tetrachlorodibenzo-*p*-dioxin (TCDD) with immune responses of rainbow trout. *Vet Immunol Immunopathol* 1986;12:263–280.
118. Spitsbergen JM, Schat KA, Kleeman JM, Peterson RE. Effects of 2,3,7,8-tetrachlorodibenzo-*p*-dioxin (TCDD) or Aroclor 1254 on the resistance of rainbow trout, *Salmo gairdneri Richardson*, to infectious hematopoietic necrosis virus. *Vet Immunol Immunopathol* 1987;13:231–235.
119. Anderson DP, Merchant B, Dixon OW, Schott CF, Lizzio EF. Flush exposure and injection immunization of rainbow trout to selected DNP conjugates. *Dev Comp Immunol* 1983;7:261–268.
120. Anderson DP, Roberson BS, Dixon OW. Immunosuppression induced by a corticosteroid or an alkylating agent in rainbow trout (*Salmo gairdneri*) administered a *Yersinia ruckeri* bacterin. *Dev Comp Immunol* 1983; 7:261–268.
121. Hoffman RE, Stehr-Green PA, Webb KB. Health effects of long-term exposure to 2,3,7,8-tetrachlorodibenzo-*p*-dioxin. *JAMA* 1986;255:2031–2038.
122. Baumann PC. PAH metabolites and neoplasia in feral fish populations. In: Varanasi U, ed. *Metabolism of polycyclic aromatic hydrocarbons in the aquatic environment*. Boca Raton, FL: CRC Press; 1989:269–289.
123. Burrell R, Flaherty DK, Sauers LJ, eds. *Toxicology of the immune system: a human approach*. New York: Van Nostrand Reinhold; 1992.
124. Faisal M, Marzouk MSM, Smith CL, Huggett RJ. Mitogen induced proliferative responses of lymphocytes from spot (*Leiostomus xanthurus*) exposed to polycyclic aromatic hydrocarbon contaminated environments. *Immunopharmacol Immunotoxicol* 1991;13:311–327.
125. Faisal M, Weeks BA, Vogelbein WK, Huggett RJ. Evidence of aberration of the natural cytotoxic cell activity in *Fundulus heteroclitus (Pisces: Cyprinodontidae)* from the Elizabeth River, Virginia. *Vet Immunol Immunopathol* 1991;29:339–351.
126. Weeks BA, Warinner JE, Mason PL, McGinnis DS. Influence of toxic chemicals on the chemotactic response of fish macrophages. *Fish Biol* 1986;28:653–658.
127. Dean JH, Luster MI, Boorman GA, Lauer LD, Luebke RW, Lawson LD. Immune suppression following exposure of mice to the carcinogen benzo[*a*]pyrene but not the non-carcinogenic benzo[*e*]pyrene. *Clin Exp Immunol* 1983;52:199–206.
128. Lakhotia RL, Stephens JF. Effects of chlortetracycline on agglutinating antibody response to *Salmonella typhimurium* in young chickens. *Avian Dis* 1972;16:1029–1034.
129. Weisberger AS, Daniel TM, Hoffman A. Suppression of antibody synthesis and prolongation of homograft survival by chloramphenicol. *J Exp Med* 1964;120:183–198.
130. Daniel TM, Suhrland LG, Weiberger AS. The effect of chloramphenicol on the anamnestic antibody response to tetanus toxoid in man. *J Lab Clin Med* 1964;64:850–851.
131. Wishkovsky A, Roberson BS, Hetrick FM. *In vitro* suppression of the phagocytic response of fish macrophages by tetracyclines. *J Fish Biol* 1987;31:61–65.
132. Rijkers GT, van Osterom RV, Van Muiswingel WB. The immune system of cyprinid fish. Oxytetracyline and the regulation of humoral immunity in carp (*Cyprinus carpio*). *Vet Immunol Immunopathol* 1981;2:281–290.
133. Grondel JL, Gloudemans AGM, Van Muiswinkel WB. The influence of antibiotics on the immune system. II. Modulation of fish leukocyte responses in culture. *Vet Immunol Immunopathol* 1985; 9:251–260.
134. Bost KL, Smith EM, Wear LB, Blalock JE. Presence of ACTH and its receptor on a B lymphocytic cell line: a possible autocrine function for a neuroendocrine hormone. *J Biol Regul Homeost Agents* 1987;1:223–225.
135. Peters GM, Faisal M, Lang T, Ahmend II. Stress caused by social interaction and its effect on the susceptibility to *Aeromonas hydrophila* infection in the rainbow trout, *Salmo gairdneri*. *Dis Aquatic Org* 1988;4:369–380.
136. Ghoneum M, Faisal M, Peters G, Ahmed II, Cooper EL. Suppression of natural cytotoxic cell activity by social aggressiveness in tilapia. *Dev Comp Immunol* 1988;12:595–602.
137. Faisal M, Chiapelli F, Weiner H, Ahmed II, Cooper EL. Role of endogenous opioids in modulating some immune functions in hybrid tilapia. *J Aquatic Anim Health* 1989;1:301–306.

138. Webb DR, Winkelstein A. Immunosuppression, immunopotentiation and anti-inflammatory drugs. In: Stites DP, Stobo JD, Fudenberg HH, Wells JV, eds. *Basic and clinical immunology*. Los Altos, CA: Lange Medical Publishers; 1982:277–292.
139. Robertson CH, Hane S, Wexler BC, Rinfret AP. The effect of hydrocortisone on immature rainbow trout (*Salmo gairdneri). Gen Comp Endocrinol* 1963;3:422–427.
140. Weinreb EL. Studies on the histology and histopathology of the rainbow trout, *Salmo gairdneri irideus*, I. Hematology: under normal and experimental conditions of inflammation. *Zoologica* 1959;43:45–52.
141. Bisset KA. The influence of adrenal cortical hormones upon immunity in cold-blooded vertebrates. *J Endocrinol* 1949; 6:99–103.
142. Sakai DK. Immunological roles of sensitive lymphocytes and resistant lymphocytes against cyclophosphamide in rainbow trout immune system reorganized by adoptive transfer. *Bull Jpn Soc Sci Fish* 1982;48:1059–1064.
143. Blazer VS, Wolke RE. The effects of α-tocopherol on the immune response and non-specific resistance factors of rainbow trout (*Salmo gairdneri Richardson*). *Aquaculture* 1984;37:1–9.
144. Hardie LJ, Fletcher TC, Secombes CJ. The effect of vitamin E on the immune response of the Atlantic salmon (*Salmo salar L.). Aquaculture* 1990;87:1–13.
145. Panush RS, Delafuente JC. Vitamins and immunocompetence. *World Rev Nutr Diet* 1985,45:97–123.
146. Chandra RK, ed. Nutrition and immunology, contemporary issues in clinical nutrition. New York: Alan R Liss; 1988.
147. Delafuente JC, Panush RS. Modulation of certain immunologic responses by vitamin C. *Int J Vitam Nutr Res* 1979;50:44–54.
148. Durve VS, Lovell RT. Vitamin C and disease resistance in channel catfish (*Ictalurus punctatus). Can J Fish Aquatic Sci* 1982;39:948–951.
149. Bonham K, Donaldon LR, Foster RF, Welander AD, Seymour AH. The effect of X-ray on mortality, weight, length and counts of erythrocytes and hematopoietic cells in fingerling chinook salmon, *Oncorhychus tschawytscha*. *Growth* 1948;12:107–110.
150. Finstad J, Fange R, Good RA. The development of lymphoid systems: immune response and radiation sensitivity in lower vertebrates in lymphatic tissue and germinal centers in immune response. In: Fiore-Donati L, Hana MG, eds. *Advances in experimental medicine and biology*. New York: Plenum Press; 1969:21–30.
151. Shechmeister IL, Watson LJ, Cole VW, Jackson LL. The effect of X-irradiation on goldfish. I. The effect of X-irradiation on survival and susceptibility of the goldfish, *Carassius auratus*, to infection by *Aeromonas salmonicida* and *Gyrodactylus* spp. *Radiat Res* 1962;16:89–95.
152. Gerber GB, Altman KI, eds. *Radiation biochemistry*. New York: Academic Press; 1970.

Immunotoxicology and Immunopharmacology, Second Edition, edited by J. H. Dean, M. I. Luster, A. E. Munson, and I. Kimber.
Raven Press, Ltd., New York © 1994.

6

Immunotoxicity of TCDD and Related Halogenated Aromatic Hydrocarbons

Nancy I. Kerkvliet and *Gary R. Burleson

*Department of Agriculture Chemistry and Environmental Health Sciences, Oregon State University, Corvallis, Oregon 97331; *Miami Valley Laboratory, Procter & Gamble, Cincinnati, Ohio 45239*

Extensive evidence has accumulated over the past 20 years that shows that the immune system is a target for the toxic effects of 2, 3, 7, 8-tetrachlorodibenzo-*p*-dioxin (TCDD) and structurally related halogenated aromatic hydrocarbons (HAHs), including other polychlorinated dibenzodioxin (PCDD), polychlorinated dibenzofurans (PCDFs), polychlorinated biphenyls (PCBs), and polybrominated biphenyls (PBBs). This evidence has derived from numerous studies in various animal species, primarily rodents, but also guinea pigs, rabbits, monkeys, marmosets, and cattle. Poisoning incidents as well as epidemiologic studies also provide evidence for the immunotoxicity of HAHs in humans. Several comprehensive reviews have been published on the immunotoxic effects of HAHs in general (1–3) and TCDD in particular (4,5). The present chapter will not reiterate this extensive, often conflicting literature, but rather, it will emphasize more recent developments in the field of HAH immunotoxicity that relate to understanding the underlying cellular, biochemical, and molecular mechanisms of HAH immunotoxicity. Gaps in our knowledge that require further research will also be identified.

ROLE OF THE Ah LOCUS IN HAH IMMUNOTOXICITY

One of the most important advances in the study of HAH toxicity in recent years has been the elucidation of a genetic basis for sensitivity to the toxicity of these chemicals, which may ultimately provide a logical explanation for much of the conflicting data in the literature regarding HAH toxicity in different species and in

---

The material presented here was modified from a document prepared by the authors for the USEPA's Health Assessment for 2,3,7,8-Tetrachlorodibenzo-*p*-dioxin (TCDD) and Related Compounds, August 1992.

different tissues of the same species. In this regard, many of the biochemical and toxic effects of HAHs appear to be mediated via binding to an intracellular protein known as the aromatic hydrocarbon (Ah) or TCDD receptor, in a process similar to steroid hormone receptor-mediated responses (6,7). Ah receptor activation follows stereospecific ligand binding; interaction of the receptor–ligand complex with dioxin-response elements (DREs) in the genome induces the transcription of the structural genes encoding messenger ribonucleic acid (mRNA) for CYP1A1 enzyme activity (i.e., cytochrome P_1450), as well as the expression of additional unidentified genes, the products of which are hypothesized to mediate HAH toxicity (8). Differences in toxic potency between various HAH congeners generally correlate with differences in Ah receptor binding affinities. The most toxic HAH congeners are approximate stereoisomers of 2,3,7,8-TCDD and are halogen-substituted in at least three of the four lateral positions in the aromatic ring system.

In mice, allelic variation at the Ah locus has been described (9,10). The different alleles code for Ah receptors that differ in their ability to bind TCDD and thus help to explain the different sensitivities of various inbred mouse strains to TCDD toxicity. Ah^{bb} C57Bl/6 (B6) mice represent the prototype "responsive" strain and are the most sensitive to TCDD toxicity, while Ah^{dd} DBA/2 (D2) mice represent the prototypic "nonresponsive" strain and require higher doses of TCDD to produce the same toxic effect. Recently, congenic Ah^{dd} mice on a B6 background were derived that differ from conventional B6 mice primarily at the Ah locus. The spectrum of biochemical and toxic responses to TCDD exposure was similar in both strains but the doses needed to bring about the responses were significantly higher in congenic mice homozygous for the Ah^{d} allele as compared to mice carrying two Ah^{b} alleles (11,12).

Two lines of evidence have been used to investigate the Ah receptor dependence of the acute immunotoxicity of TCDD and related HAHs: (a) comparative studies using PCDD, PCDF, and PCB congeners that differ in their binding affinity for the Ah receptor, and (b) studies using mice of different genetic background known to differ at the Ah locus. Vecchi et al. (13) was the first to report that the antibody response to sheep red blood cells (SRBCs) was differentially suppressed by TCDD in B6 mice as compared to D2 mice, with D2 mice requiring approximately a ten times higher dose to produce the same degree of suppression. Immunosuppression in F1 and backcross mice supported the role of the Ah locus in the expression of TCDD immunotoxicity. 2,3,7,8-TCDF was significantly less potent than TCDD and showed similar differential immunosuppressive effects in B6 and D2 mice. At the same time, Silkworth and Grabstein (14) reported a B6 versus D2 strain-dependent difference in sensitivity to suppression of the anti-SRBC response by 3,4,3′,4′-tetrachlorobiphenyl, a ligand for the Ah receptor. In comparison, the 2,5,2′,5′-tetrachlorobiphenyl isomer, which lacks affinity for the Ah receptor, was not immunosuppressive in either B6 or D2 mice. Structure–activity relationships were extended by Kerkvliet et al. (15) in studies that compared the immunosuppressive potency of the chlorinated dioxin and furan isomers that contaminate technical grade pentachlorophenol. The 1,2,3,6,7,8-hexachlorodioxin (HxCDD), 1,2,3,4,

6,7,8-heptachlorodioxin (HpCDD), and 1,2,3,4,6,7,8-heptachlorofuran (HpCDF) isomers, which bind the receptor, were all significantly immunosuppressive. The dose of each isomer that produced 50% suppression of the anti-SRBC response (ID_{50}) was 7.1, 85, and 208 μg/kg for HxCDD, HpCDD, and HpCDF, respectively, compared to an ID_{50} for TCDD of 0.65 μg/kg based on the data of Vecchi et al. (16) (Fig. 1). Similar ID_{50} values for suppression of the anti-SRBC response following acute TCDD exposure have since been reported by other laboratories (12,17–19). In contrast, octachlorodibenzo-*p*-dioxin (OCDD), which does not bind the receptor, was not immunosuppressive at a dose as high as 500 μg/kg (15). More extensive structure-dependent immunosuppressive activities of technical grade PCB mixtures (20), PCB congeners (21), and PCDF congeners (18) have also been reported.

The role of the Ah receptor in suppression of the anti-SRBC response has recently been verified in studies using B6 mice congenic at the Ah locus (12). As expected, congenic Ah^{dd}-B6 mice were significantly less sensitive to TCDD-induced immune suppression as compared to wild-type Ah^{bb}-B6 mice. Unexpectedly, however, the dose–response in congenic B6-Ah^{dd} mice appeared to be bimodal, with a portion of

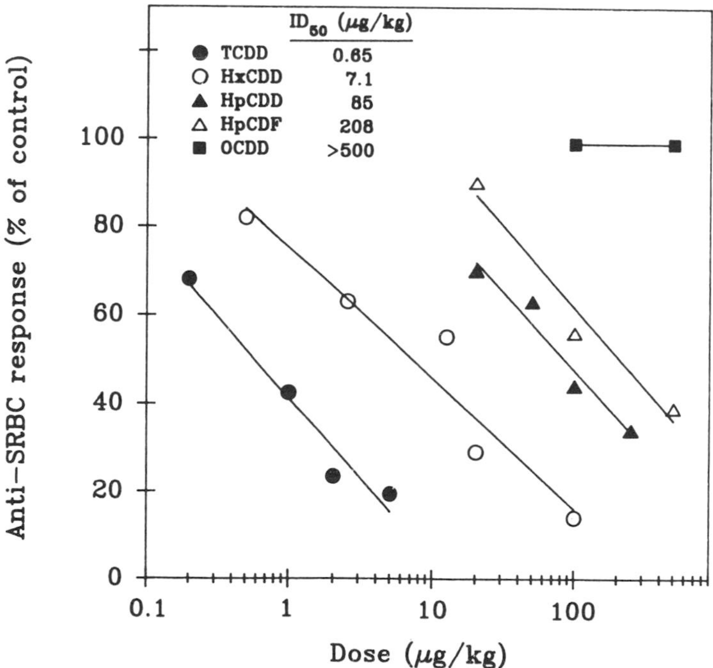

FIG. 1. Structure-dependent immunotoxicity of some polychlorinated dioxin and furan isomers. Immunotoxicity assessed by suppression of the splenic antibody response to SRBCs. (Adapted from ref. 15.)

the response sensitive to suppression by low doses of TCDD. Because of the bimodal response, the data did not permit extrapolation of an ID_{50} in the congenic mice. The results were interpreted to suggest potential non-Ah receptor-mediated immunosuppressive effects. It should be noted, however, that more recent studies using rederived congenic Ah^{dd}-B6 mice did not corroborate a bimodal dose–response in the congenic mice (19). They reported an ID_{50} of 7.5 μg/kg in congenic Ah^{dd}-B6 mice compared to an ID_{50} of 0.54 μg/kg in Ah^{bb}-B6 mice. These values are consistent with an Ah receptor-dependent mechanism of immune suppression. The issue of Ah receptor-independent immunotoxicity will be discussed in detail in a subsequent section of this chapter.

Ah receptor-dependent immunotoxicity has also been demonstrated in mice using other immunologic responses. For example, Kerkvliet et al. (12) reported that the ID_{50} for suppression of the antibody response to trinitrophenyl–lipopolysaccharide (TNP-LPS) in Ah^{bb}-B6 mice was 7.0 μg/kg compared to a significantly higher ID_{50} of 30 μg/kg in congenic Ah^{dd}-B6 mice. Since the antibody response to TNP-LPS shows little requirement for macrophages or T helper cells (22), these results suggest an Ah receptor-dependent B cell response. In regard to cytotoxic T cells, Clark et al. (23) were first to report data suggesting that TCDD and PCB isomers suppressed *in vitro* cytotoxic T lymphocyte (CTL) responses of B6 and D2 mice through an Ah receptor-dependent mechanism. Subsequently, Kerkvliet et al. (24) reported that B6 mice congenic at the Ah locus showed Ah-dependent sensitivity to suppression of the *in vivo* CTL response following exposure to either TCDD or 3,4,5,3′,4′,5′-hexachlorobiphenyl (HxCB). Furthermore, the potency of TCDD and of three HxCB congeners to suppress the CTL response of Ah^{bb}-B6 mice directly correlated with their relative binding affinities for the Ah receptor (24). The ID_{50} of TCDD for suppression of the CTL response in B6 mice was 7.0 μg/kg. [The dose of TCDD required to suppress the CTL response reported by Kerkvliet et al. (24) is significantly greater than that reported by Clark et al. (25), who reported CTL suppression following four weekly doses of 0.1 μg/kg TCDD. Clark et al. (23) also reported that doses of TCDD as low as 4 ng/kg to B6 mice suppressed the *in vitro* generation of CTLs, and that the suppression was Ah dependent. The potency of TCDD described in Clark's studies has not been corroborated by other laboratories.]

If the immunotoxicity of TCDD and structurally similar HAHs is dependent on Ah receptor-mediated mechanisms, then coexposure to subsaturating levels of more than one Ah receptor ligand should produce additive effects. Indeed, this hypothesis forms the basis of toxic equivalency factor (TEF) calculations used for hazard assessment of mixtures of Ah-receptor-binding HAHs. An additive immunotoxic interaction was demonstrated in mice coexposed to 1,2,3,6,7,8-HxCDD and 1,2,3,4,6,7,8-HpCDD, two relatively strong Ah receptor ligands (15). On the other hand, Davis and Safe (18,21) have reported that coexposure of mice to an immunotoxic dose of TCDD and a subimmunotoxic dose of different commercial Aroclors or different PCB congeners resulted in partial antagonism of TCDD suppression of the anti-SRBC response. In limited studies, an apparently similar antagonism was observed following coexposure to 2,3,7,8-TCDF (10 μg/kg) and TCDD (1.2 μg/kg)(26). The mechanism for the antagonism has not been fully elucidated, but the effects are consistent with competition for binding at the Ah receptor, since the weaker agonist was administered in excess compared to TCDD. In addition, Silkworth et al. (19,27) have shown that the immunotoxicity of TCDD can be modified by coexposure to other organic chemicals present as cocontaminants of actual environmental samples from Love Canal through non-Ah receptor-dependent mechanisms. Such interactions may preclude the use of TEFs for hazard assessment of mixtures.

In summary, the data relating TCDD immunotoxicity, at least in part, to Ah receptor-dependent events are convincing. However, it should be emphasized that all the data have been obtained from studies in inbred mice using an acute or subacute exposure regimen. Except for thymic atrophy, structure–immunotoxicity relationships in other species including rats have not been established, and inbred strains of other species with defined Ah genotype are not currently available. The importance of Ah receptor-mediated events in chronic, low-level HAH immunotoxicity is also controversial. Morris et al. (28) recently reported that the sensitivity of D2 mice to TCDD-induced suppression of the anti-SRBC response increased significantly when TCDD was administered daily over 2 weeks rather than as an acute single dose. Unfortunately, in these studies, the lowest dose of TCDD produced near-maximum suppression of the anti-SRBC response of B6C3F1 mice in the acute exposure model, precluding the detection of any similar increase in sensitivity of the B6C3F1 mice to chronic dosing. In contrast to these findings, Vecchi et al. (13) Jreported that multiple exposures to TCDD (2 μg/kg for 5 weeks or 0.5 μg/kg for 8 weeks) did not increase the sensitivity of D2 mice to suppression of the anti-SRBC response. Thus the basis for any change in potency resulting from multiple treatment or chronic exposure to TCDD and the role of Ah receptor-mediated events in the phenomenon remain to be elucidated.

CELLULAR TARGETS FOR HAH IMMUNOTOXICITY

Despite considerable investigation, the cellular basis for the suppressed immune function following HAH exposure has not been unequivocally established. The main reason for the lack of definitive progress in this area is the conflicting data reported from different laboratories regarding the ability of TCDD to suppress lymphocyte functions when examined *ex vivo* or *in vitro*. As discussed in a subsequent section, the *in vitro* effects of TCDD are greatly influenced by the *in vitro* culture conditions, which may explain the discrepancies in effects observed in different laboratories.

In contrast to *in vitro* studies, the *in vivo* immunotoxicity of TCDD, expressed in terms of suppression of the anti-SRBC response of B6 or B6C3F1 mice, is highly reproducible between laboratories. [Several laboratories have reported that the antibody response to SRBC in B6 mice is sensitive to suppression following acute exposure to TCDD either intraperitoneally (ip) or orally at doses below 1 μg/kg. In contrast, Clark et al. (25) reported that four weekly ip doses of 10 but not 1 or 0.1 μg/kg TCDD suppressed the anti-SRBC response of B6 mice. The basis for the discrepancies between the data of Clark et al. (23,25) and other laboratories regarding the potency of TCDD to suppress the anti-SRBC response is not known.] Since the magnitude of the anti-SRBC response depends on the concerted interactions of antigen-presenting cells (APCs), regulatory T cells (helper and suppressor), and B cells, this response has been used most widely to evaluate target cell sensitivity to HAHs. In addition, the antibody response to SRBCs can be modulated by many nonimmunologic factors, including hormonal and nutritional variables, and HAHs are known to affect numerous endocrine and metabolic functions. These latter effects will be apparent only in *in vivo* studies, while only direct effects of HAHs on APCs and lymphocyte functions would be evident following *in vitro* exposure to HAHs.

Kerkvliet and Brauner (29) compared the sensitivity of antibody responses to antigens that differ in their requirements for APCs and T cells as an *in vivo* approach to evaluate the cellular targets of 1,2,3,4,6,7,8-HpCDD humoral immunotoxicity. The T helper cell independent (TI) antigens, dinitrophenol (DNP)-Ficoll and TNP-LPS, were used in these studies. These TI antigens differ from each other in their requirement for APCs (higher for DNP-Ficoll) and their sensitivity to regulatory (amplifier and suppressor) T cell influence (DNP-Ficoll is sensitive, TNP-LPS is not) (30). Obviously, all antibody responses require B cell differentiation into antibody-secreting plasma cells. Although HpCDD produced dose-dependent suppression of the antibody response to all three antigens, sensitivity to suppression directly correlated with the sensitivity of the response to T cell regulation. The ID_{50} values were 53, 127, and 516 μg/kg for SRBCs, DNP-Ficoll, and TNP-LPS, respectively. These results were interpreted as follows. If one assumes that B cell function is targeted in the TNP-LPS response, then regulatory T cells and/or APCs may represent the more sensitive target in the SRBC and DNP-Ficoll responses. The difference in sensitivity between the SRBC and DNP-Ficoll responses suggests that the T helper cell may be a particularly sensitive target. The differential sensitivity of the antibody responses to TNP-LPS versus SRBCs has been corroborated in TCDD-treated mice (12,17). Thus the exquisite *in vivo* sensitivity of the antibody response to SRBCs would appear to depend on the T cell and/or APC components of the response rather than the B cell, unless the B cells that respond to SRBCs are different from the B cells that respond to TNP-LPS. Clearly, the influence of TCDD on different pathways of B cell activation is an important avenue for further study. The APC is also an unlikely target of TCDD in this model, since the ability of APCs primed *in vivo* with SRBCs to induce SRBC-specific T helper cell proliferation was unaltered by TCDD exposure (31).

These *in vivo* results contrast with the *ex vivo* data of Dooley and Holsapple (32) and Dooley et al. (33). Using separated spleen T cells, B cells, and adherent cells from vehicle- and TCDD-treated mice, they reported that B cells from TCDD-treated mice were functionally compromised in *in vitro* antibody responses but T cells and APCs were not. The basis for the different responses to TCDD *in vivo* versus *ex vivo* has not been established. However, it is possible that the effects of TCDD on T cells occur indirectly on activated T cells following antigen exposure such that removal of the cells from the TCDD environment of the host prior to antigen challenge precludes detection of T cell dysfunction. This interpretation is supported by the findings of Tomar and Kerkvliet (34) that spleen cells taken from TCDD-treated mice were not compromised in their ability to reconstitute the antibody response of lethally irradiated mice. This interpretation is also consistent with the reported lack of direct effects of TCDD and other HAHs on T cells *in vitro* (25,35,36).

While the direct effects of TCDD on T cells *in vitro* have not been demonstrated, it is clear that functional T cell responses generated *in vivo* are compromised following *in vivo* exposure. Nude mice that are congenitally T cell deficient are significantly less sensitive to HpCDD-induced suppression of the antibody response to DNP-Ficoll when compared to their T cell-competent littermates (29). Likewise, exposure to TCDD or HxCB suppresses the development of CTL activity following alloantigen challenge (24,35).

The influence of TCDD exposure on regulatory T cell functions has been addressed in a limited number of studies. Clark et al. (25) first proposed that T suppressor cells were induced by TCDD in the thymus and were responsible for the suppressed CTL response. However, increased suppressor cell activity in peripheral lymphoid tissue was not observed in mice exposed to TCDD (33) or 3,4,5,3′,4′,5′-HxCB (36). In terms of T helper cell activity, Tomar and Kerkvliet (34) reported that a dose of 5 μg/kg TCDD suppressed the *in vivo* generation of carrier-specific T helper cells. Lundberg et al. (37) reported that thymocytes from B6 mice treated with TCDD (50 μg/kg) were less capable of providing help for an *in vitro* anti-SRBC response. However, Clark et al. (23) reported in *ex vivo* studies that T cells from TCDD-treated mice produced normal levels of interleukin-2 (IL-2). The *in vivo* effects of TCDD on the production of IL-2 as well as other lymphokines important in the development of an antibody response (e.g., IL-4, IL-5) have not been reported. On the other hand, recent studies by Steppan et al. (38) have shown that the suppression of CTL development *in vivo* is correlated with a profound suppression of IL-2 and interferon-γ (IFN-γ) production in TCDD- and HxCB-treated mice.

The influence of TCDD exposure on B cell function has been addressed primarily in *in vitro* studies. The issue is difficult to address *in vivo* given that most B cell responses (except perhaps anti-LPS responses) are dependent on interactions with T cells and macrophages. *In vitro* studies have described the direct effects of TCDD on the activation and differentiation of purified B cells (39,40). These studies suggest that TCDD inhibits the terminal differentiation of B cells via alteration of an early activation event (39). Increased phosphorylation and tyrosine kinase activity in TCDD-treated B cells may underlie this B cell dysfunction (41,42).

Macrophage activities independent of their role as APCs have also been examined following TCDD exposure and generally found to be resistant to suppression by TCDD when assessed *ex vivo*. Macrophage-mediated phagocytosis, macrophage-mediated tumor cell cytolysis or cytostasis, oxidative reactions of neutrophils and macrophages, and natural killer (NK) cell activity were not suppressed following TCDD exposure at doses as high as 30 μg/kg (43,44). A potentially important exception is the reported selective inhibition of phorbol ester-activated antitumor cytolytic and cytostatic activity of neutrophils by TCDD (45).

On the other hand, it is interesting to note that the pathology associated with TCDD toxicity often includes neutrophilia and an inflammatory response in liver and skin characterized by activated macrophage and neutrophil accumulation (46–49). While these observations may simply reflect a normal inflammatory response to tissue injury, there is some experimental evidence suggesting inflammatory cells may be activated by TCDD exposure. For example, Alsharif et al. (50) recently reported that TCDD increased superoxide anion production in rat peritoneal macrophages. In addition, it has been shown that TCDD exposure results in an enhanced inflammatory response following SRBC challenge (31). This effect of TCDD was characterized by a two- to fourfold increase in the number of neutrophils and macrophages locally infiltrating the intraperitoneal site of SRBC injection. However, the kinetics of the cellular influx was not altered by TCDD. Likewise, the expression of macrophage activation markers (I-A and F4/80) and the antigen-presenting function of the peritoneal exudate cells were unaltered by TCDD. Thus the effect of TCDD appeared to reflect a quantitative rather than a qualitative change in the inflammatory response. Importantly, TCDD-induced suppression of the anti-SRBC response could not be overcome by increasing the amount of antigen used for sensitization, suggesting that enhanced antigen clearance/degradation by the increased numbers of phagocytic cells (e.g., decreased antigen load) was not responsible for the decreased antibody response in TCDD-treated mice. Thus the relationship, if any, between the inflammatory and immune effects of TCDD remain to be elucidated.

One mechanism by which TCDD and related HAHs may augment inflammatory responses is via enhanced production of inflammatory mediators such as IL-1 and tumor necrosis factor (TNF). Recent evidence suggests that the long-recognized hypersusceptibility of TCDD- and PCB-treated animals to endotoxin (LPS) (43,51–53) may be related to an increased production of TNF and/or IL-6 in the chemically treated animals (54–56). The ability of methylprednisolone to reverse the mortality associated with TCDD/endotoxin treatment is also consistent with an inflammatory response (57). Enhanced TNF activity also appears to underlie the enhanced inflammatory response to SRBCs, since treatment of the mice with a TNF receptor-soluble binding protein prevents the enhanced neutrophil response in TCDD-treated mice (58). Similarly, increased inflammatory mediator production may underlie the enhanced rat paw edema response to carrageenan and dextran in TCDD-treated rats (59,60). Serum complement activity, on the other hand, has been reported to be suppressed in dioxin-treated mice (61), although enhanced activity was reported at the lowest exposure level when 1,2,3,6,7,8-hexachlorodioxin was tested. A primary effect of TCDD on IL-1 is supported by the recent findings of Sutter et al. (62) that IL-1β gene expression in keratinocytes may be regulated by TCDD. Likewise,

Steppan and Kerkvliet (63) have reported that under some exposure conditions TCDD increased the level of mRNA for IL-1 in TCDD-treated IC21 cells, a macrophage cell line derived from B6 mice. On the other hand, House et al. (17) reported that inflammatory macrophages obtained from TCDD-treated mice produced control levels of IL-1 when examined *ex vivo*. Thus the effect of TCDD on inflammatory mediator production may be a "priming effect" and may require coexposure to antigen or LPS. The influence of TCDD on inflammatory mediator production and action is an important area for further study.

Since the rapid influx of phagocytic cells to the site of pathogen invasion is an important factor in host resistance to infection, the ability of TCDD to augment the production of inflammatory chemoattractive mediators would imply that TCDD exposure could result in enhanced host resistancc. However, since TCDD exposure is, at the same time, immunosuppressive, resulting in decreased specific immune responses generated by T and B lymphocytes, the overall impact of TCDD exposure on disease susceptibility will likely vary depending on the nature of the pathogen and the major mode of host response to the specific infectious agent. Such effects may in fact help to explain the disparate effects of TCDD in different host resistance models that have been previously reported.

INFLUENCE OF TCDD ON HOST RESISTANCE TO DISEASE

The ability of an animal to resist and/or control viral, bacterial, parasitic, and neoplastic diseases is determined by both nonspecific and specific immunologic functions. Decreased functional activity in any immunologic compartment may result in increased susceptibility to infectious and neoplastic diseases. In terms of risk assessment, host resistance is often accorded the "bottom line" in terms of relevent immunotoxic endpoints. Animal host resistance models that mimic human disease are available and have been used to assess the effect of TCDD on altered host resistance.

Several studies have shown that TCDD exposure increased susceptibility of mice and rats to challenge with the gram-negative bacterium *Salmonella* (43,64,65). TCDD exposure also resulted in a reduced resistance to *Escherichia coli* endotoxin (43,52), suggesting that the increased susceptibility to *Salmonella* caused by TCDD may be due to the endotoxin associated with the gram-negative bacterium. Rosenthal et al. (57) reported that endotoxin hypersensitivity in B6C3F1 mice was associated with hepatotoxicity and decreased clearance of the endotoxin. In addition, DBA/2 and congenic B6-Ah^{dd} mice were relatively resistant to this TCDD effect, implicating Ah receptor-dependent mechanisms in endotoxin hypersensitivity. However, endotoxin is not a prerequisite for TCDD effects since White et al. (61) have shown that TCDD treatment of mice resulted in increased mortality when challenged with *Streptococcus pneumoniae*, a gram-positive bacterium.

Under certain exposure conditions, TCDD has also been shown to increase susceptibility to *Listeria monocytogenes* infection. Hinsdill et al. (65) reported that 50 ppb TCDD in the diet increased bacteremia and mortality of Swiss Webster mice that had been injected intravenously with 10^5 *Listeria*. Similarly, exposure of pregnant B6C3F1 mice to 5.0 μg/kg TCDD at day 14 of gestation and again on days 1, 7, and 14 following birth resulted in an increased mortality in pups challenged with *Listeria* when they were 8 weeks of age (66,67). However, Vos et al. (43) reported that oral administration of 50 μg TCDD/kg once a week for 4 weeks to young Swiss mice did not alter the number of viable *Listeria* organisms per spleen, suggesting that TCDD did not affect nonspecific phagocytosis and killing of *Listeria*. Also, House et al. (17) reported that a single oral dose of TCDD up to 10 μg/kg did not enhance mortality to a *Listeria* challenge given 7 days later. Differences in study design such as TCDD dose, route, single versus multiple administrations, or mouse strain, age, and sex may contribute to these disparate effects.

Enhanced susceptibility to viral disease has also been reported after TCDD administration. Clark et al. (23) reported that TCDD treatment of B6 mice significantly enhanced mortality to *herpes simplex type II strain 33* virus. In contrast, TCDD exposure did not alter the time to death or the incidence of mortality following *herpesvirus suis* infection (64). House et al. (17) reported that TCDD treatment enhanced mortality of B6 mice challenged with *influenza/A/Taiwan/1/64 (H2N2)*. The lowest observable effect level was 0.1 μg/kg, making this one of the most sensitive endpoints for TCDD immunotoxicity. These results have recently been verified by Burleson et al. (67a). TCDD treatment of rats significantly augmented influenza virus replication in the lungs (68). This effect was correlated with a significant suppression of virus-augmented but not spontaneous NK cell activity.

TCDD exposure has also been shown to alter parasitic disease. Tucker et al. (69) studied the effects of TCDD administration on *Plasmodium yoelii 17 XNL*, a nonlethal strain of malaria, in 6- to 8-week-old B6C3F1 female mice. A single dose of TCDD at 5 or 10 μg/kg per mouth (os) resulted in increased susceptibility to *P. yoelii* as evidenced by the magnitude and duration of the peak parasitemia.

Luster et al. (66,67) demonstrated enhanced growth of transplanted tumors in offspring of mice treated with TCDD at doses of 1.0 or 5.0 μg/kg at day 14 of gestation and again on days 1, 7, and 14 following birth; host resistance studies were performed 6 to 8 weeks after weaning. This exposure protocol resulted in an increased incidence of PYB6 tumors in pups from dams receiving repeated doses of 5.0 but not 1.0 μg TCDD/kg. In contrast, Yang et al. (68) found that the metastatic spread of prostate-derived tumor cells was inhibited by acute TCDD treatment of rats at TCDD doses of 3, 10, or 30 μg/kg. When rats were treated for 14 days to a total TCDD dose of 10 μg/kg, metastases were inhibited on weeks 3 and 4 but were enhanced at week 5 post-tumor inoculation. Treatment of rats with PCBs (Aroclor 1254) also inhibited the growth of transplanted Walker 256 carcinosarcomas (70).

In summary, results from host resistance studies provide evidence that exposure to TCDD may result in increased susceptibility to bacterial, viral, parasitic, and neoplastic diseases. These effects are observed at low doses and likely result from TCDD-induced suppression of immunologic function. However, the specific immunologic functions targeted by TCDD in each of the host resistance models remain to be fully defined. Likewise, nonimmunologic mechanisms for altered host resistance should not be discounted without investigation.

IN VITRO IMMUNOTOXIC EFFECTS OF HAHs

Investigators in the field of TCDD immunotoxicity have long acknowledged the difficulties in consistently demonstrating the immunotoxicity of TCDD when cells from treated animals are tested *ex vivo* or when TCDD is added to culture *in vitro*. While effects following *in vitro* and *ex vivo* exposure to TCDD or related HAHs on lymphocyte functions have been reported (25,32,39,69), other laboratories have failed to observe suppression with *in vitro* or *ex vivo* exposure to HAHs (25,36,37; N.I. Kerkvliet, *unpublished data*). In addition, the effects of TCDD seen *in vitro* are sometimes inconsistent with those observed after *in vivo* assessment of immunotoxicity. For example, the rank order of sensitivity to suppression of T helper cell-dependent and T helper cell-independent antibody responses seen *in vivo* (12,17,29) is not seen *in vitro* (69,71), suggesting different cellular targets may be affected following *in vitro* exposure to TCDD. More importantly, some data suggest that suppression of the *in vitro* antibody response may occur independent of the Ah receptor. Tucker et al. (69) and Holsapple et al. (71) reported that direct addition of TCDD *in vitro* suppressed the antibody response to SRBCs. However, based on the response of cells from congenic mice as well as a limited structure–activity study, the data of Tucker et al. (69) supported an Ah receptor-dependent suppression while the data of Holsapple et al. (71) did not. In the latter study, the magnitude of suppression was comparable using cells from responsive B6C3F1 or congenic heterozygous (B6-Ah^{bd}) mice compared to nonresponsive D2 or homozygous B6-Ah^{dd} mice. In addition, the 2,7-dichlorodibenzo-*p*-dioxin congener, which lacks affinity for the Ah receptor, was equipotent with TCDD in suppressing the *in vitro* response (72).

In other studies, Davis and Safe (73) directly compared the *in vitro* structure–immunotoxicity relationships for a series of HAH congeners, which show more than a 14,900-fold-difference in *in vivo* immunotoxic potency. Results of these studies indicated that all the congeners were equipotent *in vitro* and produced a similar concentration-dependent suppression of the *in vitro* anti-SRBC response using cells from either B6 or D2 mice. Coexposure to the Ah receptor antagonist α-napthoflavone antagonized the immunosuppression induced by either TCDD or 1,3,6,8-TCDF (a weak Ah receptor agonist). Collectively, the results supported a mechanism of suppression *in vitro* that was *independent* of the Ah receptor.

The basis for these variable effects of TCDD *in vitro* are currently not known. However, recent studies by Morris et al. (40) demonstrated that the *in vitro* effects of TCDD on the anti-SRBC response were critically dependent on the type and concentration of the serum used in the *in vitro* culture. Only 3 of 23 lots of serum were able to support a full dose-responsive suppression, and, in serum-free cultures,

TCDD caused a 15-fold *enhancement* of the anti-SRBC response. Thus differences in medium components used in *in vitro* cultures may account for the different effects seen *in vitro* in different laboratories. Other factors such as the TCDD carrier/solvent used, the calcium content of the media, or procedures used for preparation of spleen cell suspensions may all contribute to variable effects of TCDD *in vitro*. The adaptation of *in vitro* assays to the use of autologous mouse serum may be a useful approach to reduce concern about the modifying role of calf serum components in the observed effects (74,75).

The obvious question relates to the relevance of many of the published *in vitro* findings to the *in vivo* immunotoxicity of TCDD. In this respect, it is important to note that the concentrations of TCDD required for *in vitro* suppression of immune function (1×10^{-9} to 30×10^{-9} M) of murine lymphocytes is several orders of magnitude higher than the concentration found in lymphoid tissues following exposure *in vivo* to an immunotoxic dose of TCDD (76). The amount of TCDD associated with isolated spleen cells obtained from mice 2 days following treatment with 5 μg/kg [^{3}H]-TCDD was 2×10^{-15} M per 10^7 spleen cells. Importantly, as much as 50% of the radioactivity associated with whole spleen tissue was recovered in the stromal and/or capsular material (i.e., splenic tissue that resisted passage through the mesh screens used for preparation of spleen cell suspensions). These findings suggest that (a) the most potent effects of TCDD on immune function *in vivo* may be induced indirectly by effects on nonlymphoid cells, or (b) based on the delivered dose of TCDD, this molecule is more toxic than previously thought. Alternatively, TCDD effects *in vivo* on nonlymphoid cells may amplify the direct effects of TCDD on lymphoid tissue.

INDIRECT MECHANISMS OF HAH IMMUNOTOXICITY

The difficulty in demonstrating consistent, direct effects of TCDD *in vitro* on lymphocytes, the dependence of those effects on serum components, and the requirement for high concentrations of TCDD are all consistent with an indirect mechanism of TCDD on the immune system. One potentially important indirect mechanism is via effects on the endocrine system. Several endocrine hormones have been shown to regulate immune responses, including glucocorticoids, sex steroids, thyroxine, growth hormone, and prolactin. Importantly, TCDD and other HAHs have been shown to alter the activity of all these hormones.

Kerkvliet et al. (24) reported that exposure of mice to various HxCB isomers followed by injection of P815 allogeneic tumor cells induced an Ah receptor-dependent and dose-dependent elevation of serum corticosterone (CS) concentrations, which correlated with the dose-dependent suppression of the anti-P815 CTL response. However, since adrenalectomy or treatment with the glucocorticoid receptor antagonist RU 38486 failed to protect mice from the immunosuppressive effect of HxCB (77), a role for the elevated CS in the suppression of the CTL response seems unlikely. Adrenalectomy and hypophysectomy also failed to prevent TCDD-induced thymic atrophy in rats (78).

Using the P815 allogeneic tumor model, Kerkvliet and Baecher-Steppan (35) reported that male mice were more sensitive than female mice to suppression of the CTL response by HxCB. Castration of male rats partially ameliorated the immunosuppressive effects of HxCB (77), suggesting a role for testosterone in suppression of the CTL response.

Pazdernik and Rozman (79) suggested that thyroid hormones may play a role in TCDD immunotoxicity based on the finding that radio-thyroidectomy prevented the suppression of the anti-SRBC response in rats treated with TCDD. However, since thyroidectomy alone suppressed immune function, the significance of the findings require further study.

ROLE OF THE THYMUS IN HAH IMMUNOTOXICITY

Thymic involution is one of the hallmarks of exposure to TCDD and related HAHs in all species examined. In mice, thymic involution occurs by an Ah receptor-dependent mechanism (6). Because the thymus plays a critical role in the ontogeny of T lymphocytes, thymic involution is often referred to as an immunotoxic effect. However, while an intact thymus is crucial to the developing immune system during the prenatal and early postnatal period of rodents as well as during the prenatal period of humans, the physiologic role played by the thymus in adult life has not been established. In animal models, adult thymectomy has little effect on the quantity or quality of T lymphocytes, which have already matured and populated the secondary lymphoid organs (80). Likewise, in humans, childhood and adult thymectomy produces no clearly identifiable adverse consequences in terms of altered immune function. Based on this knowledge, it is not surprising that a direct relationship between the effects of TCDD on the thymus and immune suppression has not been established in studies using adult animals. In fact, adult thymectomy prior to HAH exposure did not modify TCDD- or HpCDD-induced suppression of the anti-SRBC response (29,69). Furthermore, suppression of immune responses occurs at dose levels of HAHs significantly lower than those required to induce thymic atrophy (12,43,69,72,81). Thus it is clear that thymic involution does not represent a surrogate marker for TCDD immunotoxicity in adult animals. On the other hand, it is possible that chronic exposure to TCDD resulting in a chronic thymic atrophy may produce more delayed, subtle effects on immune function not yet identified (82).

In contrast to adult animals, congenital thymic aplasia or neonatal thymectomy results in severe reduction in the number and function of T lymphocytes and produces a potentially lethal wasting disease (80). Similarly, there is evidence from studies carried out in the 1970s that rodents exposed to TCDD or other HAHs during the pre/neonatal period are more sensitive to immune suppression as compared to rodents exposed as adults, and that the prenatal effects are more selective for cell-mediated immunity (66,67,83,84). TCDD has also been shown to alter thymocyte differentiation *in vitro* in cell cultures (85,86) and organ cultures (87,88) as well as *in vivo* following prenatal exposure to TCDD (89). These observations suggest that altered thymic T cell maturation induced by TCDD in the thymus may play an important role in the suppressed immune function of prenatally exposed animals. However, since TCDD also influences B cell development in the bursa of chick embryos (90) as well as lymphocyte stem cells in the fetal liver and bone marrow of mice (91,92), other mechanisms of developmental immunotoxicity are also likely to be important.

IMMUNOTOXICITY FOLLOWING PRE/NEONATAL EXPOSURE TO HAHs

The increased susceptibility of very young animals to HAH immunotoxicity has been reported in several studies in which immune function was examined in mice, rats, and/or guinea pigs following exposure to TCDD or PCBs during fetal development and/or via lactation (47,52,66,83). The most sensitive indicator of TCDD immunotoxicity in these studies was an increase in the growth of transplanted tumor cells in the offspring of B6C3F1 mice (Ah responsive strain) treated with 1 μg/kg TCDD at 4-week intervals. (Total TCDD dose to dam was 4 μg/kg; dose to offspring was not determined.) The offspring of Swiss mice fed a diet containing 1 ppb TCDD for 7 weeks showed enhanced mortality following endotoxin challenge, while the plaque-forming cell response to SRBC and delayed hypersensitivity response were suppressed in offspring of mice fed 5.0 ppb TCDD diets. (Estimated daily dose to 20-g dam consuming 5 g of 5 ppb TCDD diet is equivalent to 1.25 μg/kg TCDD/day.) Rats appeared to be more resistant to the immunotoxic effects of pre/neonatal exposure to TCDD based on the finding that 5 but not 1 μg/kg TCDD given four times at weekly intervals produced immunotoxicity in the offspring. Immunotoxic endpoints that were unaffected by the highest exposure levels in these studies included blastogenesis induced by LPS and serum antibody titers to SRBCs and bovine gamma globulin (BGG).

Two recent studies have examined immune function in offspring of female mice exposed to TCDD (93) or PCB (Kanechlor 500) (94) but that were cross-fostered to unexposed lactating mice at birth. Thus exposure was limited to *in utero* exposure. (It is important to recognize that rodents are born with an immature immune system that matures in the first few weeks following birth. In contrast, the human immune system is considered to be more mature at birth.) B6 mice exposed to 3.0 μg/kg TCDD on gestational days 6 to 14 gave birth to offspring that had significant thymic atrophy and hypoplasia measured on gestational day 18 or on day 6 postnatally. The thymic effects were no longer apparent by day 14. At 7 to 8 weeks postnatally, mitogen responses and antibody plaque-forming cell response to SRBCs were unaltered while the CTL response was significantly suppressed compared to controls (93). These results suggest a selectivity of prenatal TCDD on the CTLs and not the T helper cells involved in the antibody response to SRBCs. In contrast to these results, Takagi et al. (94) exposed female C3H mice per os to 50 mg/kg Kanechlor 500 twice per week for 4 weeks, at which time steady-state tissue levels were noted.

The offspring derived from mating to unexposed males had an unaltered antibody response to the T-independent antigen DNP-dextran. On the other hand, carrier-primed T helper cell activity assessed by adoptive transfer was significantly suppressed by PCB exposure when assessed 4 and 7 weeks after birth, but fully recovered by 11 weeks. Together, these studies confirm prior studies to indicate that T cell function is selectively altered by HAHs when exposure is prenatal. While both T helper cells and CTLs show altered function, T helper cell activity may recover faster than CTL function.

Fine et al. (92) reported on TCDD levels in offspring following maternal treatment with TCDD (10 μg/kg) on gestational day 14. The fetal liver had the highest concentration on gestational day 18 (235 fg/mg), which declined slightly by postnatal day 6 to around 100 fg/mg. The concentration of TCDD in the thymus on gestational day 18 was 140 fg/mg, which declined to 20 fg/mg on day 6 after birth. (These thymic TCDD concentrations are equivalent to 60 to 425 pM assuming 1 kg of tissue is equivalent to 1 liter of water.) TCDD concentrations in the spleen remained constant at about 40 fg/mg during the same time frame, while bone marrow concentrations were very low (about 3 fg/mg). These concentrations of TCDD were associated with thymic atrophy (91) and significant reduction in the ability of prothymocytes in liver and bone marrow to repopulate an irradiated thymus (93).

IMMUNOTOXICITY OF HAHs IN NONHUMAN PRIMATES

A limited number of studies using nonhuman primates as surrogate models for humans have been conducted to assess HAH immunotoxicity. Immunologic effects were described in rhesus monkeys and their offspring chronically exposed to TCDD at levels of 5 or 25 ppt for 4 years (95). In the mothers, the total number of T cells increased in monkeys fed 25 ppt TCDD, with a selective increase in CD8+ cells and a decrease in CD4+ cells. However, no significant effect on T cell function was established when assessed as proliferation response to mitogens, alloantigens, or xenoantigens. NK cell activity and production of antibodies to tetanus immunization were normal. In the offspring of TCDD-exposed dams examined 4 years after exposure, a significantly *increased* antibody response to tetanus toxoid immunization was observed, which correlated with TCDD tissue levels. The body burden of TCDD in the offspring ranged from a low of 290 ppt to a high of 1400 ppt. Interestingly, there was no strict correlation between exposure levels and resulting body burden.

In other TCDD studies, a single injection of TCDD in marmosets (*Callithrix jacchus*) resulted in a delayed decrease in the percentage of CD4+ T cells and CD20+ B cells in the blood and an increase in the percentage of CD8+ cells (96). The total number of T cells was not significantly altered by TCDD exposure. The CD4+ subset most affected was the CDw29+ "helper-inducer" or "memory" subset, with significant effects observed after a TCDD dose of 10 ng/kg. The no observable effect level (NOEL) for this effect was 3 ng/kg TCDD. Concomitant with suppression of the CDw29 subset in TCDD-treated animals, the percentage of CD4+ CD45RA+ cells increased. This subset has been classified as "suppressor-inducer" or "naive" cells. The changes in the T cell subsets were intensified following *in vitro* culture of the cells with mitogen (97). Interestingly, however, a recent study from the same laboratory reported that chronic exposure of young marmosets to very low levels of TCDD (0.3 ng/kg/wk for 24 weeks) produced the opposite effect on the CD4+CDw29+ subset, resulting in a significant increase in this population while the CD4+CD45RA+ subset decreased (98). Upon transfer of the animals to a higher dose of TCDD (1.5 ng/kg/wk) for 3 weeks, the enhancement effect was reversed, and suppression of the CD4+CDw29+ subset was observed, with maximum suppression after 6 weeks of exposure to the higher dose. In addition, the CD8+CD56+ cytotoxic T cell subset transiently increased, but normalized with continued dosing of TCDD. After discontinuation of dosing, the reduction in the percentage and absolute number of CD4+CDw29+ cells persisted for 5 weeks and only reached normal range after 7 weeks. These results led the authors to conclude that "extrapolations of the results obtained at higher doses to very low exposures is not justified with respect to the effects induced by TCDD on the immune system of marmosets."

The immunomodulatory effects of chronic low-level PCB exposure in monkeys have also been investigated. In early studies, Thomas and Hinsdill (51) reported that rhesus monkeys fed diets containing 2.5 or 5 mg/kg of Aroclor 1248 had significantly suppressed antibody response to SRBCs but not to tetanus toxoid (TT). These monkeys had chloracne, alopecia, and facial edema. Similarly, exposure of cynomolgus monkeys to Aroclor 1254 (100 or 400 μg/kg/d) for 3 months suppressed antibody responses to SRBC but not to TT (99). Suppressive effects on anti-SRBC responses were more severe in cynomolgus monkeys when the PCB mixture contained PCDFs (100).

Tryphonas et al. (101–103) reported studies in rhesus monkeys exposed chronically to Aroclor 1254 (5 to 80 μg/kg/d) for 23 or 55 months. These exposures resulted in steady-state blood PCB levels that ranged from a mean low of 0.01 ± 0.001 ppm in the 5-μg/kg group to a mean high of 0.11 ± 0.01 ppm in the 80-μg/kg group. The only consistently altered immune parameters were the primary and anamnestic antibody responses to SRBC, which were suppressed in a dose-dependent manner. In contrast, the antibody response to pneumococcus vaccine antigen measured at 55 months of exposure was not significantly altered. At 23 months, the percentage of T helper cells in the blood was significantly decreased in the 80-μg/kg group, and the percentage and absolute number of T suppressor cells were increased; however, these effects were not apparent at 55 months of exposure (103). Lymphoproliferative responses to phytohemagglutinin antigen (PHA) and concanavalin A (Con A) were not significantly altered at 23 months but were dose-dependently suppressed at 55 months. Proliferation to alloantigens was not significantly altered. Likewise, serum immunoglobulin and hydrocortisone levels did not differ between treatment groups. After 55 months, the chemiluminescent response (time to peak) of monocytes was slower in PCB-exposed leukocytes. Also noted at

55 months was a significant elevation in serum hemolytic complement levels, a dose-related increase in NK cell activity, and a dose-related increase in thymosin α-1 levels but not thymosin β-4 levels (102). Effects on IFN levels were inconsistent, and TNF production was not altered.

These studies in nonhuman primates are important from the viewpoint that the antibody response to SRBC emerged as the only immunologic parameter consistently suppressed by HAHs in several different animal species. Other immunologic endpoints such as total T cell numbers, percentages of T cell subsets, lymphoproliferative responses, and delayed-type hypersensitivity (DTH) responses are inconsistently increased or decreased in various studies. At the present time, it is not clear why the antibody response to SRBC is most consistently altered by HAH exposure in different species. The sensitivity of the anti-SRBC response did not appear to be due solely to the T cell dependency of the response since antibody responses to other T-dependent antigen (e.g., TT, BGG) were not suppressed and may be enhanced following HAH exposure. The sensitivity of the technique used to quantify the antibody response may contribute to the increased sensitivity of the SRBC model, which is most often measured as the plaque-forming cell (PFC) response rather than serum antibody titers, which are usually more variable.

IMMUNOTOXICITY OF HAH IN HUMANS

The immunotoxicity of TCDD and related HAHs in humans has been the subject of several studies following accidental and/or occupational exposures to PCBs, PBBs, and TCDD. Immunologic assessment was carried out on patients who consumed acnegenic and hepatotoxic doses of PCDF-PCB contaminated rice oil in Taiwan in 1979. Clinical symptoms were primarily related to increased frequency of various kinds of infection, especially of the respiratory tract and skin (104). Immunologic effects included decreased serum IgA and IgM, but not IgG, decreased percentage of T cells in peripheral blood related to decreased CD4+ T helper cells and increased CD8+ T suppressor cells. Suppressed dermal DTH responses to streptokinase/streptodornase and tuberculin antigens were also observed (reviewed in ref. 104). The percentage of anergy increased and the degree of induration decreased in patients with increased PCB concentration in their blood. In contrast, lymphoproliferative responses of peripheral blood lymphocytes (PBLs) to PHA, pokeweed mitogen (PWM), and tuberculin, but not Con A, were significantly augmented in PCB-exposed individuals. PCB concentrations in the blood ranged from 3 to 1156 ppb with a mean of 89 ± 6.9 ppb. The oil was contaminated at PCB concentrations of 4.8 to 204.9 ppm with a mean of 52 ± 39 ppm.

Similarly, immunotoxic effects were described in Michigan dairy farmers accidentally exposed to PBBs in 1973 via contaminated dairy products and meat (105). Like PCB-exposed individuals, the percentage and absolute numbers of T cells in peripheral blood of PBB-exposed farmers were significantly reduced compared to a control group. However, in contrast to PCBs, lymphoproliferation responses to

PHA, PWM, and allogeneic leukocytes were significantly decreased in PBB-exposed persons. Also in contrast to PCBs, skin testing using standard recall antigens indicated that PBB-exposed Michigan dairy farmers had significantly increased responses, particularly to *Candida* and Varidase. Tissue levels of PBBs in the subjects were not determined in these studies.

Webb et al. (106) reported the findings from immunologic assessment of 41 persons from Missouri with documented adipose tissue levels of TCDD resulting from occupational, recreational, or residential exposure. Of the participants, 16 had tissue TCDD levels less than 20 ppt, 13 had levels between 20 and 60 ppt, and 12 had levels greater than 60 ppt. The highest level was 750 ppt. Data were analyzed by multiple regression based on adipose tissue level and the clinical dependent variable. Increased TCDD levels were correlated with an increased percentage and total number of T lymphocytes. CD8+ and T11+ T cells accounted for the increase, while CD4+ T cells were not altered in percentage or number. Lymphoproliferative responses to Con A, PHA, PWM, or TT were unaltered as was the cytotoxic T cell response. Serum IgA, but not IgG, was increased. No adverse clinical disease was associated with TCDD levels in these subjects. Only 2 of the 41 subjects reported a history of chloracne. These findings differ from those reported for the Quail Run Mobile Home Park residents (tissue levels unknown) in which decreased T cell numbers (T3, CD4, and T11) and suppressed cell-mediated immunity were reported (107). However, subsequent retesting of these anergic subjects failed to confirm the anergy (108). On the other hand, when sera from some of these individuals were tested for levels of the thymic peptide, thymosin α-1, the entire frequency distribution for the TCDD-exposed group was shifted toward lower thymosin α-1 levels (109). The statistically significant difference between the TCDD-exposed persons and controls remained after controlling for age, sex, and socioeconomic status, with a trend for decreased thymosin α-1 levels with increased number of years of residence in the TCDD-contaminated residential area. The thymosin α-1 levels were not correlated with changes in other immune system parameters nor with any increased incidence of clinically diagnosed immune suppression. The decrease in thymosin α-1 levels in humans contrasts with the increase in thymosin α-1 seen in PCB-treated monkeys (103).

Finally, Mocarelli et al. (110) reported studies on the immune status of 44 children, 20 of whom had chloracne, who were exposed to TCDD following an explosion at a herbicide factory in Seveso, Italy. No abnormalities were found in the following parameters: serum immunoglobulin concentrations, levels of circulating complement, or lymphoproliferative responses to T and B cell mitogens. Interestingly, in a study conducted 6 years after the explosion, a different cohort of TCDD-exposed children exhibited a significant *increase* in complement protein levels, which correlated with the incidence of chloracne, as well as increased numbers of peripheral blood lymphocytes and increased lymphoproliferative responses (111). However, no specific health problems were correlated with dioxin exposure in these children.

It is readily apparent that no clear pattern of immunotoxicity to HAHs emerges from these studies in humans. In some cases T cell numbers increase; in others, they decrease. The findings are not unlike the varied and often conflicting reports found in the literature regarding animal studies of HAH immunotoxicity. The basis for the lack of consistent, significant exposure-related effects is unknown and may be dependent on several factors. Most notable in this regard is the generic difficulties in assessing subclinical immunomodulation, particularly in outbred human populations. Most immunologic assays have a very broad range of normal responses, reducing the sensitivity to detect small changes. Similarly, the assays used to examine immune function in humans exposed to TCDD and related HAHs have unfortunately been based to a greater extent on what was clinically practical (e.g., mitogen responsiveness) rather than on assays that have been shown to be sensitive to TCDD in animal studies. Thus the lack of consistent and/or significant immunotoxic effects in humans resulting from TCDD exposure may be as much a function of the assays used as the immune status of the cohort. In addition, few studies have examined the immune status of individuals with known, documented exposure to HAHs. Rather, cohorts based on presumption of exposure have been studied. There is some evidence to suggest that the lack of significant effects may sometimes be due to the inclusion of subjects that had little or no actual exposure to TCDD (106). Likewise, the important role that Ah phenotype plays in TCDD immunotoxicity has not been considered when addressing human sensitivity. Whether there are human equivalents of murine Ah^{bb} and Ah^{dd} receptor types is not known. Finally, in most studies, the assessment of immune function in exposed populations was carried out long after exposure to TCDD ceased. Thus recovery from the immunotoxic effects of TCDD may have occurred.

In summary, given the current lack of data correlating clinical immunologic endpoints with immune status in humans (except in cases of overt immune deficiencies), massive *retrospective* studies of poorly defined exposure groups cannot be justified to try to "prove" that immune modulation has occurred in these people. Rather, such efforts would be better directed toward the establishment of a broad database of normal values for the clinical immunology endpoints that may be of use in immunotoxicity assessments. In conjunction with this effort, research must focus on the definition of sensitive endpoints (i.e., biomarkers) of immune dysfunction in humans so that, in the future, emergency response teams could respond rapidly to accidental exposures to assess the immunologic status of the exposed persons. To validate these biomarkers, there is a parallel need for animal research to identify TCDD-sensitive immune endpoints in animals that can also be measured in humans in order to establish correlative changes in the biomarker and immune function. In particular, it will be important to determine in animal models how well changes in immune function in the lymphoid organs (e.g., spleen and lymph nodes) correlate with changes in the expression of lymphocyte subset/activation markers in peripheral blood. Until such correlations are established, the interpretation of changes observed in subsets/activation markers in human peripheral blood lymphocytes in terms of health risk will be limited to speculation. Research must also continue to develop well-defined animal models using multiple animal species that will lead to an understanding of the underlying mechanisms of HAH immunotoxicity. For example, there is a clear need to document Ah receptor involvement in the immunotoxicity of TCDD and related HAHs in species other than mice. These studies need to go beyond descriptive immunotoxicity assessment to determine the mechanistic basis for differences in species sensitivity to TCDD immunotoxicity following both acute and chronic exposure. In the interim, the available database derived from well-controlled animal studies on HAH immunotoxicity can be used for establishment of no effect levels and acceptable exposure levels for human risk assessment of TCDD using the same procedures that are used for other noncarcinogenic toxic endpoints. Because the antibody response to SRBCs has been shown to be dose-dependently suppressed by TCDD and related HAHs in several animal species, this database is best suited for current application to risk assessment. The validity of using TEFs to extrapolate from one HAH to another, however, remains to be established.

REFERENCES

1. Kerkvliet NI. Halogenated aromatic hydrocarbons (HAH) as immunotoxicants. In: Kende M, Gainer J, Chirigos M, eds. *Chemical regulation of immunity in veterinary medicine*. New York: Alan R. Liss; 1984:369–387.
2. Thomas PT, Faith RE. Adult and perinatal immunotoxicity induced by halogenated aromatic hydrocarbons. In: Dean J, ed. *Immunotoxicology and immunopharmacology*. New York: Raven Press; 1985:305–313.
3. Vos JG, Luster MI. Immune alterations. In: Kimbrough RD, Jensen S, eds. *Halogenated biphenyls, terphenyls, naphthalenes, dibenzodioxins and related products*. Amsterdam: Elsevier Science Publishers; 1989:295–322.
4. Holsapple MP, Morris DL, Wood SC, Snyder NK. 2,3,7,8-Tetrachlorodibenzo-*p*-dioxin-induced changes in immunocompetence: possible mechanisms. *Annu Rev Pharmacol Toxicol* 1991;31:73–100.
5. Holsapple MP, Snyder NK, Wood SC, Morris DL. A review of 2,3,7,8-tetrachlorodibenzo-*p*-dioxin-induced changes in immunocompetence: 1991 update. *Toxicology* 1991;69:219–251.
6. Poland A, Knutson JC. 2,3,7,8-Tetrachlorodibenzo-*p*-dioxin and related halogenated aromatic hydrocarbons: examination of the mechanism of toxicity. *Annu Rev Pharmacol Toxicol* 1982;22:517–554.
7. Cuthill S, Wilhelmsson A, Mason GGF, Gillner M, Poellinger L, Gustafsson J-A. The dioxin receptor: a comparison with the glucocorticoid receptor. *J Steroid Biochem* 1988;30:277–280.
8. Whitlock JP. Genetic and molecular aspects of 2,3,7,8-tetrachlorodibenzo-*p*-dioxin action. *Annu Rev Pharmacol Toxicol* 1990;30:251–277.
9. Poland A, Glover E, Taylor BA. The murine Ah locus: a new allele and mapping to chromosome 12. *Mol Pharmacol* 1987;32:471–478.
10. Poland A, Glover E. Characterization and strain distribution pattern of the murine Ah receptor specified by the Ah^{d} and Ah^{b-3} alleles. *Mol Pharmacol* 1990;38:306–312.
11. Birnbaum LS, McDonald MM, Blair PC, Clark AM, Harris MW. Differential toxicity of 2,3,7,8-tetrachlorodibenzo-*p*-dioxin (TCDD) in C57Bl/6 mice congenic at the Ah locus. *Fundam Appl Toxicol* 1990;15:186–200.
12. Kerkvliet NI, Steppan LB, Brauner JA, Deyo JA, Henderson MC, Tomar RS, Buhler DR. Influence of the Ah locus on the humoral immunotoxicity of 2,3,7,8-tetrachlorodibenzo-*p*-dioxin (TCDD) immunotoxicity: evidence for Ah receptor-dependent and Ah receptor-independent mechanisms of immunosuppression. *Toxicol Appl Pharmacol* 1990;105:26–36.
13. Vecchi A, Sironi M, Canegrati MA, Recchis M, Garattini S. Immunosuppressive effects of 2,3,7,8-tetrachlorodibenzo-*p*-dioxin in strains of mice with different susceptibility to induction of aryl hydrocarbon hydroxylase. *Toxicol Appl Pharmacol* 1983;68:434–441.

14. Silkworth JB, Grabstein EM. Polychlorinated biphenyl immunotoxicity: dependence on isomer planarity and the Ah gene complex. *Toxicol Appl Pharmacol* 1982;65:109–115.
15. Kerkvliet NI, Brauner JA, Matlock JP. Humoral immunotoxicity of polychlorinated diphenyl ethers, phenoxyphenols, dioxins and furans present as contaminants of technical grade pentachlorophenol. *Toxicology* 1985;36:307–324.
16. Vecchi A, Mantovani A, Sironi M, Luini M, Cairo M, Garattini S. Effect of acute exposure to 2,3,7,8-tetrachlorodibenzo-*p*-dioxin on humoral antibody production in mice. *Chem Biol Interact* 1980;30:337–341.
17. House RV, Lauer LD, Murray MJ, Thomas PT, Ehrlich JP, Burleson GR, Dean JH. Examination of immune parameters and host resistance mechanisms in B6C3F1 mice following adult exposure to 2,3,7,8-tetrachlorodibenzo-*p*-dioxin. *J Toxicol Environ Health* 1990;31:203–215.
18. Davis D, Safe S. Immunosuppressive activities of polychlorinated dibenzofuran congeners: quantitative structure–activity relationships and interactive effects. *Toxicol Appl Pharmacol* 1988;94: 141–149.
19. Silkworth JB, Cutler DS, O'Keefe PW, Lipinskas T. Potentiation and antagonism of 2,3,7,8-tetrachlorodibenzo-*p*-dioxin effects in a complex environmental mixture. *Toxicol Appl Pharmacol* 1993;119:236–247.
20. Davis D, Safe S. Immunosuppressive activities of polychlorinated biphenyls in C57Bl/6N mice: structure–activity relationships as Ah receptor agonists and partial antagonists. *Toxicology* 1990; 63:97–111.
21. Davis D, Safe S. Dose–response immunotoxicities of commercial polychlorinated biphenyls (PCBs) and their interactions with 2,3,7,8-tetrachlorodibenzo-*p*-dioxin. *Toxicol Lett* 1989;48:35–43.
22. Jelinek DF, Lipsky PE. Regulation of human B lymphocyte activation, proliferation, and differentiation. *Adv Immunol* 1987;40:1–59.
23. Clark DA, Sweeney G, Safe S, Hancock E, Kilburn DG, Gauldie J. Cellular and genetic basis for suppression of cytotoxic T cell generation by haloaromatic hydrocarbons. *Immunopharmacology* 1983;6:143–153.
24. Kerkvliet NI, Steppan LB, Smith BB, Youngberg JA, Henderson MC, Buhler DR. Role of the Ah locus in suppression of cytotoxic T lymphocyte (CTL) activity by halogenated aromatic hydrocarbons (PCBs and TCDD): structure–activity relationships and effects in C57Bl/6 mice. *Fundam Appl Toxicol* 1990;14:532–541.
25. Clark DA, Gauldie J, Szewczuk MR, Sweeney G. Enhanced suppressor cell activity as a mechanism of immunosuppression by 2,3,7,8-tetrachlorodibenzo-*p*-dioxin. *Proc Exp Biol Med* 1981;168: 290–299.
26. Rizzardini M, Romano M, Tursi F, et al. Toxicological evaluation of urban waste incinerator emissions. *Chemosphere* 1983;12:559–564.
27. Silkworth JB, Sack G, Cutler D. Immunotoxicity of 2,3,7,8-tetrachlorodibenzo-*p*-dioxin in a complex environmental mixture from the Love Canal. *Fundam Appl Toxicol* 1988;12:303–312.
28. Morris DL, Snyder NK, Gokani V, Blair RE, Holsapple MP. Enhanced suppression of humoral immunity in DBA/2 mice following subchronic exposure to 2,3,7,8-tetrachlorodibenzo-*p*-dioxin (TCDD). *Toxicol Appl Pharmacol* 1992;112:128–132.
29. Kerkvliet NI, Brauner JA. Mechanisms of 1,2,3,4,6,7,8-heptachlorodibenzo-*p*-dioxin (HpCDD)-induced humoral immune suppression: evidence of primary defect in T cell regulation. *Toxicol Appl Pharmacol* 1987;87:18–31.
30. Braley-Mullen H. Differential effect of activated T amplifier cells on B cells responding to thymus-independent type-1 and type-2 antigens. *J Immunol* 1982;129:484–489.
31. Kerkvliet NI, Oughton JA. Acute inflammatory response to sheep red blood cell challenge in mice treated with 2,3,7,8-tetrachlorodibenzo-*p*-dioxin (TCDD): phenotypic and functional analysis of peritoneal exudate cells. *Toxicol Appl Pharmacol* 1993;119:248–257.
32. Dooley RK, Holsapple MP. Elucidation of cellular targets responsible for tetrachlorodibenzo-*p*-dioxin (TCDD)-induced suppression of antibody responses: the role of the B lymphocyte. *Immunopharmacology* 1988;16:167–180.
33. Dooley RK, Morris DL, Holsapple MP. Elucidation of cellular targets responsible for tetrachlorodibenzo-*p*-dioxin (TCDD)-induced suppression of antibody response. 2. Role of the T lymphocyte. *Immunopharmacology* 1990;19:47–58.
34. Tomar RS, Kerkvliet NI. Reduced T helper cell function in mice exposed to 2,3,7,8-tetrachlorodibenzo-*p*-dioxin (TCDD). *Toxicol Lett* 1991;57:55–64.

35. Kerkvliet NI, Baecher-Steppan L. Suppression of allograft immunity by 3,4,5,3′,4′,5′-hexachlorobiphenyl. I. Effects of exposure on tumor rejection and cytotoxic T cell activity. *Immunopharmacology* 1988;16:1–12.
36. Kerkvliet NI, Baecher-Steppan L. Suppression of allograft immunity by 3,4,5,3′,4′,5′-hexachlorobiphenyl. II. Effects of exposure on mixed lymphocyte reactivity in vitro and induction of suppressor cells. *Immunopharmacology* 1988;16:13–23.
37. Lundberg K, Dencker L, Gronvik K-O. Effects of 2,3,7,8-tetrachlorodibenzo-*p*-dioxin (TCDD) treatment in vivo on thymocyte functions in mice after activation in vitro. *Int J Immunopharmacol* 1990;12:459–466.
38. Steppan LB, DeKrey GK, Fowles JR, Kerkvliet NI. Polychlorinated biphenyl (PCB) induced alterations in the cytokine profile in the peritoneal cavity of mice during the course of P815 tumor rejection. *J Immunol* 1993;150:134A.
39. Luster MI, Germolec DR, Clark G, Wiegand G, Rosenthal GJ. Selective effects of 2,3,7,8-tetrachlorodibenzo-*p*-dioxin and corticosteroid on in vitro lymphocyte maturation. *J Immunol* 1988;140: 928–935.
40. Morris DL, Jordan SD, Holsapple MP. Effects of 2,3,7,8-tetrachlorodibenzo-*p*-dioxin (TCDD) on humoral immunity: I. Similarities to *Staphylococcus aureus* Cowan strain I (SAC) in the in vitro T-dependent antibody response. *Immunopharmacology* 1991;21:159–170.
41. Kramer CM, Johnson KW, Dooley RK, Holsapple MP. 2,3,7,8-Tetrachlorodibenzo-*p*-dioxin (TCDD) enhances antibody production and protein kinase activity in murine B cells. *Biochem Biophys Res Commun* 1987;145:25–32.
42. Clark GC, Bland JA, Germolec DR, Luster MI. 2,3,7,8-Tetrachlorodibenzo-*p*-dioxin stimulation of tyrosine phosphorylation in B lymphocytes: potential role in immunosuppression. *Mol Pharmacol* 1991;39:495–501.
43. Vos JG, Kreeftenberg JG, Engel HWB, Minderhoud A, Van Noorle Jansen LM. Studies on 2,3,7,8-tetrachlorodibenzo-*p*-dioxin-induced immune suppression and decreased resistance to infection: endotoxin hypersensitivity, serum zinc concentrations and effect of thymosin treatment. *Toxicology* 1978;9:75–86.
44. Mantovani A, Vecchi A, Luini W, Sironi M, Candiani GP, Spreafico F, Garattini S. Effect of 2,3,7,8-tetrachlorodibenzo-*p*-dioxin on macrophage and natural killer cell mediated cytotoxicity in mice. *Biomedicine* 1980;32:200–204.
45. Ackermann MF, Gasiewicz TA, Lamm KR, Germolec DR, Luster MI. Selective inhibition of polymorphonuclear neutrophil activity by 2,3,7,8-tetrachlorodibenzo-*p*-dioxin. *Toxicol Appl Pharmacol* 1989;101:470–480.
46. Weissberg JB, Zinkl JG. Effects of 2,3,7,8-tetrachlorodibenzo-*p*-dioxin upon hemostasis and hematologic function in the rat. *Environ Health Perspect* 1973;5:119–123.
47. Vos JG, Moore JA, Zinkl JG. Effect of 2,3,7,8-tetrachlorodibenzo-*p*-dioxin on the immune system of laboratory animals. *Environ Health Perspect* 1973;5:149–162.
48. Vos JG, Moore JA, Zinkl JG. Toxicity of 2,3,7,8-tetrachlorodibenzo-*p*-dioxin (TCDD) in C57Bl/6 mice. *Toxicol Appl Pharmacol* 1974;29:229–241.
49. Puhvel SM, Sakamoto M. Effect of 2,3,7,8-tetrachlorodibenzo-*p*-dioxin on murine skin. *J Invest Dermatol* 1988;90:354–358.
50. Alsharif NZ, Lawson T, Stohs SJ. TCDD-induced production of superoxide anion and DNA single strand breaks in peritoneal macrophages of rats. *Toxicologist* 1990;10:276 (abst).
51. Thomas PT, Hinsdill RD. Effect of polychlorinated biphenyls on the immune responses of rhesus monkeys and mice. *Toxicol Appl Pharmacol* 1978;44:41–51.
52. Thomas PT, Hinsdill RD. The effect of perinatal exposure to tetrachlorodibenzo-*p*-dioxin on the immune response of young mice. *Drug Chem Toxicol* 1979;2:77–98.
53. Loose, LD, Silkworth JB, Mudzinski SP, Pittman KA, Benitz KF, Mueller W. Environmental chemical-induced immune dysfunction. *Ecotoxicol Environ Safety* 1979;2:173–198.
54. Clark GC, Taylor MJ, Tritscher AM, Lucier GW. Tumor necrosis factor involvement in 2,3,7,8-tetrachlorodibenzo-*p*-dioxin-mediated endotoxin hypersensitivity in C57Bl/6 mice congenic at the Ah locus. *Toxicol Appl Pharmacol* 1991;111:422–431.
55. Taylor MJ, Clark GC, Atkins ZZ, Lucier G, Luster MI. 2,3,7,8-Tetrachlorodibenzo-*p*-dioxin increases the release of tumor necrosis factor-alpha (TNF-α) and induces ethoxyresorufin-*o*-deethylase (EROD) activity in rat Kupffer's cells (KCs). *Toxicologist* 1990;10:276 (abst).
56. Hoglen N, Swim A, Robertson L, Shedlofsky S. Effects of xenobiotics on serum tumor necrosis factor (TNF) and interleukin-6 (IL-6) release after LPS in rats. *Toxicologist* 1992;12:290 (abst).

57. Rosenthal GJ, Lebetkin E, Thigpen JE, Wilson R, Tucker AN, Luster MI. Characteristics of 2, 3,7,8-tetrachlorodibenzo-*p*-dioxin induced endotoxin hypersensitivity: association with hepatotoxicity. *Toxicology* 1989;56:239–251.
58. Moos A, Steppan L, Kerkvliet NI. Interleukin 1 (IL-1) and tumor necrosis factor (TNF) activity in a model of 2,3,7,8-tetrachlorodibenzo-*p*-dioxin (TCDD) induced hyperinflammation. *J Immunol* 1993;150:138A.
59. Theobald HM, Moore RW, Katz LB, Peiper RO, Peterson RE. Enhancement of carrageenan and dextran-induced edemas by 2,3,7,8-tetrachlorodibenzo-*p*-dioxin and related compounds. *J Pharmacol Exp Ther* 1983;225:576–583.
60. Katz LB, Theobald HM, Bookstaff RC, Peterson RE. Characterization of the enhanced paw edema response to carrageenan and dextran in 2,3,7,8-tetrachlorodibenzo-*p*-dioxin-treated rats. *J Pharmacol Exp Ther* 1984;230:670–677.
61. White KL, Lysy HH, McCay JA, Anderson AC. Modulation of serum complement levels following exposure to polychlorinated dibenzo-*p*-dioxins. *Toxicol Appl Pharmacol* 1986;84:209–219.
62. Sutter TR, Guzman K, Dold KM, Greenlee WF. Targets for dioxin: genes for plasminogen activator inhibitor-2 and interleukin-1β. *Science* 1991;254:415–418.
63. Steppan LB, Kerkliet NI. Influence of 2,3,7,8-tetrachlorodibenzo-*p*-dioxin (TCDD) on the production of inflammatory cytokine mRNA by C57Bl/6 macrophages. *Toxicologist* 1991;11:35 (abst).
64. Thigpen JE, Faith RE, McConnell EE, Moore JA. Increased susceptibility to bacterial infection as a sequela of exposure to 2, 3, 7, 8-tetrachlorodibenzo-*p*-dioxin. *Infect Immun* 1975;12:1319–1324.
65. Hinsdill RD, Couch DL, Speirs RS. Immunosuppression in mice induced by dioxin (TCDD) in feed. *J Environ Pathol Toxicol* 1980;4(2-3):401–425.
66. Luster MI, Boorman GA, Dean JH, Harris MW, Luebke RW, Padarathsingh ML, Moore JA. Examination of bone marrow, immunologic parameters and host susceptibility following pre- and postnatal exposure to 2,3,7,8-tetrachlorodibenzo-*p*-dioxin (TCDD). *Int J Immunopharmacol* 1980;2: 301–310.
67. Luster MI, Boorman GA, Harris MW, Moore JA. Laboratory studies on polybrominated biphenyl-induced immune alterations following low-level chronic and pre-/postnatal exposure. *Int J Immunopharmacol* 1980;2:69–80.
67a. Burleson GR, Lebrec H, Yang YG, Ibanes JD, Pennington KN, Birnbaum LS. Effect of 2, 3, 7, 8-tetrachlorodibenzo-p-dioxin (TCDD) on influenza virus host resistance in mice. *Fund Appl Toxicol [in press]*.
68. Yang YG, Lebrec H, Burleson GR. Effect of 2,3,7,8-tetrachlorodibenzo-*p*-dioxin (TCDD) on natural killer (NK) activity, viral replication and tumor metastasis in rats *Fund Appl Toxicol [in press]*.
69. Tucker AN, Vore SJ, Luster MI. Suppression of B cell differentiation by 2,3,7,8-tetrachlorodibenzo-*p*-dioxin. *Mol Pharmacol* 1986;29:372–377.
70. Kerkvliet NI, Kimeldorf DJ. Antitumor activity of a polychlorinated biphenyl mixture, Aroclor 1254, in rats inoculated with Walker 256 carcinosarcoma cells. *J Natl Cancer Inst* 1977;59:951–955.
71. Holsapple MP, Dooley RK, McNerney PJ, McCay JA. Direct suppression of antibody responses by chlorinated dibenzodioxins in cultured spleen cells from (C57Bl/6 × C3H)F1 and DBA/2 mice. *Immunopharmacology* 1986;12:175–186.
72. Holsapple MP, McCay JA, Barnes DW. Immunosuppression without liver induction by subchronic exposure to 2,7-dichlorodibenzo-*p*-dioxin in adult female B6C3F1 mice. *Toxicol Appl Pharmacol* 1986;83:445–455.
73. Davis D, Safe S. Halogenated aryl hydrocarbon-induced suppression of the in vitro plaque-forming cell response to sheep red blood cells is not dependent on the Ah receptor. *Immunopharmacology* 1991;21:183–190.
74. Morris DL, Jeong HG, Stevens WD, Chun YJ, Holsapple MP. Serum modulation of the effects of TCDD on the *in vitro* antibody response and on enzyme induction in primary hepatocytes. *Immunopharmacology* 1994;27:93–105.
75. Prell RA, Neumann CM, Oughton JA, Kerkvliet NI. Autologous mouse serum enhances T cell responsiveness to anti-CD3 stimulation. *J Immunol* 1993;150:266A.
76. Neumann CM, Steppan LB, Kerkvliet NI. Distribution of 2,3,7,8-tetrachlorodibenzo-*p*-dioxin (TCDD) in splenic tissue of C57Bl/6J mice. *Drug Metab Dispos* 1992;20:467–469.
77. DeKrey GK, Steppan LB, Deyo JA, Kerkvliet NI. PCB-induced immune suppression: castration, but not adrenalectomy or RU 38486 treatment, partially restores the suppressed cytotoxic T lymphocyte response to alloantigen. *J Pharmacol Exp Ther* 1993;267:308–315.

78. van Logten MJ, Gupta BN, McConnell EE, Moore JA. Role of the endocrine system in the action of 2,3,7,8-tetrachlorodibenzo-*p*-dioxin (TCDD) on the thymus. *Toxicology* 1980;15:135–144.
79. Pazdernik TL, Rozman KK. Effect of thyroidectomy and thyroxine on 2,3,7,8-tetrachlorodibenzo-*p*-dioxin induced immunotoxicity. *Life Sci* 1985;36:695–703.
80. Benjamini E, Leskowitz S. *Immunology. A short course, 2nd ed.* New York: Wiley-Liss; 1991:26.
81. Silkworth JB, Antrim L. Relationship between Ah receptor-mediated polychlorinated biphenyl (PCB)-induced humoral immunosuppression and thymic atrophy. *J Pharmacol Exp Ther* 1985;235: 606–611.
82. Clarke AG, MacLennan KA. The many facets of thymic involution. *Immunol Today* 1986;7:204–205.
83. Vos JG, Moore JA. Suppression of cellular immunity in rats and mice by maternal treatment with 2,3,7,8-tetrachlorodibenzo-*p*-dioxin. *Int Arch Allergy* 1974;47:777–794.
84. Faith RE, Luster MI, Moore JA. Chemical separation of helper cell function and delayed hypersensitivity responses. *Cell Immunol* 1978;40:275–284.
85. Greenlee WF, Dold KM, Irons RD, Osborne R. Evidence for direct action of 2,3,7,8-tetrachlorodibenzo-*p*-dioxin (TCDD) on thymic epithelium. *Toxicol Appl Pharmacol* 1985;79:112–120.
86. Cook JC, Dold KM, Greenlee WF. An *in vitro* model for studying the toxicity of 2,3,7,8-tetrachlorodibenzo-*p*-dioxin to human thymus. *Toxicol Appl Pharmacol* 1987;89:256–268.
87. Dencker L, Hassoun E, d'Argy R, Alm G. Fetal thymus organ culture as an in vitro model for the toxicity of 2,3,7,8-tetrachlorodibenzo-*p*-dioxin and its congeners. *Mol Pharmacol* 1985;28:357–363.
88. d'Argy R, Bergman J, Dencker L. Effects of immunosuppressive chemicals on lymphoid development in foetal thymus organ cultures. *Pharmacol Toxicol* 1989;64:33–38.
89. Blaylock BL, Holladay SD, Comment CE, Heindel JJ, Luster MI. Exposure to tetrachlorodibenzo-*p*-dioxin (TCDD) alters fetal thymocyte maturation. *Toxicol Appl Pharmacol* 1992;112: 207–213.
90. Nikolaidis E, Brunstrom B, Dencker L, Veromaa T. TCDD inhibits the support of B-cell development by the bursa of Fabricius. *Pharmacol Toxicol* 1990;67:22–26.
91. Fine JS, Gasiewicz TA, Silverstone AE. Lymphocyte stem cell alterations following perinatal exposure to 2,3,7,8-tetrachlorodibenzo-*p*-dioxin. *Mol Pharmacol* 1989;35:18–25.
92. Fine JS, Gasiewicz TA, Fiore NC, Silverstone AE. Prothymocyte activity is reduced by perinatal 2,3,7,8-tetrachlorodibenzo-*p*-dioxin exposure. *J Exp Pharmacol Ther* 1990;255:1–5.
93. Holladay SD, Lindstrom P, Blaylock BL, Comment CE, Germolec DR, Heindell JJ, Luster MI. Perinatal thymocyte antigen expression and postnatal immune development altered by gestational exposure to tetrachlorodibenzo-*p*-dioxin (TCDD). *Teratology* 1991;44:385–393.
94. Takagi Y, Aburada S, Otake T, Ikegami N. Effect of polychlorinated biphenyls (PCBs accumulated in the dam's body on mouse filial immunocompetence. *Arch Environ Contam Toxicol* 1987; 16:375–381.
95. Hong R, Taylor K, Abonour R. Immune abnormalities associated with chronic TCDD exposure in rhesus. *Chemosphere* 1989;18:313–320.
96. Neubert R, Jacob-Muller U, Stahlmann R, Helge H, Neubert D. Polyhalogenated dibenzo-*p*-dioxins and dibenzofurans and the immune system. 1. Effects on peripheral lymphocyte subpopulations of a non-human primate (*Callithrix jacchus*) after treatment with 2,3,7,8-tetrachlorodibenzo-*p*-dioxin (TCDD). *Arch Toxicol* 1990;64:345–359.
97. Neubert R, Jacob-Muller U, Helge H, Stahlmann R, Neubert D. Polyhalogenated dibenzo-*p*-dioxins and dibenzofurans and the immune system. 2. In vitro effects of 2,3,7,8-tetrachlorodibenzo-*p*-dioxin (TCDD) on lymphocytes of venous blood from man and a non-human primate (*Callithrix jacchus*). *Arch Toxicol* 1991;65:213–219.
98. Neubert R, Golor G, Stahlmann R, Helge H, Neubert D. Polyhalogenated dibenzo-*p*-dioxins and dibenzofurans and the immune system. 4. Effects of multiple-dose treatment with 2,3,7,8-tetrachlorodibenzo-*p*-dioxin (TCDD) on peripheral lymphocyte subpopulations of a non-human primate (*Callithrix jacchus*). *Arch Toxicol* 1992;66:250–259.
99. Truelove J, Grant D, Mes J, Tryphonas H, Tryphonas L, Zawidzka Z. Polychlorinated biphenyl toxicity in the pregnant cynomolgus monkey: a pilot study. *Arch Environ Contam Toxicol* 1982; 11:583–588.
100. Hori S, Obana H, Kashimoto T, et al. Effect of polychlorinated biphenyls and polychlorinated quaterphenyls in cynomolgus monkey (*Macaca fasicularis*). *Toxicology* 1982;24:123–139.

101. Tryphonas H, Hayward S, O'Grady L, Loo JCK, Arnold DL, Bryce F, Zawidzka ZZ. Immunotoxicity studies of PCB (Aroclor 1254) in the adult rhesus (*Macaca mulatta*) monkey—preliminary report. *Int J Immunopharmacol* 1989;11:199–206.
102. Tryphonas H, Luster MI, Schiffman G, et al. Effect of chronic exposure of PCB (Aroclor 1254) on specific and nonspecific immune parameters in the rhesus (*Macaca mulatta*) monkey. *Fundam Appl Toxicol* 1991;16:773–786.
103. Tryphonas H, Luster MI, White KL Jr, et al. Effects of PCB (Aroclor 1254) on non-specific immune parameters in rhesus (*Macaca mulatta*) monkeys. *Int J Immunopharmacol* 1991;13:639–648.
104. Lu Y-C, Wu Y-C. Clinical findings and immunological abnormalities in Yu-Cheng patients. *Environ Health Perspect* 1985;59:17–29.
105. Bekesi JG, Anderson HA, Roboz JP, Roboz J, Fischbein A, Selikoff IJ, Holland JF. Immunologic dysfunction among PBB-exposed Michigan dairy farmers. *Ann NY Acad Sci* 1979;320:717–728.
106. Webb KB, Evans RG, Knutsen AP, et al. Medical evaluation of subjects with known body levels of 2,3,7,8-tetrachlorodibenzo-*p*-dioxin. *J Toxicol Environ Health* 1989;28:183–193.
107. Hoffman RE, Stehr-Green PA, Webb KB, et al. Health effects of long-term exposure to 2,3,7,8-tetrachlorodibenzo-*p*-dioxin. *JAMA* 1986;255:2031–2038.
108. Evans RG, Webb KB, Knutsen AP, et al. A medical follow-up of the health effects of long-term exposure to 2,3,7,8-tetrachlorodibenzo-*p*-dioxin. *Arch Environ Health* 1988;43:273–278.
109. Stehr-Green PA, Naylor PH, Hoffman RE. Diminished thymosin alpha-1 levels in persons exposed to 2,3,7,8-tetrachlorodibenzo-*p*-dioxin. *J Toxicol Environ Health* 1989;28:285–295.
110. Mocarelli PL, Marocchi A, Brambilla P, Gerthoux P, Young DS, Mantel N. Clinical laboratory manifestations of exposure to dioxin in children, a six-year study of the effects of an environmental disaster near Seveso, Italy. *JAMA* 1986;256:2687–2695.
111. Tognoni G, Bonaccorsi A. Epidemiological problems with TCDD (a critical view). *Drug Metab Rev* 1982;13:447–469.

Immunotoxicology and Immunopharmacology, Second Edition, edited by J. H. Dean, M. I. Luster, A. E. Munson, and I. Kimber.
Raven Press, Ltd., New York © 1994.

7

Mechanisms of Polycyclic Aromatic Hydrocarbon Immunotoxicity

Kimber L. White, Jr., *Thomas T. Kawabata, and †Gregory S. Ladics

*Departments of Biomedical Engineering, Pharmacology, and Toxicology, Medical College of Virginia, Virginia Commonwealth University, Richmond, Virginia 23298; *Procter & Gamble, Cincinnati, Ohio 45239; and †Department of Central Research and Development, DuPont Company, Haskell Laboratory, Newark, Delaware 19714*

Polycyclic aromatic hydrocarbons (PAHs) are ubiquitous environmental contaminants that enter the environment by various natural routes including through the decay of organic materials, during forest fires, and as a result of volcanic eruptions. Humans also contribute to the environmental levels of PAHs through the burning of fossil fuels, particularly gasoline, diesel fuel, and coal (1). It was the use of coal as an early source of home heating fuel that began the study of chemical carcinogenesis through the subsequent observations of the London surgeon, Percival Potts, of the high incidence of epithelioma of the scrotum among chimney sweeps exposed to coal residue in the form of soot. The subsequent induction of tumors in an animal model by repeated application of coal tar in studies conducted by Yamagiwa and Ichikawa ushered in the era of experimental carcinogenesis (2). Benzo[*a*]pyrene (BaP), which was the first carcinogenic compound isolated from coal tar (3), is also the prototype immunosuppressive PAH.

The PAHs represent a class of compounds that have been extensively studied for their carcinogenic and mutagenic activities. Because many of the PAHs have also been found to be potent immunosuppressants as well as environmental contaminants, this class of compounds has been well studied with regard to their effect on the immune system. The effects of PAHs on the immune system have been reviewed in detail (4,5). The most extensively studied PAHs are BaP and 7,12-dimethylbenz[*a*]anthracene (DMBA), the prototype methylated PAH. Humoral immune responses have been shown to be suppressed by BaP exposure, whereas cell-mediated immune responses and innate immunity, for example, natural killer (NK) cell activity, remain unaffected. In contrast, DMBA suppresses the cell-mediated immune responses, NK cell activity, and humoral immune responses at much lower doses than BaP. Furthermore, numerous studies have shown that many PAHs, including BaP and DMBA, are capable of suppressing immune responses of animals *in vivo* and human and animal lymphocytes *in vitro*, as well as decreasing host resistance to microbial pathogens and tumors in various animal models (6–20). While the ability of PAHs to compromise the immune system has been reported repeatedly, the mechanism(s) by which PAHs suppress the immune response has been studied to only a limited extent. This chapter focuses on the proposed mechanisms by which PAHs, particularly the prototype compounds BaP and DMBA, mediate their immunosuppressive actions.

MECHANISMS OF PAH IMMUNOTOXICITY

In reviewing the potential mechanisms by which PAHs can suppress the immune system, it is convenient to divide the mechanisms into those related to the parent compounds and those related to reactive metabolites. Obviously, this grouping is artificial and not mutually exclusive. In most of the mechanistic studies undertaken, only the parent compounds were utilized and no attempt was made to determine if the immunosuppressive moiety was the parent compound or a metabolite. As a result, those mechanisms that attribute the effect to the parent compound may, in fact, be due to a metabolite produced. As of this time the actual mechanisms of PAH-induced immunosuppression still remain to be definitively established. Various mechanisms of action have been postulated by researchers working in this field. Several of the proposed mechanisms are discussed briefly below, while the mechanism that is consistent with the established carcinogenic and mutagenic actions of PAHs (i.e., formation of reactive metabolites) is discussed in detail.

Interaction with the Ah Receptor

Many of the immunosuppressive PAHs have been shown to bind to the Ah receptor (21–23). This observation and the association of PAHs and the halogenated aromatic hydrocarbons (HAHs) to suppress the immune system have led some to postulate that the immunosuppressive action of PAHs is through Ah receptor binding and subsequent activation of the *Ah* gene complex (24). While this proposed mechanism is still under study, there are several lines of *in vitro* and *in vivo* evidence which do not support this concept. For example, in competitive binding studies with 2,3,7,8-tetrachlorodibenzo-*p*-dioxin (TCDD) (21), BaP and benzo[*a*]-anthracene were shown to have identical concentration response curves. However, BaP has been shown repeatedly to be more immunosuppressive than benz[a]anthracene in both *in vitro* and *in vivo* studies. Similarly, binding studies by Okey et al. (23) using both mouse and rat hepatic cytosols found similar Ah binding affinity for TCDD, 3-methylcholanthrene, and dibenz[*a*,*h*]anthracene. However, these compounds also differ significantly in their ability to suppress the immune response. In the *in vivo* studies of White et al. (13) using Ah response B6C3F1 mice and nonresponse DBA/2 mice, the authors reported greater immunosuppression of the antibody-forming cell (AFC) response in the DBA/2 mice following treatment with BaP, DMBA, or 3-methylcholanthrene than in the Ah responsive B6C3F1 mice. Similarly, Thurmond et al. (17), using Ah-congenic C57BL/6J (responsive B6-Ah^bAh^d and nonresponsive B6-Ah^dAh^d) and multiple immunologic endpoints, observed that the overall differences between immunosuppressive responses of splenocytes from the congenic strains treated *in vivo* with DMBA were not significantly different. Even the role of Ah receptor binding in HAH-induced immunosuppression has come under question with the reports of Ah receptor-independent mechanisms of immunosuppression by HAHs (25–27).

Membrane Perturbation Effects

Many of the PAHs have a planar structure and are highly lipophilic; this is particularly true for the immunosuppressive PAHs. Pallardy et al. (28), have suggested that some PAHs (e.g., DMBA) may exert immunomodulatory effects by entering the membrane of cells and disrupting transduction of transmembrane signals and/or altering the conformation of receptors in the membrane. In their studies using human peripheral blood mononuclear cells (PBMCs), these authors reported DMBA decreased the membrane fluidity of resting T lymphocytes. In proliferation studies, they demonstrated DMBA had to be present at the initiation of cell activation to induce immunosuppression. Furthermore, they were able to restore the proliferative ability of PBMCs, in the presence of DMBA, through the use of pharmacologic agents that bypassed receptor triggering and mimic downstream events. Additional studies with planar lipophilic PAHs, which are not immunosuppressive, such as benzo[*e*]pyrene and pyrene, are needed to help confirm this proposed mechanism of PAH-induced immunosuppression.

Alterated Interleukin (IL) Production

A proposed mechanism of action that continues to receive considerable attention and has support from several research groups is the possibility that PAHs produce immunosuppressive effects as a result of alterations in the production of various ILs. In a series of studies from the same research group (29–32), BaP was shown to have effects on production of IL-1 and IL-2 but not IL-3. The consequences of BaP-altered IL production are further addressed in a later section of this chapter in the context of the cellular target of BaP. In studies also conducted with mouse splenocytes, Pallardy et al. (33), demonstrated that DMBA inhibited the production of IL-2 and IL-2 high-affinity receptor expression *in vitro* but did not alter expression of the low-affinity IL-2 receptor. Additionally, House et al. (18), were able to restore the DMBA suppression of the cytotoxic T lymphocyte (CTL) response by the *in vitro* addition of IL-2 to the CTL cultures. While effects on IL production currently represent a viable mechanism for PAH-induced immunosuppression, additional research in this field, including studies with inactive congeners, needs to be conducted.

Disruption of Intracellular Calcium (Ca^{2+}) Mobilization

Burchiel and colleagues (20) have established a relationship between immunosuppressive PAHs and altered mobilization of intracellular (Ca^{2+}). Using the Jurkat human T cell line, they found that, with *in vitro* exposure, DMBA produced a dose- and time-dependent inhibition of Ca^{2+} mobilization and a corresponding increase in free cytoplasmic Ca^{2+} following stimulation with the T cell mitogen phytohemagglutinin (PHA). Of particular interest was their observation that benzo[*e*]pyrene and anthracene, two nonimmunosuppressive PAHs, did not alter either Ca^{2+} mobilization or free cytoplasmic Ca^{2+} levels. In studies by Davis and Burchiel (34), it was also reported that *in vivo* DMBA exposure increased Ca^{2+} levels in resting B cells and inhibited B cell activation by anti-immunoglobulin D (anti-IgD) antibodies. More recent studies have also shown that *in vivo* exposure to DMBA produces increased intracellular levels of Ca^{2+} in cells of the spleen and Peyer's patches of B6C3F1 mice. However, thymocytes did not demonstrate an elevation in intracellular levels of Ca^{2+}. DNA fragmentation was observed in each of these three organs, which led the researchers to the conclusion that DMBA produces lymphotoxicity through an apoptosis-like mechanism involving fragmentation of genomic DNA by Ca^{2+}-activated enzymes (35). While DMBA and other PAHs may produce immunosuppression by altering intracellular levels of Ca^{2+} in lymphoid tissues, which appears to be at least one mechanism of lymphocyte cytotoxicity, the *in vivo* dose levels of DMBA necessary to alter intracellular levels of Ca^{2+} are significantly greater than doses that have been shown to decrease immune functions.

Metabolic Activation to Reactive Metabolites

The carcinogenic and mutagenic actions of PAHs have been shown to be mediated by reactive electrophilic metabolites rather than the parent compound. Based on this observation, it has been hypothesized that the immunotoxicity produced by PAHs is also mediated by reactive metabolites. Metabolic activation of a PAH in immune tissues could result in the generation of reactive metabolites, which may then bind to cellular nucleophilic target sites such as deoxyribonucleic acid (DNA), ribonucleic acid (RNA), and proteins that are important in mediating an immune response and/or maintaining cellular homeostasis. The metabolism schemes of BaP (Fig. 1) and DMBA (Fig. 2) have been well established. The potential reactive mutagenic and carcinogenic metabolites have also been identified. The abbreviations for each metabolite are listed in Table 1.

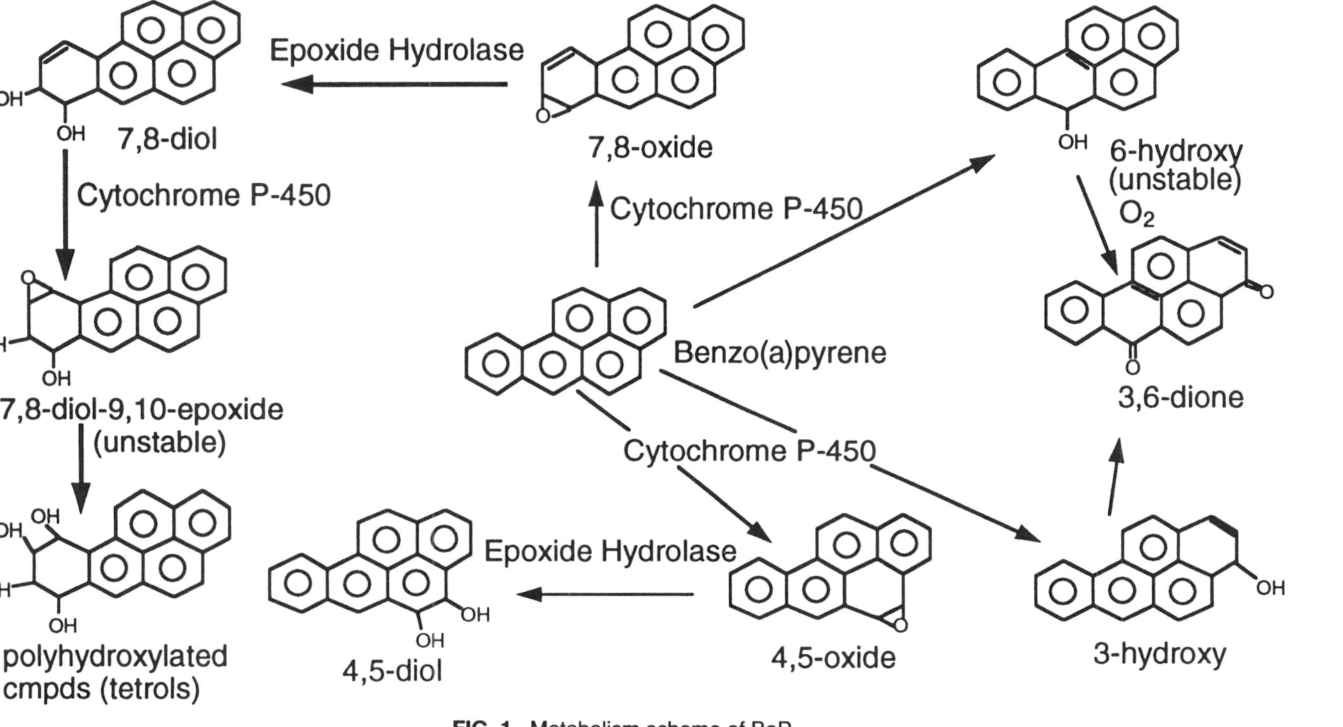

FIG. 1. Metabolism scheme of BaP.

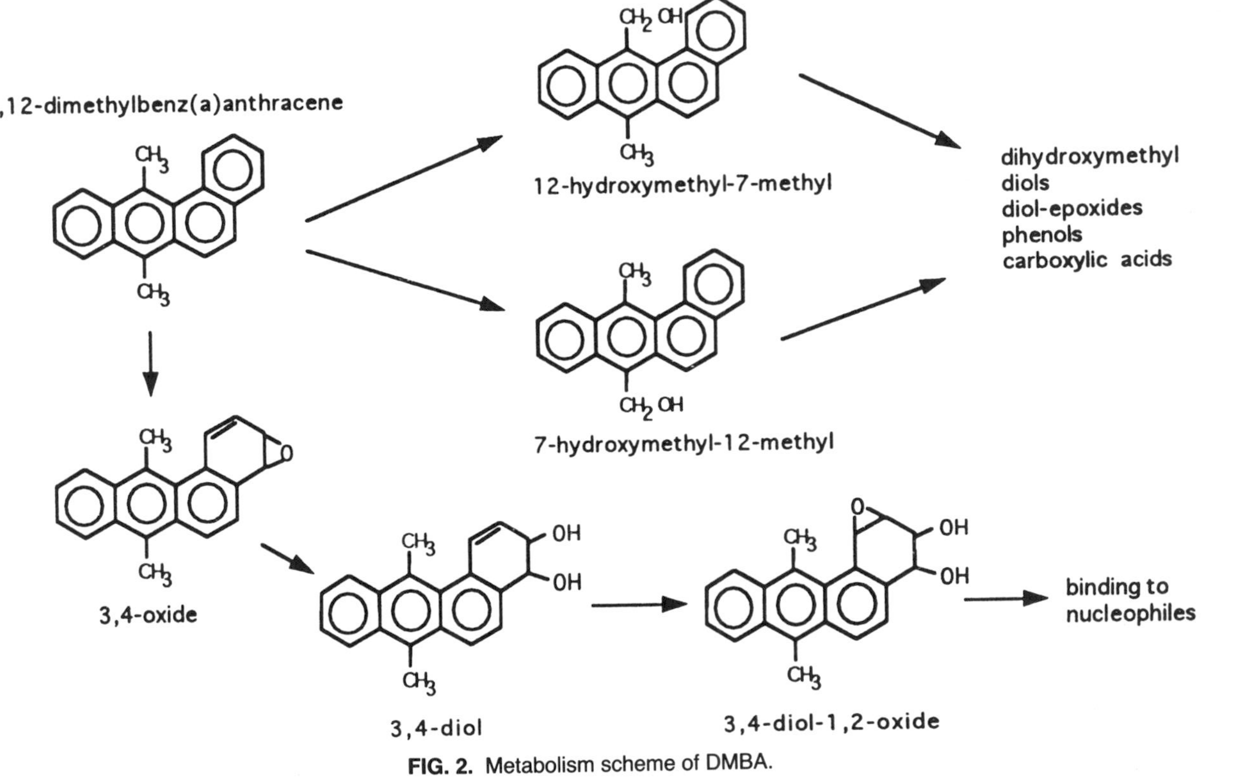

FIG. 2. Metabolism scheme of DMBA.

TABLE 1. *Abbreviations for metabolites*

Name of compound	Abbreviation
BaP-7,8-dihydroxy-7,8-dihydrodiol	BaP-7,8-diol
BaP-4,5-dihydroxy-4,5-dihydrodiol	BaP-4,5-diol
7,8-Dihydroxy-9,10-epoxy-7,8,9,10-tetrahydro-BaP	BPDE
DMBA-3,4-dihydroxy-3,4-dihydrodiol	DMBA-3,4-diol
DMBA-5,6-dihydroxy-5,6-dihydrodiol	DMBA-5,6-diol
7-Hydroxymethyl-12-methyl-benzanthracene	7-OHMe-12-Me-BA
7-Hydroxymethyl-12-hydroxy-methyl-benzanthracene	7-OHMe-12-OHMe-BA
3,4-Dihydro-1,2-epoxy-1,2,3,4-tetrahydroxy-7,12-DMBA	DMBA-3,4-diol-1,2-epoxide

In Vivo *and* In Vitro *Structure–Activity Studies*

Indirect evidence that reactive metabolites mediate the immunosuppression observed following PAH exposure has come from *in vivo* immunotoxicity structure–activity studies. In these studies (5,13), the relationship between metabolism and immunotoxicity was examined by comparing the immunosuppressive actions of a variety of carcinogenic and noncarcinogenic PAHs. The carcinogenic PAHs used in these studies had been studied extensively for their mutagenic and carcinogenic effects and were known to require metabolic activation to produce the ultimate carcinogenic and mutagenic metabolites. Conversely, the noncarcinogenic PAHs were known not to undergo metabolic activation. In an immunotoxicity study that evaluated ten PAHs, it was found that the noncarcinogenic PAHs (pyrelene, benzo[*e*]pyrene, and anthracene) did not produce immunosuppression, whereas the carcinogenic PAHs were found to suppress, to varying degrees, the *in vivo* IgM AFC response to the T-dependent antigen sheep erythrocytes (11).

A similar relationship between immunotoxicity and carcinogenic and noncarcinogenic PAHs has also been observed with *in vitro* studies. Direct addition of benzo[*e*]pyrene, anthracene, or naphthalene (13,36) to splenocyte cultures did not affect various immune responses, while BaP, DMBA, and 3-methylcholanthrene (3-MC) have been found to be immunosuppressive (4,8,11,13,15,16). DMBA was much more potent than BaP in its immunosuppressive effects, which ranks with its carcinogenic potency.

Role of Metabolism

In vitro studies have been undertaken to determine if the suppressive actions of PAHs on lymphoid cells are mediated by the parent compound or by its metabolites. It has been reported that either the addition of BaP (16) or DMBA (19) or selected metabolites to splenocyte cultures as capable of suppressing the *in vitro* AFC response to sheep red blood cells (sRBCs). The metabolites BaP-7,8-diol and DMBA-3,4-diol were found to be the most potent immunosuppressive metabolites evaluated, producing a concentration-dependent suppression of the AFC response similar to parent BaP and DMBA. In contrast, the BaP-4,5-diol and DMBA-5,6-diol metabolites did not suppress the AFC response. Others have shown that the BaP-7,8-diol and DMBA-3,4-diol undergo further metabolism to form the reactive BPDE (37–39) and 3,4-diol-1,2-epoxide-DMBA (40), whereas BaP-4,5-diol and DMBA-5,6-diol are not metabolized to reactive diol epoxides (Figs. 1 and 2), which might explain their different immunosuppressive activities. BPDE and 3,4-diol-1,2-epoxide-DMBA are the proposed ultimate carcinogenic forms of BaP (41–43) and DMBA (44–46). Direct addition of BPDE was shown to decrease the AFC response of cultured splenocytes at concentrations similar to BaP (47). These findings suggest that the *in vitro* immunosuppressive action of both BaP and DMBA were mediated by the diol epoxides.

It is also important to point out that other metabolites of BaP may act in conjunction with BPDE to produce BaP-induced immunosuppression. For example, Kawabata and White (16) also demonstrated that the 3-hydroxy, 4,5-epoxide, and 6,12-dione metabolites of BaP produced a slight but significant decrease in the AFC response without affecting cell viability. At higher concentrations, however, both cell viability and the AFC response were decreased. The 3-hydroxy-BaP can undergo further metabolism to quinone and reactive epoxide metabolites (48,49) (Fig. 1). Quinones (i.e., 6,12-dione) have been shown to undergo oxidation–reduction cycles involving quinone, hydroquinone, and molecular oxygen, resulting in the formation of oxygen radicals and semiquinone radicals (48). Macrophage peroxidases were found to catalyze the metabolic oxidation of hydroquinones to macromolecular binding metabolites (50). Such radicals may be involved in producing cellular injury and inhibition of cellular processes (51). The hydrolysis products of BPDE, the tetrol metabolites, may also contribute to the immunotoxic effects of BaP. *In vitro* studies have shown that tetrols can bind noncovalently to DNA by an intercalation mechanism (52–54).

α-*Naphthoflavone (ANF) Inhibits PAH Immunosuppression*

To further investigate the role of metabolism in PAH-induced immunosuppression, the effects of the cytochrome P450 inhibitor, ANF, on the BaP-, BaP-7,8-diol-, and DMBA-induced suppression of the *in vitro* AFC response were examined by Ladics et al. (19). These authors observed that the addition of ANF before the addition of BaP or DMBA resulted in an attenuation of the PAH-induced suppression to control levels. ANF is known to inhibit isozymes of cytochrome P450 induced by PAHs (55). This same P450 isozyme is responsible for the metabolism of BaP-7,8-diol and DMBA-3,4-diol to the diol epoxide metabolites. In contrast, Thurmond et al. (56) demonstrated that ANF was unable to reverse the DMBA-induced suppression of the *in vitro* lymphocyte proliferative immune response to concanavalin A (Con A). How ANF is able to reverse the AFC response to DMBA-induced suppression and not the proliferative response to Con A is not known.

Metabolism of PAHs by Spleen Cells

Although the metabolic capacities of extrahepatic tissue are substantially lower than the liver, metabolic activation of protoxicants like PAHs in potential target tissues, that is, those of the immune system, may play a critical role in determining their toxicity. It is well established that PAHs must be converted to reactive metabolites via cytochrome P450-dependent monoxygenase systems, in particular isozymes IA1 and IA2, to exert their carcinogenic and mutagenic effects (reviewed in refs. 37 and 39). PAH-induced immunosuppression may be mediated by reactive metabolites generated within target immune tissues, since splenocytes from numerous experimental species (12,57–60), as well as human peripheral lymphocytes (61), possess cytochrome P450, which are known to metabolize PAHs (47,62,63). Studies have also demonstrated that BaP can be metabolized to a number of metabolites by microsomal preparations of spleen cells (16,47). Metabolism was inhibited by ANF but not by SKF-525A (inhibitor of the phenobarbital-induced P450).

The metabolism of DMBA by murine splenocytes has been more difficult to demonstrate. Thurmond et al. (56) demonstrated that cultured splenocytes were unable to generate detectable metabolites for [^{14}C]DMBA. This may be due to the low specific activity of ^{14}C-labeled DMBA. In a study conducted by Kawabata and White (64) using ^{3}H-labeled DMBA (high specific activity) and splenic microsomes, detectable levels of diols and hydroxy-methyl metabolites were observed above that produced in control reactions (heat-inactivated microsomes). Since BaP and DMBA are metabolized by the same P450 isozyme, this finding is consistent with the demonstration that BaP is metabolized by splenic microsomes.

Metabolism of BaP Within Splenic Macrophages and T and B Lymphocytes

Recent studies by Ladics et al. (62,63) have shown that the macrophage population is capable of metabolizing BaP within the murine spleen (Figs. 3 and 4). Other splenic cell types examined [B and T cells, polymorphonuclear cells (PMNs), and the splenic capsule] did not produce amounts of BaP metabolites significantly above background levels. Additionally, exposure of mice to BaP (63) resulted in a significant increase in the amounts of some BaP metabolites generated by splenic macrophages. Consistent with the inability of B and T lymphocytes and PMNs to metabolize BaP, Germolec et al. (65) were unable to detect cytochrome P450 in unseparated splenic lymphocytes, while Bast et al. (59) could not detect basal or inducible aryl hydrocarbon hydroxylase (AHH) activity in peripheral blood PMNs. Additionally, freshly isolated lymphocytes were not found to contain measurable amounts of AHH activity until cultured in the presence of mitogens (66–68).

Data of Ladics et al. (62,63) are consistent with several studies examining the capability of macrophages and monocytes to metabolize PAHs and other xenobiotics. AHH activity has been shown to be present and inducible in cell types of

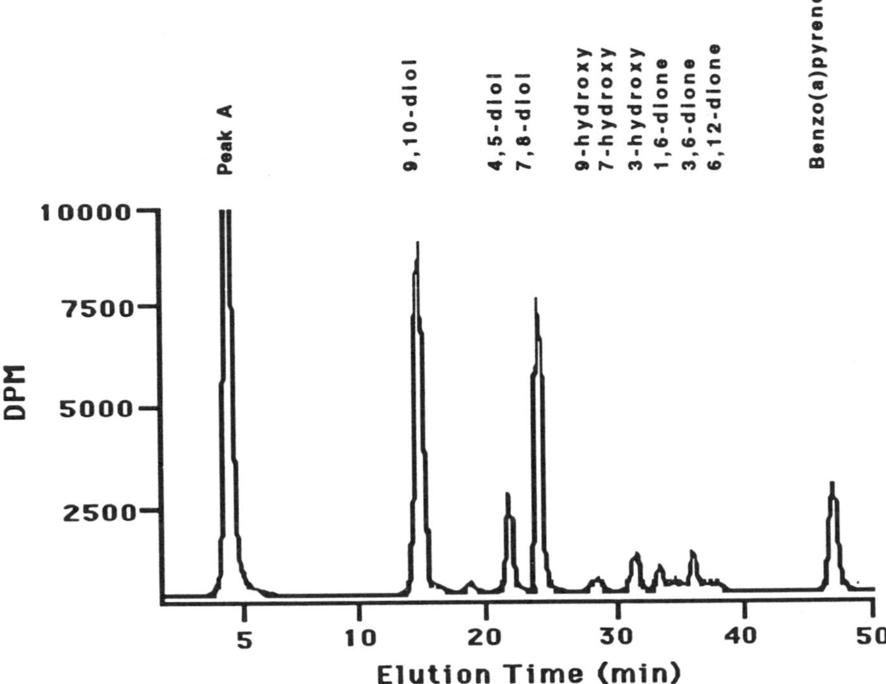

FIG. 3. Chromatogram of BaP metabolites produced by unseparated splenocytes of untreated mice. Splenocytes were incubated with [^{3}H]BaP for 24 hr and the metabolites extracted and then separated by high-performance liquid chromatography (HPLC). The number of disintegrations per minute (DPM) of the metabolites was monitored by a radiation flow detector.

the macrophage lineage of several species including Kupffer cells (69), peritoneal macrophages (70–72), and pulmonary alveolar macrophages (70,73). Tomingas et al. (70) and Palmer et al. (74) demonstrated that peritoneal macrophages could metabolize BaP and DMBA, respectively. Wickramasinghe (75) reported that splenic macrophages are capable of metabolizing certain drugs via a cytochrome P450-dependent mechanism, while Autrup et al. (76) showed that pulmonary alveolar macrophages metabolized BaP. AHH activity has also been shown to be present and inducible in monocytes (72,77,78). Lake et al. (78) demonstrated that human monocytes can metabolize BaP. Holz et al. (79) reported the presence of DNA adducts in human blood monocytes but not in unstimulated blood lymphocytes following *in vitro* incubation with BaP.

In studies by Kawabata and White (16), the relative degree of immunosuppression was BaP-7,8-diol>BaP-6,12-dione>BaP-4,5-epoxide>3-hydroxy-BaP. BaP-7,8-diol can be further oxidized to two different BPDE stereoisomers, the *anti* or *syn*, by both a cytochrome P450 pathway and an unsaturated fatty acid hydroperoxide-dependent co-oxygenation pathway via peroxyl radicals (39,80–84) (Fig.

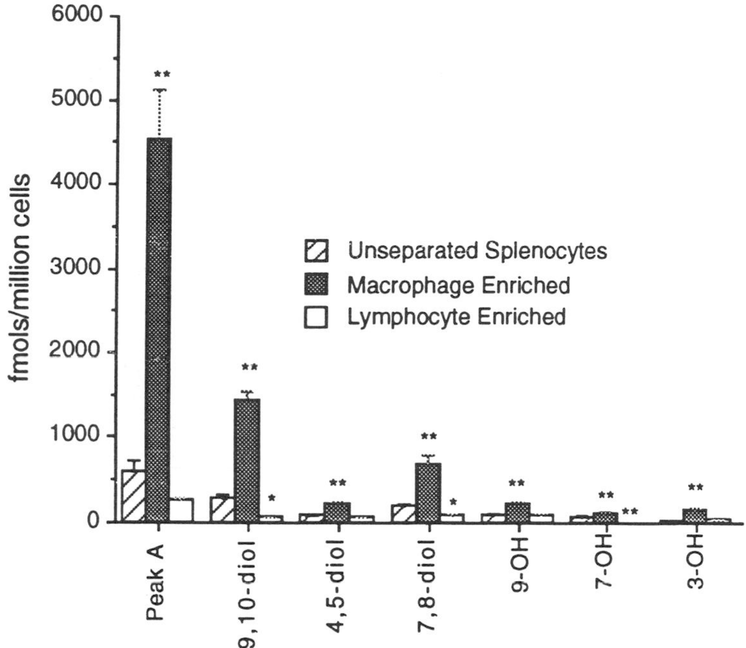

FIG. 4. The macrophage population is responsible for the metabolism of BaP within the spleen. Enriched macrophage and lymphocyte populations were incubated with [^{3}H]BaP for 24 hr. After 24 hr, BaP metabolites were isolated and then separated and quantitated by HPLC. Data are derived from three experiments. Results represent the mean ± SE with $n = 4$. *$p \leq 0.05$ versus unseparated splenocytes. **$p \leq 0.01$ versus unseparated splenocytes.

5). The two BPDEs are very unstable and undergo *cis* and *trans* addition of water to the epoxide group to form two stereoisomeric pairs of tetrol metabolites (reviewed in refs. 37 and 39). Importantly, the initial oxidation of BaP to BaP-7,8-oxide can only be mediated by cytochrome P450 because no other mammalian enzymes mediate the generation of PAH epoxides. BaP-7,8-oxide can then be hydrolyzed to BaP-7,8-diol via epoxide hydrolase (reviewed in ref. 39). Peroxyl radicals were found to only oxidize BaP to quinones (85). This finding was confirmed by Kawabata and White (47), who reported that with the addition of arachidonic acid (AA) as a cofactor in place of reduced nicotinamide adenine dinucleotide phosphate (NADPH), splenic microsomes only generated quinone metabolites when incubated with BaP. Ladics et al. (86) demonstrated that splenic macrophages were capable of generating BPDE from BaP (Fig. 6). Results further demonstrated that once macrophages generate BaP-7,8-diol, it may be metabolized to the two BPDE stereoisomers by both a cytochrome P450-dependent and -independent (peroxyl radical) pathway (86). Additionally, exposure of mice to BaP resulted in a significant increase in the amounts of each tetrol metabolite (i.e., BPDE) formed by macrophages when compared to those of vehicle-exposed animals (86).

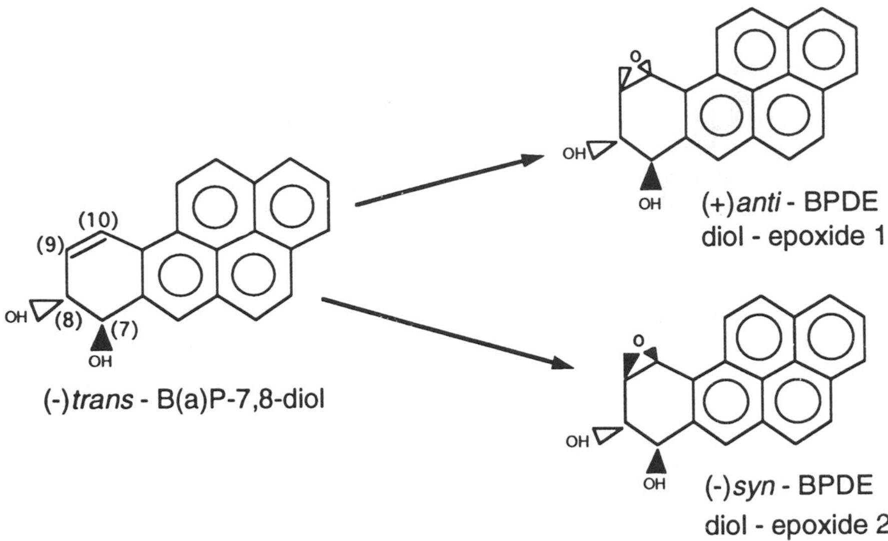

FIG. 5. Enzymatic epoxidation of the *trans*-BaP-7,8-diol to the *anti* and *syn* stereoisomers of BPDE.

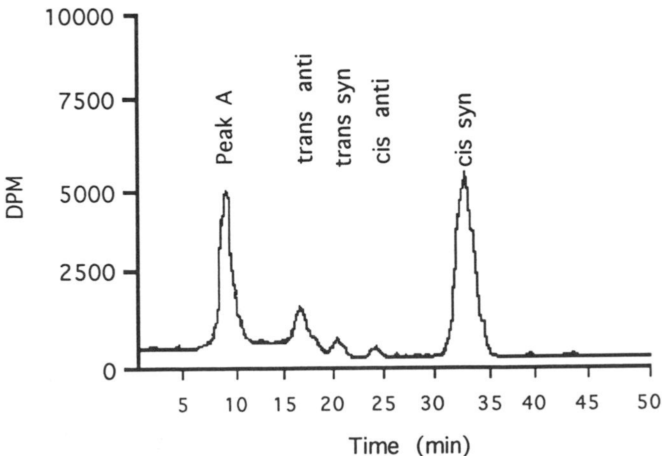

FIG. 6. Chromatogram of BaP tetrol metabolites produced by an enriched splenic macrophage population. Macrophages were incubated with [^{3}H]BaP for 24 hr and the generated tetrol metabolites (i.e., BPDE) detected via HPLC procedures. The number of DPM of the metabolites was monitored by a radiation flow detector.

BaP Metabolism and Effects on the Target Cell Population

Ladics et al. (62,63,86) demonstrated that macrophages are the cell types capable of metabolizing BaP within the murine spleen. As a result, the macrophages should be an excellent candidate as the target cell whose compromised immune functions are responsible for or contribute to PAH-induced immunosuppression. This postulate is consistent with several studies showing that the major cell type affected following BaP exposure is the macrophage. Meyers et al. (31) reported that exposure of mice to BaP decreased uptake, presentation, and/or processing of the T cell-dependent antigen, keyhole limpet hemocyanin by macrophages to antigen-primed T cells. The initiation of the T cell-dependent AFC response requires that macrophages or other accessory cells successfully process and present antigen to T helper cells in association with class II (Ia) antigens (87,88). *In vitro* time course studies have demonstrated an early requirement for BaP in culture in order to produce significant suppression of the AFC response to sRBCs (14). This early temporal requirement in the AFC response indicates possible effects on macrophage responses such as antigen processing/presentation or macrophage–lymphocyte interactions.

Ladics et al. (62) reported that the smaller, denser splenic macrophages appear to be more proficient at metabolizing BaP compared to the larger, less dense macrophages. Interestingly, in several studies where macrophages were separated based on density into several distinct subpopulations at various stages of differentiation, it was found that the small, more dense, less mature cells expressed large amounts of surface Ia, displayed peroxidase activity, and provided antigen-presenting function for T cell proliferative responses. Larger, less dense, more mature cells expressed little Ia antigen and were ineffective in antigen presentation (89–91). An intriguing possibility is that the smaller, denser macrophages, by virtue of their apparent increased capability to metabolize BaP, may be predisposed to the immunotoxic effects of BaP. Such a possibility could explain the decrease in the presentation and/or processing of antigen by macrophages following BaP exposure observed by Meyers et al. (31).

Lyte and Bick (29) demonstrated that addition of IL-1 to splenocyte cultures of BaP-treated mice attenuated the suppression of AFC responses to sRBCs to control levels. IL-1, which is produced by cells of macrophage–monocyte lineage, as well as other cell types, is critically important for the differentiation and proliferation of T and B lymphocytes in response to antigens such as the T cell-dependent antigen sRBCs (92,93). Following *in vivo* exposure of mice to BaP, the *in vitro* AFC response to both T cell-dependent and T cell-independent antigens was evaluated by Ladics et al. (63). BaP suppressed the primary AFC response to the T cell-dependent antigen sRBCs. Generation of an optimal AFC response to sRBCs is dependent on the presence of functional T lymphocytes, accessory cells (macrophages), and B lymphocytes (94–96). BaP was also found to significantly suppress the AFC response to the T cell-independent antigen dinitrophenyl–Ficoll (DNP-Ficoll) but not lipopolysaccharide (LPS). Unlike the AFC response to sRBCs or DNP-Ficoll, generation of an AFC response to LPS has been shown to require minimal participation of macrophages and T cells (97). Enumeration of splenocytes following *in vivo* exposure to BaP indicated that alterations in the *in vitro* AFC response were not due to alterations in total splenic cell number or the percentages of the various splenic cell subpopulations (macrophages, B and T cells) (63).

White and Holsapple (11) conducted *in vitro* studies where BaP was added directly to naive splenocyte cultures along with each of a number of different antigens. Addition of BaP was found to suppress the AFC response to both T cell-dependent and T cell-independent antigens but not the polyclonal response to LPS, again suggesting an effect of BaP on the macrophage population. Additionally, studies by Lyte et al. (30) and Meyers et al. (32) have demonstrated that BaP exposure results in a dose-dependent decrease in the IL-2 responsiveness of T cells (i.e., decreased IL-2 production, receptor expression, and proliferation to IL-2). As BaP-treated T cells were able to respond to IL-2 in the presence of untreated macrophages, the decrease was suggested by these authors to occur due to a defect in the capability of the macrophage to provide the necessary signals required by T cells to express IL-2 responsiveness. Following BaP exposure of mice, 2-mercaptoethanol (2-ME) was found to reverse the BaP-induced suppression of the AFC response to sRBCs (98). 2-ME is a compound believed to substitute for or enhance many macrophage functions (99,100).

Results of separation–reconstitution studies conducted by Blanton et al. (101) following a 14-day dosing regimen with 40 mg/kg BaP subcutaneously (sc) indicated that suppression of the AFC response was due to alterations in the splenic adherent (AD, macrophage) cell population. Blanton et al. (101) reported that cultures reconstituted with BaP-treated splenic AD cells + vehicle (VH)-treated nonadherent (NAD, B and T cells) cells were significantly suppressed compared to controls, while cultures containing VH-treated splenic AD + BaP-treated NAD cells were not statistically different from controls. Similarly, following exposure of mice for 4 days to 200 mg/kg BaP sc, separation–reconstitution studies by Ladics et al. (63) demonstrated that the suppression of the primary IgM antibody response was due to alterations in the splenic AD (macrophage) cell population rather than the NAD population.

Extrasplenic Metabolism in BaP-Induced Immunosuppression

A series of studies have suggested that following intraperitoneal (ip) exposure to BaP, immunosuppression *in vivo* may result from activation of BaP to BPDE in tissues (liver and lung) other than the spleen (102–104). BPDE was found to be released into the blood, sequestered and protected by the serum, and transported systemically to the spleen, where it was released and taken up by splenocytes. Similarly, others have demonstrated BPDE adducts in splenic DNA following ip exposure to BaP (105). Ginsberg et al. (104) also found that cultured splenocytes had a low capacity to generate BaP/DNA adducts and suggested that splenocytes had a low capacity to form BPDE from BaP. Based on these results, the reactive BPDE appears to be generated within the liver in contrast to the spleen. Ginsberg et al. (104), however, calculated BPDE-DNA adduct levels based on total splenic DNA. Since macrophages appear to be the cells capable of forming BPDE within the spleen (86), the majority of BPDE adducts formed would most likely be found in this cell population. Macrophages, however, make up only 4% to 8% of the total splenic cell population (106). Thus the total amount of adducts/mg DNA in the spleen would be low as found by Ginsberg and colleagues. Depending on the dose and route of administration of BaP, both hepatic and extrahepatic tissues (i.e., spleen) may play a role in generating BPDE. The biologic relevance of interorgan- versus intraorgan-generated reactive metabolites of BaP, however, has not been determined, while compounds, such as PAHs, can form many adducts with nucleophilic targets, only some of which are biologically relevant (107).

To ultimately make a correlation between the site of metabolic activation and the site of toxicity for PAHs such as BaP, studies investigating BaP adduct formation in different immune cell types need to be conducted. Also, studies examining individual adduct levels in different immune cell types and correlated with immunotoxicity are needed. These studies may not only allow for a better understanding of BaP-induced immunosuppression but may also help identify possible target cells for other immunosuppressive compounds requiring metabolic activation. While the mechanisms of PAH-induced immunosuppression still remain to be definitively established, there is a high probability that one or more of the mechanisms discussed here will be found to be responsible for or contribute to the immunosuppressive effects produced by this class of environmental contaminants.

REFERENCES

1. Baum E. Occurrence and surveillance of polycyclic aromatic hydrocarbons. In: Gelboin H, Ts'O T, eds. *Polycyclic hydrocarbons and cancer*, vol 1. New York: Academic Press; 1978;45–70.
2. Harvey RG. Polycyclic hydrocarbons and cancer. *Am Scientist* 1982;70:386–393.
3. Cook JW, Hewett CL, Heiger I. The isolation of cancer-producing hydrocarbon from coal tar. *J Chem Soc* 1933;135(1):395–405.
4. Ward EC, Murray MJ, Dean JH. Immunotoxicity of nonhalogenated polycyclic aromatic hydrocarbons. In: Dean JH, Luster MI, Munson AE, Amos H, eds. *Immunotoxicology and immunopharmacology*. New York: Raven Press; 1985:291–303.
5. White KL Jr. An overview of immunotoxicology and carciogenic polycyclic aromatic hyrdocarbons. *J Environ Sci Health* 1986;C4:163–202.
6. Stjernsward J. Effect of noncarcinogenic and carcinogenic hydrocarbons on antibody-forming cells measured at the cellular level *in vitro*. *J Natl Cancer Inst* 1966;36:1189–1195.
7. Zwilling BS. The effect of respiratory carcinogenesis on systemic humoral and cell-mediated immunity of Syrian golden hamsters. *Cancer Res* 1977;37:250–252.
8. Dean JH, Luster MI, Boorman GA, Lauer LD, Luebke RW, Lawson L. Selective immunosuppression resulting from exposure to the carcinogenic congener of benzopyrene in B6C3F1 mice. *Clin Exp Immunol* 1983;52:199–206.
9. Seidegard J, Depierre JW. Drug metabolizing enzymes in resting human lymphocytes. In: Rydstrom J, Montelius J, Bengtsson M, eds. *Extrahepatic drug metabolism and chemical carcinogenesis*. New York: Elsevier Science Publishers; 1983:209.

10. Ward EC, Murray MJ, Lauer LD, House RV, Irons R, Dean JH. Immunosuppression following 7,12-dimethylbenz[*a*]anthracene exposure in B6C3F1 mice. I. Effects on humoral immunity and host resistance. *Toxicol Appl Pharmacol* 1984;75:299–308.
11. White KL Jr, Holsapple MP. Direct suppression of *in vitro* antibody production by mouse spleen cells by the carcinogen benzo[*a*]pyrene but not the noncarcinogenic congener benzo[*e*]pyrene. *Cancer Res* 1984;44:3388–3393.
12. Wojdani A, Alfred LJ. Alterations in cell-mediated immune functions induced in mouse splenic lymphocytes by polycyclic aromatic hydrocarbons. *Cancer Res* 1984;44:942–945.
13. White KL Jr, Lysy HH, Holsapple MP. Immunosuppression by polycyclic aromatic hydrocarbons: a structure–activity relationship in B6C3F1 and DBA/2 mice. *Immunopharmacology* 1985;9:155–164.
14. Blanton RH, Lyte M, Myers MJ, Bick PH. Immunomodulation by polycyclic aromatic hydrocarbons in mice and murine cells. *Cancer Res* 1986;46:2735–2739.
15. Dean JH, Ward EC, Murray MJ, et al. Immunosuppression following 7,12-dimethylbenz[*a*]anthracene exposure in B6C3F1 mice. II. Altered cell-mediated immunity and tumor resistance. *Int J Immunopharmacol* 1986;8:189–198.
16. Kawabata TT, White KL Jr. Suppression of the *in vitro* humoral immune response of mouse splenocytes by benzo[*a*]pyrene and inhibition of benzo[*a*]pyrene-induced immunosuppression by α-naphthoflavone. *Cancer Res* 1987;47:2317–2322.
17. Thurmond LM, Lauer LD, House RV, Cook JC, Dean JH. Immunosuppression following exposure to 7,12-dimethylbenz[*a*]anthracene (DMBA) in *Ah*-responsive and *Ah*-nonresponsive mice. *Toxicol Appl Pharmacol* 1987;91:450–460.
18. House RV, Pallardy MJ, Dean JH. Suppression of murine cytotoxic T-lymphocyte induction following exposure to 7,12-dimethylbenz[*a*]anthracene: dysfunction of antigen recognition. *Int J Immunopharmacol* 1989;11:207–215.
19. Ladics GS, Kawabata TT, White KL Jr. Suppression of the *in vitro* humoral immune response of mouse splenocytes by 7,12-dimethylbenz[*a*]anthracene metabolites and inhibition of immunosuppression by α-naphthoflavone. *Toxicol Appl Pharmacol* 1991;110:31–44.
20. Burchiel SW, Thompson TA, Davis DP. Alterations in mitogen-induced calcium mobilization and intracellular free calcium produced by 7,12-dimethylbenz[*a*]anthracene in the Jurkat human T cell line. *Int J Immunopharmacol* 1991;13:109–115.
21. Poland A, Glover E, Kende AS. Stereospecific, high affinity binding of 2,3,7,8-tetrachlorodibenzo-*p*-dioxin by hepatic cytosol. *J Biol Chem* 1976;251:4936–4946.
22. Okey AB, Dube AW, Vella LM. Binding of benzo[*a*]pyrene and dibenz[*a,h*]anthracene to the Ah receptor in mouse and rat hepatic cytosols. *Cancer Res* 1984;44:1426–1432.
23. Okey AB, Vella LM, Iverson F. *Ah* receptor in primate liver: binding of 2,3,7,8-tetrachlorodibenzo-*p*-dioxin and carcinogenic aromatic hydrocarbons. *Can J Physiol Pharmacol* 1984;62:1292–1295.
24. Silkworth JB, Antrim L, Kaminsky LS. Correlations between polychlorinated biphenyl immunotoxicity, the aromatic hydrocarbon locus, and liver microsomal enzyme induction in C57BL/6 and DBA/2 mice. *Toxicol Appl Pharmacol* 1984;75:156–165.
25. Holsapple MP, McCay JA, Barnes DW. Immunosuppression without liver induction by subchronic exposure to 2,7-dichlorodibenzo-*p*-dioxin in adult female B6C3F1 mice. *Toxicol Appl Pharmacol* 1986;83:445–455.
26. Kerkvliet NI, Steppan LB, Brauner JA, Deyo JA, Henderson MC, Tomar RS, Buhler DR. Influence of the *Ah* locus on the humoral immunotoxicity of 2,3,7,8-tetrachlorodibenzo-*p*-dioxin: evidence for *Ah*-receptor-dependent and *Ah*-receptor-independent mechanisms of immunosuppression. *Toxicol Appl Pharmacol* 1990;105:26–36.
27. Davis D, Safe S. Halogenated aryl hydrocarbon-induced suppression of the *in vitro* plaque-forming cell response to sheep red blood cells is not dependent on the *Ah* receptor. *Immunopharmacology* 1991;21:183–190.
28. Pallardy M, Mishal Z, Lebrec H, Bohuon C. Immune modification due to chemical interference with transmembrane signalling: applications to polycyclic aromatic hydrocarbons. *Int J Immunopharmacol* 1992;14:377–382.
29. Lyte ML, Bick PH. Modulation of interleukin-1 production by macrophages following benzo[*a*]pyrene exposure. *Int J Immunopharmacol* 1986;8:377–381.
30. Lyte ML, Blanton RH, Myers MJ, Bick PH. Effect of *in vivo* administration of the carcinogen benzo[*a*]pyrene on interleukin-2 and interleukin-3 production. *Int J Immunopharmacol* 1987;9:307–312.

31. Meyers MJ, Schook LB, Bick PH. Mechanisms of benzo[*a*]pyrene-induced modulation of antigen presentation. *J Pharmacol Exp Ther* 1987;242:399–404.
32. Meyers MJ, Blanton RH, Bick PH. Inhibition of IL-2 responsiveness following exposure to benzo[*a*]pyrene is due to alterations in accessory cell function. *Int J Immunopharmacol* 1988;10:177–186.
33. Pallardy MJ, House RV, Dean JH. Molecular mechanism of 7,12-dimethylbenz[*a*]anthracene-induced immunosuppression: evidence for action via the interleukin-2 pathway. *Mol Pharmacol* 1989;36:128–133.
34. Davis DA, Burchiel SW. Inhibition of calcium-dependent pathways of B-cell activation by DMBA. *Toxicol Appl Pharmacol* 1992;116:202–208.
35. Burchiel SW, Davis DP, Ray SD, Archuleta MM, Thilsted JP, Corcoran GB. DMBA-induced cytotoxicity in lymphoid and nonlymphoid organs of B6C3F1 mice: relation of cell death to target cell intracellular calcium and DNA damage. *Toxicol Appl Pharmacol* 1992;113:126–132.
36. Kawabata TT, White KL Jr. Effects of naphthalene and napththalene metabolites on the in vitro humoral immune response. *J Toxicol Environ Health* 1990;30:53–67.
37. Gelboin HV. Carcinogens, enzyme induction, and gene action. *Cancer Adv Res* 1967;10:1–81.
38. Van Cantfort J, Gielen JE, Nebert DW. Benzo[*a*]pyrene metabolism in mouse liver. Association of both 7,8-epoxidation and covalent binding of a metabolite of the 7,8-diol with the Ah locus. *Biochem Pharmacol* 1985;34:1821–1826.
39. Osborne MR, Crosby NT. Benzopyrenes. In: Coombs MM, Ashby J, Newbold RF, eds. *Cambridge monographs on cancer research*. London: Cambridge University Press; 1986:1–330.
40. DiGiovanni G, Juchau MR. Biotransformation and bioactivation of 7,12-dimethylbenz[*a*]anthracene. *Drug Metab Rev* 1980;11:61–101.
41. Sims P, Grover PL, Swaisland A, Pal K, Hewer A. Metabolic activation of benzo[*a*]pyrene proceeds by a diol-epoxide. *Nature* 1974;252:326–328.
42. Thakker DR, Yagi H, Lu AYH, Levin W, Conney AH, Jerina DM. Metabolism of benzo[*a*]pyrene: conversion of (±)-*trans*-7,8-dihydroxy-7,8-dihydrobenzo[*a*]pyrene to highly mutagenic 7,8-diol-9,10-epoxides. *Proc Natl Acad Sci USA* 1976;73:3381–3385.
43. Wood AW, Chang RL, Levin W, Yagi H, Thakker DR, Jerina DM, Conney AH. Differences in mutagenicity of the optical enantiomers of the diastereomeric benzo[*a*]pyrene 7,8-diol-9,10-epoxides. *Biochem Biophys Res Commun* 1977;77:1389–1396.
44. Chou MW, Yang SK. Identification of four trans-3,4-dihydrodiol metabolites of 7,12-dimethylbenz[*a*]anthracene and their *in vitro* DNA binding activities upon further metabolism. *Proc Natl Acad Sci USA* 1978;75:5466–5470.
45. Dipple A, Tomaszewski JE, Moschel RC, Bigger CAH, Nebzydoski JA, Egan M. Comparison of metabolism-mediated binding to DNA of 7-hydroxymethyl-12-methylbenz[*a*]anthracene and 7,12-dimethylbenz[*a*]anthracene. *Cancer Res* 1979;39:1154–1158.
46. Huberman E, Chou MW, Yang SK. Identification of 7,12-dimethylbenz[*a*]anthracene metabolites that lead to mutagenesis in mammalian cells. *Proc Natl Acad Sci USA* 1979;76:862–866.
47. Kawabata TT, White KL Jr. Benzo[*a*]pyrene metabolism by murine spleen microsomes. *Cancer Res* 1989;49:5816–5822.
48. Lorentzen RS, Ts'O PO. Benzo[*a*]pyrenedione/benzo[*a*]pyrene diol oxidation reduction couples and the generation of reactive reduced molecular oxygen. *Biochemistry* 1977;16:1467–1473.
49. Owens IS, Koteen GM, Legraverend C. Mutagenesis of certain benzo[*a*]pyrene phenols *in vitro* following further metabolism by mouse liver. *Biochem Pharmacol* 1979;28:1615–1622.
50. Schlosser MJ, Kalf GF. Metabolic activation of hydroquinone by macrophage peroxidase. *Chem Biol Interact* 1989;72:191–207.
51. Lorentzen RS, Lesko SA, McDonald K, Ts'O PO. Toxicity of metabolic benzo[*a*]pyrenediones to cultured cells and the dependence upon molecular oxygen. *Cancer Res* 1979;39:3194–3198.
52. Geacintov NE, Ibanez V, Gagliano AG, Yoshida H, Harvey RG. Kinetics of hydrolysis to tetrols and binding of benzo[*a*]pyrene-7,8-dihydrodiol-9,10-oxide and its tetrol derivatives to DNA. Conformation of adducts. *Biochem Biophys Res Commun* 1980;92:1335–1342.
53. Ibanez V, Geacintov NE, Gagliano AG, Brandimarte S, Harvey RG. Physical binding of tetrols derived from BaPDE to DNA. *J Am Chem Soc* 1980;102:5661–5666.
54. Chen FM. Sequence specific binding of tetrols of BaPDE to DNA in neutral and acidic solutions. *Carcinogenesis* 1984;5:753–758.
55. Goujon FM, Nerbert DW, Gielen JE. Genetic expression of aryl hydrocarbon hydroxylase induction. IV. Interaction of various compounds with different forms of cytochrome P-450 and the effect on benzo[*a*]pyrene metabolism *in vitro*. *Mol Pharmacol* 1972;8:667–680.

56. Thurmond LM, Tucker AN, Rickert DE, Lauer LD, Dean JH. Functional and biochemical disposition of 7,12-dimethylbenz[*a*]anthracene in murine lymphoid cells. *Chem Biol Interact* 1989;72:93–104.
57. Schacter BA, Mason JI. The effect of phenobarbital, 3-methylcholanthrene, 3,4-benzopyrene, and pregnenolone-16-carbonitrile on microsomal heme oxygenase and splenic cytochrome P-450. *Arch Biochem Biophys* 1974;160:274–278.
58. Atlas SA, Boobis AR, Felton JA, Thorgeirsson SS, Nebert DW. Ontogenetic expression of polycyclic aromatic compound-inducible monooxygenase activities and forms of cytochrome P-450 in rabbit. *J Biol Chem* 1977;252:4712–4721.
59. Bast RC Jr, Miller H, Rapp HJ, Gelboin HV. Aryl hydrocarbon (benzo[*a*]pyrene) hydroxylase in guinea pig lymphoid tissue. *J Natl Cancer Inst* 1981;67:359–364.
60. Alfred LJ, Wojdani A. Effects of methylcholanthrene and benzanthracene on blastogenesis and aryl hydrocarbon hydroxylase induction in splenic lymphocytes from three inbred stains of mice. *Int J Immunopharmacol* 1983;5:123–129.
61. Okano P, Miller HN, Robinson RC, Gelboin HV. Comparison of benzo[*a*]pyrene and (−)-trans-7,8-dihydroxy-7,8-dihydrobenzo[*a*]pyrene metabolism in human blood monocytes and lymphocytes. *Cancer Res* 1979;39:3184–3193.
62. Ladics GS, Kawabata TT, Munson AE, White KL Jr. Metabolism of benzo[*a*]pyrene by murine splenic cell types. *Toxicol Appl Pharmacol* 1992;116:248–257.
63. Ladics GS, Kawabata TT, Munson AE, White KL Jr. Evaluation of murine splenic cell type metabolism of benzo[*a*]pyrene and functionality *in vitro* following repeated *in vivo* exposure to benzo[*a*]pyrene. *Toxicol Appl Pharmacol* 1992;116:258–266.
64. Kawabata TT, White KL Jr. Metabolism of 7,12-dimethylbenz[*a*]anthracene by splenic microsomes. *FASEB J* 1989;1:2199.
65. Germolec DR, Rosenthal GJ, Taylor MJ, Corsini E, Craig WA, Luster MI. A comparative assessment of metabolic enzyme levels in immune tissues. *Toxicologist* 1991;11(1):52.
66. Whitlock JP, Cooper HL, Gelboin HV. Aryl hydrocarbon (benzopyrene) hydroxylase is stimulated in human lymphocytes by mitogens and benz[*a*]anthracene. *Science* 1972;177:618–619.
67. Gurtoo HL, Minowada J, Paigen B, Parker NB, Thompson N. Factors influencing the measurement and the reproducibility of aryl hydrocarbon hydroxylase activity in cultured human lymphocytes. *J Natl Cancer Inst* 1977;59:787–798.
68. Kouri RE, McKinney CE, Slomiany DJ, Snodgrass DR, Wray NP, McLemore TL. Positive correlation between high aryl hydrocarbon hydroxylase activity and primary lung cancer as analyzed in cryopreserved lymphocytes. *Cancer Res* 1982;42:5030–5037.
69. Cantrell E, Bresnick E. Benzopyrene hydroxylase activity in isolated parenchymal and nonparenchymal cells or rat liver. *J Cell Biol* 1972;52:316–321.
70. Tomingas R, Dehnen W, Lange HU, Beck EG, Manojlovic N. The metabolism of free and soot-bound benzo[*a*]pyrene by macrophages from guinea pigs *in vitro*. *Zentralbl Bakt Hyg I Abt Orig* 1971;155:159–167.
71. Bast RC Jr, Shears BW, Rapp HJ, Gelboin HV. Aryl hydrocarbon (benzo[*a*]pyrene) hydroxylase in guinea pig peritoneal macrophages: benzo[*a*]anthracene-induced increase of enzyme activity *in vivo* and in cell culture. *J Natl Cancer Inst* 1973;51:675–678.
72. Ptashne K, Brothers L, Axline SG, Cohen SN. Aryl hydrocarbon hydroxylase induction in mouse peritoneal macrophages and blood-derived human macrophages. *Proc Soc Exp Biol Med* 1974;146:585–589.
73. Cantrell E, Busbee D, Warr G, Martin R. Induction of aryl hydrocarbon hydroxylase in human lymphocytes and pulmonary alveolar macrophages—a comparison. *Life Sci* 1973;13:1649–1654.
74. Palmer WG, Todd AJ, Tomaszewski JE. Metabolism of 7,12-dimethylbenz[*a*]anthracene by macrophages and uptake of macrophage-derived metabolites by respiratory tissues *in vitro*. *Cancer Res* 1978;38:1079–1084.
75. Wickramasinghe SN. Evidence of drug metabolism by macrophages: possible role of macrophages in the pathogenesis of drug-induced tissue damage and in the activation of environmental procarcinogens. *Clin Lab Haematol* 1987;9:271–280.
76. Autrup H, Harris CC, Stoner GD, Selkirk JK, Schafer PW, Trump BF. Metabolism of [^{3}H]benzo[*a*]pyrene by cultured human bronchus and cultured human pulmonary alveolar macrophages. *Lab Invest* 1978;38:217–224.
77. Bast RC Jr, Whitlock JP Jr, Miller H, Rapp HJ, Gelboin HV. Aryl hydrocarbon (benzo[*a*]pyrene) hydroxylase in human peripheral blood monocytes. *Nature* 1974;250:664–665.

78. Lake RS, Pezzutti MR, Kropko ML, Freeman AE, Igel HJ. Measurement of benzo[*a*]pyrene metabolism in human monocytes. *Cancer Res* 1977;37:2530–2537.
79. Holz O, Krause T, Rudifer HW. Differences in DNA adduct formation between monocytes and lymphocytes after *in vivo* incubation with benzo[*a*]pyrene. *Carcinogenesis* 1991;12:2181–2183.
80. Panthananickal A, Marnett LJ. Arachidonic acid-dependent metabolism of 7,8-dihydroxy-7,8-dihydrobenzo[*a*]pyrene to polyguanylic acid-binding derivatives. *Chem Biol Interact* 1981;33:239–252.
81. Sivarajah K, Lasker JM, Eling TE. Prostaglandin synthetase-dependent cooxidation of (±)-benzo[*a*]pyrene-7,8-dihydrodiol by human lung and other mammalian tissues. *Cancer Res* 1981;41:1834–1839.
82. Dix TA, Marnett LJ. Metabolism of polycyclic aromatic hydrocarbon derivatives to ultimate carcinogens during lipid peroxidation. *Science* 1983;221:77–79.
83. Dix TA, Fontana P, Panthani A, Marnett LJ. Hematin-catalyzed epoxidation of 7,8-dihydroxy-7,8-dihydrobenzo[*a*]pyrene (BP-7,8-diol) by polyunsaturated fatty acid hydroperoxides. *J Biol Chem* 1985;260:5358–5365.
84. Eling T, Curtis J, Battista J, Marnett LJ. Oxidation of (+)-7,8-dihydroxy-7,8-dihydrobenzo[*a*]pyrene by mouse keratinocytes: evidence for peroxyl radical- and monoxygenase-dependent metabolism. *Carcinogenesis* 1986;7:1957–1963.
85. Marnett LJ, Reed GA, Johnson JT. Prostaglandin synthetase-dependent benzo[*a*]pyrene oxidation: products of the oxidation and inhibition of their formation by antioxidants. *Biochem Biophys Res Commun* 1977;79:569–576.
86. Ladics GS, Kawabata TT, Munson AE, White KL Jr. Generation of 7,8-dihydroxy-9,10-epoxy-7,8,9,10-tetrahydro-benzo[*a*]pyrene by murine splenic macrophages. *Toxicol Appl Pharmacol* 1992;115:72–79.
87. Mosier DE. A requirement for two cell types for antibody formation *in vitro*. *Science* 1967;158:1573–1575.
88. Rosenthal AS, Shevach EM. Function of macrophages in antigen recognition by guinea pig T lymphocytes. I. Requirement for histocompatible macrophages and lymphocytes. *J Exp Med* 1973;138:1194–1212.
89. Lee KC. On the origin and the mode of action of functionally distinct macrophage subpopulations. *Mol Cell Biochem* 1980;30:39–55.
90. Lee KC. Regulation of T cell activation by macrophage subsets. *Lymphokines* 1982;6:1–23.
91. Murphy MA, Herscowitz HB. Heterogeneity among alveolar macrophages in humoral and cell-mediated immune responses: separation of functional subpopulations by density gradient centrifugation on Percoll. *J Leukoc Biol* 1984;35:39–54.
92. Hoffman MK, Mizel SB, Hirst JA. IL-1 requirement for B cell activation revealed by use of adult serum. *J Immun* 1984;133:2566–2568.
93. Dinarello CA. Interkleukin-1. *Rev Infect Dis* 1984;6:51–95.
94. Claman HN, Chaperon EA, Triplett RF. Immunocompetence of transferred thymus-marrow cell combinations. *J Immunol* 1966;97:828–832.
95. Mosier DE, Coppelson LW. A three-cell interaction required for induction of the primary immune response in vitro. *Proc Natl Acad Sci USA* 1968;61:542–547.
96. Mitchell GF, Miller JFAP. Cell to cell interaction in the immune response. II. The source of hemolysin-forming cells in irradiated mouse given bone marrow and thymus or thoracic duct lymphocytes. *J Exp Med* 1968;128:821–837.
97. Fernandez C, Severinson E. The polyclonal lipopolysaccharide response is accessory-cell dependent. *Scand J Immunol* 1983;18:279–289.
98. White KL Jr, Parrott MC, Kawabata TT. Adherent and non-adherent fractions of splenocytes are targets of benzo[*a*]pyrene [B(a)P] and 7,12-dimethylbenz[*a*]anthracene (DMBA) induced suppression of the humoral immune response. *Toxicologist* 1988;8(1):326.
99. Chen C, Hirsch JG. The effect of mercaptoethanol and of peritoneal macrophages on the antibody-forming capacity of nonadherent mouse spleen cells in vitro. *J Exp Med* 1972;136:604–617.
100. Click RE, Benck L, Atler BJ. Enhancement of antibody synthesis in vitro by mercaptoethanol. *Cell Immunol* 1972;3:156–160.
101. Blanton RH, Myers MJ, Bick PH. Modulation of immunocompetent cell populations by benzo[*a*]-pyrene. *Toxicol Appl Pharmacol* 1988;93:267–274.
102. Ginsberg GL, Atherholt TB. Transport of DNA-adducting metabolites in mouse serum following benzo[*a*]pyrene administration. *Carcinogenesis* 1989;10:673-679.

103. Ginsberg GL, Atherholt TB. DNA adduct formation in mouse tissues in relation to serum levels of benzo[*a*]pyrene-diol-epoxide after injection of benzo[*a*]pyrene or the diol-epoxide. *Cancer Res* 1990;50:1189–1194.
104. Ginsberg GL, Atherholt TB, Butler GH. Benzo[*a*]pyrene-induced immunotoxicity: comparison to DNA adduct formation *in vivo*, in cultured splenocytes, and in microsomal systems. *J Toxicol Environ Health* 1989;28:205–220.
105. Phillips DH, Hewer A, Grover PL. Aberrant activation of benzo[*a*]pyrene in cultured rat mammary cells *in vitro* and following direct application to rat mammary glands *in vivo*. *Cancer Res* 1985; 45:4167–4174.
106. van Furth R, Diesselhoff-den Dulk MMC. Dual origin of mouse spleen macrophages. *J Exp Med* 1984;160:1273–1283.
107. Setlow RB. Human carcinogenesis. In: Harris CC, Autrup HN, eds. *Human carcinogenisis*. New York: Academic Press; 1983:231–251.

Immunotoxicology and Immunopharmacology, Second Edition, edited by J. H. Dean, M. I. Luster, A. E. Munson, and I. Kimber.
Raven Press, Ltd., New York © 1994.

8

Mechanisms and Consequences of Immunomodulation by Lead

Michael J. McCabe, Jr.

Institute of Chemical Toxicology, Wayne State University, Detroit, Michigan 48201

Certain metals (e.g., zinc, copper, and iron) are essential trace elements functioning as important cofactors and structural elements in select biochemical reactions that mediate diverse molecular and cellular processes. Some of these biochemical reactions, while critical to normal immune function, do not occur exclusively in immune tissues; whereas other metal-containing enzyme reactions are unique to cells of the lymphoid or myeloid lineages. An example of the former is the ubiquitous zinc-finger-containing transcription factor, Sp1, which binds to the promoter regions of many housekeeping genes; whereas an example of the latter is the plasma cell copper-containing immunoglobulin M (IgM)-polymerizing enzyme, which catalyzes the formation of pentameric IgM. While a cataloguing of all the metal-containing enzyme reactions involved in the immune response is beyond the scope of this chapter, an obvious well-documented fact is that certain metals play an important role in the normal functioning of the immune system. This chapter focuses on a separate, perhaps less obvious, and certainly less understood issue—the toxicity to the immune system of the heavy metal lead (Pb). Pb is not considered an essential trace element nor is it considered to play a role in the normal functioning of any biologic system. On the contrary, Pb is already well recognized to be highly toxic for the central nervous, renal, and hematopoietic systems, and additional emphasis has been placed on questioning and understanding whether other tissues and organ systems, such as the immune system, are targeted by Pb. Despite prevention programs initiated in the early 1970s, Pb poisoning remains a leading childhood illness, which is more prevalent than many common childhood infectious diseases such as viral meningitis, mumps, whooping cough, and measles. It is estimated that millions of children in the United States alone exhibit excessive (i.e., $\geq$10 μg/dl of whole blood) blood lead concentrations (Pb-B). Furthermore, exposure to excessive levels of Pb in the workplace continues to be a significant occupational health hazard. The Centers for Disease Control and Prevention (CDC) has stated that Pb is the number one environmental health threat to American children and that the evidence linking low levels of Pb exposure with significant impairment of intelligence and neurobehavioral development is compelling (1). The potent neurotoxicity of Pb has dominated research over the past decade and a half, and it has given rise to passionate believers and equally passionate disbelievers of the evidence leading to the current CDC position. Against the backdrop of this fervor, when Pb poisoning is being blamed for everything ranging from lower scholastic aptitude to the fall of the Roman Empire (2,3), the issue of the immune system as a target for low-dose Pb toxicity has been raised. A growing number of publications have recognized the possibility that Pb modulates the immune system, and several reviews on the subject of the immunotoxicity of Pb and other heavy metals have been published (4–7). In this chapter, the evidence that Pb induces immune dysfunction in animals and may contribute to the pathogenesis of human disease is presented.

THE POTENTIAL FOR THE HUMAN IMMUNE SYSTEM TO BE A TARGET FOR Pb TOXICITY

Unlike the seminal research of Needleman et al. (8) linking childhood Pb exposure with diminished intelligence, no comparable epidemiologic study that extensively considers covariables and that unveils immune system dysfunction due to Pb exposure in any sizable sample of the human population has been reported. Nevertheless, several clinical and experimental studies have described adverse effects of Pb on the human immune system. For the most part, these accounts often adopted seemingly faulty experimental designs and were fraught with inconsistent conclusions. For example, numerous investigations of the effects of Pb on the human humoral immune response have relied on measurements of serum immunoglobulin (Ig) and complement levels because serum is easily obtainable. Although the occurrence of gammaglobulinemias would be indicative of overt immune dysfunction, such approaches unlikely shed light on the more subtle synergistic or antagonistic aspects of immunomodulation that may occur with Pb intoxication, such as altered host resistance upon challenge with a pathogen. Nonetheless, several investigators have examined the effects of Pb on serum immunochemistries and have reported conflicting results. Ewers et al. (9) measured the levels of serum Igs (i.e., IgM, IgG, and IgA) and C3 complement in 72 German Pb workers (mean Pb-B = 51 μg/dl) and 53 reference subjects (mean Pb-B = 12 μg/dl). There was a slight increased frequency of colds and influenza infections in the Pb-exposed group, a finding confirmed in a study of the frequency of cold infections in Japanese workers at a Pb refinery (10). Compared to the reference group, the German Pb workers had, on average, lower serum complement C3, IgM, IgG, and IgA levels. Due to the large random variations of the levels of complement C3 and Igs in the groups examined, the observed differences in these serum parameters were not statistically significant, except for serum IgM. Linear correlations between Pb-B and serum complement C3 and Ig levels were calculated for each group. Significant negative correlations were found between Pb-B and complement C3 and between Pb-B and

IgG in the Pb worker group. Also, a positive correlation was found between Pb-B and serum IgA levels, yet the same study noted a significantly lower salivary IgA level in the Pb workers relative to the reference subjects. Horiguchi et al. (11) also reported a positive correlation between Pb-B and serum IgA as well as a significantly higher number of subjects with markedly elevated serum IgE in a group exhibiting Pb-B greater than 60 μg/dl. Another study conducted by Kimber et al. (12) examined the immunologic status of individuals occupationally exposed to Pb by evaluating serum IgG, IgA, and IgM levels. At the time of testing, the Pb-exposed population had a mean Pb-B of 38 μg/dl ($n = 39$) compared with a mean Pb-B of 12 μg/dl for an age- and sex-matched control group ($n = 21$). No differences in the serum Ig levels, which all fell within normal ranges, were noted between the two study populations, and there was no apparent correlation between Pb-B and serum Ig levels. These studies clearly reach diverse conclusions regarding whether Pb intoxication correlates with impaired humoral immunity and adverse human health effects. One reason for this discrepancy may be because the reported mean Pb-B concentrations in the occupationally exposed populations differ between the investigations. A collective interpretation of the data suggests that serum Ig concentrations are relatively insensitive parameters for Pb poisoning, becoming influenced only at relatively high Pb-B (i.e., >50 μg/dl). In keeping with this notion, lower serum Ig levels were found in one Pb-exposed subject from the Kimber report with the highest Pb-B (i.e., 53 μg/dl). A second reason for the conflicting conclusions reached by these investigations may be due to other confounding variables, such as the route and duration of exposure to Pb, the form of Pb worked with, and the nature of the work environment.

In a study designed to detect deficiencies in the humoral immune systems of children with suspected exposure to airborne Pb (13), children exhibiting relatively high Pb-B (i.e., range = 22 to 42 μg/dl) showed markedly higher frequencies of abnormal serum IgM and secretory IgA values than did children from a low-lead comparison group (i.e., range = 11 to 24 μg/dl). As with the literature dealing with occupational exposures of adults, diverse conclusions regarding the influence of Pb intoxication on children's serum Ig levels have been reported. Reigart et al. (14) examined the serum levels of complement and Igs as well as the amnestic response to tetanus toxoid in 19 black, preschool-aged children. By their study criteria, 12 of these children had evidence of Pb intoxication (mean Pb-B = 45 μg/dl; range = 41 to 51 μg/dl), whereas seven children were designated as controls for comparison (mean Pb-B = 23 μg/dl; range = 14 to 30 μg/dl). No differences between the control group and the Pb-intoxicated group with respect to serum Ig or complement levels or the amnestic response to the tetanus toxoid antigen were noted. However, it should be noted that by today's CDC standards, all the children in this study would be considered Pb-intoxicated (i.e., Pb-B≥10 μg/dl). With this in mind, approximately 26% of these 19 children exhibited elevated serum IgG levels relative to published reference standards (i.e., ≥1420 mg/dl), while more than half demonstrated reduced serum C3 complement levels (i.e., ≤123 mg/dl). Furthermore, upon booster immunization with tetanus toxoid, all the children from both experimental groups exhibited excessive antitoxin levels, suggesting that aberrant immunoregulatory mechanisms may have existed in these children.

Complement deficiencies are reported in many of the investigations that have addressed the effects of occupational or pediatric Pb poisoning on humoral immunity. The complement system, which is the main effector of the humoral immune system, consists of a family of distinct, naturally occurring plasma glycoproteins. Activation of the complement system involves the interaction of specific complement components in a highly ordered enzymatic cascade that generates reaction products that ultimately facilitate antigen clearance and drive inflammatory responses. The complement system is activated by the binding of certain antibody classes (e.g., IgM and IgG, except IgG4) to tissues, bacterial cells, or enveloped viruses, by the formation of soluble antigen–antibody complexes, or by the binding of selected complement components (e.g., C3b) to bacterial cell wall constituents. The effector functions of the complement cascade include cell lysis, inflammation, opsonization of antigen, viral neutralization, and solubilization of immune complexes. Hence deficiencies in complement components may predispose an individual to recurrent infections, especially those caused by gram-negative bacteria. Furthermore, reduced serum complement may be indicative of complement consumption due to an increased formation of soluble immune complexes or to the deposition of high quantities of complement-fixing autoantibodies, both of which can occur within certain tissues indicative of autoimmune diseases such as systemic lupus erythematosus, rheumatoid arthritis, and glomerulonephritis. An autoimmune glomerulonephritis, possibly involving complement-mediated immune injury, has been described in a cohort of men working in a Pb smelting plant (15). In this study, which supports an association between occupational Pb exposure and the pathogenesis of autoimmune kidney disease, it was reported that 21 of 57 workers undergoing renal function tests had excessive body Pb burdens (i.e., mean Pb-B = 50 μg/dl) and impaired kidney function. Suitable glomerular specimens for immunofluorescent analysis were obtained from 7 of 15 workers diagnosed as having Pb nephropathy as the underlying reason for their kidney disease. In five glomeruli presented for immunofluorescent examination, fine granular deposition of IgG (with C3 in two) was detected; in one specimen, linear IgM was present in glomerular capillaries; and in one other, no immunofluorescence was seen. Most (six out of eight) proximal tubule specimens examined showed linear Ig deposition along the basement membrane, which consisted of either IgG alone, IgG plus complement, or complement alone. Deposition of IgG anti-tubule basement membrane was also detected in three out of eight biopsy specimens; however, circulating anti-tubule basement membrane antibodies were not detected by immunofluorescent studies. As will be discussed elsewhere in this chapter, several immune reactivities measured *in vitro* are enhanced by Pb. Although enhancement of immune reactivity is consistent with and may be indicative of a proclivity for autoimmune disease, the described potential correlation between Pb intoxication and autoimmune kidney disease is the only direct evidence that Pb intoxication may play a role in autoimmune pathogenesis.

Activation of the complement cascade also generates by-products that mediate a more effective inflammatory response consisting of mast cell, eosinophil, and basophil degranulation, vasodilation, chemotaxis, and extravasation of polymorphonuclear cells (i.e., neutrophils) from the blood into the tissue space. Defective neutrophil chemotaxis and respiratory burst activity have been reported in a study of 22 workers occupationally exposed to Pb (mean Pb-B = 41 μg/dl) relative to 39 healthy unexposed control subjects (mean Pb-B ≤ 10 μg/dl) (16). Impairment of neutrophil chemotaxis due to occupational Pb exposure has been confirmed in at least two other studies where the Pb-B values were appreciably elevated relative to the control subjects (17,18). Together with these observations, an *in vitro* analysis of Pb effects on human neutrophils indicating a concentration-dependent inhibition of neutrophil chemotaxis at relatively low Pb levels (i.e., 1.2 to 28 μM) has fueled claims that impairment of neutrophil function may be a sensitive biomarker for adverse health effects of Pb (19). Human peripheral blood neutrophils as well as those present at inflammatory sites have been shown to undergo cell death by the mechanism of apoptosis (20,21). Although speculative at this time, impairment of neutrophil function by Pb may be linked to apoptosis. In support of this notion, reduced granulocyte viability has been reported in children living in a Pb-polluted environment (22).

Phenotypic and functional alterations in the T lymphocyte subsets, a characteristic associated with the acquired immunodeficiency syndrome (AIDS), have also been described in Pb-exposed populations. For example, in a study of New York metropolitan area firearms instructors, who were divided into two groups based on their Pb-B levels (i.e., low-Pb group, mean Pb-B = 15 μg/dl; high-Pb group, mean Pb-B = 31 μg/dl), phenotypic parameters and the functional integrity of peripheral blood mononuclear cells were compared with healthy unexposed controls (i.e., mean Pb-B ≤ 10 μg/dl) (23). A significant decrease in the absolute numbers of peripheral blood T helper (T_H) lymphocytes (i.e., CD4+) was found without generalized lymphopenia in both of the Pb-exposed groups, suggesting that the decreased number of CD4+ T_H cells had been countered by an increase in another population and/or populations of peripheral blood mononuclear cells. Analysis of the numbers of suppressor/cytotoxic T cells (i.e., CD8+), B cells (i.e., CD20+), or natural killer (NK) cells (i.e., CD16+) failed to reveal a corresponding increase in these populations in the Pb-intoxicated subjects. Analysis of B cell function was inadequate, especially with respect to T cell regulation of B cell differentiation; however, B cell mitogenesis and spontaneous IgG secretion were intact. Since no corresponding increase in another cell population was detected, it is conceivable that the reduced numbers of CD4+ T_H cells was due either to a decreased cell surface density of CD4 or to an increase in the number of circulating monocytes, which were not accounted for in the experimental design. The latter would represent a marked monocytosis (three- to sixfold increase in monocytes depending on the Pb dose) associated with Pb intoxication. Furthermore, the decreased absolute numbers of circulating CD4+ T cells may represent a deficit in a particular functional subset of T_H cells rather than a general decrease in all CD4+ subpopulations. Functional impairment of cell-mediated immunity was assessed by T cell mitogenic responses and mixed lymphocyte responsiveness, which were both decreased in the Pb-exposed group, supporting the notion of diminished T_H cell activity or increased suppressor T cell activity.

An apparent increase in functional suppressor T cell activity has been reported in humans occupationally exposed to Pb (24). In this experimental design, which compared ten Pb workers (Pb-B range = 40 to 51 μg/dl) with ten healthy controls (Pb-B ≤ 19 μg/dl), total T cells and T cell subsets (i.e., CD4+ and CD8+) were enumerated, proliferative responses to T cell mitogens [i.e., concanavalin A (Con A) and phytohemagglutin antigen (PHA)] were assessed, and the generation of functional T cell suppression was determined. No abnormal values relative to the control group for total T cells, percentage of T_H cells, percentage of suppressor/cytotoxic T cells, CD4/CD8 ratio, or lymphocyte blast transformation were noted for the Pb-intoxicated group. However, lymphocytes obtained from the Pb-intoxicated subjects failed to exhibit suppressor cell activity in an *in vitro* assay designed to generate and detect it. Detailed data and interpretation were lacking from this report; however, the implications are that Pb intoxication may modulate T cell regulatory functions in humans.

At the present time, sweeping conclusions regarding the effect (or lack thereof) of Pb on the human immune system are unwarranted; too few hypotheses have adequately been addressed. The studies described above suggest that Pb may be a silent modulator of the human immune system, in that overt toxicity (e.g., Pb-induced agammaglobulinemia) does not occur. Although, to date, we cannot point to any human immunodeficiency or autoimmune disease where Pb can be implicated with certainty, considerable evidence obtained with animal models both *in vivo* and *in vitro* suggests that the immunomodulatory aspects of Pb intoxication are complex, and that Pb may be a potent and important immunomodulator. It has become increasingly clear that much of the uncertainty regarding both the mechanisms and consequences of Pb immunotoxicity can be attributed to the types of analyses or model systems that have been performed to evaluate Pb exposure. For example, the level of Igs in serum measures the existence of B cells, but it does not gauge their capacity to be involved in a specific humoral immune response. In fact, in culture systems using human (and animal, *vide infra*) lymphocytes, Pb increases the production of antigen-specific antibodies (25,26). This dichotomy between serum Igs and specific antibody production is clearly evident in AIDS patients who present normal or elevated serum Ig levels yet have a limited capacity to produce specific antibodies. Thus additional clinical indices of immune function may need to be included in the analysis of Pb effects on the human immune response in order to uncover the potential intricate nature of Pb immunomodulation. Furthermore, animal and cell culture models that go beyond assessing immune function solely within the framework of the 1988 National Toxicology Program interlaboratory study, which identified and standardized various immunologic assays (27), need to be employed or at least better integrated with hypothesis-driven research. Moreover, appropriate methods of monitoring Pb exposure, such as bone Pb burden, need to be factored into animal and human experimental designs since Pb-B, an indicator for short-term lead exposure, may not be the appropriate dosimeter for correlating long-term Pb exposure with immune system dysfunction. An epidemiologic analysis of the potential effects of Pb intoxication on some aspect of the immune response modeled after what has been done with epidemiologic/statistical analysis of behavioral deficits due to Pb poisoning would be useful. The inclusion of missed school days in the model might serve as an additional factor for impaired intellectual development due to Pb exposure.

EFFECTS OF LEAD ON IMMUNITY AS ASSESSED BY ANIMAL MODELS

The immunotoxic consequences of metal exposure in animals can be divided experimentally into three main categories: decreased host resistance, hypersensitivity, and increased propensity for autoimmune disease. Each of these effects depends on specific immune dysfunction.

In studies of immunomodulation by Pb, researchers have mainly sought to demonstrate that Pb intoxication alters host resistance in infectious disease models (Table 1). The immune response to pathogens (i.e., bacteria, viruses, and protozoans) depends on their location (i.e., intracellular versus extracellular, blood versus mucosal surface), involves different arms of immune defense (i.e., humoral versus cell-mediated immunity), and involves distinct regulatory cells (i.e., T_H1 versus T_H2 cells) and effector cell types and function (e.g., cytotoxic T cells versus cytophilic antibodies). Immunity to bacterial infections is achieved via humoral defense mechanisms unless the bacterium is capable of intracellular growth, in which case requisite cell-mediated immune defense mechanisms are activated. Infection by extracellular bacteria elicits the synthesis of specific antibodies or Igs, which are secreted by activated B cells and plasma cells residing in the spleen, the regional lymph nodes, as well as the submucosa of the respiratory, gastrointestinal, and urogenital tracts. Five major classes (i.e., isotypes) of Igs (IgG, IgA, IgM, IgD, and IgE), which differ in their primary structure, physicochemical and serologic properties, and biologic effector function, exist. Binding of the specific antibodies to antigens on the surface of the invading bacterium can target its destruction by two major mechanisms. First, cytophilic antibodies serve as opsonins, which facilitate clearance of the microbe by phagocytic cells. Antibodies can also neutralize bacterial toxins by opsonization. Second, activation of the complement cascade by complement-fixing antibodies leads to bacterial lysis especially of gram-negative bacteria. Certain Ig isotypes perform these effector functions with differing degrees of efficiency. For example, IgM, which is secreted as a pentamer, is the first Ig class produced in response to an antigenic challenge. The unique pentameric structure of IgM has several advantages including enhanced agglutination of particulate antigens and increased efficiency for complement-mediated cell lysis. Certain subclasses of IgG (human IgG3 $>>$ IgG1 $>$ IgG2 $>>>$ IgG4) are effective activators of the

TABLE 1. *Decreased host resistance to pathogens due to lead exposure*

Host	Pathogen	Pb exposure	Pb effect	Reference
Mouse (Swiss Webster)	*Salmonella typhimurium*	Pb-nitrate, daily 30 d, 100–250 μg ip	10-fold ↓ in LD_{50} for bacterial challenge	28
Mouse (CD-1, ♂)	Encephalomyocarditis virus	Pb-acetate, 2 wk 10–50 mM, drinking H_2O	↑ Incidence and rate of lethality	29,30
Mouse (CBA/J, ♀)	*Listeria monocytogenes*	Pb-acetate, 2 wk 0.4–10 mM, drinking H_2O	↑ Incidence and rate of lethality	31,32
Rat (Charles River, ♂)	*Escherichia coli, Straphylococcus epidermis*	Pb-acetate, 2 mg/100 g body weight iv	↑ Mortality	33
Rat (Sprague–Dawley, ♀)	Endotoxin, gram-negative species	Pb-acetate, 1–5 mg/100 g body weight iv	10^5-fold ↑ in lethality to endotoxemia	34
Rat (Sprague–Dawley, ♂)	Endotoxin (*E. coli*)	Pb-acetate, 2 mg/100 g body weight iv	10^3-fold ↑ in lethality to endotoxemia	35
Rat (Charles River, ♂)	Endotoxin, (*Salmonella enteriditis*)	Pb-acetate, 0.854 mg/100 g body weight iv	↑ Lethality to endotoxemia	36
Rabbit (New Zealand, ♂)	Pseudorabies virus	Pb-acetate, 10 wk 2500 ppm, drinking H_2O	10-fold ↓ in serum neutral activity	37

complement system, while certain subclasses of IgG (human IgG1, IgG3 > IgG4 >> IgG2) serve as efficient opsonins by interacting with high affinity with Fc receptors on phagocytic cells. Furthermore, IgG1, IgG3, and IgG4 readily cross the placenta and play an important role in protecting the developing fetus. IgA, the predominant Ig class in external secretions and mucosal tissues, serves an important effector function by inhibiting bacterial and viral attachment and colonization at portals of entry. IgE is found in extremely low quantities in serum, yet it has potent biologic activity by mediating immediate hypersensitivity (i.e., allergic) reactions via mast cell and basophil degranulation, and IgE-mediated effector functions facilitate immune defense against nematode and helminth parasites. The biologic effector function of IgD, aside from being a B cell surface antigen receptor together with monomeric IgM, is not known.

Viral infections also elicit both humoral and cell-mediated immune defense mechanisms. Antibodies to viral surface components can neutralize the adherence and/or penetration stages of viral infections. Agglutination by pentameric IgM or secretory IgA, opsonization by cytophilic antibodies and complement, or complement-mediated lysis in the case of enveloped viruses are also efficient humoral defense mechanisms against viral infections. Humoral immune mechanisms are crucial in containing the spread of viruses during the acute stages of infection; however, antibodies are not able to eliminate a virus once a chronic infection has been established. As is the case with infections caused by intracellular bacteria, chronic or latent viral infections are characterized by viral replication/residence within host cells. Thus cell-mediated immunity, regulated in large part by T_H1 cells and involving cytotoxic T lymphocytes (CTLs) and NK cell effector functions, is important for host defense against viral infections.

Numerous animal studies have demonstrated that Pb intoxication exacerbates the pathologic effects of bacterial and viral infections (Table 1). Exacerbation of disease may be due to synergistic interactions between the toxicant and the pathogen directly on the target tissue (e.g., Pb and encephalomyocarditis virus both affecting the brain). Alternatively, a toxic insult on a component of the immune system resulting in impaired defense against the invading pathogen may contribute to the disease. This toxic insult may manifest itself as a direct selective killing of a class of immunocompetent cells (e.g., CD4+ T_H cells) or as an impairment of a particular immune function (e.g., decreased levels of serum opsonins). Moreover, the toxic insult need not always be due to a decreased response; increased unregulated immune responses can be detrimental to an organism. Hence, due to the balanced nature of the immune response, hyperresponsiveness of an inappropriate arm of the immune system resulting in the activation of the wrong effector function might result in either impaired host resistance to microbes or an aberrant response to self-constituents. Additionally, the aberrant immune response can mediate the pathologic process. The contributions of an imbalanced immune response to disease have become more clear particularly from the emerging understanding of the role of the T_H1/T_H2 dichotomy in controlling immune defense mechanisms (38). For example, certain mouse strains (e.g., BALB/c) manifest excessive T_H2-mediated immunity when challenged with the intracellular protozoan *Leishmania* species, but due to the lack of an appropriate T_H1 response the mice fail to control the infection and die (39). The *T_H1/T_H2 dichotomy* by definition refers to categories of T_H cells that produce distinct cytokine panels. Aspects of this cellular/functional dichotomy have been observed in other facets of immunobiology and infectious disease including AIDS (40,41), pregnancy (42,43), aging (44,45), autoimmunity (46,47), and immunotoxicology (47–49).

Since quite different immune regulatory and effector functions are required for protection against infections by extracellular and intracellular pathogens, evaluation of host resistance is a good starting, yet incomplete, strategy to assess the immunomodulatory capacity of a toxic environmental agent. Challenge with bacteria, viruses, protozoa, or tumors stresses the animal's immune capabilities and affords an assessment of the host's protective capacity. In addition, the examination of host resistance to extracellular pathogens (e.g., *Streptococcus pneumoniae*) and intracellular pathogens (e.g., *Listeria monocytogenes*) constitutes a holistic approach, because resistance to extracellular pathogens requires T_H2 cells, B cells, and macrophage interactions for the production of specific cytophilic or complement-fixing antibodies, and resistance to intracellular pathogens requires T_H1 cells and macrophage interactions for the initiation of macrophage bactericidal activities. The most consistent finding in experimental studies evaluating the effects of Pb on host resistance is an increased susceptibility to infectious agents. Usually, these experimental studies have consisted of experimental designs whereby mortality after a sublethal challenge with an intracellular pathogen is compared between Pb-treated and control animals. Collectively, the studies outlined in Table 1 clearly point to an increased rate and/or incidence of lethality in Pb-intoxicated animals upon infection with various microbes. In hindsight, most of these investigations have focused on determining the effects of Pb intoxication on infectious agents that expectedly are controlled by the T_H1 arm of immunity. For the most part, these studies fail to document the immune indices that are modulated by Pb intoxication, except for an investigation where a neutralizing antibody titer to pseudorabies virus, as measured in a viral plaque inhibition assay, was reported (37).

In the most extensive assessment of the influence of Pb on host resistance, Lawrence showed that the mortality of *Listeria*-infected CBA/J mice was significantly increased by exposure to Pb in their drinking water, and that the recovery of viable bacteria from the spleens and livers of Pb-intoxicated mice was markedly increased (31,32). Although Pb significantly altered the resistance of these mice to *Listeria*, it did not alter the primary humoral immune response as measured by the plaque-forming cell (PFC) assay or cell-mediated immunity as measured by mixed lymphocyte reactivity and responsiveness of T cells to mitogens. Again, this exemplifies the need to understand the limitations of assays employed to assess immunotoxicity. Different experimental outcomes may arise depending on the parameter being assessed, and immunosuppression, in the classic sense of the concept, need not always be the mechanism involved.

An additional shortfall of many of the studies presented in Table 1 is that the rationale for the dose and route of Pb administration is usually unstated, precluding facile extrapolation of these data to predict risk stemming from likely human exposure situations. Host resistance models for Pb immunotoxicity need to incorporate into the experimental designs relevance to "natural" exposure. For instance, in an early and often quoted study by Hemphill and colleagues it is clearly shown that daily intraperitoneal injection of Pb-nitrate for 30 days markedly suppresses the resistance of mice to *Salmonella typhimurium* (28), an intracellular bacterium. Despite the authors' claim that no clinical signs of Pb toxicity were apparent in these mice, it is impossible to judge whether this exposure regimen is pertinent regarding Pb immunotoxicity for exposed human populations and other animal models. Similar criticisms of studies employing acute exposure to Pb followed by endotoxins can be applied.

Generation of an effective immune response to intracellular pathogens like the bacteria *L. monocytogenes* or *S. typhimurium* requires communication between macrophages and T cells, resulting in the generation of cell-mediated effector functions. As discussed, challenge of Pb-intoxicated mice with sublethal doses of *L. monocytogenes* results in a marked increase in morbidity and mortality relative to nominally Pb-free animals challenged with a similar bacterial inoculum (32). Since the immune response to *Listeria* requires both macrophage and T cell functions, it is possible that the target for Pb toxicity is selective for the function and/or development of one or both of these cell types. Effects of Pb on other indices of cell-mediated immunity such as the *in vivo* delayed-type hypersensitivity response (50,51) strongly suggest that T cell function is targeted by Pb. However, both macrophage recruitment and the interplay between macrophages and T_H cells (particularly T_H1 cells) appear to be affected by Pb.

Macrophage effector function in response to *Listeria*, as assessed by phagocytosis of the bacterium or by interleukin-1 (IL-1) production, is not influenced by Pb intoxication (52). In experiments designed to assess the effects of either *in vivo* or *in vitro* Pb exposure on the ability of unelicited peritoneal macrophages to phagocytose *Listeria*, it was found that Pb had no effect on the percentage of macrophages containing intracellular bacteria (i.e., phagocytic index), the number of *Listeria* organisms phagocytosed per macrophage (i.e., phagocytic capacity), or the production of the monokine, IL-1. These experiments also demonstrated that *in vitro* Pb exposure had no effect on the phagocytic index using splenic macrophages. Likewise, Pb reportedly did not affect the phagocytosis of opsonized or nonopsonized sheep erythrocytes *in vitro* by splenic macrophages (32). In contrast to these data, the percentage of macrophages phagocytosing IgG-opsonized sheep erythrocytes was slightly increased in *in vivo* Pb-exposed mouse mineral oil activated peritoneal macrophages (53); whereas other investigators using a comparable protocol reported that *in vivo* Pb exposure inhibited the phagocytic capacity of unelicited peritoneal macrophages (54). Furthermore, several reports have indicated that intravenous exposure to Pb impairs the ability of Kupffer cells to clear colloidal carbon and endotoxin (36,55); while opposite effects of oral Pb exposure on reticuloendothelial system (RES) functioning also have been reported (56). Because of differences in the particulate antigens used, the extent of antigen opsonization, the activation state or source of the macrophage populations, and the route of Pb exposure, it is difficult to make generalizations about the effects of Pb on macrophage phagocytic capacity or function. Having cautioned that the experimental variables make synopsis of general Pb effects on phagocytosis speculative, the data discussed above may collectively suggest that initially macrophage phagocytic function, as assessed in the studies with *Listeria*, is unaltered by Pb, but that later on in an immune response when serum opsonins are elevated, as exemplified in the studies employing IgG-coated sheep erythrocytes, Pb either stimulates or inhibits macrophage phagocytosis depending on the activation state of the responding macrophages. Hence a range of Pb effects on macrophage effector function may exist depending on the state of immune activation, and these conflicting reports may be attributed to diverse effects of Pb on distinct cell processes or populations. Diverse effects of Pb on a given cell population may also be related to the maturational state of the targeted cell lineage. For example, Pb impairs the ability of bone marrow-derived macrophages to proliferate and form colonies in response to colony-stimulating factor-1 (57), and this lack of bone marrow-derived macrophage development and/or recruitment likely contributes to the increased mortality observed with *L. monocytogenes* challenged, Pb-treated mice. Since macrophage proliferation constitutes the initial phase of the immune response against *Listeria* independent of T cells, the effects of Pb on the response of macrophage progenitors to cytokines may constitute an important effect of Pb on immune development.

A major function of macrophages in immune defense is to process phagocytosed particulate antigens and to present the appropriate antigenic peptides to antigen-specific T cells. Although peritoneal macrophages from *in vivo* Pb-exposed mice display normal phagocytic function, the capacity of these macrophages to process and/or present *Listeria* antigen to *Listeria*-primed T cells was impaired by Pb (52). Despite this impaired ability to function in an antigen-specific capacity, macrophages from Pb-intoxicated mice stimulated a nonspecific, autologous response in antigen presentation assays (52). A developing theme regarding the effects of Pb on an immune response is that Pb subtly alters immune recognition, perhaps via Pb alteration of antigen-presenting cell function, which is potentially coupled to additional direct or indirect effects of Pb on other aspects of immune response regulation such as cytokine networks. Similar to cytokines, the effects of Pb on immunocompetent cells are viewed as being pleiotropic; that is, Pb very likely has different effects on different target cells depending on the circumstances.

Lead enhances B lymphocyte differentiation to IgM-secreting cells as measured by the direct hemolytic PFC assay, causing more than a twofold increase in the number of sheep erythrocyte-specific antibody-producing cells in cultures containing either mouse splenocytes or purified splenic B cells (32,48,58–60). *In vitro* concentrations of $PbCI_2$ of 5 to 100 μM significantly enhanced the IgM PFC response (58). Optimal enhancement by Pb of the IgM PFC response, which peaks on day 5, occurred when Pb was added *in vitro* within 16 hr after culture initiation, suggesting that a relatively early event in immune activation was affected by Pb (59). This early event may be a direct effect of Pb on B cell activation [e.g., cell surface major histocompatibility complex (MHC) class II molecule expression] or an effect on B cell responsiveness to T_H cell-derived cytokines. In experiments employing membrane-segregated cultures to assess the influences of Pb on B cell differentiation in the absence of B cell–T cell contact, it was discovered that Pb enhanced both the IgM PFC response of B cells to T cell-derived factors and the production of T cell-derived factors (48). The identity of the factors responsible for this enhancement, indeed whether or not they are cytokines, remains to be determined. Hence Pb appears to have direct effects on B cells and also to enhance communication between B cells and T cells either through enhancing contact between the two cells or by modulating immunoregulatory cytokine networks. The immunoenhancing effects of Pb on humoral immunity are not limited to the antigen, sheep erythrocytes. Pb has been shown to enhance the *in vitro* primary humoral immune response to other particulate antigens (e.g., sheep erythrocytes coupled with trinitrophenol), to soluble antigens [e.g., trinitrophenyl (TNP)–keyhole limpet hemocyanin and conalbumin), and to a T cell-independent antigen (e.g., TNP–lipopolysaccharide (LPS)] (48,59). Furthermore, Pb directly influences B cell differentiation *in vitro*, as measured by secretion of polyclonal IgM into the culture medium, since it enhances LPS-induced IgM secretion in highly purified B cell cultures (61). It may be noteworthy that Pb, which markedly augments the lethality of LPS in rats, also enhances the LPS-induced production of the cytokine, tumor necrosis factor (TNF) (62). The influences of Pb on *in vitro* B cell responsiveness do not appear to be mouse strain (48) or species specific, and similar indices of immune enhancement appear to occur in cultured human cells (25,26). Single injection of Pb-acetate intravenously or intraperitoneally markedly enhances the *ex vivo* IgM PFC response in a manner comparable to that obtained with cultured splenocytes (63,64). Unlike the striking effects that *in vivo* exposure to Pb via the drinking water has on host resistance to bacterial pathogens (e.g., *L. monocytogenes*), oral exposure to Pb has little effect on *in vivo* measures of humoral immunity, unless the animals are intoxicated with Pb during prenatal and postnatal development, in which case the exposure to Pb inhibits humoral immunity perhaps by affecting the developmental maturation of T cells (65).

The MHC class II molecules (i.e., I-A and I-E in mice; DR, DQ, and DP in humans), the most polymorphic gene products known, play central roles in determining an individual's immunoresponsiveness to a particular antigen and in regulating immune function. Expression of MHC class II molecules is normally restricted to specific cell types of hematopoietic origin (e.g., B Iymphocytes, activated macrophages, dendritic cells, and activated human T cells). The MHC class II complex functions to bind peptides, which are derived from endocytosed intracellular proteolysis of extracellular antigens within an intracellular endosomal compartment, and to transport these antigenic peptide fragments to the cell surface to be recognized by antigen-specific T cells. The cell surface density of the antigen in association with the MHC class II complex, which can be regulated by select physiologic stimuli in a cell-specific manner in the absence of T cells, regulates the intensity of an immune response by controlling the frequency of interactions between antigen-presenting cells and T cells (66,67). In addition to their roles as peptide-binding proteins and restriction elements for T cell recognition, there is a growing body of evidence suggesting that the MHC class II molecules can function as signal transducing molecules (68–71). Hence the quantitative variation in the cell surface density of MHC class II molecules may regulate B cell differentiation both passively, by presenting antigen to T cells and focusing T cell help, and actively, by serving as signal transduction elements for the activation of B cell function initiated by receptor–ligand interactions. In experiments aimed at evaluating direct effects of Pb on B cells independent of T cell function, it was discovered that Pb, at concentrations as low as 1 μM, enhanced both the cell surface density and total cellular levels of I-A and I-E in highly purified B cell cultures (61,72). Although B cells constitutively express MHC class II molecules on their cell surface, the total cellular levels of MHC class II molecules as well as of the invariant chain, which targets the MHC class II complex into the endosomal compartment where it associates with proteolytically generated antigen peptide fragments (73,74), are upregulated via the activation of transcriptional, translational, and post-translational control mechanisms by the T_H cell-derived cytokine IL-4 (75).

Upregulation of B cell I-A and I-E does not occur via transcriptional activation;

hence Pb exerts its effect on the expression of MHC class II molecules by influencing translational and/or post-translational control mechanisms (72). Preliminary findings suggest that Pb alters the degradation and possibly the intracytoplasmic trafficking of the invariant chain/MHC class II complex. Inclusion of neutralizing antibodies to IL-4 does not abrogate the ability of Pb to increase I-A and I-E, indicating that the effects of Pb on the B cell are not mediated through IL-4 produced by contaminating T cells. This is an important point, as it has been reported that mercury (Hg) also increases MHC class II expression on B cells (49,76); however, in the case of Hg, upregulation of B cell surface MHC class II expression is mediated by increased IL-4. With respect to heightened MHC class II expression, it is interesting that Pb mimics rather than induces this cytokine activity. It may be that the heightened cell surface expression of MHC class II on the B cell surface is nonfunctional—that is, devoid of antigen peptide due to a defect in the intracytoplasmic trafficking of the MHC class II complex due to Pb.

The cell surface expression of the MHC class II molecules complexed with antigenic peptides initiates the immune response upon recognition by the appropriate clone of T_H cells. As such, increased cell surface MHC class II molecule expression due to Pb intoxication fits with the data describing Pb enhancement of B cell differentiation. Also, *in vitro* Pb induces the proliferation of T lymphocytes in a manner indicative of an enhancement of the autologous mixed lymphocyte response (60, 77), a response to self-MHC class II molecules either in the presence or absence of self-peptides. Given these observations, it might be predicted that Pb would enhance T cell recognition of exogenous antigens in antigen presentation assays. However, the effects of Pb on antigen presentation, like the phenomenon of antigen presentation itself, are complex. Some of the complexity may be attributed in part to the discovery of different classes of T_H cells designated T_H1 cells and T_H2 cells. Although merely a hypothesis at this stage, much of the diversity observed with the effects of Pb on the immune response may be attributed to the T_H1/T_H2 dichotomy since these cell subsets appear to control separate immune responses via diverse mechanisms at both the cellular and molecular levels.

Reports detailing alteration of immunity by Pb are often conflicting. For example, in addition to the studies discussed in detail above, other reports have indicated that Pb inhibits B cell differentiation (65,78) as well as cell-mediated immunity. For example, Luster et al. (65) reported that chronic prenatal and postnatal exposure of rats to 25 ppm Pb-acetate via the drinking water (resulting in a mean Pb-B of 29 μg/dl) resulted in depressed humoral immunity exemplified by reduced serum total IgG levels as well as by a significant reduction in the number of splenic PFCs secreting IgM antibodies to sheep erythrocytes. In retrospect, it is difficult to integrate the findings of each of these studies into a concerted understanding of immunomodulation by Pb. Nonetheless, two observations regarding immune parameters altered by Pb, which themselves appear to be conflicting on face value, appear to hold true. First, Pb intoxication suppresses resistance to intracellular bacterial infections as exemplified by the *L. monocytogenes* model. Second, Pb enhances the *in vitro* primary humoral immune response by affecting B cells both indirectly (i.e., altering the production of T_H cell-derived factors) and directly (i.e., altering the responsiveness of B cells to T cell-derived factors and increasing the cell surface density of MHC class II molecules). As far as it has been tested, the upregulation of MHC class II expression appears to be cell specific, in that, unlike its effect on B cell MHC class II, I-A and I-E are not induced by Pb in macrophages. The importance of these differential effects of Pb on the expression of MHC class II molecules by these two populations of antigen-presenting cells may be related to the growing body of evidence that the T_H cell populations (i.e., T_H1 and T_H2 cells) utilize different antigen-presenting cells to become activated (79–81). Although there is considerable debate regarding which T_H cell type couples with which antigen-presenting cell, convincing data suggest that the T_H1 cell prefers high cell surface MHC class II expression (i.e., B cells) to become activated, while the T_H2 cells require much lower levels to become activated (79,80). Interestingly, Pb displays differential effects on T_H1 and T_H2 cells in antigen presentation assays in that it inhibits antigen presentation to a series of T_H1 clones, yet it enhances antigen presentation to a series of T_H2 clones (48). Furthermore, Pb inhibits the production of IL-2, a T_H1-derived cytokine, in antigen presentation assays (82), and Pb inhibits the presentation of *Listeria*, a largely T_H1-controlled microbial infection, to *Listeria*-primed T cells (52). Since the T_H1 clones and T_H2 clones were initially defined on the basis of the cytokine profiles that they express (83), it is tempting to speculate that the differential effects of Pb on T_H1 and T_H2 activation relates to distinct effects of Pb on particular cytokines and/or cytokine receptors. T_H1 clones exclusively produce IL-2, interferon-γ (IFN-γ), and TNF-β; whereas, T_H2 clones exclusively produce IL-4, IL-5, and IL-10 (38). It is well established that the immune response to intracellular pathogens (e.g., *Listeria, Salmonella, Leishmania*) requires macrophage–T_H1 cell interactions (52,84). Activated macrophages are considered to be the primary effector cells in the host defense against these pathogens, and IFN-γ appears to be the main cytokine involved in macrophage activation. *In vivo* neutralization of IFN-γ activity with monoclonal anti-IFN-γ (85) or disruption of the IFN-γ gene (86) or IFN-γ receptor gene (87) by transgenic "knockout" technology prevents an effective cell-mediated immune response against *Listeria*. Hence inhibition of antigen presentation to T_H1 cells by Pb may be related mechanistically to the increased susceptibility of Pb-intoxicated mice to intracellular pathogens, possibly through effects of Pb on the biology of IFN-γ. Likewise, what appears to be an enhancement of T_H2 activity may be related mechanistically to enhancement of humoral immunity by Pb, since the T_H2-derived cytokines are viewed as the predominant helper factors for B cell activation and differentiation (38). Additionally, discrepancies regarding enhancement versus inhibition of B cell responses by Pb may also be related to the functional T_H cell dichotomy, since their respective cytokines differentially control Ig class switching (88). The process whereby B cells, initially expressing membrane IgD or IgM, switch to the expression/secretion of IgA, IgE, or one of the four IgG subclasses is known as *immunoglobulin class switching*. T_H cells play an important, obligatory role in regulating the Ig class switch by secreting various cytokines. Hence the switch to isotypes having the required biologic effector function is governed by cytokines produced by distinct T cell subsets designated T_H type 1 (i.e., T_H1) and T_H type 2 (i.e., T_H2) cells. For example, IL-4 derived from T_H2 cells stimulates the production of murine IgG1 (human IgG4) and IgE, IFN-γ derived from T_H1 cells stimulates the production of murine IgG2a and IgG3 (human IgG1 and IgG3, respectively), and transforming growth factor-β (TGF-β) enhances the production of murine IgA and IgG2b (human IgG2). In this respect, enhancement of humoral immunity by Pb may contribute to immunopathologies, as higher levels of an antibody of the wrong isotype and therefore having the inappropriate biologic function may be detrimental to the host. Since some T_H1- and T_H2-derived cytokines reciprocally antagonize the activity of the other cell type, the potential immunomodulatory effects of Pb on one or more cytokines could be far-reaching by indirectly influencing an entire network of cytokine signaling and cellular functioning. It is expected that the complexity of such immunomodulation would be considerable. Finally, there is evidence that the T_H1 and T_H2 clones exhibit biochemical differences with respect to signal transduction pathways. For example, T_H1 cells appear to flux calcium ions (Ca^{2+}) more readily and there also appears to be differential sensitivity of T_H1 and T_H2 clones to cyclic adenosine monophosphate (cAMP) elevating agents (79,89–92). Hence the differential effects of Pb on T_H1 and T_H2 clones may offer clues regarding the effects of Pb on biochemical signal transduction processes that may be applicable to other cells and tissues. In addition to the second messengers, cAMP and Ca^{2+}, signal transducing mechanisms involving protein kinase C and other kinases and phosphatases may be instrumental in the mechanisms of Pb immunotoxicity. There is ample literature on the effects of Pb on protein kinase C (PKC) (93–95). Whether Pb activates or inhibits particular PKC isozymes is currently being debated. Interestingly, PKC-activating phorbol esters, like Pb, inhibit neutrophil chemotaxis, suggesting that they share a common mode of action (96).

CONCLUSION

While one purpose of this chapter was to compile a comprehensive review of the data concerning the immunotoxicity of Pb, a second purpose was to highlight research areas that will bring better understanding to the mechanisms and the health consequences of immunomodulation by Pb. These areas include additional clinical and epidemiologic investigations of the effects of childhood or occupational exposure to Pb on indices of immune function, additional host resistance animal models that integrate and document the immune functions that are disrupted by Pb, additional investigations to explore the effects of Pb on inter- and intracellular communication, and the subcellular/molecular effects of Pb on processes ranging from gene expression to signal transduction. These issues are of interest to immunologists and toxicologists alike. Ironically, one of the forefathers of modern immunology—Paul Erlich, Nobel laureate and champion of the "side-chain" theory of antibody specificity—contributed significantly to the development of diagnostic tests for plumbism (97). In all likelihood these were unrelated pursuits of his—if not separated conceptually, then certainly separated chronologically. We will never know what relationships, if any, he may have pondered; nonetheless, nearly a century later, the issue of Pb influencing the immune system is beginning to be pondered in earnest.

REFERENCES

1. Centers for Disease Control and Prevention. Preventing Pb poisoning in young children: a statement by CDC. Department of Human Health Series Publication, October 1991.
2. Gilfillan SC. Lead poisoning and the fall of Rome. *J Occup Med* 1965;7:53–60.
3. Nriagu JO. Saturnine gout among Roman aristocrats: did lead poisoning contribute to the fall of the empire? *N Engl J Med* 1983;308:660–663.
4. Fischbein A, Tsang P, Luo JJ, Bekesi JG. The immune system as target for subclinical lead related toxicity. *Br J Ind Med* 1993;50:185–186.
5. Koller LD. Immunotoxicology of heavy metals. *Int J Immunopharmacol* 1980;2:269–279.
6. Kowolenko M, McCabe MJ Jr, Lawrence DA. Metal-induced alterations of immunity. In: Newcombe DS, Rose NR, Bloom JC, eds. *Clinical immunotoxicology*. New York: Raven Press; 1992: 401–419.
7. Lawrence DA. Immunotoxicity of heavy metals. In: Dean JH, Luster MI, Munson AE, Amos H, eds. *Immunotoxicology and immunopharmacology*. New York: Raven Press; 1985:341–353.
8. Needleman HL, Gunnoe C, Leviton A, Ree R, Peresie H, Maher C. Deficits in psychological and classroom performance of children with elevated dentine lead levels. *N Engl J Med* 1979;300:689–695.
9. Ewers U, Stiller-Winkler R, Idel H. Serum immunoglobulin, complement C3, and salivary IgA levels in lead workers. *Environ Res* 1982;29:351–357.
10. Horiguchi S, Endo G, Kiyota I, et al. Frequency of cold infections in workers at a lead refinery. *Osaka City Med J* 1992;38:79–81.
11. Horiguchi S, Kiyota I, Endo G, et al. Serum immunoglobulin and complement C3 levels in workers exposed to lead. *Osaka City Med J* 1992;38:149–153.
12. Kimber I, Stonard MD, Gidlow DA, Niewola Z. Influence of chronic low-level exposure to lead on plasma immunoglobulin concentration and cellular immune function in man. *Int Arch Occup Environ Health* 1986;57:117–125.
13. Wagnerovà M, Wagner V, Màdlo Z, Zavàzal V, Wokounovà D, Kñž J, Mohyla O. Seasonal variations in the level of immunoglobulins and serum proteins of children differing by exposure to air-borne lead. *J Hyg Epidemiol Microbiol Immunol* 1986;30:127–138.
14. Reigart JR, Graber CD. Evaluation of the humoral immune response of children with low level lead exposure. *Bull Environ Contam Toxicol* 1976;16:112–116.
15. Wedeen RP, Mallik DK, Batuman V. Detection and treatment of occupational lead nephropathy. *Arch Intern Med* 1979;139:53–57.
16. Queiroz MLS, Almeida M, Gallão MI, Höehr NF. Defective neutrophil function in workers occupationally exposed to lead. *Pharmacol Toxicol* 1993;72:73–77.
17. Bergeret A, Pouget E, Tedone R, Meygret T, Cadot R, Descotes J. Neutrophil functions in lead-exposed workers. *Hum Exp Toxicol* 1990;9:231–233.
18. Valentino M, Governa M, Marchiseppe I, Visonă I. Effects of lead on polymorphonuclear leukocyte (PMN) functions in occupationally exposed workers. *Arch Toxicol* 1991;65:685–688.
19. Governa M, Valentino M, Visonă I. *In vitro* impairment of human granulocyte functions by lead. *Arch Toxicol* 1987;59:421–425.
20. Martin SJ, Bradley JG, Cotter TG. HL-60 cells induced to differentiate towards neutrophils subsequently die via apoptosis. *Clin Exp Immunol* 1990;79:448–453.
21. Savill JS, Wyllie AH, Henson JE, Walport MJ, Henson PM, Haslett C. Macrophage phagocytosis of aging neutrophils in inflammation: programmed cell death in the neutrophil leads to its recognition by macrophages. *J Clin Invest* 1989;83:865–875.

22. Hager-Malecka B, Lukas A, Szczepanski Z, Frydrych J, Sliwa F, Lukas W, Romanska K. Granulocyte viability test in children from an environment with heavy metal pollution. *Acta Paed Hung* 1986;27:227–231.
23. Fischbein A, Tsang P, Luo JJ, Roboz JP, Jiang JD, Bekesi JG. Phenotypic aberrations of $CD3^+$ and $CD4^+$ cells and functional impairments of lymphocytes at low-level occupational exposure to lead. *Clin Immunol Immunopathol* 1993;66:163–168.
24. Cohen N, Modai D, Golik A, et al. Increased concanavalin A-induced suppressor cell activity in humans with occupational lead exposure. *Environ Res* 1989;48:1–6.
25. Borella P, Giardino A. Lead and cadmium at very low doses affect *in vitro* immune response of human lymphocytes. *Environ Res* 1991;55:165–177.
26. Lawrence DA, Slavik J. *In vitro* effects of metals on various reactivities of human peripheral blood and splenic mononuclear cells. *Toxicologist* 1992;12:29(abst).
27. Luster MI, Munson AE, Thomas P, et al. Development of a testing battery to assess chemical-induced immunotoxicity: National Toxicology Program's guidelines for immunotoxicity evaluation in mice. *Fundam Appl Toxicol* 1988;10:2–19.
28. Hemphill FE, Kaeberle ML, Buck WB. Lead suppression of mouse resistance to *Salmonella typhimurium*. *Science* 1971;172:1031–1032.
29. Gainer JH. Lead aggravates viral disease and represses the antiviral activity of interferon inducers. *Environ Health Perspect* 1974;7:113–119.
30. Gainer JH. Effects of heavy metals and of deficiency of zinc on mortality rates in mice infected with encephalomyocarditis virus. *Am J Vet Res* 1977;38:869–872.
31. Kowolenko M, Tracy L, Lawrence D. Early effects of lead on bone marrow cell responsiveness in mice challenged with *Listeria monocytogenes*. *Fundam Appl Toxicol* 1991;17:75–82.
32. Lawrence DA. *In vivo* and *in vitro* effects of lead on humoral and cell-mediated immunity. *Infect Immun* 1981;31:136–143.
33. Cook JA, Hoffman EO, Di Luzio NR. Influence of lead and cadmium on the susceptibility of rats to bacterial challenge. *Proc Soc Exp Biol Med* 1975;150:741–747.
34. Selye H, Tuchweber B, Bertók L. Effect of lead acetate on the susceptibility of rats to bacterial endotoxins. *J Bacteriol* 1966;91:884–890.
35. Schumer W, Erve PR. Endotoxin sensitivity of adrenalectomized rats treated with lead acetate. *J Reticuloendothel Soc* 1973;13:122–125.
36. Cook JA, Marconi EA, Di Luzio NR. Lead, cadmium, endotoxin interaction: effect on mortality and hepatic function. *Toxicol Appl Pharmacol* 1974;28:292–302.
37. Koller LD. Immunosuppression produced by lead, cadmium, and mercury. *Am J Vet Res* 1973; 34:1457–1458.
38. Street NE, Mosmann TR. Functional diversity of T lymphocytes due to secretion of different cytokine patterns. *FASEB J* 1991;5:171–177.
39. Sher A, Coffman RL. Regulation of immunity to parasites by T cells and T cell-derived cytokines. *Annu Rev Immunol* 1992;10:385–409.
40. Clerici M, Shearer GM. A TH1 to TH2 switch is a critical step in the etiology of HIV infection. *Immunol Today* 1993;14:107–111.
41. Ezzell C. AIDS' unlucky strike: when T cells would rather switch than fight. *J NIH Res* 1993;5:59–64.
42. Dudley DJ, Chen C, Mitchell MD, Daynes RA, Araneo BA. Adaptive immune responses during murine pregnancy: pregnancy-induced regulation of lymphokine production by activated T lymphocytes. *Am J Obstet Gynecol* 1993;168:1155–1163.
43. Wegmann TG, Lin H, Guilbert L, Mosmann TR. Bidirectional cytokine interactions in the maternal–fetal relationship: is successful pregnancy a TH2 phenomenon? *Immunol Today* 1993;14:353–356.
44. Kubo M, Cinader B. Polymorphism of age-related changes in interleukin (IL) production: differential changes of T helper populations, synthesizing IL2, IL3, and IL4. *Eur J Immunol* 1990;20:1289–1296.
45. Nagelkerken L, Hertogh-Huijbregts A, Dobber R, Dräger A. Age-related changes in lymphokine production related to a decreased number of $CD45RB^{hi}$ $CD4^+$ T cells. *Eur J Immunol* 1991;21:273–281.
46. Fowell D, McKnight AJ, Powrie F, Dyke R, Mason D. Subsets of $CD4^+$ T cells and their roles in the induction and prevention of autoimmunity. *Immunol Rev* 1991;123:37–63.
47. Goldman M, Druet P, Gleichmann E. TH2 cells in systemic autoimmunity: insights from allogeneic diseases and chemically-induced autoimmunity. *Immunol Today* 1991;12:223–227.

48. McCabe MJ Jr, Lawrence DA. Lead, a major environmental pollutant, is immunomodulatory by its differential effects on CD4$^+$ T cell subsets. *Toxicol Appl Pharmacol* 1991;111:13–23.
49. Ochel M, Vohr HW, Pfeiffer C, Gleichmann E. IL-4 is required for the IgE and IgG1 autoantibody formation in mice treated with mercuric chloride. *J Immunol* 1991;146:3006–3011.
50. Faith RE, Luster MI, Kimmel CA. Effect of chronic developmental lead exposure on cell-mediated immune function. *Clin Exp Immunol* 1979;35:413–420.
51. Müller S, Gillert KE, Krause C, Gross U, L'Age-Stehr J, Diamantstcin T. Suppression of delayed type hypersensitivity of mice by lead. *Experientia* 1977;33:667–668.
52. Kowolenko M, Tracy L, Mudzinski S, Lawrence DA. Effect of lead on macrophage function. *J Leukoc Biol* 1988;43:357–364.
53. Koller LD, Roan JG. Effects of lead and cadmium on mouse peritoneal macrophages. *J Reticuloendothel Soc* 1977;21:7–12.
54. Kerkvliet NI, Baecher-Steppan L. Immunotoxicology studies on lead: effects of exposure on tumor growth and cell-mediated tumor immunity after syngeneic or allogeneic stimulation. *Immunopharmacology* 1982;4:213–224.
55. Filkens JP, Bychanan BJ. Effects of lead acetate on sensitivity to shock, intravascular carbon and endotoxin clearances, and hapatic endotoxin detoxification. *Proc Soc Exp Biol Med* 1973;142:471–475.
56. Schlick E, Friedberg KD. The influence of low lead doses on the reticuloendothelial system and leucocytes of mice. *Arch Toxicol* 1981;47:197–207.
57. Kowolenko M, Tracy L, Lawrence DA. Lead-induced alterations of *in vitro* bone marrow cell responses to colony stimulating factor-1. *J Leukoc Biol* 1989;45:198–206.
58. Lawrence DA. Heavy metal modulation of lymphocyte activities. 1. *In vitro* effects of heavy metals on primary humoral immune responses. *Toxicol Appl Pharmacol* 1981;57:439–451.
59. Lawrence DA. Heavy metal modulation of lymphocyte activities. 2. Lead, an *in vitro* mediator of B cell activiation. *Int J Immunopharmacol* 1981;3:153–161.
60. Warner GL, Lawrence DA. Stimulation of murine lymphocyte responses by cations. *Cell Immunol* 1986;101:425–439.
61. McCabe MJ Jr, Lawrence DA. The heavy metal lead exhibits B cell-stimulatory factor activity by enhancing B cell Ia expression and differentiation. *J Immunol* 1990;145:671–677.
62. Honchel R, Marsano L, Cohen D, Shedlofsky S, McClain CJ. Lead enhances lipopolysaccharide and tumor necrosis factor liver injury. *J Lab Clin Med* 1991;117:202–208.
63. Koller LD, Exon JH, Roan JG. Humoral antibody response in mice after single dose exposure to lead or cadmium. *Proc Soc Exp Biol Med* 1976;151:339–342.
64. Lawrence DA, Mitchell D, Rudofsky U. Heavy metal modulation of lymphocyte and macrophage activity. In: Archer D, ed. *Proceedings of the 13th Annual Conference on Environmental Toxicology*. Springfield, VA: National Technical Information Service; 1983:63–79.
65. Luster MI, Faith RE, Kimmel CA. Depression of humoral immunity in rats following chronic developmental lead exposure. *J Environ Pathol Toxicol* 1978;1:397–402.
66. Matis LA, Glimcher LH, Paul WE, Schwartz RH. Magnitude of a response of histocompatibility-restricted T cell clones is a function of the product of the concentrations of antigen and Ia molecules. *Proc Natl Acad Sci USA* 1983;80:6019–6023.
67. Roehm NW, Leibson HJ, Zlotnik A, Kappler J, Marrack P, Cambier JC. Interleukin-induced increase in Ia expression by normal mouse B cells. *J Exp Med* 1984;160:679–694.
68. Cambier JC, Newell MK, Justement LB, McGuire JC, Leach KL, Chen ZZ. Ia binding ligands and cAMP stimulate nuclear translocation of PKC in B lymphocytes. *Nature* 1987;327:629–631.
69. Chen ZZ, McGuire JC, Leach KL, Cambier JC. Transmembrane signaling through B cell MHC class II molecules: anti-Ia antibodies induce protein kinase C translocation to the nuclear fraction. *J Immunol* 1987;138:2345–2352.
70. Corley RB, LoCascio NJ, Ovnic M, Haughton G. Two separate functions of class II (Ia) molecules: T cell stimulation and B cell excitation. *Proc Natl Acad Sci USA* 1985;82:516–520.
71. St-Pierre Y, Nabavi N, Ghogawala Z, Glimcher LH, Watts TH. A functional role for signal transduction via the cytoplasmic domains of MHC class II proteins. *J Immunol* 1989;143:808–812.
72. McCabe MJ Jr, Dias JA, Lawrence DA. Lead influences translational or posttranslational regulation of Ia expression and increases invariant chain expression in mouse B cells. *J Biochem Toxicol* 1991;6:269–276.
73. Guagliardi LE, Koppelman B, Blum JS, Marks MS, Cresswell P, Brodsky FM. Co-localization of molecules involved in antigen processing and presentation in an early endocytic compartment. *Nature* 1990;343:133–139.

74. Lotteau V, Teyton L, Peleraux A, et al. Intracellular transport of class II MHC molecules directed by invariant chain. *Nature* 1990;348:600–605.
75. Noelle RJ, Kuziel WA, Maliszewski CR, McAdams E, Vitetta ES, Tucker PW. Regulation of the expression of multiple class II genes in murine B cells by B cell stimulatory factor-1 (BSF-1). *J Immunol* 1986;137:1718–1723.
76. Dubey C, Bellon B, Hirsch F, Kuhn J, Vial MC, Goldman M, Druett P. Increased expression of class II major histocompatibility complex molecules on B cells in rats susceptible or resistant to $HgCl_2$-induced autoimmunity. *Clin Exp Immunol* 1991;86:118–123.
77. Warner GL, Lawrence DA. Cell surface and cell cycle analysis of metal-induced murine T cell proliferation. *Eur J Immunol* 1986;16:1337–1342.
78. Koller LD, Kovacic S. Decreased antibody formation in mice exposed to lead. *Nature* 1974;250: 148–149.
79. Abbas AK, Williams ME, Burstein HJ, Chang T, Bossu P, Lichtman AH. Activation and function of $CD4^+$ T cell subsets. *Immunol Rev* 1991;123:5–22.
80. Janeway CA Jr, Carding S, Jones B, et al. $CD4^+$ T cells: specificity and function. *Immunol Rev* 1988;101:39–80.
81. Schmitz J, Assenmacher M, Radbruch A. Regulation of T helper cell cytokine expression: functional dichotomy of antigen-presenting cells. *Eur J Immunol* 1993;23:191–199.
82. Smith KL, Lawrence DA. Immunomodulation of *in vitro* antigen presentation by cations. *Toxicol Appl Pharmacol* 1988;96:476–484.
83. Mosmann TR, Cherwinski H, Bond MW, Giedlin MA, Coffman RL. Two types of murine helper T cell clone. 1. Definition according to profiles of lymphokine activities and secreted proteins. *J Immunol* 1986;136:2348–2357.
84. North RJ. The relative importance of blood monocytes and fixed macrophages to the expression of cell-mediated immunity to infection. *J Exp Med* 1970;132:521–534.
85. Buchmeier NA, Schrieber ND. Requirement of endogenous interferon-γ production for resolution of *Listeria monocytogenes* infection. *Proc Natl Acad Sci USA* 1985;82:7404–7408.
86. Dalton DK, Pitts-Meek S, Keshav S, Figari IS, Bradley A, Stewart TA. Multiple defects of immune cell function in mice with disrupted interferon-γ genes. *Science* 1993;259:1739–1742.
87. Huang S, Hendriks W, Althage A, et al. Immune response in mice that lack the interferon-γ receptor. *Science* 1993;259:1742–1745.
88. Snapper CM, Mond JJ. Towards a comprehensive view of immunoglobulin class switching. *Immunol Today* 1993;14:15–17.
89. Betz M, Fox BS. Prostaglandin E_2 inhibits production of TH1 lymphokines but not of TH2 lymphokines. *J Immunol* 1991;146:108–113.
90. Gajewski TF, Schell SR, Fitch FW. Evidence implicating utilization of different T cell receptor-associated signaling pathways by TH1 and TH2 clones. *J Immunol* 1990;144:4110–4120.
91. Muñoz E, Zubiaga AM, Merrow M, Sauter NP, Huber BT. Cholera toxin discriminates between T helper 1 and 2 cells in T cell receptor-mediated activation: role of cAMP in T cell proliferation. *J Exp Med* 1990;172:95–103.
92. Novak TJ, Rothenberg EV. cAMP inhibits induction of interleukin 2 but not of interleukin 4 in T cells. *Proc Natl Acad Sci USA* 1990;87:9353–9357.
93. Laterra J, Bressler JP, Indurti RR, Belloni-Olivi L, Goldstein GW. Inhibition of astroglia-induced endothelial differentiation by inorganic lead: a role for protein kinase C. *Proc Natl Acad Sci USA* 1992;89:10748–10752.
94. Markovac J, Goldstein GW. Picomolar concentrations of lead stimulate brain protein kinase C. *Nature* 1988;334:71–73.
95. Murakami K, Feng G, Chen SG. Inhibition of brain protein kinase C subtypes by lead. *J Pharmacol Exp Ther* 1992;264:757–761.
96. Sha'afi RI, Molski TFP, Huang CK, Naccache PH. The inhibition of neutrophil responsiveness caused by phorbol esters is blocked by the protein kinase C inhibitor H7. *Biochem Biophys Res Commun* 1986;137:50–60.
97. Hektoen L. Scientific books. Paul Erlich, eine darstellung seines wissenschaftlichen wirkens. *Science* 1915;41:27–28.

Immunotoxicology and Immunopharmacology, Second Edition, edited by J. H. Dean, M. I. Luster, A. E. Munson, and I. Kimber.
Raven Press, Ltd., New York © 1994.

9

Mycotoxin-Induced Immune Modulation

James J. Pestka and *Genevieve S. Bondy

*Department of Food Science and Human Nutrition, Michigan State University, East Lansing, Michigan 48824; and *Toxicology Research Division, Food Directorate, Health Protection Branch, Health Canada, Ottawa, Ontario, K1A OL2 Canada*

Mycotoxins are a structurally diverse group of chemicals that are produced as secondary metabolites by fungi. A wide variety of biologic and toxicologic effects have been associated with these compounds (1). Mycotoxins are present in many agricultural commodities including corn, wheat, and nuts and are sometimes carried over into animal foods. Since they are recalcitrant to processing, these compounds are often detected in finished food products. Mycotoxins can also be found in the environment in association with mold spores (2,3).

It has long been recognized by veterinary clinicians that marked immunosuppression is observed in livestock ingesting mycotoxins at levels below those that cause overt toxicity (4). Mycotoxin-induced immunomodulation is significant because ingestion or inhalation of mycotoxins by humans may contribute etiologically to immune dysfunction diseases or to increased susceptibility to infectious agents and neoplasms. Altered immune function may also be closely associated with the symptoms of certain animal mycotoxicoses. Additionally, mycotoxins may predispose food-producing animals to infectious disease agents such as *Listeria* and *Salmonella* and thus result in increased animal-to-human transmission.

There are a number of reviews of immune alteration by mycotoxins (5–9). While these address much of the seminal work in this field, this chapter focuses on more recent studies using oral exposure, since this mimics natural exposure to mycotoxins. *In vitro* studies and other *in vivo* studies employing alternate exposure routes are described when they provide additional insight into the mechanistic basis of mycotoxin-induced immune alteration. For discussion purposes, it is convenient to group the mycotoxins into those elaborated by the *Aspergillus–Penicillium* and the *Fusarium* groups in plant foods during growth, harvest, or storage since these have the greatest potential impact on the food supply.

ASPERGILLUS AND *PENICILLIUM* TOXINS

Aflatoxin

The aflatoxins are a group of difuranocoumarins, produced by *Aspergillus flavus* and *A. parasiticus*, that are potent hepatotoxins and hepatocarcinogens (1). Extensive research has been done on the immunomodulatory effects of aflatoxins, particularly on the effects of aflatoxin B1 (AFB1) (reviewed in ref. 8). Recent literature supports the contention that AFB1 has the greatest effect on cell-mediated immunity (CMI). In CD-1 mice, orally exposed to AFB1 (0.145 and 0.7 mg/kg body weight), there was dose-related suppression of delayed-type hypersensitivity to keyhole limpet hemocyanin (10). C57Bl/6 mice exhibit significant decreases in splenic CD4 (T helper, TH) cell numbers at 0.75 mg/kg AFB1, and in interleukin-2 (IL-2) production by splenic lymphocytes at 0.15 and 0.75 mg/kg AFB1 (11). In guinea pigs receiving oral aflatoxin, there was reduced response to intradermal phytohemagglutinin (PHA) at 0.045 mg/kg AFB1 and a reduction in delayed cutaneous hypersensitivity to *Nocardia asteroides* at 0.042 mg/kg AFB1 (12,13).

Considerable research has focused on the effects of aflatoxin on the avian immune system since the toxin poses an economic threat to the poultry industry. Again, cell-mediated immune responses are particularly sensitive. For example, in broiler chicks receiving 1 ppm AFB1 in feed, the delayed hypersensitivity response to dinitrofluorobenzene is reduced (14), and in chickens receiving 0.3 ppm AFB1 in feed, the graft-versus-host response is suppressed (15). Other indications of a cell-mediated immune effect in chicks fed AFB1 are reduced thymus weight and reduced peripheral T lymphocyte numbers (14,16,17). Additionally, there appears to be a genetic component involved in AFB1-related CMI suppression. Studies have been done with a population of chickens selected for high plasma protein responsiveness to dietary AFB1. Oral administration of AFB1 to these chicks at 0.1 and 0.5 mg/kg results in lower peripheral blood lymphocyte proliferation responses to the T cell mitogen concanavalin A (Con A) compared to chicks with low plasma protein concentrations in response to AFB1 (18).

In vitro data indicate that T cell-mediated responses are sensitive to AFB1. In murine spleen cells cocultured with rat hepatocytes and AFB1, the T cell-dependent antibody response to sheep red blood cells (SRBCs) is more sensitive to AFB1 than antibody responses to either a polyclonal activator lipopolysaccharide (LPS) or a T cell-independent activator [dinitrophenol (DNP)–Ficoll] (19). The mitogenic response to Con A is more sensitive to AFB1 suppression than was the response to LPS or PHA in murine splenic lymphocytes cocultured with rat hepatocytes.

The effects of AFB1 on humoral immunity were not as evident as effects on CMI and are not consistent across species barriers. Bursal weight loss is significant in chicks fed AFB1 but is comparatively less than thymus weight loss (17). In swine receiving up to 500 ppm AFB1 in feed and inoculated with *Erysipelothrix rhusiopathiae* bacteria, there is no significant difference in antibody titers compared to inoculated swine receiving uncontaminated feed (20). The ability of guinea pigs to produce antibodies to *Brucella abortus* is unaffected by aflatoxin (0.045 mg/kg) administered orally (13). In rabbits receiving aflatoxin in feed (approximately 24 ppm) the antibody-forming response to SRBCs, a T cell-dependent antigen, is unchanged compared to animals receiving AFB1-free diets (21). In contrast, C57Bl/6 mice receiving up to 0.75 mg/kg AFB1 by gavage exhibit a dose-related decrease in plasma immunoglobulin M (IgM) titers to SRBCs (11). In CD-1 mice, oral AFB1 exposure (0.145 to 0.7 mg/kg) had reduced the numbers of splenic IgM-producing cells specific for SRBCs, while the number of antibody-producing cells specific for the T cell-independent antigen LPS was not altered (10). This suggested that although AFB1 can suppress B cell function, its effects were mediated by T regulatory cells.

The effects of oral AFB1 administration on spontaneous and mitogen-stimulated lymphocyte proliferation do not conclusively support the possibility of suppression of either CMI or humoral immunity. Blastogenic responses in the presence of AFB1 appears to be strain dependent in mice. In CD-1 mice receiving AFB1 orally (po) (0.03 to 0.7 mg/kg), spontaneous splenic lymphocyte blastogenesis was more sensitive than mitogen-stimulated blastogenesis, whereas in BALB/c mice, mitogen-stimulated blastogenesis was suppressed without regard for mitogen specificity (10,22). In C57Bl/6 mice, both LPS- and pokeweed mitogen (PWM)-stimulated spleen lymphocyte blastogenesis were suppressed to a greater extent than Con A- and PHA-stimulated lymphocyte proliferation, suggesting specific effects on splenic B cell function (11). A study with human peripheral blood lymphocytes (PBLs) suggested a genetic component to suppression of lymphocyte blastogenesis by AFB1. It was also interesting to note that human PBLs bearing the human leukocyte antigen (HLA)-A3 were more sensitive to *in vitro* suppression of PHA-stimulated blastogenesis than PBLs negative for HLA-A3 (23).

The phagocytic functions of macrophages and cells of the reticuloendothelial system were consistently inhibited by AFB1. For example in chicks, the percentage of nitroblue tetrazolium (NBT) positive cells in splenic tissue was depressed by AFB1 exposure (0.3 to 1.0 ppm in feed), an indicator of depressed macrophage function (14). Likewise, the clearance of circulating colloidal carbon was depressed in chicks receiving AFB1 (0.3 ppm) (15). Finally, in rats, both macrophage number and function were depressed by oral administration of AFB1 (0.35 to 0.7 mg/kg bw) (24).

In vitro data also support the suppression of phagocytic activity *in vivo* in rats and chickens by AFB1. Phagocytosis, intracellular killing of *Candida albicans*, and spontaneous oxygen (O^{-2}) production are suppressed in rat peritoneal macrophages exposed to aflatoxins *in vitro* (25). Microsomal activation of AFB1 alters adherence, morphology, and phagocytic ability of chicken and turkey peritoneal macrophages *in vitro*. In this study, the P450 inhibitor piperonyl butoxide reverses all morphologic and functional alterations, indicating that activation of AFB1 by mixed function oxidases plays a significant role in macrophage toxicity (26,27). Walsh et al. (28) determined that AFB1 depresses proliferation of mitogen-stimulated bovine blood macrophages but did not affect IL-1 production.

Other aspects of innate immunity were suppressed to varying degrees by AFB1. Natural killer (NK) cell-mediated cytolysis of YAC-1 target cells was suppressed in BALB/c mice receiving oral AFB1 at concentrations of 0.03 to 0.7 mg/kg (22), but was unaffected in C57Bl/6 mice (0.03 to 0.75 mg/kg) (11) and in rabbits (24 ppm in feed) (21). Total hemolytic serum complement activity was reduced in pigs receiving feed containing 500 ppm AFB1; however, complement activity was unaffected in pigs receiving 300 ppm AFB1 and in rabbits receiving 95 ppm AFB1 in feed (20,21).

In summary, AFB1 suppresses CMI to a greater extent than humoral immunity. Some aspects of innate immunity, especially phagocytic responses, are also inhibited by AFB1 exposure.

Ochratoxin A

The ochratoxins are a group of isocoumarin derivatives linked to phenylalanine that have been found in cereals, beans, peanuts, and rice. The early literature concerning the immunosuppressive effects of ochratoxin A (OA) has been reviewed by Thurston et al. (8). Unlike AFB1, which primarily affects CMI responses, experimental administration of OA does not appear to specifically suppress any single immune response. General signs of immunosuppression following OA ingestion include lymphocytopenia and depletion of lymphoid cells, particularly in the thymus, bursa of Fabricius, and Peyer's patches (29–31). These events indicate that OA ingestion affects both CMI and humoral immunity, which was borne out by the assessment of specific immune functions. Suppression of CMI responses in turkeys following OA ingestion (4 ppm in feed) was indicated by depressed delayed hypersensitivity to *Mycobacterium avium* and its purified protein derivative (30). In chickens, depressed humoral responses are indicated by lower serum IgM and IgG concentrations in birds receiving OA (up to 4 ppm in feed) compared to control birds (29). Intraperitoneal administration of OA to mice suppressed antibody responses to SRBCs (1 μg/kg OA) (32) and *Brucella abortus* antigen (5 mg/kg OA) (33). However, antibody responses in mice (4 ppm OA in feed) and in chicks (2 ppm OA in feed) were unaffected when OA was administered in feed (33,34). Dietary factors may account for some of the differences in OA-induced immunosuppression, since phenylalanine has been shown to attenuate immunosuppression in mice and to reduce mortality in broiler chicks receiving OA-contaminated diets (35,36).

Ochratoxin A has variable effects on innate immunity. In chickens receiving 4 to 8 mg/kg OA in feed, phagocytic activity in peripheral blood monocytes was suppressed (37). In mice receiving OA subcutaneously (sc) (up to 80 mg/kg), peritoneal macrophage phagocytosis and tumor cytolysis were increased (31); however, in mice treated with OA intraperitoneally (ip) (up to 13.4 mg/kg), there is no effect on the ability of peritoneal macrophages to develop tumoricidal activity (38). Murine peritoneal macrophage migration was inhibited to a maximum of 56.2% of control migration by concentrations of OA up to 1.7 mM *in vitro*. Addition of phenylalanine prevents OA-induced inhibition of macrophage migration (39). Dietary OA reduces total hemolytic complement activity in chickens at 2 ppm in feed but failed to suppress complement activity when administered orally to guinea pigs at concentrations of 0.45 mg/d (34,40). It remains to be determined whether differences in species, dose, route of exposure, or other experimental factors are responsible for this discordance.

The potential link between OA-induced immunosuppression and carcinogenesis has been explored. When Manolova et al. (41) tested the ability of OA to alter chromosomes in human peripheral lymphocytes *in vitro* in the presence or absence of a kidney microsomal metabolic activation system, OA induced X-chromosome aberrations that were similar to those previously detected in lymphocytes from patients suffering from endemic nephropathy. A form of tumor resistance, splenic NK cell activity, was decreased in mice ingesting OA (6.7 and 13.4 mg/kg), whereas macrophage-mediated antitumor activity and cytotoxic T lymphocyte-mediated antitumor activity were unaffected (38). The observed suppression of NK cell activity appeared to be the result of inhibition of endogenous interferon (IFN) levels.

OA inhibits lymphocyte function *in vitro*. OA was found to be more toxic to porcine blood lymphocytes than to granulocytes in a colorimetric cytotoxicity assay (42). Likewise, Con A-stimulated blastogenesis of porcine lymphocyte was inhibited by OA *in vitro* (43). Blastogenesis of both human B and T lymphocytes was inhibited by OA *in vitro* (44). In this study, both IL-2 receptor expression and IL-2 production were inhibited.

It is difficult to correlate *in vitro* inhibition of lymphocyte function by OA with immunosuppression seen in animal studies, especially since route of exposure to OA appears to influence the extent to which immunosuppression will occur. OA is known to bind to serum albumin *in vivo*; however, in porcine lymphocytes exposed to OA *in vitro* there were no marked differences in inhibition of blastogenesis in cultures with or without added bovine serum albumin (43,45). Based on naturally occurring levels of OA (46), the concentrations of OA required to induce immunosuppression experimentally are generally higher than the levels found in contaminated foods and feeds.

Citrinin

Citrinin is a quinone methide that has been found in wheat, rye, oats, and barley. Campbell et al. (47) found that cellular and humoral responses were not affected in broiler chickens receiving citrinin in feed. In mice administered citrinin ip, the toxin appears to be immunostimulatory rather than immunosuppressive (48). Peripheral lymphocyte numbers were depressed at a dose of 0.6 mg/kg citrinin, while antibody responses to SRBCs were stimulated at the same dose. Splenic lymphocyte blastogenesis with or without mitogens is stimulated at all doses tested *in vivo*. Citrinin

(45 to 3800 μM) inhibits murine peritoneal macrophage migration *in vitro* by up to 92.5% of control migration (39). Supportive data suggesting that exposure to citrinin in feed or food is immunotoxic do not exist.

Cyclopiazonic Acid

Cyclopiazonic acid is a toxic metabolite that has been found in corn, peanuts, millet, and cheese. Guinea pigs receiving cyclopiazonic acid (CPA) orally (2 mg/kg), exhibited suppressed delayed cutaneous hypersensitivity to *Nocardia asteroides* (13). Both complement activity and cutaneous hypersensitivity to *Mycobacterium tuberculosis* were unaffected in guinea pigs at CPA doses up to 2 mg/d (49). Intraperitoneal injection of CPA (0.1 to 5.0 mg/kg) in rats causes a transient depression of antibody responses to SRBCs, but at day 14 after SRBC injection antibody production was higher in CPA-treated animals than in control animals (50). There is insufficient evidence to conclude that oral exposure to CPA would have similar transient immunosuppressive effects.

Patulin

Patulin is a toxic metabolite found in apple juice and moldy feeds that can cause ulceration and hemorrhagic lesions. Oral administration of patulin has variable effects on cell-mediated and humoral activity. In mice receiving patulin orally (10 mg/kg), splenic T lymphocytes and T suppressor/cytotoxic (Ts/c) lymphocytes were significantly increased and accompanied by a depressed CD4:CD8 (T_H:T_s) ratio (51). BALB/c mice receiving a single ip injection of patulin (2 or 4 mg/kg) exhibited depressed delayed hypersensitivity response to *Bordetella pertussis* (52). In both mice and rabbits, serum IgA, IgG, and IgM concentrations were lower than in control animals (51). In contrast, oral administration of patulin (10 mg/kg) increases neutrophil numbers and resistance to *Candida albicans* infection in Swiss mice (53).

Patulin has been shown to have effects on phagocytic cells *in vitro*. Oxidative activity is depressed in mouse and rabbit leukocytes incubated with patulin (51). In peritoneal macrophages, isolated from C57BL/6J mice, *in vitro* exposure to patulin inhibited *Saccharomyces cerevisiae* killing and phagocytosis, O^{-2} production, phagosome–lysosome fusion, and lysosomal enzyme production (54). Protein synthesis was inhibited and cell membrane function was compromised in rat alveolar macrophages exposed to patulin *in vitro* (55). There was no experimental evidence indicating that the above-described immune events were affected in animals ingesting patulin.

Secalonic Acid D

Secalonic acid D (SAD) is a metabolite of *Penicillium oxalicum*. Exposure to SAD increased white blood cell (WBC) and neutrophil counts but reduced circulating lymphocyte counts in mice exposed ip at 15 to 45 mg/kg (56). Mice administered SAD ip at 35 mg/kg exhibited increased mortality from influenza virus infection and had lower antibody titers to influenza virus than control mice (57). At this time there is no experimental evidence to indicate that ingestion of low levels of SAD would be significantly immunosuppressive.

Wortmannin

The potential for immunosuppression by wortmannin, a steroid metabolite of *Penicillium wortmanni, Fursarium oxysporum*, and other fungi, was indicated by the anti-inflammatory activity of the structurally related fungal metabolite 11-desacetoxy-wortmannin (58). Ingestion of wortmannin affects both CMI and humoral immunity. Severe necrosis of the spleen, lymph nodes, and gut-associated lymphoid tissue was observed in rats receiving crude wortmannin in feed or purified wortmannin (4 to 50 mg/kg) by gavage. Gavaged rats also display severe necrosis of the thymus cortex, whereas rats receiving wortmannin in feed exhibit depletion and only mild necrosis of thymus lymphoid tissue (59).

Ingestion of wortmannin at sublethal levels (<5 ppm) in feed depresses a number of immune parameters in rats. Thymus weight and cellularity were significantly reduced, serum IgM and IgG levels were depressed, and LPS-stimulated spleen lymphocyte blastogenesis was suppressed. Additionally, the number of cells producing antibody to both a T-dependent antigen (SRBCs) and a T-independent antigen (trinitrophenol–conjugated LPS) was reduced (60). *In vitro*, phagocytic cells were also affected by wortmannin. Exposure of human neutrophils and mouse bone marrow-derived macrophages to nanomolar concentrations of wortmannin or its 11-desacetoxy analog inhibits induction of respiratory bursts during phagocytosis (61).

FUSARIUM TOXINS

Trichothecenes

The trichothecenes are a group of over 60 sesquiterpenoids that include some of the most potent protein synthesis inhibitors known (62,63). These compounds have been associated with human and animal toxicoses that are sometimes fatal (63–66). Experimentally, acute exposure to trichothecene mycotoxins causes severe damage to actively dividing cells in bone marrow, lymph nodes, spleen, thymus, and intestinal mucosa. At lower doses, these compounds can be both immunosuppressive and immunostimulatory. Vomitoxin (deoxynivalenol), nivalenol, T-2 toxin, and diacetoxyscirpenol are among the most commonly detected trichothecenes.

Repetitive exposure to the trichothecenes T-2 toxin and diacetoxyscirpenol increased susceptibility to *Mycobacterium* (67), *Candida* (68), *Cryptococcus* (69), *Listeria* (70), *Salmonella* (71–73) and herpes simplex virus type I (74). Immunosuppression was dramatically illustrated by a five log reduction in the median lethal dose (LD_{50}) for *Salmonella* observed when orally coadministered to mice with T-2 toxin (71). There was a marked increase in susceptibility to *Salmonella typhimurium* LPS when T-2 toxin was coadministered, perhaps suggesting that impaired resistance to LPS might be one mechanism for increased susceptibility to *Salmonella* (75). Taylor et al. (76,77) have hypothesized that T-2 toxin treatment enhances LPS absorption from the gut and that this produces some of the pathologic sequelae associated with T-2 toxicosis.

Cell-mediated immunity appears to be impaired by trichothecenes. A single injection of T-2 toxin depresses the delayed hypersensitivity response to *B. pertussis* (52) and increases skin graft rejection time (78). Both oral dosing and feeding studies in mice indicate that vomitoxin (deoxynivalenol) can increase susceptibility to *Listeria* and depress the delayed hypersensitivity response (79,80).

In contrast, Cooray and Jonsson (81) noted enhanced resistance to mastitis-causing pathogens when mice were administered T-2 toxin by gavage prior to experimental infection. Short-term preinoculation with T-2 enhances resistance to *Listeria*, whereas postinoculation with T-2 toxin results in immunosuppression (70,82–84). Enhanced resistance is associated with increased migration of macrophage and elevated phagocytic activity. Corrier (6) hypothesized that these latter effects may have been mediated by altered T regulatory cell activity.

Trichothecenes cause a variety of cellular effects that impact immune function. For example, *in vitro* exposure to trichothecenes resulted in toxicity to alveolar macrophages (85–87), but induced differentiation of human myeloid leukemic cells (88). Pang et al. (89) noted that inhalation of T-2 toxin in swine results in depressed alveolar macrophage phagocytosis and blastogenic responses in pulmonary lymphocytes. Dose-dependent decreases or increases in B and T cell mitogen responses were found in lymphocytes from animals exposed to T-2 toxin, vomitoxin, or various macrocyclic trichothecenes (52,74,79,90–94). In splenic cells of mice exposed to macrocyclic trichothecenes, T cell proliferation was significantly increased in the mixed lymphocyte reaction (91).

In similar fashion, *in vitro* trichothecene exposure impairs or enhances mitogen-induced proliferation (90,95–103). The rank order of potency among trichothecene classes for *in vitro* inhibition of rodent and human lymphocyte proliferation assays is macrocyclic > type A group > type B group (104–110). *In vitro* lymphotoxicity of the type A and type B trichothecenes apparently depends on the degree of acylation in substituent groups. Porcher et al. (111) determined differences in sensitivities among lymphocyte cell types and related this to both differences in uptake and metabolism to less toxic compounds.

Humoral immunity can also be both stimulated and impaired by trichothecene exposure. Rosenstein et al. (112) observed that repeated injection of T-2 toxin caused a decreased humoral response to T-dependent antigens but an increased response to T-independent antigens. *In vitro* exposure to T-2 inhibits the plaque-forming cell (PFC) response to T cell-dependent and -independent antigens (113). Tomar et al. (102,110) found that dietary exposure of CD-1 mice to 3-acetyldeoxynivalenol or T-2 toxin did not alter T cell-independent antibody responses to DNP–

Ficoll or *Escherichia coli* LPS, but at 10 ppm they enhanced the T cell-dependent response to SRBCs. Female CD-1 mice fed T-2 toxin (3 ppm) for 16 months exhibit an enhanced PFC response to SRBCs (114). Prenatal exposure to T-2 toxin on day 11 of gestation does not impair immunity in CD-1 mice (115). Macrocyclic trichothecenes depress murine antibody response to SRBCs when injected ip. Exposure to vomitoxin in the diet at a 10 ppm threshold or by gavage at 0.75 mg/kg can similarly impair the murine splenic PFC response to the SRBCs (80,93,116).

Oral gavage with T-2 toxin results in increased spontaneous antibody-producing cells for all isotypes in the spleen (117). Consistent with this latter finding, Forsell et al. (118) detected a dramatic elevation in serum IgA, but concurrent decreases in IgM and IgG, in mice fed vomitoxin. The threshold for this effect was 2 ppm, with maximal effects occurring in the 10- to 25-ppm range (119–122). Increased serum IgA appeared concomitantly with elevated IgA immune complexes and polymeric IgA. Furthermore, Peyer's patch lymphocytes and to a lesser extent splenic lymphocytes isolated from vomitoxin-fed mice produced significantly more IgA than control cultures, both with and without mitogen stimulation (96,120,123,124). This indicates that there is premature maturation of IgA-secreting cells at the Peyer's patch level and that this is reflected in the systemic compartment. Possible T cell dysregulation was suggested by an increase in CD4+ and CD4:CD8 ratios of Peyer's patches and spleens of vomitoxin-fed mice (123).

Vomitoxin-induced dysregulation was strikingly similar to human IgA nephropathy (Berger's disease), which is the most common glomerulonephritis worldwide (125,126). In addition to *in vitro* and *in vivo* IgA hyperelevation, vomitoxin-exposed mice exhibit mesangial IgA accumulation and hematuria, which are hallmarks of this disease (119). Elevated serum IgA, mesangial IgA, and hematuria persisted for up to 3 months after withdrawal of vomitoxin from the mouse diet (127). Interestingly, there was a progressive increase in serum IgE after withdrawal of vomitoxin from the diet (128). IgA nephropathy occurs to a greater extent in males than females. Recently, it was determined that in B6C3F1 mice, males exhibit a predilection for vomitoxin-induced IgA nephropathy in terms of threshold toxin dose, as well as onset and magnitude of response (129). Another common feature of the human disease and the murine model is the involvement of polyvalent "natural" IgA, which may be associated with immune complex formation and the subsequent glomerulonephritis (130,131,131a).

Suppression and stimulation of immune function by trichothecenes present a seemingly unresolvable contradiction. Clearly, most immunotoxic manifestations of mycotoxins can be attributed to alterations in T cell function. While other toxic mechanisms such as impaired membrane function (132) or altered intercellular communication (133) are possible, trichothecene-induced immunosuppression is most readily explained by the capacity of these compounds to bind to ribosomes and inhibit protein synthesis (62,134). The immunostimulatory effects are somewhat more problematic. Trichothecenes and other protein synthesis inhibitors stimulate IL-1 production by macrophages (99,135) and IL-2 formation by lymphocytes (136,137). Sherman et al. (138) identified cardiovascular lesions in rats that had received splenic cells from syngeneic rats treated with T-2 toxin and suggested that this may be mediated by IL production. Recently, we have determined that *in vitro* exposure of splenic CD4+ cells to vomitoxin can result in increased help for IgA secretion by B cells (139) as well as elevated levels of IL-4 and IL-5 production (139a). Cloned T cells also exhibit a superinduction of IL-5 when cultured with vomitoxin (139b). One plausible mechanism for trichothecene hyperelevation of IgA production is through superinduction of T_H2 cytokines. The following temporal order or events upon trichothecene exposure in a lymph node might be predicted: (a) protein synthesis inhibition, (b) enhanced T_H cytokine messenger ribonucleic acid (mRNA) expression, (c) elevated T_H cytokine production *after* vomitoxin metabolism/removal and cessation of protein synthesis inhibition, and (d) terminal differentiation of Ig-secreting cells. The Peyer's patch may be particularly prone to this type of dysregulation since it would be exposed to concentrated levels of vomitoxin in food and after enterohepatic recirculation. A potential mechanism for "superinduction of cytokines" includes interference with synthesis of high-turnover proteins that limits transcription or half-life of IL mRNA; an analogous mechanism could be proposed at the level of translation.

Fumonisin B1

Fumonisin B1 (FB1), produced by *Fusarium moniliforme*, is the causative agent of equine leukoencephalomalacia and porcine pulmonary edema and is hepatotoxic and carcinogenic to rats (140–142). At this time there are few existing studies that address possible *in vivo* immunosuppressive activity by FB1 or the structurally related fumonisin toxins. Epidemiologic evidence supports a correlation between mystery swine disease (MSD) and feeding corn contaminated with FB1 and FB2 at concentrations of 20 ppm or higher (143). In conjunction with pyrexia, anorexia, and problems with gestation and farrowing, affected swine also exhibited increased infection rates, indicating the potential involvement of an immunosuppressive agent (144). Relatedly, Haschek et al. (145) found that pigs dosed intravenously (iv) with fumonisin over a period of several days (total of 4.6 to 7.9 mg/kg) or fed 48 to 166 ppm of the toxin exhibit membranous material in pulmonary macrophages. Dombrink-Kurtzman et al. (146) noted reduced lymphocyte viability in chickens fed a diet containing 62 ppm FB1 and 15 ppm FB2.

FB1 is cytotoxic *in vitro* to several rat hepatoma cell lines and to the Madin–Darby canine kidney (MDCK) cell line (147). Although *in vitro* murine splenic lymphocyte blastogenesis is unaffected by FB1 at concentrations up to 10 μg/ml (Bondy and J. J. Pestka, *unpublished data*), other studies indicate that FB1 and FB2 are cytotoxic to turkey lymphocytes with 50% cytotoxic doses ranging between 0.3 and 2 μg/ml (148,149). Chicken peritoneal macrophages treated with FB1 (10 to 100 μg) showed morphologic alterations, reductions in cell viability, and reduced phagocytic potential (150). Tumoricidal factor production in a chicken macrophage cell line was unaffected. In addition to studies of the effects of dietary fumonisins on overall immune function, there is a need for *in vivo* data to confirm *in vitro* suppression of macrophage function, and for studies of the effects of FB1 on the immune mechanisms associated with tumor resistance.

Zearalenone

Zearalenone is an estrogenic mycotoxin produced by *Fusarium* species and found in many cereal grains. While few studies have been directed specifically at the immunologic effects of this compound, other estrogens decrease host resistance to pathogens (151,152), increase tumor susceptibility (153), alter macrophage function (154), reduce NK cell activity (155), and depress the delayed hypersensitivity response (156). Zearalenone and its derivative zearalenol can induce thymic atrophy and macrophage activation (157). Ingestion of 10 ppm zearalenone for 2 weeks decreases resistance to *Listeria* but has no effects on antibody-forming cells to SRBCs or delayed hypersensitivity responses (80). Upon comparison of zearalenone analogs in a mitogen-stimulated lymphocyte proliferation assay, it appears that the keto group or the α-hydroxyl group at position C-6′ contributes to the lymphotoxicity of the parent molecule (106). However, the thresholds for inhibition by the zearalenone analogs exceed those that would be encountered physiologically and do not correlate with the estrogenic potencies for the compounds.

Fusarochromanone

Fusarochromanone (TDP-1) is a mycotoxin produced by *Fusarium equiseti* that has been associated with tibial dyschondroplasia (TDP) in poultry. This mycotoxin was both inhibitory and stimulatory (at lower levels) in the mitogen-induced lymphocyte proliferation assay (158). Deacetylation to its metabolite, TDP-2, greatly reduces these immunotoxic manifestations. Additional studies are warranted to verify whether immunotoxicity is similarly evident *in vivo*.

RELEVANCE TO HUMAN AND ANIMAL HEALTH

The investigations described in this chapter clearly indicate that several mycotoxins may be immunosuppressive or immunostimulatory and that these effects are dependent on route of exposure, timing, and dose. While immune alteration may be detectable following multiple high-dose injections, examination of the dietary effects of mycotoxins, particularly at levels found in human food and animal feed, are most desirable. Design of feeding experiments is complicated by the likelihood that high-level exposure to mycotoxins occurs sporadically in humans and animals. Another problem is that mycotoxin mixtures are likely to occur naturally and these may alter immunity in an additive or synergistic manner. Nutritional effects associated with feed refusal may also contribute to observed immune alterations. Finally, while systemic immunity is the focus of most investigations, it is very probable that mycotoxins have their greatest effect on mucosal lymphoid tissue (particularly gut and bronchial) before they are absorbed and metabolized. This possibility is verified by the observation that vomitoxin ingestion results in IgA hyperelevation and IgA-mediated glomerulonephritis. It should be noted that additional investigation of the immune effects of inhaled mycotoxins is also of interest because of the potential for environmental exposure via grain dust or mold-contaminated air supplies (2,3,159).

Taking the above into account, there is as yet insufficient experimental data to support the possibility that citrinin, cyclopiazonic acid, patulin, secalonic acid D, wortmannin, fumonisin, fusarochromanone, or zearalenone cause specific immune dysfunction in humans or animals. However, investigations of the aflatoxins, trichothecenes, and ochratoxin A might suggest a potential role for toxin-induced immune modulation in human and animal health problems.

Clearly, dietary aflatoxin exceeding 1 ppm can exert a variety of immunosuppressive effects, specifically on cell-mediated immunity. These concentrations might be most likely encountered in animal feed that is not inspected for interstate or international commerce or in human foods grown and stored in developing countries. However, the presence of aflatoxins in human food is regulated at the low parts per billion (ppb) range (e.g., <20 ppb in the United States) in most developed countries because of their potent hepatocarcinogenicity. Thus vigilant monitoring should minimize the potential for aflatoxin-induced immunosuppression in humans.

Ochratoxin A is reportedly a renal carcinogen (160) and has been suggested to contribute to human renal and urinary tumors (161,162). Luster et al. (38) suggested that suppression of NK cell activity might be a factor in the development of tumors because (a) dose for tumor induction was similar to that required for immunosuppression, (b) immunosuppression preceded development of detectable tumors, and (c) immune alterations were consistent with those involved in tumor immunity and correlated with changes in resistance to transplantable syngeneic tumor cells. One problem with this hypothesis is that existing evidence suggests that most immunodeficiency tumors are lymphomas and leukemias rather than solid tumors as occurs with ochratoxin A. A second concern is that the studies by Luster et al. (38) were conducted with very high levels of ochratoxin A which may not be encountered naturally.

It has been demonstrated that trichothecene-induced immune suppression can potentially impact food animal production. For example, simultaneous exposure of animals to trichothecenes and pathogens such as *Salmonella* can synergistically cause enhanced mortality, increased disease severity, accelerated body weight loss, and elevated pathogen load. Increased asymptomatic infection might theoretically result in enhanced movement of pathogen reservoirs into the food chain and ultimately increase animal-to-human transmission.

A common theme for trichothecene modulation of immunity involves the potential for both suppression or stimulation, as well as T cell dysregulation. The potential for trichothecenes to induce IgA-mediated immune complex glomerulonephritis is perhaps one of the most intriguing aspects of mycotoxin-induced immune alteration that has been observed. Although little is known of the etiologic factors that contribute to human IgA nephropathy, prior mucosal infection and diet are thought to play roles (163). Vomitoxin can exist in retail grain-based human foods at levels greater than those shown to cause serum IgA hyperelevation (2 ppm) in mice (164). Understanding the mechanistic basis for vomitoxin-induced IgA nephropathy would provide insight into the potential for trichothecenes to contribute to the human disease and clarify the thresholds for stimulation versus suppression of various immune responses.

While it is apparent that certain mycotoxins can affect immune function, extrapolation of those data obtained from genetically defined animal models to actual disease in humans or food-producing animals is problematic. *In vivo* comparison and validation in livestock and poultry are feasible and future research should focus on the cellular and molecular bases for *in vivo* observations and potential species variations. Additional studies could provide possible immunologic biomarkers for prospective epidemiologic studies in geographic or environmental situations where there is high degree of mycotoxin exposure.

ACKNOWLEDGMENTS

This work was supported by U.S. Public Health Service Grant ES-03358, the National Kidney Foundation of Michigan, the Michigan State University Agricultural Experiment Station, and Institute for Environmental Toxicology.

REFERENCES

1. Pestka JJ, Casale WL. Naturally occurring fungal toxins. In: Simmons MS, Nriagu J, eds. *Food contamination from environmental sources*. New York: Wiley; 1990:613–638.
2. Miller JD. Fungi as contaminants in indoor air. International Conference on Indoor Air Quality and Climate, July 29–August 3, 1990, Toronto, Ottawa.
3. Sorenson WG, Frazer DG, Jarvis BB, Simpson J, Robinson VA. Trichothecene mycotoxins in aerosolized conidia of *Stachybotrys atra*. *Appl Environ Microbiol* 1987;53:1370–1375.
4. Richard J, Thurston JR, Pier AC. Effects of mycotoxins on immunity. In: Rosenberg P, ed. *Toxins: animal, plant and microbial*. New York: Pergamon Press; 1978:801–817.
5. CAST. Mycotoxins: economic and health risks. *Council for Agricultural Science and Technology Task Force Report* 1989;116:17–19.
6. Corrier DE. Mycotoxicosis: mechanisms of immunosuppression. *Vet Immunol Immunopathol* 1991; 30:73–87.
7. Pestka JJ, Bondy GS. Alteration of immune function following dietary mycotoxin exposure. *Can J Pharmacol Physiol* 1990;68:1009–1016.
8. Thurston JR, Richard JL, Peden WM. Immunomodulation in mycotoxicoses other than aflatoxicosis. In: Richard JL, Thurston JR, eds. *Diagnosis of mycotoxicosis*. Boston: Martinus Nijhoff Publishers; 1986:149–161.
9. Vidal DR. Proprietes immunosuppressives des mycotoxines de groupe des trichothecenes. *Bull Inst Pasteur* 1990;88:159–192.
10. Reddy RV, Taylor MJ, Sharma RP. Studies of immune function of CD-1 mice exposed to aflatoxin B_1. *Toxicology* 1987;43:123–132.

11. Hatori Y, Sharma RP, Warren RP. Resistance of C57Bl/6 mice to immunosuppressive effects of aflatoxin B_1 and relationship with neuroendocrine mechanisms. *Immunopharmacology* 1991;22: 127–136.
12. Pier AC, Varman MJ, Dahlgren RR, Belden EL, Maki LR. Aflatoxic suppression of cell-mediated immune responses and interaction with T-2 toxin. In: Steyn PS, Vieggar R, eds. *Mycotoxins and phycotoxins*. Amsterdam: Elsevier Science Publishers; 1986:423–434.
13. Pier AC, Belden EL, Ellis JA, Nelson EW, Maki LR. Effects of cyclopiazonic acid and aflatoxin singly and in combination on selected clinical, pathological and immunological responses of guinea pigs. *Mycopathologia* 1989;105:135–142.
14. Ghosh RC, Chauhan HVS, Jha GJ. Suppression of cell-mediated immunity by purified aflatoxin B_1 in broiler chicks. *Vet Immunol Immunopathol* 1991;28:165–172.
15. Kadian SK, Monga DR, Goel MC. Effect of aflatoxin B_1 on the delayed type hypersensitivity and phagocytic activity of reticuloendothelial system in chickens. *Mycopathologia* 1988;104:33–36.
16. Ghosh RC, Chauhan HVS, Roy S. Immunosuppression in broilers under experimental aflatoxicosis. *Br Vet J* 1990;146:457–462.
17. Virdi JS, Tiwari RP, Saxena M, Khanna V, Singh G, Saini SS, Vadehra DV. Effects of aflatoxin on the immune system of the chick. *J Appl Toxicol* 1989;9:271–275.
18. Scott TR, Rowland SM, Rodgers RS, Bodine AB. Genetic selection for aflatoxin B_1 resistance influences chicken T-cell and thymocyte proliferation. *Dev Comp Immunol* 1991;15:383–391.
19. Yang KH, Kim BS, Munson AE, Holsapple MP. Immunosuppression induced by chemicals requiring metabolic activation in mixed cultures of rat hepatocytes and murine splenocytes. *Toxicol Appl Pharmacol* 1986;83:420–429.
20. Panangala VS, Giamgrone JJ, Diener UL, et al. Effects of aflatoxin on the growth performance and immune responses of weanling swine. *Am J Vet Res* 1986;47:2062–2067.
21. Singh J, Tiwari RP, Singh G, Singh S, Vadehra DV. Biochemical and immunological effects of aflatoxin in rabbits. *Toxicol Lett* 1987;35:225–230.
22. Reddy RV, Sharma RP. Effects of aflatoxin B_1 on murine lymphocytic functions. *Toxicology* 1989;54:31–44.
23. Cheng-ya W, Xin-sheng Y, Jin-xin H, Tao-zhen L, Yao-qin Y. HLA related genetic control of natural killer activity and aflatoxin B_1 suppression of lymphocytic blastogenesis. *Chin Med J* 1987;100:29–33.
24. Raisuddin Singh KP, Zaidi SIA, Saxena AK, Ray PK. Effects of aflatoxin on lymphoid cells of weanling rat. *J Appl Toxicol* 1990;10:245–250.
25. Cusumano V, Costa GB, Seminara S. Effect of aflatoxins on rat peritoneal macrophages. *Appl Environ Microbiol* 1990;56:3482–3484.
26. Neldon-Ortiz DL, Qureshi MA. Direct and microsomal activated aflatoxin B_1 exposure and its effects on turkey peritoneal macrophage functions *in vitro*. *Toxicol Appl Pharmacol* 1991;109:432–442.
27. Neldon-Ortiz DL, Qureshi MA. The effects of direct and microsomal activated aflatoxin B_1 on chicken peritoneal macrophages *in vitro*. *Vet Immunol Immunopathol* 1992;31:61–76.
28. Walsh CJ, Bodine AB, Scott TR. Co-mitogenic assay for assessing the effects of aflatoxin B_1 on interleukin-1 production in bovine macrophages. *Drug Dev Res* 1991;24:157–166.
29. Dwivedi P, Burns RB. Pathology of ochratoxicosis A in young broiler chicks. *Res Vet Sci* 1984; 36:92–103.
30. Dwivedi P, Burns RB. Immunosuppressive effects of ochratoxin A in young turkeys. *Avian Pathol* 1985;14:213–225.
31. Boorman GA, Hong HL, Dieter MP, Hates HT, Pohland AE. Myelotoxicity and macrophage alteration in mice exposed to ochratoxin A. *Toxicol Appl Pharmacol* 1984;72:304–312.
32. Creppy EE, Stormer FC, Roschenthaler R, Dirheimer G. Effects of two metabolites of ochratoxin A, (4R)-4-hydroxyochratoxin A and ochratoxin α, on immune response in mice. *Infect Immun* 1983; 39:1015–1018.
33. Prior MG, Sisodia CS. The effects of ochratoxin A on the immune response of Swiss mice. *Can J Comp Med* 1982;46:91–96.
34. Campbell ML, May JD, Huff WE, Doerr JA. Evaluation of immunity of young broiler chickens during simultaneous aflatoxicosis and ochratoxicosis. *Poult Sci* 1983;62:2138–2144.
35. Gibson RM, Bailey CA, Kubena LF, Huff WE, Harvey RB. Impact of L-phenylalanine supplementation on the performance of three-week-old broilers fed diets containing ochratoxin A. 1. Effects on body weight, feed conversion, relative organ weight, and mortality. *Poult Sci* 1990; 69:414–419.

36. Haubeck H-D, Lorkowski G, Kolsch E, Roschenthaler R. Immunosuppression by ochratoxin A and its prevention by phenylalanine. *Appl Environ Microbiol* 1981;41:1040–1042.
37. Chang C-F, Hamilton PB. Impairment of phagocytosis by heterophils from chickens during ochratoxicosis. *Appl Environ Microbiol* 1980;39:572–575.
38. Luster MI, Germolec DR, Burleson GR, Jameson CW, Ackermann MF, Lamm KR, Hayes HT. Selective immunosuppression in mice of natural killer cell activity by ochratoxin A. *Cancer Res* 1987;47:2259–2263.
39. Klinkert W, Lorkowski G, Creppy EE, Dirheimer G, Roschenthaler R. Inhibition of macrophage migration by ochratoxin A and citrinin, and prevention by phenylalanine of the ochratoxin A-induced inhibition. *Tox Eur Res* 1981;3:185–189.
40. Richard JL, Thurston JR, Deyoe BL, Booth GD. Effect of ochratoxin and aflatoxin on serum proteins, complement activity, and antibody production to *Brucellus abortus* in guinea pigs. *Appl Microbiol* 1975;29:27–29.
41. Manolova Y, Manolov G, Parvanova L, Petkova-Bocharova T, Castegnaro M, Chernozemsky IN. Induction of characteristic chromosomal aberrations, particularly X-trisomy, in cultured human lymphocytes treated by ochratoxin A, a mycotoxin implicated in Balkan endemic nephropathy. *Mutat Res* 1990;231:143–149.
42. Reubel GH, Gareis M, Amselgruber WM. Cytotoxicity evaluation of mycotoxins by an MTT-bioassay. *Mycotoxin Res* 1987;3:85–96.
43. Holmberg T, Thuvander A, Hult K. Ochratoxin A as a suppressor of mitogen-induced blastogenesis of porcine blood lymphocytes. *Acta Vet Scand* 1988;29:219–223.
44. Lea T, Stelen K, Stormer FC. Mechanism of ochratoxin A-induced immunosuppression. *Mycopathologia* 1989;107:153–159.
45. Fuchs R, Hult K. Ochratoxin A in blood and its pharmacokinetic properties. *Food Chem Toxicol* 1992;30:204–210.
46. Krogh P. Role of ochratoxin in disease causation. *Food Chem Toxicol* 1992;30:213–224.
47. Campbell ML, Doerr JA, Wyatt RD. Immune status in broiler chickens during citrinin toxicosis. *Poult Sci* 1981;60:1634.
48. Reddy RV, Taylor MJ, Sharma RP. Evaluation of citrinin toxicity on the immune functions of mice. *J Food Protect* 1988;51:32–36.
49. Richard JL, Peden WM, Fichtner RE, Cole RJ. Effect of cyclopiazonic acid on delayed hypersensitivity to *Mycobacterium tuberculosis*, complement activity, serum enzymes, and bilirubin in guinea pigs. *Mycopathologia* 1986;96:73–77.
50. Hill JE, Lomax LG, Cole RJ, Dorner JW. Toxicologic and immunologic effects of sublethal doses of cyclopiazonic acid in rats. *Am J Vet Res* 1986;47:1174–1177.
51. Escoula L, Thomsen M, Bourdiol D, Pipy B, Peuriere S, Roubinet F. Patulin immunotoxicology: effect on phagocyte activation and the cellular and humoral immune system of mice and rabbits. *Int J Immunopharmacol* 1988;10:983–989.
52. Paucod J-C, Krivobok S, Vidal D. Immunotoxicity testing of mycotoxins T-2 and patulin on balb/c mice. *Acta Microbiol Hung* 1990;37:331–339.
53. Escoula L, Bourdiol D, Linas MD, Recco P, Seguela JP. Enhancing resistance and modulation of humoral immune response to experimental *Candida albicans* infection by patulin. *Mycopathologia* 1988;103:153–156.
54. Bourdiol D, Escoula L, Salvayre R. Effect of patulin on microbicidal activity of mouse peritoneal macrophages. *Food Chem Toxicol* 1990;28:29–33.
55. Sorenson WG, Simpson J, Castranova V. Toxicity of the mycotoxin patulin for rat peritoneal macrophages. *Environ Res* 1985;38:407–416.
56. Eldelb MMR, Reddy CS. Toxic effects of secalonic acid D in mice and protection by dimethylsulfoxide. *Bull Environ Contam Toxicol* 1990;44:692–699.
57. Fleischhacker DS, Akers TG, Katz SP, Palmgren MS. Enhancement of influenza virus infections by secalonic acid D. *Environ Health Perspect* 1986;66:113–118.
58. Wiesinger D, Gubler HU, Haefliger W, Hauser D. Antiinflammatory activity of the new mould metabolite 11-desacetoxy-wortmannin and of some of its derivatives. *Experientia* 1974;30:135–136.
59. Gunther R, Abbas HK, Mirocha CJ. Acute pathological effects on rats of orally administered wortmannin-containing preparations and purified wortmannin from *Fusarium oxysporum*. *Food Chem Toxicol* 1989;27:173–179.
60. Gunther R, Kishore PN, Abbas HK, Mirocha CJ. Immunosuppressive effects of dietary wortmannin on rats and mice. *Immunopharmacol Immunotoxicol* 1989;11:559–570.

61. Bagglollni M, Dewald B, Schnyder J, Ruch W, Cooper PH, Payne TG. Inhibition of the phagocytosis-induced respiratory burst by the fungal metabolite wortmannin and some analogues. *Exp Cell Res* 1987;169:408–418.
62. Bamburg JR. Biological and biochemical actions of trichothecene mycotoxins. *Prog Mol Subcell Biol* 1983;8:41–110.
63. Ueno Y. General toxicology. In: Ueno Y, ed. *Trichothecenes: chemical, biological and toxicological aspects*. New York: Elsevier Science Publishing; 1983:135–146.
64. Bhat RV, Beedu SR, Ramakrishna Y, Munshi KL. Outbreak of trichothecene mycotoxicosis associated with consumption of mould-damaged wheat products in Kashmir Valley, India. *Lancet* 1989;7:35–37.
65. Cote LM, Reynolds JD, Vesonder RF, Buck WB, Swanson SP, Coffey RT, Brown DC. Survey of vomitoxin-contaminated feed grains in midwestern United States, and associated health problems in swine. *J Am Vet Med Assoc* 1984;184:189–192.
66. Joffe A. *Fusarium poae* and *F. sporotrichoides* as principal causal agents of alimentary toxic aleukia. In: Wyllie T, Morehouse L, eds. *Mycotoxic fungi, mycotoxins, mycotoxicoses*. New York: Marcel Dekker; 1978.
67. Kanai K, Kondo E. Decreased resistance to *Mycobacterium* infection in mice fed a trichothecene compound. *Jpn J Med Sci Biol* 1984;37:97–104.
68. Salazar S, Fromentin H, Mariat F. Effects of diacetoxyscirpenol on experimental candidiasis of mice. *CR Acad Sci Ser* 1980;290:877–878.
69. Fromentin H, Salazar-Mejicanos S, Mariat F. Experimental cryptococcosis in mice treated with diacetoxyscirpenol, a mycotoxin of *Fusarium*. *Sabouraudia* 1981;19:311–313.
70. Corrier DE, Ziprin RL, Mollenhauer HH. Modulation of cell-mediated resistance to listeriosis in mice given T-2 toxin. *Toxicol Appl Pharmacol* 1987;89:323–331.
71. Tai J-H, Pestka JJ. Impaired murine resistance to *Salmonella typhimurium* following oral exposure to the trichothecene T-2 toxin. *Food Chem Toxicol* 1988;26:691–698.
72. Tai J-H, Pestka JJ. T-2 toxin impairment of murine response to *Salmonella typhimurium*: a histopathologic assessment. *Mycopathologia* 1990;109:149–155.
73. Vidal D, Mavet S. *In vitro* and *in vivo* toxicity of T-2 toxin, a *Fusarium* mycotoxin, to mouse peritoneal macrophages. *Infect Immun* 1989;57:2260–2264.
74. Friend SCE, Babluk LA, Schiefer HB. The effects of dietary T-2 toxin on the immunological function and herpes simplex reactivation in Swiss mice. *Toxicol Appl Pharmacol* 1983;69:234–244.
75. Tai J-H, Pestka JJ. Synergistic interaction between the trichothecene T-2 toxin and *Salmonella typhimurium* lipopolysaccharide in C3H/HeN and C3H/HeJ mice. *Toxicol Lett* 1988;44:191–200.
76. Taylor MJ, Smart RA, Sharma RP. Relationship of the hypothalamic–pituitary–adrenal axis with chemically induced immunomodulation. I. Stress-like response after exposure to T-2 toxin. *Toxicology* 1989;56:179–195.
77. Taylor MJ, Lafarge-Frayssinet C, Luster MI, Frayssinet C. Increased endotoxin sensitivity following T-2 toxin treatment is associated with increased absorption of endotoxin. *Toxicol Appl Pharmacol* 1991;109:51–59.
78. Rosenstein Y, Lafarge-Frayssinet, C, Lespinats G, Loisillier F, Lafont P, Frayssinet C. Immunosuppressive activity of *Fusarium* toxins. Effects on antibody synthesis and skin grafts of crude extracts, T-2 toxin and diacetoxyscirpenol. *Immunology* 1979;36:111–117.
79. Tryphonas H, Iverson F, So Y, et al. Effects of deoxynivalenol (vomitoxin) on the humoral and cellular immunity of mice. *Toxicol Lett* 1986;30:137–150.
80. Pestka JJ, Tai JH, Witt MF, Dixon DE, Forsell JH. Suppression of immune response in the B6C3F1 mouse after dietary exposure to the *Fusarium* toxins deoxynivalenol (vomitoxin) and zearalenone. *Food Chem Toxicol* 1987;25:297–304.
81. Cooray R, Jonsson P. Modulation of resistance to mastitis pathogens by pretreatment of mice with T-2 toxin. *Food Chem Toxicol* 1990;28:687–692.
82. Corrier DE, Ziprin RL. Immunotoxic effects of T-2 toxin on cell-mediated immunity to listeriosis in mice: comparison with cyclophosphamide. *Am J Vet Res* 1986;47:1956–1960.
83. Corrier DE, Ziprin RL. Enhanced resistance to listeriosis induced in mice by preinoculation treatment with T-2 mycotoxin. *Am J Vet Res* 1986;47:856–859.
84. Corrier DE, Holt PS, Mollenhauer HH. Regulation of murine macrophage phagocytosis of sheep erythrocytes by T-2 toxin. *Am J Vet Res* 1987;48:1304–1307.
85. Gerberick GF, Sorenson WG. Toxicity of T-2 toxin, a *Fusarium* mycotoxin, to alveolar macrophages *in vitro*. *Environ Res* 1983;32:260–285.

86. Gerberick GF, Sorenson WG, Lewis DM. The effects of T-2 toxin on alveolar macrophage function *in vitro*. *Environ Res* 1984;33:246–260.
87. Sorenson WG, Gerberick GF, Lewis DM, Castranova V. Toxicity of mycotoxins for the rat pulmonary macrophage *in vitro*. *Environ Health Perspect* 1986;66:45–53.
88. Samara A, Yagen B, Agranat I, Rachmillewitz E, Fibach E. Induction of differentiation in human myeloid leukemic cells by T-2 toxin and other trichothecenes. *Toxicol Appl Pharmacol* 1987;89: 418–428.
89. Pang VF, Lambert RJ, Feisburg PJ, Beasley VR, Buck WB, Haschek WM. Experimental T-2 toxicosis in swine following inhalation exposure: effects of pulmonary and systemic immunity, and morphologic changes. *Toxicol Pathol* 1987;15:308–319.
90. Hughes BJ, Taylor MJ, Sharma RP. Effects of verrucarin A and roridin A, macrocyclic trichothecene mycotoxins, on the murine immune system. *Immunopharmacology* 1988;16:79–87.
91. Hughes BJ, Hsieh GC, Jarvis BB, Sharma RP. Effects of macrocyclic trichothecene mycotoxins on the murine immune system. *Arch Environ Contam Toxicol* 1989;18:388–395.
92. Lafarge-Frayssinet C, Lespinats G, Lafont P, Loisillier F, Mousset S, Rosenstein Y, Frayssinet C. Immunosuppressive effects of *Fusarium* extracts and trichothecenes: blastogenic response of murine splenic and thymic cells to mitogen. *Proc Soc Exp Biol Med* 1979;160:301–311.
93. Robbana-Barnat S, Lafarge-Frayssinet C, Cohen H, Neish GA, Frayssinet C. Immunosuppressive properties of deoxynivalenol. *Toxicology* 1988;48:155–166.
94. Taylor MJ, Reddy RV, Sharma RP. Immunotoxicity of repeated low level exposure to T-2 toxin, a trichothecene mycotoxin, in CD-1 mice. *Mycotoxin Res* 1985;1:57–64.
95. Atkinson HAC, Miller K. Inhibitory effect of deoxynivalenol, 3-acetyldeoxynivalenol and zearalenone on induction of rat and human lymphocyte proliferation. *Toxicol Lett* 1984;23:215–221.
96. Bondy GS, Beremand MN, McCormick SP, Pestka JJ. Murine lymphocyte proliferation impaired by substituted neosolaniols and calonectrins—*Fusarium* metabolites associated with trichothecene biosynthesis. *Toxicon* 1991;29:1107–1113.
97. Cooray R. Effects of some mycotoxins on mitogen-induced blastogenesis and SCE frequency in human lymphocytes. *Food Chem Toxicol* 1984;22:529–534.
98. Hughes BJ, Jarvis BB, Sharma RP. Effects of macrocyclic trichothecene congeners on the viability and mitogenesis of murine splenic lymphocytes. *Toxicol Lett* 1990;50:57–67.
99. Miller K, Atkinson HAC. The *in vitro* effects of trichothecenes on the immune system. *Food Chem Toxicol* 1986;24:545–549.
100. Miller K, Atkinson HAC. The *in vitro* effects of trichothecenes on the immune system. *Arch Toxicol Suppl* 1987;11:321–324.
101. Tomar RS, Blakley BR, Schiefer HB, DeCoteau WE. *In vitro* effects of 3-acetyldeoxynivalenol on the immune response of human peripheral blood lymphocytes. *Int J Immunopharmacol* 1986;8: 125–130.
102. Tomar RS, Blakley BR, DeCoteau WE. Immunological responsiveness of mouse spleen cells after *in vivo* or *in vitro* exposure to 3-acetyldeoxynivalenol. *Food Chem Toxicol* 1987;25:393–398.
103. Tomar RS, Blakley BR, DeCoteau WE. *In vitro* effects of T-2 toxin on the mitogen responsiveness and antibody-producing ability of human lymphocytes. *Toxicol Lett* 1988;40:109–117.
104. Bondy G, Pestka JJ. Dietary exposure to the trichothecene vomitoxin (deoxynivalenol) stimulates terminal differentiation of Peyer's patch B cells to IgA secreting plasma cells. *Toxicol Appl Pharmacol* 1991;108:520–530.
105. Forsell JH, Kately J, Yoshizawa T, Pestka JJ. Inhibition of mitogen-induced blastogenesis in human lymphocytes by T-2 toxin and its metabolites. *Appl Environ Microbiol* 1985;49:1523–1526.
106. Forsell JH, Pestka JJ. Relation of 8-ketotrichothecene and zearalenone analog structure to inhibition of mitogen-induced human lymphocyte blastogenesis. *Appl Environ Microbiol* 1985;50:1304–1307.
107. Mekhancha-Dahel C, Lafarge-Frayssinet C, Frayssinet C. Immunosuppressive effects of four trichothecene mycotoxins. *Food Addit Contam* 1990;7:S94–S96.
108. Pestka JJ, Forsell JH. Inhibition of human lymphocyte transformation by the macrocyclic trichothecenes roridin A and verrucarin A. *Toxicol Lett* 1988;41:215–222.
109. Thompson WL, Wannemacher RW. Structure–function relationships of 12,13-epoxytrichothecene mycotoxins in cell culture: comparison to whole animal lethality. *Toxicon* 1986;24:985–994.
110. Tomar RS, Blakley BR, DeCoteau WE. Antibody producing ability of mouse spleen cells after subacute dietary exposure to T-2 toxin. *Int J Immunopharmacol* 1988;10:145–151.

111. Porcher J-M, Dehol C, Lafarge-Frayssinet C, Chu FS, Frayssinet C. Uptake and metabolism of T-2 toxin in relation to its cytotoxicity in lymphoid cells. *Food Chem Toxicol* 1988;26:587–593.
112. Rosenstein Y, Kretschner RR, Lafarge-Frayssinet C. Effect of *Fusarium* toxins, T-2 toxin and diacetoxyscirpenol on murine T-independent immune responses. *Immunology* 1981;44:555–560.
113. Holt PS, DeLoach JR, *In vitro* effect of T-2 mycotoxin on the immune response of mice. *Am J Vet Res* 1988;49:1480–1484.
114. Schiefer HB, Rousseaux CG, Hancock DS, Blakley BR. Effects of low-level long-term oral exposure to T-2 toxin in CD-1 mice. *Food Chem Toxicol* 1987;25:593–601.
115. Blakley BR, Hancock DS, Rousseaux CG. Embryotoxic effects of prenatal T-2 toxin exposure in mice. *Can J Vet Res* 1986;51:399–402.
116. Tryphonas H, O'Grady L, Arnold DL, McGuire PF, Karpinski K, Vesonder RF. Effect of deoxynivalenol (vomitoxin) on the humoral immunity of mice. *Toxicol Lett* 1984;23:17–24.
117. Cooray R, Lindahl-Kiessling K. Effect of T-2 toxin on the spontaneous antibody-secreting cells and other non-lymphoid cells in the murine spleen. *Food Chem Toxicol* 1987;25:25–29.
118. Forsell JH, Witt FM, Tai J-H, Jensen R, Pestka JJ. Effects of chronic exposure to dietary deoxynivalenol (vomitoxin) and zearalenone on the growing B6C3F1 mouse. *Food Chem Toxicol* 1986; 24:213–219.
119. Dong W, Sell JE, Pestka JJ. Quantitative assessment of mesangial immunoglobulin A (IgA) accumulation, elevated circulating IgA immune complexes, and hematuria during vomitoxin-induced IgA nephropathy. *Fundam Appl Toxicol* 1991;17:197–207.
120. Pestka JJ, Moorman MA, Warner R. Dysregulation of IgA production and IgA nephropathy induced by the trichothecene vomitoxin. *Food Chem Toxicol* 1989;27:361–368.
121. Pestka JJ, Moorman MA, Warner R. Altered serum immunoglobulin response to model intestinal antigens during dietary exposure to vomitoxin (deoxynivalenol). *Toxicol Lett* 1990;50:75–84.
122. Pestka JJ, Moorman MA, Warner RL, Witt MF, Forsell JH, Tai J-H. Immunoglobulin A nephropathy as a manifestation of vomitoxin (deoxynivalenol) immunotoxicity. In: Pohland AE, Dowell VR, Richard JL, eds. *Cellular and molecular mode of action of selected microbial toxins in foods and feeds*. New York: Plenum Press; 1990:427–440.
123. Pestka JJ, Dong W, Warner RL, Rasooly L, Bondy GS, Brooks KH. Elevated membrane IgA$^+$ and CD4$^+$ (T helper) populations in murine Peyer's patch and splenic lymphocytes during dietary administration of the trichothecene vomitoxin (deoxynivalenol). *Food Chem Toxicol* 1990;28:409–420.
124. Pestka JJ, Warner RL, Dong W, Rasooly L, Bondy GS. Effects of dietary administration of the trichothecene vomitoxin (deoxynivalenol) on IgA and IgG secretion by Peyer's patch and splenic lymphocytes. *Food Chem Toxicol* 1990;28:693–699.
125. Berger J. IgA glomerular deposits in renal disease. *Transplant Proc* 1969;1:939–941.
126. D'Amico GD. The commonest glomerulonephritis in the world: IgA nephropathy. *Q J Med* 1987; 247:709–727.
127. Dong W, Pestka JJ. Persistent dysregulation of IgA production and IgA nephropathy in the B6C3F1 mouse following withdrawal of dietary vomitoxin (deoxynivalenol). *Fundam Appl Toxicol* 1993;20:38–47.
128. Pestka JJ, Dong W. Progressive serum IgE hyperelevation in the B6C3F1 mouse following withdrawal of dietary vomitoxin (deoxynivalenol). *Fund Appl Toxicol* 1994;314–316.
129. Greene DM, Azcona-Olivera JI, Pestka JJ. Vomitoxin (deoxynivalenol)-induced IgA nephropathy in the B6C3F1 mouse: dose response and male predilection. *Toxiciology* 1994 (*in press*).
129a. Greene DM, Bondy GS, Azcona-Olivera JI, Petska JJ. Role of gender and strain in vomitoxin-induced dysregulation of IgA production and IgA nephropathy in the mouse. *J Toxicol Environ Health* 1994 (*in press*).
130. Rasooly L, Pestka JJ. Vomitoxin-induced dysregulation of serum IgA, IgM and IgG reactive with gut bacterial and self antigens. *Food Chem Toxicol* 1992;30;499–504.
131. Rasooly L, Pestka JJ. Polyclonal autoreactive IgA increase and mesangial deposition during vomitoxin-induced IgA nephropathy in BALB/c mouse. *Food Chem Toxicol* 1994 (*in press*).
131a. Rasooly L, Abouzied MM, Brooks KH, Pestka JJ. Polyspecific and autoreactive IgA secreted by hybridomas derived from Peyer's patches of vomitoxin-fed mice: characterization and possible pathogenic role in IgA nephropathy. 1994 (*in press*).
132. Bunner DL, Morris ER. Alteration of multiple cell membrane functions in L-6 myoblasts by T-2 toxin: an important mechanism of action. *Toxic Appl Pharmacol* 1988;92:113–121.
133. Jone C, Erickson L, Trosko JE, Chang CC. Effect of biologic toxins on gap-junctional intercellular communication in Chinese hamster V79 cells. *Cell Biol Toxicol* 1987;3:1–15.

134. Rosenstein Y, Lafarge-Frayssinet C. Inhibitory effect of *Fusarium* T-2 toxin on lymphoid DNA and protein synthesis. *Toxicol Appl Pharmacol* 1983;70:283–288.
135. Mizel SB, Mizel DJ. Purification to apparent homogeneity of murine interleukin 1. *J Immunol* 1981; 126:834–837.
136. Efrat S, Zelig S, Yagen B, Kaempfer R. Superinduction of human interleukin-2 messenger RNA by inhibitor of translation. *Biochem Biophys Res Commun* 1984;123:842–848.
137. Holt PS, Corrier DE, DeLoach JR. Suppressive and enhancing effect of T-2 toxin on murine lymphocyte activation and interleukin 2 production. *Immunopharmacol Immunotoxicol* 1988;10: 365–385.
138. Sherman Y, More R, Yagen B, Yarom R. Cardiovascular pathology induced by passive transfer of splenic cells from syngeneic rats treated with T-2 toxin. *Toxicol Lett* 1987;36:15–22.
139. Warner R, Brooks K, Pestka JJ. *In vitro* exposure to vomitoxin (deoxynivalenol) enhances T cell-mediated IgA secretion by splenic B cells. *FASEB J* 1992; 6:A1875.
139a. Warner RL, Brooks K, Pestka JJ. *In vitro* effects of vomitoxin (deoxynivalenol) or lymphocyte function: enhanced T cell interleukin production and help for IgA secretion. *Food Chem Toxicol* 1994 (*in press*).
139b. Dong W, Azcona-Olivera JI, Brooks KA, Linz JE, Pestka JJ. Elevated gene expression and production of interleukins 2, 4, 5, and 6 during exposure to vomitoxin (deoxynivalenol) and cycloheximide in the EL-4 thymoma. *Toxicol Appl Pharmacol* 1994 (*in press*).
140. Colvin BM, Harrison LR. Fumonisin-induced pulmonary edema and hydrothorax in swine. *Mycopathologia* 1992;117:79–82.
141. Gelderblom WCA, Kriek NPJ, Marasas WFO, Thiel PG. Toxicity and carcinogenicity of the *Fusarium moniliforme* metabolite, fumonisin B_1, in rats. *Carcinogenesis* 1991;12:1247–1251.
142. Kellerman TS, Marasas WFO, Thiel PG, Gelderblom WCA, Cawood M, Coetzer JAW. Leucoencephalomalacia in two horses induced by oral dosing of fumonisin B_1. *Onderstepoort J Vet Res* 1990;57:269–275.
143. Bane DP, Neumann EJ, Hall WF, Harlin KS, Slife FLN. Relationship between fumonisin contamination of feed and mystery swine disease. *Mycopathologia* 1992;117:121–124.
144. Moore C, Bilodeau R, Wiseman B. Clinical aspects and consequences of mystery swine disease in nursery and grow-finish pigs. In: *Proceedings of the Mystery Swine Disease Committee Meeting*, Denver, CO. Madison, WI: Public Livestock Conservation Institute; 1990:41–51.
145. Haschek WM, Motelin G, Ness DK, et al. Characterization of fumonisin toxicity in orally and intravenously dosed swine. *Mycopathologia* 1992;117:83–96.
146. Dombrink-Kurtzman MA, Bennett GA, Richard JL. Avian lymphocytes as *in vitro* models to predict fumonisin cytotoxicity. *FASEB J* 1992;6:A2007.
147. Shier WT, Abbas HK, Mirocha CJ. Toxicity of the mycotoxins fumonisins B_1 and B_2 and *Alternaria alternata* f. sp. *lycopersici* (AAL) in cultured mammalian cells. *Mycopathologia* 1991;116: 97–104.
148. Dombrink-Kurtzman MA, Bennett GA, Richard JL. Cytotoxicity of fumonisins in avian lymphocytes. *Abstracts of the 106th Association of Official Analytical Chemists Annual Meeting*; 1992b,p145.
149. Dombrink-Kurtzman MA, Javed T, Bennett GA, Richard JL, Cote LM, Buck WB. Lymphocyte cytotoxicity and erythrocyte abnormalities induced in broiler chicks by fumonisins B_1, and B_2 and moniliformin from *Fusarium* proliferatum. In: *Abstracts of the 106th Association of Official Analytical Chemists Annual Meeting*; 1992:233.
150. Qureshi MA, Hagler WM. Effect of fumonisin-B_1 exposure on chicken macrophage function *in vitro*. *Poult Sci* 1992;71:104–112.
151. Pung OJ, Luster MI, Hayes HT, Rader J. Influence of steroidal and nonsteroidal sex hormones on host resistance in mice: Increased susceptibility to *Listeria monocytogenes* after exposure to estrogenic hormones. *Infect Immun* 1984;46:301–307.
152. Pung OJ, Tucker AN, Vore SJ, Luster MI. Influence of estrogen on host resistance: Increased susceptibility of mice to *Listeria monocytogenes* correlates with depressed production of interleukin 2. *Infect Immun* 1985;50:91–96.
153. Dean JH, Luster MI, Boorman GA, Luebke RW, Lauer LD. The effect of adult exposure to diethylstilbestrol in the mouse, alterations in tumour susceptibility and host resistance parameters. *J Reticuloendothel Soc* 1980;28:571–583.
154. Boorman GA, Luster MI, Dean JH, Wilson RD. The effect of adult exposure to diethylstilbestrol in the mouse on macrophage functions and numbers. *Res J Reticuloendothel Soc* 1980;28:547–560.

155. Kalland T, Campbell T. Effects of diethylstilbestrol on human natural killer cell *in vitro*. *Immunopharmacology* 1984;8:19–25.
156. Luster MI, Boorman GA, Dean JH, Luebke RW, Lawson LD. The effect of adult exposure to diethylstilbestrol in the mouse: alterations in immunological functions. *J Reticuloendothel Soc* 1980;28:561–569.
157. Luster MI, Boorman GA, Lorach KS, Dieter MP, Hong L. Myelotoxicity toxicity resulting from exogenous estrogens: evidence for bimodal mechanism of action. *Int J Immunopharmacol* 1984; 6:287–297.
158. Minervini F, Lucivero G, Visconti A, Bottalico C. Immunomodulatory effects of fusarochromanones TDP-1 and TDP-2. *Nat Toxins* 1992;1:15–18.
159. Croft WA, Jarvis BB, Yatawara CS. Airborne outbreak of trichothecene toxicosis. *Atmos Environ* 1986;20:549–552.
160. Bendele AM, Carlton WW, Krogh P, Lillehoj EB. Ochratoxin A carcinogenesis in the (C57BL/6J × C3H) F_1 mouse. *J Natl Cancer Inst* 1985;75:733–742.
161. Austwick PC. Balkan nephropathy. *Practitioner* 1981;225:1031–1038.
162. Radovanovic Z, Naunovic T, Velimirovic D. Clustering of the upper urothelial tumors in a family. *Oncology (Basel)* 1984;41:396–398.
163. Coppo R, Roccatello D, Amore A, et al. Effects of gluten-free diet in primary IgA nephropathy. *Nephrology* 1990;33:72–86.
164. Abouzied MM, Azcona JI, Braselton WE, Pestka JJ. Immunochemical assessment of mycotoxins in 1989 grain foods: evidence for deoxynivalenol (vomitoxin) contamination. *Appl Environ Microbiol* 1991;57:672–677.

Immunotoxicology and Immunopharmacology, Second Edition, edited by J. H. Dean, M. I. Luster, A. E. Munson, and I. Kimber.
Raven Press, Ltd., New York © 1994.

10

Organic Solvents

Carroll A. Snyder

Department of Environmental Medicine, New York University Medical Center, Tuxedo, New York 10987

Through the efforts of a number of investigators, it has become increasingly apparent that the immune system is exquisitely sensitive to perturbation by exposures to a wide variety of toxicants. The sensitivity of the immune system seems to reside in the complex interactions that occur when immune defenses are mobilized. These interactions involve the recognition and processing of antigen, the synthesis and release of cytokines, followed by cellular proliferation, differentiation, and activation. Disruption of any one of these processes can markedly alter the normal responses of the immune system.

There is limited but sufficient evidence that exposures to some organic solvents can adversely affect various aspects of the immune system. Yet it must be understood that one of the most important properties of solvents is their relative unreactivity. Their function is to dissolve materials but not to alter them. This reduced chemical reactivity exhibited by most organic solvents probably contributes to the truncated literature concerning the immunotoxic potential of these compounds. It also must be noted that commercial solvents are frequently composed of mixtures of compounds and that any immunotoxic properties of commercial solvents may be due to minor constituents in these mixtures.

For the purposes of this chapter, organic solvents are defined as carbon-based compounds that are liquids at room temperature and pressure and that are used to dissolve other materials. Three general categories of solvents are discussed: the hydrocarbons, the halogenated hydrocarbons, and the hydroxyethers.

HYDROCARBONS

Benzene

Although it possesses excellent solvent properties, the use of benzene as a solvent has diminished because of its hematotoxic and leukemogenic properties. Lymphocytes are particularly susceptible to the toxic effects of benzene (1) and, for this reason, these cells have frequently been used to study the underlying mechanisms of benzene-induced cytotoxicity (2). Since lymphocytes are particularly vulnerable to the toxic effects of benzene, it is not surprising that benzene is a powerful immunotoxicant. Benzene exposure alters aspects of both humoral and cell-mediated immunity as well as the production of cytokines. Specifically, the humoral immunotoxic effects of benzene include suppression of B cell mitogenesis (3–5) and suppression of antibody production toward a T cell-dependent antigen (sheep red blood cells, SRBCs) (5,6). The cell-mediated immunotoxic effects of benzene include suppression of T cell mitogenesis (3–5), mixed lymphocyte reactions (5,7), tumor lytic activity by cytotoxic T cells (5,7), and host resistance to tumor challenge (7) and to T cell-dependent bacterial challenge (8). Benzene exposure has also been found to elevate the production of tumor necrosis factor-α (TNF-α) and interleukin-1 (IL-1) (9) but to decrease the production of IL-2 (5,10).

Toluene

There is little evidence that toluene represents a severe immunotoxic hazard. Although some immunomodulating effects of toluene exposure have been observed (11–13), these effects generally occur at high doses. For example, mice exhibited decreased IL-2 production when exposed to high levels of toluene (405 mg/liter in drinking water), an exposure concentration that also produced elevated corticosterone levels. At lower exposure concentrations (17 and 80 mg/liter in drinking water), neither decreased IL-2 production nor increased corticosterone levels were observed (10). The authors postulate that the decreased IL-2 production was induced by the elevated corticosterone levels, an event that occurred only at the highest toluene concentration tested. In addition, there is evidence that toluene attenuates the immunotoxic effects of benzene (5). This occurs because coincident administration of toluene and benzene reduces the rate of benzene metabolism, probably due to competition for sites on the metabolizing enzymes (14), and the consequent benzene toxicity (15). Clearly, compared to benzene, toluene has a relatively benign effect on immune-associated processes since it is able to moderate the immunotoxic effects of benzene.

Straight-Chain Alkanes

Immunotoxicologic data on straight-chain alkanes is scarce. Exposure to these compounds is associated with neurotoxicity and respiratory tract injury (16,17). At least part of the respiratory tract injury induced by these compounds is believed to be due to injury to pulmonary macrophages with subsequent release of lysosomal enzymes (18). Since injury to pulmonary macrophages can lead to decreased resistance to airborne infectious agents, the action of straight-chain alkanes on these cells is considered here.

One study has provided evidence for a relationship between chain length and the cytotoxicity of alkanes toward pulmonary macrophages (18). Alkanes of 7 or 8 carbon length are more toxic to these cells than alkanes composed of either 6, 9, or 10 carbons. In addition, C_7 and C_8 alkanes are also more toxic toward pulmonary macrophages than either benzene or toluene (18). Cytotoxicity in this study was measured by cell death, release of lysosomal enzymes, loss of cell respiration, and increases in lipid peroxidation.

There is evidence that 2,5-hexanediol, a metabolite of *n*-hexane, is immunotoxic in mice. Exposures of male, Swiss albino mice to hexanediol at 20% of the oral median lethal dose (LD_{50}) induced marked impairment in the following immune function tests: delayed hypersensitivity reaction, plaque-forming cell assay, serum antibody titer against SRBCs, and resistance to endotoxin. It should be noted that this dose was sufficiently toxic to cause reduced cellularities in lymphoid organs (19).

Hydrocarbon Mixtures

Solvent grade hydrocarbons are usually composed of mixtures of compounds. Thus the results of studies concerned with the immunotoxic effects of solvents used in the workplace frequently reflect the effects due to hydrocarbon mixtures. It is difficult to "tease out" the effects that might be due to one component in the mixture since combinations of compounds can have very different immunotoxic effects than those of the individual components. For example, we have already seen that toluene attenuates the immunotoxic effects of benzene. When dealing with workplace exposure to hydrocarbon solvents, at least for now, it is best to consider the mixture as an entity.

Two studies have demonstrated that occupational exposures to organic solvents decrease circulating antibody levels (20,21). In these studies the effects of both cigarette smoking and solvent exposure were considered. Both cigarette smoking alone and solvent exposure alone depressed circulating antibody levels. Those workers who smoked cigarettes and who were also exposed to solvents containing benzene and its homologs exhibited greater decreases in circulating antibody levels than either solvent-exposed workers who did not smoke or smokers who were not exposed to solvents (20). In another study, depressed levels of IL-1 production and depressed levels of CD3+ lymphocytes were found in refinery workers presumably exposed to a number of different hydrocarbon compounds (22). The results of these three studies indicate that immunologic parameters may provide a useful biomarker of exposure for workers occupationally exposed to hydrocarbon solvents.

HALOGENATED HYDROCARBONS

Halogenated hydrocarbon solvents are more noted for hepatic toxicity and nephrotoxicity than for immunotoxicity. Nevertheless, there is evidence that some of these compounds represent immunologic hazards.

Carbon Tetrachloride

In two studies using B6C3F1 mice, carbon tetrachloride was found to inhibit the T cell-dependent antibody response to SRBCs, the cell-mediated response in the mixed lymphocyte reaction, and the mitogen-induced proliferations of B and T cells (23,24). These studies employed a wide range of doses [25 to 5000 mg/kg, delivered daily intraperitoneally (ip) or orally (po) for 7 to 30 days]. Induction of cytochrome P450 activity by ethanol pretreatment was found to enhance the CCl_4-induced suppression of the antibody response to SRBCs while treatment with the P450 competitive inhibitor, aminoacetonitrile, reversed this suppression (23). In contrast, F-344 rats given ten daily po doses of carbon tetrachloride of up to 40 mg/kg showed no immunotoxic effects in the T cell-dependent antibody response to SRBCs or in a number of other immune-associated processes including mitogen-induced proliferation, mixed lymphocyte reaction, and the lytic activities of cytotoxic T cells and of natural killer (NK) cells (25). The absence of responses in these immune function assays was observed at dosages that produced histologically observable hepatotoxicity. The results of these studies taken as a whole indicate that the immunotoxic properties of CCl_4 are mediated via its metabolism and that for rats, at least, this compound represents a greater hazard to the liver than to the immune system.

Trans-1,2-Dichloroethylene

Male and female CD-1 mice were given dichloroethylene in the drinking water for 90 days. Doses were calculated to deliver 17, 175, and 387 mg/kg to the males and 23, 224, and 452 mg/kg to the females. Males, but not females, exhibited depressed abilities to produce antibody against SRBCs. In contrast, females, but not males, exhibited decreased macrophage function as indicated by the reduced ability of thioglycollate-recruited peritoneal exudate cells to phagocytize SRBCs (26).

1,2-Dichloroethane

A single 3-hr inhalation exposure of female CD-1 mice to 10 ppm 1,2-dichloroethane (DCE) decreased pulmonary bactericidal activity toward inhaled *Klebsiella pneumoniae* and increased mortality in these mice due to respiratory infection. A single exposure to 5 ppm DCE also increased mortality due to respiratory infection although alveolar macrophage activity in these mice as measured by inhibition of tumor cell proliferation or by phagocytosis of SRBCs was not affected by single 3-hr exposures of either 10 or 100 ppm DCE. In contrast, no increased mortality or decrement in bactericidal activity was observed in male, Sprague–Dawley rats given single-5 hr exposures to either 100 or 200 ppm DCE (27).

Dichloromethene, Tetrachloroethene, and Trichloroethene

The responses of mice to inhaled *Klebsiella pneumoniae* infection were also used to assess the immunotoxic potential of the three compounds listed above. A single 3-hr exposure to 100 ppm dichloromethene or 50 ppm trichloroethene or 50 ppm tetrachloroethene increased respiratory infections in female CD-1 mice (28). The dichloromethene and tetrachloroethene exposures also suppressed pulmonary bactericidal activity.

Halogenated Hydrocarbon Mixtures

One of the more famous cases involving exposures to mixtures of halogenated hydrocarbons and immune system abnormalities concerned residents in the town of Woburn, Massachusetts. Residents were exposed to well water contaminated with trichloroethylene, tetrachloroethylene, *trans*-dichloroethylene, 1,1,1-trichloroethane, and chloroform (29). The incidence of childhood leukemia in the town was 2.5 times the average for the U.S. population and there was a correlation between access to the well water and the incidence of this type of leukemia (29). In addition, there were significant increases in the incidences of pulmonary and urinary infections in the children in East Woburn. These children received the highest concentration of the water from the contaminated wells (29). These increases in infection spurred an immunologic assessment of 25 surviving family members of the leukemia patients (30). These assessments were initiated 5 years after closure of the wells and were repeated at 1 month and 18 months thereafter. The family members exhibited a lymphocytosis accompanied by elevations in the numbers of CD4+ and CD8+ cells. Helper/suppressor ratios, however, were depressed in these individuals. These changes were not persistent. Reanalysis 18 months later showed that all these parameters had returned to control levels (30).

Since the immunologic profiles were performed 5 years after closure of the wells, it is possible that alterations in the profiles were more severe in the subjects during and immediately after exposures. There is indirect evidence to support this contention. For a year or two after closure of the wells, more than half of the subjects who participated in the immunologic profile assays presented with recurrent maculopapular rashes (30). No obvious causes could be established but it is known that rashes are associated with industrial exposures to trichloroethylene (31).

HYDROXYETHERS

There is very good evidence that 2-methoxyethanol (2ME) is an immunotoxicant in rats. Oral treatment of rats (50 to 200 mg/kg/d) with 2ME produced a number of immunotoxic responses including a reduction in thymus weight, reduced proliferative responses to several mitogens [phytohemagglutinin (PHA), concanavalin A (Con A), and pokeweed (PWM)] and reduced responses to T cell-dependent and T cell-independent antigens (32). Additional studies showed that many of the immunotoxic effects of 2ME could be produced in rats by oral administration of 2-methoxyacetic acid (2MAA), the principal metabolite of 2ME (33). In addition, it was found that treatment with 4-methylpyrazole, an inhibitor of the conversion of 2ME to 2MAA, could reverse the 2ME-induced suppression of antibody response to a T cell-independent antigen (33). These results strongly suggest that the immunotoxic effects of 2ME are due to its metabolite, 2MAA.

In contrast to these studies with rats, studies employing B6C3F1 mice exposed orally to 2ME or to 2MAA showed no immune effects except reductions in thymus weights (34). These contrasting results may imply that rats are more sensitive to 2ME than mice.

Finally, there is some evidence for structure–activity effects among the hydroxyethers as 2ME was found to be more immunotoxic than 2-butoxyethanol when the compounds were delivered at equal doses (35).

IMPLICATIONS FOR NEPHROTOXICITY

It appears that organic solvents are, for the most part, not potent immunotoxic compounds. With certain exceptions, solvents must be administered in relatively high doses to induce immune-modulating effects. However, one intriguing aspect of the immunotoxicity of solvents is that the immunomodulating effects of these compounds may play a role in the induction of nephrotoxicity. Solvent exposure is associated with an increased risk of kidney damage (36). There is evidence that circulating immune complexes (perhaps formed by hapten–antibody reactions) trapped or formed *in situ* in the glomeruli may play a role in the nephrotoxic effects of solvents. It is hypothesized that the exposure to these complexes must be protracted and that kidney damage in addition to the accumulation of immunocomplexes must be present for the production of severe glomerulonephritis (37). Thus, although solvents may not be potent immunotoxicants, perhaps even subtle immune-altering effects of these compounds may play a role in their nephrotoxicity.

REFERENCES

1. Snyder CA. Benzene. In: Snyder R, ed. *Ethel Browning's toxicity and metabolism of industrial solvents*, 2nd ed. Amsterdam: Elsevier; 1987:3–37.
2. Pfeifer R, Irons R. Inhibition of lectin-stimulated lymphocyte agglutination and mitogenesis by hydroquinone: reactivity with intracellular sulfhydryl groups. *Exp Mol Pathol* 1981;35:189–198.
3. Rozen M, Snyder CA, Albert R. Depressions in B- and T-lymphocyte mitogen-induced blastogenesis in mice exposed to low concentrations of benzene. *Toxicol Lett* 1984;20:343–349.
4. Rozen M, Snyder CA. Protracted exposure of C57BL/6 mice to 300 ppm benzene depresses B- and T-lymphocyte numbers and mitogen responses. Evidence for thymic and bone marrow proliferation in response to the exposures. *Toxicology* 1985;37:13–26.
5. Hsieh G, Parker R, Sharma R, Hughes B. Subclinical effects of groundwater contaminants. *Arch Toxicol* 1990;64:320–328.
6. Aoyama K. Effects of benzene inhalation on lymphocyte subpopulations and immune response in mice. *Toxicol Appl Pharmacol* 1986;85:92–101.

7. Rosenthal G, Snyder CA. Inhaled benzene reduces aspects of cell-mediated tumor surveillance in mice. *Toxicol Appl Pharmacol* 1987;88:35–43.
8. Rosenthal G, Snyder CA. Modulation of the immune response to *Listeria monocytogenes* by benzene inhalation. *Toxicol Appl Pharmacol* 1985;80:502–510.
9. Maceachern L, Laskin D. Increased production of tumor necrosis factor-α by bone marrow leukocytes following benzene treatment of mice. *Toxicol Appl Pharmacol* 1992;113:260–266.
10. Hseih G, Sharma R, Parker R. Hypothalamic–pituitary–adrenocortical axis activity and immune function after oral exposure to benzene and toluene. *Immunopharmacology* 1991;21(1):23–31.
11. Fishbein L. An overview of environmental and toxicological aspects of aromatic hydrocarbons II. Toluene. *Sci Total Environ* 1985;42:267–288.
12. Aranyi C, O'Shea W, Sherwood R, Graham J, Miller F. Effects of toluene inhalation on pulmonary host defenses of mice. *Toxicol Lett* 1985;25:103–110.
13. Hsieh G, Sharma R, Parker R. Immunotoxicologic evaluation of toluene exposure via drinking water in mice. *Environ Res* 1989;49:93–103.
14. Sato A, Nakajima T. Dose-dependent metabolic interaction between benzene and toluene *in vivo* and *in vitro*. *Toxicol Appl Pharmacol* 1979;48:249–256.
15. Kalf G, Rushmore T, Snyder R. Benzene inhibits RNA synthesis in mitochondria from liver and bone marrow. *Chem Biol Interact* 1982;42:353–370.
16. Spencer P, Schaumberg H, Sabri M, Veronise B. The enlarging view of hexacarbon neuropathy. *CRC Crit Rev Toxicol* 1980;7:279–356.
17. Baldachin B, Melmed R. Clinical and therapeutic aspects of kerosine poisoning, 200 cases. *Br Med J* 1964;2:28–30.
18. Suleiman S. Petroleum hydrocarbon toxicity *in vitro*: effect of *n*-alkanes, benzene and toluene on pulmonary alveolar macrophages and lysosomal enzymes of the lung. *Arch Toxicol* 1987;59:402–407.
19. Kannan K, Singh K, Goel S, Shanker R. Effect of 2,5-hexanediol on immunocompetence of mice. *Environ Res* 1985;36:14–25.
20. Moszczynski P, Slowinski S, Moszczynski P. Synergistic effect of organic solvents and tobacco smoke on the indicators of humoral immunity in humans. *Gig Tr Prof Zabol* 1991;3:34–36.
21. Moszczynski P, Lisiewicz J, Slowinski S. Synergistic effect of organic solvents and tobacco smoke on serum immunoglobulin levels in humans. *Med Pr* 1989;40(6):337–341.
22. Zeman K, Tchorzewski H, Baj Z, et al. The effects of occupational exposure to hydrocarbons on some immune parameters of workers in the phenol division of a petrochemical plant. *Pol J Occup Med* 1990;3(4):399–407.
23. Kaminski N, Barnes D, Jordan S, Holsapple M. The role of metabolism in carbon tetrachloride-mediated immunosuppression: *in vivo* studies. *Toxicol Appl Pharmacol* 1990;102:9–20.
24. Kaminski N, Jordan S, Holsapple M. Suppression of humoral and cell-mediated immune responses by carbon tetrachloride. *Fundam Appl Toxicol* 1989;12:117–128.
25. Smialowicz R, Simmons J, Luebke R, Allis J. Immunotoxicologic assessment of subacute exposure of rats to carbon tetrachloride with comparison to hepatotoxicity and nephrotoxicity. *Fundam Appl Toxicol* 1991;17:186–196.
26. Shopp G, Sanders V, Munson A. Humoral and cell-mediated immune status of mice exposed to *trans*-1,2-dichloroethylene. *Drug Chem Toxicol* 1985;8(5):393–407.
27. Sherwood R, O'Shea W, Thomas P, Ratajczak H, Aranyi C, Graham J. Effects of inhalation of ethylene dichloride on pulmonary defenses of mice and rats. *Toxicol Appl Pharmacol* 1987;91:491–496.
28. Aranyi C, O'Shea W, Graham J, Miller F. The effects of inhalation of organic chemical air contaminants on murine lung host defenses. *Fundam Appl Toxicol* 1986;6:713–720.
29. Lagakos S, Wessen B, Zelen M. An analysis of contaminated well water and health effects in Woburn, Massachusetts. *J Am Stat Assoc* 1986;81:583–614.
30. Byers V, Levin A, Ozonoff D, Baldwin R. Association between clinical symptoms and lymphocyte abnormalities in a population with chronic domestic exposure to industrial solvent-contaminated domestic water supply and a high incidence of leukemia. *Cancer Immunol Immunother* 1988;27:77–81.
31. Waters E, Gerstner H, Huff J. Trichloroethylene I: an overview. *J Toxicol Environ Health* 1977; 2:671–707.
32. Smialowicz R, Riddle M, Luebke R, et al. Immunotoxicity of 2-methoxyethanol following oral administration in Fischer 344 rats. *Toxicol Appl Pharmacol* 1991;109:494–506.

33. Smialowicz R, Riddle M, Rogers R, Copeland A, Luebke R, Andrews D. Evaluation of the immunotoxicity of orally administered 2-methoxyacetic acid in Fischer 344 rats. *Fundam Appl Toxicol* 1991;17:771–781.
34. House R, Lauer L, Murray M, Ward E, Dean J. Immunological studies in B6C3F1 mice following exposure to ethylene glycol monomethyl ether and its principal metabolite methoxy acetic acid. *Toxicol Appl Pharmacol* 1985;77:358–362.
35. Exon J, Mather G, Bussiere J, Olson D, Talcott P. Effects of subchronic exposure of rats to 2-methoxyethanol or 2-butoxyethanol: thymic atrophy and immunotoxicity. *Fundam Appl Toxicol* 1991;16:830–840.
36. Daniell W, Couser W, Rosenstock L. Occupational solvent exposure and glomerulonephritis. *JAMA* 1988;259(15):2280–2283.
37. Ravnskov U. Non-systemic glomerulonephritis: exposure to nephrotoxic and immunotoxic chemicals predispose to immunologic harassment. *Med Hypotheses* 1989;30:115–122.

Immunotoxicology and Immunopharmacology, Second Edition, edited by J. H. Dean, M. I. Luster, A. E. Munson, and I. Kimber.
Raven Press, Ltd., New York © 1994.

11

Pesticides

John B. Barnett and *Kathleen E. Rodgers

*Departments of Microbiology and Immunology, West Virginia University School of Medicine, Morgantown, West Virginia 26506; and *Department of Obstetrics and Gynecology, University of Southern California, Livingston Research Center, Los Angeles, California 90033*

Pesticides are xenobiotics that are by definition biocidal. That is, they are deliberately added to the environment for the purpose of killing a form of life. The pesticides are designed to be selective to the species to be killed through metabolism or targeting of a site that is specific to the target organism. Within the pesticides is a group of compounds that includes a large assortment of insecticides, herbicides, fungicides, and so on. This classification includes such a large and diverse group of compounds that the discussion in this chapter is limited to the immunotoxicity of selected members of the organochlorine and organophosphate classes (Fig. 1) of insecticides to allow more depth in coverage.

The organochlorine insecticides, comprised of a basic chlorinated hydrocarbon structure, are further subdivided depending on whether they have a cyclodiene structure (e.g., chlordane, heptachlor, aldrin, dieldrin), dichlorodiphenyltrichloroethane (DDT) or analog structure, a benzene hexachloride structure (e.g., lindane), or are toxaphenes. The organochlorine insecticides reviewed in this chapter include aldrin, dieldrin, endrin, chlordane, heptachlor, hexachlorocyclohexane isomers, and DDT. The exposure of humans to these compounds initially came as a result of their extensive use in agriculture, structure protection, vector control, and, in one case, as a directly applied medicine (i.e., lindane). Initially, there was widespread use of these pesticides; however, since the early 1970s, the use of many of these insecticides is either restricted or banned altogether. DDT continues to be used outside North America to control medically important insect vectors (e.g., mosquitoes); however, the emergence of DDT-resistant insect species limits its effectiveness. The only member of this group of compounds that is deliberately applied directly to humans is lindane, to control body and head lice, and it is also being replaced by permethrin (Elimite, Herbert Laboratories).

Although the use of many of the organochlorine pesticides is severely restricted, or banned altogether, most of these agents continue to be a potential human health

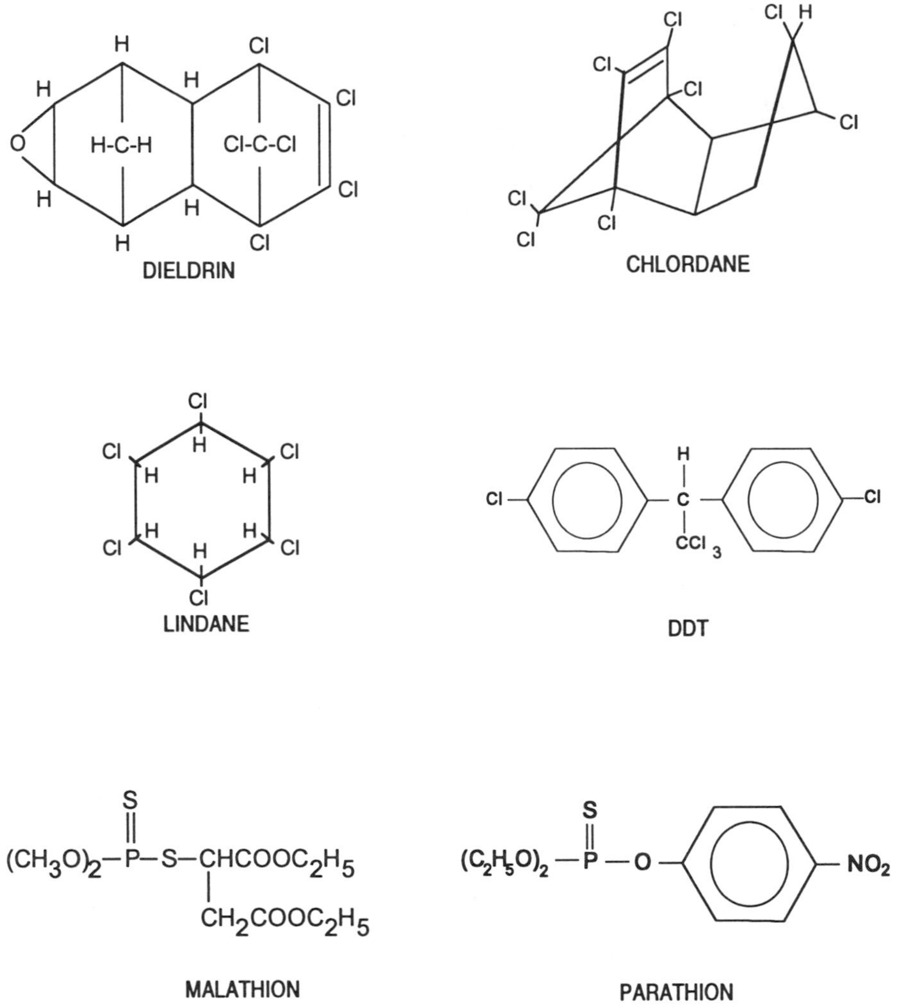

DIELDRIN CHLORDANE

LINDANE DDT

MALATHION PARATHION

FIG. 1. Chemical structures of the organochlorine and organophosphate pesticides reviewed in this chapter.

and environmental problem because of their extremely long half-life in soil, ability to enter the groundwater supplies, and propensity to be concentrated in adipose tissue and thus enter the food chain. The concentrations of all these agents in human adipose tissues are monitored in many different countries. One such survey by the U.S. Environmental Protection Agency (EPA), the National Human Adipose Tissue Survey (NHATS) (summarized in ref. 1), indicates that while the levels of some pesticides dropped during the years 1970 to 1983 (e.g., dieldrin), others remained very stable during that period (e.g., oxychlordane). There are numerous reports of measured organochlorine pesticide levels in both adult and infant human adipose tissue and the milk of mothers. For example, in a 1991 study, mean 1,1-dichloro-2,2′-bis(*p*-chlorophenyl)ethylene (DDE) (metabolite of DDT) levels of 2276 and 2270 ng per gram of human milk were measured in mothers of two Italian towns (2).

Organophosphate insecticides represent another chemical class of pesticides. Unlike the organochlorine pesticides, organophosphate pesticides are still widely used in the United States. Malathion and parathion are the most extensively used members of this class of pesticides and our discussion of the organophosphate pesticides is largely limited to these compounds. Malathion has the principal virtue of having fairly potent insecticide activity and relatively low mammalian toxicity, whereas parathion, while being more potent, is also more toxic (3–5). This low toxicity of malathion is attributed to its rapid detoxification to nontoxic monoacid derivatives by mammalian carboxylesterases present in liver and other tissues (4,6–8). For this reason, malathion is widely used in situations where the public would be exposed (9). This compound was used extensively in the aerial spraying for fruit flies in California and Florida where large urban populations were exposed (10). Malathion is also used by both agricultural workers and consumers in the control of certain pests on fruit, vegetables, and ornamental plants (11,12). It is used in the control of house flies, mosquitoes, and lice as well as on pests affecting domesticated animals. Parathion, on the other hand, is largely used in agricultural settings due to its toxicity. Since the potential for not only environmental but also personal contamination is therefore present, the determination of the immunotoxic effects and mechanism of these effects is of interest.

GENERAL TOXICITY (NONIMMUNE)

The most commonly noted nonimmune toxic effects of the organochlorine pesticides relate to hepatotoxicity and neurotoxicity, with some differences in the actual symptoms produced by a given agent or isomer of that agent. These toxic effects are well described by Murphy (13) and are not repeated here. It should be noted, however, that in addition to the neuro- and hepatotoxicity, acute exposure to chlordane or heptachlor is reported to be associated with a self-limited refractory megaloblastic anemia (14), other blood dyscrasias, and childhood tumors (15).

Malathion and parathion are absorbed through the gut, skin, and lung, then transported to the liver, where it undergoes metabolism to many derivatives including nontoxic monoderivative and toxic oxygen metabolites (5,16). Acute poisoning by organophosphates leads to inhibition of acetylcholinesterase through phosphorylation of the esterase active site, resulting in an accumulation of acetylcholine, a neurotransmitter in the sympathetic and parasympathetic fibers, neuromuscular junctions, and some synapses within the central nervous system (17). Malaxon, a metabolite of and an impurity in malathion, and paraoxon are thought to be the active esterase inhibitors. Signs of acute intoxication include nausea, vomiting, diarrhea, mitositis, bradycardia, and lacrimation (16).

IMMUNOTOXICITY

Organochlorine Pesticides

Aldrin/Dieldrin/Endrin

Aldrin is metabolized to dieldrin by mammals, soil microorganisms, plants, and insects; therefore studies on dieldrin are pertinent to aldrin. Like many organochlorine pesticides, dieldrin bioconcentrates in adipose tissue. However, endrin is epoxidized to isodrin and, although it has a high acute toxicity, shows little tendency to become stored in adipose tissue (18).

An especially enlightening group of reports on dieldrin's immunotoxicity are provided by Fornier, Kyzystyniak, Hugo, Bernier, and colleagues. These reports provide a degree of consistency in methodology that is difficult to achieve when comparing data among groups of scientists. Throughout these investigations, most experiments use a dieldrin dose of 0.6 LD_{50}, where LD_{50} is the median lethal dose. Building on the earlier reports by Loose (19) and Kaminsky et al. (20) of a dieldrin-induced decrease in macrophage (mϕ) activity, the effects of dieldrin on mouse hepatitis virus type 3 (MHV3) resistance was determined (21–25). Mϕs are the main target cell for MHV3 (26). The first of these studies reports the effect of dieldrin on MHV3 resistance in three strains of mice: a susceptible strain (C57B1/6), a resistant strain (A/J), and the F1 hybrid, which has an intermediate level of resistance. Dieldrin treatment of the susceptible C57B1/6 strain causes a significant decrease in mean time to death after MHV3 infection. Anti-MHV3 immunoglobulin G (IgG) antibody titers in sera and spleen cell supernatants are also reduced in the C57B1/6 strain. Several experiments confirm that the dieldrin is affecting the mϕs and not interfering with viral replication, absorption, and so on. They recognize that it is difficult from these data to definitively determine whether the apparent resistance of the A/J strain to dieldrin-induced increased MHV3 sensitivity is due to this mouse strain's inherent insensitivity to the virus or whether the dieldrin is not being metabolized to a toxic component in the resistant strain (26). However, lymph node cells from dieldrin-treated A/J mice show a decrease in potential to induce a graft-versus-host reaction (GvHR) in a histoincompatible strain (27). This decrease in GvHR is not due to the direct cytotoxicity of the dieldrin on the transferred lymph node cells or to a change in the T cell subpopulations contained in the transferred cells. These results imply that the lack of effect in the A/J strain is due to its inherent resistance to the virus.

Although A/J are resistant to lethal challenge with MHV3, infection of this strain results in mϕ activation manifested by restriction of MHV3 replication in mϕ cultures after *in vitro* rechallenge with virus. Dieldrin treatment of the A/J mice abrogates this inherent resistance to the virus (22). In addition, mϕs from dieldrin-treated mice infected *in vivo* show higher levels of cytopathic effect, MHV3 antigen, and virulent MHV3 than control animals. Other parameters of mϕ functional status [i.e., superoxide generation, adherence to plastic, sheep red blood cell

(SRBC) phagocytosis, and cell viability] show no detrimental effect of dieldrin exposure. The attachment and uptake of ^{3}H-labeled MHV3 virions by activated mϕs are also not affected. Because MHV3 infections in this resistant strain of mice are closely correlated with an "innate" resistance of mϕs, it is concluded that the noted differences in dieldrin-treated and control animals are due to a specific effect of dieldrin on the mϕs. However, it should be noted that there are also reductions in anti-MHV3 IgG antibody pointing to possible defects in immune elements other than the mϕs or that the antigen processing and presenting capabilities of the mϕs are affected.

The effect of dieldrin on other cellular immune parameters, such as mixed lymphocyte responses (MLRs) either with (23) or without (28) a combined MHV3 infection, is also noted. The MLRs in C57B1/6 mice without a MHV3 infection are depressed at 7 days after dieldrin treatment; however, the MLR is essentially normal at 4 or 24 days after treatment (28). The noted decrease (at 7 days) is not due to an effect on total lymphoid or T cell subtype ratios. Combined dieldrin treatment with MHV3 infection shows no synergistic decrease in MLR due to virus-induced decrease in lymphoproliferation (23).

In addition to the anti-viral antibody responses, antibody responses to SRBCs, *Salmonella typhimurium*, or lipopolysaccharide (LPS) were measured to determine if the noted effect on the humoral response could be pinpointed to a T cell-dependent or T cell-independent response. Antibody responses to both types of antigens were depressed (29,30). However, since both of these response types require the cooperation of an antigen-presenting cell (APC), the effect of the dieldrin still could primarily be due to an effect on mϕs.

More direct measurements of the effect of dieldrin on mϕs to determine the *ex vivo* ability of dieldrin-treated mϕs to phagocytose and kill *S. typhimurium* show that mϕs from dieldrin-treated animals have depressed phagocytic (24,30) and bactericidal (30) capabilities. As previously stated, the reduced cidal activity is not attributed to a reduction in superoxide generation (24). Recent studies on mϕ function indicate that arginine-dependent production of nitrate/nitrite is an important cytotoxic mechanism of mϕs (for review, see ref. 31). The reduced killing capacity could therefore be due to a reduction in these agents. However, the effect of oral endrin administration on rat peritoneal mϕ function shows an increase in *ex vivo* nitrate/nitrite production (32). Differences in species and the more acute toxicity of endrin (1) make it imprudent to make direct comparisons between the two studies; however, it would be informative to measure either the mϕs nitrate/nitrite production in mice after dieldrin treatment or superoxide levels, phagocytosis, and killing after oral endrin adminstration.

It appears that with MHV3, antigen presentation and processing by the mϕs are paramount in the humoral response to the virus. Krzystyniak et al. (33) and Bernier et al. (25) address possible affects of dieldrin on antigen processing and presentation using an avidin model. Peritoneal mϕs from dieldrin-treated animals show less uptake of avidin and release of processed antigen than control animals (25,33). The ability of "processed" antigen to induce normal lymph node cell proliferation is used as a measure of this antigen to induce an immune response (33). However, inasmuch as this is soluble or released processed antigen and not antigen presented in context with the major histocompatibility complex (MHC) class II, it is not clear whether these studies accurately represent the normal *in vivo* activity.

These studies *in toto* implicate the mϕ as the primary target of dieldrin-induced immunotoxicity in mice. Additional studies on the molecular or subcellular effects of dieldrin on the mϕ would be very informative and interesting, as would studies on the effects of dieldrin on host resistance to viruses that specifically target other types of immune cells. From separate studies, it is known that dieldrin stimulates calcium-dependent superoxide release from rat neutrophils *in vitro* (34) and the role of any possible effects on neutrophils in mice does not appear to have been addressed. In addition, the specificity of the dieldrin for the mϕ should also be investigated by challenging other APCs, such as the Langerhans' cell.

Chlordane/Heptachlor

Commercial preparations of chlordane are a mixture of closely related compounds, the chlordane isomers, heptachlor, as well as transnonachlor. Therefore immunotoxicity of these agents is discussed together. One of the earliest indicators of chlordane's immunotoxicity is a 1976 report of significant hematologic changes and recurring fevers in a human after documented exposure to chlordane (14). However, the first definitive immunotoxicologic study is by Spyker-Cranmer and others (35) in 1982.

Numerous developmental immunotoxicologic studies on model organochlorine insecticides are published; however, chlordane is the most extensively studied for its effects on the developing immune system. Spyker-Cranmer and co-workers (35) report that the offspring of dams treated with chlordane throughout gestation show a profound deficit in contact hypersensitivity response (CHR) to a contact allergen, oxazolone, without measurable adverse effects on their humoral immune response [anti-SRBC plaque-forming cells (PFCs)] The initially observed decrease in CHR was interpreted as an indication of a possible T cell defect; however, extensive investigations on T cell efferent functions such as mitogen responses to concanavalin A (Con A) and phytohemagglutinin (PHA) (36), antigen-specific T cell blastogenesis (36), and cytotoxic T lymphocyte (CTL) function (37) show these functions to be normal. Another cellular response, natural killer (NK) cell activity, is also not affected (38). Thus prenatal chlordane exposure does not appear to affect the T cell response as judged by these functional assays.

Host resistance studies on chlordane-exposed offspring with virulent influenza virus [A/PR8/34] demonstrate that the offspring of chlordane-treated dams can withstand a higher infectious dose of virus (39). In mice, the delayed-type hypersensitivity (DTH) response contributes to the pathology of an influenza infection, and the ultimate outcome of the infection depends on a balance between the immunoprotective effects of CTLs and the degree of pulmonary damage mediated by

T_{DTH} cells (40,41). Influenza-specific DTH responses are severely depressed in chlordane-treated offspring (37) and it follows that reduced DTH-induced pathology damage coupled with normal CTL responses in the chlordane-exposed offspring will increase the LD_{50} to this infectious agent.

Continuing studies on the mechanism of the decreased DTH function focus on the mϕ, which functions both in the afferent portion in antigen processing and presentation and the efferent portion as an effector cell influenced by numerous T cell cytokines. Mϕs undergo a series of phenotypically definable changes during progression from the resident state to the fully activated state (for review see ref. 42). As mϕs proceed toward activation, significant modulation of secretory products (43,44) and expression of cell surface receptors (45,46) become readily apparent. The mϕs are thought to play a central role in the host response to tumor cells, and one endpoint of the activation scheme is the attainment of the ability to lyse tumor target cells (e.g., P815 mastocytoma cells). Initial studies on the ability of peritoneal mϕs from adult mice exposed *in utero* to chlordane (hereafter referred to as chlordane-mϕs) to become tumoricidal show that there is a lag in the peak time of cytotoxicity. Inflammatory control-mϕs, stimulated with interferon-γ (IFN-γ) and LPS, demonstrate significant cytotoxicity at 2 and 24 hr of culture, while stimulated inflammatory chlordane-mϕs show no tumoricidal activity until 48 hr (47). However, the level of cytotoxicity by chlordane-mϕs at the 48-hr time point is equivalent to that of the control-mϕs. Studies on TNF-α levels show a similar lag in chlordane-mϕs, while nitrate/nitrite levels show no demonstrable lag (48). Further studies on the levels and timing of second messenger molecules critical to the mϕ activation events (e.g., inositol triphosphate) also show this temporal delay with subsequent recovery to control levels (49). Additional studies on enzymatic and receptor-expression events that characterize the activation state of mϕs indicate that the chlordane-mϕs appear to reside in a more elevated state of activation than control-mϕs (49). It is not known at this time whether or how this heightened state of activation is related to the increase in response time required by chlordane mϕs. The ability of chlordane-mϕs to reach a similar level of activation as control mϕs, with sufficient time, however, explains why no overt adverse effects on the health of the animal are noted.

The prenatal exposure route data also prompted studies on the effect of chlordane on the various stem cell populations. The work published thus far has focused on the pluripotent colony-forming unit (CFU-S) and multipotent granulocyte–macrophage colony-forming unit (GM-CFU) stem cell populations. With both cell populations, a significant depression is noted in their ability to either reconstitute an irradiated host (CFU-S) or respond to exogenous mouse lung conditioned media as a source of granulocyte–macrophage colony-stimulating factor (GM-CSF) (50,51). These effects were measured in cells from fetal liver (gestation day 18) and adult bone marrow cells at ages up to 300 days. Although prenatal exposure to chlordane affects the ability of myeloid stem cell populations to respond to exogenous growth factors, a cause–effect relationship between the stem cell effects and the deficits noted in the mϕ population is yet to be determined.

Johnson et al. (52) exposed adult (C57B1/6 × C3H)F1 (B6C3F1) mice to graded doses of chlordane for 14 days and measured a number of standard immunologic functions. These functional assays include anti-SRBC PFC, mitogen-induced blastogenic responses, MLRs, and DTH. Neither the antibody responses nor the B cell mitogen responses are affected by exposure to ≤8.0 mg/kg of chlordane. Although Con A responses and MLRs of chlordane-treated splenocytes are reported to be increased in treated animals, *in vivo* DTH responses are not significantly affected by the chlordane treatment. It is concluded by these authors that chlordane causes no significant biologic immunotoxicity in adult mice.

A recent report on the effects of chlordane in 27 humans, exposed to chlordane either at home or occupationally from 0.33 to 10 years past (53), provides conflicting data to that described above. For some individuals, pesticide exposure is quantified by fat biopsy measurements for oxychlordane (metabolite of chlordane), transnonachlor, and heptachlor epoxide. Flow cytometric measurements of 14 different CD membrane markers, CD4:CD8 ratios, as well as several functional assays are included in this study. Expression of CD1, found on thymocytes and Langerhans' cells (unknown function), and CD45RA on CD4+ cells is reduced in exposed individuals. CD45RA is associated with naive T cells and is thought to have a role in signal transduction via tyrosine phosphokinase. Kappa and lambda light chains are found more frequently on the B cells of the chlordane-exposed group than controls. Functional studies include measuring NK cell and Fc-mediated antibody-dependent cell-mediated cytotoxicity (ADCC) as well as MLRs and mitogen responses. NK cell function is not changed in the chlordane-exposed individuals, whereas ADCC responses are significantly depressed. MLRs and mitogen responses are also depressed in the exposed individuals. Antibody levels to nuclear antigen (ANA), deoxyribonucleic acid (DNA), and smooth muscle are used as an index of possible autoimmunity. Twelve individuals demonstrate measurable levels of these antibodies, indicating some degree of autoimmunity. However, examination of the data provided in the report shows no obvious positive correlation between adipose tissue levels or duration of exposure and autoantibody titers (no statistical comparison is provided). Thus it is not clear whether the exposure of these individuals to chlordane, apparently solely as an adult, is the single cause of their diminished immune capacity. However, this study provides some evidence linking human adult exposure to demonstrable immunotoxicity.

There are numerous *in vitro* studies on the effects of chlordane exposure. Chlordane or oxychlordane (at 0.6 to 10 μM; dissolved in ethanol) causes significant reductions in both humoral and cell-mediated immune functions (54). Furthermore, it is shown that although chlordane reduces antibody responses it does not alter the kinetics of the response and must be added to the culture during the early stages of the response to cause the suppression. In a separate study, Chuang et al. (55) show that *in vitro* concentrations of 10 to 40 μM of chlordane or heptachlor cause significant increases in mitogen-induced blastogenic responses and IL-2 production in rhesus monkey peripheral blood monocytes (PBMs). The solvent used to dilute the pesticides is not indicated and all assays are conducted in the presence of serum.

Johnson et al. (54) note that the inclusion of serum into the culture media abrogates the depression of mitogen responses. Perhaps the different results in these two studies are related to the inclusion of serum in one group of experiments and not the other. In addition, Chuang et al. (55) do not appear to control for carryover of the chlordane or heptachlor from primary cell culture media to the IL-2 bioassay with cytotoxic T lymphocyte line (CTLL) cells.

Chlordane and heptachlor, *in vitro*, also induce numerous changes in guinea pig neutrophils (56). These changes include stimulation of superoxide generation, altered membrane potential, and increased intracellular calcium levels ($[Ca^{2+}]_i$). The increase in $[Ca^{2+}]_i$ is attributed both to an acceleration of extracellular Ca^{2+} penetration and to Ca^{2+} release from the intracellular pool. The chlordane-induced lag in superoxide generation is somewhat reminiscent of the temporal retardation in mϕs cytotoxicity and second messenger production noted by Theus et al. (47,49) after prenatal exposure to chlordane.

The *in vitro* effects of chlordane or heptachlor on Madin–Darby canine kidney (MDCK) cells (57), African green monkey kidney (AGMK) cells (57), and human myeloblastic leukemia (ML-1) cells (58) are also known. *In vitro* exposure of MDCK or AGMK cells to chlordane (0.5 to 10 ppm in ethanol) causes a significant reduction in the ability of influenza virus but not herpes simplex type 1 virus to infect these cells (57). This appears to be due to an effect of chlordane on the membrane of the target cell and not to any direct effect of chlordane on the viruses themselves. Chuang et al. (58) report that heptachlor [2.6 nM to 2.6 μM in dimethylsulfoxide (DMSO)] induces growth stimulation, cell adherence, and formation of extended cytoplasmic pseudopodia in ML-1 cells. Similar effects are caused by 12-*O*-tetradecanoylphorbol-13-acetate (TPA); however, these studies do not provide evidence that TPA and heptachlor operate in the same manner.

Based on the numerous reports of chlordane/heptachlor contamination of groundwater, human milk, adipose tissue, and so on and the recent report by McConnachie and Zahalsky (53), these agents are still of immunotoxicologic concern. Although *in vitro* studies are important to our understanding of the effects of these agents, more definitive cellular and molecular *ex vivo* studies should be a high priority. The studies of Theus et al. (47) and Gregory et al. (59) also indicate that functional studies that look relatively "long-term" to the initial stimulatory events, that is, in excess of 24 to 48 hr, are probably not sensitive enough to detect important immunotoxic effects. Further investigations using these techniques on adults as well as prenatal exposures are warranted.

Lindane

Five isomers of 1,2,3,4,5,6-hexachlorocyclohexane (HCH), *alpha* (α), *beta* (β), *gamma* (γ), *delta* (δ) and *epsilon* (ϵ), were originally contained in a commercial preparation of HCH known as benzene hexachloride (BHC). BHC is no longer marketed (since 1978); however, a commercially available insecticide, lindane, contains 99% γ-HCH as opposed to other isomers (1). The interpretion of the studies on the effect of HCH is confused by the failure of some investigators to indicate which isomer of HCH is being studied.

Prenatal exposure to lindane (isomer composition unspecified) alters DTH, mitogen-induced blastogenesis, and anti-SRBC antibody responses (60). Ten-day-old Swiss albino mice, exposed *in utero* to 10 mg/kg maternal body weight (m.b.w.), showed significant enhancement of the DTH and anti-SRBC responses over the controls. However, at a higher (100 mg/kg m.b.w.) dose, the DTH response is significantly decreased, while no effect on the mitogen or antibody responses is noted.

In vivo lindane treatment of adult mice induces numerous immunomodulating effects. André et al. (61) show that subchronic and chronic lindane (isomer composition unspecified) exposure affects humoral immunity and the duration of primary *Giardia muris* infection. Animals fed lindane-spiked diet for 4 weeks show no effect on the anti-SRBC IgM responses after parenteral immunization; however, serum IgG2b anti-SRBC levels are elevated subsequent to an intragastic immunization. Animals fed a lindane-spiked diet for 10 weeks are unable to resist a *G. muris* infection, whereas all control animals eliminate the infection. The lindane-treated animals also produce anti-*Giardia* antibodies while the control animals do not. Cornacoff et al. (62), using the β-HCH isomer, show that IgM and IgG anti-SRBC responses are not affected by a 30-day subchronic exposure to 100 mg/kg of β-HCH. However, animals fed a higher 300-mg/kg dose of β-HCH show significant decreases in several cellular parameters including lymphoproliferative responses as well as CTL and NK responses.

A curious effect is reported by Meera et al. (63) during and after a 24-week *in vivo* exposure to γ-HCH. Three subtoxic doses (0.012, 0.12, 1.2 mg/kg) of γ-HCH are administered in feed and animals are assayed each month from the beginning of the exposure period. Cell-mediated immunity (CMI) and humoral immune components are assessed using DTH responses, Con A- and LPS-induced lymphoproliferative responses, and anti-SRBC and anti-LPS IgM PFC responses. These assays uniformly show a biphasic response characterized by an initial stimulation at 4 and 8 weeks, followed by a period of no difference (12 weeks) and at later times (16 to 24 weeks) suppression in a dose-responsive manner. Mφ phagocytosis and killing are not affected at any time or dose level. The results at the earlier points (4 and 8 weeks) reported by Meera et al. (63) appear to be in accordance with those of André et al. (61) at similar time points (4 and 10 weeks), although André et al. (61) administered a much higher dose (150 ppm). The similarity of results with such disparate doses may partially be explained if these results are specific for γ-HCH and if André et al. (61) used technical-grade HCH. Technical-grade HCH may contain only 14% to 15% γ-HCH (62). There does not appear to be a systematic *in vivo* study that compares the immunotoxic effects of the different isomers of HCH; however, the results of Cornacoff et al. (62), utilizing β-HCH for 4 weeks and finding no decreases in antibody responses, indicate that the different isomers can produce distinct effects.

Several investigators report the effects of *in vitro* exposure to various isomers of HCH (64–68). Roux et al. (64) report that γ-HCH at doses of $\geq 10^{-4}$ M inhibits ribonucleic acid (RNA) synthesis but not protein synthesis in mouse mφs. In a subsequent study, Roux et al. (67) show similar effects of γ-HCH on protein and RNA synthesis in nonstimulated and PHA-stimulated human lymphocytes. It is their conclusion that because of the concentrations of γ-HCH needed, these effects are probably caused by membrane perturbations. Meade et al. (68) show an increase in arachidonic acid production and concomitant reduction of phosphatidylinositol turnover from γ-HCH-treated (63 to 250 μM) mφs. β-HCH is without effect at these concentrations. It also appears that γ-HCH favored stimulation of the lipoxygenase pathway over the cyclooxygenase pathway as the primary arachidonic acid metabolite was leukotriene C_4. γ-HCH, at much lower concentrations (0.005 to 20 μM), acts synergistically with a phorbol ester, TPA, to induce prostaglandin, leukotriene, and chemiluminescence production (66). Forgue et al. (66) note a similarity between the effects of γ-HCH + TPA and A23187 ($[Ca^{2+}]_i$ agonist) + TPA, leading them to speculate that γ-HCH may be operating by a similar mechanism. Thus it is apparent that γ-HCH has a profound effect on mφ function, probably at the membrane level.

In vitro exposure of bovine lymph node cells to α-HCH at 5- to 50-μM concentrations in conjunction with PHA results in an enhancement of lymphoproliferation (69). α-HCH by itself is not mitogenic and brief exposure early in the culture period provided the greatest enhancement. Other isomers of HCH are either not costimulatory (β-HCH) or toxic at very low concentrations (γ-HCH or δ-HCH; ≥10 μM). A follow-up study by this group (65) shows that γ-HCH or δ-HCH could prevent Con A + TPA-induced capping of bovine lymphocytes. The α-HCH or β-HCH isomers have no effect. Furthermore, it is shown that cytochalasin B, which is known to affect microfilaments, prevents the active dispersion of preformed lymphocyte caps by γ-HCH or δ-HCH, which again implies that the γ-HCH or δ-HCH is acting at the membrane level. It is interesting that Kensler and Mueller (69) find concentrations of ≥10 μM γ-HCH to be toxic to bovine lymphocytes, while Meade et al. (68) and Forgue et al. (66) do not report any toxicity on mouse mφs at 20 and 250 μM, respectively.

As stated earlier, the literature on HCH immunotoxic effects is confused by apparent differences in effect mediated by the different isomers of HCH. Given the continuing use of lindane, a systematic study on the effects of, at least, γ-HCH on *in vivo*, *ex vivo*, and *in vitro* immune responses is warranted. Finally, the differential results of André et al. (61) on the humoral response with intragastric versus parenteral immunization should be expanded to look at mucosal responses.

Dichlorodiphenyltrichloroethane (DDT)

DDT is one of the oldest pesticides in use. It was first licensed for use in the early 1940s and has been used extensively since that time. Its current use is restricted in the United States and many other countries; however, because of its high efficacy and low mammalian toxicity, it is still used for mosquito vector control for malaria prevention.

DDT is also one of the first pesticides studied for its effect on the immune system. Wassermann et al. (70) report that rats receiving 200 ppm DDT in drinking water for 35 days show a 35% reduction in their anti-ovalbumin serum antibody titers. Subsequently, Gabliks et al. (71) demonstrate that DDT treatment of guinea pigs results in a reduction in anaphylactic shock induction without a measurable effect on serum antibody levels to diphtheria toxoid. This is the result of reduced numbers of mast cells (72). Gabliks et al. (73) also show a similar phenomenon in rats. The mechanism of how DDT results in this apparent selective reduction of a particular cell population is not explained.

Street and Sharma (74) report no detrimental effect of up to 57 days of DDT treatment (≤6.54 mg/kg/d) on anti-SRBC hemagglutinin or hemolysin titers in rabbits after SRBC–Freund's complete adjuvant immunization at day 33. Banerjee et al. (75), however, report that mice fed a DDT-spiked diet of 20, 50, or 100 ppm daily for 3 to 12 weeks show a decrease in primary anti-SRBC IgM serum antibody on the 12th week. Secondary anti-SRBC IgM and IgG titers are reduced with the highest dose of DDT (100 ppm) at 3, 6, 8, and 12 weeks of dosing. Only secondary direct PFCs are reduced at the 100-ppm dose at 3 weeks of treatment; however, increased exposure times result in a time- and dose-dependent decrease in both primary and secondary PFCs. Rao and Glick (76) also show a decrease in serum anti-SRBC IgG with a concomitant increase in serum anti-SRBC IgM in chickens fed a DDT-spiked diet (100 ppm) *ad libitum* from hatching to 40 days of age. Thus, in at least one mammalian and one avian species, DDT treatment causes decreased humoral immune responses.

There is a relative paucity of immunotoxicologic studies on DDT and, as just described, there are some obvious discrepancies in the results of the different investigators, likely due to species and methodologic differences. The continued use of DDT would indicate that more extensive studies are warranted, especially mechanistic and CMI functional studies. However, the demonstration of low mammalian toxicity of DDT may be contributing to a lack of interest—the use of DDT was restricted because of its adverse effects on avian reproduction and aquatic species, not because of concern for the health of humans or other mammals. The results of Rao and Glick (76), however, indicate that the effects of DDT extend beyond its reproductive effects and again indicate a need for more extensive studies, particularly on avian species indigenous to areas in which DDT is heavily used.

Organophosphate Pesticides

In general, there is relatively little information available on the effects of organophosphate compounds on the immune system. Malathion and parathion are the organophosphate pesticides most extensively studied.

Malathion

Most studies of the effects of organophosphate compounds on the immune system have been conducted in laboratory animals. Those studies conducted in humans are for the most part epidemiologic in nature and lack adequate exposure information. One study involved the deliberate exposure of humans to malathion. In this study, technical grade malathion was administered in a 10% solution under an occluded patch for 2 days (77). After this exposure, 43% of the people developed "contact sensitivity." In this study, however, no measure of the formation of IgE antibodies to malathion was conducted (although formation of such antibodies is unlikely since there was no previous exposure). These data may be explained by the animal studies described below. In contrast, in this study, very few persons developed a classic hypersensitivity response (i.e., rash formation) after challenge with very low doses of technical grade malathion. In the literature, repeated exposure to malathion was shown to result in allergic response in guinea pigs, rats, and mice (78–80). However, malathion was not shown to be a potent sensitizer (as determined by the formation of IgE antibodies to malathion) in these animal studies.

Administration of several low doses of malathion for prolonged periods of time, which results in an overall high-dose exposure, was shown to result in a decrease in the level of humoral immune responses. For example, administration of 5 to 10 mg/kg/d malathion to rabbits for 5 to 6 weeks significantly decreased the serum antibody titers generated in response to *Salmonella typhi* vaccination (81). In addition, a single cholinergic dose of malathion 2 days after immunization with SRBCs suppressed a primary IgM response. However, this study indicated that administration of multiple low doses of malathion did not suppress an IgG response to SRBCs. These studies suggest that the cholinergic poisoning may have resulted in a stress-related suppression of the immune response (82).

The effects of *in vitro* exposure to malathion on the generation of an immune response were also determined. *In vitro* exposure of human mononuclear cells (either pretreated or continuously treated) or murine splenocytes to malathion suppressed the proliferative response to mitogens (83,84). In addition, *in vitro* exposure of murine splenocytes to malathion inhibited the generation of a CTL response to alloantigen (85,86). *In vitro* exposure of murine peritoneal cells to malathion inhibited the respiratory burst activity of these cells in response to phorbol esters (84). Further studies indicated that when malathion was coincubated with a reduced nicotinamide adenine dinucleotide phosphate (NADPH) regenerating S-9 liver enzyme system, the metabolites of malathion were no longer able to block the generation of an allogenic CTL response or a proliferative response to malathion (84–86). *In vitro* exposure of murine peritoneal cells or human peripheral blood mononuclear cells to metabolized malathion elevated the respiratory burst activity of these cells.

In describing the immunotoxicity of a compound, the emphasis is frequently on a decrease in immune function; however, enhancement of immune function can also be the result of exposure to this agent. Such is the case after oral administration of noncholinergic doses (acute and subacute) of malathion in which the generation of cellular, humoral, and mitogenic responses was examined (87). Acute (50% LD_{50}) or subacute (10% LD_{50} per day for 14 days) administration of malathion *in vivo* did not affect the *in vitro* generation of a CTL response to allogeneic tumor. However, 5 days after acute administration of malathion, there was an increase in humoral immune responsiveness. Acute treatment with purified malathion (50% LD_{50}) did not affect body weight, splenic cell number, thymic size, or serum cholinesterase. However, the proliferative response to mitogens was significantly enhanced on all days tested following acute administration of malathion. In contrast, subacute administration of malathion did not affect mitogenic response but led to a significant decrease in thymic cell number.

In order to investigate the mechanism of action of malathion, cell separation and reconstitution experiments were conducted after acute administration of high noncholinergic doses of malathion. These studies showed that malathion affected the function of the adherent cell population (84). Further studies showed that acute administration of malathion elevated the respiratory burst of peritoneal leukocytes. The lowest observed acute effect level (LOAEL) and the no observed acute effect level (NOAEL) for the effect of acute administration of malathion on the respiratory burst of peritoneal leukocytes were shown to be 0.25 and 0.1 mg/kg malathion, respectively (88). The upper limit calculated for acute exposure to malathion during the recent aerial spraying with malathion in southern California was approximately 0.5 mg/kg [total for dermal, oral, and respiratory using several health protective assumptions) (8).

Further mechanistic studies through the microscopic examination of peritoneal cells showed that peritoneal mast cells were degranulated within 4 hr after malathion administration (88). In addition, the percentage of phagocytic peritoneal cells ingesting mast cell granules and the number of granules ingested per cell were elevated. Studies reported in the literature indicate that mast cell products can modulate leukocyte activity (89). Therefore malathion may enhance the respiratory burst of peritoneal cells through the degranulation of peritoneal mast cells and the subsequent exposure of peritoneal cells to mast cell mediators (90). *In vitro* exposure of RBL-1 cells, a rat basophilic leukemia cell line, to paraoxon led to the release of β-hexosaminidase, a measure of degranulation (88). Paraoxon is the toxic oxygen intermediate of parathion that is most reactive in binding to acetylcholinesterase. These data correspond with a report in the literature that diisopropyl fluorophosphate, an organophosphate compound that is an irreversible inhibitor of serine esterase, caused mast cell degranulation in the absence of IgE antibody (91).

The available evidence on malathion immunotoxicity reviewed above suggests that metabolism is an important consideration in the examination of malathion immunotoxicity and that malathion may act on mast cells through phosphorylation of a serine esterase. One hypothesis is that malathion or a metabolite of malathion binds to an esterase on the surface of basophilic cells and leads to degranulation of these cells in the absence of antigen-specific IgE antibody. The degranulation leads to the release of mast cell products, such as histamine and heparin, and these products interact with leukocytes, elevating leukocyte function and thereby nonspecifically enhancing the generation of an immune response. This hypothesis is consistent with the observations of Milby and Epstein (77) that "contact sensitivity" develops after a single exposure to a 10% solution of technical grade malathion.

There are several avenues that future studies into the effects of malathion on the immune system can take. These include assessment of the effect of organophosphate compounds on host resistance in animal models, studies of humans exposed in an occupational setting, and analysis of the molecular site of action of malathion on the immune system.

In summary, malathion suppresses the generation of an immune response at high, cholinergic doses. This may be due to effects of malathion on the nervous system *per se*, direct effects of malathion on the immune system, or simply the effects of the stress of such a toxic exposure. At low, noncholingeric doses, malathion elevates the immune response. The alterations in the immune response are a result of enhanced function of the adherent population. Malathion may indirectly enhance mϕ function through effects on the mast cell and subsequent exposure of the mϕ to mast cell products.

Parathion

Parathion is more acutely toxic than malathion and thus its immunotoxic potential has attracted some attention. The ability of subacute *in vivo* administration of parathion to block the generation of humoral (92) and cellular immune responses (92,93) in mice is reported. Other investigators also show that parathion suppresses the humoral immune response of mice following acute and subacute exposure (82,94). However, Desi et al. (81) show that methyl parathion administered over 4 weeks does not affect the generation of humoral or cellular immune responses in rabbits.

Host resistance to infectious agents frequently involves an interplay of multiple immune responses and thus serves as an important immunotoxicity test. Parathion appears to affect host resistance to infectious agents. Peroral dosing of parathion to mice with a cytomegalovirus infection elevates mortality (95) and methyl parathion increases the virulence of *S. typhimurium* infection in rabbits (96,97). However, in light of the lack of immunotoxicity after *in vivo* administration of methyl parathion in rabbits discussed above, it is difficult to draw cause-and-effect conclusions on the mechanism of this decreased resistance to infectious agents. Similarly, although *in vivo* host resistance provides an important holistic immunotoxicity test, the impact of infectious agents across many immune functions often makes drawing mechanistic conclusions from host resistance studies difficult.

In vitro exposure experiments provide additional evidence of the immunotoxicity of parathion (83,86,98–100). The proliferative response of human lymphocytes to mitogens is suppressed following *in vitro* exposure to paraoxon (99), and paraoxon and two structurally related compounds also inhibit the production of IL-2 by rat splenocytes (100). In addition, *in vitro* exposure of mouse splenocytes to parathion

TABLE 1. *Summary of* in vivo *immunotoxic effects of organochlorine and organophosphate pesticides*

Pesticide[a]	Species	Significant effect seen	Reference
Organochlorines			
Dieldrin (postnatal)	Mouse	↓ mϕ Activity	19–30
Dieldrin (postnatal)	Rat	↑ PMN superoxide	34
Endrin (postnatal)	Rat	↑ mϕ Nitrate/nitrite	32
Chlordane (prenatal)	Mouse	↓ DTH/CHR	35
Chlordane (prenatal)	Mouse	↑ Resistance to influenza virus	39
Chlordane (prenatal)	Mouse	Delayed mϕ activity	47–49
Chlordane (prenatal)	Mouse	↓ Stem cell numbers	50,51
Chlordane (postnatal)	Human	↓ ADCC, MLR and Mito	53
Lindane (prenatal)	Mouse	↑ At low/ ↓ at high dose—DTH and PFCs	60
Lindane (postnatal)	Mouse	↓ Resistance to *Giardia muris*	61
β-HCH (postnatal)	Mouse	↓ At high dose—CTLs, NK, and Mito	62
γ-HCH (postnatal)	Mouse	↑ Early and ↓ late—CMI and antibody	63
DDT (postnatal)	Rat	↓ Serum antibody	70
DDT (postnatal)	Guinea pig	↓ Anaphylaxis, ↓ mast cell numbers	71,72
DDT (postnatal)	Mouse	↓ Antibody	75
DDT (postnatal)	Chicken	↓ Antibody	76
Organophosphates			
Malathion (postnatal)	Various	Contact sensitivity	77–80
Malathion (postnatal)	Rabbit	↓ Serum antibody	81
Malathion (postnatal)	Mouse	↓ Serum IgM	82
Malathion (postnatal)	Mouse	↑ Antibody, Mito	84,87
Malathion (postnatal)	Mouse	↑ Respiratory burst of peritoneal leukocytes	84,88
Malathion (postnatal)	Mouse	↑ Peritoneal mast cell degranulation	88
Parathion (postnatal)	Mouse	↓ Antibody	82,94
Parathion (postnatal)	Rabbit	↓ Host resistance	96,97
Methyl parathion (postnatal)	Mouse	↓ Host resistance	95
Parathion (postnatal)	Mouse	↓ Stem cell activity	101

[a]Time of exposure.

PMN, neutrophil; mϕ, macrophage; DTH, delayed-type hypersensitivity; CHR, contact hypersensitivity reaction; ADCC, antibody-dependent cell-mediated cytotoxicity; MLR, mixed leukocyte reaction; Mito, mitogen-induced blastogenesis; PFCs, plaque-forming cells (antibody); CTLs, cytotoxic T lymphocytes; NK, natural killer cells; CMI, cell-mediated immunity. ↓, Decreased; ↑, increased.

and methyl parathion blocks the generation of a cell-mediated immune response (86). However, others report that *in vitro* exposure of human peripheral blood monocytic cells to methyl parathion does not affect their proliferative response to mitogen but does decrease their chemotactic response (83). Thus, although it appears that *in vitro* exposure to parathion does affect cell functions, some differences in the effects are seen by different investigators.

An effect of parathion on hematopoiesis is also documented. Gallichio et al. (101) show that oral administration of parathion for 14 days, at a dose that did not

TABLE 2. *Summary of* in vitro *immunotoxic effects of organochlorine and organophosphate pesticides*

Pesticide	Cell type	Significant effect seen	Reference
Organochlorines			
Chlordane or heptachlor	Rhesus PBM	↑ Mito, IL-2 production	55
Chlordane	Guinea pig PMN	↑ Superoxide, $[Ca^{2+}]_i$ levels	56
Chlordane	MDCK	↓ Influenza infectivity	57
Chlordane	AGMK	↓ Influenza infectivity	57
Heptachlor	ML-1	↑ Growth, adherence, and pseudopodia	58
Chlordane	Mouse spleen	↓ MLR, Mito, antibody production*	54
Oxychlordane	Mouse spleen	↓ Antibody production*	54
γ-HCH	Mouse mϕ	↓ RNA synthesis	64
γ-HCH	Mouse l'cyte	↓ RNA synthesis	67
γ-HCH	Mouse mϕ	↑ LT_4 production, ↓ PI turnover	68
γ-HCH	Mouse mϕ	↑ PG, LT, and chemiluminescence	66
α-HCH	Bovine l.n.	↑ PHA mitogenesis	69
α-HCH or δ-HCH	bovine l.n.	↓ Con A + phorbol-induced capping	65
Organophosphates			
Malathion	Human PBM	↓ Mito	83,84
Malathion	Mouse spleen	↓ Mito, CTLs	84–86
Malathion	Mouse p.c.	↓ Phorbol-induced respiratory burst	84
Malathion metabolite	Mouse p.c.	↑ Phorbol-induced respiratory burst	84–86
Malathion metabolite	Human PBM	↑ Phorbol-induced respiratory burst	84–86
Paraoxon	Human l'cyte	↓ Mito	99
Paraoxon	Rat spleen	↓ IL-2 production	100
Parathion and methyl parathion	Mouse spleen	Block CMI generation	86
Methyl parathion	Human PBM	↓ Chemotoxis	83
Parathion	Human b.m.	↓ BFU-E, CFU-E, and CFU-GM	102

**In vitro*-induced antibody production.

PBM, peripheral blood mononuclear cells; MDCK, Madin–Darby canine kidney cells; AGMK, African green monkey cells; ML-1, human myeloblastic leukemia cells; PMN, neutrophil; mϕ, macrophage; l'cyte, lymphocyte; l.n., lymph node cells; p.c., peritoneal cells; b.m., bone marrow; Mito, mitogen-induced blastogenesis; MLR, mixed leukocyte reaction; $[Ca^{2+}]_i$, intracellular calcium levels; CMI, cell-mediated immunity; PG, prostaglandin; LT, leukotriene; PI, phosphoinositol; CTLs, cytotoxic T lymphocytes; ↓ decreased; ↑, increased.

affect the body weight or generate cholinergic symptoms, altered the bone marrow-derived stem cell colonies in mice for up to 2 weeks after the last dose of parathion. *In vitro* exposure of human bone marrow cells to paraoxon or malaoxon significantly depresses the generation of colonies of burst-forming units–erythroid (BFU-E), colony forming unit–erythroid (CFU-E), and CFU-GM (102).

Overall, these studies are difficult to correlate due to the differences in exposure route, immune parameters studied, and the species studied. In general, however, parathion appears to be immunosuppressive, but the mechanism of these effects is unknown. Further studies should be conducted to determine the mechanism of action of parathion on the immune system.

CONCLUSION

Pesticides continue to be a health concern because of their continued use or persistence in the environment. Tables 1 and 2 provide a summary of the *in vivo* and *in vitro* immunotoxic effects of members of the organochlorine and organophosphate classes of pesticide. However, frequently, important mechanistic studies are lacking and the dearth of these subcellular and cellular mechanistic studies hampers the reconciliation of divergent data as well as extrapolation of these data to human risk assessment. And finally, although the discussion in this chapter has been limited to two classes of insecticides, immunotoxicity is not limited to these two types of pesticides and the data on many of the other pesticides also suffer from a lack of subcellular and cellular mechanistic studies.

REFERENCES

1. Kutz FW, Wood PH, Bottimore DP. Organochlorine pesticides and polychlorinated biphenyls in human adipose tissue. *Rev Environ Contam Toxicol* 1991;120:1–82.
2. Franchi E, Focardi S. Polychlorinated biphenyl congeners, hexachlorobenzene and DDTs in human milk in central Italy. *Sci Total Environ* 1991;102:223–228.
3. Frawley JP, Fuyat HN, Hagan EC, Blake JR, Fitzhugh OG. Marked potentiation in mammalian toxicity from simultaneous administration of two anticholinesterease compounds. *J Pharmacol* 1957;121:96.
4. Umetsu N, Grose FH, Allahyari R, Abu-El-Haj S, Fukuto TR. Effect of impurities on mammalian toxicity of technical malathion and acephate. *J Agric Food Chem* 1977;25:946–953.
5. March RB, Fukuto TR, Metcalf RL, Maxon MG. Fate of p32-labelled malathion in the laying hen, white mouse and American cockroach. *J Econ Entomol* 1956;49:185–195.
6. Umetsu N, Mallipudi NM, Toia RF, March RB, Fukuto TR. Toxicologic properties of phosphorothioate and related esters present in organophosphate insecticides. *J Toxicol Environ Health* 1981,7:481–497.
7. Aldridge WN, Miles TW, Mount DL, Vershoyle RD. The toxicologic properties of impurities in malathion. *Arch Toxicol* 1979;42:95.
8. Mallipudi NM, Talcott RE, Ketterman A, Fukuto TR. Properties and inhibition of rat malathion carboxylesterases. *J Toxicol Environ Health* 1980;6:585–596.
9. NIOSH. *Occupational exposure to malathion*. US Dept Health Education and Welfare Publ #76-205;1976.
10. Exposure estimation. In: *Health risk assessment of aerial application of malathion-bait*. Los Angeles: California Department of Health Services; 1991:7-1–7-65.
11. Hayes WJ Jr. *Clinical handbook on economic poisons—emergency information for treating poisoning*, PHS Bulletin No 476. Atlanta: US Department of Health, Education and Welfare; 1963.
12. Clyne RM, Shaffer CB. *Toxicological information—cyanamide organophosphate pesticides*. Princeton: American Cyanamide Co; 1970.
13. Murphy SD. Toxic effects of pesticides. In: Klaassen CD, Amdur MO, Doull J, eds. *Toxicology. The basic science of poisons*, 3rd ed. New York: Macmillan; 1986:519–581.

14. Furie B, Trubowitz S. Insecticides and blood dyscrasias. Chlordane exposure and self-limited refractory megaloblastic anemia. *JAMA* 1976;235:1720–1722.
15. Infante PF, Epstein SS, Newton WA. Blood dyscrasias and childhood tumors and exposure to chlordane and heptachlor. *Scand J Work Environ Health* 1978;4:137–150.
16. Holmstedt BA Pharmacology of organophosphorus cholinesterase inhibitors. *Pharmacol Rev* 1959; 11:567–688.
17. Koelle GB. Neurohumoral transmission and the autonomic nervous system. In: Goodman-Gilman A, ed. *The pharmacologic basis of therapeutics*, 4th ed. New York: Macmillan; 1970.
18. Brooks, GT. *Chlorinated insecticides*. Cleveland: CRC Press; 1974.
19. Loose LD. Macrophage induction of T-suppressor cells in pesticide-exposed and protozoan-infected mice. *Environ Health Perspect* 1982;43:89–97.
20. Kaminski NE, Roberts JF, Guthrie FE. The effects of DDT and dieldrin on rat peritoneal macrophages. *Pestic Biochem Physiol* 1982;17:191–195.
21. Krzystyniak K, Hugo P, Flipo D, Fournier M. Increased susceptibility to mouse hepatitis virus 3 of peritoneal macrophages exposed to dieldrin. *Toxicol Appl Pharmacol* 1985;80:397–408.
22. Krzystyniak K, Bernier J, Hugo P, Fournier M. Suppression of MHV3 virus-activated macrophages by dieldrin. *Biochem Pharmacol* 1986;35:2577–2586.
23. Fournier M, Chevalier G, Nadeau D, Trottier B, Krzystyniak K. Virus–pesticide interactions with murine cellular immunity after sublethal exposure to dieldrin and aminocarb. *J Toxicol Environ Health* 1988;25:103–118.
24. Krzystyniak K, Troffler B, Jolicoeur P, Fournier M. Macrophage functional activities versus cellular parameters upon sublethal pesticide exposure. *Mol Toxicol* 1987;1:247–259.
25. Bernier J, Fournier M, Blais Y, Lombardi P, Chevalier G, Krzystyniak K. Immunotoxicity of aminocarb. I. Comparative studies of sublethal exposure to aminocarb and dieldrin in mice. *Pestic Biochem Physiol* 1988;30:238–250.
26. Bang FB, Warwick A. Mouse macrophages as host cells for the mouse hepatitis virus and the genetic basis of their susceptibility. *Proc Natl Acad Sci USA* 1960;46:1065–1075.
27. Hugo P, Bernier J, Krzystyniak K, Potworowski EF, Fournier M. Abrogation of graft-versus-host reaction by dieldrin in mice. *Toxicol Lett* 1988;41:11–22.
28. Hugo P, Bernier J, Krzystyniak K, Fournier M. Transient inhibition of mixed lymphocyte reactivity by dieldrin in mice. *Toxicol Lett* 1988;41:1–9.
29. Bernier J, Hugo P, Krzystyniak K, Fournier M. Suppression of humoral immunity in inbred mice by dieldrin. *Toxicol Lett* 1987;35:231–240.
30. Jolicoeur P, Fournier M, Krzystyniak K. Suppression of microbicidal activity of peritoneal exudate by sublethal dieldrin exposure of outbred and inbred mice. *Pestic Biochem Physiol* 1988;31:203–212.
31. Nathan C. Nitric oxide as a secretory product of mammalian cells. *FASEB J* 1992;6:3051–3064.
32. Akubue PI, Stohs SJ. Endrin-induced production of nitric oxide by rat peritoneal macrophages. *Toxicol Lett* 1992;62:311–316.
33. Krzystyniak K, Flipo D, Mansour S, Fournier M. Suppression of avidin processing and presentation by mouse macrophages after sublethal exposure to dieldrin. *Immunopharmacology* 1989;18: 157–166.
34. Hewett JA, Roth RA. Dieldrin activates rat neutrophils *in vitro*. *Toxicol Appl Pharmacol* 1988; 96:269–278.
35. Spyker-Cranmer JM, Barnett IB, Avery DL, Cranmer MF. Immunoteratology of chlordane: cell-mediated and humoral immune responses in adult mice exposed *in utero*. *Toxicol Appl Pharmacol* 1982;62:402–408.
36. Barnett JB, Holcomb D, Menna JH, Soderberg LS. The effect of prenatal chlordane exposure on specific anti-influenza cell-mediated immunity. *Toxicol Lett* 1985;25:229–238.
37. Barnett JB, Soderberg LS, Menna JH. The effect of prenatal chlordane exposure on the delayed hypersensitivity response of BALB/c mice. *Toxicol Lett* 1985;25:173–183.
38. Blaylock BL, Soderberg LSF, Gandy J, Menna JH, Denton R, Barnett JB. Cytotoxic T-lymphocyte and NK responses in mice treated prenatally with chlordane. *Toxicol Lett* 1990;51:41–49.
39. Menna JH, Barnett JB, Soderberg LS. Influenza type A virus infection of mice exposed *in utero* to chlordane; survival and antibody studies. *Toxicol Lett* 1985;24:45–52.
40. Wyde P, Peavy D, Cate T. Morphological and cytochemical characterization of cells infiltrating mouse lungs after influenza infection. *Infect Immun* 1978;21:140–146.
41. Leung FN, Ada GL. Cells mediating delayed-type hypersensitivity in the lungs of mice infected with an influenza A virus. *Scand J Immunol* 1980;12:393–400.

42. Adams DO, Hamilton TA. Molecular basis of macrophage activation: diversity and origins. In: Lewis CA, McGee JO'D, eds. *The macrophage*. New York: IRL Press; 1992:75–114.
43. Nathan CF. Secretory products of macrophages. *J Clin Invest* 1987;79:319.
44. Tabor DR, Burchett SK, Jacobs RF. Enhanced production of monokines by canine alveolar macrophages in response to endotoxin-induced shock. *Proc Exp Biol Med* 1988;187:408.
45. Tabor DR, Azadegan AA, Schell RF, Lefrock JL. Inhibition of macrophage C3b-mediated ingestion by symphilitic hamster T cell-enriched fractions. *J Immunol* 1984;135:2698–2699.
46. Vogel SN, Finbloom DS, English KE, Rosenstreich DL, Langreth SG. Interferon induced enhancement macrophage Fc receptor expression: a-interferon treatment of C3H/HeJ macrophage results in increased numbers and density of Fc receptors. *J Immunol* 1983;130:1210.
47. Theus SA, Tabor DR, Soderberg LSF, Bamett JB. Macrophage tumoricidal mechanisms are selectively altered by prenatal chlordane exposure. *Agents Actions* 1992;37:140–146.
48. Theus SA, Tabor DR, Barnett JB. Alteration of macrophage TNF production by prenatal chlordane exposure. *FASEB J* 1991;5:A1347.
49. Theus SA, Lau KA, Tabor DR, Soderberg LSF, Barnett JB. *In vivo* prenatal chlordane exposure induces development of endogenous inflammatory macrophages. *J Leukoc Biol* 1992;51:366–372.
50. Barnett JB, Blaylock BL, Gandy J, Menna JH, Denton R, Soderberg LSF. Long-term alteration of adult bone marrow colony formation by prenatal chlordane exposure. *Fundam Appl Toxicol* 1990; 14:688–695.
51. Barnett JB, Blaylock BL, Gandy J, Menna JH, Denton R, Soderberg LSF. Alteration of fetal liver colony formation by prenatal chlordane exposure. *Fundam Appl Toxicol* 1990;15:820–822.
52. Johnson KW, Holsapple MP, Munson AE. An immunotoxicological evaluation of gamma-chlordane. *Fundam Appl Toxicol* 1986;6:317–326.
53. McConnachie PR, Zahalsky AC. Immune alterations in humans exposed to the termiticide technical chlordane. *Arch Environ Health* 1992;47:295–301.
54. Johnson KW, Kaminski NE, Munson AE. Direct suppression of cultured spleen cell responses by chlordane and the basis for differential effects on *in vivo* and *in vitro* immunocompetence. *J Toxicol Environ Health* 1987;22:497–515.
55. Chuang LF, Liu Y, Killam K Jr, Chuang RY. Modulation by the insecticides heptachlor and chlordane of the cell-mediated immune proliferative responses of rhesus monkeys. *In Vivo* 1992;6:29–32.
56. Suzaki E, Inoue B, Okimasu E, Ogata M, Utsumi K. Stimulative effect of chlordane on the various functions of the guinea pig leukocytes. *Toxicol Appl Pharmacol* 1988;93:137–145.
57. Beggs M, Menna JH, Barnett JB. Effect of chlordane on influenza type A virus and herpes simplex type 1 virus replication in vitro. *J Toxicol Environ Health* 1985;16:173–188.
58. Chuang LF, Hinton DE, Cheung ATW, Chuang RY. Induction of differentiation of human myeloblastic leukemia ML-1 cells by heptachlor, a chlorinated hydrocarbon insecticide. *Toxicol Applied Pharmacol* 1991;109:98–107.
59. Gregory SH, Barczynski LK, Wing EJ. Effector function of hepatocytes and Kupffer cells in the resolution of systemic bacterial infections. *J Leukoc Biol* 1992;51:421–424.
60. Das SN, Paul BN, Saxena AK, Ray PK. Effect of *in utero* exposure to hexachlorocyclohexane on the developing immune system of mice. *Immunopharmacol Immunotoxicol* 1990;12:293–310.
61. André F, Gillon J, André C, Lafont S, Jourdan G. Pesticide-containing diets augment anti-sheep red blood cell nonreaginic antibody responses in mice but may prolong murine infection with *Giardia muris*. *Environ Res* 1983;32:145–150.
62. Cornacoff JB, Lauer LD, House RV, et al. Evaluation of the immunotoxicity of beta-hexachlorocyclohexane (β-HCH). *Fundam Appl Toxicol* 1988;11:293–299.
63. Meera P, Rao PR, Shanker R, Tripathi O. Immunomodulating effects of γ-HCH (lindane) in mice. *Immunopharmacol Immunotoxicol* 1992;14:261–282.
64. Roux F, Puiseux-Dao S, Treich I, Fournier E. Effect of lindane on mouse peritoneal macrophages. *Toxicology* 1978;11:259–269.
65. Kwong CH, Mueller GC. Effects of hexachlorocyclohexane isomers on concanavalin A "capping" in bovine lymphocytes. *Biochim Biophys Acta* 1979;586:501–511.
66. Forgue MF, Pinelli E, Beraud M, Souqual MC, Pipy B. Chemiluminescence response and arachidonic acid metabolism of macrophages induced by gamma-hexachlorocyclohexane (lindane). *Food Addit Contam* 1990;7(Suppl1):S97–S99.
67. Roux F, Treich I, Brun C, Desoize B, Fournier E. Effect of lindane on human lymphocyte responses to phytohemagglutinin. *Biochem Pharmacol* 1979;28:2419–2426.

68. Meade CJ, Harvey J, Boot JR, Turner GA, Bateman PE, Osborne DJ. Gamma-hexachlorocyclohexane stimulation of macrophage phospholipid hydrolysis and leukotriene production. *Biochem Pharmacol* 1984;33:289–293.
69. Kensler TW, Mueller GC. Effects of hexachlorocyclohexane isomers on the mitogenic response of bovine lymphocytes. *Biochem Pharmacol* 1978;27:667–671.
70. Wassermann M, Wassermann D, Gershon Z, Zellermayer L. Effects of organochlorine insecticides on body defense systems. *Ann NY Acad Sc* 1969;160:393–401.
71. Gabliks J, Askari EM, Yolen N. DDT and immunological responses. I. Serum antibodies and anaphylactic shock in guinea pig. *Arch Environ Health* 1973;26:305–309.
72. Askari EM, Gabliks J. DDT and immunological responses. II. Altered histamine levels and anaphylactic shock in guinea pigs. *Arch Environ Health* 1973;26:309–312.
73. Gabliks J, Al-zubaidy T, Askari E. DDT and immunological responses. 3. Reduced anaphylaxis and mast cell population in rats fed DDT. *Arch Environ Health* 1975;30:81–84.
74. Street JC, Sharma RP. Alternation of induced cellular and humoral immune responses by pesticides and chemicals of environmental concern: quantitative studies of immunosuppression by DDT, Aroclor 1254, carbaryl, carbofuran, and methylparathion. *Toxicol Appl Pharmacol* 1975;32: 587–602.
75. Banerjee BD, Ramachandran M, Hussain QZ. Sub-chronic effect of DDT on humoral immune response in mice. *Bull Environ Contam Toxicol* 1986;37:433–440.
76. Rao DSVS, Glick B. Pesticide effects on the immune response and metabolic activity of chicken lymphocytes. *Proc Soc Exp Biol Med* 1977;154:27–29.
77. Milby TH, Epstein WL. Allergic contact sensitivity to malathion. *Arch Environ Health* 1964;9: 434–437.
78. Centeno ER, Johnson WJ, Sehon AW. Antibodies to two common pesticides, DDT and malathion. *Int Arch Allergy Appl Immunol* 1970;37:1–13.
79. Vijay HM, Mendoza CE, Lavergne G. Production of homocytotropic antibodies (IgE) to malathion in the rat. *Toxicol Appl Pharmacol* 1978;44:137–142.
80. Cushman JR, Street JC. Allergic hypersensitivity to insecticide malathion in BALB/c mice. *Toxicol Appl Pharmacol* 1983;70:29.
81. Desi TF, Varga G, Judet CG. Immunosuppressive effects of chlorinated hydrocarbon and organophosphate pesticide administration. *Hyg Sanit* 1976;20:358.
82. Casale GP, Cohen SD, DiCapua RA. The effects of organophosphate-induced cholinergic stimulation on the antibody response to sheep erythrocytes in inbred mice. *Toxicol Appl Pharmacol* 1983; 68:198–205.
83. Lee TP, Moscati R, Park BH. Effects of pesticides on human leukocyte functions. *Res Commun Chem Pathol Pharmacol* 1979;23:597–609.
84. Rodgers KE, Ellefson DD. Modulation of respiratory burst activity and mitogenic response of human peripheral blood mononuclear cells and murine splenocytes and peritoneal cells by malathion. *Fundam Appl Toxicol* 1990;14:309–317.
85. Rodgers KE, Grayson MH, Imamura T, Devens BH. *In vitro* effects of malathion and O,O,S-trimethyl phosphorothioate on cytotoxic T-lymphocyte responses. *Pestic Biochem Physiol* 1985; 24:260–266.
86. Rodgers KE, Leung N, Devens BH, Imamura T. Rapid *in vitro* screening assay for immunotoxic effects of organophosphorus and carbamate pesticides on the generation of cytotoxic T lymphocyte responses. *Pestic Biochem Physiol* 1986;26:292.
87. Rodgers KE, Leung N, Ware CF, Devens BH, Imamura T. Lack of immunosuppressive effects of acute and subacute administration of malathion. *Pestic Biochem Physiol* 1986;25:358.
88. Rodgers KE, Ellefson DD. Mechanism of modulation of murine peritoneal cell function and mast cell degranulation by low doses of malathion. *Agents Actions* 1992,35:57.
89. Baggiolini M, Horisberger U, Martin U. Phagocytosis of mast cell granules by mononuclear phagocytes, neutrophils and eosinophils during anaphylaxis. *Int Arch Allergy Appl Immunol* 1982; 67:219.
90. Yoffe JR, Taylor DJ, Wooley DE. Mast cell products and heparin stimulate the production of mononuclear cell factor by cultured human monocytes/macrophages. *Biochem J* 1985;230:83.
91. Kazimierczak W, Muir HL, MacGlashan DW, Lichtenstein LM. An antigen-activated DFP-inhibitable enzyme controls basophil desensitization. *J Immunol* 1984;132:399.
92. Wiltrout RW, Ercegovich CD, Ceglowski WS. Humoral immunity in mice following oral administration of selected pesticides. *Bull Environ Contam Toxicol* 1978;20:423.

93. Dandliker WB, Hides AN, Levinson SA. Effects of pesticides on the immune response. *USNITS PBRep PB80-811* 1980:532, 14.
94. Bartholomew PM, Casale GP, Duggan WJ. Effect of repeated parathion exposure on the primary IgM response and bone marrow stem cells in C57B1/6 mice. *Toxicologist* 1984;4:159.
95. Raise BT. Role of adaptive immune defense mechanisms. In: Rouse BT, Lopez C, eds. *Immunobiology of herpes simplex virus infection*. Boca Raton, FL: CRC Press; 1983:69–73.
96. Fan A, Street JC, Nelson RM. Immunosuppression in mice administered methyl parathion and carbofuran by diet. *Toxicol Appl Pharmacol* 1984;45:235.
97. Fan AMM. Effects of pesticides on immune competency: influence of methyl parathion and carbofuran on immunologic response to *Salmonella typhimurium*. *Diss Abst Int B* 1981;41:2962.
98. Duggan QJ, Casale GP, Cohen SD. Paraoxon induced suppression of the *in vitro* response of murine spleen cells to sheep red blood cells. *Toxicologist* 1984;4:159.
99. Waterhouse J, Tourney T. The effects of organophosphorus and carbamate cholinesterase inhibitors on *in vitro* immune responses. *Toxicologist* 1984;4:159.
100. Pruett SB, Chambers JB. Effects of paraoxon, *p*-nitrophenol, phenyl saligenin cyclic phosphate and phenol on the rat interleukin 2 system. *Toxicol Lett* 1988;40:11.
101. Gallichio VS, Casale GP, Bartholomew PM, Watts TD. Altered colony forming activities of bone marrow hematopoietic stem cells in mice following short-term *in vivo* exposure to parathion. *Int J Cell Cloning* 1987;15:231.
102. Gallichio VS, Casale GP, Watts TD. Inhibition of human bone marrow-derived stem cell colony formation (CFU-E, BFU-E, and CFU-GM) following *in vitro* exposure to organophosphates. *Exp Hematol* 1987;15:1099.

Immunotoxicology and Immunopharmacology, Second Edition, edited by J. H. Dean, M. I. Luster, A. E. Munson, and I. Kimber.
Raven Press, Ltd., New York © 1994.

12

Immunotoxicology of Arsenic

Leigh Ann Burns, *David G. LeVier, and *Albert E. Munson

*Department of Immunology, Mayo Clinic and Foundation, Rochester, Minnesota 55905; and *Department of Pharmacology and Toxicology, Medical College of Virginia, Virginia Commonwealth University, Richmond, Virginia 23298*

Arsenic is an ubiquitous metal that occurs naturally in our environment. The concentration of arsenic in the soil is estimated to be less than 2 mg/kg, although this value is dependent on the location and content of the soil/bedrock (1). Concentrations of arsenic in the drinking water also vary with location and bedrock content. Most sources of drinking water contain small quantities of arsenic (less than 0.01 mg/liter) (2). However, this concentration is dependent on the community in question as concentrations of 0.05 mg/liter have been reported in Nova Scotia, where the arsenic content of the bedrock is high. Greater levels have been seen in communities around mineral springs such as those in California, the former Soviet Union, and New Zealand (0.4 to 1.3 mg/liter) (3) with more extreme values observed in Japan (1.7 mg/liter) (4) and Argentina (3.4 mg/liter) (2). Although the speciation of arsenic in the water source is largely unknown, one report indicated that in surveyed groundwaters, 25% to 50% of the arsenic was in the form of As^{3+} (2).

Arsenic is also present in many food items and an extensive list has previously been published (1). The content of arsenic in foodstuffs is generally below 0.25 mg/kg (2,5). This value is influenced by the natural content of arsenic in the soil, the species of plant and its uptake of arsenic, and by the quantity of arsenic-containing herbicides and insecticides that are used. Values for arsenic (primarily trivalent) of 0.5 mg/liter have been reported in wine and were attributable to the insecticides used to spray the grapes (6). By far, however, the highest concentrations of arsenic in foodstuffs are found in the marine life and seaweed that are consumed. Concentrations may vary from 10 mg As/kg in bony fishes to over 100 mg As/kg in crustaceans and other bottom-dwelling marine flora and fauna (2,7). The average daily intake of arsenic has been estimated to be 0.05 to 0.1 mg per individual and is greatly influenced by the amount of seafood consumed in the diet.

Although the vast majority of arsenic exposure comes from dietary intake, exposure to arsenic may also occur in the occupational setting. Persons employed in copper, zinc, and lead smelters, in the manufacture and spraying of pesticides, and in the production of wood treated with chromated copper arsenate are at risk from occupational exposure to arsenic. The U.S. Environmental Protection Agency (EPA) has mandated that the maximum 24-hr concentrations of arsenic in these industries not exceed 0.1 to 1 $\mu g/m^3$. More recently, individuals employed in the semiconductor industry, producing gallium arsenide (GaAs) or indium arsenide (InAs), have also been determined to be at risk. Because their high-speed performance is superior to other compounds used for the same purposes, GaAs and InAs have recently become the materials of choice in this and other industries. Although the manufacture of GaAs requires the use of arsine gas (one of the most deadly gases known to humans), in the industrial setting the primary route of exposure to GaAs is inhalation of GaAs particles generated in the sawing and polishing of the GaAs wafers. It has been estimated that between 50% and 60% of the GaAs crystals are converted into GaAs dust in this step of processing (8). The toxicity of GaAs only began to be investigated in a limited number of laboratories in the past decade and thus the degree of risk that workers in these industries assume is not clear. In 1983, Willardson reported that manufacturing processes used 5 to 10 tons of arsenic in GaAs devices and that production was expected to increase three- to tenfold by the year 1990. Presently, GaAs is regulated on the basis of inorganic arsenic toxicity data (Code of Federal Regulations, 1985) with a recommended exposure limit (REL) of 2 $\mu g/m^3$ for a maximum of 15 min (9). Although it has been shown recently that GaAs dissociates into its component metals, gallium and arsenic, following intratracheal instillation or oral exposure in rats (10) and intratracheal exposure in mice (11), the actual levels of arsenic exposure in GaAs-exposed workers remains unknown.

Characterizing the toxicity of arsenic is difficult because it exists in both inorganic and organic forms, in both the trivalent (As^{3+}) and pentavalent (As^{5+}) species. Inorganic arsenic is transformed in the body to monomethyl- and dimethylarsenic acid and rapidly excreted. Much of the basis of our current understanding of the mechanism of arsenic toxicity comes from toxicity studies from the late 1800s, development of arsenical drugs, and the need to develop antidotes for arsenical warfare agents such as Lewisite. These studies have been reviewed extensively in the literature (2,12–14). Whereas a single exposure to arsenic may or may not induce any overt toxicity, chronic exposure may lead to neurologic and central nervous system effects including sensory alterations, paresthesias, and muscle weakness. Peripheral neuropathy is also possible, leading ultimately to the demyelination of nerves. Long-term chronic exposure may result in hepatic injury and peripheral vascular disease.

The potential of arsenic as a human carcinogen has been reviewed (15,16) and this metal has been classified as such based on epidemiologic studies of the action of arsenic on airways and skin (2,17,18). The U.S. Public Health Service (USPHS) adopted a standard of 50 μg As/liter in the drinking water several years ago. However, based on epidemiologic studies, there is a one in five million lifetime probability of developing cancer from a daily intake $\geq$30 ng. The mechanism by which arsenic is carcinogenic is not clear but several possibilities exist. Arsenite (As^{3+})

can interfere with deoxyribonucleic acid (DNA) synthesis and repair (2,14,19,20) while arsenate (As^{5+}) may substitute for phosphate and form unstable esters in DNA (2,14). More importantly, exposure to arsenic may compromise immunologic integrity and suppress the natural immune surveillance, which aids in protecting the body from the development of neoplasms. This issue is the focus for the remainder of this chapter.

IMMUNOMODULATION BY ARSENIC COMPOUNDS

Specific immunotoxic consequences of metal exposure are well documented in the literature and have been reviewed elsewhere (see the chapter by McCabe). It is evident that they may exert many immunomodulatory actions that are directly dependent on the exposure level. At high concentrations most metals exert immunosuppressive activity (21,22). However, at lower concentrations immunoenhancement may be seen. This is true for several metals including arsenic (20,23,24).

The current literature is frought with inconsistencies concerning the immunotoxic potential of arsenic. Several factors must be taken into account when evaluating these studies. First, arsenic occurs in both organic and inorganic forms. Additionally, numerous salts exist for each of these forms of arsenic and have been examined by various routes of administration. The variations in the toxicokinetics for each arsenic compound and the route of administration may account for some of the variable results obtained. Second, the speciation of arsenic in the compounds evaluated may also play a primary role in the observed differences. It is generally accepted that trivalent arsenic (As^{3+}) is the more toxic form of arsenic when compared to the pentavalent species (As^{5+}). Additionally, their cellular and biochemical mechanisms of toxicity appear to be somewhat different (2,14). Third, immunotoxicity studies have been conducted in several species including the calf (20), human (19,20,25–27), and various strains of mice including the Swiss mouse (28–30), C57B1/6 (24,25,31), C3H (23), BALB/c (28,29), CD-1 (28,29), and the B6C3F1 (11,32–42). Because immune responses involve some genetic control, the variation in mouse strain may also be a factor contributing to mixed results in arsenic immunotoxicology. Finally, discrepancies in the literature may be related to acute versus chronic administration of the arsenic compounds. Since there are relatively few published reports concerning arsenic immunotoxicity (compared to other metals such as lead, cadmium, and mercury), none of these reasons currently stands out as a primary contributor.

Host Resistance

Until recently, investigations concerning the immunotoxic potential of arsenic primarily focused on arsenic-induced alterations in host resistance. In an elaborate series of studies involving various times of exposure of mice to sodium arsenite ($NaAsO_2$) in the drinking water (0.002 M) or subcutaneously (3.13 to 6.25 mg/kg),

Gainer and Pry (28) determined that exposed mice had a two- to ninefold increase in mortality rate to pseudorabies, encephalomyocarditis, and St. Louis encephalitis viruses. In contrast, mortality to Western encephalitis virus was increased if mice received $NaAsO_2$ after viral inoculation intraperitoneally (ip) and was decreased if arsenic exposure occurred prior to inoculation. Concomitant studies by Gainer (29) showed that exposure to $NaAsO_2$, Na_2HAsO_4 (sodium arsenate), roxarsone, and *p*-arsenilic acid inhibited the production and dose-dependently inhibited the activity of interferon (IFN) in mouse embryo cells. Additionally, the inhibition of activity was cell mediated and time dependent. These studies suggest that arsenic exposure increases susceptibility to viral disease by inhibiting IFN production and activity.

In contrast to the studies by Gainer (29) and Gainer and Pry (28), Schrauzer and Ishmael (23) and Kerkvliet et al. (24) reported different observations. C3H/St mice exposed to $NaAsO_2$ in the drinking water (10 ppm for 15 months) demonstrated a 68% decrease in the development of spontaneous tumors (23). Although there was a decreased incidence, the tumors that did develop grew at a much faster rate and the mean survival time after the appearance of tumors was decreased 50% in arsenic-exposed mice when compared with controls. Similar results were noted for transplanted mammary tumors (injection into the gland) as well. Kerkvliet et al. (24) reported comparable observations in mice exposed to Na_2HAsO_4 in the drinking water (2.5 to 100 ppm for 10 to 12 weeks) and injected intramuscularly (im) in the leg with moloney sarcoma virus (MSV) sarcoma cells. In those studies there was also a decreased incidence of tumors despite an increased mortality rate and enhanced growth rate of more mature tumors. No alterations in cell-mediated immunity could be demonstrated. These investigators proposed that arsenic-induced inhibition of viral transformation may account for the significant growth of late tumors since both the MSV and the sarcomas used by Schrauzer both have a viral etiology. This would not explain, however, the results observed by Gainer.

Following a single intratracheal exposure to the semiconductor material gallium arsenide (GaAs), Sikorski et al. (34) and Burns et al. (41) evaluated host resistance to several infectious agents including *Streptococcus pneumoniae, Listeria monocytogenes*, and the B16F10 melanoma. Investigations by Sikorski demonstrated that 14 days after intratracheal exposure to GaAs (50 to 200 mg/kg) there was an increased incidence and growth of the B16F10 tumor in the lungs of these animals. In contrast, there was no change in susceptibility to *S. pneumoniae* and there was protection against *L. monocytogenes* infection [intravenous (iv) inoculation]. Burns et al. (41) examined host resistance 24 hr after GaAs exposure (50 to 200 mg/kg) and noted similar results to Sikorski with the exception that resistance to *S. pneumoniae* was enhanced. Burns et al. (11) previously demonstrated the presence of detectable concentrations of dissociated gallium and arsenic in the blood, lungs, and spleen of mice 2 to 24 hr after exposure to GaAs (200 mg/kg). Using the arsenic chelator *meso*-2,3-dimercaptosuccinic acid (DMSA), it was determined that arsenic was the primary immunosuppressive component of GaAs. Arsenicals were once widely used as chemotherapeutic agents (such as Fowler's and Donovan's solutions, asiatic pills, atoxyl, sodium cacodylate, and arsphenamine) before the development of more specific and less toxic agents with higher therapeutic indices. Serial dilutions of GaAs (0.039 to 5 mg/ml) in brain–heart infusion (BHI) broth inoculated with either *S. pneumoniae* or *L. monocytogenes* slowed the growth of both organisms with a minimal inhibitory concentration (MIC) of 0.625 mg/ml (41). Furthermore, sera from mice collected at various time intervals after exposure to GaAs (200 mg/kg) were also capable of retarding the growth of both organisms with the maximal inhibition noted 24 hr after exposure. However, sera from GaAs-exposed mice (24 hr after exposure) were incapable of slowing the growth of the B16F10 melanoma. Addition of DMSA to sera from mice exposed to GaAs followed by inoculation with *L. monocytogenes* resulted in growth of this organism, which was comparable to growth observed in vehicle cultures. These studies demonstrate that arsenic in the sera of GaAs-exposed mice is capable of exerting chemotherapeutic effects on *S. pneumoniae* and *L. monocytogenes*. These results are important to the area of immunotoxicology because they are among the first to directly demonstrate the intricate interplay between the host, the pathogen, and exposure to a xenobiotic. While certain microbes appear to be sensitive to growth inhibition by arsenic, the B16F10 tumor in those studies was not. The reason for this contradiction is unknown but may lie in the metabolic difference between normal and transformed cells. This explanation may be applicable to the studies of Schrauzer and Ishmael (23) as well as those of Kerkvliet et al. (24).

Humoral and Cell-Mediated Immunity

Although Kerkvliet et al. (24) could not demonstrate any changes in cell-mediated immunity following exposure to sodium arsenate in the drinking water (2.5 to 100 ppm for 10 to 12 weeks), other studies examining immunocompetence have shown that there are changes in immune function following exposure to arsenic compounds. In 1980, Blakely et al. (30) exposed mice to $NaAsO_2$ in the drinking water for 3 weeks (0.5 to 10 ppm). *In vivo* evaluation of the primary immunoglobulin M (IgM) and secondary immunoglobulin G (IgG) immune responses showed significant immunosuppression (50% and 40%, respectively) at all concentrations. These results were not, however, dose related. Arsine gas is a recognized industrial hazard that produces toxicity at >30 ppm. Immunotoxicology studies conducted following inhalation exposure (0.5, 2.5, and 5 ppm) 6 hr/d for 14 days demonstrated a dose-dependent increase in spleen weight (32,33) and hemolysis in conjunction with a suppression of bone marrow erythroid precursors (32). Rosenthal et al. (33) showed that, despite the observed splenomegaly, there was also a significant depletion in splenic lymphocytes (83.4% in controls to 45.6% in animals dosed with 5 ppm arsine). T cells appeared to be more sensitive than B cells to the effects of arsine gas. However, the *in vivo* T cell-dependent antibody response was significantly enhanced by arsine exposure. There were dose-dependent decreases in natural killer (NK) cell and cytotoxic T lymphocyte (CTL) functions but no remarkable differences in lymphoproliferative activity [phytohemagglutinin (PHA), concanavalin A (Con A), lipopolysaccaride (LPS), mixed lymphocyte reaction (MLR)]. Similar to the host resistance studies with GaAs (34,43), exposure to arsine gas produced variable changes in host resistance including an increased susceptibility to *L. monocytogenes* (opposite of results for GaAs) and *Plasmodium yoelii* and no effect on resistance to influenza virus or the B16F10 tumor.

Studies examining *in vitro* exposure to arsenic have shown two effects on the immune system, which are dependent on dose: immunoenhancement is generally seen at low concentrations and immunosuppression at higher concentrations. Sodium arsenite exposure augments the proliferative response of human and bovine peripheral blood lymphocytes to mitogens at arsenic concentrations of 1 μM but suppresses proliferation at 4 μM (20). Exposure to Na_2HAsO_4 also showed similar results with enhancement at 20 μM (bovine) and 5 μM (human) and suppression at 70 μM (bovine) and 40 μM (human). Yoshida et al. (31,44) have shown enhancement by $NaAsO_2$ of the *in vitro*-generated antibody-forming cell (AFC) response to sheep red blood cells (SRBCs) at low concentrations (50 ng/ml) and suppression at higher concentrations (between 100 and 500 ng/ml). Also, addition of arsenic (50 ng/ml) at the time of immunization or 96 hr later enhanced the AFC response while addition of arsenic 24, 48, or 72 hr after immunization had no effect on antibody formation. The findings of Yoshida et al. (44) suggest arsenic exposure may result in the depletion of precursors of suppressor T cells from normal spleen and, in so doing, enhances the immune response.

More studies are needed on the action of arsenicals on human immunocompetence. Investigations involving human peripheral blood lymphocytes stimulated with PHA revealed that exposure to arsenic resulted in inhibition of proliferation and arrest of the cells in S and G2 phases (19,45). More recently, Yoshida et al. (26) demonstrated that workers employed in the semiconductor industry who had been exposed to arsenic dust exhibited enhanced lymphoproliferative responses (PHA) in the absence of clinical symptoms. In another study, Ostrosky-Wegman et al. (27) evaluated urinary arsenic concentrations, mutagenicity, and lymphocyte proliferation kinetics in two groups of individuals from Coahuila, Mexico, a rural area with chronic arsenic contamination in the drinking water. In arsenic-exposed persons (water containing 0.39 mg As/liter; 98% As^{5+}, 2% As^{3+}), there was a tenfold higher concentration of arsenic excreted in the urine (as methylated or demethylated organic arsenic) and a decreased proliferative response of lymphocytes compared with the control group (0.019 to 0.06 mg As/liter). There were, however, no differences in chromosome aberrations or sister chromatid exchange frequencies between the two groups of individuals. These data support the data of other investigators (19,20,46) and strongly suggest that the carcinogenic potential of arsenic may not lie in the mutagenicity of arsenic itself, but in the alterations in immunocompetence induced by arsenic exposure, which allow transformed or damaged cells to escape natural immune surveillance. This is supported by the observation that the skin cancers reported in immunosuppressed patients (47) are similar to those observed in individuals chronically exposed to arsenic (48,49).

Gallium Arsenide

There are several lines of evidence in the literature that indicate that gallium arsenide (GaAs) represents a health hazard as a result of systemic arsenic exposure. Webb et al. (10) reported partial dissolution of GaAs in buffers of various ionic strength. These investigations have been confirmed by other laboratories as well (50,51). In studies by Webb et al. (52), intratracheal administration of GaAs (10, 30, and 100 mg/kg) in rats resulted in detection of blood arsenic concentrations of 5.5, 14.3, and 53.6 ng/ml by flame atomic absorption spectrophotometry. Oral administration of GaAs showed similar results. No gallium was detected, in contrast to studies by Burns et al. (11), which found gallium to accumulate over 14 days in the blood and spleen of mice exposed intratracheally to GaAs. These data suggest GaAs dissociates into gallium and arsenic species when administered orally or intratracheally. Qualitative and quantitative alterations in urinary porphyrins were reported as well (10). Similar alterations in urinary porphyrins were found when inorganic arsenic was administered to rats (53). Further investigations by Webb et al. (52) confirmed GaAs dissolution 14 days following a single intratracheal administration of 100 mg/kg GaAs in rats. Gallium trioxide and arsenic trioxide were also evaluated and revealed that gallium trioxide produced little biologic activity. Arsenic trioxide produced some of the same qualitative effects as those noted when GaAs was tested (increased dry lung weight, protein, DNA, and lipid content).

Yamauchi et al. (50) also showed that organic products of arsenic metabolism (dimethylarsenic acid and methylarsenic acid) were found in urine and other tissues of hamsters exposed either orally (10 to 1000 mg/kg) or intraperitoneally (100 mg/kg) to GaAs or to indium arsenide (InAs, 100 mg/kg) (54). Comparison of metabolism and excretion following intratracheal exposure to GaAs, arsenic (III) oxide, and arsenic (V) oxide at 5 mg/kg revealed that GaAs is metabolized in the hamster to the same compounds as arsenite and arsenate, showing a metabolic profile most similar to that observed for sodium arsenite (55). Taken together, the toxicology data collected on GaAs indicate the likelihood of systemic arsenic exposure.

Studies evaluating cellular and humoral immunity following exposure to GaAs are numerous and represent a large portion of the current literature on arsenic immunotoxicity. The effects of GaAs exposure on host resistance have been discussed above and related to the chemotherapeutic potential of arsenic. Although a role for gallium in immunosuppression induced by GaAs has not been unequivocally eliminated, studies by Burns et al. (11) convincingly demonstrated that arsenic is the primary immunosuppressive moiety of GaAs following both *in vivo* and *in vitro* exposures. This model of arsenic exposure is quite unique in that the lung appears to act as a depot for the slow release of dissociated gallium and arsenic. The result is a prolonged (at least 14 days) systemic exposure to both metals (11).

Gallium arsenide has been demonstrated to produce dose-dependent immunosuppressive effects 14 days following intratracheal exposure of mice to concentrations between 50 and 200 mg/kg (34,42). Studies by Sikorski et al. (34) show the IgG and

IgM antibody responses (humoral immunity) were decreased 48% and 66%, respectively, at the 200-mg/kg exposure. The delayed hypersensitivity and mixed lymphocyte responses were also dose-dependently decreased. Analysis of peritoneal exudate cells (PECs) revealed a dose-dependent decrease in total number and a cell population shift consisting of an increase in monocytes from 53% to 81% and a decrease in lymphocytes from 46% to 20% following exposure to GaAs.

McCay et al. (42) demonstrated a dose-dependent decrease in thymus weight and an increase in spleen weight in GaAs-exposed mice. Histopathologic evaluation of spleen and lung showed gross changes in the lung indicative of an acute inflammatory response. There were no changes in the spleen. Blood glucose levels in these mice were decreased dose-dependently while serum glutamic–pyruvic transaminase (SGPT) levels were elevated (247%) at the 200-mg/kg exposure. Gallium oxide, gallium nitrate, and sodium arsenite were all found to suppress the antibody response. Arsenic trioxide did not suppress the AFC response and this may be related to metabolism and excretion over the 14 days following a single exposure. These studies indicate that the primary target organs for GaAs following a single intratracheal exposure are the lung and immune system, and that GaAs (as well as its component metals, gallium and arsenic) suppress humoral immune function.

In vivo administration of GaAs dose-dependently suppresses the *in vitro*-generated primary antibody response to the T cell-dependent antigen SRBCs and to the T cell-independent antigen dinitrophenyl (DNP)–Ficoll (35). Fluorescence-activated cell sorter (FACS) analysis showed decreased total numbers of T cells, B cells, and macrophages in GaAs-exposed splenocytes, but percentages of these cells were unchanged when compared to vehicle-exposed splenocytes. Separation and reconstitution studies indicated that GaAs affects all cells involved in the generation of a primary antibody response (macrophage, T cell, and B cell). Investigations involving the adherent population (macrophages) demonstrated that the suppression could be enhanced by titrating GaAs-exposed macrophages into reconstituted wells containing control adherent and nonadherent cells (T cells and B cells). This suppression was not due to induction of suppressor macrophages or release of prostaglandins.

Mechanistic studies on the macrophage revealed that phagocytosis of latex covaspheres and interleukin-1 (IL-1) production were not decreased in GaAs-exposed macrophages (36). However, exposed macrophages were impaired in their ability to present SRBCs to SRBC-primed lymph node T cells. Presentation of soluble antigens such as keyhole limpet hemocyanin (KLH), pigeon cytochrome *c*, and DASP (the synthetic fragment of cytochrome *c*) by GaAs-exposed macrophages to T cells primed for each antigen were not suppressed. Flow cytometric analysis showed that although the number of GaAs-exposed macrophages expressing the class II molecule Ia^k (required for proper interaction of the macrophage with the T cell) was not different from vehicle-exposed macrophages, the total amount of Ia^k on any individual GaAs-exposed macrophage was decreased. From these data it was concluded that GaAs alters splenic macrophage function by altering a step or steps involved in the processing or presentation of particulate antigens.

Investigations designed to determine the immunosuppressive component of GaAs (11) used graphite atomic absorption spectrophotometry to evaluate concentrations of gallium and arsenic in various organs of mice following a single GaAs intratracheal instillation of 200 mg/kg. In these studies, arsenic was found in the blood at 2 hr after exposure and remained elevated (200 ng/ml) through 48 hr. Gallium concentrations (undetected in previous studies) (10) were detected at 2 hr as well (350 ng/ml). By 14 days the arsenic concentrations had returned to baseline; however, gallium concentrations were significantly elevated (600 ng/ml). Similar results were noted in the spleen, where arsenic concentrations peaked at 1250 ng/ml by 24 hr. Gallium concentrations at this time were 750 ng/ml. Unlike the blood, arsenic concentrations in the spleen remained elevated at 800 ng/ml at 14 days while gallium concentrations continued to rise (12,000 ng/ml at 14 days). Because the concentrations of gallium and arsenic in each of the organs evaluated did not occur in a 1:1 ratio, it was concluded that GaAs must be dissociating in the lung into gallium and arsenic species.

In vitro studies with GaAs showed GaAs directly suppressed the *in vitro*-generated AFC response in a dose-dependent (6.25 to 75 μM) and time-dependent (addition up to 36 hr after immunization) manner. Both $NaAsO_2$ and $Ga(NO_3)_3$ suppressed the AFC response dose- and time-dependently when added to the *in vitro* system. However, based on IC_{50} (concentration that inhibits 50%) values for each salt, the role of the gallium component in the immunosuppression appears weak. The arsenic chelator DMSA dose-dependently blocked GaAs-induced immunosuppression *in vitro*, while the gallium chelator oxalic acid (OA) had no effect. The metal-binding compounds were determined to be specific for the metals used in these studies and did not cross-react with one another. DMSA was also able to block GaAs-induced suppression of the AFC response (*in vivo* exposure) when given subcutaneously (sc) every 4 hr beginning 1 hr prior to GaAs exposure. It was concluded that arsenic was the primary immunosuppressive component of GaAs following both *in vivo* and *in vitro* GaAs exposure.

Exposure (24 hr) to a single intratracheal administration of GaAs (200 mg/kg) has been shown to suppress antibody production as well as other T cell-mediated immunologic functions (34; B. Shrisuchart and A.E. Munson, *unpublished data*). GaAs has also been shown to exert toxic effects on events occurring early in the AFC response, which may include lymphocyte activation and proliferation (11). Extensions of those observations revealed that GaAs (200 mg/kg) decreased the ability of whole splenocytes to proliferate in response to antigen stimulation when compared to control cultures (37). Isolated GaAs-exposed T cells were significantly suppressed in their ability to proliferate when stimulated by Con A, PHA, anti-$CD3_{\epsilon}$, and IL-2 while isolated B cells exhibited no difference between vehicle- and GaAs-exposed cells in proliferative capacity when introduced to various stimuli. Analysis of surface receptors revealed that expression of CD25 (the IL-2 receptor), leukocyte function antigen-1 (LFA-1), and intercellular adhesion molecule-1 (ICAM-1) in GaAs-exposed mice were significantly below those of vehicle-exposed mice (36%, 18%, and 18%, respectively). Although expression of these molecules was upregulated by T cell reactivity (TCR) and IL-2 stimulation, a level of expression equal to vehicle was never obtained (39). These data support the studies of Petres et al. (19), Wen et al. (46), McCabe et al. (20), and Ostrosky-Wegman et al. (27), which also indicate that GaAs selectively inhibits T cell proliferation, possibly by interfering with primary and secondary signals involved in mitogenic and antigen-driven responses.

In addition to modulating T cell proliferative capacity, exposure to GaAs also alters production of soluble factors, which are critical for the proper generation of a primary immune response (38,39). Supernatants from *in vivo* and *in vitro* vehicle-exposed splenocyte cultures dose- (25% to 100%) and time-dependently (24 to 36 hr after immunization) reversed GaAs-induced suppression of the *in vitro*-generated primary AFC response produced by both *in vitro* (50 μM) and *in vivo* (200 mg/kg) exposure to GaAs. Concentration of 24-hr vehicle supernatants and treatment with proteinases revealed the reversing factors were protein in nature with molecular weights of 5000 to 50,000 daltons. This molecular weight (MW) range encompasses many of the lymphokines known to be necessary for the generation of an immune response. Evaluation of antibody cultures demonstrated that GaAs exposure (50 μM or 200 mg/kg) alters production of IL-2, IL-4, IL-5, and IL-6. Interestingly, the alterations in lymphokine production differed between the *in vivo* and *in vitro* exposure regimes. IL-2 (6.25 to 50 ng/ml) was able to dose-dependently reverse GaAs-induced suppression (*in vivo* exposure) and was also dependent on the concentration of GaAs (50 to 200 mg/kg). It would appear from these and previous data that IL-2 and/or its receptor is a primary target for GaAs following *in vivo* exposure. This action of an arsenical on lymphokine production was seen previously by Gainer (29), where $NaAsO_2$ and *p*-arsenilic acid decreased both the production and activity of IFN. In the GaAs studies, it is not known whether the compound is altering production or activity of IL-2.

Concerns with the studies involving GaAs are the contribution of pulmonary inflammation to the observed immunotoxicity (as a result of instillation of a particulate agent in the lung) and the induction of corticosterone as a result of respiratory problems. Corticosterone is valued in medical practice for its potent immunosuppressive activity. Investigations utilizing the glucocorticoid antagonist RU-486 (Mifepristone, Hoecht-Rousell) and tantalum (an inert particulate compound) showed clearly that (a) the presence of a particulate in the lung does not alter spleen or thymus weight, lymphocyte subpopulations, or the AFC response; and (b) a high concentration of serum corticosterone results from GaAs exposure (50 to 200 mg/kg; 491 to 757 ng/ml corticosterone compared to 86 ng/ml in controls), which is responsible for the observed decrease in spleen and thymus cellularity. This elevated corticosterone level does not appear to contribute, however, to the GaAs-induced suppression of the AFC response (43). These data indicate that GaAs (presumably the arsenic component) exerts a direct immunosuppressive effect that is independent of the induction of endogenous corticosteriods and that is not a result of pulmonary inflammation.

CONCLUSION

From the studies presented in this chapter it is clear that exposure to arsenic (in its various chemical forms) represents a potential health hazard. This risk is associated not only with the obvious overt toxicity of arsenical compounds but also with subtle to profound changes in the immune system, which compromise immunologic integrity and may result in suppression of natural immunosurveillance. More studies involving occupational exposure of human subjects are needed in order to determine the actual risk these workers assume in industries that manufacture and/or utilize arsenicals. Those studies, in conjunction with the data presented in this chapter, would also aid in the determination of threshold limit values for exposure to various forms of arsenic including GaAs and InAs.

REFERENCES

1. National Academy of Sciences. *Arsenic. Medical and biological effects of environmental pollutants.* Washington, DC: National Research Council; 1977.
2. Squibb KS, Fowler BA. The toxicity of arsenic and its compounds. In: Fowler BA, ed. *Biological and environmental effects of arsenic.* Amsterdam: Elsevier Science Publishers; 1983:233–269.
3. Schroeder HA, Balassa JJ. Abnormal trace metals in man: arsenic. *J Chron Dis* 1966;19:85–106.
4. Goyer RA. Toxic effects of metals. In: Amdur MO, Doull J, Klaassen CD, eds. *Cassarett and Doull's toxicology. The basic science of poisons*, 4 ed. Oxford: Pergamon Press; 1991:630.
5. Jelinek CF, Corneliussen PE. Levels of arsenic in the United States food supply. *Environ Health Perspect* 1977;19:83–87.
6. Crecelius EA. Changes in the chemical speciation of arsenic following ingestion by man. *Environ Health Perspect* 1977;19:147–150.
7. Munro IC, Charbonneau SM, Sandi E, Spemcer K, Bruce F, Grice HC. In: *Proceedings of the 13th Annual Meeting of the Society of Toxicology*, Washington, DC, March 1974:1–9.
8. Briggs TM, Owens TW. *Industrial hygiene characterization of the photovoltaic cell industry.* NIOSH Technical Report, DHEW (NIOSH) publication 80-112. Cincinnati, OH: US Department of Health, Education and Welfare; 1980.
9. NIOSH. NIOSH testimony to U.S. Department of Labor: comments at the OSHA arsenic hearing, July 14, 1982. NIOSH policy statement. Cincinnati, OH: US Department of Health and Human Services, PHS, CDC, NIOSH, 1982.
10. Webb DR, Sipes IG, Carter DE. *In vitro* solubility and *in vivo* toxicity of gallium arsenide. *Toxicol Appl Pharmacol* 1984;76:96–104.
11. Burns LA, Sikorski EE, Saady J, Munson AE. Evidence for arsenic as the primary immunosuppressive componant of gallium arsenide. *Toxicol Appl Pharmacol* 1991;110:157–169.
12. Webb JL. Arsenicals. In: Webb JL, ed. *Enzyme and metabolic inhibitors*, vol. 3. New York: Academic Press; 1966:595–793.
13. Fowler BA, Ishinishi N, Tsuchiya K, Vahter M. Arsenic. In: Friberg L, ed. *Handbook on the toxicology of metals.* New York: Elsevier; 1979:293–319.
14. Aposhian HV. Biochemical toxicology of arsenic. *Rev Biochem Toxicol* 1989;10:265–299.
15. WHO. *Environmental health criteria: arsenic*, vol 19. Geneva: EHE/EHC, World Health Organization; 1981.
16. EPA. *Special report on ingested inorganic arsenic: skin cancer and nutritional essentiality. Risk assessment form.* Washington, DC: US Environmental Protection Agency; 1987.
17. Hindmarsh JT, McCurdy RF. Clinical and environmental aspects of arsenic toxicity. *CRC Crit Rev Clin Lab Sci* 1986;23:315–347.
18. Wu MM, Kuo TB, Hwang Y, Chen CJ. Dose–response relation between arsenic concentration in well water and mortality from cancers and vascular diseases. *Am J Epidemiol* 1987;130:1123–1132.

19. Petres J, Baron D, Hagedorn M. Effects of arsenic on cell metabolism and cell proliferation: cytogenetic and biochemical studies. *Environ Health Perspect* 1977;19:223–227.
20. McCabe M, Maguire D, Nowak M. The effects of arsenic compounds on human and bovine lymphocyte mitogenesis *in vitro*. *Environ Res* 1983;31:323–331.
21. Koller LD. Immunotoxicology of heavy metals. *Int J Immunopharmacol* 1980;2:269–279.
22. Vos JG. Immune suppression as related to toxicology. *CRC Crit Rev Toxicol* 1977;5:67–101.
23. Shrauzer GN, Ishmael D. Effects of selenium and of arsenic on the genesis of spontaneous mammary tumors in inbred C3H mice. *Ann Clin Lab Sci* 1974;4:441–446.
24. Kerkvliet NI, Steppan, LB, Koller LD, Exon JH. Immunotoxicology studies of sodium arsenate—effects of exposure on tumor growth and cell-mediated tumor immunity. *J Environ Pathol Toxicol* 1980;4:65–79.
25. Yoshida T, Shimamura T, Shigeta S. Enhancement of the immune response *in vitro* by arsenic. *Int J Immunopharmacol* 1987;9:411–415.
26. Yoshida T, Shimamura T, Shigeta S. Immunotoxicity of arsenic: immunological changes observed in the workers contacting with arsenic and in mice exposed to it, and their possible mechanisms. Presented at the 5th International Conference on Immunpharmacology. *Int J Immunopharmacol* 1991;13(6):772.
27. Ostrosky-Wegman P, Gonsebatt ME, Montero R, et al. Lymphocyte proliferation kinetics and genotoxic findings in a pilot study on individuals chronically exposed to arsenic in Mexico. *Mutat Res* 1991;250:447–482.
28. Gainer JH, Pry TW. Effects of arsenicals on viral infections in mice. *Am J Vet Res* 1972;33:2299–2307.
29. Gainer JH. Effects of arsenicals on interferon formation and action. *Am J Vet Res* 1972;33:2579–2586.
30. Blakely BR, Sisodia CS, Mukkur TK. The effect of methylmercury, tetraethyl lead, and sodium arsenite on the humoral immune response in mice. *Toxicol Appl Pharmacol* 1980;52:245–254.
31. Yoshida T, Shimamura T, Shigeta S. Immunological effects of arsenic compound on mouse spleen cells *in vitro*. *Tokai J Exp Clin Med* 1986;11:353–359.
32. Hong HL, Fowler BA, Boorman GA. Hematopoietic effects in mice exposed to arsine gas. *Toxicol Appl Pharmacol* 1989;97:173–182.
33. Rosenthal GJ, Fort MM, Germolec DR, et al. Effect of subchronic arsine inhalation on immune function and host resistance. *Inhal Toxicol* 1989;1:113–127.
34. Sikorski EE, McCay JA, White KL, Bradley SG, Munson AE. Immunotoxicity of the semiconductor gallium arsenide in female B6C3F1 mice. *Fundam Appl Toxicol* 1989;13:843–858.
35. Sikorski EE, Burns LA, Stern ML, Luster MI, Munson AE. Splenic cell targets in gallium arsenide-induced suppression of the primary antibody response. *Toxicol Appl Pharmacol* 1991;110:129–142.
36. Sikorski EE, Burns LA, McCoy KL, Stern M, Munson AE. Suppression of splenic accessory cell function in mice exposed to gallium arsenide. *Toxicol Appl Pharmacol* 1991;110:143–156.
37. Burns LA, Munson AE. Reversal of gallium arsenide-induced suppression of the AFC response by vehicle supernatants. I. Pharmacokinetics following *in vitro* and *in vivo* exposure. *J Pharmacol Exp Ther* 1993;265:144–149.
38. Burns LA, Munson AE. Reversal of gallium arsenide-induced suppression of the AFC response by vehicle supernatants. II. Nature and identification of reversing factors. *J Pharmacol Exp Ther* 1993; 265:150–158.
39. Burns LA, Munson AE. Gallium arsenide selectively inhibits T cell proliferation and alters expression of CD25 (IL-2R/p55). *J Pharmacol Exp Ther* 1993;265:178–186.
40. Burns LA, Butterworth LF, Munson AE. Reversal of gallium arsenide-induced suppression of the antibody response by a mixed disulfide metabolite of *meso*-2,3-dimercaptosuccinic acid. *J Pharmacol Exp Ther* 1993;264(2):695–701.
41. Burns LA, MeCay JA, Munson AE. Arsenic in the sera of gallium arsenide-exposed mice inhibits bacterial growth and increases host resistanee. *J Pharmacol Exp Ther* 1993;265:795–800.
42. McCay JA, Sikorski EE, White KL, Page DG, Lysy HH, Musgrove DL, Munson AE. The toxicology of gallium arsenide in female B6C3F1 mice exposed by the intratracheal route (*in preparation*).
43. Burns LA, Spriggs TL, Munson AE. Gallium arsenide-induced increase in serum corticosterone is not responsible for suppression of the IgM antibody response *J Pharmacol Exp Ther* 1994:268:740–746.
44. Yoshida T, Shimamura T, Kitagawa H, Shigeta S. The enhancement of the proliferative response of peripheral blood lymphocytes of workers in semiconductor plant. *Ind Health* 1987;25(1):29–33.

45. Baron D, Kunick I, Frischmuth I, Petres J. Further *in vitro* studies on the biochemistry of the inhibition of nucleic acid and protein synthesis induced by arsenic. *Arch Dermatol Res* 1975;253: 15–22.
46. Wen W-N, Lieu T-L, Chang H-J, Wuu SW, Yau M-L, Jan KY. Baseline and sodium arsenite-induced sister chromatid exchanges in cultured lymphocytes from patients with Blackfoot disease and healthy persons. *Hum Genet* 1981;59:201–203.
47. Walder BK, Robertson MR, Jeremy J. Skin cancer and immunosuppression. *Lancet* 1971;2:1282–1283.
48. Cebrian ME, Albores A, Aguilar M, Blakeley E. Chronic arsenic exposure in the north of Mexico. *Hum Toxicol* 1983;2:121–133.
49. Cebrian ME. Some potential problems in assessing the effects of chronic arsenic exposure in north Mexico. Presented at the Americal Chemical Society, Division of Environmental Chemistry, 194th Meeting. 1987.
50. Yamauchi H, Takahashi K, Yamamura Y. Metabolism and excretion of orally and intraperitoneally administered gallium arsenide in the hamster. *Toxicology* 1986;40:237–246.
51. Pierson B, Wagenen SV, Nebesny KW, Fernando Q, Scott N, Carter DE. Dissolution of crystalline gallium arsenide in aqueous solutions containing complexing agents. *Am Ind Hyg Assoc J* 1989; 50(9):455–459.
52. Webb DR, Wilson SE, Carter DE. Comparative pulmonary toxicity of gallium arsenide, gallium (III) oxide, or arsenic (III) oxide intratracheally instilled into rats. *Toxicol Appl Pharmacol* 1986; 82:405–416.
53. Woods JS, Fowler BA. Altered regulation of mammalian hepatic heme biosynthesis and urinary porphyrin excretion during prolonged exposure to sodium arsenate. *Toxicol Appl Pharmacol* 1978; 43:361.
54. Yamauchi H, Takahashi K, Yamamura Y, Fowler BA. Metabolism of subcutaneous administered indium arsenide in the hamster. *Toxicol Appl Pharmacol* 1992;116:66–70.
55. Rosner MH, Carter DE. Metabolism and excretion of gallium arsenide and arsenic oxides by hamsters following intratracheal instillation. *Fundam Appl Toxicol* 1987;9:730–737.

Immunotoxicology and Immunopharmacology, Second Edition, edited by J. H. Dean, M. I. Luster, A. E. Munson, and I. Kimber.
Raven Press, Ltd., New York © 1994.

13

Immunopharmacology of Recombinant Cytokines

James E. Talmadge and *Jack H. Dean

*Departments of Pathology and Microbiology, University of Nebraska Medical Center, Omaha, Nebraska 68198; and *Drug Development, Sterling Winthrop Pharmaceuticals Research Division, Sterling Winthrop Inc., Collegeville, Pennsylvania 19426*

Immunoregulatory and hematoaugmenting cytokines have come into their own as novel therapeutic compounds for diverse indications including oncology, infectious disease, and a wide variety of congenital diseases. Indeed, it is astonishing to observe the rapidity with which new cytokines and growth factors are identified, cloned, and moved into clinical development. The current emphasis is on recombinant proteins, due to their focused bioactivity. Immunopharmacologic analyses of structure–activity relationships, toxicology, pharmacokinetics, and immunopharmacodynamics have yielded information contributing to the more effective use of these agents in disease models. Current avenues of immunotherapy suggest that the ultimate use of these drugs will be as adjuvants in combination with other therapies for immunodeficiencies, cancer, and infections. Nonetheless, perhaps the most exciting and rapidly advancing area of oncology is the use of biologic adjuvants together with more traditional forms of anticancer therapy. This chapter discusses the recombinant biologics that are currently either licensed or in active clinical trials in the United States, Europe, and Asia. In addition to providing a compendium of immunologically active agents that are either licensed or in clinical trials, we have also attempted to address some of the strategies for the development of these pharmacophores as well as the difficulties and scientific–clinical challenges for their development.

RECOMBINANT PROTEINS

Cytokines and growth factors are relatively low molecular weight proteins that are secreted in minute quantities and act in either an autocrine fashion on the cell from which they are secreted or in a paracrine manner on adjacent cells. The isolation of complementary deoxyribonucleic acid (cDNA) clones for cytokines and growth factors has permitted their production in large and reproducible quantities, which in turn has accelerated the preclinical and clinical study of their function and therapeutic attributes. The ability to cut and rejoin DNA at any desired site or to introduce point mutations at directed sites has resulted in the development and clinical use of mutant as well as chimeric therapeutic proteins. Thus we can now utilize proteins that are either exact or mutated forms of the naturally occurring ones, or design proteins that are composed of various polypeptide structures derived from different sequences, that is, the humanized monoclonal antibodies. The use of various point mutations has resulted in drugs with decreased toxicity, better production capabilities, or higher expression levels such as the mutant interleukin-2 (IL-2), IL-3, or granulocyte colony-stimulating factor (G-CSF) molecules (1–4), where, for example, serines are substituted for cysteines to reduce the development of aberrant tertiary structures. Furthermore, there is the development of chimeric cytokines expressing properties associated with multiple parent structures such as PIXY, which is a single biologically active drug comprised of IL-3 and granulocyte–macrophage colony-stimulating factor (GM-CSF) (5–7).

Therapeutic proteins including the cytokines and growth factors have emerged as an important class of drugs for the treatment of cancer, immunodepression, and infectious disease (8). However, their development has been slowed by our limited understanding of predictive models, their intended pharmacology, and their mechanism of action. To facilitate the development of these immunoregulatory proteins, additional information is needed on their pharmacology (9,10). One approach to the development of these proteins is to identify a clinical hypothesis based on the preclinical identification of a therapeutic surrogate(s). Notably this strategy was recently formally accepted by the Food and Drug Administration (FDA) (11). A surrogate for clinical efficacy may be phenotypic, biochemical, enzymatic, functional (immunologic, molecular, or hematologic), or quality of life measurement, which is believed to be associated with therapeutic activity. Phase I clinical trials can then be designed to identify the optimal and maximum tolerated dose and regime or treatment schedule for protein administration, which maximizes the augmentation of the surrogate endpoint(s). Subsequent phase II/III trials can then be established to determine if the changes in the surrogate levels correlate with therapeutic activity. Table 1 lists the immunologically and hematologically active drugs that are approved for general use in the United States. The proteins that are currently in clinical trials are listed in Table 2 along with the indications under investigation.

In contrast to strategies based on the identification of surrogates for efficacy, many protocols for these recombinant proteins have been predicted on practices developed for conventional low molecular weight drugs and may not be advantageous for the development of proteins. This is because of the unique pharmacologic attributes of proteins, which require selective or targeted delivery to the desired site (i.e., the bone marrow, spleen, or tumor) (12,13). To optimally administer proteins as drugs and assure their targeting are the primary challenges for their development. One further difficultly in the development of a recombinant protein is that in many instances there is little relationship between the dose administered and

TABLE 1. *Approved biotechnology drugs*

Product type	Abbreviated indication	U.S. status
Interferon-γ1b	Chronic granulomatous disease	Dec. 1990
Interferon-αn3	Genital warts	Oct. 1989
Epoetin-α	Anemia of chronic renal failure	June 1989
Epoetin-α	Anemia of chronic renal failure	Dec. 1990
Interferon-α2b	Hairy cell leukemia	June 1986
	Genital warts	June 1986
	AIDS-related Kaposi's sarcoma	Nov. 1988
	Non-A, non-B hepatitis	Feb. 1991
Sargramostin (GM-CSF)	Autologous bone marrow transplant	Mar. 1991
Sargramostin (GM-CSF)	Autologous bone marrow transplant	Mar. 1991
Filgrastim (r-G-CSF)	Chemotherapy-induced neutropenia	Feb. 1991
Interferon-α2a	Hairy cell leukemia	June 1986
	AIDS-related Kaposi's sarcoma	Nov. 1988
Aldesleukin (IL-2)	Renal cell carcinoma	May 1992

biologic effect. Indeed, in some instances there is a nonlinear dose–response relationship that has been described as bell shaped (14). This dose–response relationship, or lack thereof, may be due to (a) the nonlinear way in which the drug is dispersed in the body, (b) a poor ability to enter into a saturable receptor-mediated transport process, (c) chemical instability, (d) sequence of administration with other agents or an incorrect time of administration, and (e) an inappropriate location and response of the target cells. Furthermore, a bell-shaped dose–response curve could be associated with the tachyphylaxis of receptor expression or a signal transduction mechanism whereby the cells become refractory to subsequent receptor-mediated augmentation. Because the regulation of biologic control can and likely will lead to numerous physiologically untoward events, it is important that both the physicochemical structure and the mechanism of administration of recombinant proteins be tailored so as to ensure that the required physiologic activity occurs.

INTERFERON-α (IFN-α): IMMUNOMODULATORY AND THERAPEUTIC PROPERTIES

The initial clinical studies with IFN-α were the subject of much enthusiasm, and these nonrandomized studies suggested therapeutic activity against malignant melanoma, osteosarcoma, and various lymphomas (15–21). However, subsequent randomized trials with IFN-α demonstrated significant therapeutic activity only against less common tumor histiotypes, including hairy cell leukemia, chronic myelogenous leukemia (CML) (15,16), and a few types of lymphoma (17), including low grade non-Hodgkin's lymphoma (21) and cutaneous T cell lymphoma (19). Recently, the list of responding tumor histiotypes has expanded to include renal cell carcinoma (20,22), acquired immunodeficiency syndrome (AIDS) and Kaposi's

TABLE 2. *Biotechnology drugs in development*

Product type	Abbreviated indication	U.S. status
Colony-stimulating factors		
GM-CSF	Adjuvant to chemotherapy	Phase I/II
GM-CSF	Low blood cell counts	Submitted
Sargramostim (GM-CSF)	Allogeneic bone marrow transplants, chemotherapy adjuvant	Phase III
	Adjuvant to AIDS therapy	Phase II
M-CSF	Cancer, fungal disease	Phase I
M-CSF	Cancer, hematologic neoplasms, bone marrow transplants	Phase I
Filgrastim (r-G-CSF)	AIDS, leukemia, aplastic anemia	Submitted
Sargramostim (GM-CSF)	Neutropenia to secondary chemotherapy	Phase III
PIXY	Neutropenic	Phase I/II
Stem cell factor	Neutropenia/thrombocytopenia	Phase I
Erythropoietins		
Epoetin-β	Anemia secondary to kidney disease	Submitted
	Autologous transfusion	Phase II/III
Epoetin-α	Anemia of cancer and chemotherapy	Submitted
	Anemia of surgical blood loss, autologous transfusion	Phase III
Interferons		
Interferon-α1b	Small-cell lung cancer, atop dermatitis	Phase III
	Trauma-related infections, renal cell carcinoma	Phase II
	Asthma and allergies	Phase I
Interferon-αn3	ARC, AIDS	Phase I/II
Interferon-β	Multiple sclerosis	Phase III
	Cancer	Phase I/II
Interferon-γ	Rheumatoid arthritis	Phase II/III
	Venereal warts	Phase II
Interferon consensus	Cancer, infectious disease	Phase II/III
Interferon-γ	Cancer, infectious disease	Phase II
Interferon-α2b	Superficial bladder cancer, basal cell carcinoma, chronic hepatitis B, delta hepatitis	Submitted
	Acute hepatitis B, delta hepatitis, acute, chronic myelogenous leukemia	Phase III
	HIV (with Retrovir)	Phase I
Interferon-β	Unresponsive malignant diseases	Phase I
Interferon-α2a	Colorectal cancer (with 5-FU) chronic, acute hepatitis B; non-A, non-B hepatitis; chronic myelogenous leukemia; HIV positive; ARC; AIDS (with Retrovir)	Phase II
Interleukins		
PEG IL-2	AIDS (with Retrovir)	Phase I
Aldesleukin (IL-2)	Cancer	Phase II/III
	Kaposi's sarcoma (with Retrovir)	Phase I
Human IL-1α	Bone marrow suppression (chemo-, radiotherapy)	Phase I/II
Human IL-1β	Bone marrow suppression, melanoma, immunotherapy	Phase I/II
	Wound healing	Phase II
Human IL-2	Cancer immunotherapy	Phase III
Human IL-2	Cancer immunotherapy (with Roferon-A)	In clinical trials
Human IL-3	Bone marrow failure, platelet deficiencies, autologous marrow transplant, chemotherapy adjuvant	Phase I/II

TABLE 2. *Continued.*

Product type	Abbreviated indication	U.S. status
	Peripheral stem cell transplant	Phase I
Human IL-4	Immunodeficient disease, cancer therapy, vaccine adjuvant, immunization	Phase I/II
Human IL-4	Cancer immunomodulator	Phase II
Human IL-6	Platelet deficiencies	Phase I/II
Human IL-11	Thrombocytopenia	Phase I
Tumor necrosis factors		
TNF	Cancer	Phase II
Others		
Anakinra (IL-1 receptor antagonist)	AML, CML, inflammatory bowel disease, rheumatoid arthritis, sepsis, septic shock	Phase II
TNF-β	Cancer	Phase II

ARC, acquired immunodeficiency syndrome-related complex; AML, acute myeloid leukemia.

sarcoma (23–26), hepatitis, and bladder papillomatosis (27). It is now agreed that most patients with hairy cell lymphoma respond to low doses of chronically administered IFN-α. However, it is clear that, despite IFN-α activity against specific leukemias and lymphomas, it has limited activity against solid tumors.

Thus it has taken almost three decades to translate the concept of IFN-α as an antiviral to its routine utility in clinical oncology. Despite extensive clinical studies, the development of IFN-α is still in its early stages, and such basic parameters as optimal dose and therapeutic schedule remain to be determined (17,18,28,29). The mechanism of activity is also controversial since IFN-α has been shown to have dose-dependent antitumor activities *in vitro*, yet it is active at low doses for hairy cell leukemia (17,18,28,29). Immunomodulation as the mechanism of therapeutic activity with IFN-α is perhaps best supported by its activity against hairy cell leukemia. Treatment with IFN-α is associated with a 90% to 95% response rate; however, this is not achieved until the patients have been on protocol for a year and it appears that low doses of IFN-α are as active as higher doses—that is $(0.3 \text{ to } 0.4) \times 10^6$ U/M^2 versus the maximal tolerated dose (MTD) of $(5 \text{ to } 20) \times 10^6$ U/M^2 (28–30). The toxicity of IFN-α is both dose and possibly peak level dependent (59). In contrast to the clinical result, IFN-α is most active *in vitro* when added to tumor cells as a continuous low-dose exposure (31). Phase II clinical trials have shown that significant objective results can be achieved with IFN-α following continuous infusion of low doses of IFN-α over a 28-day period (18). In contrast, chronic administration of high doses of IFN-α does not appear to augment immune reactivity and may reduce stem cell and natural killer (NK) cell activity (30,32).

Initial dose finding studies by Quesada and co-workers determined that a dose of 12×10^6 U/M^2 of r-IFN-α was not tolerable in patients with hairy cell leukemia (33,34). Subsequently, they demonstrated that a dose of 2×10^6 U/M^2 was both well tolerated and effective when administered three times per week (62). In a recent study by Smalley et al. (34), they demonstrated that highly purified natural IFN-α at a dose of 2×10^6 U/M^2 when administered for 28 days was well tolerated in most patients with hairy cell leukemia but suggested that this dose might be myelosuppressive in some patients as well as neurotoxic or cardiotoxic in other patients. In their studies, a lower dose of 200,000 U/M^2 was also administered for 28 days and it was found that this dose was better tolerated and also induced improvements in peripheral neutrophil and platelet counts as rapidly as the standard dose. In this trial substantial clinical improvement, primarily in terms of increased platelet or neutrophil count, was observed within the first 4 to 8 weeks of treatment in patients receiving the low dose of IFN-α. This gain was obtained with an improved quality of life—a concomitant depression in cardiac and neurologic toxicity, flu-like syndrome, myelosuppression, the need for platelet transfusion, and incidence of bacterial infections. They suggested that once such an improvement has been obtained at 200,000 U/M^2, and patients have become tolerant to the acute toxicity associated with IFN-α, the dose could then be increased to the standard 2×10^6 U/M^2 to obtain the significantly greater antileukemia effect of the higher dose. In their study, Smalley et al. (34) escalated the dose following 6 months of low-dose treatment. However, they suggested that this dosage escalation could occur earlier, perhaps 3 months after induction therapy. Their results confirmed previous reports (35), which demonstrated a low dose effect of IFN-α on platelet and neutrophil counts. It appears that comparable improvement in thrombocytopenia and neutropenia can rapidly be induced in the majority of patients when low and minimally toxic doses of IFN-α are used. However, there is also a therapeutic dose–response effect, whereby higher doses of IFN-α will induce a quantitatively greater antileukemic response than that observed with low doses of IFN-α. We should note that the mechanism of action of IFN-α remains obscure. It potentially may act as an antiproliferative, immunoaugmenting, or differentiation induction agent. Alternatively, it may function via multiple mechanisms; however, it is clear that it continues to have new potential not only as a single agent but also in synergy with other biologics.

INTERFERON-γ: IMMUNOMODULATORY AND THERAPEUTIC PROPERTIES

Preclinical studies have revealed that murine r-IFN-γ has significant therapeutic activity in animal models of experimental and spontaneous metastasis, which occurs with a reproducible bell-shaped dose–response curve (14). Furthermore, studies of macrophage activation in normal animals have revealed that the same bell-shaped dose–response curve occurs for the augmentation of macrophage tumoricidal activity. Studies by Golomb et al. (35), to identify the mechanism of activity of r-Mu-IFN-γ in tumor-bearing animals, treated mice with r-IFN-γ and at various times thereafter monitored levels of effector cell activity at various sites. Optimal therapeutic activity was observed with the three time per week intravenous (iv) administration of r-IFN-γ for the treatment of experimental and spontaneous melanoma metastasis. The dosage optimum was 30 to 50,000 units per animal with significantly less therapeutic activity at lower and higher doses. In these studies, they noted a significant and inverse correlation between macrophage augmentation in the lung of the pulmonary metastasis-bearing mice and therapeutic efficacy (35). The results suggested that immunologic augmentation provides an indirect mechanism for the therapeutic effect of r-IFN-γ and supports the hypothesis that treatment with the MTD of r-IFN-γ may not be optimal in an adjuvant setting.

The preclinical hypothesis of a bell-shaped dose–response curve for r-IFN-γ has been confirmed in numerous clinical studies of the immunoregulatory effects of r-IFN-γ and defined an optimal immunomodulatory dose (OID) (36–38). In general, the OID for r-IFN-γ has been found to be between 0.1 and 0.3 mg/M^2 following iv or intramuscular (im) injection. In contrast, the MTD for r-IFN-γ may range from 3 to 10 mg/M^2 depending on the source of the r-IFN-γ and/or the clinical center. The identification of an OID for r-IFN-γ in patients with minimal tumor burden has resulted in the development of clinical trials to test the hypothesis that the immunologic enhancement induced by r-IFN-γ will result in prolongation of the disease-free state and overall survival of patients in an adjuvant setting (38). However, it should be noted that r-IFN-γ was found on an empirical basis to have therapeutic activity in chronic granulomatous disease (CGD) (23,24) and it was for this indication that the FDA approved r-IFN-γ. Thus despite the use of a rational developmental strategy, r-IFN-γ was initially licensed predicated on an empirical developmental strategy. These studies in CGD suggested that the mechanism of therapeutic activity for IFN-γ was associated with enhanced phagocytic oxidase activity and increased superoxide production by neutrophils. However, more recent data suggest that the majority of CGD patients obtained clinical benefit by prolonging IFN-γ therapy, and the mechanism of action may not be due to enhanced neutrophil oxidase activity but rather may be due to the correction of a respiratory burst deficiency in a subset of monocytes (39,40).

IFN-γ has a relatively mild toxicity profile compared to other cytokines such as IL-2 (discussed later), tumor necrosis factor (TNF), or IL-1. The MTD appears to be about 8 MU/M^2, a dose at which almost all patients experience fever greater than 40 °C, elevated serum glutamic–oxaloacetic transaminase (SGOT) levels greater than six times normal, and reversible hypotension. In addition, patients at this dose would typically experience severe chills and confusion. The clinical toxicity suggests a dose–response relationship with fever normally beginning 1 to 2 hr after initial injection, peaking at 4 to 6 hr, and resolving by 24 hr. Tachyphylaxis to fever usually develops within 1 week. Acetaminophen will partially ameliorate the fever. In addition to the fever, fatigue, myalgia, and influenza-like syndrome occur frequently and are considered to be the primary chronic toxicity for most patients. On discontinuation of IFN-γ administration, such side effects are reversible. In addition, cardiovascular toxicity is observed with the hypotension occurring in approximately 50% to 60% of patients. Peak hypotension occurs 3 to 8 hr after initial dosing and often antedates the fever peak. IFN-γ also has hematopoietic activities with the induction of granulocytopenia and occasionally thrombocytopenia.

INTERLEUKIN-2: STUDIES OF PHARMACOKINETICS, IMMUNOMODULATORY ACTIVITY, AND TOXICITY

IL-2 is first and foremost a T cell proliferative agent. In addition, it is a potent NK cell augmenting agent and can activate what is termed lymphokine activate killer (LAK) cells *in vitro* or *in vivo* following chronic (72-hr) interaction with lymphoid cells and is required for T cell proliferation. As such, it is important in all facets of T cell as well as NK cell augmentation and proliferation. In addition, IL-2 can augment monocyte–macrophage activities. IL-2 has recently been approved for use as a single agent, although it is also administered in conjunction with LAK or T cell-infiltrating lymphocytes (TILs). However, it has been questioned whether the adoptive transfer of LAK cells is necessary or adds to the clinical efficacy of r-IL-2. Indeed, from the initial clinical trials, there has been little indication of an improved therapeutic effect by r-IL-2 plus LAK cells versus IL-2 alone (41,42). When the clinical trials with IL-2 are rigorously examined, neither strategy has impressive (as opposed to significant) therapeutic activity (42,43). The overall response rate with r-IL-2 is 7% to 14%, which is also associated with considerable toxicity (44). One unanticipated clinical observation (45) post-treatment with r-IL-2 was a rapid depletion of peripheral blood lymphocytes with a subsequent rebound at 4 to 7 days (45–49). The rebound results in a twofold increase in peripheral blood lymphocytes, increased numbers of r-IL-2 receptor-positive lymphocytes (4- to 15-fold increase), and an increase in NK-like (anti-K-562) and LAK-like activity. In the initial study (45), partial responses were observed in 4 out of 31 patients. Interestingly, these partial responders did not correspond to the patients with increased LAK or NK cell activity. However, the partial responder could be due to an antitumor effect mediated by *in situ* LAK cells that are not represented in the peripheral population. The functional difference between LAK cells and TILs is not clear since LAK cells are present among TILs as shown in several studies using both functional and phenotypic criteria (41,44,45). The antitumor effect of both of these cell types could be due to a direct activity or could be secondary to the generation of other cytokine mediators acting in concert with the immune effective cells and/or upon the tumor cells. The latter is suggested by the observation that r-IL-2-stimulated lymphocytes produce IFN-α and TNF as well as other cytokines and that the therapeutic activity of r-IL-2 may be synergistic with both cytokines.

The r-IL-2 augmented activity *in vivo*, be it NK or LAK cell, is transient and dependent on recent exposure to IL-2. This is consistent with the requirement for continuous exposure to r-IL-2 to augment NK cells in culture (50). The *in vitro* augmentation of maximal NK cell cytotoxicity, by IL-2, requires receptor occupancy for 16 to 24 hr at approximately 100 units/ml (50). To achieve these parameters clinically, either a continuous IL-2 infusion or multiple daily injections of high IL-2 doses by push administration are required (51). Clinical trials have demonstrated that iv bolus injections of r-IL-2 at doses sufficient to achieve a continuous low serum level result in appreciable toxicity (47). It appears that the pharmacologically appropriate route of administration is continuous infusion and that significantly less protein/M^2 is required (42,47,52–65), although this remains controversial (56). The route of administration of r-IL-2 is important because of its influence on the bioavailability and serum half-life of the r-IL-2. The preclinical observation of therapeutic activity at low doses by continuous infusion suggests that r-IL-2 might be therapeutically effective using this less toxic protocol (42,47–49,52–56). Indeed, the lymphoid hyperplasia and therapeutic activity that are observed with continuous administration of r-IL-2 suggest that *ex vivo* LAK cell induction, cultivation, and infusion technology may be unnecessary (52,57,58). Similar therapeutic and immunomodulatory activity has been shown preclinically with low doses of r-IL-2 when it was delivered chronically by solid phase (59) or mini-pellet administration (60).

The hypothesis that moderate doses of r-IL-2 when administered by continuous infusion will have decreased toxicity with the retention of therapeutic activity has been examined in the clinic. There are some indications that continuous infusion may be associated with lower toxicity than iv bolus administration and yet have comparable immunoregulatory activity *in vivo* (48,58,61,62). The observation of decreased toxicity with a similar response rate has also been reported with continuous infusion versus iv bolus studies with r-IL-2 in combination with LAK cell therapy (41,61–63). In a preliminary report by West et al. (41), responses were found in 9 of 16 available melanoma patients, and it has been suggested that maintenance administration of r-IL-2 by continuous infusion for 1 week each month following two cycles of r-IL-2 and LAK therapy may prolong the response as compared to two or three cycles of r-IL-2 and LAK. Because the acute toxicity of r-IL-2 is rapidly reversed following cessation of treatment, continuous infusion provides a safer way of regulating dosage and avoiding the hypotension that usually terminates treatment when r-IL-2 is given by the intensive push schedule (q 8 hr). Indeed, by using continuous infusion, only 6 of the 40 patients of West et al. (41) could not be managed on an ordinary ward. Toxicity was further diminished with a regular temporal interruption of infusion (46). Additional phase I/II clinical trials with this protocol using r-IL-2 alone have reported response rates similar to r-IL-2 and LAK protocols (47,50–52). Several studies in the United States and Europe have revealed that immune parameters are significantly enhanced by repetition(s) of r-IL-2 cycles beyond the first week of therapy and that bolus r-IL-2 has less immunostimulatory activity than continuous r-IL-2 administration. It appears that the toxicity by r-IL-2 is dose dependent and immunomodulation is maximal by continuous infusion compared with 2- or 8-hr infusion or three times a day (tid) push injections (40). Lastly, r-IL-2 induces a rebound lymphocytosis that is directly related to dose following continuous infusion. In such studies, continuous infusion of r-IL-2 initially produces leukopenia but later results in lymphoid hyperplasia in the peripheral blood and increased LAK cell activity as determined *ex vivo*.

Many of the trials of continuous iv infusion of IL-2 with or without LAK cell therapy in metastatic renal cell carcinoma have used a MTD of IL-2 [i.e., (3 to 6) $\times 10^6$ U/M^2/d]. A recent study by Thompson et al. (64) compared maintenance IL-2 therapy at the MTD of 6×10^6 U/M^2/d to 2×10^6 U/M^2/d. They found that it was possible to maintain the patients for a median of 4 days at 6×10^6 U/M^2/d but in the presence of severe hypotension and capillary leak syndrome. In the lower dose protocol none of the patients experienced severe hypotension or capillary leak syndrome and the median duration of maintenance IL-2 therapy was 9 days. In the lower dose protocol there was a total response rate of 41%. This is in contrast to the higher dose protocol (with a shorter duration of administration), which had a 22% response rate. These investigators suggest that it is unlikely that a dose–response relationship exists between continuous iv infusion of IL-2 and LAK cells and antitumor activity and that there may be an improved therapeutic activity associated with a longer maintenance protocol at lower doses, which is associated with significantly less toxicity. In a number of clinical studies, IL-2 has shown a very significant toxicity profile. Typically, at doses of 3×10^5 U/M^2/d, the clinical toxicity profile is relatively mild and rarely requires pharmacologic intervention. Nonetheless, even at this low dose IL-2 may have toxicities including hypotension, weight gain, and mild azotemia. Higher doses of IL-2 (3×10^6 U/M^2/d) induce a more severe toxicity profile with flu-like syndromes consisting of fevers, chills, and myalgias that increase in severity over a course of infusion, resolving within 72 hr post-discontinuation of administration. In most cases, a combination of acetaminophen, diphenhydramine, and meperidine can alleviate the symptoms. In higher dose groups, there are also severe hemodynamic effects including marked fluid retention, prerenal azotemia, and oliguria. These symptoms typically require clinical support including iv fluids, low-dose dopamine, and albumin. In addition, anorexia is not unusual and is observed over the first few days of the course of therapy including nausea and vomiting. A transient confusion is also observed although at a lesser frequency and does not normally require medication or psychiatric intervention. Eosinophilia is observed in most treatment groups perhaps due to the upregulation of IL-5.

Combination therapy with IL-2 and LAK cells is also associated with significant cardiorespiratory effects including what is termed a leaky capillary syndrome. The most significant toxicities include severe peripheral edema and significant ascites or plural effusions. Severe respiratory distress is also experienced and in some instances requires intubation. Cardiovascular effects include tachycardia and hypotension requiring vasopressor administration and intravenous fluid administration. Arrhythmias that are observed are primarily superventricular and in a limited percentage of patients angina or an ischemic change is noted. In addition, with approximately a 1% incidence, myocardial infarctions have been observed.

COLONY-STIMULATING FACTORS (CSFs): AN EXAMPLE OF COMBINATION THERAPY

In contrast to IFN-α, and due in part to experience gained with IFN-α and IFN-γ, IL-2, and TNF, there has been a rapid development of the CSFs. These growth factors have shown marked efficacy in improving the myelosuppression found in many clinical conditions, including bone marrow transplantation, aggressive chemotherapy, and various forms of congenital or iatrogenic cytopenia. Indeed, this class of proteins (i.e., myelorestorative agents) may prove to be the first that are applicable in humans for a wide variety of indications. The CSFs, which are cytokines with growth factor-like activity for bone marrow stem cells, have marked efficacy for decreasing the toxicity and potential for increasing the therapeutic index of chemotherapeutic and irradiation protocols used in the treatment of neoplasia. The importance of chemotherapeutic dose intensity has been shown in both retrospective and prospective studies, in that the more aggressive use of chemotherapeutic agents increases their therapeutic activity (65–67). Increased dose intensity of chemotherapeutic agents can be achieved, in part, by preventing or decreasing the neutropenia associated with their aggressive use. A decrease in neutropenia can be achieved with stem cell transplantation (bone marrow transplantation, BMT) and the administration of agents that facilitate the outgrowth of stem cells and thereby reduce or prevent neutropenia and thrombocytopenia (i.e., CSFs).

The CSFs also have rate-limiting pharmacokinetics similar to that experienced with r-IL-2. Following a single iv push, an initial high blood level of GM-CSF has been reported (T_α half-life of 3 to 5 min) that is followed by a fairly rapid decrease (T_β half-life of 150 min) with the expected two-compartment model (109). Following subcutaneous (sc) injection, detectable serum levels are observed within 15 to 30 min and sustained serum levels are observed for varying periods of time depending on the dose administered. Serum levels greater than 1 ng/ml can be maintained for longer than 12 hr following a single sc injection of GM-CSF at 10 ug/kg. This corresponds to a concentration of GM-CSF that supports near-maximal *in vitro* proliferation. Thus sc administration or, preferentially, continuous infusion either intravenously or subcutaneously results in optimal pharmacokinetics for hematorestoration with the CSFs (68). Recently, Neidhart et al. (69) examined whether the sc administration or continuous iv administration of GM-CSF had the best capabilities to support a dose-intensive chemotherapy regime. They found that the optimal regime of GM-CSF was 500 $\mu g/M^2$ given by continuous iv infusion. The duration of leukopenia was 5.9 days as opposed to 13.2 and 10.2 days in the control arms. Other studies by Cebon et al. (70) compared the iv administration of GM-CSF by bolus or 2-hr infusion as opposed to sc administration. GM-CSF was more effective following sc as compared to either iv bolus or 2-hr iv infusion. They found that the duration of GM-CSF concentrations in the serum at levels greater than 1 ng/ml and the area under the concentration–time curve provided a significant correlation with an increased leukocyte count. In contrast, there was no correlation between leukocyte count and peak serum GM-CSF level. However, there was a significant correlation between toxicity as characterized by hypoxemia and hypotension, which was associated with a high C_{max} and iv administration. Thus not only does a low dose of GM-CSF administered by continuous infusion or sc administration express increased biologic activity, but it also has less toxicity than that observed following a high dose and/or bolus iv administration (70).

It is apparent that the successful utilization of the CSFs is dependent on the schedule and timing of their administration. It is believed, as discussed above, that if CSFs are administered too soon after injection of a chemotherapeutic agent, increased toxicity or a lack of activity may be observed (71). In contrast, if the myelorestorative drug is administered after complete metabolism of the agent, either alone or with autologous bone marrow transplantation (AuBMT), accelerated myeloid reconstitution will occur. Recently, Meropol et al. (72) reasoned that there might be a protective effect of continuously administered G-CSF on the oral mucosa in those patients receiving fluorouracil (5-FU) and low-dose leucovorin. This patient population commonly has dose-limiting mucositis, although severe myelosuppression is uncommon with this regime. In this study, three of the first four patients develop grade IV neutropenia with an absolute neutrophil count of less than 500/min^3. This is in contrast to patients who did not receive G-CSF in combination with 5-FU and leucovorin and who had a 6.8% incidence of leukopenia. In subsequent studies, they administered G-CSF 5 days following the administration of a cycle of 5-FU and leucovorin without the induction of any neutropenia. This provides an unfortunate, but fairly convincing, demonstration of the potential dangers associated with chemotherapy and growth factor administration.

Several CSFs have been tested clinically including r-GM-CSF (71,72), r-G-CSF (73,74), and partially purified natural or recombinant macrophage colony-stimulating factor (M-CSF) (75,76) and all have demonstrated clinical efficacy. As a generality, these agents have shown as high as 100-fold increase in the number of circulating progenitor cells of a variety of lineages, including granulocytic–monocytic, granulocytic, monocytic, and, to a lesser extent, erythroid and megakaryocytic precursors. These progenitors remain elevated for up to 3 days after the cessation of therapy. r-GM-CSF has also induced marked increases in eosinophils. Reconstitution of hematopoietic parameters in the peripheral blood as well as increased bone marrow myeloid/erythroid ratio and total medullary cellularity has been observed with CSFs following aggressive chemotherapy with or without bone marrow reconstitution and in chronic neutropenia (74), myelodysplastic syndromes (71), hairy cell leukemia associated neutropenia (77), patients immunodepressed with AIDS (78), and aplastic anemia (79). Associated with the increase in the absolute neutrophil counts, there has been a trend for a significant reduction in the number of days per patient in which the absolute neutrophil counts are less than 500 to 1000, a reduction in the number of days in which patients need to be on antibiotics to treat fever and neutropenia, and the percentage of patients who are qualified to receive planned chemotherapy as per previously determined schedules. Finally, there is a significant decrease in the incidence of mucositis and iatrogenic mortality.

At present, there are five additional cytokines undergoing clinical development. These include IL-3, which to date have shown less myeloid restorative activity as compared to G-CSF or GM-CSF (80), IL-4 as both a hematoregulator and immunoregulator (81), IL-1 (82), IL-6, IL-11, and stem cell factor (SCF). IL-1 has the ability to treat interdermal/subcutaneous tumors in rodents and has potent radio- or chemotherapy protective properties in rodents as well as myelostimulatory properties. It has not, to date, in the preliminary phase I trials (82) shown significant therapeutic properties. In contrast, IL-1 has shown marked toxicity with or without support by indomethacin to reduce hypotension. The administration of IL-1, in addition to showing dose-limited toxicities of hypotension, myocardial infarction, confusion, severe abdominal pain, and renal insufficiency, has demonstrated a dose-related increase in total white blood cell (WBC) count and bone marrow cellularity. It should be noted that all doses including ones as low as 0.1 μg/kg have shown no dose-limiting toxicities such as fever, chills, fatigue, and nausea. Recently, IL-6 has also entered clinical trials as an agent to reduce thrombocytopenia. Clinical trials have also been initiated with IL-11 and SCF to reduce thrombocytopenia and/or neutropenia. Preclinical evidence has suggested that IL-11 might not only have effects on neutropenia but might also be similar to IL-6 in its activities on thrombocytopenia. Initial clinical trials with SCF have shown an impact on neutropenia and preclinical results strongly suggests that it would have synergistic activity together with other hematopoietic cytokines. Thus a number of immunoregulatory and hematoregulatory cytokines are entering into clinical trials and it is hoped that hypothesis-based clinical trials will be initiated with these exciting new proteins.

BIOLOGY AND PHARMACOLOGY OF IL-4

Native IL-4 has properties that exemplify many of the characteristics of immune recognition-induced lymphokines (83). It is produced principally, although not exclusively, by activated (CD4+) T lymphocytes (84) and mediates much of its pharmacologic action across short distances between target cells and IL-4-producing cells. As with most molecules whose biologic functions were initially detected by *in vitro* assays, a question still remains as to the major physiologic action of IL-4, although it is now well recognized that it has a wide range of biologic functions (85). It is clear that IL-4 does express at least one critical *in vivo* function and in the mouse it is principally responsible for the production of immunoglobulin E (IgE) in response to a variety of stimuli that elicit Ig class switching (86). *In vitro* analysis has indicated functions of IL-4 on B cells, T cells, macrophages, hematopoietic precursors, and stromal cells, although the biologic relevance of some of these findings *in vivo* has yet to be determined. IL-4 was described initially because of its ability to enhance DNA synthesis by resting B lymphocytes stimulated with anti-IgM antibodies and was thus designated B cell growth factor (BCGF). This was superseded by the name IL-4, which was proposed at the time of the derivation of cDNA clones and because of the recognition of its pleiotropic action on non-B-cell targets. It also enhances hematopoiesis and it is synergistic with G-CSF and erythropoietin (EPO) and enhances the release of other CSFs. IL-4 induces differentiation of marrow pre-B-cells and stimulates the clonal proliferation of resting B cells. It also increases Ig production *in vitro* as well as regulates the CD23 receptor.

It is known that resting human T cells do not respond directly to the addition of r-hu-IL-4, but do so if they have been activated previously with mitogen [phytohemagglutinin (PHA) or concanavalin A (Con A)] or selective stimuli (anti-CD3 or PMA) (87). IL-4 enhances antigen-specific T cell-mediated cytotoxicity (88) and may augment the growth of tumor infiltrating lymphocytes (TILs) in the presence of IL-2 (89). However, it does inhibit antigen-unrestricted LAK cell production. Because of its potential to enhance several functions of the immune system thought to be relevant for preventing neoplasia, it is considered a candidate for the treatment of refractory cancer.

It is now clear that cells of the immune system communicate, at least in part, via a network of interacting cytokines. In the mouse, and more recently shown in humans, T helper (T_H) cells have been divided into two major subsets (T_H1 and T_H2) based on distinct cytokine secretion patterns (90). T_H1 cells produce IL-2, IFN-γ, and lymphotoxins, whereas T_H2 cells predominantly secrete IL-4, IL-5, IL-6, and IL-10 (90, 91). Because in most instances immunization with a strong immunogen not only activates T_H1 but also T_H2 cells, the question has arisen as to whether T_H1 cells may be subjected to regulatory effects by the cytokines produced by T_H2 cells. It appears that there is a reciprocal inhibitory relationship between T_H1 and T_H2 cells. IL-10, which is produced by T_H2 cells and was originally known as cytokine synthesis inhibitory factor, has been shown to inhibit synthesis of most cytokines produced by T_H1 cells (92). A recent report (93) examined the possibility that IL-4, a T_H2 product, may negatively regulate delayed-type hypersensitivity (DTH) and inhibited a model of contact hypersensitivity. It was found that IL-4 partially blocked the efferent phase of hapten-specific contact sensitization but had no effect on the afferent phase of the response. It also appears that IL-4 inhibits the expression of TNF-β and interferon-inducable protein-10 (IP-10) messenger RNA in macrophages treated with culture supernatants from immune lymph node cells. Thus IL-4 exhibits anti-inflammatory activity, which may act by inhibiting cytokine secretion by mononuclear cells. Similarly, IL-4 has been shown to inhibit IL-1α induced GM-CSF expression in murine B lymphocyte cell lines via the downregulation of RNA (94). In other studies from the laboratory of Ogura (95) it was shown that IL-4 could downregulate not only cytokine production but also the activation of human alveolar macrophages to the tumoricidal state. Recent studies have also shown that IL-4 can also upregulate the immune response to a tumor vaccine. In studies from several laboratories (96,97) it has been demonstrated that genetically engineered renal carcinoma cells, which secreted IL-4, have a significant increase in adjuvancy and subsequent protection to tumor challenge. In preliminary assessments, r-hu-IL-4 has been shown to have a direct antiproliferative effect on tumor cells, including specimens from most B cell chronic lymphatic leukemia (CLL) and 50% of the specimens of adult T cell leukemia. Likewise, r-hu-IL-4 has inhibited the proliferation of melanoma patient cells and lymphoma patient tumor specimens. Because of this pharmacologic profile, IL-4 is being pursued for its anti-tumor potential in humans. The effectiveness of IL-4 on cytotoxic cells is highly variable and dependent on their phenotype and state of activation (98). IL-4 inhibits the induction of cytotoxic T cells from resting cells if added before alloantigen (99), antagonizes the ability of IL-2 to induce NK cells to develop LAK cell activity (99–

101), and inhibits the antiproliferative effects of monocytes on melanoma cells *in vitro* (102) as described previously. On the other hand, IL-4 accounts for most of the non-IL-2 cytotoxicity-inducing factor activity present in T cell culture supernatant (103), acts with IL-2 to augment the proliferation and cytolytic activity of alloantigen-specific cytotoxic T lymphocytes or TILs derived from melanoma (104–106), and has therapeutic activity such that antigen-specific cytotoxic tumor may contribute to tumor regression *in vivo*. Initial studies by Tepper et al. (97) suggested that IL-4 exhibits antitumor activity *in vivo*. They demonstrated that tumor cells transfected with cDNA for IL-4 were less tumorigenic than the parental line and that this inhibitory effect could be blocked with the coadministration of an antibody to IL-1. In addition to its effects on cytolytic cells, IL-4 has been shown to strongly inhibit the induction of both IL-1 and TNF synthesis by a variety of stimuli (107–109). These two pyrogenic cytokines are felt to be responsible for many of the side effects observed with high-dose cytokine therapy; thus, there is the potential that IL-4 activates cytotoxic cells without inducing the release of these "negative" cytokines, making IL-4 an attractive agent for clinical investigation. In a phase I evaluation of IL-4, and due to its rapid excretion and poor pharmokinetics, a thrice daily IL-4 administration regime was used (98). In these initial studies toxic symptoms were noted at the dose level of 15 mg/kg of IL-4 and included nasal congestion, diarrhea, nausea and vomiting, fatigue, anorexia, headache, dysaphia, and capillary leak syndrome. Fever with sustained hypotension did not occur and there was a decrease in the lymphocyte count and Ig levels in the patients. Phenotypic analysis of the peripheral blood lymphocytes (PBLs) showed a decrease in the frequency of circulating CD16 and CD14 positive cells. Plasma TNF and IL-1β levels were unaffected, whereas serum C reactive protein concentrations increased slightly and plasma IL-1 receptor antagonist levels increased markedly. In this initial phase I trial, no tumor responses were observed, although one might not expect this to occur in such a preliminary study. It was concluded, based on these preliminary results, that 15 mg/kg of IL-4 is the MTD using this protocol of administration.

CONCLUSION

In the last 20 years, nonspecific immunostimulation has progressed from the initial trials with crude microbial mixtures and extracts to more sophisticated uses with a large collection of immunopharmacologically active compounds (only some of which are discussed here) having diverse actions on various aspects of the immune system. Extensive immunopharmacologic evaluation has followed and a number of classifications have been derived to characterize these agents. A body of immunopharmacologic knowledge has evolved, which shows substantial divergence from conventional pharmacology, particularly in terms of the relationship of dosing schedules to immunopharmacodynamics. This knowledge is important in evaluating agents and predicting appropriate use. While much remains to be learned and new compounds to be extracted and/or cloned, the future of immunotherapy seems bright, particularly in the context of immunorestoration in secondary or iatrogenic cellular immune deficiency.

The major opportunities for the exploitation of immunoregulatory proteins with therapeutic activities are likely to be predicated on combination treatments. Such strategies include the combination of proteins that are clinically efficacious with cytotoxic agents or antibiotics (e.g., IFN-α or IFN-β, zidovudine, and GM-CSF) (4), or a combination of proteins such as IFN-α or IL-2 and TNF. It should be noted that although the growth factors prevent or reduce the depth or duration of neutropenia and reduce the morbidity and mortality associated with secondary infection, there does not appear to be any increased therapeutic efficacy of such combination protocols. Nonetheless, there remains the potential for increased therapeutic efficacy due to an increased number of chemotherapy cycles or dose intensity associated with the support of myeloid augmentation by growth factors.

In summary, a number of the cytokines have been licensed having shown significant therapeutic activity in humans. However, they have as a class general deficiencies including pharmacokinetic liabilities, which have stimulated an interest in the development of orally active peptide mimetics. In theory, synthetic biologic response modifiers (BRMs) would have significant pharmacologic advantages in that they have a potential to be orally active. While synthetic peptides may not have the same high level of biologic activity that the cytokines and growth factors induce, their lower level of activity is compensated by the ease of administration as well as the potential to induce *in situ* the "correct" cocktail of cytokines for optimal immunoregulatory or hematostimulatory activity. Clearly, the latter "hypothesis" has not been adequately tested; regardless, it is becoming clear that combinations of growth factors, cytokines, and BRMs will have optimal activity when used as adjuvants with more traditional therapeutic modalities.

REFERENCES

1. Kuga T, Komatsu Y, Yamasaki M, et al. Mutagenesis of human granulocyte colony stimulating factor. *Biochem Biophys Res Comm* 1989;159:103–111.
2. Rosenberg SA, Grimm E, McGrogan M, Doyle M, Kawasaki E, Koths K, Mark DF. Biological activity of recombinant human interleukin-2 produced in *Escherichia coli*. *Science* 1984;223: 1412–1415.
3. Lu HS, Boone TC, Souza LM, Lai P-H. Disulfide and secondary structures of recombinant human granulocyte colony stimulating factor. *Arch Biochem Biophys* 1989;268:81–92.
4. Krown SE, Paredes J, Buindow D, Polsky B, Gold JWM, Flomemberg N. Interferon-B, zidovudine, and granulocyte-macrophage colony-stimulating factor: a phase I AIDS clinical trials group study in patients with Kaposi's sarcoma associated with AIDS. *J Clin Oncol* 1992;10:1344–1351.
5. Williams DE, Broxmeyer HE, Curtis BM, et al. Enhanced biological activity of a human GM-CSF/IL-3 fusion protein (abst). *Exp Hematol* 1990;18:615.
6. Bruno E, Briddell RA, Cooper RJ, Brandt JE, Hoffman R. Recombinant GM-CSF/IL-3 fusion protein: its effect on in vitro human megakaryocytopoiesis. *Ex Hematol* 1992;20:494–499.
7. Bhalla K, Tang C, Lbrado AM, et al. Granulocyte–macrophage colony-stimulating factor/interleukin-3 fusion protein (pIXY 321) enhances high-dose ara-C-induced programmed cell death or apoptosis in human myeloid leukemia cells. *Blood* 1992;80:2883–2890.
8. Oldham RK. Biological response modifiers program. *J Biol Response Modifiers* 1982;1:81–100.

9. Talmadge JE, Herberman RB. The preclinical screening laboratory. Evaluation of immunomodulatory and therapeutic properties of biological response modifiers. *Cancer Treat Rep* 1986;70:171–182.
10. Mihich E. Future perspectives for biological response modifiers: a viewpoint. *Semin Oncol* 1986; 13:234–254.
11. FDA okays surrogate markers. *Science* 1993;259:171–172.
12. Tomlinson E. Site-specific drugs and delivery systems: toxicological and regulatory implications. In: Breimer DD, Crommelin DJA, Midha KK, eds. *Topics in pharmaceutical sciences*. The Hague: Federation International Pharmaceutic; 1989:661–671.
13. Tomlinson E. Site-specific proteins. In: Hider RC, Barlow D, eds. *Polypeptide and protein drugs: production, characterization and formulation*. Chichester: Ellis Horwood Ltd; 1991:251–364.
14. Talmadge JE, Tribble HR, Pennington RW, Phillips H, Wiltrout RH. Immunomodulatory and immunotherapeutic properties of recombinant γ-interferon and recombinant tumor necrosis factor in mice. *Cancer Res* 1987;47:2563–2570.
15. Misset JL, Mathe G, Gastiaburu J, et al. Treatment of leukemias and lymphomas by interferons: II. Phase II of the trial treatment of chronic lymphoid leukemia by human interferon α^+. *Biomed Pharmacol Ther* 1982;39:112–116.
16. Foon KA, Bottino G, Abrams PG. Phase II trial of recombinant leukocyte A interferon in patients with advanced chronic lymphocytic leukemia. *Am J Med* 1985;78:216–220.
17. Golomb HM, Fefer A, Golde DW, et al. Report of a multi-institutional study of 193 patients with hairy cell leukemia treated with interferon-α 2b. *Semin Oncol* 1988;15:7–9.
18. Quesada JR, Reuben J, Manning JT, Hersh E, Gutterman JU. Alpha interferon for induction of remission in hairy-cell leukemia. *N Engl J Med* 1984;310:15–18.
19. Bunn PA, Foon KA, Ihde DC, et al. Recombinant leukocyte A interferon: an active agent in advanced cutaneous T-cell lymphomas. *Annu J Int Med* 1984;101:484–487.
20. Muss HB. Interferon therapy for renal cell carcinoma. *Semin Oncol* 1987;14:36–42.
21. O'Connell MJ, Colgan JP, Oken MM, Ritts RE Jr, Kay NE, Itri LM. Clinical trial of recombinant leukocyte A interferon as initial therapy for favorable histology non-Hodgkin's lymphomas and chronic lymphocytic leukemia. An Eastern Cooperative Oncology Group pilot study. *J Clin Oncol* 1986;4:128–136.
22. Quesada JR, Rios A, Swanson D, Trown P, Gutterman JU. Antitumor activity of recombinant-derived interferon alpha in metastatic renal cell carcinoma. *J Clin Oncol* 1985;3:1522–1528.
23. Lane HC, Feinberg J, Davey V, et al. Anti-retro-viral effects of interferon-α in AIDS-associated Kaposi's sarcoma. *Lancet* 1988;2(8622):1218–1222.
24. Bhalla K, Birkhofer M, Grant S, Graham G. The effect of recombinant human granulocyte–macrophage colony-stimulating factor (rGM-CSF) on 3′-deoxythymidine (AZT)-mediated biochemical and cytotoxic effects on normal human myeloid progenitor cells. *Exp Hematol* 1989; 17:17–20.
25. Rios A, Mansell P, Newell GR, Reuben JM, Hersh EM, Gutterman JU. Treatment of acquired immunodeficiency syndrome-related Kaposi's sarcoma with lymphoblastoid interferon. *J Clin Oncol* 1985;3:506–512.
26. Groopman JE, Gottlieb MS, Goodman J, et al. Recombinant α-2 interferon therapy for Kaposi's sarcoma associated with the acquired immunodeficiency syndrome. *Ann Intern Med* 1984;100: 671–676.
27. Torti FM, Shortliffe LD, Williams RD, et al. Alpha-interferon in superficial bladder cancer: a Northern California Oncology Group study. *J Clin Oncol* 1988;6:476–483.
28. Moormeier J, Ratain M, Westbrook C, Vardiman J, Daly K, Golomb HM. Low dose interferon in the treatment of hairy cell leukemia. *Proc Am Assoc Cancer Res* 1988;29:215.
29. Jones GJ, Itri LM. Safety and tolerance of recombinant interferon alpha-2a (Roferon-A) in cancer patients. *Cancer* 1986;57:1709–1715.
30. Teichmann JV, Sieber G, Ludwig WD, Ruehl H. Modulation of immune functions by long-term treatment with recombinant interferon-α2 in a patient with hairy-cell leukemia. *J Interferon Res* 1988;8:15–24.
31. Cantell K, Hirvonen S. Preparation of human leukocyte interferon for clinical use. *Tex Rep Biol Med* 1977;35:138–144.
32. Maluish AE, Ortaldo JR, Conlon JC, et al. Depression of natural killer cytotoxicity after in vivo administration of recombinant leukocyte interferon. *J Immunol* 1983;37:236–244.
33. Quesada JR, Reuben NJ, Manning JT, Hersh EM, Gutterman JU. Alpha interferon for induction of remission in hairy cell leukemia. *N Engl J Med* 1984;310:15.

34. Smalley RV, Anderson SA, Tuttle RL, et al. A randomized comparison of two doses of human lymphoblastoid interferon-α in hairy cell leukemia. *Blood* 1991;78:3133–3141.
35. Golomb HM, Fefer A, Golde DW, et al. Report of a multi-institutional study of 193 patients with hairy cell leukemia treated with interferon-α 2b. *Semin Oncol* 1988;15:7–9.
36. Maluish AE, Urba WJ, Longo DLO, et al. The determination of an immunologically active dose of interferon-gamma in patients with melanoma. *J Clin Oncol* 1988;6:434–445.
37. Kleineman ES, Kurzrock R, Wyatt D, Quesada JR, Gutterman JU, Fidler IG. Activation or suppression of the tumoricidal properties of monocytes from cancer patients following treatment with human recombinant γ-interferon. *Cancer Res* 1986;46:5401–5405.
38. Jaffe HS, Herberman RB. Rationale for recombinant human IFN-a adjuvant immunotherapy for cancer (editorial). *J Natl Cancer Inst* 1988;80:616–619.
39. Talpaz M, Kantarjian HM, McCredie K, Trujillo JM, Keating MJ, Gutterman JV. Hematologic remission and cytogenic improvement induced by recombinant human interferon alpha A in chronic myelogenous leukemia. *N Engl J Med* 1986;314:1065–1069.
40. Woodman RC, Richard W, Rae J, Jaffe HS, Curnutte JT. Prolonged recombinant interferon-γ therapy in chronic granulomatous disease: evidence against enhanced neutrophil oxidase activity. *Blood* 1992;79:1558–1562.
41. West WH, Tauer KW, Yannelli JR, Marshall GD, Orr DW, Thurman GB, Oldham RK. Constant-infusion recombinant interleukin-2 plus lymphokine-activated killer cells in metastatic renal cancer. *N Engl J Med* 1987;316:898–905.
42. Oldham O, Maleckar J, West W, Yannelli J. IL-2 and cellular therapy: lymphokine-activated killer cells and tumor-derived activated cells. *Int J Cancer* 1989;43:410–414.
43. Negrier S, Philip T, Stoter G, et al. Interleukin 2 with or without LAK cells in metastatic renal cell carcinoma: a report of a European multicentre study. *Eur J Cancer Clin Oncol* 1989;25:21.
44. Lotze MT, Chang AE, Seipp CA, Simpson C, Vetto SJ, Rosenberg SA. High-dose recombinant interleukin 2 in the treatment of patients with disseminated cancer. Responses, treatment-related morbidity and histologic findings. *JAMA* 1986;256:3117–3124.
45. Ghosh AK, Dazzi H, Thatcher N, Moore M. Lack of correlation between peripheral blood lymphokine-activated killer (LAK) cell function and clinical response in patients with advanced malignant melanoma receiving recombinant interleukin 2. *Int J Cancer* 1989;43:410–414.
46. Sosman JA, Kohler PC, Hank JA, Moore KH, Bechhofer R, Storer B, Sondel PM. Repetitive weekly cycles of interleukin-2. II. Clinical and immunologic effects of dose, schedule, and addition of indomethacin. *J Natl Cancer Inst* 1988;80:1451–1461.
47. Sano T, Saijo N, Sasaki Y, et al. Three schedules of recombinant human interleukin-2 in the treatment of malignancy: side effects and immunologic effects in relation to serum level. *Jpn J Cancer Res (Gann)* 1988;79:131–143.
48. Creekmore SP, Harris JE, Ellis TM, et al. A phase I clinical trial of recombinant interleukin-2 by periodic 24-hour intravenous infusions. *J Clin Oncol* 1989;7:276–284.
49. Sondel PM, Kohler PC, Hank JA, et al. Clinical and immunological effects of recombinant interleukin-2 given by repetitive weekly cycles to patients with cancer. *Cancer Res* 1988;48:2561–2567.
50. Talmadge JE, Phillips H, Schindler J, Tribble H, Pennington R. Systematic preclinical study on the therapeutic properties of recombinant human interleukin-2 for the treatment of metastatic disease. *Cancer Res* 1987;47:5725–5732.
51. Mottel CG. On lymphokines, cytokines and breakthroughs. *JAMA* 1986;256:1341.
52. Thompson JA, Lee DJ, Lindgren CG, Benz LA, Collins C, Levitt D, Fefer A. Influence of dose and duration of infusion of interleukin-2 on toxicity and immunomodulation. *J Clin Oncol* 1988; 6:669–678.
53. Herberman RB. Interleukin-2 therapy of human cancer: potential benefits versus toxicity. *J Clin Oncol* 1989;7:1–4.
54. Herberman RB. Clinical cancer therapy with IL-2. *Cancer Invest* 1989;7:515–516.
55. Stevenson HC, Creekmore S, Stewart M, et al. Interleukin-2 and lymphokine-activated killer cell therapy: analysis of bolus interleukin 2 and a continuous infusion interleukin 2 regimen. *Cancer Res* 1990;50:7343–7350.
56. Alper J. Cetus' proleukin in cancer—the excitement grows. *SCRIP* 1988;1363:24.
57. Konrad MW, Hamstreet G, Hersh EM, Mansell PWA, Mertelsmann R, Kolitz JE, Bradley EC. Pharmacokinetics of recombinant interleukin-2 in humans. *Cancer Res* 1990;50:2009.
58. Lu HS, Boone TC, Souza LM, Lai P-H. Disulfide and secondary structures of recombinant human granulocyte colony stimulating factor. *Arch Biochem Biophys* 1989;268:81–92.

59. Crum ED, Kaplan DR. In vivo activity of solid phase interleukin 2. *Cancer Res* 1991;51:875.
60. Jujjwara T, Sakagami K, Matsuoka J, et al. Application of an interleukin-2 slow delivery system to the immunotherapy of established murine colon 26 adenocarcinoma liver metastases. *Cancer Res* 1990;50:7003.
61. Vlasveld LT, Rankin EM, Hekman A, et al. A phase I study of prolonged continuous infusion of low dose recombinant interleukin-2 in melanoma and renal cell cancer. Part I: clinical aspects. *Br J Cancer* 1992;65:744–750.
62. Lim SH, Newland AC, Kelsey S, et al. Continuous intravenous infusion of high-dose recombinant interleukin-2 for acute myeloid leukaemia-a phase II study. *Cancer Immunol Immunother* 1992; 34:337–342.
63. Clark JW, Smith JW II, Steis RG, et al. Interleukin-2 and lymphokine-activated killer cell therapy: analysis of a bolus interleukin-2 and a continuous infusion interleukin-2 regimen. *Cancer Res* 1990;50:7343–7350.
64. Thompson JA, Shulman KL, Benyunes MC, et al. Prolonged continuous intravenous infusion interleukin-2 and lymphokine-activated killer-cell therapy for metastatic renal cell carcinoma. *J Clin Oncol* 1992;10:960–968.
65. Bush HW. The importance of dose intensity in chemotherapy of metastatic breast cancer (review). *J Clin Oncol* 1984;2:1281–1288.
66. Hryniuk W, Levine MN. Analysis of dose intensity for adjuvant chemotherapy trials in stage II breast cancer. *J Clin Oncol* 1986;4:1162–1167.
67. Tannock IF, Boyd NF, DeBoer G, et al. A randomized trial of two dose levels of cyclophosphamide, methotrexate, and fluorouracil chemotherapy for patients with metastatic breast cancer. *J Clin Oncol* 1988;6:1377–1387.
68. Herrmann F, Schulz G, Lindemann A, Meyenburg W, Krumwieh D, Mertelsmann R. Yeast-expressed granulocyte–macrophage colony-stimulating factor in cancer patients; a phase 1b clinical study. *Behring Inst Mitt* 1988;83:107–118.
69. Neidhart JA, Mangalik A, Stidley CA, Tebich SL, Sarmiento LE, Pfile JE. Dosing regimen of granulocyte–macrophage colony-stimulating factor to support dose-intensive chemotherapy. *J Clin Oncol* 1992;10:1460–1469.
70. Cebon J, Lieschke GJ, Bury RW, Morstyn G. The dissociation of GM-CSF efficacy toxicity according to route of administration: a pharmacodynamic study. *Br J Hematol* 1992;80:144–150.
71. Meisenberg BR, David TA, Melaragno AJ, Stead R, Monroy RL. A comparison of therapeutic schedules for administering granulocyte colony-stimulating factor to nonhuman primates after high-dose chemotherapy. *Blood* 1992;79:2267–2272.
72. Meropol MJ, Miller LL, Korn EL, Braitman LE, MacDermott ML, Schuchter LM. Severe myelosuppression resulting from concurrent administration of granulocyte colony-stimulating factor and cytotoxic chemotherapy. *J Natl Cancer Inst* 1992;84:1201–1203.
73. Gabrilove JL, Jakubowski A, Scher H, et al. Effect of granulocyte colony-stimulating factor on neutropenia and associated morbidity due to chemotherapy for transitional-cell carcinoma of the urothelium. *N Engl J Med* 1988;318:1414–1422.
74. Morstyn G, Souza LM, Keech J, et al. Effect of granulocyte colony stimulating factor on neutropenia induced by cytotoxic chemotherapy. *Lancet* 1988;26:667–671.
75. Komiyama A, Ishiguro A, Kubo T, et al. Increases in neutrophil counts by purified human urinary colony-stimulating factor in chronic neutropenia of childhood. *Blood* 1988;71:41–45.
76. Sanda MG, Yang JC, Topalian SL, et al. Intravenous administration of recombinant human macrophage colony-stimulating factor to patients with metastatic cancer: a phase I study. *J Clin Oncol* 1992;10:1643–1649.
77. Bronchud MH, Potter MR, Morgenstern G, et al. In vitro and in vivo analysis of the effects of recombinant human granulocyte colony-stimulating factor in patients. *Br J Cancer* 1988;58:64–69.
78. Gutterman J. Clinical studies of granulocyte–macrophage colony stimulating factor. *Semin Oncol* 1988;15:52–53.
79. Kaplan SS, Basford RE, Wing EJ, Shadduck RK. The effect of recombinant human granulocyte macrophage colony stimulating factor on neutrophil activation in patients with refractory carcinoma. *Blood* 1989;73:636–638.
80. Brugger W, Frisch J, Schulz J, Pressler K, Mertelsman R, Kanz L. Sequential administration of interleukin-3 and granulocyte–macrophage colony stimulant factor following standard dose combination chemotherapy with etoposide, ifosfamide and cisplatin. *J Clin Oncol* 1994;10:1452–1459.
81. Wong HL, Lotze MT, Wahl LM, Wahl SM. Administration of recombinant IL-4 to humans regu-

lates gene expression, phenotype, and function in circulating monocytes. *J Immunol* 1992;148: 2118–2125.
82. Smith JW II, Urba WJ, Curti BD, et al. The toxic and hematologic effects of interleukin-1 alpha administered in a phase I trial to patients with advanced malignancies. *J Clin Oncol* 1992;10:1141–1152.
83. Dean JH, Comacoff JB, Barbolt TA, Gossett KA, LaBrie T. Pre-clinical toxicity of IL-4: a model for studying protein therapeutics. *Int J Immunopharmacol* 1992;14:391–397.
84. Ben-Sasson SZ, LeGros G, Conrad DH, Finkelman FD, Paul WE. IL-4 production by T cells from naive donors. IL-2 is required for IL-4 production. *J Immunol* 1990;140:1127.
85. Paul WE. Interleukin 4/B cell stimulatory factor 1: one lymphokine, many functions. *FASEB J* 1988;1:456.
86. Finkelman FD, Holmes J, Katona IM, et al. Lymphokine control of in vivo immunoglobulin isotope selection. *Annu Rev Immun* 1990;8:303.
87. Mitchell LC, Davis LS, Lipsky P. Promotion of human T lymphocyte proliferation by IL-4. *J Immun* 1989;142:1548–1557.
88. Spits H, Yssel H, Paliard X, Kastelein R, Rigdor C, DeVries JE. IL-4 inhibits IL-2 mediated induction of human lymphokine-activated killer cells, but not the generation of antigen-specific cytotoxic T lymphocytes in mixed leukocyte cultures. *J Immunol* 1988;141:29.
89. Kawakami Y, Rosenberg SA, Lotze MT. Interleukin-4 promotes the growth of tumour-infiltrating lymphocytes cytotoxic for human autologous melanoma. *J Exp Med* 1988;168:2183–2191.
90. Mosmann TR, Cherwinski H, Bond MW, Giedlin MA, Coffman RL. Two types of murine helper T cell clone. 1. Definition according to profiles of lymphokine activities and secreted proteins. *J Immunol* 1986;136:23–48.
91. Mosmann TR, Moore KW. The role of IL-10 in crossregulation of Th1 and Th2 responses. *Immunol Today* 1991;12:A49.
92. Florentino DF, Bond MW, Mosmann TR. Th2 clones secrete a factor that inhibits cytokine production by Th1 clones. *J Exp Med* 1989;170:2081.
93. Subhash C, Gautam CNF, Hamilton TA. Anti-inflammatory action of IL-4. *Am Assoc Immunologists* 1992;148:1411–1415.
94. Akahane K, Pluznik DH. Interleukin-4 inhibits interleukin-1α-induced granulocyte–macrophage colony-stimulating factor gene expression in a murine B-lymphocyte cell line via downregulation of RNA precursor. *Blood* 1992;79:3188–3195.
95. Nishioka Y, Sone S, Orino E, Nii A, Ogura T. Down-regulation by interleukin 4 of activation of human alveolar macrophages to the tumoricidal state. *Cancer Res* 1991;51:5526–5531.
96. Golumbek PT, Lazenby AJ, Levitsky HI, Jaffee LM, Karasuyama H, Baker M, Pardoll DM. Treatment of established renal cancer by tumor cells engineered to secrete interleukin-4. *Science* 1991;254:713–716.
97. Tepper RI, Pattengale PK, Leder P. Murine interleukin-4 displays potent anti-tumor activity in vivo. *Cell* 1989;57:503–512.
98. Atkins MB, Vachino G, Tilg HJ, Karp DD, Robert NJ, Kappler K, Mier JW. Phase I evaluation of thrice-daily intravenous bolus interleukin-4 in patients with refractory malignancy. *J Clin Oncol* 1992;10:1802–1809.
99. Horohov DW, Crim JA, Smith PL, et al. IL-4 (B cell stimulatory factor 1) regulates multiple aspects of influenza virus-specific cell-mediated immunity. *J Immunol* 1988;141:4217–4223.
100. Kawakami Y, Custer MC, Rosenberg SA, et al. IL-4 regulates IL-2 induction of lymphokine-activated killer activity from human lymphocytes. *J Immunol* 1989;142:3452–3461.
101. Spits H, Yssel H, Paliard X, et al. IL-4 inhibits IL-2-mediated induction of human lymphokine-activated killer cells, but not the generation of antigen-specific cytotoxic T lymphocytes in mixed leukocyte cultures. *J Immunol* 1988;141:29–36.
102. Te Velde AA, Klomp JPG, Yard BA, et al. Modulation of phenotypic and functional properties on human peripheral blood monocytes. *J Immunol* 1988;140:1548–1554.
103. Garman RD, Fan DP. Characterization of helper factors distinct from IL-2 necessary for the generation of allospecific cytotoxic T lymphocytes. *J Immunol* 1983;130:756–762.
104. Lotze MT, Zeh HJ III, Elder EM, et al. Use of T-cell growth factors (interleukins 2, 4, 7, 10, and 12) in the evaluation of T-cell reactivity to melanoma. *J Immunother* 1992;12(3):212–217.
105. Kawakami Y, Rosenberg SA, Lotze MT. Interleukin-4 promotes the growth of tumor-infiltrating lymphocytes cytotoxic for human autologous melanoma. *J Exp Med* 1988;168:2183–2191.

106. Widmer MD, Acres RB, Sassenfeld HM, et al. Regulation of stimulatory factor 1 (interleukin 4). *J Exp Med* 1987;166:1447–1451.
107. Essner R, Rhoades K, McBride WH, et al. IL-4 down-regulates IL-1 and TNF gene expression in human monocytes. *J Immunol* 1989;142:3857–3861.
108. Te Velde AA, Huijbens RJF, Heije K, et al. Interleukin-4 (IL-4) inhibits secretion of IL-1B, TNF alpha, and IL-6 by human monocytes. *Blood* 1990;76:1392–1397.
109. Kotik A, Mier JW. Selective cytokine in mRNA destabilization: a contributing factor in IL-4 mediated suppression of IL-2-induced IL-1β synthesis. *Int J Immunopathol Pharmacol* 1992;4: 123.

Immunotoxicology and Immunopharmacology, Second Edition, edited by J. H. Dean, M. I. Luster, A. E. Munson, and I. Kimber.
Raven Press, Ltd., New York © 1994.

14

Immunotoxicologic Manifestations of AIDS Therapeutics

Gary J. Rosenthal and *Michael Kowolenko

*Department of Drug Development, Somatogen, Inc., Boulder, Colorado 80301; and *Department of Pre-Clinical Biology, Miles Pharmaceutical Company, West Haven, Connecticut 06516*

Therapeutic development and treatment for acquired immunodeficiency syndrome (AIDS) has proven to be a formidable task with respect to selectivity for the invader and toxicity to the host. The very nature of an immunodeficiency disease begs consideration of the impact of the potential therapeutic on immune system components (Table 1). While previous therapeutic dogma considered suppression of immune function an undesirable adverse effect in AIDS, current clinical thinking favors an approach of immune upregulation for cytotoxic T lymphocytes and an overall suppression of other aspects of immune activity. It is hypothesized that this type of immune targeting would help maintain the CD4+ response to infection, primarily in the T helper type 1 (T_H1) cells and it would activate the cytotoxic T lymphocyte response. At the same time a reduction in inflammatory cytokines might also help to prevent already infected cells from expressing the virus and recruiting uninfected cells to anergy and apoptosis.

Rationale drug design for preventing the infection or replication of human immunodeficiency virus 1 (HIV-1) in host cells employs several strategies that interrupt various steps in the life cycle of the virus. To minimize toxicity, the pharmacologic agent should preferentially modulate biochemical processes unique to the virus without interfering with the normal cells' biochemistry. Unfortunately, because the virus utilizes end products of biochemical pathways of the host cell, it has proven to be exceptionally difficult to design compounds that prevent viral replication without affecting the host. Current treatment of HIV-1 infections includes inhibiting the infectivity of HIV-1 by altering the binding of the virion to the CD4 molecule or interference with virus-specific regulatory or structural enzymes.

To date, drug development for AIDS has largely been focused on two viral targets: reverse transcriptase and, more recently, viral protease. Reverse transcriptase

TABLE 1. *Major abnormalities of immune function in AIDS*

Leukopenia
Selective loss of CD4+ (helper/inducer T cell subset)
Suppressed cellular immunity *in vivo*
Increased susceptibility to opportunistic infections and certain neoplasms
Decreased delayed-type hypersensitivity response
Impaired CTL function
Suppressed CD4+ cell function in response to T cell mitogens
Suppressed lymphokine (IL-2, IFN-γ)
Polyclonal B cell activation
Hypergammaglobulinemia and increased levels of circulating immune complex
Altered monocyte or macrophage function
Decreased chemotaxis and Ia antigen expression

is a viral enzyme that enables the ribonucleic acid (RNA) of the virus to be transcribed into a deoxyribonucleic acid (DNA) fragment that can be inserted into the host cell. Reverse transcriptase is an appealing drug target because its inactivation would prevent the virus from integrating its DNA and thus reproducing itself. In addition, it was theorized that toxicity would be low because the enzyme is not present in normal human cells. While a number of reverse transcription inhibitors are now in clinical use and marketed, at the time of this writing, no protease inhibitors are on the market.

To design effective treatments, it is necessary to understand the life cycle of the virus. Infection of the host cell by HIV-1 is accomplished as follows. The virion binds to CD4 antigen on target cells via its envelope glycoprotein gp-120 (1). This is followed by fusion or endocytosis of the virion (2). Following internalization, there is a release of viral RNA, viral reverse transcriptase, and integrase within the cytoplasm of the host cell (3). Each enzyme is essential for viral integration. Viral reverse transcriptase utilizes the viral RNA as a template and synthesizes its corresponding double-stranded DNA using nucleoside triphosphates generated by the metabolic machinery of the host cell (4,5). Each complementary strand of viral DNA is synthesized with long terminal repeats (LTRs) on each 5′ end for use by the viral integrase as well as to serve as recognition sequences for viral regulatory proteins. Viral integrase and cDNA are transported to the nucleus where integration into genomic DNA occurs. Integration of viral cDNA results in the proviral form of HIV-1 (6).

Transcriptional activation of the provirus occurs following activation of the host cell (7,8) and leads to increased production of the nucleoid and structural proteins with virion assembly and budding from the infected cell. Control of viral reproduction is dependent on host cell activation but is enhanced by the production of regulatory proteins coded for by the integrated virus, primarily *tat*, but also including nef and *rev* (6). Structural proteins (gag) and polymerase (pol) are reportedly regulated by *rev* (9) and are upregulated following the interaction of *tat* with the LTRs (10). These regulatory and structural proteins are unique to the virus and are attractive targets for pharmacologic intervention.

AGENTS INFLUENCING HIV-1 INTERACTION WITH TARGETS

Soluble CD4

Soluble CD4 (sCD4) is a recombinant protein that represents a truncated form of the human CD4 molecule (11). Modifications include removal of the transmembrane and C-terminal region of the molecule (11). In phase I clinical trials, sCD4 was administered as an intravenous (iv), subcutaneous (sc), or intramuscular (im) injection with patients receiving doses daily for up to 10 days followed by a washout period and subsequent dosing three times a week for 8 weeks (12). Dosages ranged from 1 to 300 μg/kg. Immunologic parameters monitored included total leukocyte counts, total CD4+ and CD8+ cells, and anti-CD4+ antibody formatiom, serum immunoglobulin, and total complement levels. No drug-related effects were observed on any of the immunologic parameters assessed.

In a dose-escalation study, patients were treated with sCD4 at doses of 9 or 30 mg/d in three divided doses, intramuscularly for 28 days (13). Lymphocyte phenotyping (CD3, CD4, and CD8) and anti-sCD4 formation were assessed as an indication of immunotoxicity and efficacy. No significant changes were observed in the distribution or number of lymphocytes obtained from treated patients. Anti-sCD4 antibody formation was observed in 1 of 11 patients. Based on these data, it would appear that sCD4 treatment does not alter immune function. Unfortunately, there did not appear to be amelioration of the severity of infection in these early clinical trials.

A second-generation of modified sCD4 molecules synthesized with the purpose of destroying HIV-1-infected cells are the sCD4 immunoadhesins or the sCD4 immunotoxins. In the case of the immunoadhesins, the CD4 molecule has been modified by the addition of the hinge and Fc regions of a human immunoglobulin G (IgG) antibody. This provides greater activity and increased serum half-life when compared to the truncated sCD4 molecule (14). In a phase I dose-escalation study, doses of up to 1000 μg/kg weekly for 12 weeks had no effect on lymphocyte CD4 counts, suggesting that there is no overt immunotoxicity with this compound (12).

An immunotoxin consisting of ricin-A chain and recombinant CD4 is under investigation. This compound is targeted at infected cells expressing the viral gp-120 protein. *In vitro* assays of immune function indicate that sCD4–ricin-A failed to inhibit B cell activation or T cell responsiveness in the mixed lymphocyte reaction (15).

Assessment of the immunotoxicity of sCD4 poses several technical difficulties. Use of preclinical animal models may not provide an accurate representation of the immunomodulatory effect of this compound. As a recombinant human protein, sCD4 could be expected to be a potent immunogen in rodents and, to a lesser extent, in primates. Anti-sCD4 antibody formation possesses another safety concern—generation of these antibodies could lead to targeting of CD4+ cells, leading to further destruction of an already depleted cell population.

Based on its interaction with the major histocompatibility complex (MHC) of antigen-presenting cells (as a prerequisite for antigen-specific responsiveness), there is the potential of sCD4 to interfere with immune function. Binding of sCD4 to the MHC molecules of antigen-presenting cells would be expected to interfere with normal antigen presentation. However, *in vitro* data indicate that antigen presentation is not inhibited by the presence of sCD4 (16). Further clinical trials are required in order to determine the safety and efficacy of this form of treatment.

AGENTS TARGETING HIV-1 REPLICATION

The discovery that viral reverse transcriptase (DNA polymerase) has a higher affinity for dideoxynucleotides than deoxynucleotides along with the knowledge that mammalian DNA polymerase α and β had rather low affinity for dideoxynucleotides led to the use of these compounds in the treatment of HIV-1 infection (17–19). The primary mechanism of action of the dideoxynucleotides is to serve as substrates for reverse transcriptase that, if incorporated into viral DNA, result in chain termination. Viral DNA, like mammalian DNA, requires the formation of $5' \rightarrow 3'$ phosphodiester bonds. By modifying the $3'$ position of the nucleoside sugar so that chain elongation is terminated, viral replication is halted. In addition, these compounds appear to inhibit the activity of viral reverse transcriptase (20–22).

Zidovudine

Zidovudine (3′-azido-3′-deoxythymidine, AZT), a pyrimidine analog, was the first reverse transcriptase inhibitor shown to be clinically effective in the treatment of HIV-1 (23,24). Typical treatment consists of 20 mg/kg administered three to four times daily (23). Unfortunately, the major dose-limiting toxicity of this compound observed in the clinic is myelotoxicity characterized by macrocytic megaloblastic anemia and granulocytopenia (23,25).

Conversion of AZT to its active moiety AZT triphosphate (AZT-TP) requires the sequential phosphorylation of AZT to AZT monophosphate (AZT-MP) by thymidine kinase followed by its conversion to the diphosphate form by thymidylate kinase. This second step in the activation is reported to be the rate-limiting AZT-TP synthesis. Cell lines cultured in the presence of AZT show an accumulation of AZT-MP with relatively lower concentrations of the di- and triphosphates (26,27). The effective concentration of AZT-TP required for inhibition of HIV reverse transcriptase is 0.16 to 0.45 μM (27).

While the most pronounced toxicity of AZT is on innate immunity, there appears to be little effect of this compound on acquired immunity. In preclinical studies, B6CDF1 mice were treated with up to 400 mg/kg daily for 22 days by oral gavage. Assessment of the antibody response, mixed leukocyte response, cytotoxicity assays, and clonogenic hematopoietic assays were performed along with hematologic analysis of peripheral blood (28,29). The data obtained displayed a slight macrocytic anemia. However, there was no corresponding decrease in bone marrow colony formation. Plaque-forming cell (PFC) response to sheep red blood cells

(SRBCs) and cell-mediated cytotoxicity [cytotoxic T lymphocyte (CTL), natural killer (NK) cell, and macrophage-mediated] were affected.

Numerous clinical studies (17,23,30,31) have shown that treatment with AZT increases the number of circulating CD4+ cells. This has been accepted as a surrogate marker for an improvement in the immunologic status of patients infected with HIV-1. To further support its lack of immunotoxicity, Glaser et al. (32) have demonstrated that AZT treatment enhances the response to pneumococcal vaccine, suggesting that AZT does not interfere with the ability of the immune system to generate antigen-specific antibodies.

In an effort to determine the effect of AZT on the cellular immune response in humans treated with AZT, Rinaldo et al. (33) assessed lymphocyte subsets, proliferative response to phytohemagglutinin (PHA), cytomegalovirus (CMV), herpes simplex 1, and interleukin-2 (IL-2), NK cell-mediated cytotoxicity, and interferon-γ (IFN-γ) production. These results suggest a transient stimulation of cellular immunity following AZT treatment that did not appear to be dose related. Mitogenic responses and IFN-γ production following PHA-induced blastogenesis were somewhat elevated compared to pretreatment values, as was the response to CMV and NK cell activity. In each case, the increases were transient, occurring 10 to 20 weeks after therapy, and returned to baseline 40 weeks after treatment (33).

The myelotoxicity of AZT has been observed in a number of *in vitro* and *in vivo* systems. The IC_{50} (concentration that inhibits 50%) of AZT in a human clonogenic bone marrow assay using granulocyte–macrophage colony-stimulating factor (GM-CSF) is reported to be approximately 1.0 μm (34). Similar values have been obtained from murine bone marrow cells (35,36). Erythroid colonies appear to be more sensitive with the IC_{50} reported to be approximately 0.1 μm (37) following continuous exposure to AZT. The marrow toxicity observed has been attributed to perturbation of the nucleotide pool as a result of the accumulation of AZT-MP. Perturbation of the nucleotide pool has long been associated with lymphocyte toxicity (e.g., adenosine deaminase and purine nucleoside phosphorylase deficiencies). Frick et al. (38) have shown that incubation of HL-60, H-9, and K-562 human cell lines in the presence of 200 μm AZT results in inhibition of thymidylate kinase with subsequent depletion of dTTP. Investigators have reported reversal of the *in vitro* myelotoxicity of AZT by co-culturing bone marrow cells with deoxycytidine (39) or uridine (40). Exposure of cells to AZT and deoxycytidine produces an increase in deoxythymidine triphosphate (dTTP) and deoxycytidine triphosphate (dCTP) pools. Deoxycytidine monophosphate (dCMP) is converted to deoxyuridine triphosphate (dUTP) by dCMP deaminase with conversion to deoxythymidine monophosphate (dTMP); dTMP can compete with AZT-MP for thymidylate kinase, thereby reducing toxicity.

However, Sommadossi et al. (34) have demonstrated that human bone marrow exposed to pharmacologically relevant concentrations of AZT (10 μm) had minimal decrease in the dTTP pool. Furthermore, in the same study, AZT was shown to be incorporated into host DNA in a manner consistent with chain termination.

The metabolites of AZT may also play a pivotal role in the myelotoxicity of AZT.

Cretton et al. (41) have shown that AZT was converted to 3′-amino-3′-deoxythymidine (AMT) in human bone marrow, which was five- to sevenfold more toxic than AZT in a human bone marrow clonogenic assay. AMT has been shown to be a potent inhibitor of DNA polymerase α with an IC_{50} of approximately 1 μm (42). Interestingly, Fischer et al. (43) demonstrated that the *in vitro* cytotoxicity of 3′-AMP can be reversed by dideoxycytidine (dCyd), perhaps by competing with AMT as a substrate for thymidylate kinase in a manner analogous to that observed with AZT.

Based on experimental data, the myelotoxicity of AZT may not be an exclusive event since a combination of factors may contribute. These include the incorporation and termination of DNA synthesis, its metabolism to AMT, a potent inhibitor of DNA polymerase α, and, to a lesser extent, the depletion of dTTP pools within the host cell.

2′, 3′-Didehydro-2′, 3′-dideoxythymidine

A second pyrimidine analog currently in clinical trials is d4T (2′, 3′-didehydro-2′, 3′-dideoxythymidine, stavudine). Like AZT, this thymidine derivative lacks a 3′ hydroxy group, thus resulting in chain termination. However, unlike AZT, the rate-limiting step in the activation of d4T to its active triphosphate form is its conversion from d4T to d4T monophosphate (d4T-MP) by thymidine kinase (27). The IC_{50} for d4T is reported to be 0.33 μm (44).

In a 30-day toxicology study, CD-1 mice were dosed with up to 1000 mg/kg d4T daily, by gavage. Erythrocytopenia was observed as was leukopenia and absolute lymphopenia (44). To determine if the decrease in leukocyte counts was associated with alterations in immune function, B6C3F1 mice were treated with 500 mg/kg daily for 30 days by gavage. At the end of treatment, animals were assessed for alterations in lymphocyte subsets, mitogenic response, antibody formation, bone marrow responsiveness to IL-3, and host resistance to *Listeria monocytogenes*. These results indicate no effect on any parameter measured (M. Kowolenko, *unpublished data*).

Luster et al. (29) have demonstrated similar findings in mice treated with 500 mg/kg d4T for 30 days, which failed to show any alteration in the generation of CTLs, NK cell activity, PFC response, or mixed lymphocyte response. These investigators observed a decrease in the number of erythroid colonies (CFU-E) formed from bone marrow of C57BL/6 mice (Ah^+) in response to erythropoietin while DBA mice (Ah low) failed to display a decrease in the CFU-E assay, implying that differences in metabolism of d4T may account for the toxicity observed.

In clinical trials, where the anticipated clinical doses are 0.5 to 1 mg/kg/d, the dose-limiting toxicity of d4T appears to be a sensory peripheral neuropathy rather than a myelotoxicity as observed with AZT (45). The circulating levels of CD4+ increased in patients receiving d4T, implying that this compound may improve the immunologic status of these patients (45).

As stated previously, the rate-limiting reaction in the activation of d4T is formation of d4T-MP, which does not appear to inhibit thymidylate kinase or alter dTTP pools as does AZT. There is evidence that d4T is incorporated into host DNA at a much lower rate than AZT and that metabolism of d4T differs considerably from AZT (46). Zhu et al. (46) have shown that d4T is degraded to thymine followed by formation to thymidine (dThd), which is excised from host DNA while AZT is not. This may account for the difference in myelotoxicity observed between AZT and d4T.

2′, 3′-Dideoxycytidine

A third pyrimidine analog that has recently been approved for use is ddC (2′, 3′-dideoxycytidine, zalcitabine). Like AZT and d4T, its antiviral activity is associated with inhibition of viral reverse transcriptase and chain termination (47). Metabolic activation requires the conversion of the ddC to ddC monophosphate (ddC-MP) by deoxycytidine kinase followed by phosphorylation to its di- and triphosphate forms. The IC_{50} for ddC is 0.046 to 0.6 μm (48). Clinical doses range from 0.03 to 0.75 mg/kg/d with the dose-limiting toxicity being peripheral neuropathy (49).

In order to determine the immunotoxic effect of ddC, Luster et al. (28,29) treated C57Bl/6 mice with up to 600 mg/kg daily, by gavage for 30 days and evaluated clinical hematology, antibody response, mixed lymphocyte response, cytotoxicity, and hematopoietic function. These studies found no significant effects on immune function following ddC exposure. There appeared to be a decreased erythrocyte count in the 300- and 600-mg/kg dose groups, although marrow cellularity and myeloid colony formation were unaltered. *In vitro* exposure of bone marrow cells to ddC inhibited stromal cell colony formation at concentrations ranging from 5 to 50 μm. Likewise, other investigators have shown a concentration-dependent inhibition of bone marrow colony formation by ddC (50). Clinically, there appears to be no significant myelotoxicity (31,51–53). Clinical studies have demonstrated that ddC improves the CD4+ count and restores cellular immunity as assessed by skin testing, implying that there is improvement in the immunologic status of these HIV-infected patients. Due to dose-limiting toxicity of peripheral neuropathy with ddC and the hematotoxicity associated with AZT, current protocols call for the clinical combination of these two agents at lower dosages or on a rotational schedule (31,54,55).

2′, 3′-dideoxyinosine

The first purine analog that has been approved for treatment of HIV-1 infection is ddI (2′, 3′-dideoxyinosine, videx). Following administration, ddI is converted to ddI monophosphate (ddI-MP) by 5′-nucleotidase, which in turn is converted to dideoxyadenosine monophosphate (ddA-MP) with subsequent formation to ddA-TP (18,56,57). Initially, ddA was considered as an antiviral agent; however, in the low pH of the stomach it is rapidly converted to free adenine. The metabolism of adenine results in the formation of insoluble 2,8-dihydroxyadenine that precipitates in renal tubules, leading to renal failure. While free ddI is also cleaved in the gut to its base and sugar, the catabolism of inosine results in increased levels of uric acid (58,59). At clinical doses of 8 to 12 mg/kg/d, the dose-limiting toxicity for ddI has been peripheral neuropathy and pancreatitis (60–62).

Preclinical studies have shown that ddI, when administered at a dose of 1050 mg/kg/d for 30 days to B6C3F1 mice, produced a decrease in the PFC response to SRBCs (29). Cao et al. (63), using ddA, have shown a dose-dependent decrease in the PFC response. The mechanism of this toxicity has been attributed to chain termination or purine cytotoxicity as a result of the accumulation of adenosine (63). No other alterations in immune function have been observed with either ddI or ddA.

Clinical studies have demonstrated the effectiveness of ddI in improving CD4 counts and restoring cellular immunity as determined by reversal of anergy, increased blastogenic response to pokeweed mitogen (PWM), and increased *ex vivo* antigen-specific responses (64). In addition, HIV-1-associated myelosuppression has also been reversed following ddI treatment (65).

AGENTS TARGETING OPPORTUNISTIC DISEASES

One of the most insidious aspects of AIDS is the plethora of opportunistic pathogens that are most often ultimately responsible for the high rate of mortality (66) (Table 2). Opportunistic infections such as *Pneumocystis carinii*, which rarely affects healthy individuals, is seen in approximately 50% of cases. A variety of other (often multiple) opportunistic infections, including CMV, candidiasis, toxoplasmosis, and herpesvirus infections, have also been found in AIDS patients. In addition, recent studies have identified a variety of bacterial infections as well, presumably related to defects in humoral immunity (67). In addition, neoplasia, primarily in the form of Kaposi's sarcoma, manifests in about 25% of patients (68). These superimposed disease states present the clinician with difficult choices in treating AIDS and often result in multiple therapeutic regimens. Below are representative examples of therapeutic agents currently used to target opportunistic pathogens.

Pentamidine Isethionate

Pneumocystis carinii pneumonia is a frequent cause of morbidity and mortality in immunocompromised patients and afflicts more than 50% of patients with AIDS (66). Pentamidine has been used since the 1930s as an antiprotozoal agent (69) and is now widely used for the treatment of infection due to *P. carinii*, particularly in patients with AIDS (70). While a high risk of toxicity occurs with parenteral administration of the drug (71), administration via inhalation has been used successfully for the treatment and prophylaxis of *P. carinii* pneumonia in AIDS patients (72). The exact mechanism of action for pentamidine on *P. carinii* pneumonia is unclear,

TABLE 2. *Selected secondary infections and neoplasms found in patients with HIV infection*

Protozoal or helminthic infections
Cryptosporidiosis
Pneumocystis carinii
Toxoplasmosis
Fungal infections
Candidiasis
Cryptococcosis
Histoplasmosis
Bacterial infections
Mycobacteriosis
Salmonella
Viral infections
Cytomegalovirus
Herpesvirus
Malignant neoplasms
Burkitt's lymphoma
Kaposi's sarcoma

although impairment of oxidative phosphorylation, nucleic acid synthesis, glucose metabolism, or dihydrofolate reductase in the parasite have been suggested to contribute to its efficacy (71).

In light of the dramatic increase in the use of pentamidine within the past 5 years, a significant effort has been made to understand the potential immunotoxicity, both *in vitro* and *in vivo*. While the impaired immune status of patients receiving pentamidine for AIDS has made clinical evaluation of its immunotoxicity difficult, a number of animal and *in vitro* studies have shed some light on its potential for immunomodulation. Rosenthal et al. (73) demonstrated that pentamidine inhibits the release of IL-1 from alveolar macrophages at pharmacologic concentrations through impairment of post-translational processing. Further studies demonstrated that other inflammatory cytokines including IL-6 and tumor necrosis factor (TNF) were similarly suppressed by pentamidine both *in vivo* (74) and *in vitro* (75,76). Since TNF has been shown to be influential in eradication of the *P. carinii* organism, such suppression by pentamidine may be considered adversative. However, other immunosuppressant drugs, including corticosteroids, have proved beneficial in AIDS-related *P. carinii* pneumonia; consequently, it is debatable whether such a suppression of inflammatory cytokines can be assessed as a toxicity or perhaps a mechanism of pharmacologic action.

Interferon-α (IFNα)

While the pathogenesis of Kaposi's sarcoma (KS) in the context of AIDS is not completely understood, the particularly aggressive nature of this neoplastic disease underscores the importance of effective therapeutic strategies. IFN-α has been used with substantial success in the treatment of KS (68). Although the precise mechanism for its action remains to be elucidated, its immunomodulatory capacity such as the rise in the number of CD4+ cells, the increase in β_2-microglobulin, and the well-known stimulation of NK cell activity may all play a role (68). Toxicologically, human studies have been hampered by the confounding factors of altered immune responsiveness from the disease process itself (i.e., cancer, AIDS). For example, Einhorn et al. (77) have shown that the levels of 2′,5′-oligoadenylate synthetase, a cellular enzyme increased in the antiviral action of IFNs and associated with decreased lymphoid proliferation, was elevated in lymphocytes from cancer patients prior to IFN treatment. The mitogenic responsiveness of those patients was also suppressed when compared with the healthy donor group in the absence of IFN treatment, and under these conditions it would be possible to miss IFN-induced effects on lymphocytes.

In addition to clinically observed hematotoxicity, IFN-α has been implicated as an inhibitor of myelopoiesis (78), a finding that has been supported by *in vitro* studies (79). Unfortunately, the high degree of species specificity associated with both natural and recombinant human IFN-α has limited the information available from preclinical animal toxicology studies, resulting in a number of uncertainties concerning the adverse effects of IFN on myelopoiesis. Rosenthal et al. (80) demonstrated that IFN-α administered ip at doses of 1000, 10,000, and 100,000 units/d for 10 days demonstrated a reduction in lymphocytes in both the bone marrow and spleen. In addition, the proliferative capacities of splenic B and T lymphocytes were significantly suppressed. Erythroid cells decreased in the marrow but increased in the spleen, an observation that suggests that the microenvironment may play a significant role in the effect of IFN-α. While NK cell stimulation is a well-known effect of IFN-α, it has been shown that multiple administration can result in a form of tolerance and perhaps suppressed NK cell activity (81).

AGENTS TARGETING OTHER MANIFESTATIONS OF AIDS

Granulocyte-Macrophage Colony Stimulating Factor

The progression of HIV-1 infection to the symptomatic AIDS patient often is accompanied by decreased hematopoiesis. This may manifest itself as thrombocytopenia, anemia, and leukopenia (82,83). In addition, the prolonged use of AZT, with its effects on myelopoiesis, amplifies the hematopoietic deficiencies associated with AIDS. In order to improve the hematopoietic status of these patients, antiviral treatment may be supplemented with hematopoietic growth factors such as GM-CSF.

Recombinant human GM-CSF, depending on the source, is a glycosylated protein with a molecular weight ranging from 18,000 to 30,000 that induces proliferation and differentiation of neutrophils and monocytes (84). It should be noted that its activity is not restricted to proliferation. *In vitro*, GM-CSF has been shown to intensify phagocytosis and cytotoxicity of monocytes and neutrophils (85). Fc receptor expression is enhanced on neutrophils and these cells appear to be "primed" for enhanced generation of superoxide radicals (86). Other effects on neutrophil function include inhibition of migration and increased adhesion, mostly like the result of increased expression of CD11b (87). Macrophage differentiation is also affected by GM-CSF with increased production of IL-1 and TNF observed (88). Antibody-dependent cell-mediated cytotoxicity is enhanced as is MHC class II expression (89,90).

Preclinical studies of GM-CSF have not revealed any alterations in immune function. Primates treated with GM-CSF daily for 28 days presented with increased leukocytosis characterized by increased numbers of neutrophils with moderate increases in monocytes, lymphocytes, and reticulocytes (91).

In patients with HIV-1, GM-CSF has been shown to improve the circulating neutrophil count without a concomitant increase in viral replication (83). This is especially noteworthy since *in vitro* studies of macrophage cell lines infected with HIV-1 have demonstrated increased viral replication (92). The side effects associated with GM-CSF treatment are an extension of its effect on the immune system. Local inflammation at the site of injection, fever, and malaise have been observed in HIV-1-infected patients treated with GM-CSF (93). Unfortunately, while GM-CSF is pharmacologically active in this patient population, the increase in circulating neutrophil counts does not prevent the occurrence of infection (94). Whether GM-CSF prolongs life or minimizes the toxicity of nucleoside analogs has not been determined, necessitating further studies.

ERYTHROPOIETIN (EPO)

Apart from targeting the HIV-1 infection or opportunistic infections, other manifestations of AIDS warrant therapeutic consideration. As an example, anemia is a frequent complication of AIDS and of AIDS related complex (95) of which the incidence and severity in patients with AIDS may be increased by therapy with AZT (96). In the trial of the Wellcome Collaborative Group (96) the hemoglobin concentration decreased to 7.5 g/dl in 31% of AZT-treated patients with AIDS, with 47% requiring transfusion during the 24-week study. It has been suggested that if AZT remains the principal means of treating AIDS, and if this prevalence of anemia is extrapolated to the population with AIDS, more than 100,000 patients will be receiving AZT and at least 40% of them may have anemia severe enough to require frequent transfusions. Consequently, therapies that reverse anemia have been integral to current AIDS therapy regimens. In view of the more than 95% rate of response to recombinant human erythropoietin (rEPO) in patients with anemia associated with chronic renal failure, a number of clinical studies have been conducted to assess the potential of EPO in treating the anemia in AIDS patients. Taken together, these studies have demonstrated that EPO is highly effective in circumventing AIDS and/or AZT-induced anemia.

While proven effective, the use of EPO is not without safety concerns. An adverse effect demonstrated in animals is the potential of EPO to induce bone marrow fibrosis (97). However, myelofibrosis in humans is not generally considered clinically relevant at the doses used for chronic renal insufficiency or AIDS-related anemia. There do appear to be some effects of EPO on immune system elements but whether these are necessarily adverse remains open to debate. In renal failure patients (98) the influence of rEPO on NK cell activity and the mitogenic response to concanavalin A (Con A) were assessed. While rEPO did not affect NK cell activity, mitogen-driven proliferation was significantly improved following rEPO therapy. Similar effects were observed in patients receiving open heart surgery by Hasatomi et al. (99), who also found an increase in lymphocyte activation (assessed by PHA-induced blast formation) after EPO therapy. These observations may be secondary to the reported increase in IL-2 by EPO (99), which may be a function of the recent discovery of significant similarities of the EPO receptor and the IL-2 receptor (beta chain) (100).

While its immunostimulatory capacity on cell-mediated immunity has been described in greater detail than humoral immunity, Kimata et al. (101) describe the potential of EPO to directly stimulate B cell immunoglobulin production and proliferation. This stimulatory effect was not manifested in small resting B cells but was markedly induced in activated and differentiated B cells. While this effect was blocked by antibodies to EPO, no speculation was given on the mechanism of these effects. Overall, the immunomodulatory data relating to EPO use would suggest an immunopotentiating effect, which is likely to be a beneficial response in the majority of clinical settings. However, since its use in AIDS-related anemia is relatively recent, the influence of these effects in immunodeficiency disorders awaits further assessment.

CONCLUSION

Antiviral therapies have not been uniformly successful in their attempts to cure viral infections. Unlike bacteria, which offer multiple metabolic targets, viruses are intracellular parasites attacking the host's genetic apparatus. Consequently, to kill the virus, the infected cells would have to be killed. As the therapeutic strategies in treating AIDS have become more sophisticated, it is clear that selective stimulation and suppression of immune system components represent a strategy with profound utility. As medical science develops new therapeutic strategies, either individual agents or convergent or combination therapy, an adequate understanding of the immunotoxicologic impact of these novel modalities will be a key to successful new antiviral agents.

REFERENCES

1. Dalgleish AG, Beverly PCL, Clapham PR, Crawford DH, Greaves MF. The CD4 (T4) antigen is an essential component of the receptor for the AIDS retrovirus. *Nature* 1984;342:816–819.
2. Stein BS, Gowda SD, Lifson JD, Penhallow RC, Bensch KG, Engleman EG. pH-independent HIV

entry into CD4-positive T cells via virus envelope fusion to the plasma membrane. *Cell* 1987; 49(5):659–668.

3. Ellison V, Abrams H, Roc T, Lifson J, Brown P. Human immunodeficiency virus integration in a cell-free system. *J Virol* 1990;64(6):2711–2715.
4. Varmus H. Reverse transcription. *Sci Am* 1987;257(3):56–59.
5. Varmus H. Retroviruses. *Science* 1988;240(4858):1427–1435.
6. Cullen BR. Regulation of human immunodeficiency virus replication. *Annu Rev Microbiol* 1991;45:219–250.
7. Nabel G, Baltimore D. An inducible transcription factor activates expression of human immunodeficiency virus in T cells. *Nature* 1987;326(6114):711–713. [Published erratum appears in *Nature* 1990;344(6262):178.]
8. Stevenson M, Stanwick TL, Dempsey MP, Lamonica CA. HIV-1 replication is controlled at the level of T cell activation and proviral integration. *EMBO J* 1990;9(5):1551–1560.
9. Sodroski J, Goh WC, Rosen C, Dayton A, Terwilliger E, Haseltine W. A second post-transcriptional trans-activator gene required for HTLV-III replication. *Nature* 1986;321(6068):412–417.
10. Pomerantz RJ, Trono D, Feinberg MB, Baltimore D. Cells nonproductively infected with HIV-1 exhibit an aberrant pattern of viral RNA expression: a molecular model for latency. *Cell* 1990; 61(7):1271–1276.
11. Daar ES, Li XL, Moudgil T, Ho DD. High concentrations of recombinant soluble CD4 are required to neutralize primary human immunodeficiency virus type 1 isolates. *Proc Natl Acad Sci USA* 1990;87(17):6574–6578.
12. Kahn JO, Allan JD, Hodges TL, et al. The safety and pharmacokinetics of recombinant soluble CD4 (rCD4) in subjects with the acquired immunodeficiency syndrome (AIDS) and AIDS-related complex. A phase I study. *Ann Intern Med* 1990;112(4):254–261.
13. Schooley RT, Merigan TC, Gaut P. Recombinant soluble CD4 therapy in patients with the acquired immunodeficiency syndrome (AIDS) and AIDS-related complex. A phase I-II escalating dosage trial. *Ann Intern Med* 1990;112(4):247–253.
14. Harris RJ, Wagner KL, Spellman MW. Structural characterization of a recombinant CD4-IgG hybrid molecule. *Eur J Biochem* 1990;194(2):611–620.
15. Ghctic V, Till MA, Ghctic MA, et al. Preparation and characterization of conjugates of recombinant CD4 and deglycosylated ricin A chain using different cross-linkers. *Bioconjug Chem* 1990; 1(1):24–31.
16. Weber S, Traunecker A, Karjalainen K. Constitutive expression of high levels of soluble mouse CD4 in transgenic mice does not interfere with their immune function. *Eur J Immunol* 1993; 23(2):511–516.
17. Hirsch MS. Chemotherapy of human immunodeficiency virus infections: current practice and future prospects. *J Infect Dis* 1990;161(5):845–857.
18. De Clercq E. HIV inhibitors targeted at the reverse transcriptase. *AIDS Res Hum Retroviruses* 1992;8(2):119–134.
19. De Clercq E. Antiviral agents: characteristic activity spectrum depending on the molecular target with which they interact. *Adv Virus Res* 1993;42(55):1–55.
20. Izuta S, Saneyoshi M, Sakurai T, Suzuki M, Kojima K, Yoshida S. Mechanisms of inhibitions of DNA polymerase gamma by nucleotide analogues having anti-HIV activities. *Nucleic Acids Symp Ser* 1991;25(80):79–80.
21. Copeland WC, Chen MS, Wang TS. Human DNA polymerases alpha and beta are able to incorporate anti-HIV deoxynucleotides into DNA. *J Biol Chem* 1992;267(30):21459–21464.
22. Orr DC, Figueiredo HT, Mo CL, Penn CR, Cameron JM. DNA chain termination activity and inhibition of human immunodeficiency virus reverse transcriptase by carbocyclic 2′,3′-didehydro-2′,3′-dideoxyguanosine triphosphate. *J Biol Chem* 1992;267(6):4177–4182.
23. Yarchoan R, Klecker RW, Weinhold KJ. Administration of 3′-azido-3′-deoxythymidine, an inhibitor of HTLV-III/LAV replication, to patients with AIDS or AIDS-related complex. *Lancet* 1986; 1(8481):575–580.
24. Yarchoan R, Mitsuya H, Myers CE, Broder S. Clinical pharmacology of 3′-azido-2′,3′-dideoxythymidine (zidovudine) and related dideoxynucleosides. *N Engl J Med* 1989;321(11):726–738. [Published erratum appears in *N Engl J Med* 1990;322(4):280.]
25. Yarchoan R, Mitsuya H, Broder S. Clinical and basic advances in the antiretroviral therapy of human immunodeficiency virus infection. *Am J Med* 1989;87(2):191–200.

26. Balzarini J, Herdewijn P, De Clercq E. Differential patterns of intracellular metabolism of 2′,3′-didehydro-2′,3′-dideoxythymidine and 3′-azido-2′,3′-dideoxythymidine, two potent anti-human immunodeficiency virus compounds. *J Biol Chem* 1989;264(11):6127–6133.
27. Ho HT, Hitchcock MJ. Cellular pharmacology of 2′,3′-dideoxy-2′,3′-didehydrothymidine, a nucleoside analog active against human immunodeficiency virus. *Antimicrob Agents Chemother* 1989;33(6):844–849.
28. Luster MI, Germolec DR, White K Jr, et al. A comparison of three nucleoside analogs with antiretroviral activity on immune and hematopoietic functions in mice: in vitro toxicity to precursor cells and microstromal environment. *Toxicol Appl Pharmacol* 1989;101(2):328–339.
29. Luster MI, Rosenthal GJ, Cao W, et al. Experimental studies of the hematologic and immune system toxicity of nucleoside derivatives used against HIV infection. *Int J Immunopharmacol* 1991;13(1):99–107.
30. Fischl MA, Richman DD, Grieco MH, et al. The efficacy of azidothymidine (AZT) in the treatment of patients with AIDS and AIDS-related complex. A double-blind, placebo-controlled trial. *N Engl J Med* 1987;317(4):185–191.
31. Merigan TC. Treatment of AIDS with combinations of antiretroviral agents. *Am J Med* 1991; 90(4A):8S–17S.
32. Glaser JB, Volpe S, Aguirre A, Simpkins H, Schiffman G. Zidovudine improves response to pneumococcal vaccine among persons with AIDS and AIDS-related complex. *J Infect Dis* 1991; 164(4):761–764.
33. Rinaldo C, Huang XL, Piazza P. Augmentation of cellular immune function during the early phase of zidovudine treatment of AIDS patients. *J Infect Dis* 1991;164(4):638–645.
34. Sommadossi JP, Carlisle R, Zhou Z. Cellular pharmacology of 3′-azido-3′-deoxythymidine with evidence of incorporation into DNA of human bone marrow cells. *Mol Pharmacol* 1989;36(1):9–14.
35. Gallicchio VS, Doukas MA, Hulette BC, Hughes NK, Gass C. Protection of 3′-azido-3′-deoxythymidine induced toxicity to murine hematopoietic progenitors (CFU-GM, BFU-E and CFU-MEG) with interleukin-1. *Proc Soc Exp Biol Med* 1989;192(2):201–204.
36. Gallicchio VS, Hughes NK, Hulette BC, Noblitt L. Effect of interleukin-1, GM-CSF, erythropoietin, and lithium on the toxicity associated with 3′-azido-3′-deoxythymidine (AZT) in vitro on hematopoietic progenitors (CFU-GM, CFU-MEG, and BFU-E) using murine retrovirus-infected hematopoietic cells. *J Leukoc Biol* 1991;50(6):580–586.
37. Gallicchio VS, Hughes NK, Tse KF. Comparison of dideoxynucleoside drugs (DDI and zidovudine) and induction of hematopoietic toxicity using normal human bone marrow cells in vitro. *Int J Immunopharmacol* 1993;15(2):263–268.
38. Frick LW, Nelson DJ. Effects of 3′-azido-3′-deoxythymidine on the deoxynucleoside triphosphate pools of cultured human cells. *Adv Exp Med Biol* 1989;94:389–394.
39. Bhalla K, Birkhofer M, Li GR, et al. 2′-Deoxycytidine protects normal human bone marrow progenitor cells in vitro against the cytotoxicity of 3′-azido-3′-deoxythymidine with preservation of antiretroviral activity. *Blood* 1989;74(6):1923–1928.
40. Sommadossi JP, Carlisle R, Schinazi RF, Zhou Z. Uridine reverses the toxicity of 3′-azido-3′-deoxythymidine in normal human granulocyte–macrophage progenitor cells in vitro without impairment of antiretroviral activity. *Antimicrob Agents Chemother* 1988;32(7):997–1001.
41. Cretton EM, Xie MY, Bevan RJ, Goudgaon NM, Schinazi RF, Sommadossi JP. Catabolism of 3′-azido-3′-deoxythymidine in hepatocytes and liver microsomes, with evidence of formation of 3′-amino-3′-deoxythymidine, a highly toxic catabolite for human bone marrow cells. *Mol Pharmacol* 1991;39(2):258–266.
42. Chen MS, Woods KL, Prusoff WH. Molecular basis of the antineoplastic activity of 3′-amino-3′-deoxythymidine. *Mol Pharmacol* 1984;25(3):441–445.
43. Fischer PH, Lin T-S, Prusoff WH. Reversal of the cytotoxicity of 3′-amino-3′-deoxythymidine by pyrimidine deoxyribonucleosides. *Biochem Pharmacol* 1979;31:991–994.
44. Mansuri MM, Hitchcock MJ, Buroker RA, et al. Comparison of in vitro biological properties and mouse toxicities of three thymidine analogs active against human immunodeficiency virus. *Antimicrob Agents Chemother* 1990;34(4):637–641.
45. Browne MJ, Mayer KH, Chafee SB, et al. 2′,3′-Didehydro-3′-deoxythymidine (d4T) in patients with AIDS or AIDS-related complex: a phase I trial. *J Infect Dis* 1993;167(1):21–29.
46. Zhu Z, Hitchcock MJ, Sommadossi JP. Metabolism and DNA interaction of 2′,3′-didehydro-2′,3′-dideoxythymidine in human bone marrow cells. *Mol Pharmacol* 1991;40(5):838–845.

47. Balzarini J, Cooney DA, Dalal M, et al. 2′,3′-Dideoxycytidine: regulation of its metabolism and anti-retroviral potency by natural pyrimidine nucleosides and by inhibitors of pyrimidine nucleotide synthesis. *Mol Pharmacol* 1987;32(6):798–806.
48. Whittington R, Brogden RN. Zalcitabine. A review of its pharmacology and clinical potential in acquired immunodeficiency syndrome (AIDS). *Drugs* 1992;44(4):656–683.
49. Broder S, Yarchoan R. Dideoxycytidine: current clinical experience and future prospects. A summary. *Am J Med* 1990;88(5B):31S–33S.
50. Du DL, Volpe DA, Grieshaber CK, Murphy M Jr. In vitro myelotoxicity of 2′,3′-dideoxynucleosides on human hematopoietic progenitor cells. *Exp Hematol* 1990;18(7):832–836.
51. Broder S. Dideoxycytidine (ddC): a potent antiretroviral agent for human immunodeficiency virus infection. An introduction. *Am J Med* 1990;88(5B):315–335.
52. Merigan TC, Skowron G. Safety and tolerance of dideoxycytidine as a single agent. Results of early-phase studies in patients with acquired immunodeficiency syndrome (AIDS) or advanced AIDS-related complex. Study Group of the AIDS Clinical Trials Group of the National Institute of Allergy and Infectious Diseases. *Am J Med* 1990;88(5B):11S–15S.
53. Shelton MJ, O'Donnell AM, Morse GD. Zalcitabine. *Ann Pharmacother* 1993;27(4):480–489.
54. Skowron G, Merigan TC. Alternating and intermittent regimens of zidovudine (3′-azido-3′-deoxythymidine) and dideoxycytidine (2′,3′-dideoxycytidine) in the treatment of patients with acquired immunodeficiency syndrome (AIDS) and AIDS-related complex. *Am J Med* 1990;88(5B):20S–23S.
55. Meng TC, Fischl MA, Boota AM, et al. Combination therapy with zidovudine and dideoxycytidine in patients with advanced human immunodeficiency virus infection. A phase I/II study [see comments]. *Ann Intern Med* 1992;116(1):13–20.
56. Fridland A, Johnson MA, Cooney DA, Ahluwalia G, Marquez VE, Driscoll JS, Johns DG. Metabolism in human leukocytes of anti-HIV dideoxypurine nucleosides. *Ann NY Acad Sci* 1990; 616(16):205–216.
57. Gao WY, Shirasaka T, Johns DG, Broder S, Mitsuya H. Differential phosphorylation of azidothymidine, dideoxycytidine, and dideoxyinosine in resting and activated peripheral blood mononuclear cells. *J Clin Invest* 1993;91(5):2326–2333.
58. Gelb AB, Fye KH, Tischfield JA, Sahota AS, Sparks JW, Hancock DC, Sibley RK. Renal insufficiency secondary to 2,8-dihydroxyadenine urolithiasis. *Hum Pathol* 1992;23(9):1081–1085.
59. Fye KH, Sahota A, Hancock DC, et al. Adenine phosphoribosyltransferase deficiency with renal deposition of 2,8-dihydroxyadenine leading to nephrolithiasis and chronic renal failure. *Arch Intern Med* 1993;153(6):767–770.
60. Yarchoan R, Mitsuya H, Thomas RV, et al. In vivo activity against HIV and favorable toxicity profile of 2′,3′-dideoxyinosine. *Science* 1989;245(4916):412–415.
61. Dolin R, Lambert JS, Morse GD, et al. 2′,3′-Dideoxyinosine in patients with AIDS or AIDS-related complex. *Rev Infect Dis* 1990;12(5):S540–S549.
62. LeLacheur SF, Simon GL. Exacerbation of dideoxycytidine-induced neuropathy with dideoxyinosine. *J Acquir Immune Defic Syndr* 1991;4(5):538–539.
63. Cao W, Sikorski EE, Fuchs BA, Stern ML, Luster MI, Munson AE. The B lymphocyte is the immune cell target for 2′,3′-dideoxyadenosine. *Toxicol Appl Pharmacol* 1990;105(3):492–502.
64. Yarchoan R, Pluda JM, Thomas RV, et al. Long-term toxicity/activity profile of 2′,3′-dideoxyinosine in AIDS or AIDS-related complex. *Lancet* 1990;336(8714):526–529.
65. Rozencweig M, McLaren C, Beltangady M, et al. Overview of phase I trials of 2′,3′-dideoxyinosine (ddI) conducted on adult patients. *Rev Infect Dis* 1990;12(5):S570–S575.
66. MMWR. Update: acquired immunodeficiency syndrome. *MMWR Morb Mortal Wkly Rep* 1985; 34:245–248.
67. Witt DJ. Bacterial infections in adult patients with the acquired immune deficiency syndrome and AIDS related complex. *Am J Med* 1987;82:900.
68. de Wit R. AIDS related Kaposi's sarcoma and the mechanisms of interferon alpha's activity: a riddle within a puzzle. *J Intern Med 1992;231:321–325.*
69. Schoenbach EB. The pharmacology, mode of action and therapeutic potentialities of stilbamidine, pentamidine, propamidine and other diamidines: a review. *Medicine* (*Baltimore*) 1948;27:327–377.
70. Sands M, Kron MA, Brown RB. Pentamidine: a review. *Rev Infect Dis* 1985;7:625–634.
71. Goa KL, Campoli-Richards DM. Pentamidine isethionate, a review of its antiprotozoal activity, pharmacokinetic and therapeutic use in *Pneumocystis carinii* pneumonia. *Drugs* 1987;33:242–258.

72. Monk JP. Inhaled pentamidine: an overview of its pharmacological properties and a review of its therapeutic use in *Pneumocystis carinii* pneumonia. *Drugs* 1990;39:741–756.
73. Rosenthal GJ, Corsini E, Craig W, Comment C, Luster MI. Pentamidine: an inhibitor of interleukin 1 that acts via a post translational event. *Toxicol Appl Pharmacol* 1991;107:555–561.
74. Rosenthal GJ, Craig W, Corsini E, Taylor M, Luster M. Pentamidine blocks the pathophysiologic effects of endotoxemia through inhibition of cytokine release. *Toxicol Appl Pharmacol* 1992;112: 222–228.
75. Corsini E, Craig W, Rosenthal GJ. Modulation of tumor necrosis factor release from alveolar macrophages treated with pentamidine isethionate. *Int J Immunopharmacol* 1992;14:121–130.
76. Corsini E, Dykstra C, Craig W, Tidwell R, Rosenthal GJ. *Pneumocystis carinii* induction of tumor necrosis factor by alveolar macrophages: modulation by pentamidine isethionate. *Immunol Lett* 1992;34:303–308.
77. Einhorn S, Ling P, Einhorn N, Strander H, Wasserman J. Influence of interferon therapy on blood lymphoid cells. *Cancer Immunol Immunother* 1987;24:190–196.
78. Neumann HA, Fauser AA. Effect of interferon on pluripotential hemopoietic progenitors (CFU-GEMM) derived from human bone marrow. *Exp Hematol* 1982;10:587–594.
79. Broxmeyer HE, Lu L, Platzer E, Feit C, Juliano L, Rubin BY. Comparative analysis of the influence of human gamma, alpha, and beta interferons on human multipotential (CFU-GEMM) erythroid (BFU-E) and granulocyte-macrophage (CFU-GM) progenitor cells. *J Immunol* 1983; 131:1300–1305.
80. Rosenthal GJ, Stranahan RP, Thompson M, et al. Organ specific hematopoietic changes induced by a recombinant human interferon alpha in mice. *Fundam Appl Toxicol* 1990;14:666–675.
81. Brunda MD, Rosenberg D. Modulation of murine natural killer cell activity in vitro and in vivo by recombinant human interferons. *Cancer Res* 1984;44:597–601.
82. Groopman JE, Feder D. Hematopoietic growth factors in AIDS. *Semin Oncol* 1992;19(4):408–414.
83. Groopman JE. The use of growth hematopoietic factors in AIDS. *Pathol Biol* 1992;39(9):874–875.
84. Moore MA. The clinical use of colony stimulating factors. *Annu Rev Immunol* 1991;9:159–191.
85. Braun DP, Siziopikou KP, Casey LC, Harris JE. The in vitro development of cytotoxicity in response to granulocyte/macrophage-colony-stimulating factor or interferon gamma in the peripheral blood monocytes of patients with solid tumors: modulation by arachidonic acid metabolic inhibitors. *Cancer Immunol Immunother* 1990;32(1):55–61.
86. Edwards SW, Watson F, MacLeod R, Davies J. Receptor expression and oxidase activity in human neutrophils: regulation by granulocyte–macrophage colony-stimulating factor and dependence upon protein biosynthesis. *Biosci Rep* 1990;10(4):393–401.
87. Maurer D, Fischer GF, Felzmann T, et al. Ratio of complement receptor over Fc-receptor III expression; a sensitive parameter to monitor granulocyte–macrophage colony-stimulating factor effects on neutrophils. *Ann Hematol* 1991;62(4):135–140.
88. Essner R, Rhoades K, McBride WH, Morton DL, Economou JS. Differential effects of granulocyte–macrophage colony-stimulating factor and macrophage colony-stimulating factor on tumor necrosis factor and interleukin-1 production in human monocytes. *J Clin Lab Immunol* 1990;32(4): 161–166.
89. Baldwin GC, Chung GY, Kaslander C, Esmail T, Reisfeld RA, Golde DW. Colony-stimulating factor enhancement of myeloid effector cell cytotoxicity towards neuroectodermal tumour cells. *Br J Haematol* 1993;83(4):545–553.
90. Chantry D, Turner M, Brennan F, Kingsbury A, Feldmann M. Granulocyte–macrophage colony stimulating factor induces both HLA-DR expression and cytokine production by human monocytes. *Cytokine* 1990;2(1):60–67.
91. Donahue RE, Wang EA, Stone DK, et al. Stimulation of haematopoeisis in primates by continuous infusion of recombinant human GM-CSF. *Nature* 1986;321:872–875.
92. Perno CF, Cooney DA, Gao WY, et al. Effects of bone marrow stimulatory cytokines on human immunodeficiency virus replication and the antiviral activity of dideoxynucleosides in cultures of monocyte/macrophages. *Blood* 1992;80(4):995–1003.
93. Krown SE, Paredes J, Bundow D, Polsky B, Gold JW, Flomenberg N. Interferon-alpha, zidovudine, and granulocyte–macrophage colony-stimulating factor: a phase I AIDS Clinical Trials Group study in patients with Kaposi's sarcoma associated with AIDS. *J Clin Oncol* 1992; 10(8):1344–1351.

94. Mitsuyasu RT. Use of recombinant interferons and hematopoietic growth factors in patients infected with human immunodeficiency virus [see comments]. *Rev Infect Dis* 1991;13(5):979–984.
95. Fischl MGJE, Levine D, Groopman E, et al. Recombinant human erythropoietin for patients with AIDS treated with zidovudine. *N Engl J Med* 1990;322(21):1488–1493.
96. Richman DD, Grieco MH, Gottlieb MS, et al. The toxicity of azidothymidine (AZT) in the treatment of patients with AIDS and AIDS-related complex. A double-blind, placebo-controlled trial. *N Engl J Med* 1987;317:192–197.
97. Bader R, Bode G, Rebel W, Lexa P. Stimulation of bone marrow by administration of excessive doses of recombinant human erythropoietin. *Pathol Res Pract* 1992;188:676–679.
98. Singh AB, Palekar S, Levy S, Nunn C, Mann RA. The effects of recombinant human erythropoietin on the cell mediated immune response of renal failure patients. *J Med* 1992;23(5):289–302.
99. Hasatomi K, Yasunaga H, Isomura T, Fukunaga S, Hirano A, Kosuga K, Oishi K. The changes of the cell mediated immunity in patients with administration of recombinant erythropoietin. *Nippon Geka Gakkai Zasshi* 1992;93:518–522.
100. D'Andrea AD, Fasman G, Lodish HF. Erythropoietin receptor and interleukin-2 receptor beta chain: a new receptor family. *Cell* 1989;58:1023–1024.
101. Kimata H, Yoshida A, Ishioka C, Masuda S, Mikawa H. Human recombinant erythropoietin directly stimulates B cell immunoglobulin production and proliferation in serum free medium. *Clin Exp Immunol* 1991;85:151–156.

Immunotoxicology and Immunopharmacology, Second Edition, edited by J. H. Dean, M. I. Luster, A. E. Munson, and I. Kimber.
Raven Press, Ltd., New York © 1994.

15

Transplantation Agents

Bernhard Ryffel, Bruce D. Car, Hans-Pietro Eugster, and Gaetane Woerly

Institute of Toxicology, University of Zürich, CH-8603 Schwerzenbach ZH, Switzerland

HISTORICAL REVIEW OF ORGAN TRANSPLANTATION

The replacement of a failing organ with its healthy counterpart was the therapeutic dream of clinical medicine for many years. The first important steps toward this goal were made by pioneers of experimental surgery, who developed the necessary techniques first with vascular anastomoses in animals. In 1902, Ullmann and Carrel, despite having had successfully transplanted kidneys that afterward attained normal renal function, were thwarted by a gradual loss of function that could not be explained by their knowledge of infarction or infection (reviewed in ref. 105). The reason for this failure was not of technical nature but due to graft rejection by the immune system of the host. At this time the immunologic basis of events involved in graft rejection was unknown. The notion of histocompatibility antigens and their differences between individuals had not yet emerged. Successful allotransplantation was performed between identical twins as early as 1950. Irradiation and chemical immunosuppression were first attempted as adjunct therapies in the early 1960s. The milestones of the exciting story of renal transplantation are summarized in Table 1.

The discovery of azathioprine and its combined use with glucocorticosteroids hailed the beginning of a new era in organ transplantation. Surgeons, encouraged by results with chemical immunosuppression, attempted the transplantation of several other organs, including the liver and heart. Rejection crises were treated with high doses of glucocorticosteroids and/or antilymphocyte serum. An important limitation of the treatment was the toxicity of the immunosuppressants: leukopenia induced by the purine analog azathioprine and Cushing's syndrome induced by chronic glucocorticosteroid excess.

The discovery of cyclosporin A (CsA) (1) and its introduction into the clinic in 1978 (2) heralded a therapeutic breakthrough that enabled controlled immunosuppression to be employed in transplant patients. CsA proved to be much more selective for the immune system and devoid of adverse effects on the hematopoietic

TABLE 1. *Milestones of kidney transplantation*

1902	Experimental kidney transplantation (Ullmann)
1906	Xenotransplantation into human (Jaboulay)
1954	Kidney transplantation between twins (Murray and co-workers)
1960	Azathioprine immunosuppression (Calne, Zukoski)
1967	Antilymphocyte globulin (Starzl)
1978	Cyclosporine (Calne)
1983	OKT-3 antibody (Cosimi)
1990	FK506 (Starzl)

system (3). Despite the excellent results achieved, clinicians retain reservations concerning the use of CsA for at least two reasons: renal dysfunction is a major side effect, and CsA fails to induce lasting immunologic tolerance (2).

The roles of new immunosuppressants emerging from microbiologic research, such as the macrolide-structured molecules FK506 and rapamycin (4–6), and a few novel chemicals are also discussed.

IMMUNOBIOLOGY OF TRANSPLANT REJECTION

A simplified scheme of cellular events occurring during the interaction between the grafted organ and its host is given in Fig. 1. Schematically, three phases may be distinguished: first, an afferent phase, which includes the recognition of foreign tissue (i.e., the allograft); second, a central phase occurring within the immune system, comprising the differentiation of alloantigen-specific lymphocytic clones into effector cells; and third, the efferent phase, characterized by cellular and humoral effector mechanisms, leading to the ultimate rejection of the allograft (reviewed in refs. 7 and 8).

Genetic differences between the donor and the host are defined by histocompatibility complex molecules expressed on the cell membrane. Donor cells with histocompatibility molecules differing from those of the host are recognized by the host's immune system. Continuous alloantigenic stimulation results in profound activation of T helper (T_H) cells with the release of several cytokines leading ultimately to the maturation of effector immune cells, for example, cytotoxic T cells, activated macrophages, natural killer (NK) cells, and plasma cells. Graft rejection results from the combined effect of activated effector cells and cytokines; for example, interferons that increase the class II expression within the graft, tumor necrosis factor (TNF) with its direct cytotoxic effect, and specific antibodies. The recent characterization and cloning of a series of cytokines and the identification of their specific membrane receptors will allow a better understanding of the molecular events of the graft rejection (9,10).

We have investigated the effects of several immunosuppressants on the acceptance of allografts in rats. The effects of a daily administration of CsA at 5 mg/kg

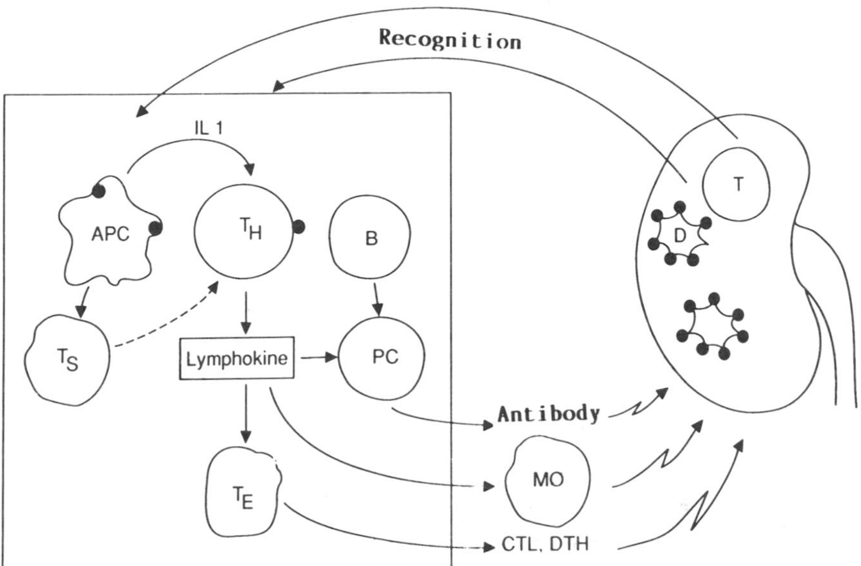

FIG. 1. Cellular events leading to graft rejection. Afferent limb: alloantigen from the graft is presented by dendritic cells (D). Central part: recognition of alloantigen by host immune system, activation of antigen-presenting cells (APC), T cells, and B cells. Efferent limb: activated lymphocytes (T effector cells, T_E; plasma cells, PC), antibodies and complement, macrophages (Mo), killer cells (CTL), and lymphokines destroy the graft.

over 2 weeks on long-term survival of orthotopic renal allotransplants are striking (reviewed in ref. 1). The microscopic appearance of rat allograft rejection, demonstrating infiltration by effector cells, is illustrated in Fig. 2. The administration of CsA at the time of surgery prevented the cellular infiltration by inhibiting the synthesis of cytokines, thereby allowing the long-term functioning of the graft. The detailed cellular events have been reviewed elsewhere (7,8).

POSSIBLE SITES OF IMMUNOLOGICAL INTERVENTION

The interaction of the antigen-presenting cell (APC) with the antigen receptor on the T_H lymphocyte surface is the central event leading to the activation of the immune system (Table 2) (reviewed in ref. 3). The activation of the T_H cells results in the synthesis and release of several cytokines, which promote the maturation of effector cells with cytotoxic function (Tc, NK cells) and of B lymphocytes (Fig. 3). In the induction of immunosuppression, the first potential site of intervention in the host immune system would be at the level of antigen uptake, followed by processing and final assembly into the host class II antigen of APCs. While such specificity is possible *in vitro*, it may be difficult to achieve *in vivo*. Agents that inhibit the

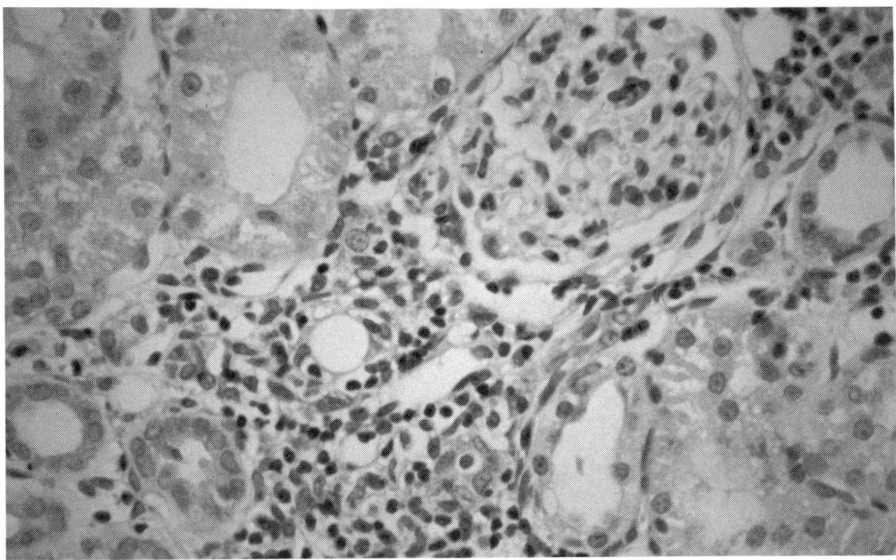

FIG. 2. Microscopic appearance of renal allograft rejection in rats. Kidneys from Fischer rats were transplanted into previously uninephrectomized Wistar–Furth rats.

activation of APCs and their release of cytokines [e.g., interleukin-1 (IL-1), IL-6, or TNF], however, may have a profound effect on subsequent T cell activation. The T cell receptor (TcR), consisting of heterodimeric antigen-recognition domain and several invariant associated chains, known as the CD3 complex, is a potential site of immunointervention, which could theoretically prevent recognition of the antigenic signal (112). Antibodies directed against the TcR or CD3 complex may block the access of the processed antigen presented by the class II molecules. Instead of antibodies, irrelevant peptides can also compete for the class II site, thereby preventing correct recognition by the TcR. The interaction of the TcR with the specific

TABLE 2. *Potential sites of immunosuppression: macrophage/T_H cell*

Antigen presentation	Inhibition of antigen processing, presentation on MHC class II antigen, bioengineered xenotransplants
Signal recognition	Blocking antibodies against TcR, accessory molecule of T cell activation, specific peptides
Signal transduction	Inhibition of specific kinases or phosphatases: fyn-, lck kinase, CD45 phosphatase, calcineurin, PLCγ, MAP kinase, G-proteins
Gene transcription	Inhibition of cytokine or receptor, modulation of regulatory gene (myc, myb, rb, p53, cyclins)
Cytokine action	Neutralizing antibodies against cytokine or cytokine receptor, soluble receptors
Inhibition of cell cycle	Antimetabolites

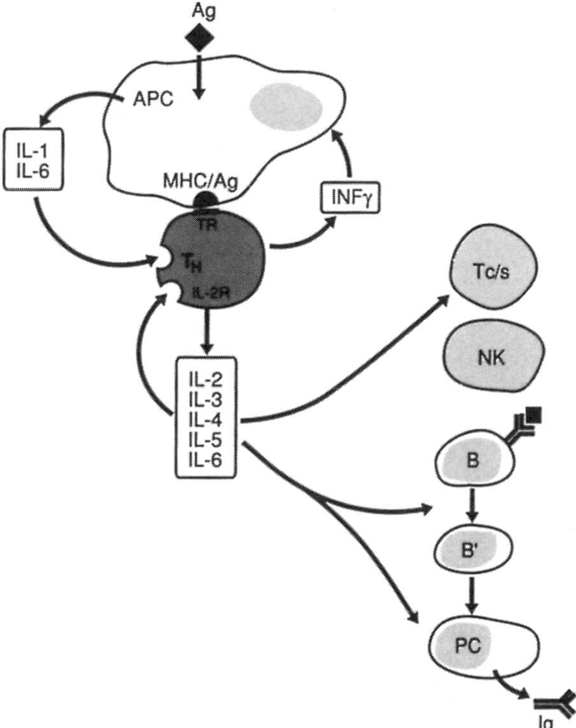

FIG. 3. Central role of T_H lymphocyte, cellular interactions. Antigen (Ag) is processed by antigen-presenting cells (APC) and presented within the major histocompatibility complex (MHC) molecules to the T cell receptor (TcR). Activated APC release IL-1, IL-6, and TNF, while activated T_H cells synthesize several ILs, which have multiple regulatory effects; for example, autocrine stimulation of T_H cells, differentiation of cytotoxic and suppressor T cells ($T_{c/s}$), and B cell differentiation into antibody-secreting (Ig) plasma cells (PC).

antigenic peptide presented by class II molecules provides the specificity of the reaction but alone is insufficient for T cell activation. Other membrane molecules such as CD4/8 and several adhesion molecules are necessary to increase the affinity of the cellular interaction; thus prevention of these additional contact sites, predominantly by antibodies, is another potential avenue for inhibition of T cell activation. Upon recognition by the TcR, the antigenic signal is transduced through complex biochemical pathways, which include the activation of several enzymes (e.g., phospholipase Cγ), kinases (e.g., fyn, lck, and MAP kinase), and phosphatases (e.g., CD45 and calcineurin). A key feature of this transduction is the release of inositol-3-phosphate, which mobilizes intracellular calcium and which, combined with diacylglycerol, activates protein kinase C. Recent reports concerning CsA and FK506 have concluded that the phosphatase calcineurin plays an important role through dephosphorylating of the nuclear factor of activated T cells (NFAT). Upon dephosphorylation, NFAT is translocated into the nucleus where it binds to the IL-2 promotor resulting in IL-2 gene transcription (see below). However, other factors (e.g., NFKB and AP-1) were shown to be necessary for IL-2 gene activation. The control of IL-2 gene activation/transcription is an area of intense research.

The genetic program induced by antigen stimulation is complex and includes the active transcription of at least 70 genes (100). The inhibition of gene expression of molecules such as cytokine receptors, interferons (IFNs), and TNF must also be considered for the induction of immunosuppression.

Pharmacologic modulation of antigenic processing within the APC is also a potential avenue to immunosuppression that remains unexplored.

OVERVIEW OF IMMUNOSUPPRESSIVE AGENTS

A variety of immunosuppressants are presently in use with widely varying mechanisms of action (Table 3).

Azathioprine. Azathioprine is an imidazole derivative of 6-mercaptopurine—a purine analog with antimetabolite properties, inhibiting primary immune responses. Since azathioprine immunsuppression is mediated by inhibition of cell proliferation, it is not surprising that other systems, especially the hematopoietic system, are also adversely affected. Leukopenia is the main dose-limiting side effect.

Anti-lymphocyte Antibodies. Polyclonal antibodies raised against human lymphocytes in rabbit or horse are in clinical use for the treatment of transplant rejection. These antisera bind to circulating lymphocytes, causing a sequestration in the spleen and resulting in subsequent lympholysis. Monoclonal antibodies (anti-CD3) have the advantage of being homogenous products, in contrast to the antisera. Although acting similarly to the polyclonal antibodies, an important difference is the mitogenic activity of anti-CD3 monoclonal antibodies on T cells, which leads to their activation, resulting in fever due to the release of cytokines.

TABLE 3. *Overview of immunosuppressant agents for transplantation: chemical and biologicals*

Drug	Mode of action	Side effects
Azathioprine	Antimetabolite, inhibition of purine biosynthesis	Myelotoxicity
CsA	Inhibition of IL-2 gene transcription	Nephrotoxicity
Glucocorticosteroids	Inhibition of IL-1 synthesis	Cushing syndrome
FK506	Inhibition of IL-2 gene transcription	Nephrotoxicity
Rapamycin	Inhibition of IL-2 signal transduction, inhibition of S6 kinase	NA
Deoxyspergualin	Inhibition of IL-2 signal transduction?	NA
RS 61443	Inhibition of *de novo* purine synthesis	NA
Brequinar	Inhibition of *de novo* purine synthesis	NA
Ciamexone	Inhibition of antibody-mediated response	NA
OKT3	Activation and sequestration of T lymphocytes	Fever
Antibodies	MHC class II; IL-2R; ICAM-1, LFA-1, CD4; IFN-γ, TNF	

NA, none associated.

Glucocorticosteroids. Steroids inhibit T lymphocyte activation by blocking the release of IL-1 from macrophages and subsequent IL-2 synthesis. Furthermore, steroids cause the lysis of lymphocytes. Steroids have pleiotropic actions on other systems in the body; they inhibit inflammation and have profound effects on metabolism. The adverse metabolic effects of chronic therapy, manifesting as Cushing's syndrome, are usually dose-limiting.

CsA. CsA is a fungal peptide, which inhibits IL-2 gene transcription. Recent investigations revealed that CsA confers immunosuppression by inhibiting calcineurin phosphatase. It is assumed that deficient dephosphorylation of NFAT prevents its nuclear translocation and IL-2 gene transcription (1).

FK506 and Rapamycin. These two novel molecules are potent immunosuppressants with macrolide structure. While FK506 has a similar mode of action to CsA (e.g., inhibition of IL-2 gene transcription by affecting calcineurin phosphatase), rapamycin is the prototype of a novel class of immunosuppressants. Rapamycin does not effect IL-2 gene expression but potently blocks IL-2 signal transduction by inhibition of the S6 kinase as discussed below (2,5,6).

CsA: NEW INSIGHTS INTO MODE OF ACTION

CsA is a member of the cyclic undecapeptides (Fig. 4), which have immunosuppressive properties (1). It has been used successfully to prevent allograft rejection and to treat several autoimmune diseases (2). Molecular studies on its mode of action have revealed that CsA prevents T lymphocyte activation at the level of cytokine gene transcription (reviewed in refs. 3–5). Recent investigations with macrolide immunosuppressants showed that FK506 has the same effect on cytokine gene transcription as CsA, thereby inhibiting T lymphocyte activation (6–10). These findings provoked investigations at the molecular level designed to identify possible common pathways for both immunosuppressants. Such studies have provided important insights into the regulation of cytokine gene activation.

Cellular Uptake of CsA. Specific, saturable, and reversible binding was shown for CsA with murine and human mononuclear blood leukocytes utilizing a [^{3}H]-CsA derivative. An affinity constant of 10^{-7} M (K_d) with about 10^6 bound molecules per cell was calculated from kinetic and equilibrium-binding studies (12). Furthermore, CsA uptake was independent of active cellular metabolism (13). Investigations over a broader concentration range in erythrocytes and in several nucleated cell types revealed two components of cell binding (3): a saturable cytosolic binding component at low CsA concentrations and a nonsaturable, nonspecific partitioning into the membrane at higher CsA concentrations. These findings, together with evidence for CsA accumulation within the cell, suggest the existence of an intracellular binding protein (14).

Cyclophilin (CPH) Receptor Family. The discovery of cyclophilin A (CPH-A), an 18-kDa protein that specifically binds CsA, was a seminal contribution to the understanding of CsA-mediated events (15), opening many avenues of research.

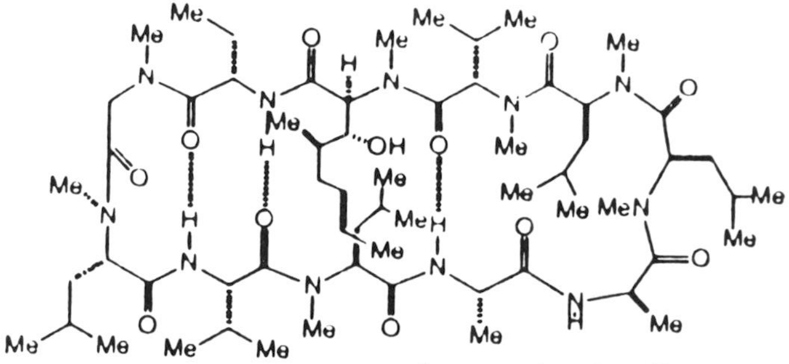

cyclosporin A (CsA)

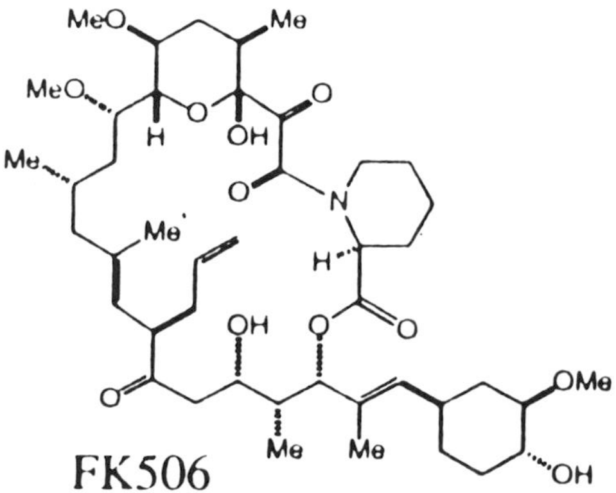

FK506

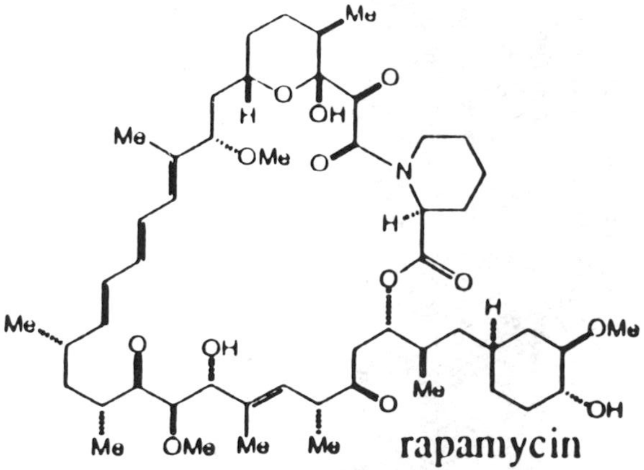

rapamycin

FIG. 4. Chemical structure of immunosuppressants: CsA, FK506, and rapamycin.

The amino acid sequence of CPH-A was apparently not related to any known protein (16); however, it was later established that CPH-A was homologous to a prolyl-peptidyl cis-trans-isomerase, also known as rotamase (17,18). This provided a new perspective on the mode of CsA action, as active cyclosporines were shown to bind to CPH-A (19) and inhibit its rotamase activity. Thus it was speculated that immunosuppression might be due to the impaired folding of a protein factor central to T lymphocyte activation, which might be rate-limiting.

Specificity of CsA–CPH-A Interaction. The specificity of CsA–CPH-A binding was investigated by hydrophobic interactions using an LH-20 column (16), a competitive solid-phase enzyme-linked immunoadsorbent assay (ELISA) (20,21), and photoaffinity labeling (22). Binding to CPH-A correlated with the immunosuppressive activity of CsA analogs. Amino acids 1, 2, 10, and 11 of the CsA molecule were found to be essential for CPH-A binding. Subtle changes in these residues reduced both the affinity for CPH-A and *in vitro* immunosuppressive activity (21,23).

The synthesis of a photoaffinity labeled CsA analog allowed the identification of several additional CsA binding proteins (22,24,25). In the T cell line Jurkat, labeled proteins of 21, 25, 40, and 60 kDa were identified (11). The labeled proteins at 21 and 25 kDa were identical with CPH-A and CPH-B (Fig. 5). CPH-B is a second CsA binding protein, which has an endoplasmic reticulum retention signal (26–28). Two new members of this family were also identified: CPH-C, which reportedly has a restricted tissue distribution (29), and CPH-D (30). These latter proteins are less abundant than CPH-A and have a molecular mass of approximately 22 kDa; thus they were not distinguishable from CPH-B by photoaffinity labeling. Kieffer et al. (31) purified a 40-kDa protein (CPH-40) by affinity chromatography; the partial sequence analysis showed homology with CPH-A. CPH-40 antiserum did not cross-react with CPH-A in immunoblot analysis. A phosphorylated 45-kDa CsA binding protein has been reported but not further characterized (32).

CPH Distribution and Function. All members of the CPH family have rotamase (prolyl-peptidyl cis-trans-isomerase) activity, which is inhibited by CsA (30,33). CPH-A exhibits the highest specific activity and is most sensitive to CsA inhibition. Macrolide-derived immunosuppressants, however, do not affect this CPH rotamase activity. All CPHs, with the possible exception of CPH-C, are highly abundant in both lymphoid and nonlymphoid tissues. The subcellular localization of CPH proteins has been investigated by biochemical cell fractionation studies and immunoelectron microscopy. CPH-A and CPH-B were found in both cytosol and nucleus and demonstrated no specific association with organellar structures (34–36). CPH-B and CPH-D possess a membrane localization signal and are found in the endoplasmic reticulum membrane fraction. The relative abundance and high conservation between the domain of CPHs suggest a role in normal cell function (15, 34,43,48). The search for an endogenous ligand of CPH has been hitherto unsuccessful. The initial uptake and intracellular concentration of active cyclosporines at cytosolic and/or nuclear sites (14), followed by inhibition of rotamase activity, are two potential roles for CPH-A in CsA-mediated immunosuppression.

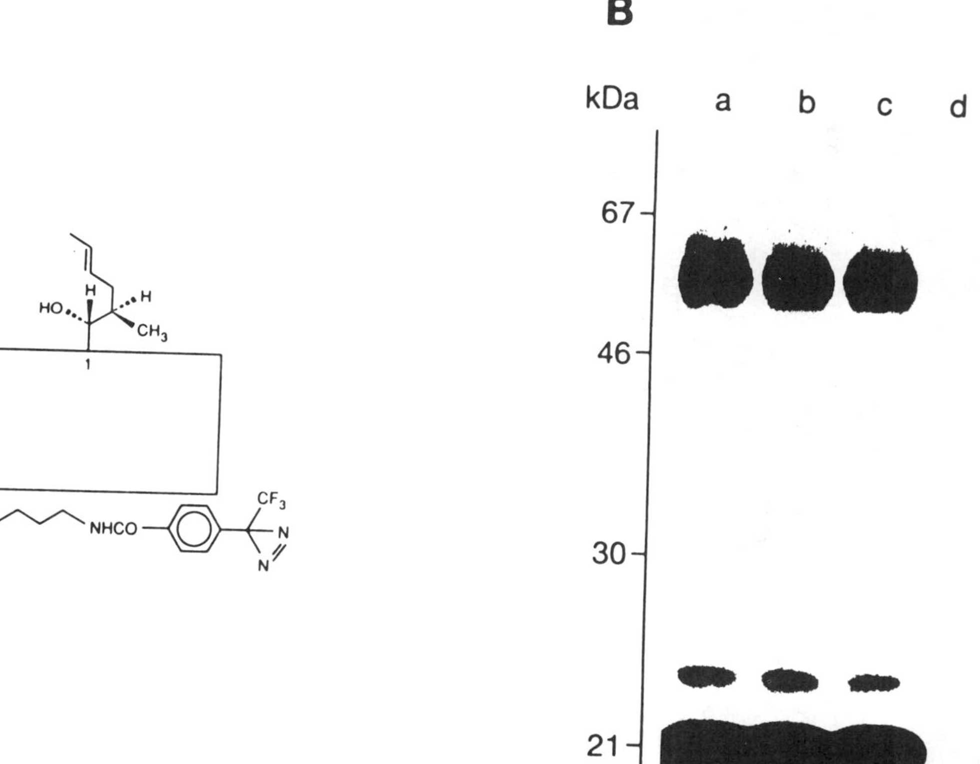

FIG. 5. A: *In vivo* detection of CsA receptor proteins. **B:** Structure of photoaffinity label derivative. The human T cell line Jurkat is incubated with titrated photoaffinity label probe. After ultraviolet (UV) cross-linking, the labeled cellular proteins are separated by sodium dodecyl sulfate–polyacrylamide gel electrophoresis (SDS-PAGE) and the proteins detected by fluoroautoradiography (**a**). The specificity of binding is defined by competition with ten times molar excess CsA (**d**) or by lack of competition by inactive CsH (**b**) or FK506 (**c**).

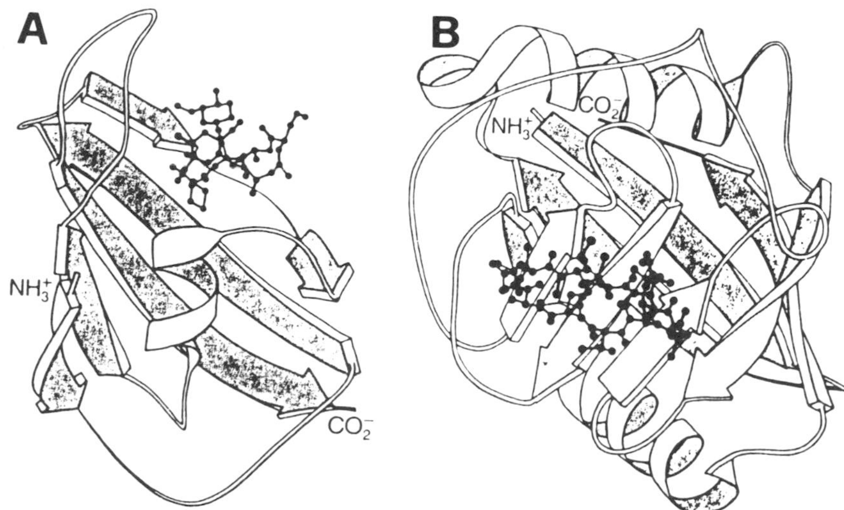

FIG. 6. Three-dimensional structure of the complex of human FKBP (**a**) with FK506 and human CPH-A with CsA (**b**). The data were obtained by x-ray and NMR analyses. (Reproduced from refs. 51 and 72 with permission.)

A role for rotamase inhibition by CsA has been questioned, since the IL-2 gene transcription is fully inhibited at just 1% occupancy of CPH-A. Thus the model linking the inhibition of cellular rotamase to inhibition of gene transcription is rather unlikely (see below).

CsA–CPH Binding Site. The CsA–CPH complex was investigated by x-ray and nuclear magnetic resonance (NMR) techniques (49–53). CPH-A exhibits a β-barrel shape with a radius of 17 Å. The main structural elements are two perpendicular four-stranded β-sheets and two well defined α-helices (Fig. 6A). Most of the hydrophobic side chains are packed in a hydrophobic core. Other hydrophobic residues occur in the contact region between the two helices, the β-sheets, and in the CsA binding site. Replacement of the two cysteines (Cys 62 and 115) by alanine neither affected CsA binding nor rotamase activity. The sole tryptophane residue (Trp 121) is, however, necessary for binding (54). The macrolide binding protein, FKBP (see below), has no significant homology with CPH-A. Common three-dimensional surface structures that could preexist or be induced by CsA or FK506 on their respective immunophilins are presently an area of intense research. Other CsA binding proteins occurring in different cell types include the gp170 membrane transporter (24,25), the bile-salt transporter and Na^+-D-glucose cotransporter in the kidney (57,58), and calmodulin (59). The latter has not been confirmed by others (60,61). Although a membrane receptor has been postulated, the molecular nature has not been identified yet (12,62,63).

Calcineurin as a Target of CsA–CPH Complex. The above arguments render the rotamase model improbable. As shown in Fig. 5 the photolabile CsA derivative labeled not only CPH but also a 60-kDa protein in Jurkat T cells, which is most likely calcineurin. It was recently demonstrated that the phosphatase calcineurin forms a complex with the drug and immunophilin (29,79). The complex was only formed in the presence of the CsA and CPH together with calmodulin and calcium.

Calcineurin consists of catalytic (A) and regulatory (B) subunits. Calcineurin B has a molecular weight (MW) of 19 kDa and high homology to calmodulin. Calcineurin A, the 61-kDa subunit, contains the catalytic domain of the serine–threonine phosphatase. Calcineurin occurs ubiquitously in the body and is a highly conserved protein. Two isozymes of calcineurin A (type I and II) are formed as the result of alternative splicing events (80). The C terminus contains an inhibitory domain and an adjacent calmodulin binding domain, which are rapidly removed by limited proteolysis. The central part of the protein, being resistant to proteolysis, harbors the catalytic domains and is identical for the two isozymes of calcineurin. This region shows extensive similarities to the catalytic subunits of protein phosphatases 1 and 2B, which define a distinct family of protein phosphatases. The 40 amino acid N-terminal fragment, which is specific for calcineurin, contains 11 successive prolines, possibly important for the binding to CPH-A/B or to FKBP. Preliminary results show that CsA binds to the catalytic domain of calcineurin A, thereby inhibiting its phosphatase activity.

Role of Calcineurin in IL-2 Gene Transcription. Calcineurin is abundant in lymphoid cells (81). Fruman et al. (82) demonstrated calcineurin phosphatase activity in lysates of Jurkat T cells. CsA inhibited cellular calcineurin activity at concentrations that inhibit IL-2 synthesis in activated T cells. These findings, taken together, suggest that calcineurin plays a role in T cell activation. Another approach chosen to investigate the role of calcineurin in T cell activation was the cotransfection of an IL-2 promotor-linked reporter-gene construct together with murine calcineurin A into Jurkat cells. As expected, the overexpression of calcineurin caused relative resistance to the immunosuppressants, necessitating higher concentrations in order to achieve the same immunosuppressive effect (82–89). These results implicate calcineurin as a component of the TcR signal transduction pathway. The present understanding of the molecular events leading to the inhibition of IL-2 gene transcription is depicted in Fig. 7.

FK506 AND RAPAMYCIN, MACROLIDES INTERRUPTING DISTINCT PATHWAYS

The macrolide immunosuppressants are a structurally distinct family of immunosuppressants, comprised of FK506 and rapamycin (Fig. 4). While FK506 inhibits cytokine gene transcription in a manner identical to that of CsA, rapamycin has a completely different mode of action (46,70).

Cellular Receptors. Both FK506 and rapamycin bind to a 12-kDa cytosolic protein, FKBP-12 (37,64–67). FKBP12 has no homology to any known protein, but it has rotamase activity comparable to that of the CPHs. The rotamase activity of FKBP12 is inhibited by FK506 and rapamycin but is not affected by CsA. Since

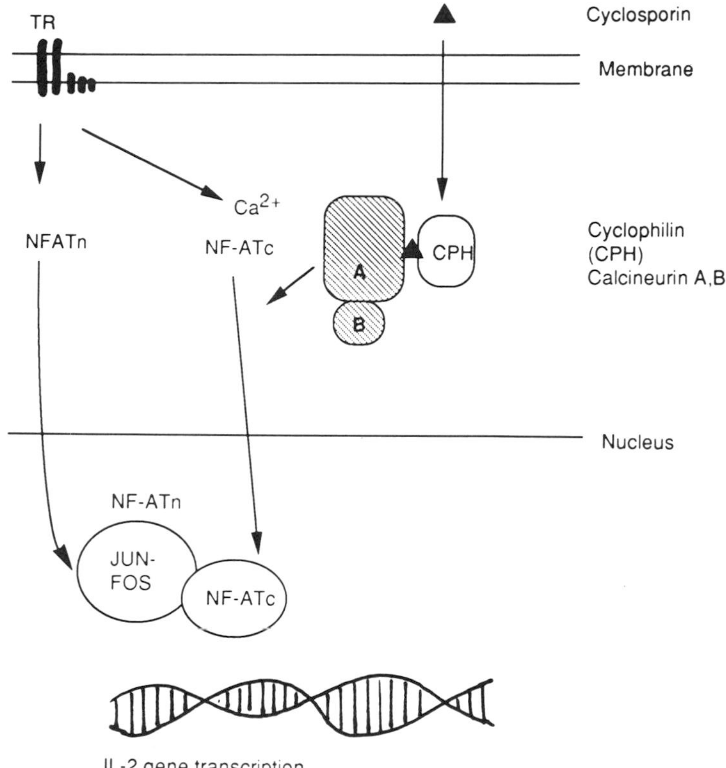

FIG. 7. Schematic representation of the drug–immunophilin complex, binding and inhibition of the calcineurin phosphatase, thus inhibiting the translocation of the cytosolic subunit of the nuclear factor of T cell activation (NFATc).

both FK506 and rapamycin have similar inhibitory effects on FKBP12, inhibition of the rotamase fails to explain the different actions of the two drugs. Additional members of the family with binding specificity for the macrolide immunosuppressants were sought (Table 4). FKBP13, a membrane form like CPH-B, was reported by Jin (68). FKBP13 has similar properties to the cytosolic form, FKBP12, in that it binds to both FK506 and rapamycin.

The discovery of FKBP25 proved to be interesting in that it appears to selectively bind rapamycin (69). The N-terminal 101 amino acids of FKBP25 are unrelated to those of the FKBP proteins and consists of an α-helix. The C-terminal 114 amino acids are homologous to FKBP12, except for a nuclear targeting sequence. The selective inhibition of the S6 kinase pathway by rapamycin (70), but not by FK506 or CsA, in lieu of the selectivity of rapamycin for FKBP25 and its special structural features, leads to the suggestion that FKBP25 may be important in the signaling of this pathway.

Finally, FKBP59, binding both rapamycin and FK506, was identified and shown

TABLE 4. *Properties of CsA and FK506 binding proteins (immunophilins)*

Name	Molecular weight (kDa)	Homology (%)	Cellular location[a]	Rotamase activity	References
Cyclophilins					
CPH-A	18	—	c	+	3,10,11,13,15–18, 20,23,33,38–41, 54,92–95
CPH-B	22	64	m	+	13,26,27,28,33,42, 44,45,83,97,98
CPH-C	23	?	?	+	29,30
CPH-D	22	72	m	+	30
CPH-40	40	?	c	+	31
CPH-45	45	?			32
FKBPs					
FKBP12	12		c	+	56,64–67,72–74,99
FKBP13	13	60	m	+	68
FKBP25	25	40	n	+	69
FKBP59	59		n?	+	71

[a]c, cytosol; m, membrane; n, nucleus.

to be related to and associated with heat shock proteins and the corticosteroid receptor (71). It is important to note that there is no sequence homology between members of the CPH and FKBP families. Finally an association of FKBP12 with calcium release channel theryanodine receptor was reported, the physiological significance of its findings is unclear (94).

The three-dimensional structure was investigated by NMR and x-ray crystallography (Fig. 6B). The main structural elements are a five-stranded antiparallel β-sheet that wraps around a short helix without any similarity to CPH-A. FK506 binds in a shallow cavity between the α-helix and the β-sheet, half of the ligand being buried in the receptor protein. The binding site is composed of conserved aromatic residues (for review see ref. 4).

Inhibition of Rotamase Activity Cannot Explain Immunosuppression. Since it was shown that the rotamase activity was also inhibitable by nonimmunosuppressant macrolides and that the rotamases have no absolute substrate specificity, it was suggested that the FKBPs and immunophilins in general may have a "dominant" function: binding of the drug to the cognate immunophilin may thus result in a gain of function (11). Proline binding by immunophilins might be an important property for the association with common target proteins.

Calcineurin as a Common Target of Drug–Immunophilin Complex. The demonstration that the phosphatase calcineurin forms a complex not only with CsA–CPH but also with FK506–FKBP was an exciting observation, possibly explaining the identical mode of action (29,79). The complex only forms in the presence of the drug, its cognate immunophilin, calmodulin, and calcium. Rapamycin bound to FKBP does not form a complex with calcineurin. The immunosuppressants CsA and FK506 inhibit calcineurin phosphatase activity in the presence of their specific immunophilins and calcium.

FK506, but Not Rapamycin, Blocks IL-2 Gene Transcription by Inhibiting the Calcineurin Phosphatase. Fruman et al. (82) demonstrated that calcineurin phosphatase activity in lysates from Jurkat T cells was inhibited by CsA and FK506, with rapamycin having no effect. Cotransfection of an IL-2 promotor-linked reporter-gene construct together with murine calcineurin A into Jurkat cells caused relative resistance to the immunosuppressants CsA and FK506 (84,85). These results implicate calcineurin as a component of the TcR signal transduction pathway. A likely substrate of calcineurin is the nuclear factor of activated T cells (NFAT), a cytoplasmic phosphoprotein. It is hypothesized that, upon T cell activation, NFAT is dephosphorylated and translocated into the nucleus, where it binds to the IL-2 promotor region. Thus it may be assumed that inhibition of the calcineurin phosphatase prevents this dephosphorylation and subsequent IL-2 gene transcription (Fig. 7).

Rapamycin Inhibits Signal Transduction Through S6 Kinase Activation. It is well established that rapamycin has no effect on calcineurin activity and does not inhibit IL-2 gene transcription. The discovery that rapamycin completely and rapidly inhibits IL-2-induced phosphorylation and activation of p70 S6 kinase was a major breakthrough in the understanding of the differing modes of action of the closely related molecules. The selective blockade of the p70 S6 kinase activation by rapamycin implicates this signaling pathway in the regulation of T cell entry into the S phase. In addition, Chung et al. (90) showed that rapamycin blocked phosphorylation and activation of p70 S6 kinase in a variety of animal cells of nonlymphoid origin. These studies demonstrate that a growth factor-induced signaling event, not merely restricted to T cells, may be impinged on by rapamycin through the induction of a blockade of entry into the S phase. Rapamycin, which binds to the same immunophilin as FK506, FKBP12, neither associates nor inhibits calcineurin phosphatase. Importantly, rapamycin has no effect on IL-2 gene transcription. An interesting observation was the recent discovery of FKBP25 (Table 4), a rapamycin-specific receptor. It may be speculated that FKBP25 targets rapamycin to the rapamycin-sensitive S6 kinase. In contrast to CsA and FK506, rapamycin inhibits the activation process at a later stage, for example, the IL-2 receptor-induced entry into S phase and subsequent T cell proliferation (76,77,89). Kuo et al. (70) presented evidence that IL-2 selectively induces the phosphorylation and activation of the p70 S6 kinase.

AZATHIOPRINE AND STEROIDS: OLD, YET STILL USEFUL THERAPEUTIC MODALITIES

Azathioprine, an imidazole derivative of 6-mercaptopurine, was the first successful immunosuppressant used in renal transplantation. Azathioprine was synthesized by Hitching and Elion and was found to be more potent than 6-mercaptopurine (105). Both compounds are purine analogs and inhibit cell replication. The importance and relative specificity of the inhibited pathway of purine metabolism for lymphocytes are clearly demonstrated by the profound immune incompetence associated with adenosine deaminase deficiency. Azathioprine proved to be a potent immunosuppressant and was useful in preventing allograft rejection, but it has no therapeutic effect in acute rejection episodes. Azathioprine combined with steroids is a most effective immunsuppressive combination. In this combination 1-year graft survival is on the order of 50%. The main dose-limiting effect of azathioprine is myelosuppression (113–120), which relates to its general inhibitory effect on cell replication.

Glucocorticosteroids, which are normally produced by the adrenal cortex, have a broad spectrum of activity including metabolic, anti-inflammatory, and immunosuppressive activities. Their anti-inflammatory and immunosuppressive properties are used to therapeutic advantage in several clinical conditions including autoimmune diseases, allergic reactions, and allograft rejection. The effect of steroids on the immune system are fairly well established. Steroids inhibit the release of the macrophage-derived IL-1, thereby blocking the IL-1-dependent activation of T lymphocytes and synthesis of IL-2, the central T cell growth factor. Steroids also produce lysis of T lymphocytes, an effect that is more profound in murine than in human lymphocytes (121,122).

At low doses steroids are useful as adjunct immunosuppressants and are of prime importance in rejection therapy. For rejection therapy, high dose intravenous (iv) bolus injections of methylprednisolone (up to 1 g) are given in combination with antilymphocyte serum or anti-CD3 antibody.

NOVEL, EXPERIMENTAL IMMUNOSUPPRESSANTS: HOPE FOR THE FUTURE

15-Deoxyspergualin. 15-Deoxyspergualin was isolated from *Bacillus laterosporus* and has an analogous structure to the antitumor drug spergualine. 15-Deoxyspergualin inhibits alloantigen- and mitogen-induced murine and human lymphocyte proliferation. It has no effect on IL-2 production but inhibits IL-2-dependent growth. 15-Deoxyspergualin binds to heat shock proteins and may interfere with a pathway common to that of steroids. 15-Deoxyspergualin prolongs the *in vivo* survival of different types of allografts in several species. Although preventing longer-term rejection, 15-deoxyspergualin does not inhibit acute rejection reactions. The most promising area for this drug is xenotransplantation, where it is highly efficacious (124–134) (Table 3).

RS 61443. RS 61443 is a mycophenolic acid derivative of fungal origin with antitumor, antiviral, and immunosuppressant activities. RS 61443 inhibits two key enzymes of the *de novo* biosynthetic pathway of guanosine. As lymphocytes lack this salvage pathway for purine synthesis, which is present in most other cells, and depend on the *de novo* synthesis, they are therefore inhibited by RS 61443. Lack of guanosine monophosphate (GMP) inhibits the cell cycle progression of lymphocytes but has no effect on IL synthesis. RS 61443 inhibits allograft rejection but has low activity in mice due to rapid metabolism. A synergism with CsA has been reported (135–144) (Table 3).

Brequinar. The sodium salt of brequinar is a novel antitumor agent that inhibits cell proliferation in general by blocking dihydroorotate dihydrogenase in mitochondria. Lymphocyte proliferation is suppressed by its cytostatic activity. Brequinar is effective in the prevention of rat allograft rejection and in prolonging cardiac xenograft survival from hamsters in rats (145–149) (Table 3).

Bredinin. Also known as mizoribine, bredinin is an imidazole nucleoside antimetabolite isolated from *Eupenicillium brefeldianum,* which inhibits the biosynthesis of purine. Bredinin inhibits T lymphocyte proliferation and prevents graft rejection in experimental models when given with CsA (150) (Table 3).

Ciamexone. Ciamexone is a 2-cyan-aziridine derivative with immunomodulatory properties. Ciamexone does not inhibit antigen- or mitogen-induced lymphoproliferation and has no direct effects on T cell function. *In vivo,* however, ciamexone suppresses antibody formation, inhibits graft-versus-host disease, and inhibits several forms of experimental autoimmune disease (151) (Table 3).

Antibodies. Several antibodies directed against the TcR or associated membrane receptor molecules (MHC class II, ICAM-1, LFA-1, CD4) are presently being developed to block T cell activation. The experimental results on transplantation rejection are very promising and clinical trials are ongoing (152–154) (Table 3). In view of the central role of IL-2 in T cell activation, the use of inhibitory antibodies to IL-2R to block cell activation were considered for use in therapy early on. IL-2 receptor-inhibitory antibody may play a role in the treatment of rejection crises. In addition to IL-2, several other cytokines are released during an immune response. The administration of neutralizing antibodies to TNF, IFN-γ, and so on may therefore represent yet another way to block or mitigate an ongoing immune response (155).

SIDE EFFECTS OF IMMUNOSUPPRESSIVE THERAPY

Any form of immunosuppression bears the risk of infections and secondary tumor development. The incidence of infection depends on the dose and the specificity of the immunosuppressant. Viral infections are presently the most frequent complications. With respect to tumor development one may distinguish between direct genetic damage and indirect or epigenetic mechanisms (91,104). Although alkylating agents predominantly comprise the first group, any type of immunosuppressant increases the risk of tumor development due to a weakening of immune surveillance. The tumor types found in immunosuppressed patients include lymphomas, skin tumors, and occasionally brain tumors (104). The risk of these complications may be reduced by minimal dosed immunosuppressive therapies.

Other side effects of immunosuppressive therapy are fever and malaise after

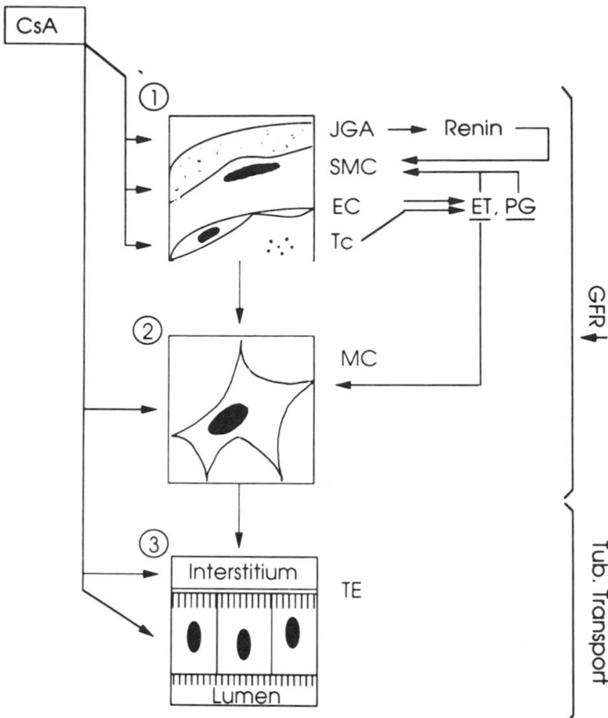

FIG. 8. Possible role of calcineurin in CsA nephrotoxicity. The cellular targets of CsA comprise: (*1*) components of the glomerulus juxtaglomerular apparatus (JGA), endothelial cells (EC), smooth muscle cells (SMC), and thrombocytes (Tc); (*2*) mesangium cells (MC); and (*3*) tubular epithelium (TE)–interstitial cells. Targeting of the immunophilin–drug complex to calcineurin in the kidney results in increased synthesis and release of renin, endothelin (ET) and prostaglandin (PG), with subsequent reduction of glomerular filtration rate (GFR).

OKT3 therapy (known as cytokine release syndrome), leukopenia after azathioprine, Cushing's syndrome following steroids, and renal dysfunction after treatment with CsA or FK506.

The molecular mechanisms responsible for nephrotoxicity warrant further discussion. At immunosuppressive doses, CsA causes a reduction of glomerular filtration rate (GFR) and slight arterial hypertension (101,102). The present knowledge of the pathogenesis of this renal dysfunction is summarized in Fig. 8. CsA may affect renal mesangial cells directly, resulting in reduction of GFR. In addition, endothelial cells and smooth muscle cells, especially of the afferent arterioles, may respond directly to CsA and release further vasoactive mediators. At higher concentrations, tubular epithelial cells themselves may develop degenerative changes.

The abundance of CPH-A, CPH-B, and calcineurin, as determined by Western blot analysis, does not differ between drug-sensitive (lymphocytes and kidney) and drug-resistant organs. Friedman and Weissman (29) claimed that CYP-C is produced only in immune cells and the kidney. CPH-C could therefore provide a rationale for the relative tissue specificity of CsA action and perhaps account for the specificity of organ toxicity (i.e., nephrotoxicity). These findings have yet to be confirmed by other investigators.

Attempts have been made by several groups to correlate the ability of several cyclosporine derivatives to bind CPH with their immunosuppressive and toxic activity *in vivo* (10). However, available *in vitro* data do not confirm such a relationship. The formation of drug–immunophilin complexes with calcineurin is very likely to occur in renal target cells, although these complexes have not yet been demonstrated *in vivo*. A further challenging question is the substrate specificity of the renal calcineurin–immunophilin complex and whether it differs from that of lymphocytes. Possible candidate substrates include the suspected effector peptides of toxicity or factors upstream leading to other mature effectors. Presently, peptides considered important for the development of nephrotoxicity are endothelin, renin, tissue factor, and tumor growth factor-β (TGF-β).

Despite initial enthusiastic reports, FK506 was shown to cause a similar form of nephrotoxicity to CsA in controlled clinical trials. The related macrolide rapamycin, with its different mode of immunosuppression, is devoid of nephrotoxic side effects (B. Ryffel *unpublished data*). One possible explanation is that rapamycin neither binds to calcineurin nor inhibits calcineurin phosphatase activation. These findings suggest that the immunophilin–drug–calcineurin complex may be involved in the development of the nephrotoxicity for both CsA and FK506.

PERSPECTIVE: TOLERANCE AND XENOTRANSPLANTATION

In recent years rapid progress has been made in the understanding of the control of T lymphocyte activation, fostered by the introduction of several investigative tools, including steroids, azathioprine, antilymphocyte sera, CsA, and the macrolide immunosuppressants FK506 and rapamycin.

An important step facilitating this progress was the discovery by Borel (1,92) of the immunosuppressive properties of the fungal-derived undecapeptide CsA. The initial observations by Borel (e.g., high selectivity for the immune system, reversible mode of action, and absence of myelotoxicity) were not only confirmed by many scientists but allowed the development of a clinically invaluable immunosuppressant.

The discovery that CsA inhibits the transcription of the IL-2 gene along with other cytokine genes after T cell activation stimulated investigation into the regulatory regions of the IL-2 enhancer and nuclear transcription factors. Several sites within the IL-2 enhancer region affected by CsA have been identified (4,7,9). The sites that are most sensitive to CsA are the binding sites for NFAT and octamer-associated proteins (OAPs).

NFAT is only expressed in activated T cells and is composed of at least two components: an inducible nuclear (NFATn) component and a constitutively expressed cytoplasmic (NFATc) component. NFATn was recently shown to be identical to the AP-1 complex comprising the heterodimer of JUN and FOS protein (93). The formation of the AP-1 complex was repeatedly shown to be CsA resistant. NFATc is a preformed cytosolic protein (of about 80 kDa), which is translocated upon T cell activation. Flanagan et al. (86) made the important observation that CsA and FK506 inhibited the nuclear translocation of NFATc, thus preventing the formation of a functional NFAT complex necessary for binding to the IL-2 gene enhancer. An important question, which has not yet been answered, is how CsA inhibits the nuclear translocation of NFATc. The discovery of the cytosolic CsA receptor by Handschumacher et al. (15) initiated much fruitful research, resulting in the identification of several binding proteins for CsA and macrolides, collectively termed the immunophilins (11). An intriguing common feature of the immunophilins is their rotamase activity.

Although the immunophilins specifically bind CsA and FK506 and clearly facilitate their intracellular accumulation, the relationship of the inhibition of immunophilin–rotamase activity to the immunosuppressive effect is unlikely. New models of action result from the discovery that the drug–immunophilin complex binds calcineurin—a ubiquitous phosphatase—inhibited by CsA and FK506. This discovery clearly stimulated a search for tissue-specific substrates. In the absence of hard data it has been hypothesized that activation of calcineurin might be important for the translocation of NFATc and thus IL-2 gene transcription.

While many research groups are focusing on the search for calcineurin substrates, other proteins should be considered as targets to which the drug–immunophilin complex might bind, with ensuing functional alterations. The association of FKBP with the glucocorticosteroid receptor and/or of deoxyspergualin to heat shock are such examples. The discovery of FKBP25, a rapamycin-specific receptor, may be important to the understanding of the mode of rapamycin action on S6 kinase. Selective inhibition of the S6 kinase by rapamycin together with the selective receptor FKBP25 is also a field that may provide new insights into the biochemical mechanisms of the cytokine signal pathways.

Mechanistic studies with these and other novel experimental immunosuppressants should provide new insight into pathways of gene activation. Since some of these agents have promise in the prevention of xenograft rejection, it is quite possible that novel pathways will be unraveled. The ultimate goal is the induction of transplant tolerance, a goal that is presently only achievable in rodent models.

With the advent of novel immunosuppressive agents and technical improvements in transplant surgery, xenotransplantation is being considered in light of the shortage of human kidneys, so that more patients might benefit from organ replacement therapy. The rejection of discordant xenografts is very different from classic cell-mediated allograft rejection. It appears to involve the binding of naturally occurring host antibodies to xenograft antigens, followed by the activation of complement (157).

Xenotransplantation of healthy organs with tolerance induction is the ultimate goal of pharmaceutical intervention in the immune system. Although impressive theoretical and experimental advances in the area of tolerance have been achieved (156), the clinical applications are still far off.

REFERENCES

1. Borel JF. Pharmacology of cyclosporin (Sandimmune). *Pharmacol Rev* 1989;42:260–372.
2. Morris PJ. Cyclosporine, FK506 and other drugs in organ transplantation. *Curr Opinion Immunol* 1991;3:748–751.
3. Ryffel B. Pharmacology of cyclosporine. Cellular activation: regulation of intracellular events by cyclosporin. *Pharmacol Rev* 1989;41:407–421.
4. Schreiber S, Crabtree G. The mechanism of action of cyclosporin A and FK506. *Immunol Today* 1992;13:136–142.
5. Sigal N, Dumont FJ. Cyclosporin A, FK-506 and rapamycin: pharmacological probes of lymphocyte signal transduction. *Annu Rev Immunol* 1992;10:519–560.
6. Thomson AW, Starzl TE. New immunosuppressive drugs: mechanistic insights and potential therapeutic advances. *Immunol Rev* 1993;136:71–98
7. Dunnill MS. Histopathology of rejection in renal transplantation. In: Morris PJ, ed. *Kidney transplantation: principles and practice*. Philadelphia: Saunders; 1989.
8. Olsen TS. Pathology of allograft rejection. In: Burdick JF, Racusen LC, Solez K, Williams GM, eds. *Kidney transplant rejection: diagnosis and treatment*. New York: Marcel Dekker; 1992.
9. Young PR. Protein hormones and their receptors. *Biotechnology* 1992;3:408–421.
10. Akira S, Kishimoto T. Mechanisms of soluble mediators. *Immunology* 1992;4:307–313.
11. Schreiber S. Chemistry and biology of the immunophilines and their immunosuppressive ligands. *Science* 1991;251:283–287.
12. Ryffel B, Goetz U, Heuberger B. Cyclosporin receptors on human lymphocytes. *J Immunol* 1982; 129:1978–1982.
13. Foxwell B, Frazer G, Winters M, Hiestand P, Wenger R, Ryffel B. Identification of cyclophilin as the erythrocyte cyclosporin-binding protein. *Biochim Biophys Acta* 1988;938:447–455.
14. Merker M, Handschumacher R. Uptake and nature of the intracellular binding of cyclosporin A in a murine thymoma cell line BW5147. *J Immunol* 1984;132:3064–3070.
15. Handschumacher R, Harding M, Rice J, Drugge R. Cyclophilin: a specific cytosolic binding protein for cyclosporin A. *Science* 1984;226:544–547.
16. Harding M, Handschumacher R, Speicher D. Isolation and amino acid sequence of cyclophilin. *J Biol Chem* 1986;261:8547–8555.
17. Fischer G, Wittmann-Liebold B, Lang K, Kiefhaber T, Schmid FX. Cyclophilin and peptidyl-prolyl cis-trans isomerase are probably identical proteins. *Nature* 1989;337:473–476.
18. Takahashi N, Hayano T, Suzuki M. Peptidylprolyl cis-trans isomerase is the cyclosporin A-binding protein cyclophilin. *Nature* 1989;337:473–475.
19. Quesniaux VFJ. Pharmacology of cyclosporine (Sandimmune). III. Immunochemistry and monitoring. *Pharmacol Rev* 1989;41:249.
20. Quesniaux VFJ, Schreier MH, Wenger RM, Hiestand PC, Harding M, Van Regenmortel MHV. Cyclophilin binds to the region of cyclosporin involved in its immunosuppressive activity. *Eur J Immunol* 1987;17:1359–1365.
21. Quesniaux VFJ, Schreier MH, Wenger RM, Van Regenmortel MHV. Molecular characteristics of cyclophilin–cyclosporin interaction. *Transplantation* 1988;46:23S–27S.
22. Foxwell B, Woerly G, Husi H, et al. Identification of several cyclosporin binding proteins in lymphoid and non-lymphoid cells in vivo. *Biochim Biophys Acta* 1992;1138:115–121.
23. Hsu V, Heald S, Harding M, Handschumacher R, Armitage I. Structural elements pertinent to the interaction of cyclosporin A with its specific receptor protein, cyclophilin. *Biochem Pharmacol* 1990;40:131–140.
24. Foxwell B, Mackie A, Ling V, Ryffel B. Identification of the multi-drug resistance related p-glycoprotein as a cyclosporin binding protein. *Mol Pharmacol* 1989;36:543–546.
25. Wenger RM. Cyclosporin: conformation and analogues as tools for studying its mechanisms of action. *Transplant Proc* 1988;20:313–318.

26. Caroni P, Rothenfluh A, McGlynn E, Schneider C. S-cyclophilin, new member of the cyclophilin family associated with the secretory pathway. *J Biol Chem* 1991;266:10739–10742.
27. Hasel KW, Glass JR, Godbout M, Suthcliffe JG. An endoplasmatic reticulum-specific cyclophilin. *Mol Cell Biol* 1991;11:3484–3491.
28. Price ER, Cidowski LD, Jin M, Baker CH, McKion FD, Walsh CHT. Human cyclophilin B, a second cyclophilin gene encodes a peptidyl-prolyl isomerase with a signal sequence. *Proc Natl Acad Sci USA* 1991;88:1903–1907.
29. Friedman J, Weissman I. Two cytoplasmic candidates for immunophilin action are revealed by affinity for a new cyclophilin: one in the presence and one in the absence of CsA. *Cell* 1991;66: 799–806.
30. Bergsma DJ, Eder C, Gross M, et al. The cyclophilin multigene family of peptidyl-prolyl isomerases. *J Biol Chem* 1991;266:23204–23214.
31. Kieffer LJ, Thalhammer T, Handschumacher RE. Isolation and characterization of a 40-kDa cyclophilin-related protein. *J Biol Chem* 1992;267:1–5.
32. Foxwell B, Hiestand P, Wenger R, Ryffel B. A comparison of cyclosporin binding by cyclophilin and calmodulin and the identification of a novel 45KD cyclosporin-binding phosphoprotein in Jurkat cells. *Transplantation* 1988;46:35S–40S.
33. Schönbrunner ER, Mayer S, Tropschug M, Fischer G, Takahashi N, Schmid FX. Catalysis of protein folding by cyclophilins from different species. *J Biol Chem* 1991;266:3630–3635.
34. Marks WH, Harding MW, Handschumacher R, Marks C, Lorber MI. The immunochemical distribution of cyclophilin in normal mammalian tissues. *Transplantation* 1991;52:340–345.
35. McDonald ML, Ardito T, Marks WH, Kashgarian M, Lorber MI. The effect of cyclosporine administration on the cellular distribution and content of cyclophilin. *Transplantation* 1992;53:460–466.
36. Ryffel B, Foxwell G, Gee A, Greiner B, Woerly G, Mihatsch MJ. Cyclosporin-relationship of side effects to mode of action. *Transplantation* 1988;46:90S–96S.
37. Standaert RF, Galat A, Verdine GL, Schreiber SL. Molecular cloning and overexpression of the human FK506-binding protein FKBP. *Nature* 1990;346:671–674.
38. Danielson P, Forss-Petter S, Brown M, Calavetta L, Douglass J, Milner R, Suthcliffe J. p1B15: a cDNA clone of the rat mRNA encoding cyclophilin. *DNA* 1988;7:261–267.
39. Haendler B, Hofer-Warbinek R, Hofer E. Complementary DNA for human T-cell cyclophilin. *EMBO J* 1987;6:947–950.
40. Haendler B, Keller R, Hiestand P, Kocher H, Wegmann G. Yeast cyclophilin. Isolation and characterization of the protein, cDNA and gene. *Gene* 1989;83:39–46.
41. Hasel KW, Suthcliff JG. Nucleotide sequence of a cDNA coding for mouse cyclophilin. *Nucleic Acids Res* 1990;18:4019.
42. Iwai N, Inagami T. Molecular cloning of a complementary DNA to rat cyclophilin-like protein mRNA. *Kidney Int* 1990;37:1460–1465.
43. Koletsky A, Harding M, Handschumacher R. Cyclophilin: distribution and variant properties in normal and neoplastic tissues. *J Immunol* 1986;137:1054.
44. Tropschug M, Nicholson D, Hartl F, Koeler H, Pfanner N, Wachter E, Neupert W. Cyclosporin A-binding protein (cyclophilin) of *Neuraspora crassa*. *J Biol Chem* 1988;263:14433–14440.
45. Tropschug M, Bathelmess IB, Neupert W. Sensitivity to cyclosporin A is mediated by cyclophilin in *Neurospora crassa* and *Saccharomyces cerevisiae*. *Nature* 1989;342:953–955.
46. Shieh BH, Stamnes MA, Seavelb S, Harris GL, Zuker CS. The nina A gene required for visual transduction in *Drosophila* encodes a homologue of cyclosporin A-binding protein. *Nature* 1989; 338:67–70.
47. Sherry B, Yarlett N, Strupp A, Cerami A. Identification of cyclophilin as a proinflammatory secretory product of lipopolysaccharide-activated macrophages. *Proc Natl Acad Sci USA* 1992;89: 3511–3515.
48. Ryffel B, Woerly G, Greiner B, Haendler B, Mihatsch MJ, Foxwell B. Distribution of the cyclosporin binding protein cyclophilin in human tissues. *Immunology* 1991;72:399–404.
49. Fesik SW, Gampe RT Jr, Holzman TF, et al. Isotope-edited NMR of cyclosporin A bound to cyclophilin: evidence for a trans 9,10 amide bond. *Science* 1990;250;1406–1409.
50. Kallen J, Spitzfaden C, Zurini MG, Wider, G, Widmer H, Wüthrich K, Walkinshaw MD. Structure of human cyclophilin and its binding site for cyclosporin A determined by X-ray crystallography and NMR spectroscopy. *Nature* 1991;353:276–279.
51. Ke H, Zydowsky L, Liu J, Walsh C. Crystal structure of recombinant human T-cell cyclophilin A at 2.5 Å resolution. *Proc Natl Acad Sci USA* 1991;88:9483–9487.

52. Spitzfaden C, Weber HP, Braun W, et al. Cyclosporin A-cyclophilin complex formation: a model based on X-ray and NMR data. *FEBS Lett* 1992;300:291–300.
53. Wüthrich K, von Freyberg B, Weber C, Wider G, Traber R, Widmer H, Braun W. Receptor-induced confirmation, change of the immunosuppressant cyclosporin A. *Science* 1991;254:953–955.
54. Liu J, Albers MW, Chen CM, Schreiber SL, Walsh CT. Cloning expression and purification of human cyclophilin in *Escherichia coli* and assessment of the catalytic role of cysteines by site-directed mutagenesis. *Proc Natl Acad Sci USA* 1990;87:2304–2308.
55. Tamai I, Safa AR. Azidopine noncompetitively interacts with vinblastine and cyclosporin A binding to P-glycoprotein in multidrug resistant cells. *J Biol Chem* 1991;266:16796–16800.
56. Van Duyne GD, Standaert RF, Karplus PA, Schreiber SL, Clardy J. Atomic structure of FKBP–FK506, an immunophilin–immunosuppressant complex. *Science* 1991;252:839–842.
57. Ziegler K, Frimmer M, Fritzsch G, Koepsell H. Cyclosporin binding to a protein component of the renal Na^+-D-glucose cotransporter. *J Biol Chem* 1990;265:3270–3277.
58. Ziegler K, Frimmer M, Koepsell H. Photoaffinity labeling of membrane proteins from rat liver and pig kidney with cyclosporin diazirine. *Transplantation* 1988;46:s15–s20.
59. Colombani P, Robb A, Hess A. Cyclosporin A binding to calmodulin: a possible site of action on T lymphocytes. *Science* 1985;228:337–339.
60. Foxwell B, Wong WC, Borel JF, Ryffel B. A comparison of cyclosporin binding by cyclophilin and calmodulin. *Transplant Proc* 1989;21:873–875.
61. LeGrue SJ, Turner R, Weisbrodt N, Dedman JR. Does the binding of cyclosporin to calmodulin result in immunosuppression? *Science* 1986;234:68–71.
62. Cacalano NA, Chen BX, Cleveland WL, Erlanger BF. Evidence for a functional receptor for cyclosporin A on the surface of lymphocytes. *Proc Natl Acad Sci USA* 1992;89:4353–4357.
63. Cacalano N, Cleveland W, Erlanger B. Characterization of a monoclonal anti-idiotypic antibody that mimics cyclosporin A in a single binding system. *J Immunol* 1991;147:3012–3017.
64. Harding WM, Galat A, Uehling DE, Speicher DW. A receptor for the immunosuppressant FK506 is a cis-trans peptidyl-prolyl-isomerase. *Nature* 1989;341:758–760.
65. Lane WS, Galat A, Harding MW, Schreiber SL. Complete amino acid sequence of the FK506 and rapamycin binding protein, FKBP, isolated from calf thymus. *J Protein Chem* 1991;10:151–160.
66. Maki N, Sekiguchi F, Nishimaki J, Miwa K, Hayano T, Takahashi N, Suzuki M. Complementary DNA encoding the human T-cell FK 506-binding protein, a peptidylprolyl cis-trans isomerase distinct from cyclophilin. *Proc Natl Acad Sci USA* 1990;87:5440–5443.
67. Siekierka JJ, Hung SHY, Poe M, Lin CS, Sigal NH. A cytosolic binding protein for the immunosuppressant FK506 has peptidyl-prolyl isomerase activity but is distinct from cyclophilin. *Nature* 1989;341:755–757.
68. Jin YJ, Albers MW, Lane WS, Bierer BE, Schreiber SL, Burakoff SJ. Molecular cloning of a membrane-associated human FK 506- and rapamycin-binding protein, FKBP-13. *Proc Natl Acad Sci USA* 1991;88:6677–6681.
69. Galat A, Lane WS, Standaert RF, Schreiber SL. A rapamycin-selective 25-kDa immunophilin. *Biochemistry* 1992;31:2427–2434.
70. Kuo CJ, Chung J, Florentino DF, Flanagan WM, Blenis J, Crabtree GR. Rapamycin selectively inhibits interleukin-2 activations of p70 S6 kinase. *Nature* 1992;358:70–73.
71. Tai PK, Albers MW, Chang H, Faber LE, Schreiber SL. Association of a 59-kilodalton immunophilin with the gluco-corticoid receptor complex. *Science* 1992;256:1315.
72. Michnick SW, Rosen, MK, Wandless TJ, Karplus M, Schreiber SL. Solution structure of FKBP, a rotamase enzyme and receptor for FK 506 and rapamycin. *Science* 1991;252:836–839.
73. Moore JM, Peattie DA, Fitzgibbon MJ, Thomson JA. Solution structure of the major binding protein for the immunosuppressant FK506. *Nature* 1991;351:248–250.
74. Van Duyne GD, Staendert RF, Galat A, Clardy J. Atomic structure of the rapamycin human immunophilin FKBP-12 complex. *J Am Chem Soc* 1991;113:7433–7434.
75. Gething M, Sambrook J. Protein folding in the cell. *Nature* 1992;355:33–45.
76. Bierer BE, Mattila P, Standaert, R, Herzenberg L, Burakoff S, Crabtree G, Schreiber SL. Two distinct signal transmission pathways in T lymphocytes are inhibited by complexes formed between an immunophilin and either FK506 or rapamycin. *Proc Natl Acad Sci USA* 1990;87:9231–9235.
77. Bierer BE, Somers P, Wandless T, Burakoff S, Schreiber SL. Probing immunosuppressant action with a nonnatural immunophilin ligand. *Science* 1990;250:556–559.
78. Rosen MK, Standaert RF, Galat A, Nakatsuka M, Schreiber SL. Inhibition of FKBP rotamase activity by immunosuppressant FK506: twisted amide surrogate. *Science* 1990;248:863–866.

79. Liu J, Farmer JD, Lane WS, Friedman J, Weissman I, Schreiber SL. Calcineurin is a common target of cyclophilin–cyclosporin A and FKBP–FK506 complexes. *Cell* 1991;66:807–815.
80. Guerini A, Klee CB. Cloning of human calcineurin A. Evidence for two isozymes and identification of a polyproline structural domain. *Proc Natl Acad Sci USA* 1989;56:9183–9187.
81. Kincaid RL, Takayama H, Billingsley ML, Sitkovsky V. Differential expression of calmodulin-binding proteins in B, T lymphocytes and thymocytes. *Nature* 1987;330:176–178.
82. Fruman DA, Klee CB, Bieber BA, Burakoff SJ. Calcineurin phosphatase activity in T lymphocytes is inhibited by FK 506 and cyclosporin A. *Proc Natl Acad Sci USA* 1992;89:3686–3690.
83. Swanson KH, Born T, Zydowsky LD, Cho H, Chang HY, Walsh CT, Rusnak F. Cyclosporin-mediated inhibition of bovine calcineurin by cyclophilins A and B. *Proc Natl Acad Sci* 1992;89:3741–3745.
84. Clipstone NA, Crabtree GR. Identification of calcineurin as a key signalling enzyme in T-lymphocyte activation. *Nature* 1992;357:695.
85. O'Keefe SJ, Tamura J, Kincaid RL, Tocci MJ, O'Neill EA. FK-506- and CsA-sensitive activation of the interleukin-2 promoter by calcineurin. *Nature* 1992;357:692–694.
86. Flanagan WM, Corthésy B, Bram R, Crabtree GR. Nuclear association of a T-cell transcription factor blocked by FK-506 and cyclosporin A. *Nature* 1991;352:803–806.
87. Flanagan WM, Crabtree GR. In vitro transcription faithfully reflecting T-cell activation requirements. *J Biol Chem* 1992;267:399–406.
88. Moll T, Tebb G, Surana U, Robitsch H, Nasmyth K. The role of phosphorylation and the CDC28 protein kinase in cell cycle-regulated nuclear import of the *S. cerevisiae* transcription factor SW15. *Cell* 1991;66:743–758.
89. Staruch M, Sigal N, Dumont F. Differential effects of the immunosuppressive macrolides FK-506 and rapamycin on activation-induced T-cell apoptosis. *Int J Immunopharmacol* 1991;13:677–685.
90. Chung J, Kuo CJ, Crabtree GR, Blenis J. Rapamycin–FKBP specifically blocks growth-dependent activation of and signaling by the 70 kd S6 protein kinases. *Cell* 1992;69:1227–1236.
91. Ryffel B. The carcinogenicity of cyclosporin. *Toxicology* 1992;73:1–22.
92. Borel JF, Feurer C, Gubler H, Staehelin H. Biological effects of cyclosporin A: a new anti-lymphocytic agent. *Agents Action* 1976;6:468–475.
93. Jain J, McCaffrey PG, Valga-Archer VE, Rao A. Nuclear factor of activated T cells contains Fos and Jun. *Nature* 1992;356:801.
94. Jayarama T, Brillantes AM, Timerman AP, Fleischer S, Erdjument-Bromage H, Tempst P, Marks AR. FK506 binding protein associated with the calcium release channel (rynodine receptor). *J Biol Chem* 1992;267:9474–9477.
95. Quesniaux VFJ, Tees R, Schreier MH, Wenger RM, Van Regenmortel MHV. Fine specificity and cross-reactivity of monoclonal antibodies to cyclosporin. *Mol Immunol* 1987;24:1159–1168.
96. Quesniaux VFJ, Tees R, Schreier MH, Maurer G, Van Regenmortel MHV. Fine specificity and cross-reactivity of monoclonal antibodies to improve therapeutic monitoring of cyclosporin. *Clin Chem* 1987;33:32–37.
97. Ryffel B, Woerly G, Quesniaux V, Husi H, Foxwell B. Covalent binding of cyclosporin inhibits irreversible T-lymphocyte activation. *Biochem Pharmacol* 1992;43:953–960.
98. Spik G, Haendler B, Delmass O, et al. A novel secreted cyclophilin-like protein (SCYLT). *J Biol Chem* 1991;266:10735–10738.
99. Fretz H, Albers MW, Galat A, et al. Rapamycin and FK506 binding protein (immunophilins). *J Am Chem Soc* 1991;113:1409–1411.
100. Crabtree GR. Contingent genetic regulatory events in T lymphocyte activation. *Science* 1989; 243:355–361.
101. Mason J. Pathophysiology and toxicology of cyclosporine in humans and animals. *Pharmacol Rev* 1989;41:423–434.
102. Mihatsch MJ, Thiel G, Ryffel B. Renal side-effects of cyclosporin A with special reference to autoimmune diseases. *Br J Dermatol* 1990;36:101–115.
103. Ryffel B. Toxicology: experimental studies. *Prog Allergy* 1986;38:181–192.
104. Penn I. The price of immunotherapy. *Curr Probl Surg* 1981;18:681.
105. Hamilton D. Kidney transplantation: a history. In: Morris PJ, ed. *Kidney transplantation: principles and practice*. Philadelphia: Saunders; 1989.
106. Calne RY, White DJG, Thiru S, et al. Cyclosporin A in patients receiving renal allografts from cadaver donors. *Lancet* 1978;2:1323–1326.
107. Burdick JF, Racusen LC, Solez K, Williams GM, eds. *Kidney transplant rejection: diagnosis and treatment*. New York: Marcel Dekker; 1992.

108. Allison AC, Eugui EM. Immunosuppressive and other effects of mycophenolic acid and ester prodrug, mycophenolate mofetil. *Immunol Rev* 1993;136:5–28.
109. Kahan BD. Toward a rational design of clinical trials of immunosuppressive agents in transplantation. *Immunol Rev* 1993;136:29–50.
110. Häyry P, Isoniemi H, Ylmaz S. Chronic allograft rejection. *Immunol Rev* 1993;134:33–82.
111. Fellström BC, Larson E. Pathogenesis and treatment perspectives of chronic graft rejection. *Immunol Rev* 1993;134:83–99.
112. Janeway CA. The T cell receptor as a multicomponent signalling machine: CD4/CD8 coreceptors and CD45 in T cell activation. *Annu Rev Immunol* 1992;10:645–674.
113. Elion GB, Callahan S, Bieber S, Hitchings GH, Rundles RW. *Cancer Chemother Rep* 1961; 14:93–98.
114. Calne RY, Alexandre GPJ, Murray JE. *Ann NY Acad Sci* 1962;99:743–761.
115. Murray JE, Merrill JP, Damin GJ, Dealy JB, Alexandre GPJ, Harrison JH. *Ann Surg* 1962; 156:337–355.
116. Bach JF, ed. *The mode of action of immunosuppressive agents*. Amsterdam: North-Holland; 1975.
117. Min DI, Monaco AP. Complications associated with immunosuppressive therapy and their management. *Pharmacotherapy* 1991;11:119S–125S.
118. Walker RG, d'Apice AJF, Mathew TH, Jacob C, Hardie IR, Menzies BO, Miach PJ. Combination immunosuppressive therapy in cadaveric renal transplantation: initial experience with a flexible regimen. *Transplant Proc* 1987;19:2834–2836.
119. Mussche MM, Ringoir SGM, Lamiere NN. *Nephron* 1976;16:289–291.
120. d'Apice AJF, Becker GJ, Kincaid-Smith P, et al. A prospective randomized trial of low-dose versus high-dose steroids in cadaveric renal transplantation.*Transplantation* 1984;37:373–377.
121. Cupps TR, Fauci AS. Corticosteroid-mediated immunoregulation in man. *Immunol Rev* 1982; 65:133–155.
122. Claman HN. Corticosteroids and lymphoid cells. *N Engl J Med* 1972;287:388–394.
123. Morris RE. Rapamycins: antifungal, antitumor, antiproliferative, and immunosuppressive macrolides. *Transplant Rev* 1992;6:39–87.
124. Okubo M, Amemiya K, Kamata K, et al. Toxicological and immunological evaluation of the immunosuppressant 15-deoxyspergualin in BALB/c mice: an in vivo and in vitro study. *Immunopharmacology* 1991;21:99–107.
125. Krzymanski M, Waaga AM, Ulrichs K, Muller-Ruchholtz W. Long standing rat kidney graft survival by a combination of organ perfusion with MHC class II monoclonal antibody and immunosuppression with reduced doses of 15-deoxyspergualin. *Immunol Invest* 1991;20:253–256.
126. Takasu S, Sakagami K, Morisaki F, et al. Immunosuppressive mechanism of 15-deoxyspergualin on sinusoidal lining cells in swine liver transplantation: suppression of MHC class II antigens and interleukin-1 production. *J Surg Res* 1991;51:165–169.
127. DeMasi R, Araneda D, Gross U, et al. Improved xenograft survival with continuous infusion deoxyspergualin and RATG. *J Invest Surg* 1991;4:59–67.
128. Okubo M, Umetani N, Inoue K, Kamata K, Shimoda Y, Uchiyama T, Aoyagi T. Reversal of established nephropathy in New Zealand B/W F1 mice by 15-deoxyspergualin. *Nephron* 1991; 57:99–105.
129. Nemoto K, Hayashi M, Ito J, et al. Deoxyspergualin in lethal murine graft versus host disease. *Transplantation* 1991;51:712–715.
130. Fukao K, Iwasaki H, Yuzawa K, et al. Immunosuppressive effect and toxicity of 15-deoxyspergualin in cynomolgus monkey. *Transplant Proc* 1991;23:556–558.
131. Hibasami H, Tsukada T, Suzuki R, et al. 15-deoxyspergualin, an antiproliferative agent for human and mouse leukemia cells shows inhibitory effects on the synthetic pathway of polyamines. *Anticancer Res* 1991;11:325–330.
132. Yabuuchi H, Nakajima Y, Segawa M, et al. Prominent prolongation of islet xenograft survival in combination therapy with FK 506 and 15-deoxyspergualin. *Transplant Proc* 1991;23:859–861.
133. Carobbi A, Araneda D, Patselas T, Thomas J, Mosca F, Thomas F. Effect of splenectomy in combination with FK 506 and 15-deoxyspergualin on cardiac xenograft survival. *Transplant Proc* 1991;23:549–550.
134. Nadler SG, Tepper MA, Schacter B, Mazzucco CE. Interaction of the immunosuppressant deoxyspargualin with a member of the Hsp70 family of heat shock proteins. *Science* 1992;258:484–486.
135. Platz KP, Eckhoff DE, Hullett DA, Sollinger HW. RS-61443 studies: review and proposal. *Transplant Proc* 1991;23:33–35.

136. Simmons RL, Wang SC. New horizons in immunosuppression. *Tansplant Proc* 1991;23:2152–2156.
137. Morris RE, Wang J, Blum JR, et al. Immunosuppressive effects of the morpholinoethyl ester of mycophenolic acid (RS-61443) in rat and nonhuman primate recipients of heart allografts. *Transplant Proc* 1991;23:19–25.
138. Allison AC, Almquist SJ, Muller CD, Eugui EM. In vitro immunosuppressive effects of mycophenolic acid and an ester pro-drug, RS-61443. *Transplant Proc* 1991;23:10–14.
139. Allison AC, Eugui EM. Immunosuppressive and long acting anti-inflammatory activity of mycophenolic acid and derivative, RS-61443. *Br J Rheumatol* 1991;30:57–61.
140. Platz KP, Bechstein WO, Eckhoff DE, Suzuki Y, Sollinger HW. RS-61443 reverses acute allograft rejection in dogs. *Surgery* 1991:110:736–741.
141. Hao L, Calcinaro F, Lafferty KJ, Allison AC, Eugui EM. Tolerance induction in adult mice: cyclosporine inhibits RS-61443 induced tolerance. *Transplant Proc* 1991;23:733–734.
142. Platz KP, Sollinger HW, Hullett DA, Eckhoff DE, Eugui EM, Allison AC. RS-61443 a new, potent immunosuppressive agent. *Transplantation* 1991;51:27–31.
143. Eugui EM, Mirkovich A, Allison ACC. Lymphocyte-selective antiproliferative and immunosuppressive activity of mycophenolic acid and its morpholinoethyl ester (RS-61443). *Transplant Proc* 1991;23:15–18.
144. Burlingham WEJ, Grailer AP, Hullett DA, Sollinger HW. Inhibition of both MLC and in vitro IgG memory response to tetanus toxoid by RS-61443. *Transplantation* 1991;51:545–547.
145. Cramer DV, Chapman FA, Jaffee BD, Eiras-Hreha G, Yasunaga C, Wu GD, Makowka L. The effect of a new immunosuppressive drug, brequinar sodium, on concordant hamster to rat cardiac xenografts. *Transplant Proc* 1992;24:720–721.
146. Cramer DV, Chapman FA, Jaffee BD, Jones EA, Knoop M, Hreha-Eiras G, Makowka L The effect of a new immunosuppressive drug, brequinar sodium, on heart, liver and kidney allograft rejection in the rat. *Transplantation* 1992;53:303–308.
147. Lakaschus G, Loffler M. Differential susceptibility of dihydroorotate dehydrogenase/oxidase to brequinar sodium (NSC 368 390) in vitro. *Biochem Pharmacol* 1992;43:1025–1030.
148. Chen SF, Perrella FW, Behrens DL, Papp LM. Inhibition of dihydroorotate dehydrogenase activity by brequinar sodium. *Cancer Res* 1992;52:3521–3527.
149. Loffler M. The "anti-pyrimidine effect" of hypoxia and brequinar sodium (NSC 368390) is of consequence for tumor cell growth. *Biochem Pharmacol* 1992;43:2281–2287.
150. Dayton JS, Turka LA, Thompson CB, Mitchell BS. Comparison of the effects of mizoribine with those of azathioprine, 6-mercaptopurine, and mycophenolic acid on T lymphocyte proliferation and purine ribonucleotide metabolism. *Mol Pharmacol* 1992;41:671.
151. Baier J, Neumann HA, Ricken O. No inhibition of interferon gamma release in human lymphocytes by ciamexone. *Cancer Immunol Immunother* 1991;32:311–314.
152. Gruber SA. Locoregional immunosuppression of organ transplants. *Immunol Rev* 1992;129:5–30.
153. Shizuru JA, Alters SE, Fathman CG. Anti-CD4 monoclonal antibodies in therapy: creation of nonclassical tolerance in the adult. *Immunol Rev* 1992;129:105–130.
154. Cobbold SP, Qin S, Leong LYW, Martin G, Waldmann H. Reprogramming the immune system for peripheral tolerance with CD4 and CD8 monoclonal antibodies. *Immunol Rev* 1992;129:165–201.
155. Waldmann TA. Immune receptors: targets for therapy of leukemia/lymphoma, autoimmune diseases and for the prevention of allograft rejection. *Annu Rev Immunol* 1992;10:675–704.
156. Lo D. T cell tolerance: *Curr Opin Immunol* 1992;4:711–715.
157. Platt JL, Vercellotti GM, Dalmasso AP, Matas AJ, Bolman RM, Najarian JS, Bach FH. Transplantation of discordant xenografts: a review of progress. *Immunol Today* 1990;11:450–456.

Immunotoxicology and Immunopharmacology, Second Edition, edited by J. H. Dean, M. I. Luster, A. E. Munson, and I. Kimber.
Raven Press, Ltd., New York © 1994.

16

Cytoreductive Drugs

Jacques G. Descotes and Thierry Vial

Laboratory of Fundamental and Clinical Immunotoxicology, INSERM U80, Alexis Carrel Faculty of Medicine, 69008 Lyon, France

Cytoreductive drugs are used in the treatment of cancer because of their ability to impair neoplastic cell growth. As a side effect, they have been shown to interfere with the immune system in a number of ways (1–3). Because of their cytotoxic effects on proliferating cells, most anticancer drugs possess intrinsic immunosuppressive properties. At low concentration, augmentation of the immune response has also been documented (4).

In addition, some cytoreductive drugs, in particular, azathioprine, cyclophosphamide, and methotrexate, have been found to be effective immunosuppressive agents in preventing allograft rejection and to treat various immunopathologic conditions.

Apart from direct toxicity to the bone marrow, resulting in neutropenia and a decreased ability to fight infection (5), cytotoxic drugs exert marked effects on the immune system. For this reason they are generally considered as prototype immunotoxic agents. In treated patients, the direct immunotoxicity of these drugs is often expressed as opportunistic infections and lymphomas. Azathioprine, cyclophosphamide, and methotrexate will be considered more extensively in this chapter as the clinical experience gained with these drugs allows for a better correlation between immunosuppressive properties and reported side effects.

AZATHIOPRINE

Immunopharmacologic Properties

Along with corticosteroids and cyclosporin A, azathioprine (AZA) is the most commonly prescribed immunosuppressive drug. AZA, or methyl-nitroimidazolyl-6-mercaptopurine, is a derivative of 6-mercaptopurine (6MP) with a nitroimidazole chain resulting in a longer duration of action than intact 6MP. Soon after its discovery, 6MP was found to possess potent immunosuppressive properties (6). 6MP is phosphorylated intracellularly to thioinosine monophosphate (TMP). Then TMP inhibits the conversion of inosine monophosphate (IMP) to adenylosuccinate by the enzyme hypoxanthine guanine phosphoribosyltransferase (HGRPT) and of IMP to xanthine monophosphate by the enzyme IMP dehydrogenase. Rapidly dividing cells are particularly sensitive to the resulting blockade in purine biosynthesis.

The cytotoxic mechanism of action of AZA is similar to that of 6MP. However, it remains to be ascertained whether the cytotoxic effects account for all the immunopharmacologic properties of the substance.

In animals, AZA can affect a variety of immune responses (6). Overall, the degree of suppression depends on numerous factors, including the nature and dose of antigen, the dose, timing, and duration of AZA treatment, and the type of immune response assessed. Delayed-type hypersensitivity (DTH), graft-versus-host reaction, and allograft rejection are markedly suppressed by AZA, whereas the lupus disease in NZB × NZW mice is less affected than experimental allergic encephalomyelitis or thyroiditis. Humoral immune responses are less sensitive while immunoglobulin G (IgG) production is more susceptible to AZA suppression than IgM production. AZA lowers the total number of lymphocytes in the bone marrow and the thymus. Interestingly, cortisone-sensitive cells of the thymic cortex appear to be more sensitive than cortisone-resistant cells of the thymic medulla. In addition, AZA is endowed with potent anti-inflammatory activity, which is likely to interfere with the expression of various immune responses.

The immunosuppressive effects of AZA in humans are more potent for T lymphocytes than B lymphocytes. *In vitro*, the concentrations required to inhibit T cytotoxic cells are in the range of 0.1 to 1.0 μg/ml, whereas concentrations about 300 times higher are required to inhibit the humoral immune response to T cell-independent antigens. Peripheral lymphocytes are relatively insensitive to AZA. Interestingly, at therapeutic doses, AZA suppressed T lymphocyte functions without destroying the cells. Patients treated with AZA have a reduced antibody-dependent cell-mediated cytotoxicity (ADCC) and natural killer (NK) cell activity (7). AZA can inhibit the humoral immune responses under particular circumstances and the synthesis of IgG is more significantly affected than that of IgM.

The basis of AZA selectivity for T cells is unclear (8). AZA has been shown to preferentially bind receptor sites on T lymphocytes. The immunosuppressive properties of AZA have been considered to depend on the formation of intracellular thiopurine ribonucleotides, but this observation was later challenged by studies showing that the mixed lymphocyte response (MLR) is inhibited by AZA only if the drug is added during the first 24 hr of incubation. This suggests that AZA may act on the first step of the immune response (e.g., antigen recognition). As the *in vivo* metabolism of AZA in mice did not generate more immunosuppressive metabolites (9), it is likely that the pharmacologic properties of AZA are due to the parent molecule. Interestingly, AZA has been shown to be 34% more potent than 6MP on MLR suppression (10). While AZA inhibited MLR in HGPRT-deficient patients, the formation of intracellular nucleotides was considered to be unnecessary and the alkylation of thiol groups on T lymphocyte membranes resulting in changes of antigen-recognition sites was suggested to account for the immunosuppressive effects of AZA (11). That AZA exerts more pronounced immunosuppressive effects than other cytotoxic agents may be explained in part by the nitroimidazole group. Indeed, niridazole, an antiparasitic drug with a nitroimidazole group, was also shown to be immunosuppressive (12).

Due to its potent immunosuppressive properties, AZA was the standard treatment for preventing kidney allograft rejection prior to the introduction of cyclosporin A (8).

Clinical Immunotoxicity

Infectious complications and secondary neoplasm have been described in patients undergoing AZA treatment (13,14). Patients on AZA are at a higher risk from infection arising as a result of dose-related immunosuppression. Opportunistic infections (e.g., listeriosis, candidiasis, and *Pneumocystis carinii* pneumonia) are common and accounted for death in 3% to 12% of transplant recipients (15–17). However, the contributing role of combination therapy with corticosteroids or other immunosuppressive drugs must be stressed since patients with rheumatoid arthritis or Crohn's disease and on low-dose AZA treatment alone developed fewer infections than control subjects (14,18).

Secondary neoplasms have also been described in patients on long-term AZA treatment. Transplant patients on AZA and corticosteroid treatment were reported to have a 100 times higher risk of developing malignancies, among which were non-Hodgkin's lymphomas, squamous cell cancers of the skin, and primary liver tumors (19,20). However, several recent studies in patients with rheumatoid arthritis or lupus erythematosus failed to confirm that low-dose AZA treatments increase the incidence of malignancies (14,21–23).

CYCLOPHOSPHAMIDE

Immunopharmacologic Properties

Cyclophosphamide (CY), a noncytotoxic molecule, is rapidly converted to highly cytotoxic metabolites, particularly 4-hydroxycyclophosphamide (4OH-CY). The active metabolites of CY are potent bifunctional alkylating agents leading to misreading of the deoxyribonucleic acid (DNA) code and impaired replication.

The immunosuppressive effects of CY have been studied extensively in animals and humans (24,25). CY is toxic for rapidly proliferating lymphoid cells resulting in thymic shrinkage and marked depletion of B cell relative to T cell areas in lymphoid tissue (26). As expected, antibody production and cell-mediated immunity are suppressed. The formation of antibodies to both thymus-dependent and thymus-independent antigens is inhibited, which suggests that CY influences T and B lymphocyte functions. The inhibition of humoral response is maximal when CY is injected near or at the time of antigen injection and a dose–response curve was observed. Various cell-mediated responses have been shown to be suppressed by CY, including DTH, graft-versus-host reaction, and allograft survival (24).

However, depending on the dose and time of injection, CY can augment both humoral and cellular immune responses. The injection of CY prior to immunization or together with the antigen provoked a marked increase in antibody production, an enhanced expression of contact sensitivity, a slowed tumor growth, or the induction of immunologic tolerance (4).

In humans, CY was found to exert preferential effects on B lymphocytes at therapeutic doses, whereas both B and T cells were destroyed at high doses (27,28). The administration of CY was followed by a 40% to 80% reduction in circulating lymphocytes. The chronic treatment of patients with autoimmune diseases resulted in a marked inhibition of the mitogen-induced proliferative response of lymphocytes and impaired antibody production to various antigens [e.g., keyhole limpet hemocyanin (KLH) and flagellin]. Impaired DTH response in CY-treated patients has been described even though most studies lacked appropriate controls.

At low doses, an immune enhancing effect of CY on cell-mediated immunity and antibody production has been described in humans, but the therapeutic relevance of these findings remains to be established since clinical studies have been limited (29).

The mechanism generally accepted to explain the immunopharmacologic properties of CY is a selective toxicity on suppressor T cells, whereas data on mononuclear phagocytes are limited (11,24). Animal studies showed augmented cellular immune response when CY was injected in the immediate vicinity of sensitization, which supports the hypothesis that precursors of suppressor T cells are more sensitive to CY. In addition, precursors of suppressor T cells were found to be more sensitive *in vitro* following *in vivo* CY treatment than are precursors of cytotoxic T cells (30).

Clinical Immunotoxicity

In addition to the treatment of various lymphoproliferative disorders and carcinomas, CY is increasingly used to treat autoimmune diseases. A complication of CY treatment is neutropenia and increased susceptibility of patients to pathogens (31). An increased incidence of herpes zoster, disseminated coccidiomycosis, and *P. carinii* infections have been reported in patients treated with CY alone or CY plus prednisone for rheumatoid arthritis or lupus erythematosus.

Neoplasms associated with long-term CY treatment were mostly skin and bladder cancers, with lymphoproliferative disorders (i.e., non-Hodgkin's lymphomas) being very uncommon (32,33).

METHOTREXATE

Immunopharmacologic Properties

Methotrexate (MTX) is a potent inhibitor of folic acid, an essential cofactor in *de novo* DNA synthesis. MTX binds to and inactivates the enzyme dihydrofolate reductase, which is required to reduce dihydrofolate to tetrahydrofolate, hence impairing thymidine synthesis and normal DNA synthesis. Although MTX is one of the oldest cytotoxic drugs in use to treat cancer, it was not used until recently in the treatment of autoimmune diseases.

Animal studies showed that MTX is a potent immunosuppressive agent (3). It can inhibit both humoral and cellular responses but was suggested to be more potent on humoral than cellular responses as well as on responses to thymic-dependent than thymic-independent antigens and on IgG responses than IgM responses. However, no suppression is observed when MTX is injected immediately prior to antigen and augmentation is seen when MTX is injected for several days prior to the antigen (34). DTH, allograft survival, and adjuvant arthritis are all influenced in relation to MTX-induced immunosuppression (35). By contrast, *in vivo* administration of MTX does not reduce peripheral blood lymphocyte counts.

Early studies in humans showed that MTX can inhibit many immune responses (3). Recent findings in patients treated with rheumatoid arthritis showed that the number of B cells, CD4+ and CD8+ cells, and the mitogen-induced proliferative response of lymphocytes were not affected (36), whereas a significant decrease in IgG, IgM, and IgA serum levels was described (37).

The decreased synthesis of thymidine resulting from the inhibition of folic acid by MTX is likely to play a critical role but the mechanism of action at the molecular level is largely unknown. MTX was recently suggested to interfere with T cell and macrophage activation (38).

Clinical Immunotoxicity

The recent extensive use of MTX to treat various immune diseases was associated with reports of adverse effects related to the immunosuppressive properties of the substance.

Infections have commonly been described in patients on MTX. Thus herpes zoster infection (39), *P. carinii* pneumonia (40–44), disseminated histoplasmosis (45), cryptococcosis (46), and nocardiosis (47,48) have recently been reported in patients with rheumatoid arthritis (49), psoriasis, or severe asthma given low-dose, long-term MTX treatment. An unexpected decrease in the number of CD4+ cells has been suggested to be predictive of the risk for *P. carinii* infection (50) as CD4+ and CD8+ cells are normally unaffected by MTX.

Lymphoproliferative disorders, in particular non-Hodgkin's lymphomas, have been reported in MTX-treated patients (24,51–53) even though some controversy still exists regarding the connection between MTX use and lymphoma. Interestingly, most cases of MTX-induced Epstein–Barr virus (EBV)-associated lymphomas were reversible after MTX cessation.

OTHER CYTOREDUCTIVE DRUGS

In this chapter, AZA, CY, and MTX received particular attention because of their extensive use clinically as immunosuppressive drugs in the treatment of a variety of non-neoplastic disorders (e.g., autoimmune diseases). However, a number of additional cytotoxic agents interfere with the immune system as well (3).

The alkylating agent *chlorambucil* exerts toxic properties similar to those of CY, but lympholytic effects develop later. *Cytosine arabinoside*, an analog of deoxycytidine, was initially developed as an antiviral drug and proved to exert marked immunosuppressive properties. Comparatively, cytosine arabinoside is more active on humoral than cellular immune responses. The vinca alkaloids, *vincristine* and *vinblastine*, are potent immunosuppressive agents. Their primary site of action is believed to be the reticuloendothelial system and antibody production is relatively unaffected. The cytotoxicity of the pyrimidine antagonist *5-fluorouracil* is primarily directed against cells in the S phase of mitosis. Antibody production, both primary and secondary, and DTH responses were found to be inhibited in treated patients. *Adriamycin* and its analog *daunomycin* are anthracycline compounds, which are cell cycle specific. Adriamycin is markedly more potent as an immunosuppressive agent. Even though these cytoreductive agents overall exert marked immunosuppressive effects, this did not result in their extensive therapeutic use to treat immune diseases.

Although most of the available information regarding the immunopharmacologic properties of cytoreductive agents was obtained years ago, several recent studies focused on their influence on cytokine release. Adriamycin, 4OH-CY, and vincristine *in vitro* at the noncytotoxic concentrations of 1 and 10 μg/ml did not affect the release of tumor necrosis factor from rat peritoneal exudate cells (54). By contrast, all three drugs inhibited interleukin-6 release from lipopolysaccharide-stimulated human peripheral blood mononuclear leukocytes *in vitro* (55), whereas adriamycin and vincristine but not 4OH-CY inhibited interleukin-3 release from concanavalin A-stimulated mouse splenocytes *in vitro* at noncytotoxic concentrations (56). Another recent issue deals with the influence of cytotoxic agents on apoptosis (or programmed cell death), which is involved in various critical immune processes such as lymphocyte activation, cell-mediated cytotoxicity or tolerance induction. Various anticancer drugs can induce apoptosis (57). Further studies are likely to contribute to a better understanding of the interference of cytotoxic agents with the immune system.

CONCLUSION

The use of cytoreductive agents for the treatment of malignant and autoimmune disorders has been associated with a number of adverse consequences, the most frequent and severe being infections and, to a lesser extent, lymphoproliferative disorders. As cytoreductive agents are markedly immunosuppressive, these clinical consequences are illustrative of the adverse effects of direct immunotoxicity. However, little information has been gained in the recent past on the immune changes in patients treated with such drugs, particularly at low doses. Such information would greatly improve our understanding of the quantitative and qualitative immune changes most likely to be associated with clinical adverse consequences.

REFERENCES

1. Ehrke MJ. Effects of cancer therapy on host response and immunobiology. *Curr Opin Oncol* 1991;3:1070–1077.
2. Ehrke MJ, Mihich E. Immunologic effects of anticancer drugs. In: Kuemmerle MP, *Clinical chemotherapy, vol. 3*. Stuttgart: Thieme; 1984:475–499.
3. Winkelstein A. Immune suppression resulting from various cytotoxic agents. *Clin Immunol Allergy* 1984;4:295–315.
4. Ehrke MJ, Mihich E, Berd D, Mastrangelo MJ. Effects of anticancer drugs on the immune system in humans. *Semin Oncol* 1989;16:230–253.
5. Peterson PK. Host defense abnormalities predisposing the patient to infection. *Am J Med* 1984; 76:2–10.
6. Winkelstein A. The effects of azathioprine and 6MP on immunity. *J Immunopharmacol* 1979; 1:429–454.
7. Prince HE, Ettenger RB, Dorey FJ, Fine RN, Fahey JL. Azathioprine suppression of natural killer activity and antibody-dependent cellular cytotoxicity in renal transplant recipients. *J Clin Immunol* 1984;4:312–318.
8. Chan GLC, Canafax DM, Johnson CA. The therapeutic use of azathioprine in renal transplantation. *Pharmacotherapy* 1987;7:165–177.
9. Abraham RT, Benson LM, Jardine I. Influence of hepatic oxidative metabolism on the immunosuppressive activities of 6-thiopurines. *J Pharmacol Exp Ther* 1986;234:670–676.
10. Al-Safi SA, Maddocks JL. Azathioprine and 6-mercaptopurine (6-MP) suppress the human mixed lymphocyte reaction (MLR) by different mechanisms. *Br J Clin Pharmacol* 1984;17:417–422.
11. Szawlowski PWS, Al-Safi SA, Dooley T, Maddocks JL. Azathioprine suppresses the mixed lymphocyte reaction of patient with Lesch–Nyhan syndrome. *Br J Clin Pharmacol* 1985;20:489–491.
12. Solbach W, Wagner H, Röllinghoff M. Effect of niridazole on cellular immunity in vivo and in vitro. *Clin Exp Immunol* 1978;32:411–418.
13. Lawson DH, Lovatt GE, Gurton CS, Hennings RC. Adverse effects of azathioprine. *Adv Drug React Acute Pois Rev* 1984;3:161–171.
14. Singh G, Fries JF, Spitz P, Williams CA. Toxic effects of azathioprine in rheumatoid arthritis. *Arthritis Rheum* 1989;32:837–843.
15. Hall CL, Sansom JR, Obeid ML, et al. Results of 250 consecutive cadaver kidney transplants. *Br Med J* 1976;1:547–550.
16. MacGeown MG, Douglas JF, Brown WA, et al. Advantage of low-dose steroid from the day after renal transplantation. *Transplantation* 1980;29:287–289.
17. Sellers AL, Llach F, Franklin S, Gordon A, Fichman M. Renal transplantation in a community hospital. *JAMA* 1976;236:2866–2869.
18. Singleton JW, Law DH, Kelley ML, Mekjian HS, Sturdevant RAL. National Cooperative Crohn's Disease Study: adverse reactions to study drugs. *Gastroenterology* 1979;77:870–882.

19. Krueger TC, Tallent MB, Richie RE, et al. Neoplasia in immunosuppressed renal transplant patients: a 20-year experience. *South Med J* 1985;78:501–506.
20. Phillips T, Salisbury J, Leigh I, Baker H. Non-Hodgkin's lymphoma associated with long-term azathioprine therapy. *Clin Exp Dermatol* 1987;12:444–445.
21. Mateson EL. Long term follow-up study of neoplasia in the rheumatoid arthritis registry. *Arthritis Rheum* 1990;33:82.
22. Wessel G, Abendroth K, Wisheit M. Malignant transformation during immunosuppressive therapy (azathioprine) of rheumatoid arthritis and systemic lupus erythematosus. A retrospective study. *Scand J Rheumatol. Suppl.* 1988;67:73–75.
23. Mastrangelo MJ, Berd D, Maguire H. The immunoaugmenting effects of cancer chemotherapeutic agents. *Semin Oncol* 1986;13:186–194.
24. Shand FL. The immunopharmacology of cyclophosphamide. *Int J Immunopharmacol* 1979;1:165–171.
25. Turk JL, Parker D. Effect of cyclophosphamide on immunological control mechanisms. *Immunol Rev* 1982;65:99–113.
26. Turk JL, Poulter LW. Selective depletion of lymphoid tissue by cyclophosphamide. *Clin Exp Immunol* 1972;10:285–296.
27. Cupps TT, Edgar LC, Fauci AS. Suppression of human B lymphocyte function by cyclophosphamide. *J Immunol* 1982;128:2453–2457.
28. Hurd ER, Giuliano VJ. The effect of cyclosphamide on B and T lymphocytes in patients with connective tissue disease. *Arthritis Rheum* 1975;18:67–75.
29. Berd D, Mastrangelo MJ. Active immunotherapy of human melanoma exploiting the immunopotentiating effects of cyclophosphamide. *Cancer Invest* 1988;6:337–349.
30. Ferguson RM, Simons RL. Differential cyclophosphamide sensitivity of suppressor and cytotoxic cell precursors. *Transplantation* 1978;25:36–38.
31. Bradley JD, Brandt KD, Katz BP. Infectious complications of cyclophosphamide treatment for vasculitis. *Arthritis Rheum* 1989;32:45-53.
32. Fraiser LH, Kanekal S, Kehrer SP. Cyclophosphamide toxicity. Characteristics and avoiding the problem. *Drug Safety* 1991;42:781–795.
33. Uhl GS, Williams JE, Arnett FC. Intracerebral lymphoma in a patient with central nervous system lupus on cyclophosphamide. *J Rheumatol* 1974;1:282–286.
34. Orbach-Arbouys S, Castes MB. Augmentation of immune responses after methotrexate administration. *Immunology* 1979;36:265–269.
35. Shiroky JB, Frosp A, Skelton JD, et al. Complications of immunosuppression associated with weekly low dose methotrexate. *J Rheumatol* 1991;18:1172–1175.
36. Olsen NJ, Callahan LF, Pincus T. Immunologic studies of rheumatoid arthritis patients treated with methotrexate. *Arthritis Rheum* 1987;30:481–488.
37. Andersen PA, West SG, O'Dell JR, Via CS, Claypool, RG, Kotzin BL. Weekly pulse methotrexate in rheumatoid arthritis. *Ann Intern Med* 1985;103:489–496.
38. Weinstein GD, Jeffes E, McCullough JL. Cytotoxic and immunologic effects of methotrexate in psoriasis. *J Invest Dermatol* 1990;95:49S–52S.
39. Antonelli MAS, Moreland LW, Brick JE. Herpes zoster in patients with rheumatoid arthritis treated with weekly, low-dose methotrexate. *Am J Med* 1991;90:295–298.
40. Carmicheal AJ, Ryatt KS. *Pneumocystis carinii* pneumonia following methotrexate. *Br J Dermatol* 1990;122:291.
41. Flood DA, Chan CK, Pruzanski W. *Pneumocystis carinii* pneumonia associated with methotrexate therapy for rheumatoid arthritis. *J Rheumatol* 1991;18:1254–1256.
42. Kuiert LM, Harrison AC. *Pneumocystis carinii* pneumonia as a complication of methotrexate treatment of asthma. *Thorax* 1991;46:936–937.
43. Vallerand H, Cossart C, Milosevic D, Lavaud F, Leone J. Fatal *Pneumocystis* pneumonia in asthmatic patients treated with methotrexate. *Lancet* 1992;339:1551.
44. Wallis PJW, Ryatt KS, Constable TJ. *Pneumocystis carinii* pneumonia complicating low dose methotrexate treatment for psoriatic arthropathy. *Ann Rheum Dis* 1989;48:247–249.
45. Witty LA, Steiner F, Curtmen M, Webb D, Wheat J. Disseminated histoplasmosis in patients receiving low-dose methotrexate therapy for psoriasis. *Arch Dermatol* 1992;128:91–93.
46. Altz-Smith M, Kendall LG, Stamm AM. Cryptococcosis associated with low-dose methotrexate arthritis. *Am J Med* 1987;83:179–181.

47. Cornelissen JJ, Bakker LJ, Van der Veen MJ, Rozenberg-Arska M, Bijilsma JWJ. *Nocardia asteroides* pneumonia complicating low dose methotrexate treatment of refractory rheumatoid arthritis. *Ann Rheum Dis* 1991;50:642–644.
48. Keegan JM, Byrd JW. Nocardiosis associated with low dose methotrexate for rheumatoid arthritis. *J Rheumatol* 1988;15:1585–1586.
49. Salinier L, De Jaureguiberry JP, Carloz E, et al. Cytomegalovirus pneumopathy during rheumatoid arthritis treated with low dose methotrexate. *Rev Med Intern* 1992;13:S223.
50. Kane GC, Troshinsky MB, Peters SB, Israel HL. *Pneumocystis carinii* pneumonia associated with weekly methotrexate: cumulative dose of methotrexate and low CD4 cell count may predict this complication. *Respir Med* 1993;87:153–155.
51. Ellman MH, Hurwitz H, Thomas C, Kozloff M. Lymphoma developing in a patient with rheumatoid arthritis taking low dose weekly methotrexate. *J Rheumatol* 1991;18:1741–1743.
52. Kamel OW, Van de Rijn M, Weiss LM, et al. Reversible lymphoma associated with Epstein–Barr virus occurring during methotrexate therapy for rheumatoid arthritis and dermatomyositis. *N Engl J Med* 1993;328:1317–1321.
53. Kingsmore SF, Hall BD, Allen NB, Rice JR, Caldwell DS. Association of methotrexate, rheumatoid arthritis and lymphoma: report of 2 cases and literature review. *J Rheumatol* 1992;19:1462–1465.
54. Hassan SI, Ahmed K, Turk JL. Effect of anticancer drugs on the release of tumor necrosis factor in vitro. *Cancer Immunol Immunother* 1990;30:363–366.
55. Hasan SI, Blaney BA, Turk JL. Effects of anticancer drugs on the release of interleukin-6 in vitro. *Cancer Immunol Immunother* 1992;34:228–232.
56. Hasan SI, Turk JL. Effect of anticancer drugs on the release of interleukin-3 in vitro. *Int J Immunopharmacol* 1991;13:1177–1185.
57. Hickman JA. Apoptosis induced by anticancer drugs. *Cancer Metastasis Rev* 1992;11:121–139.

Immunotoxicology and Immunopharmacology, Second Edition, edited by J. H. Dean, M. I. Luster, A. E. Munson, and I. Kimber.
Raven Press, Ltd., New York © 1994.

17

Drugs of Abuse and the Immune System

Herman Friedman,* Steven C. Shivers, and Thomas W. Klein

*Department of Medical Microbiology and Immunology, University of South Florida College of Medicine, Tampa, Florida 33612; *Bone Marrow Transplant Program, H. Lee Moffitt Cancer Center and Research Institute, Tampa, Florida 33612*

The problem of drug abuse in the United States has gained increased attention over the last few years, especially because of an association of this practice with the acquired immunodeficiency syndrome (AIDS). It is widely believed that the abuse of recreational drugs may be a cofactor in the progression of human immunodeficiency virus (HIV) infection. There has been a large amount of literature published over the last few decades concerning the clinical aspects of the misuse of drugs such as heroin, cocaine, marijuana, and alcohol. However, the overall impact on public health of abusing drugs is incompletely understood. In this regard, many studies concerning the effects of such drugs on human physiology have been performed. It would be desirable to perform the myriad of toxicologic and cell biologic studies required to determine the nature and mechanism of how drugs of abuse impact on human physiology. However, because of difficulties in standardizing these studies in humans, investigators have increasingly turned to experimental animal models, especially mice and rats, to assess the biologic influences of recreational drugs. Rodents, of course, do not abuse drugs normally and a direct comparison of the effects of such drugs on these animals with the effects on humans is difficult to ascertain, especially when dosing of the drugs is usually based on body weight rather than surface area. Nevertheless, studies with rodents offer some advantages because the genetic background and "lifestyle" of the test subjects can readily be controlled using animals. This reduces some of the biologic variations inherent in studies of human populations and thus facilitates data interpretation.

A variety of tissues and organs can readily be obtained from rodents, including tissues for study in culture. During the last decade, the number of studies examining the influence of drugs of abuse on cells involved in host resistance mechanisms has increased dramatically. In humans, peripheral blood is the principal source of such cells. More extensive studies designed to study the *in vivo* effects of various drugs of abuse on diverse cell systems have been accomplished more readily in mice and rats, as compared with humans. However, the data obtained should be interpreted with caution because of the many physiologic differences between rodents and humans. Despite such problems, laboratory studies on the effects of drugs of abuse on murine and rat systems have contributed significantly to our understanding of the effects of these substances on host resistance mechanisms and specifically the immune response. For example, in recent years there have been many studies concerning the influence of opiates, especially morphine, on the immune response in experimental animals. Similar studies have been reported in animal models examining the effects of cocaine on the immune response, both *in vivo* and *in vitro*. A number of informative studies performed over the last dozen years have dealt with host immunity and marijuana, especially its major psychoactive component, tetrahydrocannabinol (THC). The following is a selective review of the effects of marijuana and its components on immune responses.

Ingredients in the marijuana plant, *Cannabis sativa*, amount to over 400 separate chemical entities. Of this total, over 60 are cannabinoids, a term that is used for the typical C21 group of compounds that have in common the C ring of olivatol. Δ^9-THC is the major psychoactive cannabinoid in marijuana. Most of the cannabinoid derivatives are not psychoactive but may alter the effects of Δ^9-THC. Many clinical and basic science studies performed over the last two decades have been concerned with possible detrimental effects of marijuana, especially Δ^9-THC, on host immunity and resistance to infectious agents. Throughout this chapter, the term THC will be used to refer to the Δ^9 form, unless otherwise noted.

EFFECTS OF MARIJUANA ON HOST RESISTANCE AND IMMUNITY

Effects of Marijuana on Resistance to Infections: Mouse Studies

The overall purpose of the effector functions of immune cells, including those involved in antibody production and cell-mediated immunity, is to mediate host resistance to tumors and infectious agents. Very few studies have been reported to date examining the effects of cannabinoids on host resistance mechanisms to infectious diseases. This is in part due to the complexity of the available experimental models of infection, which makes these studies difficult to manage by pharmacologists and basic immunologists working independently. In spite of this, several early reports indicated that cannabinoids may influence the responsiveness of mice to infectious agents. For example, Morahan et al. (1) reported modified host resistance to bacterial (*Listeria monocytogenes*) and viral (herpes simplex virus, HSV, type II) infections in mice treated with various cannabinoids. Both of these infectious agents require an intact T cell-mediated immune response. The cannabinoids tested were THC, Δ^8-THC, cannabidiol, 1-methyl-Δ^8-THC, and a marijuana extract. Mice that were infected with the infectious agents and then treated on days 1 and 2 following infection with an intraperitoneal injection of the various cannabinoids showed increased susceptibility to the infections. The number of *Listeria* organisms required to kill 50% of the mice (LD_{50}) was significantly reduced by treatment with cannabidiol, 1-methyl-Δ^8-THC, THC, or the marijuana extract. For THC, the most potent in this regard, a dose range of 150 to 200 mg/kg was required to reduce resistance to *Listeria*. This is a dose range somewhat higher than that observed in human subjects who smoke one marijuana cigarette (2,3). Similar results were observed for HSV infection, except the cannabinoid-induced suppression was less than that for *Listeria* infection. Also, the marijuana extract was not suppressive in the HSV model.

In general, these studies were consistent with and supported previous observations that cannabinoids administered to mice in relatively high doses could interfere with either B or T cell-associated phenomena, such as antibody production and cell-mediated immunity. Bradley, et al. (2) also reported that THC administration to mice increased the susceptibility of the animals to bacterial endotoxin. Similarly, recent studies in our laboratory (3) have shown that infection with *Legionella pneumophila*, an opportunistic intracellular bacterium, may be potentiated in mice treated with marijuana prior to either primary or secondary challenge with the organism. Furthermore, injection of the mice with THC 1 day before and 1 day after challenge with nonlethal concentrations of viable *Legionella* resulted in a rapid toxic-like death of the animals. This observation might be related to the ability of THC to enhance the production of inflammatory cytokines such as interleukin-1 (IL-1), interleukin-6 (IL-6), and tumor necrosis factor (TNF), which normally develop in lower amounts in mice infected with opportunistic gram-negative bacteria such as *Legionella*. This toxic shock-like death only occurred when mice were given THC 1 day prior to and 1 day following infection with *Legionella* and was associated with an extremely high level of the inflammatory cytokines in the sera of the animals.

Effects of Marijuana on Resistance to Infections: Human Studies

Marijuana use in the United States is a major problem due to both its illegal status and potential health hazards. According to surveys by the National Institutes on Drug Abuse, nearly one-third of Americans over the age of 12 have smoked marijuana and about 10% are chronic users. Due to its relatively low cost and general availability, marijuana continues to be used illegally by a significant segment of the population. In addition, pharmaceutical forms of marijuana, especially nabellone (Cesemet) and dronabinol (Marinol), are often prescribed as antiemetics to cancer patients receiving radiation and chemotherapy or as an appetite stimulant for AIDS patients.

Many experimental studies have shown that cannabinoids can be immunosuppressive in animals. Although there is no conclusive evidence that human marijuana smokers are more susceptible to infections, several studies suggest that marijuana use may cause immunomodulation, which might predispose users to increased risks of infection or cancer. For example, there are a number of reports that demonstrate increased incidences of chronic diseases related to smoking marijuana. These diseases include recurrent HSV infection (4), upper respiratory tract and lung cancers (5), tongue carcinoma, and head and neck cancers (6). The occurrence of such diseases is often attributed to compounds in marijuana smoke that have not yet been described definitively.

Studies that attempted to dissect the potential suppressive effects of marijuana on specific immune responses have demonstrated, however, that marijuana smokers often show a variety of altered immune response parameters. For example, in an early study by Mann et al. (7), it was reported that alveolar macrophages from subjects who smoked marijuana showed structural and functional differences compared with macrophages from nonsmokers. Nahas et al. (8) first reported there was a decreased leukocyte blastogenic response of lymphocytes from marijuana smokers. When peripheral blood lymphocytes from marijuana smokers were stimulated with phytohemagglutinin (PHA) or allogeneic cells, they showed decreased thymidine incorporation compared with blood leukocytes from controls. The reported decreases were similar to those observed for blood cells from immunocompromised individuals, including patients with cancer or autoimmune diseases, or other patients with suppressed T lymphocyte functions. Subsequently, Nahas et al. (9) studied subjects with a history of chronic use of marijuana by evaluating serum immunoglobulin (Ig) levels. Marijuana smokers showed lower levels of IgG and IgD than control subjects. However, the smokers still showed IgG levels that fell within the lower normal range for adults.

Further studies were performed with human volunteers comparing lymphocyte numbers in marijuana smokers by measuring erythrocyte rosette formation. Cushman and Khurana (10) reported that the number of T lymphocytes was decreased significantly in about 40% of 23 marijuana smokers when compared with an equal number of controls. Further examination suggested that only the “early active” T rosettes were decreased in the marijuana users. This subpopulation of T lymphocytes comprises about 10% of the total T cell population and was shown to return to normal levels within 72 hr of cessation of smoking marijuana. The authors could not correlate this change in T lymphocyte subpopulation with any clinical effect. A study by Peterson et al. (11) examined peripheral blood lymphocyte responses to PHA and enumerated T lymphocyte numbers by rosette formation with erythrocytes. Both the PHA responses and T cell numbers were altered in the marijuana smoking group. However, the authors commented on the variability of the marijuana effect seen in humans and concluded these effects may not be associated exclusively with marijuana.

Studies attempting to show a relationship between marijuana use and malignancy suggested that some components of marijuana may be directly carcinogenic while others may have immunomodulatory effects that suppress innate anticancer immune mechanisms. Such immunosuppression may be related to the effects of marijuana on immune surveillance mechanisms, which normally prevent unchecked growth and progression of early tumor cells. Carcinogenesis seen in marijuana users may also result from combination effects between carcinogenic and immunosuppressive agents present in marijuana smoke.

Effects of Marijuana on Lymphoid Organs

Early studies designed to examine the biologic effects of administering marijuana to mice suggested that the cells and organs involved in the immune response were affected by cannabinoid treatment. Thompson et al. (12) were the first to report detailed changes in animals exposed chronically to marijuana or its active components. Fischer rats were fed Δ^9-THC, Δ^8-THC, or crude marijuana extracts emulsified in sesame oil. The drugs were administered for up to 119 consecutive days at doses 30 to 300 times the usual dose in humans. They reported a biotoxicity pattern characterized by depression of cardiac function in the first week of administration followed by hyperactivity thereafter. A lethal dose produced death within the first 1 to 3 days of treatment. Cannabinoid-induced death was characterized by hypothermia and bradypnea. All drug-treated animals showed a decrease in growth rate, which was found to be associated with a depletion of abdominal fat storage, in spite of increased food and water intake. Various organs, including the spleen, were also affected by drug treatment. A decrease in relative spleen weight was associated with a decrease in the number of tissue lymphocytes. The leukocyte count in the blood was also decreased following administration of each of the three cannabinoid substances. This type of hypocellularity might be related to immune deficiency, but this subject was not studied.

Effects of Marijuana on Antibody-Mediated Immunity

Leukocytes and their progenitors are essential for the production and release of antibody, which is protective in various situations, especially against infectious agents such as bacteria, viruses, and fungi. A decade ago, several reports indicated that THC injection into rodents suppressed the capacity to form antibody against sheep erythrocytes. For example, Lefkowitz and Chiang (13) injected Swiss Webster mice intraperitoneally with relatively high concentrations of THC prior to, during, and after injection with erythrocytes. The spleens of the animals were then analyzed for anti-erythrocyte antibody-forming capacity. Mice injected with 100 mg/kg THC, beginning 1 day before and continuing 4 days after immunization with erythrocytes, showed a significant reduction in body and spleen weight and in spleen cell number. The animals also showed reduced antibody responses relative to saline-injected controls. Injection of 50 mg/kg THC into mice had no effect. Rosenkrantz et al. (14) reported on the suppression of antibody formation by THC administered orally to rats. In contrast to the study of Lefkowitz and Chiang, their study tested lower doses of THC ranging from 1 to 10 mg/kg. Anti-erythrocyte antibody production was assessed both by the hemolytic plaque assay and by hemagglutination. In these studies, THC was found to suppress antibody formation and reduce the spleen weight of the animals. The greatest effect was in animals immunized with erythrocytes on day 1 and treated with THC on days 1 through 5. These results suggested that drug treatment interfered with lymphocyte clonal expansion following stimulation by antigen. After correction for body surface area, the THC doses used in these studies were equivalent to those found in humans who have consumed hashish, a potent form of marijuana.

Zimmerman et al. (15) reported similar effects of multiple doses of THC in mice. Mice injected intraperitoneally on four consecutive days with various doses of THC, ranging from 1 to 10 mg/kg, showed reduced numbers of antibody-forming cells, decreased serum antibody levels, and lower spleen weights. To determine the possibility that nonpsychoactive components of marijuana may also affect antibody formation, Smith et al. (16) tested the relative potency of various cannabinoids, including Δ^9-THC, Δ^8-THC, abnormal Δ^8-THC, and 1-methyl-Δ^8-THC on the immune response to sheep erythrocytes. Two days after immunization with erythrocytes, different groups of mice were injected intraperitoneally with various doses of the different cannabinoids. The number of antibody plaque-forming cells in the spleen was determined 4 to 6 days afterward. The data showed that nonpsychoactive cannabinoids, such as 1-methyl-Δ^8-THC and abnormal Δ^8-THC, were more potent in suppressing antibody formation than the psychoactive substances, Δ^9-THC and Δ^8-THC. The authors concluded that the effects of the drug on the central nervous system were not necessary for immunosuppression.

A number of studies have suggested that chronic oral ingestion of THC by rodents may result in the development of tolerance to the immunosuppressive effects of the drug. In one attempt to confirm this phenomenon, Luthra et al. (17) treated rats orally with 6 or 12 mg/kg THC for 1 to 26 days, followed by a challenge with sheep erythrocytes. Reductions in spleen weight, the number of antibody-forming cells, and the level of serum antibody all occurred in the animals treated chronically with THC, suggesting that tolerance to the immunosuppressive effects of THC did not occur. Although other investigators have reported studies in mice that demonstrate a reduced capacity of cannabinoid-induced suppression of antibody formation, many differences exist between these studies, which prevent direct comparison of the data. However, it is possible that factors that contribute to drug tolerance, such as changes in biotransformation rates and drug distribution and absorption, alter the drug tissue concentration in many cell systems, including the immune system.

Baczynsky and Zimmerman (18) demonstrated an effect of cannabinoids on the antibody-forming capability of spleen cells in culture. In these studies, antigen-primed spleen cells were obtained from mice immunized previously with sheep erythrocytes. The cells were then cultured in the presence of sheep erythrocytes as a secondary challenge *in vitro*, along with various concentrations of Δ^9-THC, cannabinol, or cannabidiol. The drugs were present either during the entire culture period (1 to 6 days) or during the first 24 hr of culture only. Δ^9-THC was found to be more potent than cannabinol or cannabidiol in its ability to suppress the antibody plaque-forming response of the spleen cells. Furthermore, Δ^9-THC appeared to be suppressive only when present during the early phase of the culture (first 24 hr) and much less suppressive when present late in the response. The authors concluded that their data supported the view that a suppressive factor induced by cannabinoids affects earlier proliferative events which occur during antibody formation.

Studies by Klein et al. (19) showed that Δ^9-THC suppressed the antibody response of spleen cell cultures that received a primary immunization of sheep erythrocytes *in vitro*. 11-Hydroxy-THC was also found to be suppressive. The observed suppression occurred in the concentration range of 6 to 32 mM, which was higher than the 5-mM THC concentration reported by Baczynsky and Zimmerman. The studies by Klein and co-workers also examined the influence of combination drug treatment on antibody formation. In these studies, splenocyte cultures were treated with sheep erythrocytes and various drugs or drug combinations. It was found that the number of antibody-forming cells developing in culture after 5 days of incubation was not affected by the addition of either Δ^9-THC or 11-hydroxy-THC at a 5-μg/ml dose. However, the combination of the two cannabinoids together significantly suppressed the antibody-forming capacity at this lower dose. The effect was essentially equivalent to that obtained in cultures exposed to 10 μg/ml of the individual cannabinoids. These results suggest that cannabinoids in combination have additive effects on the suppression of lymphocyte function.

Effects of Marijuana on Cell-Mediated Immunity

An important cell-mediated immune function resulting from the activation of lymphocytes is the delayed hypersensitivity response. This response is important in host defense mechanisms and requires participation of lymphokine-secreting T cells, possibly of the T helper type 1 (T_H1) subtype, and cells of the monocyte/macrophage lineage. Smith et al. (16) used the cell-mediated immune response to sheep erythrocytes to evaluate the effects of various cannabinoids on cell-mediated immune potential in THC-treated mice. After the animals were presensitized with sheep erythrocytes, they were given various drugs or vehicle alone on day 0 and day 3. The mice were then challenged for a foot pad swelling response to sheep erythrocytes on days 4 and 5. The authors reported that the various cannabinoids, administered subcutaneously at a dose of 100 mg/kg, affected the cell-mediated hypersensitivity response. For example, abnormal Δ^8-THC suppressed the response by about one-third, whereas Δ^8-THC suppressed the response two-thirds. A lower dose of cannabinoids was less suppressive. Watson et al. (20) also reported inhibitory effects of THC on the delayed hypersensitivity response in mice. Instead of sheep erythrocytes as antigen, they measured the ear swelling response to dinitrofluorobenzene (DNFB). Suppression was observed in animals that received 30 mg/kg of drug on the day of sensitization with DNFB and for 4 days thereafter. Paradoxically, higher doses were less suppressive than the dose of 30 mg/kg. However, as in the previous study, multiple doses of the cannabinoid were required to obtain a minimal inhibitory effect. Levy and Heppner (21) reported that haloperidol treatment had no effect on the delayed hypersensitivity response to DNFB in mice. However, unlike the studies described earlier, the haloperidol was given only as a single dose 24 hr before sensitization, rather than as multiple doses given from sensitization to challenge. The results of these studies suggest that cannabinoids, when administered in multiple doses, may suppress the delayed hypersensitivity response. However, it is not clear whether the drugs are affecting T_H cell activation and proliferation, cytokine production, or macrophage responsiveness.

Effects of Marijuana on Lymphocyte Functions

Lymphocyte Proliferation

A fundamental aspect of the activation of the immune response is the rapid proliferation of lymphocytes following exposure to antigen. Studies performed in our laboratory showed that, when added to cultures of mouse lymphocytes, Δ^9-THC and 11-hydroxy-THC inhibited lymphoproliferative responses to both T and B cell mitogens (22). This suppression was generally similar to that first observed for human peripheral blood cells. Incubation of murine spleen cells with THC suppressed the proliferative response to all mitogens tested, including B and T cell mitogens, suggesting that both types of lymphocytes were susceptible to the suppressive effects of the cannabinoids. However, T lymphocyte proliferation appeared more resistant to THC-induced immunosuppression than did B lymphocyte responses. It should be noted that, *in vivo*, THC is metabolized to 11-hydroxy-THC by hepatic microsomal enzymes. It was found that in the concentration range of 1 to 10 μg/ml 11-hydroxy-THC, there was very little effect on lymphocyte responsiveness to T cell mitogens, although there was some suppression of the response to lipopolysaccharide (LPS), suggesting that B lymphocytes are somewhat more affected by this cannabinoid.

Signal Transduction

The biochemical events in the early phases of lymphocyte activation following stimulation with a mitogen or antigen are under intense investigation. Lymphocytes are activated by the binding of ligands to surface receptors, triggering events that ultimately lead to the proliferation of the cells and the generation of effector cells. The transduction of an early signal resulting from ligand–receptor interaction is facilitated at least partially by a class of guanine nucleotide-dependent proteins. Activation of these G proteins facilitates activation of a phospholipase C enzyme, which in turn hydrolyses phosphatidylinositol-4,6-bisphosphate to yield inositol triphosphate (ITP). ITP then triggers a release of calcium from intracellular sources, thus raising the concentration of cytoplasmic calcium. Since THC effectively inhibits mitogen-induced proliferation, studies were performed in our laboratory (23) to determine whether THC can also affect calcium mobilization, presumably because of effects on signal transduction. Lymphoid cells were pretreated for a very short period of time with THC, followed by mitogenic challenge. These cells showed a substantial suppression of the expected mitogen-induced increase in intracellular calcium concentration. Inhibition of calcium mobilization by THC appeared to be related to its suppression of the mitogen responsiveness of the cells, at least *in vitro*.

Interleukin-2 Production and Interleukin-2 Receptor Expression

In the early biochemical events associated with T cell activation, signal transduction is followed by a series of intermediate events related to changes in gene transcription. IL-2 receptor (IL-2R) messenger ribonucleic acid (mRNA) can be detected within hours of lymphocyte simulation, followed by IL-2R expression on the cell surface. These cell surface receptors are required to promote T cell proliferation. Thus expansion of a T lymphocyte population in response to mitogens or other ligands requires synthesis of IL-2 as well as expression of IL-2R. As indicated earlier, THC has been found to downregulate T cell proliferation in response to mitogens. Thus studies were performed in our laboratory to examine the possibility that THC affects IL-2 production and/or biologic function. We found that THC inhibited IL-2-driven proliferation of T lymphocytes in a dose-dependent manner (24). We found also that THC interfered with the mitogen-stimulated production of IL-2 by T lymphocytes from mice, humans, and other species. In addition, THC inhibited the cytolytic activity of both T cells and natural killer (NK) cells, which are activated by IL-2. Furthermore, THC treatment of T cells *in vitro* decreased the surface expression of high- and intermediate-affinity IL-2R, while the expression of low-affinity (Tac protein) IL-2R was increased on the cell surface (25). Thus THC was shown to have marked effects on the ability of T lymphocytes to both produce IL-2 and to express IL-2R.

Interferon Production

There are many types of cytokines produced and released by a variety of cells in response to certain stimuli. These proteins bind to specific surface receptors and induce appropriate responses in the target cells. Cytokines are considered extremely important in regulating the differentiation and function of lymphocytes, macrophages, NK cells, and other cells involved in host defenses. It is now widely believed that interruption of the communicating and regulating activity of these molecules by environmental agents, including marijuana and other drugs of abuse, can significantly impact on the ability of a host to respond to infectious agents and tumors. There have been several studies dealing with the influence of marijuana and other drugs of abuse on the production and function of cytokines such as interferons (IFNs), ILs, and TNF.

Cabral et al. (26) were the first to report an influence of THC on IFN production in response to various stimuli. They injected mice intraperitoneally with THC at doses ranging from 5 to 100 mg/kg on consecutive days prior to challenge with the IFN inducers poly I:C or HSV type II. The mice were bled at 4 to 24 hr post-challenge, and IFN levels in the sera were determined by a viral plaque reduction assay. The class of IFN was characterized by acid treatment and by specific antisera. Doses of THC as low as 5 mg/kg suppressed serum IFN levels in response to poly I:C, while IFN levels in response to HSV infection were suppressed by doses of 15 mg/kg or higher. A single dose of THC, given only 1 hr prior to IFN induction with poly I:C, also suppressed the IFN response. The authors concluded that short-term exposure of mice to THC induced a state of IFN hypoproduction, and this hyporesponsive state might be related to the animal's higher susceptibility to infection.

Similar studies were performed by Blanchard et al. (27) to examine the effects of IFN production after long-term chronic exposure of mice to THC. The effect of THC on IFN production *in vitro* was also examined. For the *in vivo* studies, mice were injected intraperitoneally at selected time intervals with either THC (15 mg/kg) or vehicle alone and spleens were removed at various times, up to 56 days. The splenocytes were tested in culture for their ability to produce IFN in response to mitogens, which are known to induce predominately either IFN-γ or IFN-α/β. By the 26th day of THC treatment, the splenocytes began to show a tendency for reduced responsiveness to both types of IFN inducers. By 46 days, cells from the THC-treated animals were producing only 20% to 30% of the level of IFN produced by the controls. Thus long-term exposure of mice to THC affected the interferon-forming capacity of the animals.

The effects of THC on the IFN-producing capacity of normal splenocytes *in vitro* were also examined. For this purpose, spleen cells from normal mice were cultured for 24 hr in the presence of various mitogens and either THC or vehicle. The vehicle had no effect on IFN production in response to either IFN-γ inducers, such as PHA or *Legionella*, or to the IFN-α/β inducer, LPS. In both cases, THC at a concentration of 5 μg/ml markedly suppressed IFN production in response to PHA or LPS. These results, as well as those of Cabral et al. (26), indicate that THC has an immediate and cumulative adverse effect on the production of various types of IFNs by lymphoid cells in the mouse.

Effects of Marijuana on Macrophage Functions

Phagocytosis and Bactericidal Activity

Macrophages are also a prominent cell type in host inflammatory and immune defense mechanisms. In addition to their function as wandering phagocytes, which is important for the elimination of foreign substances in the body, they are also involved in antigen presentation and cytokine secretion. In the lungs, macrophages provide an initial barrier to pulmonary infection. It has been suggested that smoking marijuana may significantly affect pulmonary alveolar macrophages, thus compromising host defenses. In animal studies, Huber et al. (28) obtained alveolar macrophages from rats by bronchoalveolar lavage and tested the effects of various marijuana substances on the bactericidal activity of the macrophages *in vitro*. The addition of either marijuana or tobacco smoke was reported to suppress the bactericidal activity against *Staphylococcus albus*. Furthermore, the suppressive substances in these smokes were identified as water-soluble substances in the gas phase. Interestingly, addition of purified THC to cultures for several hours had no effect on the bactericidal capacity of the cells. These studies were extended to experiments involving drug treatment of the whole animal. Alveolar macrophages obtained from rats exposed for 30 consecutive days to either marijuana smoke or tobacco smoke showed very little deficiency in their ability to phagocytose radiolabeled staphylococci as compared to nontreated controls. The drug-treated animals failed to gain weight normally but the cellular content of the pulmonary lavage fluid varied little with respect to the number of cells and the ability of the recovered cells to adhere to plastic surfaces was not altered. However, marijuana treatment suppressed the ability of the cells to exhibit normal oxygen metabolism when challenged with a phagocytic load.

Purified THC has also been reported to affect the function of mouse macrophages. Raz and Goldman (29) treated cultured mouse peritoneal macrophages with THC or other cannabinoids and reported that the cells displayed a pattern of vacuolization similar to that observed in cells from the lungs of hashish smokers. The cell changes appeared within 15 min following exposure to 100 μM THC. Studies by Lopez-Cepero et al. (30) showed that even lower concentrations of THC could affect the functions of mouse peritoneal macrophages in culture. Significant changes in macrophage spreading ability occurred with very low doses of THC and decreased phagocytic ability was observed at THC concentrations well below those needed to invoke toxicity of the macrophages. These data suggest that cell membrane phenomena, such as cell spreading, are quite sensitive indicators of cannabinoid effects. Phagocytosis *in vitro* also appeared to be a sensitive indicator.

Interleukin-1 Production

The role of IL-1 in the regulation of the inflammatory and immune responses has been recognized for many years. More recently, however, this cytokine has been identified as a product of many cell types other than those in the immune system. It is now understood that IL-1 has broad biologic effects on many cells other than those involved directly in host defenses. Since previous studies have shown that THC suppresses the function of monocyte/macrophages, our laboratory performed studies to determine whether THC affects IL-1 production. Peritoneal macrophages were obtained from mice and cultured *in vitro* in the presence of microbial antigens, which stimulate IL-1 production. After 24 hr incubation, culture supernatants were assayed for IL-1 activity by the comitogen thymocyte proliferation assay (31). Surprisingly, we found that instead of suppressing IL-1 production, THC significantly augmented the appearance of this cytokine in the culture supernatants. This enhancement effect of the drug was observed particularly for cultures stimulated with bacterial LPS in the presence of drug concentrations as low as 2 μg/ml.

The observation that THC augments the production of a cytokine, which plays a central role in the regulation of the immune response, suggests that marijuana may be more appropriately considered an immunomodulator, since its effects are not necessarily immunosuppressive. The augmentation of IL-1 production and/or release by THC might also increase an inflammatory response, since IL-1 also plays an important role in inflammation. The basis for the THC-induced enhancement of IL-1 release may be related to previously reported effects of this drug on cellular arachidonic acid metabolism. The influence of THC and other cannabinoids on the metabolism of arachidonic acid and production of prostaglandins has been examined in a variety of biologic systems (32). Cannabinoid treatment of some cell types results in enhancement of prostaglandin production while on other cell types there is an inhibition or no effect. However, in lymphoid cells, THC has been reported to increase the accumulation of free arachidonic acid, an effect that may be due to a stimulation of phospholipase A_2 (33) and/or to inhibition of lysophosphatidylcholine acyltransferases (34). Such findings may be related to THC-induced increases in macrophage IL-1 production because synthesis and release of this cytokine have been reported to be regulated by arachidonic acid metabolites (35).

Tumor Necrosis Factor Production

TNF was originally described by Carswell et al. (36) as a factor produced by macrophages in response to endotoxin challenge. This factor was toxic to neoplastic cells but not to normal cells. The described induction model involved presensitizing animals with bacille Calmette–Guérin (BCG) and then injecting them with endotoxin. Within 30 min after endotoxin challenge, the sera of the mice contained TNF activity. It was of particular interest that during the period from 30 min to 4 hr after endotoxin injection, the mice were in a state of shock and many died, even though they had been injected with only sublethal doses of endotoxin.

Independent of these studies, other investigators were examining factors involved in the state of cachexia, which often accompanies the invasion of mammals by infectious agents or tumors. Cachexia is a severe wasting syndrome, characterized by a depletion of energy stores, tissue damage, multiple organ system failure, shock, and finally death. Cachexia can reduce an animal's body mass by 50%. The factor responsible for this condition was identified and termed cachectin. Cachectin was shown to be a substance secreted by macrophages in response to endotoxin treatment. Beutler et al. (37) demonstrated that cachectin contained a strong sequence homology to TNF. Today, TNF and cachectin are considered to be the same molecule and the biologic relevance of this substance and its interactions with other cytokines are extremely important.

A frequently observed condition in rodents chronically treated with marijuana substances is a decrease in body weight gain (i.e., failure to grow) and a decrease in the relative weight of certain organs, such as the spleen. Huy et al. (38) also reported this phenomenon in guinea pigs and showed that chronically treated animals displayed significantly reduced levels of fatty acids in their sera. These symptoms may result from the influence of marijuana on the immunologic cells that produce TNF. Specifically, the drug may induce changes in the production and distribution of this cytokine. Recent studies have suggested that THC may influence the formation and release of TNF. This phenomenon was recently observed in a mouse model with a sublethal *Legionella* infection (3). In animals given THC immediately before and after the organisms, there was a rapid death of the animals, which appeared to be due to shock similar to that induced by TNF. Indeed, the levels of TNF in the sera of the animals treated with the THC and the *Legionella* were extremely high. Serum IL-6 levels were also elevated in the THC-treated animals. Both TNF and IL-6 are considered to be proinflammatory cytokines and related to toxic shock.

To determine whether THC can influence TNF levels, mouse spleen cells were treated with endotoxin *in vitro* to induce TNF. Cotreatment of these cells with graded amounts of THC *in vitro* enhanced the TNF levels in the culture supernatants (*unpublished observation* in our laboratory). Other experiments, however, have shown that in mouse spleen cells pretreated *in vitro* with IFN, which enhances macrophage function and responsiveness to endotoxin, THC treatment depresses TNF production (39). Thus, under one condition, in which endotoxin only was added to macrophages, THC appeared to enhance TNF production, but in the situation where endotoxin plus IFN was used to activate macrophages, THC suppressed production of this cytokine. Additional studies concerning the effects of THC on macrophage production of inflammatory cytokines such as TNF are being continued.

Effects of Marijuana on Natural Killer Cell Functions

NK cells are large granular lymphocytes with special capabilities for cytotoxicity against a variety of naturally occurring target cells. NK cells are believed to be important in host resistance to tumor cells and to a variety of infectious agents. They have been shown to be responsive to cytokines and also to produce cytokines. NK cells are found both in lymphoid tissue and circulating in the blood of humans and rodents. Patel et al. (40) were the first to show an effect by marijuana on splenic NK activity. Rats were injected subcutaneously on a daily basis for 25 days with 3 mg/kg of THC, followed by evaluation of serum hormone levels and splenic NK cell activity. Chronic drug treatment suppressed the NK cell activity of the rat splenocytes and reduced the serum levels of epinephrine, norepinephrine, and corticosterone. However, the serum levels of β-endorphin were enhanced. Administration of naloxone along with marijuana treatment ameliorated the THC-induced suppression of NK cell activity, suggesting that the marijuana was affecting NK cell activity through the endogenous opiate system. However, a direct effect of cannabinoids on NK cell function was not ruled out.

Subsequently, studies by Klein and co-workers demonstrated a direct effect of cannabinoids on purified NK cells from mouse spleens (41) and on a cloned cell line with NK cell activities (42). NK cells were purified from splenocyte populations by discontinuous Percoll gradient centrifugation. NK cells treated in culture for 4 hr with either THC or 11-hydroxy-THC were found to be suppressed in their cytolytic capability. 11-Hydroxy-THC appeared to be more potent than THC in its ability to suppress NK cell activity. However, the ability of the effector cells to form conjugates with target cells was not affected by drug treatment. These and similar data suggest that while cannabinoids directly affect NK cell cytolytic activity, they do not prevent effector cells from binding to targets, but rather inhibit cytolysis at a postbinding stage. The cytolytic activity of cloned cells with NK cell activity was also found to be suppressed by both THC and 11-hydroxy-THC.

An important feature of NK cell activity is augmentation of the response by cytokines such as IL-2. Such lymphokine-activated killer (LAK) cells were described originally by Grimm et al. (43), and their biology has recently been reviewed (44). The importance of the LAK cell phenomenon is that cytokines apparently can activate NK cells, making them both quantitatively and qualitatively more cytolytic. In this regard, Kawakami et al. (24) demonstrated that the LAK cell phenomenon was also suppressed by cannabinoids. LAK cells were generated by preincubation of NK cells with IL-2 and then exposed to THC at various concentrations prior to being tested for cytolytic activity. Cytotoxic activity against erythroleukemia (EL-4) target tumor cells, which are highly susceptible to LAK cells, was suppressed by 7 μg/ml of THC. The killing of YAC-1 cells, a non-IL-2-dependent NK cell target, was much less affected by THC treatment. Thus it is possible that cytolytic changes induced by IL-2 treatment, which account for the LAK cell phenomenon, may be more sensitive to the modulating effects of THC.

The Role of a Putative Tetrahydrocannabinol Receptor on Immune Cells

Since it is apparent that THC can affect various immune responses of human and animal cells, both *in vivo* and *in vitro*, it is likely that a specific receptor to which THC binds may be present on lymphoid cells. It has recently been reported that such a receptor is present on neurologic cells (45), and a complementary deoxyribonucleic acid (cDNA) probe has become available to detect expression of this receptor (46). Using this cDNA probe, the presence of the receptor gene was not initially found in rat spleen or other lymphoid cells. However, additional studies using a similar probe were able to detect the presence of mRNA for the putative THC receptor in mouse lymphoid cells (47). Also, indirect evidence of a THC receptor on immunologic cells was provided by experiments that showed that a radiolabeled THC analog was bound preferentially by certain types of lymphoid cells. Devane et al. (48) have recently identified the natural ligand for the putative THC receptor on neurologic cells as a previously undefined derivative of arachidonic acid, arachidonylethanolamine, which they have termed anandamide. This finding has interesting implications for the possible involvement of THC in the modulation of arachidonic acid metabolism.

Effects of Marijuana on Behavior: The Role of Cytokines

Drugs of abuse interact with the central nervous system and modify behavior. Experimental work with animals has shown that marijuana in particular induces in rodents a very specific behavior pattern known as catalepsy. The cataleptic properties of marijuana have been studied in detail by behavioral scientists and physiologists. It has been reported that prostaglandins administered prior to THC treatment can abort the cataleptic reaction and arachidonic acid metabolites have been implicated as somehow mediating the cataleptic reaction (49). Recent studies by Gibertini in our laboratory (*unpublished observations*) have shown that monoclonal antibodies to cytokines can also prevent the cataleptic reaction in mice injected with THC. For these experiments, a typical cataleptic monitoring technique was used, permitting quantitation of the effect of THC in inducing a state of nonresponsiveness in the mice. When the animals were first treated with a cocktail of monoclonal antibodies to cytokines, including IL-1, IL-6, TNF, and IFN-γ, catalepsy was prevented. Furthermore, antibodies to the individual cytokines IL-1, IL-6, or TNF had partial effects. It is widely acknowledged these cytokines are involved in a cascade of reactions, possibly involving arachidonic acid metabolism. Thus it seems likely that there is a role for cytokines in behavioral modifications induced by drugs of abuse and this strengthens the belief of a linkage between the nervous and immune systems in terms of the effects of a drug such as marijuana.

SUMMARY AND CONCLUSIONS

Animal experiments reported from various laboratories over the last several decades have shown that a variety of drugs of abuse may affect the function of lymphocytes and macrophages *in vivo* and *in vitro* (Table 1). *In vivo*, the size and architecture of lymphoid organs are affected and such changes can be related to drug-induced alterations in a variety of cell functions, including cytokine production. The addition of drugs of abuse to cultures of mouse or rat lymphocytes readily suppresses cell proliferation in a dose-dependent manner. These lymphocytes also show evidence of being deficient in their ability to produce antibodies, respond to IL-2, and produce cytokines, especially IFN. Thus it seems possible that drugs of abuse may interfere with early events in lymphocyte signal transduction. Injection of marijuana components into mice or rats often results in suppression of their antibody-forming capacity as well as their capacity to develop delayed hypersensitivity responses. These animals may also be unable to resist challenge by otherwise sublethal infections with a virus or bacterium. It has also been reported that repeated injections of high doses of drugs of abuse usually result in an even greater suppressive effect, possibly due to neurologic hormones in an individual "stressed" by such repeated injections. This has been postulated because there is often little correlation between the psychoactive potential of some drugs of abuse and the observed immunosuppression. Furthermore, both the cytolytic activity and respon-

TABLE 1. *Effects of Δ⁹-THC on immune function*

Immune parameter	Effect[a]
Human studies	
Macrophage spreading	↓
B lymphocyte blastogenesis	—
T lymphocyte blastogenesis	↓
NK cell cytotoxicity	↓
NK cell target binding	—
LAK cell cytotoxicity	↓
LAK cell, target binding	—
IL-2 receptor expression	↓
Murine studies	
Macrophage spreading	↓
Antibody production	↓
B lymphocyte blastogenesis	↓
T lymphocyte blastogenesis	↓
NK cell cytotoxicity, spleen cells	↓
NK cell cytotoxicity, cloned cell line	↓
NK cell target binding	—
IL-1 production	↑
TNF production	↑
IFN production	↓
IL-2 production	↓
IL-2 receptor expression, cloned cell line	↓

[a] ↓, Function decreased; —, no effect; ↑, function increased.

siveness to cytokines of murine and human NK cells can readily be suppressed by a number of drugs of abuse, especially marijuana, morphine, and cocaine. This may be related to the effects of the drugs on the cytokine binding to cell surface receptors and/or other events involved in signal transduction and cell activation.

Most studies concerning the effects of drugs of abuse on immunity have been performed with adults and subjects who display normal immune function (Table 1). Recently, it has been found that marijuana and its components are more markedly suppressive for the immune responsiveness of immature individuals. For example, THC has been found to be more immunosuppressive for 1- or 2-week-old-mice, equivalent to children who are newborn or infants. Furthermore, THC has also been found to be markedly immunosuppressive for lymphoid cells from older mice equivalent to humans who are 50 to 70 years old or more. THC has also been shown to be much more suppressive for lymphocytes in the thymus as compared to lymphocytes in the spleen or lymph nodes. The thymus is thought to be more important in immunoregulation than peripheral lymphoid organs. The greater sensitivity of thymocytes to the immunosuppressive effects of THC suggests that this component of marijuana has a greater immunomodulatory potential for immature lymphocytes.

However, treatment of animals or lymphoid cells with marijuana or its components does not always result in immunosuppression. Sometimes an immunoenhancement occurs and this is often related to the use of a relatively low concentration of the drug. Production of at least one important cytokine, IL-1, is augmented in animals or macrophage cultures following exposure to THC. Cachectin/TNF production has also been found under certain circumstances to be enhanced both *in vitro* and *in vivo* following THC exposure. Immune cell functions, which are dependant on arachidonic acid metabolic pathways, appear to be enhanced but, under certain circumstances, they may be suppressed by cannabinoids.

It is important to recognize that the clinical information obtained to date indicates that marijuana or other drugs of abuse may not increase acute disease incidence or cause marked depression of immunity in normal individuals. Marijuana use, however, may be related to increased susceptibility to chronic diseases. The observed alterations of immune function by concentrations of THC close to those readily observed in the blood of drug abusers probably have little impact on the development of systemic acute disease in normal, healthy individuals. However, the laboratory observations (Table 1) made by a number of investigators over the last two decades suggest the possibility that localized disease in areas where drugs of abuse concentrate in the body may be significantly impacted. Such observations suggest that the biologic impact of a drug of abuse such as marijuana on immune mechanisms may have especially negative effects on a host by increasing susceptibility to chronic infections and/or tumors. More importantly, individuals with already compromised immune systems, due to the presence of existing tumors or immunosuppression caused by an infection, may be at higher risk for these drug effects than healthy individuals. For example, individuals with HIV infection could have an increased risk for developing active AIDS when smoking marijuana or taking other drugs of abuse, including heroin or cocaine. Furthermore, individuals using drugs of abuse may be at higher risk for infection with certain opportunistic bacteria, fungi, or viruses. It should be noted that cancer patients who use marijuana to negate the nauseating effects of chemotherapy could be at increased risk for immunosuppression, creating a greater risk of tumor re-emergence during therapy. Likewise, bone marrow transplantation patients who have been given a THC-containing product to relieve nausea may be at increased risk for opportunistic infections.

In some cases, the immunosuppressive activities of THC might also have desirable effects by increasing the potential of a host to resist disease. For example, by downregulating the production of an antitumor blocking factor, which protects a tumor from immune recognition, THC treatment may allow the destruction of the tumor. Recently, it has been reported that THC given to experimental rats blocked the induction of allergic encephalomyelitis resulting from sensitization with neurologic tissue. It was postulated this occurred because THC has immunosuppressive effects and could inhibit the autoimmune response to the neurologic tissue, which would normally induce the autoimmune disease. However, no studies have yet been performed to determine whether marijuana or other drugs of abuse given in a clinical setting have an effect on the general well-being of a patient.

Published studies to date provide little information about the mechanism of immunomodulation induced by drugs of abuse. Nevertheless, newer studies concerning the effects of these drugs on the molecular aspects of immune responses are emerging. Future investigations will undoubtedly focus more on the molecular mechanisms by which drugs of abuse affect immune cell function, not only in experimental animal systems but also in humans.

REFERENCES

1. Morahan PS, Klykken PC, Smith SH, Harris LS, Munson AE. Effects of cannabinoids on host resistance to *Listeria monocytogenes* and herpes simplex virus. *Infect Immun* 1979;23:670–674.
2. Bradley SG, Munson AE, Dewey WL, Harris LS. Enhanced susceptibility of mice to combinations of delta-9-tetrahydrocannabinol and live or killed gram-negative bacteria. *Infect Immun* 1977;17:325.
3. Klein TW, Newton C, Widen R, Friedman H. Marijuana and bacterial infections. In: Friedman H, Klein TW, Specter S, eds. *Drugs of abuse, immunity and AIDS*. New York: Plenum Press 1993.
4. Juel-Jensen BE. Cannabis and recurrent herpes simplex. *Br Med J* 1972;4:296.
5. Gong H, Fligiel S, Tashkin DP, Barbers RG. Tracheobronchial changes in habitual, heavy smokers of marijuana with and without tobacco. *Am Rev Respir Dis* 1987;136:142–149.
6. Donald PJ. Marijuana smoking possible cause of head and neck carcinoma in young patients. *Otolaryngol Head Neck Surg* 1986;94:517–521.
7. Mann PEG, Cohen AB, Finley TH, Ladman AL. Alveolar macrophages: structural and functional differences between nonsmokers and smokers of marijuana and tobacco. *Lab Invest* 1971;25:111–120.
8. Nahas CG, Suciu-Poca N, Armand JP, Morishima A. Inhibition of cellular immunity in marijuana smokers. *Science* 1974;183:419–420.
9. Nahas CG, Davies M, Osserman EF. Serum immunoglobulin concentration in chronic marijuana smokers. *Fed Proc Soc Exp Biol Med* 1979;38:591.
10. Cushman P, Khurana R. Marijuana and T lymphocyte rosettes. *Clin Pharmacol Ther* 1976;19:310–317.
11. Peterson BH, Graham J, Lemberga L. Marijuana, tetrahydrocannabinol and T-cell function. *Life Sci* 1976;19:395–400.
12. Thompson GR, Mason M, Rosenkranz H, Braude M. Chronic oral toxicity of cannabinoids in rats. *Toxicol Appl Pharmacol* 1973;25:373–390.
13. Lefkowitz SS, Chiang CY. Effects of Δ^9-tetrahydrocannabinol on mouse spleens. *Res Commun Chem Pathol Pharmacol* 1975;11:659–662.
14. Rosenkrantz H, Miller AJ, Esber HJ. Δ^9-Tetrahydrocannabinol suppression of the primary immune response in rats. *J Toxicol Environ Health* 1975;1:119–125.
15. Zimmerman S, Zimmerman AM, Cameron IL, Lawrence HL. Δ^1-Tetrahydrocannabinol, cannabidiol and cannabinol effects on immune respone of mice. *Pharmacology* 1986;15:10–23.
16. Smith SH, Harris LS, Uwaydah IM, Munson AE. Structure–activity relationships of natural and synthetic cannabinoids in suppression of humoral and cell-mediated immunity. *J Pharmacol Exp Ther* 1978;207:165–170.
17. Luthra YK, Esber HJ, Lariviere DM, Rosenkrantz H. Assessment of tolerance to immunosuppressive activity of Δ^9–tetrahydrocannabinol in rats. *J Immunopharmacol* 1980;2:245–256.
18. Baczynsky WOT, Zimmerman AM. Effects of delta-9-tetrahydrocannabinol, cannabinol and cannabidiol on the immune system in mice. *Pharmacology* 1983;26:12.
19. Klein TW, Friedman H. Modulation of murine immune cell function by marijuana. In: Watson RR, ed. Drugs of abuse and immune function. Boca Raton, FL: CRC Press; 1990:87–111.
20. Watson ES, Murphy JC, ElSohly HN, ElSohly MA, Tuma CE. Effects of the administration of coco alkaloids on the primary immune responses of mice: interaction with delta-9-tetrahydrocannabinol and ethanol. *Toxicol Appl Pharmacol* 1983;71:1.
21. Levy JA, Heppner GH. Alterations of immune reactivity by haloperidol and delta-9-tetrahydrocannabinol. *J Immunopharmacol* 1981;3:93.
22. Klein TW, Newton CA, Widen R, Friedman H. The effects of Δ^9-tetrahydrocannabinol and 11-hydroxy-Δ^9-tetrahydrocannabinol on T-lymphocyte and B-lymphocyte mitogen responses. *J Immunopharmacol* 1985;7:451–466.

23. Yebra M, Klein TW, Friedman H. Δ^9-Tetrahydrocannabinol suppresses concanavalin A induced increase in cytoplasmic free calcium in mouse thymocytes. *Life Sci* 1992;51:151–160.
24. Kawakami Y, Klein TW, Newton C, Djeu JY, Specter S, Friedman H. Suppression by Δ^9-tetrahydrocannabinol of interleukin 2-induced lymphocyte proliferation and lymphokine-activated killer cell activity. *Immunopharmacology* 1988;10:485–488.
25. Zhu W, Igarashi T, Qi ZT, Newton C, Widen R, Friedman H, Klein T. Δ^9-Tetrahydrocannabinol (THC) decreases the number of high and intermediate affinity IL-2 receptors of the IL-2 dependent cell line NKB61A2. *Int J Immunopharmacol* 1993;16:742–749.
26. Cabral GA, Lockmuller JC, Mishkin EM. Δ^9-Tetrahydrocannabinol decreases α/β-interferon response to herpes simplex virus type 2 in the B6C3F1 mouse. *Proc Soc Exp Biol Med* 1986;181:305–311.
27. Blanchard DK, Newton C, Klein TW, Stewart WE II, Friedman H. *In vitro* and *in vivo* suppressive effects of Δ^9-tetrahydrocannabinol on interferon production by murine spleen cells. *Int J Immunopharmacol* 1986;8:819–824.
28. Huber GL, Simmons GA, McCarthy CR, Cutting MB, Laguarda R, Pereira W. Depressant effect of marijuana smoke on antibacterial activity of pulmonary alveolar macrophages. *Chest* 1975;68:769–773.
29. Raz A, Goldman R. Effect of hashish compounds on mouse peritoneal macrophages. *Lab Invest* 1976; 34:69–76.
30. Lopez-Cepero M, Friedman M, Klein T, Friedman H. Tetrahydrocannabinol-induced suppression of macrophage spreading and phagocytic activity *in vitro*. *J Leukoc Biol* 1986;39:679–686.
31. Klein TW, Newton CA, Blanchard DK, Widen R, Friedman H. Induction of interleukin 1 by *Legionella pneumophila* antigens in mouse and human mononuclear leukocyte cultures. *Zentralbl Bakt Hyg A* 1987;265:462–471.
32. Martin BR. Cellular effects of cannabinoids. *Pharmacol Rev* 1986;38:45–74.
33. Laychock SG, Hoffman JM, Meisol E, Bilgin S. Pancreatic islet arachidonic acid turnover and metabolism and insulin release in response to Δ^9-THC. *Biochem Pharmacol* 1986;35:2003–2008.
34. Greenberg JH, Mellors A. Specific inhibition of an acyltransferase by Δ^9-tetrahydrocannabinol. *Biochem Pharmacol* 1978;27:329–333.
35. Kunkel SL, Chensue SW, Spengler M, Geer J. Effects of arachidonic acid metabolites and their metabolic inhibitors on interleukin-1 production. In: Kluger MJ, Oppenheim JJ, Powanda MC, eds. *The physiologic, metabolic and immunologic actions of interleukin-1*. New York: Alan R Liss; 1985:297–307.
36. Carswell EA, Old LJ, Kassel RL, Green S, Fiore N, Williamson B. An endotoxin-induced serum factor that causes necrosis of tumors. *Proc Natl Acad Sci USA* 1975;72:3666–3670.
37. Beutler B, Greenwald D, Hulmes JD, et al. Identity of tumor necrosis factor and the macrophage-secreted factor cachectin. *Nature* 1985;342:552–554.
38. Huy ND, Gailis L, Cote G, Roy PE. Effects of chronic administration of Δ^9-tetrahydrocannabinol (Δ^9-THC) in guinea pigs. *Int J Clin Pharmacol Biopharmacol* 1975;12:284–289.
39. Zheng Z-M, Specter S, Friedman H. Inhibition by delta-9-tetrahydrocannabinol of tumor necrosis factor alpha production by mouse and human macrophages. *Int J Immunopharmacol* 1992;14:1445–1452.
40. Patel V, Borysenko M, Kumar MSA, Millard WS. Effects of acute and subchronic Δ^9-tetrahydrocannabinol administration on the plasma catecholamine, β-endorphin, corticosterone levels and splenic natural killer cell activity in rats. *Proc Soc Exp Biol Med* 1985;180:400–404.
41. Klein TW, Newton C, Friedman H. Inhibition of natural killer cell function by marijuana components. *J Toxicol Environ Health* 1987;20:321–332.
42. Kawakami Y, Klein TW, Newton C, Djeu JY, Dennert G, Specter S, Friedman H. Suppression by cannabinoids of a cloned cell line with natural killer cell activity. *Proc Soc Exp Biol Med* 1988; 187:355–359.
43. Grimm EA, Mazumder A, Zhang HZ, Rosenberg SA. Lymphokine activated killer cell phenomenon. Lysis on natural killer-resistant fresh solid tumor cells by interleukin 2-activated autologous human peripheral blood lymphocytes. *J Exp Med* 1982;155:823–830.
44. Herberman RB. Lymphokine-activated killer cell activity. *Immunol Today* 1987;8:178.
45. Devane WA, Dysarz FA III, Johnson MR, Melvin LS, Howlett AC. Determination and characterization of a cannabinoid receptor in rat brain. *Mol Pharmacol* 1988;34:605–613.
46. Matsuda LA, Lolait SJ, Brownstein MJ, Young AC, Bonner TI. Structure of a cannabinoid receptor and functional expression of the cloned cDNA. *Nature* 1990;346:561–564.

47. Kaminski NE, Abood ME, Kessler FK, Martin BR, Schatz AR. Identification of a functionally relevant cannabinoid receptor on mouse spleen cells involved in cannabinoid-mediated immune modulation. *Mol Pharmacol* 1992;42:736–742.
48. Devane WA, Hanus L, Breuer A, et al. Isolation and structure of a brain constituent that binds to the cannabinoid receptor. *Science* 1992;258:1946–1949.
49. Fairbain JW, Pickens JT. The effect of conditions influencing endogenous prostaglandins on the activity of Δ^1–THC in mice. *Br J Pharmacol* 1980;69:491–493.

Immunotoxicology and Immunopharmacology, Second Edition, edited by J. H. Dean, M. I. Luster, A. E. Munson, and I. Kimber.
Raven Press, Ltd., New York © 1994.

18

Immunotoxic Effects of Ethanol

Thomas R. Jerrells and *Stephen B. Pruett

*Department of Cellular Biology and Anatomy, Louisiana State University Medical Center, Shreveport, Louisiana 71130; and *Department of Biological Sciences, Mississippi State University, Mississippi State, Mississippi 39762*

A number of observations have led to the belief that alcohol abuse and alcoholism are associated with detrimental effects on the immune system. Among these observations is the finding that alcoholics, when compared with nonalcoholics, are more susceptible to opportunistic infections, infectious diseases in general, and certain tumors (1–5). The bases of these and future observations of the effects of alcohol lie in defining the immunosuppressive role of alcohol in human beings.

In this chapter we provide a review of evidence relating specifically to the role of ethanol (ETOH) in infections in alcoholics. We then describe methods of administration and models of investigation in animals that are used to elucidate in general the effects of ETOH on the immune system. This review focuses on the effects of ETOH on the components of the immune system that would result in an inability to mediate a specific immune response to foreign material. The applicability of findings obtained from rodent models to human beings is highlighted. Finally, we highlight the effects of ETOH in relation to observed neuroendocrine changes.

ASSOCIATION OF ETOH IN INFECTIONS IN ALCOHOLICS

Increased Susceptibility

The association between chronic consumption of ETOH and increased susceptibility to infections has been recognized by clinicians for some time. Results of clinical studies, as well as of studies with experimental animals, suggest impairment of cell-mediated and humoral immunity as a consequence of long-term alcohol use (1,4,5–9). Adams and Jordan (1) have presented an extensive review of the clinical observations and studies pertaining to alcohol abuse and infection. Pulmonary infections, particularly pneumonia and tuberculosis, have the strongest association with alcoholism. The incidence of pulmonary infection is higher with, and the prognosis appears to be affected adversely by, extensive ETOH use.

Results of a study of mortality rates in patients with pneumonia admitted to Cook County Hospital demonstrated an increase in mortality with an increase in alcohol consumption. The mortality rate in abstainers or light drinkers was 22%, whereas that in the heavy drinking population and moderate drinkers was 50% and 34%, respectively (10). The mortality rate was determined in 6478 patients admitted for treatment to the Toronto Clinic of the Addiction Research Foundation, and the observed versus expected mortality rates of alcoholic patients with pneumonia were 3.01 and 7.14 times the expected rate for women and men, respectively (11). In an extensive prospective study, the incidence of bacterial pneumonia was evaluated in 900 consecutive admissions to Yale–New Haven Hospital. The incidence of pneumonia was 15.5% in alcoholic patients, compared with 6.5% in nonalcoholic patients (12). An increased risk of pulmonary disease was also demonstrated with longitudinal studies in which morbidity of alcoholic career navy men was compared with that of nonalcoholic cohorts. The incidence of respiratory disease was noted in the first year of service of young alcoholics. The older career men had a rate of pneumonia twice that of their nonalcoholic cohorts (13).

Results of a number of studies have also indicated a higher than expected rate of tuberculosis in alcoholic patients studied in Australia, Scandinavia, and the United States (14–19). Treatment has been reported to be less effective in alcoholic patients, particularly a consequence of poor compliance by the alcoholic patient in taking the prescribed drugs (20). In an extensive study of 2641 clients of the New York City Human Resources Administration, 400 clients were identified as meeting preestablished criteria for alcohol abuse, defined as consumption of at least 58 ml of ethyl alcohol per day for at least 1 month. Also identified were 246 individuals who abused both alcohol and nonprescription drugs. The rate of tuberculosis in individuals who abused only alcohol was 45 times that for an age-matched New York City general population (21).

Extrapulmonary infections also appear at a higher rate in alcoholic patients. Both spontaneous bacterial peritonitis and spontaneous bacteremia are seen among patients with cirrhosis of liver and are particularly prevalent in those with alcoholic cirrhosis (22–24). Shunts develop in the alcoholic patient with liver disease (Laennec's cirrhosis), which allow the circulation to bypass the hepatic capillary beds and consequently the reticuloendothelial system. Thus the clearance of bacteria from the blood is impaired (25). The incidence of spontaneous bacteremia in alcoholic patients is not great, and most cases of bacteremia in these patients are associated with bacterial entry from either the gastrointestinal tract or genitourinary tract (26).

Increased Exposure

In all likelihood, many of the infections associated with alcoholism are due, at least in part, to the rate of exposure in an alcoholic versus that in the general population. An exceptionally high incidence of markers of hepatitis B viral infection is seen in patients with alcoholic liver disease, and it has been suggested that this is the result of repeated exposure to the hepatitis B virus through multiple hospital admissions and unhygienic living conditions, rather than to a direct effect of ETOH (27–29). The outbreaks of diphtheria that occurred from 1972 to 1982 in a group of alcoholics in Seattle, Washington, were also considered to be due to high rates of exposure to the causative organism (i.e., *Corynebacterium diphtheriae*), rather than to general impairment of immune function (30). The impairment of mechanical defenses that occurs in association with acute intoxication is another mechanism by which an alcoholic patient's exposure to infectious organisms is increased. Loss of consciousness can inhibit closure of the glottis, which allows aspiration of particulate matter or oropharyngeal secretions into the lower respiratory tract and is thought to contribute to anaerobic lung disease often associated with alcoholism (31).

The determination of the relative importance of ETOH-impaired immune response, as opposed to other complications of alcoholism as contributors to the increased incidence and severity of infection, has been difficult to evaluate from clinical studies. Complications, such as cirrhosis, malnutrition, and increased exposure to infective organisms (either through living conditions or trauma because of higher accident rates in intoxicated individuals), may contribute to infections in the alcoholic patient (31). Although environmental factors contribute to infections in the alcoholic patient, results of several studies indicate that ETOH is directly immunosuppressive. This is particularly prominent when changes in immune system components are examined.

INVESTIGATORY METHODS AND MODELS IN ANIMALS

Rodent Models for Investigating the Effects of Alcoholism on the Immune System

Criteria

The criteria for an ideal rodent model for alcoholism to be used in immunologic studies should be slightly different from those suggested by Cicero (32) for use in neurologic or behavioral studies. Any model of alcoholism should consistently produce clinically relevant blood alcohol levels representative of those noted in human alcoholics (32). The model should also permit consistent ETOH exposure for at least several days or weeks. Long-term (≥4 weeks) ETOH exposure, which is often used to induce tolerance, dependence, or pathologic changes in neurologic or biochemical studies, may unnecessarily complicate immunologic studies. Thus many investigators have chosen short-term (several days to a few weeks) ETOH exposure to prevent extensive physiologic changes that might indirectly affect the immune system (33–38). Long-term ETOH exposure has also been used to characterize the immunologic effects of ETOH (39–41). Long-term exposure is valid in terms of providing a representation of human alcoholism, but the causes of immunologic changes noted in these models may depend less immediately on ETOH *per se* than they do in short-term models. In addition, some pathologic changes that are common in human alcoholics (e.g., severe alcoholic liver disease) and that are associated with suppression of immune functions (42) do not occur in rodent models (43). Thus rodent models are not useful in assessing the role of such changes in immunosuppression. Finally, in view of the profound effects that nutritional deficits can have on the immune system (44), it seems reasonable to exert greater care in controlling for and evaluating nutritional factors in immunologic studies than may be necessary in neurologic or behavioral studies.

Route of ETOH Administration: Oral, Intragastric, or Other

Administration of ETOH by the oral or intragastric route is preferred by many investigators, because this is the typical route of exposure in human beings. This may be more than a trivial consideration in view of evidence that soluble factors produced by the gastric mucosa in response to ETOH can affect the immune system (45). Thus administration of ETOH by injection or inhalation may not induce the full range of immunologic changes produced when ETOH is administered by the oral or intragastric route. Furthermore, physiologic changes (e.g., mild inflammatory responses in the lungs or peritoneum) that are not typically produced when human beings ingest ETOH may be induced with injection or inhalation of ETOH. Thus it is not surprising that the immunologic effects of ETOH in the rat depend somewhat on the route of administration (46). The use of inhalation or injection will undoubtedly be appropriate for some purposes, but results should be confirmed in an oral or intragastric study before they are assumed to be applicable to human beings.

In the following sections we describe methods of ETOH administration that have been used in studies designed to investigate the effects of ETOH on immune parameters. This is not an exhaustive description of all available methods.

Liquid Diet

Administration of ETOH in a liquid diet preparation that provides the sole source of water and nutrients is widely used in studies of the effects of ETOH on the immune system, and this route generally satisfies the criteria noted earlier. Liquid diet preparations, which are based on the formulation of Lieber and DeCarli (47), are available commercially. Generally, control animals are pair-fed an isocaloric liquid diet preparation in which ETOH is replaced with dextrin–maltose. This method overcomes the natural aversion to ETOH exhibited by most mammals and permits achievement of relevant blood ETOH levels [0.1% to 0.2% in rats (43); 0.3% to 0.5% in mice (34)]. It also allows adequate nutrition to be maintained for long periods (43). In addition, the Lieber–DeCarli diet includes 35% fat, an amount consistent with the average American diet (43). A Lieber–DeCarli diet preparation in which 36% of calories are supplied by ETOH approaches the average value for human alcoholics (50% of calories derived from ETOH) (43). Mice (34) and rats (43) voluntarily consume sufficient quantities of 6% to 7% (wt/vol) ETOH in a Lieber–DeCarli diet to permit growth. Rats or mice maintained on such a diet, as well as pair-fed control animals, are slightly undernourished and grow more slowly than animals given liquid diet *ad libitum* (34,43). ETOH- and pair-fed animals, however, are not malnourished (43).

Although malnutrition or extreme undernutrition can be immunosuppressive (44), rodents maintained on a reduced-calorie diet have increased longevity and decreased incidence of cancer (48,49). Thus there is no indication that mild restriction of caloric intake adversely affects host resistance to infectious disease or cancer. This is supported further by the results of a study in which pair-fed mice and mice given free access to standard laboratory chow were compared and found to be indistinguishable with regard to several immune parameters (34). Some immune functions, however, can be modulated by undernutrition (50,51), and appropriate controls should be included to account for this possibility.

Intubation

Administration of ETOH to rats by intubation every 4 to 6 hr can be used to induce ETOH tolerance and dependence (52), and this method has been used in several immunologic studies. This approach allows maintenance of relevant blood alcohol levels, and ETOH is often infused as a 20% solution in a Lieber–DeCarli diet or other commercially available nutrient mixture to provide adequate nutrition. Control animals are usually fed the same nutrient mixture in which sucrose or glucose replaces ETOH to produce an isocaloric suspension. Administration of ETOH by intubation ensures that all animals receive equal amounts of ETOH at the same time or that they maintain similar levels of intoxication (52). This approach may eliminate the large variations in blood ETOH levels usually noted when an ETOH liquid diet is consumed voluntarily (34,40). In addition, blood ETOH levels attained by this method (0.2% to 0.4%) (36) are generally higher than those attained by voluntary consumption in rats, and these higher levels may be more representative of the levels observed in human alcoholics (53). The nutritional effects of administration of ETOH by intubation, however, have not been investigated as thoroughly as those associated with voluntary consumption of the ETOH-containing Lieber–DeCarli diet. Thus appropriate controls for nutritional effects are important when intubation is used.

Drinking Water

ETOH can also be administered to rodents in their drinking water. This method does not permit maintenance of blood ETOH levels representative of those seen in human alcoholics (43,50), but it may be useful for studies of immunologic parameters that seem particularly sensitive to the effects of ETOH or those that are suppressed by undernutrition. For example, Blank and colleagues (50) used this approach in conjunction with unrestricted and restricted diets to evaluate the contributions of undernutrition and ETOH in the suppression of splenic natural killer (NK) cell activity (50).

Study Results

As rodent models for alcoholism have become more consistent from one laboratory to another, the reported immunologic effects have also become more consistent. Results from several laboratories also indicate many similarities in the immunologic effects of ETOH in rats and mice, as well as when ETOH is administered by voluntary consumption in a liquid diet or water or by frequent intubation (33,34,36–38,54). Some differences in the number and severity of immunologic deficits reported by various groups might be accounted for by differences in blood alcohol levels attained by different modes of intragastric or oral administration in rats or mice.

Although reasonably consistent results have been reported in a number of studies with the use of rats and mice and various protocols for oral or intragastric ETOH administration, most investigators have used the same sex (male) and strain (Sprague–Dawley rats; C57BL/6 mice) of animal. Immunosuppression, however, has also been reported in female rats (36) and mice (55). Thus the effects of ETOH on the immune system do not seem to be strictly sex dependent. This does not exclude the possibility of sex-related differences (56), however. Very similar immunologic effects have also been noted in studies with two different rat strains (Sprague–Dawley and Lewis) (33,36). Substantial differences may exist among mouse strains, however, depending on the protocol for ETOH administration. For example, C57BL/6 mice voluntarily consume larger quantities of ETOH than do most other strains (57). Differences between strains in this regard can be profound. Attempts to evaluate the immunologic effects of voluntary consumption of 7% ETOH in a Lieber–DeCarli diet in C57BL/6 versus B6C3F1 mice were unsuccessful, because the mice would not consume sufficient diet to maintain body weight and normal immune parameters during a 5- to 7-day experiment (S. B. Pruett, *unpublished data*). There are also substantial differences among mouse strains in several neurologic and behavioral responses (58). Thus it would not be surprising to find strain differences in ETOH-induced immunologic changes, particularly if some of these changes are mediated by neuroendocrine responses to ETOH.

Rodent Models for Assesssing the Effects of Binge Drinking on the Immune System

Evidence of Binge Drinking Effects

Occasional binge drinking is probably more prevalent than alcoholism (59), but relatively little is known of the effects of binge drinking on the immune system.

There are indications that a single drinking episode can suppress the immune system. As early as 1938, suppression of host resistance to *Streptococcus pneumoniae* was reported after acute administration of ETOH to rabbits (60). In human beings, the chemotactic response of leukocytes after dermabrasion was measured by using a chamber secured over the abraded area. Chemotaxis in persons given 50 to 75 ml of ETOH (as a 20% solution) during a 20-min period was suppressed as profoundly as in persons who were comatose because of septic shock or shock after myocardial infarction (61). Very similar results were reported more than 50 years ago in a rat model (62) and were confirmed recently in a model in which ETOH (3.0 g/kg) was administered by gavage to rats. These animals had blood ETOH levels of approximately 0.2%, and the chemotactic response of their neutrophils to *N*-formyl-methionyl-leucyl-phenylalanine *in vivo* was significantly suppressed (63). These and other similar results (35) indicate consistent, rapid suppression of important functions of phagocytic cells *in vivo* after acute administration of ETOH.

Data are very limited regarding the effects of acute administration of ETOH on immunologic parameters other than phagocyte chemotaxis and function. Results of studies with rodents (63) and human beings (64) indicate no suppression of lymphocyte mitogenic response *in vitro* after acute ETOH exposure *in vivo*. Few other parameters, however, have been evaluated. Findings in recent studies by one of us (S. B. P.) indicate that thymic atrophy and suppression of the antibody response to a T cell-dependent antigen (sheep red blood cells, SRBCs) occur in female B6C3F1 mice after a single dose of ETOH administered by gavage (Fig. 1). The ETOH doses in these experiments are higher than those typically used in neurologic or behavioral studies in which ETOH is administered by intraperitoneal injection. These intragastric doses, however, do produce a range of behavioral changes not unlike those noted in human binge drinkers (mild ataxia at 5.0 g/kg to unresponsiveness at 6.5 to 7.0 g/kg). Results of subsequent experiments indicate that administration of a 50% ETOH solution at these dosages causes focal necrosis and inflammation in the stomach or duodenum (or both), but similar immunologic effects have been noted in several experiments with the use of 32% ETOH solutions, which do not generally cause histopathologic changes (S. B. Pruett, *unpublished data*). These results suggest the possibility that binge drinking may affect several immunologic parameters.

Rodents do not voluntarily drink ETOH solutions rapidly enough to permit intoxication within a period of several minutes to several hours as required in a binge drinking model (34). Therefore most investigators interested in neurologic, behavioral, and metabolic effects of binge drinking have administered ETOH by intraperitoneal injection (65–69). As already noted, this may not be the most appropriate route of administration for investigation of immunologic effects. Options for administration by a route more representative of human exposure include intragastric administration (by intubation or gavage) and schedule-induced polydipsia. Each of these approaches has advantages and disadvantages.

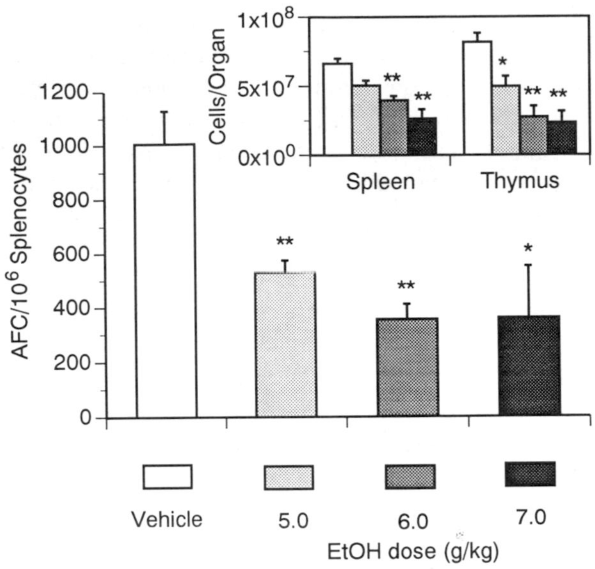

FIG. 1. Thymus and spleen cellularity and *in vitro* humoral immune response 36 hr after a single dose of ETOH in female B6C3F1 mice. The indicated doses of ETOH were administered by gavage. The vehicle control group received water. Thirty-six hours after dosing, the spleen and thymus were removed from each mouse, and nucleated cells were enumerated by using a Coulter counter (Coulter Electronics, Hialeah, FL). Splenocytes were placed in Mishell–Dutton cultures and stimulated with sheep erythrocytes. Five days later, antibody-forming cells (AFCs) were quantified by using a plaque assay. Values shown are means ± SE for groups of five mice, and values significantly different (by ANOVA followed by Dunnett's test) from vehicle controls are indicated by $^*p<0.05$ or $^{**}p<0.01$.

Intubation or Gavage

Intubation and gavage allow precise control of ETOH administration, but they are mildly stressful. Although this stress is generally not sufficient to affect most immunologic parameters, it may contribute to the stress-inducing action of ETOH in rodents and to subsequent immunologic changes. (The relationship between stress responses and ETOH-induced immunosuppression is considered further in a later section.) Few studies have been conducted with regard to the possible interactions between psychogenic and chemical stressors, but Balfour and colleagues (70) found that the combined effects of a psychogenic stressor (elevation on a small platform) and nicotine were no greater than the effects of either stressor alone. Thus it should not be assumed that all stressors act additively or synergistically. If handling and dosing contribute significantly to ETOH-induced stress responses, they must be considered in interpreting results of immunologic studies in which such models are used. This would not necessarily invalidate this mode of administration as a model for human binge drinking. Psychogenic stress seems to result in an increase in ETOH consumption (69), and it is likely that many human beings simultaneously experience psychogenic stress and binge drinking.

Schedule-Induced Polydipsia

An alternative mode of ETOH administration that may deserve consideration for use in immunologic studies is schedule-induced polydipsia. Rodents that are placed on a restricted diet and fed only at discrete time points spontaneously drink large quantities of water during the time between delivery of each food pellet during a feeding session (71). This method does not require handling or forced administration of ETOH and would therefore prevent the stress associated with these treatments. It does, however, require undernourishment (72). In addition, food presentation to food-deprived animals can suppress glucocorticoid responses to stressors (73). Because this event could alter the immunologic effects of ETOH, it should be assessed when schedule-induced polydipsia is used in immunologic studies.

Study Results and Applicability of Findings in Rodent Models to Human Beings

The applicability to human beings of the data obtained in rodent models of ETOH-induced immunosuppression is an important issue. Results of the studies reviewed in this section suggest that the immunosuppressive effects of ETOH on the immune system are quite dose dependent. It is probably not appropriate to compare doses of ETOH in human beings and rodents on a gram-per-kilogram basis, because equal doses would probably not produce equal blood alcohol levels. In addition, equal blood alcohol levels do not produce comparable behavioral effects in rodents and human beings. For example, rats lose the righting reflex at blood ETOH levels of approximately 0.5% (52). This level, however, is greater than the average lethal dose for human beings (74). Most investigators who study the neurologic and behavioral effects of ETOH in rodent models have tacitly adopted the assumption of Majchrowicz (52). That is, the most appropriate strategy is to use doses of ETOH in rodents that produce neurologic or behavioral changes comparable to those noted in human alcoholics or binge drinkers, regardless of the doses or blood levels required to achieve these effects in rodents. This strategy also seems appropriate for studies of the immunologic effects of ETOH. It should be recognized, however, that the comparative sensitivities of the rodent and human immune systems to mechanisms of ETOH action other than neuroendocrine modulation are not known. Thus it is possible that results from rodent models could overestimate or underestimate the effects of ETOH on the human immune system.

DEMONSTRATED EFFECTS OF ETHANOL ON THE IMMUNE SYSTEM

Effects of Ethanol on Components of the Immune System

Lymphocytes

Lymphocytes can be classified into several broad categories on the basis of their function, and the ultimate expression of immunity to a number of agents depends on the cellular interaction of these various categories of cells. In this chapter we discuss the thymus-derived lymphocyte (T cell), the lymphocyte that ultimately produces antibodies (B cell), nonspecific cytotoxic cells (NK cells), and various subpopulations of these broad groups. ETOH may affect immunity through a number of mechanisms, including depletion of one or all of these cell types, alteration of cellular function, or changes in the ability of the cell to leave the bloodstream and enter the local environment where the immune response occurs.

Lymphocyte Numbers

Results obtained from a number of studies have shown that ETOH abuse by human beings or administration of ETOH to experimental animals leads to a depletion of mononuclear cells (33,75–78). By necessity the studies that were done with human beings involved cellular changes in the peripheral blood (61,75,79–81). This effect of ETOH is probably the most consistent finding in various models of ETOH abuse. As will be discussed later, a number of mechanisms for cell depletion (killing) exist. It remains to be determined, however, whether ETOH depletes lymphocytes from the peripheral blood simply by affecting the ability of cells to traffic normally. ETOH affects the ability of polymorphonuclear neutrophils (granulocytes) to demarginate and thus to increase their number in the peripheral blood (33,61,82). It is not unlikely that ETOH, perhaps through its effect on the endothelium, somehow alters the ability of lymphocytes to enter the bloodstream through the endothelium.

Results of a number of studies, in which experimental animal model systems of ETOH abuse have been used, have established that a reproducible effect of ETOH is depletion of lymphoid cells from the spleen and thymus (33,34,46,76,78,83). In the rodent, the spleen is structurally organized to produce primary immune responses to antigenic material removed from the bloodstream (84) and is thus a major location for T and B cells and an important organ for immunity. ETOH has been shown to deplete this organ of cells regardless of the animal model system studied. The spleen is also a hematopoietic organ in rodents, and it is still unclear to what extent the stem cells are depleted in response to ETOH. Nevertheless, it has been determined that both T and B cells are depleted from the spleen after administration of ETOH to experimental animals (78,85). Although some controversy exists in the literature as to the relative extent ETOH influences lymphocyte numbers (38,86), apparently B cells are lost in greater numbers than are T cells (78,85). Findings from one study have established that the spleen loses about 50% of its cellularity, but immunohistologic analyses showed that the basic structural architecture is not changed (78). It remains to be seen whether the structures of the spleen that are important in immune responses (i.e., germinal centers) are altered in function. Although the studies have been limited, it appears that a significant proportion of T cells are lost from human peripheral blood (87). It should be noted, however, that the majority of peripheral blood lymphocytes are T cells.

Another lymphoid organ that is affected by ETOH is the thymus. This organ is the site of T lymphocyte maturation; that is, the primary site of production of T cells that are involved in cell-mediated immune responses. The thymus is affected more profoundly by ETOH than is the spleen, and most study results show that nearly 90% of the cells are lost (33,34,78,83). Recent study results indicate that the immature (CD4+/CD8+) thymocyte is most affected in these model systems (78). In later stages of ETOH administration, the mature T cell (CD4+/CD8− or CD4−/CD8+) is lost from the thymus (78). In contrast to the spleen, the architecture of the thymus is profoundly changed, and few histologic landmarks can be identified (78). It remains to be seen whether the functional aspects of cell types in the thymus other than the lymphocytes are changed as a result of ETOH.

It would appear that lymph nodes are also affected by ETOH in terms of cell loss (38). No data are available, however, to determine which cell types are lost, and further studies are required to determine the nature of the cells that are lost. One preliminary study has been performed. Findings have been interpreted to indicate that administration of ETOH to mice results in changes in the number and composition of lymphocytes in the lymphoid structures in the gastrointestinal tract (D. Sibley, and T. R. Jerrells, *unpublished data*). Because of the obvious importance of the lymphatic system and the lymphoid structures in the gastrointestinal tract, further work is necessary to address the effects of ETOH on this system.

Very little is known regarding the mechanisms that result in cell depletion from the spleen and thymus. Results of one study performed with the use of animals depleted of glucocorticosteroids (88) showed that the production of steroids is an important factor in the depletion of cells from the thymus and of somewhat lesser importance in cell depletion from the spleen. Findings in this study did show that animals depleted of corticosteroids by adrenalectomy still lost cells from the thymus, and corticosteroid depletion was confirmed by a lack of serum corticosteroids measured by a sensitive radioimmunoprecipitation assay. These findings support the suggestion that factors other than a stress response associated with ETOH itself (89) or associated with withdrawal from ETOH (33,88) may be important in the observed loss of cells related to ETOH. It would appear that acute exposure to ETOH administered by gavage also results in cell loss from the spleen and thymus. This cell loss, however, is due almost entirely to the effects of corticosteroids (see later section on ETOH-Induced Neuroendocrine Changes), based on the reversal of cell loss observed by concomitant treatment with a steroid inhibitor. Chronic exposure to ETOH may result in cell depletion by a combination of corticosteroids and other undefined mechanisms.

The consequences of the described changes in cell numbers, regardless of the mechanisms, can be predicted to have major effects on the host's ability to produce immune responses. For example, to generate immune responses to infectious agents or tumors in tissues, cells must leave the bloodstream in reaction to chemotactic factors and enter sites of inflammation within the tissue. If the peripheral blood is depleted of lymphocytes, it will be more difficult to get the appropriate cells into these sites of inflammation, and the immune response will necessarily be delayed or absent if the depletion is severe enough. A similar situation exists for the spleen. If sufficient numbers of cells are depleted from this organ, the ability of an individual to produce an immune response will be severely limited.

Changes in the thymus have much more potential to produce long-term changes in the immune system. Two very important aspects of the immune system have been described recently that contribute to the production of appropriate immune responses. The cells in peripheral lymphoid organs, such as lymph nodes and the spleen, must be of the appropriate type and express the appropriate T cell antigen receptor to recognize foreign antigens. It is also critical that cells with reactivity to self-antigens (autoantigens) be deleted from the pool of cells that leave the thymus to populate the peripheral organs. These two selection processes are performed in the thymus and are termed positive and negative selection, respectively. [See reviews by Winoto (90) and Scollay (91).] It is believed that these two critical functions somehow involve the thymic epithelium. If ETOH affects the thymic epithelium, dramatic changes in the ability of an individual to make immune responses may occur, and perhaps holes in the immune repertoire will occur. A failure of negative selection processes has been postulated to result in autoimmune diseases, and some of the autoimmune phenomena observed in alcoholics may be due to a defect similar to the one postulated earlier.

Lymphocyte Function

The observed defects in immune responses described earlier could also be due to an effect of ETOH on the function of the various populations of lymphocytes. This aspect of the effects of ETOH on the immune system has been studied most; the mechanisms of impaired cellular function, however, remain undefined. The production of an efficient immune response requires the interaction of many cell types and depends critically on the ability of cells to produce and respond to soluble mediators called cytokines. The cytokine network is complex, and very little is known about how ETOH affects this network. Nevertheless, sufficient information is available to make some general statements in terms of ETOH-associated changes in cell function.

The majority of work in this area has been done with the use of T cells and *in vitro* assays of responses. The direct application of ETOH at pharmacologic levels to cultured lymphocytes usually results in little change in responses to nonspecific stimuli of T cell proliferation (77), although this finding is somewhat controversial (92). On the other hand, lymphocytes exposed to ETOH in the experimental animal or human being respond poorly to nonspecific stimuli (33,34,93–97). Usually mitogens such as concanavalin A (Con A) or phytohemagglutinin (PHA) have been used to stimulate T cell responses to define the effects of ETOH. These reagents stimulate the majority of T cells to proliferate and produce cytokines. As referenced earlier, the most common finding has been that cells obtained from ETOH-treated animals or alcoholic human beings do not proliferate as well to these agents as do cells obtained from control animals or subjects. Interestingly, a similar finding has not been obtained with the study of B cell stimulation (34,77,98). Although the B cell is lost from lymphoid organs in greatest numbers (78,85), the response of rodent spleen cells to stimulation is not changed (34,54,88). As will be discussed later, the response to direct stimulation *in vivo* is also not affected by ETOH. Some data have been described that suggest that B cell responses can be affected directly by ETOH (99,100). These studies were done with the use of *in vitro* culture systems and B cell tumor cells, and the results may not necessarily reflect what occurs *in vivo*.

Very little information exists regarding the mechanisms involved in the effects of ETOH on T cells. The presence of other disease appears to be necessary for the noted impairments in immune responses in alcoholic human beings (8,101). It can easily be appreciated how severe liver disease can influence the general immune system, but findings obtained from careful study of systems in which marked changes in liver function do not occur have shown that changes in the immune system are still evident (34,88). Differences may exist between species, and ETOH may affect the immune system through different mechanisms in human beings, rodents, guinea pigs, and other species.

Lymphocytes obtained from ETOH-treated animals produce sufficient levels of interleukin-2 (IL-2), which is a critical growth factor for T cell proliferation (102, 103). Furthermore, cells apparently express appropriate numbers of high-affinity receptors for IL-2 but do not respond to IL-2 (102–104). On the basis of these data, it has been hypothesized that ETOH somehow alters the intracellular signaling events that are generated after IL-2 and IL-2 receptor interactions and that ultimately result in cellular division. The most profound effect of ETOH on T cell proliferation has been demonstrated with the use of stimuli that act through the T cell receptor. In previous studies, the response to alloantigens on foreign cells in a mixed lymphocyte response assay has been used to demonstrate the effects of ETOH (34). In more recent studies, T cells from ETOH-treated mice were stimulated in culture with a monoclonal antibody that recognizes a molecule that is associated with the T cell receptor termed CD3. Study findings indicate that stimulation of spleen cells with anti-CD3 added as a soluble reagent was not affected by ETOH treatment, but the response of purified T cell to insoluble anti-CD3 was reduced in cells from ETOH-treated animals (105). The response to insoluble anti-CD3 is independent of accessory cell function, and this finding supports the idea that ETOH is associated with a direct T cell defect that could perhaps be overcome if accessory cells were also stimulated by the same reagent (e.g., anti-CD3). To extend this idea, ETOH may affect the T cell, rather than the accessory cell, at least in terms of the production of cytokines or other factors that are necessary for T cell responses. This is obviously speculation.

Several groups have attempted to determine the effect of age and ETOH on the immune system (106–108). Because of the known effect of age on the immune system (immunosenescence) it is important to determine whether ETOH potentiates the decline of immune responsiveness that is associated with the aging process. Future studies with these models may provide insight into the effects of ETOH.

Immunity to viruses, some bacteria, and tumors is thought to be mediated by subpopulations of lymphocytes that have been characterized by their cytotoxic ability. These cells can be subdivided into those that show specificity in their antigenic responses and those that are nonrestricted. A great deal of work has been done in which the effects of ETOH on the nonspecific cytotoxic cells termed NK cells have been examined. This may be the most controversial area of research on the effects of ETOH on the immune system. Results of several studies have shown that ETOH (1) has no effect on or increases NK cell activity (109,110) or (2) decreases NK cell activity. It would appear from the literature that the most reproducible effect of ETOH in carefully controlled studies is a decrease in NK cell function (50,111–115). It remains to be seen whether this effect is due to a direct effect of ETOH on cytotoxic effector mechanisms or simply to a decrease in NK cell numbers. From data obtained from a limited number of studies (80,116) it would appear that ETOH also affects the function of specific cytotoxic cells. These studies have some serious consequences in terms of host defenses to viruses and tumors, and the studies need to be expanded to determine the relevance of these findings.

Some data exist to support the contention that corticosteroids may play a critical role in changes in lymphocyte function (88), although it is still not clear whether this is the only factor contributing to defects in cellular responses. It can be argued that B cells, which are very susceptible to corticosteroids, should equally be affected by ETOH, and this clearly is not the case in animals treated chronically with ETOH (34,54,88). Obviously, more research is required to determine the extent of the effects of ETOH on lymphocyte function, as well as the mechanisms involved in the effects of ETOH on the immune system.

Antibody Production

Paradoxical information exists regarding the effects of ETOH on the production of immunoglobulins (antibodies). Alcoholics, especially those with cirrhosis of the liver, have elevated serum immunoglobulin (Ig) levels, especially those of the IgA class. A number of theories have been put forth to explain this finding, including the presence of high levels of circulating antigens related to translocation of intestinal bacteria and bacterial endotoxin. The normal production of IgA by the liver also may be affected by ETOH, with hyperproduction of this Ig occurring as a result. Another possibility is that ETOH-associated immunosuppression results in an increased incidence of infections that ultimately results in high Ig levels. On the other hand, a number of groups have shown that ETOH treatment of experimental animals is associated with a defect in antibody production to certain antigens (33,34, 54,77). It is interesting to note that these study results have shown that the defect in antibody production is seen only when antigens that require T cell help for antibody production by B cells are used. The response to antigens that are independent of T cell help is not affected in ETOH-treated animals. These data have been used to argue that the effects of ETOH are relatively specific for T cell function and at least some subpopulations of B cells are not as sensitive to the effects of ETOH. As mentioned earlier, a large proportion of the B cells in the spleen are depleted in ETOH-treated animals, and the specific B cells that respond to T cell help may be depleted. Further studies are required to address this point. One of the more important questions regarding the effects of ETOH on Ig production is the effect on the production of secretory IgA at mucosal surfaces. Alcoholics are more susceptible than nonalcoholics to respiratory infections because of a variety of factors (5,117–119), and this may involve a defect in IgA or IgM production at the local site of infection. This important question is obviously in need of further study.

In Vivo *Immune Responses*

Very little work has been done to examine the effects of ETOH with the use of *in vivo* techniques. This is probably related to the complexity of the immune response and the difficulty in studying this system *in vivo*. It obviously is easier to isolate various components of the immune response, but these studies mostly ignore the various interactions among aspects of the immune system. It is important to determine the impact of ETOH on *in vivo* host defense mechanisms that require these complicated interactions and to devise methods to unravel these effects. A number of anecdotal study findings, including those in a number of case reports (120), clearly support the idea that ETOH has a profound effect on resistance to infectious diseases and tumors (121), and these studies underline the importance of understanding these effects. In the studies that have been done, either microorganisms or tumors have been used. Most of these studies have been complicated by the inclusion of either other drugs of abuse or another immunosuppressive viral agent such as the murine acquired immunodeficiency syndrome (MAIDS) virus (86,122). The work that has been done with the use of tumor model systems is somewhat less complicated, and results generally show that the resistance to tumor spread is adversely affected by ETOH (123,124). In at least one study, attempts have been made to determine the effects of ETOH on the induction of tumors after administration of a carcinogen (125), and the effects of ETOH may be due to activation of carcinogens (126) as well as decreasing immune responses to tumor antigens. The role of ETOH may be as a cocarcinogen, such as that described for ETOH and tobacco smoke. This effect and the noted effect of ETOH on the immune system would be predicted to increase the incidence of tumors. It remains to be shown whether ETOH increases tumor incidence in naturally occurring tumor systems such as the mouse mammary tumor virus system or others.

Study findings that have been obtained with the use of microorganisms are clearer. ETOH has been shown to affect the ability of mononuclear phagocytes to control the growth of the facultative intracellular bacterium *Mycobacterium avium* (127). *In vivo* resistance to a related organism has also been shown to be affected by ETOH (128,129). Together these observations would support the suggestion that ETOH increases susceptibility to opportunistic species of *Mycobacterium*. It has been reported that alcoholics have an increased incidence of tuberculosis (1,4,5,14–

21). It is likely that similar mechanisms are operative in the increased incidence of this pathogenic *Mycobacterium*, although this remains to be determined.

In a recent study, the effects of ETOH on resistance of mice to *Listeria monocytogenes* were examined (130). Histologic examination findings showed that mice fed an ETOH-containing diet had more severe liver lesions that were characterized by more obvious necrosis of hepatocytes, when compared with findings for these parameters in mice fed a non-ETOH-containing diet. In contrast to the latter (i.e., control diet-fed) mice, the ETOH-fed animals were unable to control the growth of the bacteria in the liver. The responses of control animals were characterized by the production of granulomas by about 5 days after infection and essentially complete clearance of the bacteria. These results could be due to an inability of the mice that were fed ETOH to produce an effective immune response to the bacteria, an inability of the inflammatory cells (especially macrophages) to enter the liver and respond to cytokines to become activated for bacterial killing, or a combination of these factors. To address some of these concerns, histologic preparations were examined to determine the relative numbers of cells and cell types that responded to the liver infection in the above study. The early lesion (abscess) in both groups was similar, and perhaps the ETOH-fed animals had more granulocytes and resulting larger lesions. These data are in contrast to data that were the basis for the suggestion that ETOH inhibits chemotactic activity of granulocytes (3,131,132). This is clearly not the case in the murine model of ETOH consumption used in the recent study. The lesions in the liver of ETOH-treated mice contained large numbers of macrophages late in the infection, showing that the noted susceptibility to this organism is not due to an inability of appropriate cells to respond to the infection and produce an inflammatory response. It is interesting to note that mice immune to *L. monocytogenes* were similarly susceptible to challenge if fed an ETOH-containing diet, and these data led to the suggestion that ETOH may be inhibiting the function of immune cells. A recent study was designed to determine the effects of ETOH on the production of interferon (IFN), and the investigators showed that IFN-γ production was adversely affected (133). Production of tumor necrosis factor (TNF) is also affected by ETOH (35,134–136). Both of these cytokines are important in the immune response to *L. monocytogenes,* and the effect of ETOH on cytokine production may be important. It is also possible that the cells that respond to the infection are unresponsive to cytokines, as has been shown for IL-2 (102–104).

Recent study results have shown that ETOH-fed mice have a defect in their ability to respond to synthetic antigens as measured by delayed-type hypersensitivity tests (C. Waltenbaugh, *personal communication*). This effect of ETOH has also been described in human beings who abuse ETOH (79,93,101). Because delayed-type hypersensitivity depends on T cells for cytokine production and a resulting influx of macrophages into the lesion, these data would support the suggestion that lymphocyte function is affected by ETOH to suppress these important responses.

Other effects of ETOH *in vitro*, such as those on regulatory circuits, T and B cell development, and subpopulations, have not been studied well or not at all. In an interesting preliminary study it was shown that feeding ETOH to mice that normally are unresponsive to a synthetic polymeric antigen resulted in conversion of these mice to responders (C. Waltenbaugh, *personal communication*). These results raise the possibility that ETOH affects some aspect of immunoregulation, and this possibility requires further study.

Prenatal Ethanol Exposure

Some data exist that have led to the suggestion that exposure of the developing immune system to ETOH *in utero* leads to relatively long-lived alterations in the immune system (137,138). Work by Ewald and colleagues (40,139–142) has shown that prenatal exposure to ETOH induces relatively profound changes in the thymus, although with time after birth these changes disappear. Several groups have shown that prenatal exposure of rats to ETOH leads to impairments in cellular immune responses measured by *in vitro* lymphocyte responses to mitogenic stimulation (37,104,143,144). Interestingly, the effects of prenatal ETOH exposure in rat models occur only in male animals (144). It has also been suggested that the changes in lymphocyte function are transient and recover as animals age (143). It remains to be shown whether prenatal ETOH exposure alters other aspects of immunity, including antibody responses, tumor production, and resistance to infectious diseases.

Ethanol-Induced Neuroendocrine Changes

It is well known that ETOH causes numerous changes in neuroendocrine parameters (145–147), some of which could be at least partially responsible for some of the effects of ETOH on the immune system. The major systemic neuroendocrine effect of ETOH is activation of the hypothalamic–pituitary–adrenal axis and production of a stress-like response (145,147). Stress responses induced by a variety of physical and psychologic stimuli can be immunosuppressive (148–152), and several stress-related neuroendocrine mediators can modulate immunologic parameters (148,153).

Blood Glucocorticoid Concentration as a Primary Indicator of Stress Response

Glucocorticoid concentration in the blood is frequently used as an indicator of neuroendocrine stress responses in ETOH-treated rodents (145,147,154), and glucocorticoids are unquestionably immunosuppressive if present at sufficient concentrations for a sufficient period (152,155). It has been difficult, however, to establish conclusively cause-and-effect relationships between the induction of increased glucocorticoid levels by ETOH or other chemicals and immunosuppression (152,156).

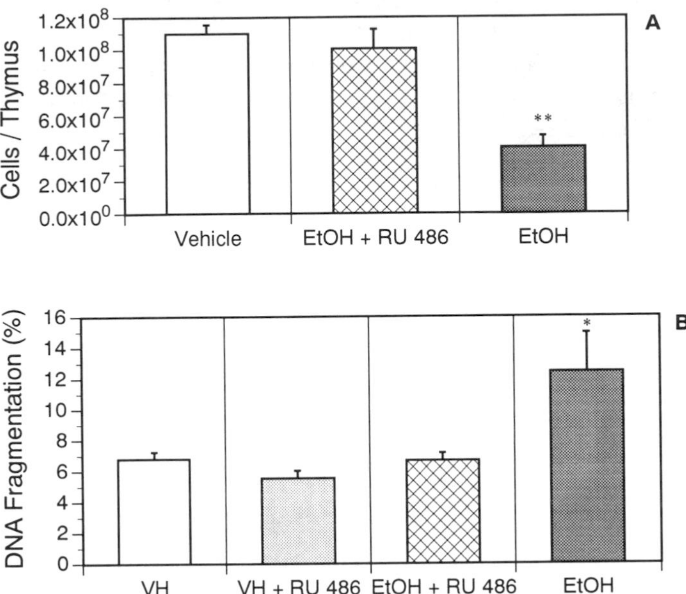

FIG. 2. Role of glucocorticoids in ETOH-induced thymic atrophy. The glucocorticoid antagonist RU 486 (100 mg/kg by gavage, 3 hr before ETOH) blocks thymic atrophy and deoxyribonucleic acid (DNA) fragmentation induced by ETOH. **A:** Mice were given a single dose of ETOH (6.7 g/kg by using a 32% ETOH solution), and thymus cellularity was measured 36 hr later. **B:** Mice were given a single dose of ETOH (6.0 g/kg by using a 32% ETOH solution), and DNA fragmentation was assessed. (RU 486 kindly provided by Roussel-Uclaf, Paris.)

Indirect, glucocorticoid-mediated mechanisms have been implicated in the suppression of several immunologic parameters by comparing the effects of ETOH in normal and adrenalectomized rats (77,88). Some of the immunologic parameters examined were substantially suppressed in ETOH-treated, adrenalectomized rats suggesting that glucocorticoids are not totally responsible for suppression of these parameters (88). For example, administration of ETOH by intermittent intubation for 4 days caused thymic hypoplasia in normal rats, and only slightly less hypoplasia was noted in adrenalectomized rats (88). In contrast, thymic hypoplasia caused by a single dose of ETOH in a mouse model for binge drinking can be suppressed completely by administration of the glucocorticoid antagonist RU 486 (Fig. 2A). The ETOH-induced DNA fragmentation [an indicator of glucocorticoid-induced programmed cell death (157)] is also completely blocked by RU 486 (Fig. 2B). Indirect immunologic effects of ETOH that are not mediated by glucocorticoids (88) may be caused by other ETOH-modulated neuroendocrine mediators [e.g., endogenous opioids or prolactin (145,154)], which can also affect the immune system (148).

Study Results and Applicability of Neuroendocrine Changes in Rodent Models to Human Beings

Moderate to high doses of ETOH increase serum cortisol concentrations in human beings (158,159). These increases seem to depend roughly on blood alcohol level (158). Although the magnitude and duration of increased glucocorticoid levels are important determinants of immunologic outcome (152), it is difficult to compare data obtained from human beings and rodents in this regard. The major adrenal steroids are different in these two species (cortisol in human beings; corticosterone in rodents). In addition, rodents are generally referred to as glucocorticoid sensitive, and human beings are referred to as glucocorticoid resistant on the basis of the differing sensitivities of human and rodent thymocytes to the cytotoxic effects of glucocorticoids (160). The sensitivity of lymphocytes to other critical effects of glucocorticoids such as the suppression of IL-2 production and responsiveness, however, is essentially the same for human beings, mice, and rats (161). In addition, it is clear that glucocorticoids suppress a variety of immune responses (not just inflammatory responses) in human beings (155). Thus it is likely that the elevated glucocorticoid levels that occur in human beings after consumption of ETOH functionally affect the immune system, although the extensive lymphocyte depletion noted in rodents would not be expected.

SUMMARY

Human consumption of ETOH, even in the absence of liver disease, is associated with adverse effects on the immune system. Administration of ETOH to experimental animals by a variety of methods convincingly causes changes in many aspects of the immune system, including nonspecific host mechanisms and the ability of an animal to generate specific immune responses. Interestingly, *in utero* exposure to ETOH in animals induces similar changes, but most obviously in males. Information regarding the mechanisms of these changes is sparse. Recent efforts by many groups, however, should add insight in this area.

ACKNOWLEDGMENTS

Thomas R. Jerrells is partially supported by grants AA07731 and AA00129. Stephen B. Pruett is partially supported by grants ES05371-03 and CR819682-01-1. The editorial assistance of Janice Jerrells is appreciated.

REFERENCES

1. Adams HG, Jordan C. Infections in the alcoholic. *Med Clin North Am* 1984;68:179–200.
2. Smith FE, Palmer DL. Alcoholism, infection and altered host defenses: a review of clinical and experimental observations. *J Chronic Dis* 1976;29:35–49.
3. MacGregor RR. Alcohol and immune defense. *JAMA* 1986;256:1474–1479.

4. Eckardt MJ, Harford TC, Kaelber CT, et al. Health hazards associated with alcohol consumption. *JAMA* 1981;246:648–666.
5. Louria DB. Susceptibility to infection during experimental alcohol intoxication. *Trans Assoc Am Physicians* 1963;76:102–110.
6. Eichner ER. The hematologic disorders of alcoholism. *Am J Med* 1973;54:621–630.
7. Johnson WD Jr. Impaired defense mechanisms associated with acute alcoholism. *Ann NY Acad Sci* 1975;252:343–347.
8. Caiazza SS, Ovary Z. Effects of ethanol intake on the immune system of guinea pigs. *J Stud Alcohol* 1976;37:959–964.
9. Di Luzio NR, Williams DL. Enhancement of host susceptibility to *Staphylococcus aureus* infection by chronic ethanol ingestion—modification by glucan immunostimulation. *Alcohol Clin Exp Res* 1980;4:254–260.
10. Capps JA, Coleman GH. Influence of alcohol on prognosis of pneumonia in Cook County Hospital. *JAMA* 1923;80:750–752.
11. Schmidt W, De Lint J. Causes of death of alcoholics. *Q J Stud Alcohol* 1972;23:171–185.
12. Nolan JP. Alcohol as a factor in the illness of university service patients. *Am J Med Sci* 1965; 249:135–142.
13. Kolb D, Gunderson EK. Alcohol-related morbidity among older career navy men. *Drug Alcohol Depend* 1982;9:181–189.
14. Brown KE, Campbell AH. Tobacco, alcohol and tuberculosis. *Br J Dis Chest* 1961;55:150–158.
15. Holmdahl S-G. Four population groups with relatively high tuberculosis incidence in Göteborg 1957–1964. *Scand J Respir Dis* 1967;48:308–320.
16. Hudolin V. Tuberculosis and alcoholism. *Ann NY Acad Sci* 1975;252:353–364.
17. Jones HW Jr, Roberts J, Brantner J. Incidence of tuberculosis among homeless men. *JAMA* 1954; 155:1222–1223.
18. Lewis JG, Chamberlain DA. Alcohol consumption and smoking habits in male patients with pulmonary tuberculosis. *Br J Prev Soc Med* 1963;17:149–152.
19. Olin JS, Grzybowski S. Tuberculosis and alcoholism. *Can Med Assoc J* 1966;94:999–1001.
20. Cheung OT. Some difficulties in the treatment of tuberculous alcoholics. *Can J Public Health* 1965;54:281–284.
21. Friedman LN, Sullivan GM, Bevilaqua RP, Loscos R. Tuberculosis screening in alcoholics and drug addicts. *Am Rev Respir Dis* 1987;136:1188–1192.
22. Conn HO, Fessel JM. Spontaneous bacterial peritonitis in cirrhosis: variations on a theme. *Medicine (Baltimore)* 1971;50:161–197.
23. Conn HO. Spontaneous peritonitis and bacteremia in Laënnec's cirrhosis caused by enteric organisms. A relatively common but rarely recognized syndrome. *Ann Intern Med* 1964;60:568–580.
24. Correia JP, Conn HO. Spontaneous bacterial peritonitis in cirrhosis: endemic or epidemic? *Med Clin North Am* 1975;59:963–981.
25. Beeson PB, Brannon ES, Warren JV. Observations on the sites of removal of bacteria from the blood in patients with bacterial endocarditis. *J Exp Med* 1945;81:9–23.
26. Whipple RL Jr, Harris JF. *B. coli* septicemia in Laënnec's cirrhosis of the liver. *Ann Intern Med* 1950;33:462–466.
27. Villa E, Baldini G, Di Stabile S, et al. Alcohol and hepatitis B virus infection. *Acta Med Scand Suppl* 1985;703:97–101.
28. Villa E, Baldini GM, Pasquinelli C, et al. Risk factors for hepatocellular carcinoma in Italy. Male sex, hepatitis B virus, non-A non-B infection, and alcohol. *Cancer* 1988;62:611–615.
29. Villa E, Rubbiani L, Barchi T, et al. Susceptibility of chronic symptomless HBsAg carriers to ethanol-induced hepatic damage. *Lancet* 1982;2:1243–1244.
30. Harnisch JP, Tronca E, Nolan CM, Turck M, Holmes KK. Diphtheria among alcoholic urban adults. A decade of experience in Seattle. *Ann Intern Med* 1989;111:71–82.
31. Sternbach GL. Infections in alcoholic patients. *Emerg Med Clin North Am* 1990;8:793–803.
32. Cicero TJ. Alcohol self-administration, tolerance, and withdrawal in humans and animals: theoretical and methodological issues. In: Rigter H, Crabbe JC, eds. *Alcohol tolerance and dependence*. Amsterdam: Elsevier–North-Holland Biomedical Press; 1980;1–52.
33. Jerrells TR, Marietta CA, Eckardt MJ, Majchrowicz E, Weight FF. Effects of ethanol administration on parameters of immunocompetency in rats. *J Leukoc Biol* 1986;39:499–510.
34. Jerrells TR, Smith W, Eckardt MJ. Murine model of ethanol-induced immunosuppression. *Alcohol Clin Exp Res* 1990;14:546–550.

35. Nelson S, Bagby GJ, Bainton BG, Summer WR. The effects of acute and chronic alcoholism on tumor necrosis factor and the inflammatory response. *J Infect Dis* 1989;160:422–429.
36. Pavia CS, Bittker S, Cooper D. Immune response to Lyme spirochete *Borrelia burgdorferi* affected by ethanol consumption. *Immunopharmacology* 1991;22:165–173.
37. Redei E, Clark WR, McGivern RF. Ethanol induced alteration of immune function may involve hormones of the hypothalamic–pituitary–adrenal axis. *Prog Clin Biol Res* 1990;325:313–320.
38. Watson RR, Prabhala RH, Abril E, Smith TL. Changes in lymphocyte subsets and macrophage functions from high, short-term dietary ethanol in C57BL/6 mice. *Life Sci* 1988;43:865–870.
39. Bagasra O, Howeedy A, Kajdacsy-Balla A. Macrophage function in chronic experimental alcoholism. I. Modulation of surface receptors and phagocytosis. *Immunology* 1988;65:405–409.
40. Ewald SJ, Walden SM. Flow cytometric and histological analysis of mouse thymus in fetal alcohol syndrome. *J Leukoc Biol* 1988;44:434–440.
41. Watson RR, Odeleye OE, Darban HR, Lopez MC. Modification of lymphoid subsets by chronic ethanol consumption in C57BL/6 mice infected with LP-BM5 murine leukemia virus. *Alcohol Alcohol* 1992;27:417–424.
42. Spinozzi F, Bertotto A, Rondoni F, Gerli R, Scalise F, Grignani F. T-lymphocyte activation pathways in alcoholic liver disease. *Immunology* 1991;73:140–146.
43. Lieber CS, DeCarli LM. Review. Liquid diet technique of ethanol administration: 1989 update. *Alcohol Alcohol* 1989;24:197–211.
44. Gershwin ME, Beach RS, Hurley LS. *Nutrition and immunity*. New York: Academic Press; 1985.
45. Elgebaly SA, Kozol RA, Kreutzer DL. Alcohol and immune system: role of gastric tissue. *Prog Clin Biol Res* 1990;325:75–78.
46. Marietta CA, Jerrells TR, Meagher RC, Karanian JW, Weight FF, Eckardt MJ. Effects of long-term ethanol inhalation on the immune and hematopoietic systems of the rat. *Alcohol Clin Exp Res* 1988;12:211–214.
47. Lieber CS, DeCarli LM. The feeding of ethanol in liquid diets. *Alcohol Clin Exp Res* 1986;10:550–553.
48. Weindruch R, Walford RL. Dietary restriction in mice beginning at 1 year of age: effect on life-span and spontaneous cancer incidence. *Science* 1982;215:1415–1418.
49. Yu BP, Masoro EJ, Murata I, Bertrand HA, Lynd FT. Life span study of SPF Fischer 344 male rats fed *ad libitum* or restricted diets: longevity, growth, lean body mass, and disease. *J Gerontol* 1982;37:130–141.
50. Blank SE, Duncan DA, Meadows GG. Suppression of natural killer cell activity by ethanol consumption and food restriction. *Alcohol Clin Exp Res* 1991;15:16–22.
51. Weindruch R, Devens BH, Raff HV, Walford RL. Influence of dietary restriction and aging on natural killer cell activity in mice. *J Immunol* 1983;130:993–996.
52. Majchrowicz E. Induction of physical dependence upon ethanol and the associated behavioral changes in rats. *Psychopharmacologia* 1975;43:245–254.
53. Mello NK, Mendelson JH. Experimentally induced intoxication in alcoholics: a comparison between programmed and spontaneous drinking. *J Pharmacol Exp Ther* 1970;173:101–116.
54. Bagasra O, Howeedy A, Dorio R, Kajdacsy-Balla A. Functional analysis of T-cell subsets in chronic experimental alcoholism. *Immunology* 1987;61:63–69.
55. Shahbazian LM, Darban HR, Darban JR, Stazzone AM, Watson RR. Influence of the level of dietary ethanol in mice with murine AIDS on resistance to *Streptococcus pneumoniae*. *Alcohol Alcohol* 1992;27:345–352.
56. Grossman CJ, Roselle GA, Mendenhall CL. Sex steroid regulation of autoimmunity. *J Steroid Biochem Mol Biol* 1991;40:649–659.
57. McClearn GE, Rodgers DA. Differences in alcohol preference among inbred strains of mice. *Q J Stud Alcohol* 1959;20:691–695.
58. Belknap JK. Genetic factors in the effects of alcohol: neurosensitivity, functional tolerance and physical dependence. In: Rigter H, Crabbe JC, eds. *Alcohol tolerance and dependence*. Amsterdam: Elsevier–North-Holland Biomedical Press; 1980:157–180.
59. Room R. Measuring alcohol consumption in the United States. In: Kozlowski LT, Annis HM, Cappell HD et al., eds. *Advances in alcohol and drug problems*, vol 10. New York: Plenum Press; 1990;39–80.
60. Pickrell KL. The effect of alcoholic intoxication and ether anesthesia on resistance to pneumococcal infection. *Bull Johns Hopkins Hosp* 1938;63:238–260.
61. Brayton RG, Stokes PE, Schwartz MS, Louria DB. Effect of alcohol and various diseases on

leukocyte mobilization, phagocytosis and intracellular bacterial killing. *N Engl J Med* 1970; 282:123–128.

62. Klepser RG, Nungester WG. The effect of alcohol upon the chemotactic response of leukocytes. *J Infect Dis* 1939;65:196–205.
63. Kawakami M, Meyer AA, Johnson MC, Rezvani AH. Immunologic consequences of acute ethanol ingestion in rats. *J Surg Res* 1989;47:412–417.
64. Spagnuolo PJ, MacGregor RR. Acute ethanol effect on chemotaxis and other components of host defense. *J Lab Clin Med* 1975;86:24–31.
65. Alkana RL, Finn DA, Bejanian M, Crabbe JC. Genetically determined differences in ethanol sensitivity influenced by body temperature during intoxication. *Life Sci* 1988;43:1973–1982.
66. Deimling MJ, Schnell RC. Circadian rhythms in the biological response and disposition of ethanol in the mouse. *J Pharmacol Exp Ther* 1980;213:1–8.
67. Ellis FW. Effect of ethanol on plasma corticosterone levels. *J Pharmacol Exp Ther* 1966;153:121–127.
68. Finn DA, Bejanian M, Jones BL, Syapin PJ, Alkana RL. Temperature affects ethanol lethality in C57BL/6, 129, LS, and SS mice. *Pharmacol Biochem Behav* 1989;34:375–380.
69. Pohorecky LA. Interaction of ethanol and stress: research with experimental animals—an update. *Alcohol Alcohol* 1990;25:263–276.
70. Balfour DJK, Khullar AK, Longden A. Effects of nicotine on plasma corticosterone and brain amines in stressed and unstressed rats. *Pharmacol Biochem Behav* 1975;3:179–184.
71. Falk JL, Tang M. Schedule induction of drug intake: differential responsiveness to agents with abuse potential. *J Pharmacol Exp Ther* 1989;249:143–148.
72. Ogata H, Ogato F, Mendelson JH, Mello NK. A comparison of techniques to induce alcohol dependence and tolerance in the mouse. *J Pharmacol Exp Ther* 1972;180:216–230.
73. Heybach JP, Vernikos-Danellis J. Inhibition of the pituitary–adrenal response to stress during deprivation-induced feeding. *Endocrinology* 1979;104:967–973.
74. Rall TW. Hypnotics and sedatives: ethanol. In: Gilman AG, Rall TW, Nies AS, Taylor P, eds. *Goodman and Gilman's the pharmacological basis of therapeutics*. New York: Pergamon Press; 1990:370–378.
75. Gilhus NE, Matre R. In vitro effect of ethanol on subpopulations of human blood mononuclear cells. *Int Arch Allergy Appl Immunol* 1982;68:382–386.
76. Slone FL, Smith WI Jr, Van Thiel DH. The effects of alcohol and partial portal ligation on the immune system of the rat. *Gastroenterology* 1977;72:1133(abst).
77. Jerrells TR, Peritt D, Marietta C, Eckardt MJ. Mechanisms of suppression of cellular immunity induced by ethanol. *Alcohol Clin Exp Res* 1989;13:490–493.
78. Saad AJ, Jerrells TR. Flow cytometric and immunohistochemical evaluation of ethanol-induced changes in splenic and thymic lymphoid cell populations. *Alcohol Clin Exp Res* 1991;15:796–803.
79. Smith WI Jr, Van Thiel DH, Whiteside T, et al. Altered immunity in male patients with alcoholic liver disease: evidence for defective immune regulation. *Alcohol Clin Exp Res* 1980;4:199–206.
80. Stacey NH. Inhibition of antibody-dependent cell-mediated cytotoxicity by ethanol. *Immunopharmacology* 1984;8:155–161.
81. Young GP, Van der Weyden MB, Rose IS, Dudley FJ. Lymphopenia and lymphocyte transformation in alcoholics. *Experientia* 1979;35:268–269.
82. MacGregor RR, Gluckman SJ, Senior JR. Granulocyte function and levels of immunoglobulins and complement in patients admitted for withdrawal from alcohol. *J Infect Dis* 1978;138:747–755.
83. Tennenbaum JI, Ruppert RD, St Pierre RL, Greenberger NJ. The effect of chronic alcohol administration on the immune responsiveness of rats. *J Allergy* 1969;44:272–281.
84. Jacob J, Kassir R, Kelsoe G. In situ studies of the primary immune response to (4-hydroxy-3-nitrophenyl)acetyl. I. The architecture and dynamics of responding cell populations. *J Exp Med* 1991;173:1165–1175.
85. Meadows GG, Wallendal M, Kosugi A, Wunderlich J, Singer DS. Ethanol induces marked changes in lymphocyte populations and natural killer cell activity in mice. *Alcohol Clin Exp Res* 1992;16:474–479.
86. Watson RR, Prabhala RH, Darban HR, Yahya MD, Smith TL. Changes in lymphocyte and macrophage subsets due to morphine and ethanol treatment during a retrovirus infection causing murine AIDS. *Life Sci* 1988;43:v–xi.
87. Bernstein IM, Webster KH, Williams RC Jr, Strickland RG. Reduction in circulating T lymphocytes in alcoholic liver disease. *Lancet* 1974;2:488–490.

88. Jerrells TR, Marietta CA, Weight FF, Eckardt MJ. Effect of adrenalectomy on ethanol-associated immunosuppression. *Int J Immunopharmacol* 1990;12:435–442.
89. Tabakoff B, Jafee RC, Ritzmann RF. Corticosterone concentrations in mice during ethanol drinking and withdrawal. *J Pharm Pharmacol* 1978;30:371–374.
90. Winoto A. Regulation of the early stages of T-cell development. *Curr Opin Immunol* 1991;3:199–203.
91. Scollay R. T-cell subset relationships in thymocyte development. *Curr Opin Immunol* 1991;3:204–209.
92. Roselle GA, Mendenhall CL. Alteration of in vitro human lymphocyte function by ethanol, acetaldehyde, and acetate. *J Clin Lab Immunol* 1982;9:33–37.
93. Gluckman SJ, Dvorak VC, MacGregor RR. Host defenses during prolonged alcohol consumption in a controlled environment. *Arch Intern Med* 1977;137:1539–1543.
94. Roselle GA, Mendenhall CL, Muhleman AF, Chedid A. The ferret: a new model of oral ethanol injury involving the liver, bone marrow, and peripheral blood lymphocytes. *Alcohol Clin Exp Res* 1986;10:279–284.
95. Roselle GA, Mendenhall CL, Grossman CJ. Age dependent alterations of host immune response in the ethanol-fed rat. *J Clin Lab Immunol* 1989;29:99–103.
96. Mutchnick MG, Lee HH. Impaired lymphocyte proliferative response to mitogen in alcoholic patients. Absence of a relation to liver disease activity. *Alcohol Clin Exp Res* 1988;12:155–158.
97. Ericsson CD, Kohl S, Pickering LK, Davis J, Glass GS, Faillace LA. Mechanisms of host defense in well nourished patients with chronic alcoholism. *Alcohol Clin Exp Res* 1980;4:261–265.
98. Jancar S, Braquet P, Sirois P. Release of eicosanoids in rat peritoneal cavity stimulated with platelet-activating factor (PAF). Effect of the PAF-antagonist BN-52021. *Prostaglandins Leukot Essent Fatty Acids* 1989;37:23–24.
99. Aldo-Benson M, Kluve-Beckerman B, Hardwick J, Lockwood M. Ethanol inhibits production of messenger ribonucleic acid for kappa-chain in stimulated B lymphocytes. *J Lab Clin Med* 1992; 119:32–37.
100. Aldo-Benson M. Mechanisms of alcohol-induced suppression of B-cell response. *Alcohol Clin Exp Res* 1989;13:469–475.
101. Berenyi M, Straus B, Cruz D. In vitro and in vivo studies of cellular immunity in alcoholic cirrhosis. *Dig Dis* 1974;13:199–205.
102. Jerrells TR, Perritt D, Eckardt MJ, Marietta C. Alterations in interleukin-2 utilization by T-cells from rats treated with an ethanol-containing diet. *Alcohol Clin Exp Res* 1990;14:245–249.
103. Kaplan DR. A novel mechanism of immunosuppression mediated by ethanol. *Cell Immunol* 1986; 102:1–9.
104. Norman DC, Chang MP, Castle SC, Van Zuylen JE, Taylor AN. Diminished proliferative response of Con A-blast cells to interleukin 2 in adult rats exposed to ethanol in utero. *Alcohol Clin Exp Res* 1989;13:69–72.
105. Domiati-Saad R, Jerrells TR. The influence of age on blood alcohol levels and ethanol-associated immunosuppression. *Alcohol Clin Exp Res* 1993;17:382–388.
106. Chang MP, Norman DC. Immunotoxicity of alcohol in young and old mice. II. Impaired T cell proliferation and T cell-dependent antibody responses of young and old mice fed ethanol-containing liquid diet. *Mech Ageing Dev* 1991;57:175–186.
107. Chang MP, Norman DC, Makinodan T. Immunotoxicity of alcohol in young and old mice. I. In vitro suppressive effects of ethanol on the activities of T and B immune cells of aging mice. *Alcohol Clin Exp Res* 1990;14:210–215.
108. Abel EL, York JL. Age-related differences in response to ethanol in the rat. *Physiol Psychol* 1979;7:391–395.
109. Rice C, Hudig D, Lad P, Mendelsohn J. Ethanol activation of human natural cytotoxicity. *Immunopharmacology* 1983;6:303–316.
110. Saxena QB, Mezey E, Adler WH. Regulation of natural killer activity in vivo. II. The effect of alcohol consumption on human peripheral blood natural killer activity. *Int J Cancer* 1980;26:413–417.
111. Abdallah RM, Starkey JR, Meadows GG. Alcohol and related dietary effects on mouse natural killer-cell activity. *Immunology* 1983;50:131–137.
112. Abdallah RM, Starkey JR, Meadows GG. Toxicity of chronic high alcohol intake on mouse natural killer cell activity. *Res Commun Chem Pathol Pharmacol* 1988;59:245–258.
113. Meadows GG, Blank SE, Duncan DA. Modulation of natural killer cell activity by alcohol consumption and nutritional status. *Prog Clin Biol Res* 1990;325:181–190.

114. Meadows GG, Blank SE, Duncan DD. Influence of ethanol consumption on natural killer cell activity in mice. *Alcohol Clin Exp Res* 1989;13:476–479.
115. Markovic SN, Murasko DM. Anesthesia inhibits poly I:C induced stimulation of natural killer cell cytotoxicity in mice. *Clin Immunol Immunopathol* 1990;56:202–209.
116. Walia AS, Lamon EW. Ethanol inhibition of cell-mediated lysis of antibody-sensitized target cells at a calcium-dependent step. *Proc'Soc'Exp'Biol'MedFS 1989;192:177–181.*
117. Dorio RJ, Forman HJ. Ethanol inhibition of signal transduction in superoxide production by rat alveolar macrophages. A proposed mechanism for ethanol related pneumonia. *Ann Clin Lab Sci* 1988;18:190–194.
118. Dorio RJ, Hoek JB, Ruhin E, Forman HJ. Ethanol modulation of rat alveolar macrophage superoxide production. *Biochem Pharmacol* 1988;37:3528–3531.
119. Chomet B, Gach BM. Lobar pneumonia and alcoholism: an analysis of thirty-seven cases. *Am J Med Sci* 1967;253:300–304.
120. Smith GW, Walker DH. Disseminated infection with *Aspergillus flavus* in an alcoholic patient. *South Med J* 1982;75:1148–1150.
121. Hakulinen T, Lehtimaki L, Lehtonen M, Teppo L. Cancer morbidity among two male cohorts with increased alcohol consumption in Finland. *J Natl Cancer Inst* 1974;52:1711–1714.
122. Watson RR, Nguyen TH. Suppression by morphine and ethanol of tumor cell cytotoxic activity released by macrophages from retrovirally infected mice upon in vitro stimulation by beta carotene. *Prog Clin Biol Res* 1990;325:79–91.
123. Batkin S, Tabrab FL. Ethanol vapour modulation of Lewis lung carcinoma, a murine pulmonary tumour. *J Cancer Res Clin Oncol* 1990;116:187–189.
124. Griciute LA, Monceviciute-Eringiene EV, Characiejus DA, Domkiene V, Barauskaite SV. Influence of ethanol on some host reactions in the early stages of N-nitrosamine carcinogenesis. *IARC Sci Publ* 1983;51:197–203.
125. Barratt G, Tenu JP, Yapo A, Petit JF. Preparation and characterisation of liposomes containing mannosylated phospholipids capable of targeting drugs to macrophages. *Biochim Biophys Acta* 1986;862:153–164.
126. Farinati F, Zhou Z, Bellah J, Lieber CS, Garro AJ. Effect of chronic ethanol consumption on activation of nitrosopyrrolidine to a mutagen by rat upper alimentary tract, lung, and hepatic tissue. *Drug Metab Dispos* 1985;13:210–214.
127. Bermudez LE, Young LS. Ethanol and survival of *Mycobacterium avium* complex within macrophages. *Prog Clin Biol Res* 1990;325:383–391.
128. Bermudez LE, Young LS. Ethanol augments intracellular survival of *Mycobacterium avium* complex and impairs macrophage responses to cytokines. *J Infect Dis* 1991;163:1286–1292.
129. Mendenhall CL, Grossman CJ, Roselle GA, et al. Host response to mycobacterial infection in the alcoholic rat. *Gastroenterology* 1990;99:1723–1726.
130. Saad AJ, Domiati-Saad R, Jerrells TR. Ethanol ingestion increases susceptibility of mice to *Listeria monocytogenes. Alcohol Clin Exp Res* 1993;17:75–85.
131. Gluckman SJ, MacGregor RR. Effect of acute alcohol intoxication on granulocyte mobilization and kinetics. *Blood* 1978;52:551–559.
132. MacGregor RR, Spagnuolo PJ, Lentnek AL. Inhibition of granulocyte adherence by ethanol, prednisone, and aspirin, measured with an assay system. *N Engl J Med* 1974;291:642–646.
133. Chadha KC, Stadler I, Albini B, Nakeeb SM, Thacore HR. Effect of alcohol on spleen cells and their functions in C57BL/6 mice. *Alcohol* 1991;8:481–485.
134. Nelson S, Bagby G, Andresen J, Nakamura C, Shellito J, Summer W. The effects of ethanol, tumor necrosis factor, and granulocyte colony-stimulating factor on lung antibacterial defenses. *Adv Exp Med Biol* 1991;288:245–253.
135. Nelson S, Bagby G, Summer WR. Alcohol suppresses lipopolysaccharide-induced tumor necrosis factor activity in serum and lung. *Life Sci* 1989;44:673–676.
136. Nelson S, Bagby GJ, Summer WR. Alcohol-induced suppression of tumor necrosis factor—a potential risk factor for secondary infection in the acquired immunodeficiency syndrome. *Prog Clin Biol Res* 1990;325:211–220.
137. Monjan AA, Mandell W. Fetal alcohol and immunity: depression of mitogen-induced lymphocyte blastogenesis. *Neurobehav Toxicol* 1984;2:213–215.
138. Johnson S, Knight R, Marmier DJ, Steele RW. Immune deficiency in fetal alcohol syndrome. *Pediatr Res* 1981;15:908–911.

139. Ewald SJ. T lymphocyte populations in fetal alcohol syndrome. *Alcohol Clin Exp Res* 1989; 13:485–489.
140. Ewald SJ, Frost WW. Effect of prenatal exposure to ethanol on development of the thymus. *Thymus* 1987;9:211–215.
141. Ewald SJ, Huang C. Lymphocyte populations and immune responses in mice prenatally exposed to ethanol. *Prog Clin Biol Res* 1990;325:191–200.
142. Ewald SJ, Huang C, Bray L. Effect of prenatal alcohol exposure on lymphocyte populations in mice. *Adv Exp Med Biol* 1991;288:237–244.
143. Norman DC, Chang MP, Wong CM, Branch BJ, Castle S, Taylor AN. Changes with age in the proliferative response of splenic T cells from rats exposed to ethanol in utero. *Alcohol Clin Exp Res* 1991;15:428–432.
144. Weinberg J, Jerrells TR. Suppression of immune responsiveness: sex differences in prenatal ethanol effects. *Alcohol Clin Exp Res* 1991;15:525–531.
145. Cicero TJ. Neuroendocrinological effects of alcohol. *Annu Rev Med* 1981;32:123–142.
146. Deitrich RA, Dunwiddie TV, Harris RA, Erwin VG. Mechanism of action of ethanol: initial central nervous system actions. *Pharmacol Rev* 1989;41:489–537.
147. Kalant H. Stress-related effects of ethanol in mammals. *Crit Rev Biotechnol* 1990;9:265–272.
148. Ader R, Felten D, Cohen N. Interactions between the brain and the immune system. *Annu Rev Pharmacol Toxicol* 1990;30:561–602.
149. Dantzer R, Kelley KW. Stress and immunity: an integrated view of relationships between the brain and the immune system. *Life Sci* 1989;44:1995–2008.
150. Dohms JE, Metz A. Stress—mechanisms of immunosuppression. *Vet Immunol Immunopathol* 1991;30:89–109.
151. Harbuz MS, Lightman SL. Stress and the hypothalamo–pituitary–adrenal axis: acute, chronic, and immunological activation. *J Endocrinol* 1992;134:327–339.
152. Pruett SB, Ensley DK, Crittenden P. The role of stress responses in chemical-induced immunosuppression: a review of quantitative associations and cause–effect relationships between chemical-induced stress responses and immunosuppression. *J Toxicol Environ Health* 1993;39:163–192.
153. Weigent DA, Blalock JE. Interactions between the neuroendocrine and immune systems: common hormones and receptors. *Immunol Rev* 1987;100:79–108.
154. Thiagarajan AB, Mefford IN, Eskay RL. Single-dose ethanol administration activates the hypothalamic–pituitary–adrenal axis: exploration of the mechanism of action. *Neuroendocrinology* 1989;50:427–432.
155. Cupps TR, Fauci AS. Corticosteroid-mediated immunoregulation in man. *Immunol Rev* 1982; 65:133–155.
156. Sanders VM, Fuchs BA, Pruett SB, Kerkvliet NI, Kaminski NE. Symposium overview. Symposium on indirect mechanisms of immune modulation. *Fundam Appl Toxicol* 1991;17:641–650.
157. Compton MM, Caron LA, Cidlowski JA. Glucocorticoid action on the immune system. *J Steroid Biochem* 1987;27:201–208.
158. Mendelson JH, Ogata M, Mello NK. Adrenal function and alcoholism. I. Serum cortisol. *Psychosom Med* 1971;33:145–157.
159. Merry J, Marks V. Plasma-hydrocortisone response to ethanol in chronic alcoholics. *Lancet* 1969; 1:921–923.
160. Claman HN, Moorhead JW, Benner WH. Corticosteroids and lymphoid cells *in vitro*. I. Hydrocortisone lysis of human, guinea pig, and mouse thymus cells. *J Lab Clin Med* 1971;78:499–507.
161. Gillis S, Crabtree GR, Smith KA. Glucocorticoid-induced inhibition of T cell growth factor production. I. The effect on mitogen-induced lymphocyte proliferation. *J Immunol* 1979;123:1624–1631.

Immunotoxicology and Immunopharmacology, Second Edition, edited by J. H. Dean, M. I. Luster, A. E. Munson, and I. Kimber.
Raven Press, Ltd., New York © 1994.

19

Mechanisms of Immune Modulation by Cannabinoids

Norbert E. Kaminski

Departments of Pharmacology and Toxicology, Michigan State University, East Lansing, Michigan 48824

The immunoinhibitory properties of cannabinoids, both natural and synthetic, have been widely established in a variety of animal models and experimental systems (reviewed in ref. 1). The focus of this chapter is to critically discuss these findings as well as those from nonimmunologic model systems, which provide insight into the mechanism by which cannabinoids modulate the immune system. It is important to emphasize that although there have been numerous studies conducted to evaluate the effects of delta-9-tetrahydrocannabinol (Δ^9-THC), the primary psychoactive component in marijuana, as well as other cannabinoids on immunocompetence, until recently very little has been known regarding the actual mechanism by which this class of compounds alters immune function. In fact, some of the most critical observations pertaining to the elucidation of a mechanism for biologic activity for cannabinoids have been forthcoming from central nervous system (CNS)-derived models, the results of which are also discussed briefly.

Interest in developing an understanding of the mechanism of action by cannabinoids can be attributed to a number of factors. One aspect pertains to ongoing attempts to develop cannabinoid-derived therapeutic agents. The greatest clinical potential to date for this class of agents has been as an antiemetic agent for patients undergoing cancer chemotherapy and for the treatment of glaucoma. Cannabinoids are very effective in decreasing the nausea produced by cancer chemotherapy and are capable of decreasing markedly the intraoccular pressure responsible for the onset of glaucoma. Recent evidence suggests also that cannabinoids may be effective in decreasing bronchoalveolar constriction associated with asthma. This is especially interesting in light of the fact that currently the etiology of asthma is believed to be at least in part autoimmune based. Unfortunately, due to CNS-associated side effects coupled with the societal stigma associated with cannabinoids, their therapeutic application has been extremely limited. The wide use of marijuana as a recreational drug and the potential short- and long-term health effects resulting from this activity have also been a driving force behind cannabinoid research. Although there is no evidence to suggest that marijuana use is life threatening, from an immunologic standpoint based on the immunoinhibitory effects observed in various animal models, one would predict that marijuana users may exhibit a greater susceptibility to common pathogens. An additional concern pertaining to drug abuse is the fact that many individuals, who abuse drugs, abuse more than one kind of drug. Immune inhibition by opiates as well as cocaine has also been widely established and presently it is unclear what effects on immunocompetence these various agents produce when abused in combination.

CANNABINOIDS AND THE IMMUNE SYSTEM

It is clear that cannabinoids can markedly alter immune function, both humoral and cell-mediated immunity. This has been established through the use of a variety of *in vivo* and *in vitro* immune function assays. However, what is less clear is whether cannabinoids exhibit selectivity with respect to the immunocompetent cell types they target and the actual mechanism by which these changes occur. What follows is a brief summary of the reported effects produced by cannabinoids on the immune system.

Humoral Immunity

Inhibition of humoral immune responses as measured by the immunoglobulin M (IgM) antibody-forming cell (AFC) response has been demonstrated by a number of laboratories. The majority of these studies have been performed using various inbred mouse strains. *In vivo*, inhibition of the AFC response has been observed at Δ^9-THC concentrations as low as 10 mg/kg, following 5 consecutive days of drug administration in ICR-SCH Swiss mice (2) and at doses as high as 300 mg/kg [median effective dose (ED_{50}) was 70 mg/kg], following a single exposure in BDF1 mice (3). Oral administration of Δ^9-THC at concentrations as low as 50 mg/kg for 7 consecutive days in the B6C3F1 mouse strain produced approximately a 40% inhibition of the sheep red blood cell (SRBC) IgM AFC response (4). In all three of these studies, Δ^9-THC was administered after antigen sensitization. In contrast, mice that received 25 mg/kg of Δ^9-THC, orally, for 8 consecutive days and sensitized with SRBCs on day 17 (10 days following the last Δ^9-THC treatment) exhibited no humoral immune suppression, suggesting that reversal of antibody response inhibition occurs quite rapidly once administration of Δ^9-THC is terminated (5). The profile of activity with respect to the actual doses required to induce inhibition of humoral immunity has been somewhat varied between reports and is most likely attributable to at least three factors: (a) route of Δ^9-THC administration, (b) differences in sensitivity to Δ^9-THC between mouse strains, and the most critical (c) temporal difference between drug administration and antigen sensitization. This third aspect is especially critical in light of recent findings from *in vivo* kinetics studies, which demonstrated that the greatest magnitude of suppression by Δ^9-THC, 25 mg/kg administered orally for 3 consecutive days, is achieved when the drug is administered at times surrounding antigen sensitization (4). What is important to emphasize is that without exception, all the findings described earlier were derived from studies using SRBCs as the sensitizing antigen, a T cell-dependent antigen. Therefore it is unclear whether humoral immunity in these studies was decreased due to direct inhibitory effects on B cell function or whether inhibition occurred at the level of altered accessory cell function [i.e., T helper (T_H) cell and/or macrophage]. Recent studies in fact suggest that B cell function is probably not sufficiently altered by Δ^9-THC to account for a decrease in the IgM AFC response. *In vivo* responses to the T cell-independent antigen dinitrophenyl (DNP)–Ficoll, which requires only macrophage accessory cell cooperativity, were not inhibited by doses of Δ^9-THC as high as 200 mg/kg (4). These findings suggest that antigen presentation as well as other accessory cell functions performed by macrophages during this response are not significantly altered by Δ^9-THC and that, at least with respect to humoral response, the T cell is the primary cellular target. This conclusion is further supported by *in vitro* Δ^9-THC direct addition studies in which various defined antigens requiring differential cellular cooperativity were utilized. Suppression of T cell-dependent humoral responses was exhibited in naive spleen cells treated with cannabinoids under *in vitro* conditions. The SRBC response was readily inhibited by Δ^9-THC (3.2 to 22 μM) in a dose-related manner, whereas responses to DNP–Ficoll or the polyclonal B cell activator lipopolysaccharide (LPS) were unaffected over this same Δ^9-THC concentration range (4). *In vitro* kinetics studies also indicated that suppression of the SRBC response was not due to a shift in the peak day of the response. Additionally, temporal addition studies clearly showed that Δ^9-THC must be added during the first 120 min following antigen sensitization in order to inhibit the SRBC response (6), suggesting that the mechanism of immune inhibition by cannabinoids is mediated through the inhibition of an early phase of T cell activation.

Cell-Mediated Immunity (CMI)

In light of the critical role CMI plays with respect to tumoricidal and antiviral activities, studies of immunosuppression by the Δ^9-THC have focused predominantly on T cell function. From these investigations it is clear that cannabinoids inhibit T cell blastogenesis. Both Δ^9-THC and its metabolite 11-OH-Δ^9-THC markedly inhibit mouse splenic and thymic T cell blastogenic responses (7). However, the magnitude of this inhibition is at least partially dependent on the specific T cell mitogen. Interestingly, blastogenic responses to phytohemagglutinin (PHA) are significantly more sensitive to inhibition by Δ^9-THC and 11-OH-Δ^9-THC than to concanavalin A (Con A). This differential sensitivity, which has been observed with different mitogens, has also been described following fluorescence-activated cell sorter (FACS) analysis. Following mitogenic stimulation in the presence of Δ^9-THC

(3 to 7 μg/ml) there was a selective decrease in the number of Ly 2+ cytotoxic T cells/suppressor T cells (T_c/T_s), but not L3T4+ (T_H) cells, as compared to mitogen-stimulated controls. Once again, greater sensitivity to inhibition by Δ^9-THC was observed following stimulation by PHA than with Con A (8). These findings suggest that certain T cell subpopulations in the mouse may exhibit a differential sensitivity to inhibition of proliferation by cannabinoids. It is also important to note that T cell blastogenic responses by cannabinoids is highly dependent on cell density with the greatest magnitude of inhibition occurring at low cell densities (4,7). The basis for this sensitivity on cell density is unknown but may in part be mediated through a partial inhibition of cytokine release by activated T cells, which would be most conspicuous at low rather than high cell densities. It is also unclear from these studies whether inhibition of blastogenic responses to T cell mitogens is due to a direct effect by cannabinoids on T cells or through the inhibition of required antigen-presenting accessory cells. However, recent findings utilizing immobilized anti-CD3 antibody, a T cell activation signal not requiring antigen-presenting cells, was also dose dependently inhibited by Δ^9-THC, suggesting that T cell inhibition is directly mediated by cannabinoids.

Similar results have been obtained with human peripheral blood lymphocytes (HPBLs) in primary culture when treated with cannabinoids. Both Δ^9-THC and 11-OH-Δ^9-THC inhibited HPBL blastogenesis to PHA and Con A but not to pokeweed mitogen (PWM) (stimulates B cells and T cells). Direct addition of interleukin-2 (IL-2) to cannabinoid-treated cells did not reverse this inhibition (9). However, washing HPBLs following a 3-hr treatment with Δ^9-THC was found to be sufficient to abrogate the inhibitory effects on either Con A or PHA blastogenesis (9). These results are interesting with respect to two points. First, the inability of IL-2 to reverse cannabinoid-induced inhibition of proliferation suggests that the induced alteration is not due to inhibition of IL-2 secretion and would further suggest that the cannabinoid-induced alteration occurs prior to IL-2 release. This is consistent with results by Schatz et al. (6), which point to the critical event occurring during the first 120 min following T cell activation. Second, the observation that the inhibitory effect produced by cannabinoid treatment can be "washed out" is somewhat paradoxical in light of the fact that cannabinoids are highly lipophilic. However, this observation may partially explain why in a number of studies HPBLs isolated from chronic marijuana or hashish smokers did not exhibit significant functional deficiencies (10–12). The lack of an effect in these individuals may very likely be attributable to the fact that isolation of HPBLs from whole blood requires numerous *in vitro* manipulations including density gradient centrifugation most often utilizing Ficoll–Hypaque followed by multiple washing steps similar to the conditions described by Specter et al. (9). We have similarly observed this phenomenon in which the effects of cannabinoids can readily be abrogated by simply washing the treated cells with fresh medium several times in mouse splenocytes (N. E. Kaminski, *unpublished data*).

Cannabinoids also inhibit secretion by and the responsiveness of T cells to cytokines. Mitogenic stimulation of spleen cells from untreated mice with either LPS, Con A, or PHA, in the presence of Δ^9-THC (5 to 10 μg/ml) markedly decreased the induction of interferons (IFNs) (13). Similarly, T cell responsiveness to IL-2 was significantly diminished by Δ^9-THC as well as the appearance of the lymphokine-activated killer (LAK) cell phenomenon in IL-2-treated spleen cell preparations (12). However, as discussed above, if the inhibitory event by cannabinoids is produced early during T cell activation, clearly all subsequent events downstream of the activation process will also be altered (e.g., cytokine secretion, IL-2 receptor expression, proliferation, differentiation).

Other CMI processes that appear to be inhibited by cannabinoids include cytolytic function by both T cells and natural killer (NK) cells. A decrease in cytolytic activity was reported against YAC-1 target cells following Δ^9-THC treatment, suggesting that Δ^9-THC also inhibits NK cell function (12). Interestingly, follow-up studies by Kawakami et al. (12) showed that the inhibition of NK cells by Δ^9-THC and 11-OH-Δ^9-THC was likely due to direct inhibition of NK cell cytolytic activity in the postbinding stage. This inhibition of cytotoxic activity was also highly reversible by extensive washing of the cells following cannabinoid pretreatment as well as partially reversible by overnight treatment with exogenous recombinant IL-2 (14). Interestingly, IL-2 treatment was most effective in reversing the cannabinoid-mediated effects when added simultaneously with Δ^9-THC to NK cell cultures and less effective if added at times following Δ^9-THC treatment. Although the ability of IL-2 to reverse cannabinoid-mediated inhibition in NK cells appears to be more effective than with T cells, nonetheless, once again the results exhibit a trend in which the later in a given immune response cells are exposed to Δ^9-THC, the less marked the inhibition. As with NK cell activity, cytolytic T lymphocyte (CTL) function was also inhibited markedly both *in vivo* and *in vitro* by Δ^9-THC and 11-OH-Δ^9-THC, which suggests an effect on the CTL response subsequent to target cell binding (15,16). It is important to emphasize that this inhibition of CTL activity was believed to be at least partially mediated through an inhibition of CTL effector maturation. Consistent with cannabinoid-mediated inhibition of CMI, Δ^9-THC markedly inhibited the mixed leukocyte reaction both in mouse spleen cells (6) and with HPBLs (N. E. Kaminski, *unpublished data*).

Cannabinoids also produce changes in macrophage morphology, certain functions, and motility; however, the impact of these changes on immunocompetence is not altogether clear. Alveolar macrophages isolated from rhesus monkeys subjected to chronic marijuana smoke exposure (1 year, 1 marijuana cigarette/day followed by a 7-month rest period) exhibited irregular cell surface morphology, increased vacuolization, and a spherical conformation upon adherence to plastic as compared to sham smoke controls (17). Recent studies also indicate that Δ^9-THC selectively inhibits macrophage extrinsic but not intrinsic antiviral activity. Macrophage uptake of herpesvirus (intrinsic activity) was unaffected by Δ^9-THC as measured in a number of macrophage cell lines including RAW264.7, J774A.1, and P388D1, whereas the ability of macrophages to elicit an IFN-independent, cell contact-dependent reduction of virus growth in infected cells (extrinsic activity) was markedly inhibited (18). Gel protein profiles from macrophages activated in the presence of Δ^9-THC exhibited altered protein expression (17). Presently, it is unclear whether cannabinoids also alter antigen processing and presentation by macrophages.

CANNABINOID RECEPTOR

Biologic activity for cannabinoids has historically been attributed to their lipophilic properties and presumably their ability to disrupt membrane processes through intercalation into the lipid bilayer of the cell membrane. However, studies primarily utilizing neuronal tissue preparations and CNS-derived cell lines during the past decade have provided a number of compelling lines of evidence that argue against a nonspecific mechanism of action such as mere membrane disruption. In fact, at least four lines of evidence strongly support the existence of cannabinoid receptors in the CNS: (a) the existence of specific tertiary structural requirements for cannabinoid activity as identified by structure–activity relationship (SAR) studies, (b) the stereoselectivity exhibited by cannabinoid compounds with respect to a broad variety of cannabimimetic effects, (c) the identification of specific cannabinoid binding sites first identified in CNS-associated tissues and more recently in non-CNS tissues as demonstrated by radioligand-binding analysis, and (d) the identification and nucleotide sequencing of the putative G-protein coupled cannabinoid receptor located in regions of the brain as well as non-CNS tissues.

Through SAR studies, primarily utilizing synthetically derived cannabinoids, important functional groups and structural features for biologic activity have been identified. From these studies, a model of three-point contact between the agonist and the putative cannabinoid receptor for mediating analgesia was formulated (19, 20). This model was based on the observation that three parts of the cannabinoid molecule were critical for activity: (a) the C ring hydroxyl, (b) the phenolic A ring hydroxyl, and (c) the A ring alkyl side chain (Fig. 1). This model was supported primarily by studies utilizing bicyclic synthetic cannabinoids lacking the tricyclic benzopyran nucleus but still possessing strong similarity to the naturally occurring cannabinoid structure. Interestingly, this class of agent, commonly referred to as nonclassic cannabinoids, exhibited even greater analgesic potency than that observed with Δ^9-THC (21). One of the most extensively characterized of this group of synthetic congeners is the bicyclic molecule, CP-55940 (Fig. 1). The significance of these findings is that they clearly demonstrate the strict tertiary requirements for cannabinoid activity, a property normally exhibited in receptor-mediated mechanisms.

Although the identification of critical functional groups for cannabinoid activity suggested a receptor-mediated mechanism, the observation that cannabinoids possessed stereoselective activity was critical evidence supporting the existence of cannabinoid receptors. In the case of cannabinoid enantiomers (i.e., structurally mirror

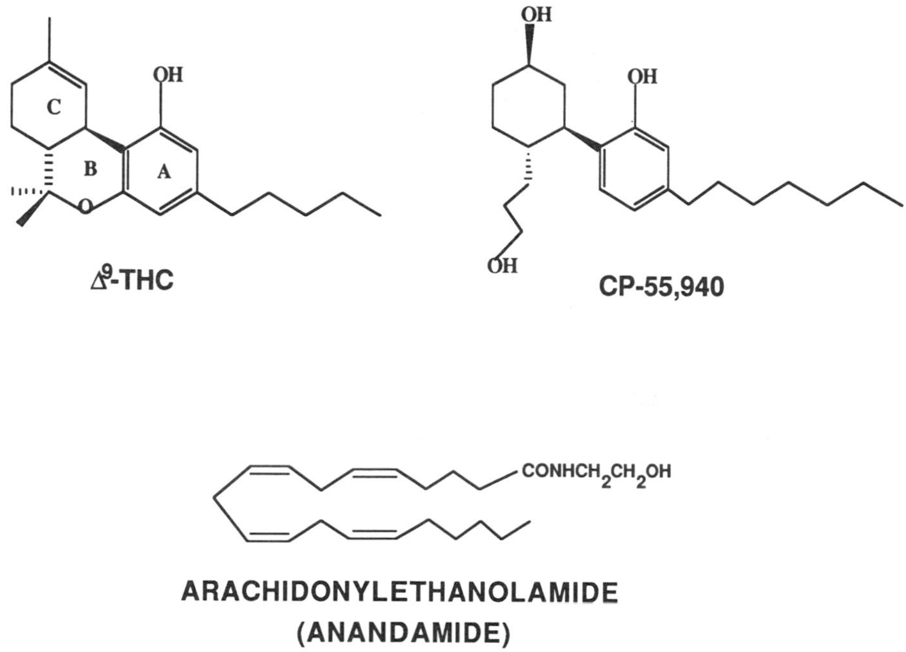

Δ^9-THC

CP-55,940

ARACHIDONYLETHANOLAMIDE (ANANDAMIDE)

FIG. 1. Chemical structures: Δ^9-tetrahydrocannabinol (Δ^9-THC) is the primary psychoactive constituent present in marijuana. Cis-3-[2-hydroxy-4-(1,1-dimethylheptylphenyl]-trans-4(3-hydroxypropyl)cyclohexanol (CP-55940) is a synthetic bicyclic cannabinoid developed by Pfizer Pharmaceutical, which exhibits potent cannabinoid activity and high affinity for the cannabinoid receptor. CP-55940 is one of several cannabinoids widely utilized for ligand binding analysis to the cannabinoid receptor. Anandamide (arachidonylethanolamide) is an arachidonic acid derivative isolated from porcine brain, which exhibits specific binding to the cannabinoid receptor. It has been speculated that anandamide may be an endogenous ligand for the cannabinoid receptor.

images), the (−) isomeric orientation generally exhibits markedly greater activity than those in the (+) orientation. This enantiospecificity has been demonstrated with a variety of cannabinoid compounds using different assay systems and various animal species (22–26). These findings are significant because (+) and (−) enantiomers are equally lipophilic and should not exhibit differences in potency if their activity is solely mediated through lipophilic properties. These stereoselective properties for cannabinoids were characterized further in comprehensive SAR studies by Thomas et al. (27) in which little correlation between the lipophilicity of cannabinoid compounds and their pharmacologic activity was found, thus providing additional evidence against a mechanism of action based solely on lipophilicity.

Critical to the formulation of a receptor-mediated mechanism for cannabinoids was the observation that Δ^8-THC and Δ^9-THC significantly inhibited adenylate cyclase activity in N18TG2 neuroblastoma cell membrane preparations (28). This inhibition was found to be rapid, noncompetitive, reversible, and greatest at micromolar concentrations of Mg^{2+} or Mn^{2+}. Additionally, basal and forskolin-activated adenylate cyclase activity (forskolin acts by directly stimulating the enzyme) was inhibited. This enzyme catalyzes the conversion of adenosine triphosphate (ATP) to cyclic adenosine monophosphate (cAMP), which in turn is involved in cell regulation through cAMP-dependent signal transduction pathways. Interestingly, pertussis toxin, which inactivates G_i through an adenosine 5′-diphosphate (ADP)-ribosylation modification, was found to abrogate the inhibitory effects of cannabimimetic agents as measured by forskolin-stimulated increases in intracellular cAMP levels in N18TG2 cells (29). These studies were the first to suggest that the cannabinoid receptor is associated with, and results in the activation of the G_i protein, which ultimately causes decreased intracellular cAMP via inhibition of adenylate cyclase. Also in agreement with these findings were SAR studies that indicated a good correlation between previously reported pharmacologic activity for cannabinoid compounds and their ability to decrease intracellular cAMP levels in N18TG2 cells (24). Thermodynamic data also suggested that inhibition of adenylate cyclase by Δ^9-THC is not related to membrane fluidization (30). In summary, the inhibition of adenylate cyclase by cannabinoids also strongly suggests the existence of cannabinoid receptors.

Another important and compelling line of direct evidence for the existence of cannabinoid receptors was the identification of cannabinoid binding sites in rat brain. Bidaut-Russell and co-workers (31) reported a high degree of specific binding by [^{3}H]CP-55940—a bicyclic synthetic cannabinoid now known to possess high affinity for the cannabinoid receptor—in rat cortex, cerebellum, hippocampus, and striatum using rat brain slice preparation. Additionally, the cannabinoid desacetyllevonanthradol was found to decrease forskolin-stimulated cAMP accumulation in the hippocampus, frontal cortex, and striatum, while, in the cerebellum, the response was biphasic, resulting in a decrease at low concentration and an increase at higher concentrations. In agreement with results obtained using N18TG2 cell preparations, pertussis toxin attenuated the modulation of cAMP accumulation by desacetyllevonanthradol. Recently, [^{3}H]CP-55940 was used to characterize the distribution of cannabinoid receptors in brain slices (32). Autoradiography of brain sections derived from several mammalian species, including human, revealed a unique distribution; binding is most dense in outflow nuclei of the basal ganglia and in the hippocampus and cerebellum. The densities associated with the forebrain and cerebellum implicate roles for cannabinoids in cognition and movement. Additionally, the potencies of a series of natural and synthetic cannabinoids as competitors of [^{3}H]CP-55940 binding closely correlated with their relative potencies in a number of biologic systems (32).

In light of these various avenues of direct and indirect evidence, the existence of cannabinoid receptors was confirmed by the isolation of a cDNA from rat brain cortex that encodes a G-protein-coupled receptor, which (a) was more responsive to psychoactive cannabinoids than to nonpsychoactive cannabinoids, (b) demonstrated enantiomer selectivity, (c) modulated adenylate cyclase, (d) was pertussis toxin sensitive, (e) exhibited a high degree of specific binding by [^{3}H]CP-55940, and (f) was present in brain and neuronal cell lines. Based on the evidence discussed above, the existence of cannabinoid receptors is presently widely accepted.

CANNABINOID RECEPTOR AND THE IMMUNE SYSTEM

With the recent identification of cannabinoid receptors in the CNS, attention has now focused to other tissues in the periphery. The immune system is of significant interest based on the fact that cannabinoids exhibit strong immunomodulatory activity. As with the CNS, multiple lines of indirect as well as direct evidence now exist to support the existence of functional cannabinoid receptors associated with the immune system. Interestingly, as in neuronal tissues, immunoinhibitory concentrations of Δ^9-THC (6) and CP-55940 (33) also inhibit markedly the adenylate cyclase activity (40% to 60%) as measured by forskolin-stimulated cAMP accumulation in mouse spleen cells. Additionally, cannabinoids exhibit stereoselective immune inhibition with the (−) enantiomers possessing significantly greater activity than the (+) enantiomers (26). Similarly, the cannabinoid receptor radioligand, [^{3}H]CP-55940, demonstrates saturation and a high degree of specific binding (45% to 65%) to mouse spleen cells (26). Scatchard analysis reveals a K_D of approximately 1 nM and a B_{max} of approximately 1000 receptors/cell. Presently, it is unclear whether this receptor is expressed selectively on a subpopulation of splenocytes at a higher density than 1000/cell, or whether there is low-density expression on all spleen cells. More recently, radioligand analysis of human leukocytes using [^{3}H]CP-55940 indicates a K_D of 0.1 nM and a B_{max} of approximately 525 fmol/mg protein (34). Competitive binding between [^{3}H]CP-55940 and a number of cannabinoids, including its less active stereoisomer, CP-56667, indicates a positive correlation between binding affinity to mouse splenocytes and immunosuppressive potency (N. E. Kaminski *unpublished data*). However, one intriguing aspect revealed by the binding analyses, in lymphoid and a variety of nonlymphoid tissues, is that despite the relatively high affinity of binding of various cannabinoids for the cannabinoid receptor, comparatively high concentrations of these same agents are required to produce functional effects in biologic systems. This perplexing relationship has been demonstrated in N18TG2 neuroblastoma cells (28,35), rat brain preparations (32,36), Sertoli cells (37), and mouse spleen cells (6). One possible explanation supported by recent cell biodistribution studies in culture using [^{3}H]CP-55940 is that the highly lipophilic cannabinoids added to culture rapidly adsorb to the lipid and protein constituents present in culture media (i.e., fetal bovine serum) as well as to the plastic of the culture vessel. This nonspecific binding significantly diminishes the amount of free drug capable of interaction with the cellular fraction (~2% to 5%) (N. E. Kaminski, *unpublished data*).

The low number of receptors expressed on mouse spleen cells, approximately 1000/cell, is the primary reason why only recently has cannabinoid receptor messenger ribonucleic acid (mRNA) been detected in lymphoid organs (26,34,38). Earlier examinations of splenic tissue from a variety of animal species including rat, mouse, and dog, by Northern analysis, were unsuccessful in detecting the presence of cannabinoid receptor mRNA (39,40). It was only through the application of more sensitive techniques such as RT-PCR and solution hybridization that cannabinoid receptor mRNA was detected. Cannabinoid receptor transcripts have also been identified by RT-PCR in human spleen, tonsils, and peripheral blood leukocytes (34). The rank order of mRNA levels in human blood cell subpopulations from these studies indicated: B cells>NK cells≥polymorphonuclear neutrophils≥CD8 cells>monocytes>CD4 cells. These findings are especially interesting in light of studies in the mouse suggesting that B cells are relatively insensitive to inhibition by cannabinoids and T cells appear to be highly sensitive, especially T_H cells (CD4 cells) (4). Additionally, the first cannabinoid receptor subtype was recently reported following its identification on macrophages from the marginal zone of human splenic monocytes (38). This novel cannabinoid receptor exhibits approximately 44% homology to that originally identified by Matsuda et al. (39). Taken together with the biochemical and immune function results, there is little doubt that functional cannabinoid receptors are expressed on lymphoid cells.

SIGNAL TRANSDUCTION THROUGH THE CANNABINOID RECEPTOR AND EFFECTS ON IMMUNOCOMPETENCE

Signal transduction through the cannabinoid receptor is mediated through inhibition of the adenylate cyclase/cAMP second messenger pathway. This has been well established in neuronal tissue model systems (28,29,41–43) and recently in mouse spleen cells (6). The central question is how the inhibition of adenylate cyclase in lymphoid cells interferes with normal cellular processes. This is an especially intriguing question in light of the generally held view that formation of cellular cAMP is primarily a downregulating signal in lymphoid cells. This view is primarily supported by the observation that membrane permeable cAMP analogs added directly to activated lymphocyte cultures markedly inhibit cell cycle progression. Both B and T cells have been shown to be arrested in transition from G_1 to S phase following experimental elevation of cytosolic cAMP: in T cells by high concentrations of cAMP analogs, 250 to 500 μM (44); or in B cells following stimulation with the diterpine adenylate cyclase activator, forskolin (45). From this standpoint, it is difficult to explain why inhibition of adenylate eyclase by cannabinoids is immunoinhibitory. However, it must be emphasized that the immune inhibition described earlier by cAMP analogs can only be demonstrated at extremely high nonphysiologically relevant concentrations of cAMP (in excess of 250 μM). Adding to this confusion is a significant body of historical data as well as recent findings that, in fact, suggest that a modest transient rise in cellular cAMP within minutes following the activation stimulus (i.e., antigen, phorbol ester plus calcium ionophore) may be a required event for lymphocyte activation. This view is supported by a number of studies that have demonstrated that early during lymphocyte activation there occurs a modest two- to five-fold transient enhancement of cytosolic cAMP, which can persist for up to approximately 30 min after the initial activating signal (46–48). This enhancement in cellular cAMP has been shown to be accompanied by corresponding protein kinase A (PKA)-associated phosphorylation events in which the greatest magnitude of PKA-mediated phosphorylation also occurs during the first 30 min following lymphocyte activation (49).

The functional relevance of adenylate cyclase inhibition by cannabinoids in lymphoid cells is presently being investigated by a number of laboratories. Cannabinoid inhibition of both the spleen cell proliferative responses to phorbol myristate acetate (PMA) plus ionomycin as well as the SRBC antibody response can be reversed by low Bt_2cAMP concentrations (10 to 50 μM) (33). Temporal addition studies revealed that the reversal of the SRBC response by Bt_2cAMP was restricted to the first 30 min following antigen sensitization, suggesting the involvement of an early activation event. Likewise, pretreatment of spleen cells for 24 hr with pertussis toxin prior to treatment with cannabinoids effectively abrogated any inhibitory influences associated with either Δ^9-THC or CP-55940 on the SRBC AFC response. This pertussis toxin pretreatment also blocks the inhibitory effects of both Δ^9-THC and CP-55940 on adenylate cyclase activity. Similar findings with pertussis toxin treatment have been reported in cell membrane preparations isolated from neuroblastoma cell lines (29).

SUMMARY

The existence of receptors on lymphoid cells capable of binding cannabinoids has now been confirmed by at least three independent laboratories. These findings are especially significant because they provide the first major step toward establishing a mechanism by which cannabinoids modulate the immune system. Many questions remain unanswered including: What is the endogenous ligand for this receptor? and Why is this receptor present on lymphoid cells? Although the results are very preliminary, it has recently been reported that arachidonylethanolamide (Fig. 1), an arachidonic acid derivative isolated from porcine brain, exhibits binding properties to the cannabinoid receptor and is capable of mimicking some of the biologic properties attributed to cannabinoids (50). Whether arachidonylethanolamide is the endogenous ligand or only one of a number of endogenous ligands for the cannabinoid receptor is not yet clear; however, further characterization of this novel receptor will provide important information toward this end. The long-term goal of cannabinoid research has primarily been directed toward the development of therapeutic agents. With the identification of endogenous cannabinoid receptors in the CNS as well as peripheral tissues, this goal and others now appear to be attainable.

ACKNOWLEDGMENTS

The author would like to acknowledge that this work was partially supported by research grants RO1DA08351 and RO1DA07908 from the National Institute on Drug Abuse.

REFERENCES

1. Munson AE, Fehr KO. Immunological effects of cannabis. In: Fehr KO, Kalant H, eds. *Adverse health and behavioral consequences of cannabis use*. Toronto: Addiction Research Foundation; 1983;257–353.
2. Watson E, Murphy J, Elsohly H, Elsohly M, Turner C. Effects of the administration of coca alkaloids on the primary immune responses of mice: interaction with Δ^9-tetrahydrocannabinol and ethanol. *Toxicol Appl Pharmacol* 1983;71:1–13.
3. Smith SH, Harris LS, Uwaydah IM, Munson AE. Structure–activity relationships of natural and synthetic cannabinoids in suppression of humoral and cell-mediated immunity. *J Pharmacol Exp Ther* 1978;207:165–170.
4. Schatz AR, Koh WS, Kaminski NE. Δ^9-tetrahydrocannabinol selectively inhibits T-cell dependent humoral immune responses through direct inhibition of accessory T-cell function. *Immunopharmacology* 1993;26:129–137.
5. Lefkowitz S, Klager K. Effect of Δ^9-tetrahydrocannabinol on in vitro sensitization of mouse splenic lymphocytes. *Immunol Commun* 1978;7:557–566.
6. Schatz AR, Kessler FK, Kaminski NE. Inhibition of adenylate cyclase by Δ^9-tetrahydrocannabinol in mouse spleen cells: a potential mechanism for cannabinoid-mediated immunosuppression. *Life Sci* 1992;51:25–30.
7. Pross S, Newton C, Klein T, Friedman H. Age-associated differences in cannabinoid-induced suppression of murine spleen, lymph node and thymus cell blastogenic responses. *Immunopharmacology* 1987;14:159–168.
8. Pross SH, Klein TW, Newton C, Smith J, Widen R, Friedman H. Age-related suppression of murine lymphoid cell blastogenesis by marijuana components. *Dev Comp Immunol* 1990;14:131–137.
9. Specter S, Lancz G, Hazelden J. Marijuana and immunity: tetrahydrocannabinol mediated inhibition of lymphocyte blastogenesis. *Int J Immunopharmacol* 1990;12:261–267.
10. White SC, Brin SC, Janicki BW. Mitogen-induced blastogenic responses of lymphocytes from marijuana smokers. *Science* 1975;188:71–72.
11. Rachelefsky G, Opelz G, Mickey M, et al. Intact humoral and cell-mediated immunity in chronic marijuana smoking. *J Allergy Clin Immunol* 1976;58:483–490.
12. Kawakami Y, Klein TW, Newton C, Djeu JY, Specter S, Friedman H. Suppression by delta-9-tetrahydrocannabinol of interleukin 2-induced lymphocyte proliferation and lymphokine-activated killer cell activity. *Int J Immunopharmacol* 1988;10:485–488.
13. Blanchard D, Newton C, Klein T, Stewart W, Friedman H. In vitro and in vivo suppressive effects of delta-9-tetrahydrocannabinol on interferon production by murine spleen cells. *Int J Immunopharmacol* 1986;8:819–824.
14. Specter S, Rivenbark M, Newton C, Kawakami Y, Lancz G. Prevention and reversal of delta-9-tetrahydrocannabinol induced depression of natural killer cell activity by interleukin-2. *Int J Immunopharmacol* 1989;11:63–69.
15. Klein T, Kawakami Y, Newton C, Friedman H. Marijuana components suppress induction and cytolytic function of murine cytotoxic T cells in vitro and in vivo. *J Toxicol Environ Health* 1991; 32:465–477.
16. Fischer-Stenger K, Updegrove AW, Cabral GA. Delta-9-tetrahydrocannabinol decreases cytotoxic T lymphocyte activity to herpes simplex virus type 1-infected cells. *Proc Soc Exp Biol Med* 1992; 200:422–430.
17. Cabral GA, Stinnett AL, Bailey J, et al. Chronic marijuana smoke alters alveolar macrophage morphology and protein expression. *Pharmacol Biochem Behav* 1991;40:643–649.
18. Cabral GA, Vasquez R. Delta 9-tetrahydrocannabinol suppresses macrophage extrinsic antiherpesvirus activity. *Proc Soc Exp Biol Med* 1992;199:255–263.

19. Johnson MR, Melvin LS, Milne GM. Prototype cannabinoid analgetics, prostaglandins, and opiates—a search for points of mechanistic interaction. *Life Sci* 1982;31:1703–1706.
20. Melvin LS, Johnson MR, Harbert CA, Milne GM, Weissman A. A cannabinoid derived prototypical analgesic. *J Med Chem* 1984;27:67–74.
21. Johnson MR, Melvin SL. The discovery of nonclassical cannabinoid analgetics. In: Meehoulam R, ed. *Cannabinoids as therapeutic agents*. Boca Raton, FL: CRC Press, 1986:121–145.
22. Martin BR, Balster RL, Razdan RK, Harris LS, Dewey WL. Behavioral comparisons of the stereoisomers of tetrahydrocannabinols. *Life Sci* 1981;29:565–574.
23. Razdan RK. Structure–activity relationships in cannabinoids. *Pharmacology* 1986;38:75–149.
24. Howlett AC, Johnson MR, Melvin LS, Milne GM. Nonclassical cannabinoid analgetics inhibit adenylate cyclase: development of a cannabinoid receptor model. *Mol Pharmacol* 1988;33:297–302.
25. Titishov N, Mechoulam R, Zimmerman AM. Stereospecific effects of (−)- and (+)-7-hydroxy-delta-6-tetrahydrocannabinol-dimethylheptyl on the immune system of mice. *Pharmacology* 1989; 39:337–349.
26. Kaminski NE, Abood ME, Kessler FK, Martin BR, Schatz AR. Identification of a functionally relevant cannabinoid receptor on mouse spleen cells involved in cannabinoid-mediated immune modulation. *Mol Pharmacol* 1992;42:736–742.
27. Thomas BF, Martin BR. In vitro metabolism of (−)-cis-3-[2-hydroxy-4(1,1-dimethylheptyl)phenyl]-trans-4-(3-hydroxypropyl)cyclohexanol, a synthetic bicyclic cannabinoid analog. *Drug Metab Dispos* 1990;18:1046–1054.
28. Howlett AC. Cannabinoid inhibition of adenylate cyclase. Biochemistry of the response in neuroblastoma cell membranes. *Mol Pharmacol* 1985;27:429–436.
29. Howlett AC, Qualy JM, Khachtrian LL. Involvement of Gi in the inhibition of adenylate cyclase by cannabimimetic drugs. *Mol Pharmacol* 1985;29:307–313.
30. Howlett AC, Scott DK, Wilken GH. Regulation of adenylate cyclase by cannabinoid drugs. Insights based on thermodynamic studies. *Biochem Pharmacol* 1989;38:3297–3304.
31. Bidaut-Russell M, Devane WA, Howlett AC. Cannabinoid receptors and modulation of cyclic AMP accumulation in the rat brain. *J Neurochem* 1990;55:21–26.
32. Herkenham M, Lynn AB, Little MD, et al. Cannabinoid receptor localization in brain. *Proc Natl Acad Sci USA* 1990;87:1932–1936.
33. Kaminski NE, Koh WS, Yang KH, Lee M, Kessler FK. Immune suppression by cannabinoids is mediated through the inhibition of adenylate cyclase by a pertussis toxin-sensitive G-protein coupled cannabinoid receptor. *Biochem Pharmacol* [*in press*].
34. Bouaboula M, Rinaldi M, Carayon P, et al. Cannabinoid-receptor expression in human leukocytes. *Eur J Biochem* 1993;214:173–180.
35. Devane WA, Dysarz FA, Johnson MR, Melvin LS, Howlett AC. Determination and characterization of a cannabinoid receptor in rat brain. *Mol Pharmacol* 1988;34:605–613.
36. Little P, Martin BR. The effects of Δ^9-tetrahydrocannabinol and other cannabinoids on cAMP accumulation in synaptosomes. *Life Sci* 1991;48:1133–1141.
37. Heidel JJ, Keith WB. Specific inhibition of FSH-stimulated cAMP accumulation by Δ^9-tetrahydrocannabinol in cultures of rat Sertoli cells. *Toxicol Appl Pharmacol* 1989;101:124–134.
38. Munro S, Thomas KL, Abu-Shaar M. Molecular characterization of peripheral receptor for cannabinoids. *Nature* 1993;365:61–65.
39. Matsuda LA, Lolait SJ, Brownstein MJ, Young AC, Bonner TI. Structure of a cannabinoid receptor and functional expression of the cloned cDNA. *Nature* 1990;346:561–564.
40. Gerard CM, Mollereau C, Vassart G, Parmentier M. Nucleotide sequence of a human cannabinoid receptor cDNA. *Nucleic Acids Res* 1990;18:7142.
41. Howlett AC, Fleming RM. Cannabinoid inhibition of adenylate cyclase. Pharmacology of the response in neuroblastoma cell membranes. *Mol Pharmacol* 1984;26:532–538.
42. Howlett AC. Cannabinoid inhibition of adenylate cyclase. Relative activity of constituents and metabolites of marijuana. *Neuropharmacology* 1987;26:507–512.
43. Bidaut-Russell M, Howlett AC. Cannabinoid receptor-regulated cyclic AMP accumulation in the rat striatum. *J Neurochem* 1991;57:1769–1773.
44. Johnson KW, Davis BH, Smith KA. cAMP antagonizes interleukin 2-promoted T-cell cycle progression at a discrete point in early G_1. *Proc Natl Acad Sci USA* 1988;83:6072–6076.
45. Maraguchi A, Miyazaki K, Fauci AS. Inhibition of human B cell activation by diterpine forskolin: interference with B cell growth factor-induced G1 to S transition of the B cell cycle. *J Immunol* 1984;133:1283–1287.

46. Smith JW, Steiner AL, Newberry WM, Parker CW. Cyclic adenosine 3′,5′-monophosphate in human lymphocytes. Alteration after phytohemagglutinin. *J Clin Invest* 1971;50:432–441.
47. Hadden JW, Hadden EM, Haddox MK, Goldberg ND. Guanosine 3′:5′-cyclic monophosphates: a possible intracellular mediator of mitogenic influences in lymphocytes. *Proc Natl Acad Sci USA* 1972;69:3024–3027.
48. Russell DH. Type I cyclic AMP-dependent protein kinase as a positive effector of growth. *Adv Cyclic Nucleotide Res* 1978;9:493–506.
49. Cross ME, Ord MG. Changes in histone phosphorylation and associated early metabolic events in pig lymphocyte culture transformed by phytohaemagglutinin or 6-N,2′-O-dibutyryladenosine 3′:5′-cyclic monophosphate. *Biochem J* 1971;124:241–248.
50. Devane WA, Hanus L, Breuer A, et al. Isolation and structure of a brain constituent that binds to the cannabinoid receptor. *Science* 1992;258:1946–1949.

Immunotoxicology and Immunopharmacology, Second Edition, edited by J. H. Dean, M. I. Luster, A. E. Munson, and I. Kimber.
Raven Press, Ltd., New York © 1994.

20

Asbestos and Other Fibers in the Lung

David B. Warheit and *Thomas W. Hesterberg

*DuPont Haskell Laboratory for Toxicology and Industrial Medicine, Newark, Delaware 19714; and *Department of Health, Safety, and Environment, Schuller International, Inc., Littleton, Colorado 80162*

The pathogenetic mechanisms underlying the pulmonary fibrogenic and carcinogenic effects of inhaled asbestos fibers have not been elucidated, although a number of studies have established that fiber dimension and chemical composition play an important role in the ability of these fibers to induce lung disease. Immunobiologic responses may also play a significant role in the pathogenesis of these disorders. As a consequence, it will be important to determine whether selected individuals develop an immunologically hyperactive response following inhalation of fibers. Indeed, the possible role of immunity in the development of asbestos-related tumors has been recognized for 20 years, when the Report of the Advisory Committee on Asbestos Cancer to the Director of the International Agency for Research on Cancer (1) recommended inquiries into the immunocompetence of asbestos-exposed populations. It is therefore pertinent to discuss the immunologic alterations reported in asbestos-exposed patients in an attempt to confirm the connection between altered immune status and the development of asbestos-related diseases. The possible mechanisms of pulmonary immunopathologic responses in asbestos-exposed animals are discussed in a later section of this chapter.

IMMUNOLOGIC STUDIES IN ASBESTOS: EXPOSED POPULATIONS

It is widely considered that alterations of humoral and cellular immune responses occur in patients with asbestosis. Some of these changes include enhanced prevalence of autoantibodies, including anti-nuclear antibodies and rheumatoid factor (2–5). In addition, some but not all studies have reported augmented levels of the immunoglobulins IgA, IgM, IgG, IgE or complement components 3 and 4 in patients with asbestosis (6–10) as well as idiopathic interstitial pulmonary fibrosis, suggesting common immunologic effects. The mechanisms responsible for the increase in serum Igs have not been described but could be related to the adjuvant-like action of asbestos described by Miller and co-workers (11), or possibly reduced suppressor T lymphocyte function, which could exert specific feedback control on antibody synthesis by B lymphocytes (12). However, this effect may not be unique to asbestos, as it appears that a variety of mineral dusts including silica, coal, and cement may stimulate components of the Ig system, following interactions with cells of the respiratory tract. These perturbations would be epiphenomenal, unrelated to the pathogenesis of asbestosis itself, and therefore would provide little value in detecting those individuals predisposed to the development of neoplasms.

Cell-mediated immunity deficits have been reported in many clinical studies of patients with asbestosis. In this regard, patients have demonstrated significantly fewer responses to standard test antigens used to assess immunologic recall when challenged with delayed hypersensitivity skin tests (9,10). In one study, subjects with documented asbestos exposure had decreased numbers of CD4+ (helper or inducer) and CD8+ (suppressor/cytotoxic) cells relative to controls (6); while in another study, decreased levels of CD8+ cells but not CD4+ cells were measured using monoclonal antibody markers in subjects with long-term asbestos exposure (13). A dose–response effect was noted in this latter study. The reduction in T lymphocytes as well as the observation of a diminished capacity to generate suppressor activity by lymphocytes obtained from asbestos-exposed subjects (14) indicates impairment of T cell function. Numerous investigators have reported a significant impairment of lymphocyte responsiveness to T cell mitogens such as phytohemagglutinin (PHA); PHA-induced cytotoxic effector cell function and natural killer (NK) cell function have also been found to be diminished in patients with asbestosis when compared to controls (6,9,15,16). It is intriguing to note that alterations in T cell number and function have been reported also in patients with pleural effects. In this regard, differences in T lymphocyte function were measured in subjects with pleural plaques, but without corresponding evidence of bronchoalveolar reactions (17). In a majority of subjects, PHA-induced cytotoxic cell function was markedly diminished. Moreover, a significant decrease in lymphocyte responsiveness to PHA was also demonstrated in the group with pleural plaques compared to those with similar exposure but no evidence of pleural reactions.

The results of these studies on asbestos exposure suggest a possible connection between diminished (or altered) T lymphocyte function and the development of progressive interstitial fibrosis following asbestos exposure. The finding of impaired T lymphocyte function in some subjects with no evidence of fibrosis suggests that such immune changes may be an early contributory factor in the pathogenesis of disease or may be an unrelated consequence of asbestos exposure. The alterations in immune function in asbestos-exposed individuals might relate to preexisting, asbestos-related cell membrane changes, or to a depletion of functional T helper (T_H) lymphocytes resulting from activation of the immune system secondary to alveolar macrophage activation by asbestos (18,19).

With regard to the development of asbestos-related cancers, there seems to be little evidence that impaired T cell function, as measured by the assays described above, exists or plays a significant role in asbestos-associated malignancy. In studies of patients with pleural mesothelioma, the majority of patients were reported to have normal T lymphocyte responses, both *in vitro* and *in vivo*, despite diminished numbers of circulating lymphocytes (15).

There remains conflicting evidence regarding the association of immunologic alterations and the development of mesothelioma. Moderate to severe immunosuppression has been observed in a significant number of untreated mesothelioma patients, with only 30% of these subjects exhibiting normal lymphocyte responses to PHA (20). This suggests that exposure to asbestos may contribute to a condition of immunodeficiency, thus rendering the host susceptible to the development of tumors. It should be noted that there is a paucity of data relating the immunologic status of individuals with asbestos-related cancers (21). At present, the available studies demonstrate conflicting results regarding the association between immunologic defects and mesothelioma, and that the significance of these changes in the causation of this disease remains unclear. Similarly, the association between immune alterations and lung cancer has not been well established. Whether any direct association exists between immune alterations and the development of asbestos-associated malignancies remains to be determined.

ROLE OF COMPLEMENT IN MACROPHAGE CLEARANCE OF INHALED FIBERS

The role of complement in mediating immunologic responses has been recognized for nearly a century (22–24). The complement system consists of plasma proteins found in normal serum, which reacts sequentially along two distinct but interrelated pathways and is activated both by immunologic and nonimmunologic stimuli. The better known classic pathway may be activated by IgM and IgG-containing immune complexes, polynucleotides, and some viruses. Activators of the alternative complement pathway include plant, fungal, and bacterial polysaccharides, organic and inorganic particles, and fibers. Activation of either pathway produces a diversity of biologic effects including complement-mediated cytolysis, the production of potent mediators of inflammation, and particle opsonization (22–24).

With regard to the lung, complement proteins are normal components of pulmonary fluids and are present in biologically active concentrations on alveolar surfaces (25,26). The functional importance of the complement system in host resistance reactions to infectious agents is well established (22–24). In this respect, complement modulates inflammatory and bacterial clearance responses in the lungs of exposed animals and humans (27). In particular, the fifth component of complement (C5) and its phlogistic cleavage fragments, C5a and C5a des arg, mediate the recruitment of macrophages and neutrophils into alveolar regions of the lung (28).

Alveolar macrophages (AMs) play an important role in clearing microorganisms and inhaled particulate matter from the lung (29). Although it is known that phagocytosis of inhaled particles and bacteria by macrophages is critical for maintaining the integrity of the alveolar compartment, the mechanisms through which AMs are recruited to inhaled particulates on distal lung surfaces following deposition are not well understood. Particle identification by AMs is a prerequisite for phagocytosis because particulates must be encountered by phagocytes before phagocytosis and clearance can occur.

In experimental studies designed to investigate the early events of fiber clearance, it was reported that significant numbers of alveolar macrophages accumulated at sites of chrysotile asbestos fiber deposition (i.e., alveolar duct bifurcations) within 48 hr following a 1-hr exposure. In contrast, duct bifurcation surfaces of sham-exposed animals were essentially devoid of macrophages (Fig. 1) (30). Histologic examination of asbestos-exposed lung tissue of rats sacrificed 48 hr after exposure revealed that the increase in tissue volume was accounted for, in part, by the presence of macrophages that adhered to the type I epithelium, which comprises the duct bifurcation surface (31).

In attempting to establish the mechanism(s) through which macrophages are preferentially recruited to alveolar duct bifurcations, it was postulated that AMs are recruited to sites of asbestos deposition by a chemotactic factor generated by the inhaled fibers on alveolar surfaces. This idea was consistent with the knowledge that administration of asbestos fibers *in vitro* activates the alterative complement pathway in serum, resulting in the generation of C5a, a potent chemotactic factor for neutrophils and macrophages (24,32,33).

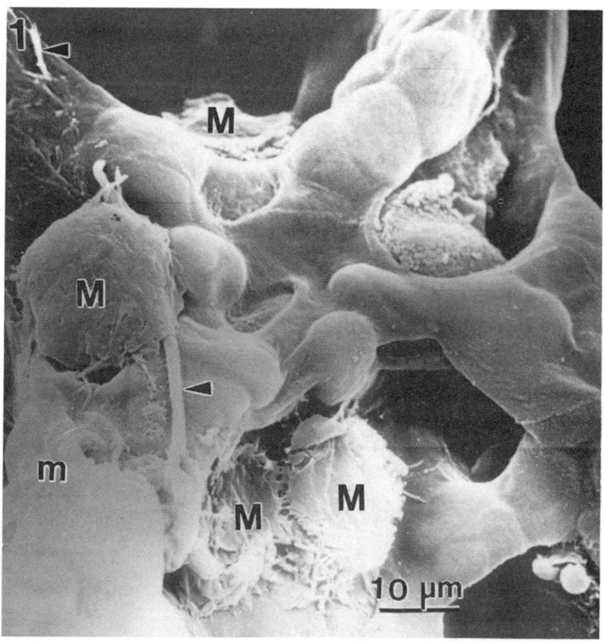

FIG. 1. Scanning electron micrograph of an alveolar duct bifurcation 48 hr after a 1-hr exposure to chrysotile asbestos. Alveolar macrophages (*M*) have accumulated at these sites to phagocytose inhaled fibers (*arrows*).

TABLE 1. *AM accumulation at sites of asbestos fiber deposition—alveolar duct bifurcations*

Strain	Number of mice	Number of bifurcations examined	Mean number of macrophages on bifurcations ($x \pm SD$)
$C5^+$ ASB 3/0	3	23	0.9 ± 0.3
$C5^-$ ASB 3/0	2	19	0.2 ± 0.4
$C5^+$ SHAM 3/48	3	24	0.4 ± 0.6
$C5^-$ SHAM 3/48	2	9	0.1 ± 0.3
$C5^+$ ASB 3/48	4	22	4.1 ± 2.5[a]
$C5^-$ ASB 3/48	4	39	1.4 ± 1.4
Treatment	**Number of rats**	**Number of bifurcations examined**	**Mean number of macrophages on bifurcations ($x \pm SD$)**
ASB 3/48	5	21	4.3 ± 3.0
CVF-ASB 3/48	4	17	1.2 ± 0.9[b]
SHAM 3/48	4	18	0.1 ± 0.3[b]

$C5^+$, mouse strain B10.D2/nSnj; $C5^-$, mouse strain B10.D2/oSnj; SHAM 3/48, 3-hr sham exposure to air and a 48-hr recovery period; ASB 3/0, 3-hr chrysotile asbestos exposure with no recovery; ASB 3/48, 3-hr chrysotile asbestos exposure and a 48-hr recovery; CVF-ASB 3/48, cobra venom-treated rats exposed to chrysotile asbestos for 3 hr and a 48-hr recovery period.
[a] $p < 0.001$ when compared with $C5^-$ ASB 3/48.
[b] $p < 0.01$ when compared with ASB 3/48.

To test the hypothesis, a series of *in vitro* chemotaxis as well as inhalation studies were carried out with rats and mice (31,34). AM chemotaxis was utilized as a bioassay for complement activation. In support of the hypothesis, the results showed that incubation of chrysotile asbestos fibers with rat serum or unexposed lavaged proteins produced enhanced macrophage chemotactic responses compared to controls. Moreover, this finding was confirmed *in vivo* where it was demonstrated that fluids lavaged from the lungs of asbestos-exposed rats contained increased chemotactic activity for macrophages, and this activity was detected in the molecular weight (MW) range of C5a (31). To further investigate the role of C5 in facilitating the asbestos-induced AM clearance response, congenic strains of complement-normal (C5+) and complement-deficient (C5−) mice, as well as normal and decomplemented rats [i.e., rats treated with cobra venom factor (CVF) to reduce serum complement], were exposed to chrysotile asbestos for brief periods. The numbers of AMs that were recruited to sites of fiber deposition were significantly reduced in the C5− mice and CVF-treated rats (Table 1). Time course studies showed that chemoattractant generation preceded the macrophage migration response and that macrophage phagocytosis of inhaled asbestos fibers was reduced in complement-deficient animals. In addition, it was shown that the depletion of measurable levels of hemolytic complement in lung fluids lavaged from asbestos-exposed rats coincided with the presence of a chemotactic factor, suggesting that complement components were consumed during the 3-hr asbestos exposure. The results of these studies demonstrated clearly that asbestos activated complement,

TABLE 2. *Rat AM chemotactic* in vitro *responses to particulate-activated sera*

Serum	Numbers of migrating macrophages/20 HPF		
	1%	5%	10% PAS
Normal heated sera	30 ± 5	62 ± 15	109 ± 15
Fiberglass	67 ± 8	159 ± 40[a]	282 ± 17[a]
Crocidolite asbestos	78 ± 16	127 ± 15[a]	227 ± 18[a]
Chrysotile asbestos	79 ± 20	190 ± 26[a]	368 ± 51[a]
Wollastonite	61 ± 8	113 ± 26[b]	163 ± 18[b]
Decomplemented sera + fiberglass	26 ± 15	38 ± 3	53 ± 14
Mount St. Helens ash	37 ± 11	64 ± 15	115 ± 24
Carbonyl iron	69 ± 18	112 ± 20[b]	138 ± 15[b]

PAS, particulate-activated sera; *N*, a minimum of nine for each particulate tested.
[a] $p < 0.01$ when compared to Mount St. Helens or normal heated sera.
[b] $p < 0.05$ when compared to Mount St. Helens or normal heated sera.

generating C5a as a by-product of this reaction, and this chemoattractant induced migration of AMs to sites of fiber deposition (31,34).

These findings have been extended to demonstrate that numerous particle or fiber types, which activate complement *in vitro* and deposit at alveolar duct bifurcations when inhaled, will generate complement-mediated chemoattractants *in vivo* following inhalation exposure. To this extent, it has been shown that chrysotile and crocidolite asbestos fibers, glass fibers, iron-coated chrysotile asbestos, wollastonite fibers, and carbonyl iron particles activated complement in rat serum and in lung fluids (Table 2). Mount St. Helens volcanic ash particles, tested through a broad range of concentrations, produced no chemotactic activity. It has been concluded that activation of complement by particulates with a variety of physical characteristics facilitates lung clearance of inhaled materials by providing a mechanism through which macrophages can detect and phagocytose particulates on alveolar surfaces (35–37).

STUDIES ON THE MECHANISMS OF ASBESTOS-INDUCED LUNG INJURY

Animal models of asbestosis have been developed in rats (38,39), mice (40), guinea pigs (41), and sheep (42,43) exposed chronically to the fibers. The chronic inhalation models are important for assessing the anatomic patterns of disease. A major limitation associated with chronic exposure models, however, is the inability to ascertain the initiating pathogenetic events. For example, the association between initial fiber deposition patterns and the subsequent cellular events that lead to asbestos-induced lung injury has not been addressed. Similarly, the role of the AM in the early development of asbestosis has not been well established. As a consequence, a rat model of asbestos-induced lung disease was developed wherein rats were exposed for 1 hr to an aerosol of chrysotile asbestos fibers and early cellular events were evaluated at 48 hr and 1 month postexposure (30,44).

Following brief inhalation exposures to asbestos, fibers were observed to have deposited preferentially on alveolar duct bifurcations (44,45) and were cleared from epithelial surfaces by AM-mediated clearance or fiber translocation. In the latter circumstance, fibers migrated from airspace to pulmonary interstitium via type I epithelial cells, where they were phagocytosed primarily by fibroblasts or interstitial macrophages (44,46). The presence of these fibers within fibroblasts induced the formation of intracellular microcalcifications, a form of nonspecific cellular injury (46). On the alveolar side, AMs rapidly accumulated at sites of fiber deposition to phagocytose fibers (30). The mechanism for AM recruitment to alveolar duct bifurcations is associated with complement activation by the inhaled fibers and consequent generation of chemotactic factors as discussed earlier. Histologic examination of exposed lung tissue indicated that proximal alveolar duct bifurcations were prominent in asbestos-exposed animals sacrificed 48 hr after exposure. Using ultrastructural morphometric techniques, Chang and co-workers (47) demonstrated that the influx of recruited pulmonary macrophages formed a component of an early lesion, which was characterized by increases in the volumes of the epithelial and interstitial compartments of the bifurcations. In addition, the numbers of AMs, interstitial macrophages, and type I and type II epithelial cells were all significantly elevated. One month after the 1-hr exposure, the numbers of AMs on bifurcation surfaces no longer exceeded the normal level but the volume of the interstitium was still significantly enhanced by 67% over sham controls. This was accounted for by an increase in the volume of noncellular interstitial matrix, concomitant with an accumulation of interstitial cells, including macrophages, myofibroblasts, fibroblasts and smooth muscle cells (47). It was concluded that acute structural changes measured at 48 hr after a 1-hr exposure were followed by a progressive response, evidenced by increased numbers of interstitial cells and localized interstitial fibrosis measured at 1 month postexposure (47).

The demonstration of an early lesion of asbestosis measured 48 hr and 1 month after a 1-hr exposure and identification of the target cell types have provided a basis for studying the mechanisms associated with the asbestos-related pathologic response. The finding of alterations in the cellular and noncellular interstitial compartments combined with the subsequent development of fibrosis implicates the involvement of fibroblasts in proliferating and synthesizing matrix components such as collagen, elastin, and glycosaminoglycans. The rate of collagen accumulation is likely to be a function of both the number of fibroblasts (i.e., fibroblast proliferation) as well as the rate of collagen synthesis by individual cells and degradation by protease-secreting cells. Recent studies have suggested that fibroblast proliferation and connective tissue formation are complex processes and may be independently regulated (48–50). Moreover, although fibroblasts are frequently regarded as responding passively to the products of effector cells, it seems clear that these cell types play a more active role in directing the course of fibrosis. Noting the complexity of potential responses in the interstitial microenvironment, it is still attractive to postulate that asbestos-exposed AMs or interstitial macrophages synthesize and secrete mitogenic factors that stimulate interstitial cells to increase in number and elaborate greater amounts of connective tissue.

FIBER-INDUCED INFLAMMATION

Inhalation of fibers may cause a pulmonary inflammatory response characterized by cytotoxicity, increased lung epithelial permeability, and an influx of inflammatory cells (neutrophils, interstitial macrophages/monocytes, or lymphocytes). An association between inflammation and the development of pulmonary fibrosis has been postulated but has not been sufficiently elucidated. Crouch (51) has concluded that inflammation and the release of inflammatory mediators are necessary, but not always sufficient, for the development of fibrosis. This conclusion is predicated on the observation that pulmonary inflammation always appears to precede fibrosis. However, the role of inflammation as a prerequisite for the development of fiber-induced pulmonary fibrosis has not been studied in sufficient detail.

Reactive oxidants released by activated phagocytes cause tissue damage and may be linked to inflammation, fibrosis, and possibly genotoxic effects. Moreover, the production of oxygen radicals by cells may result in their own death. Goodglick and Kane (52) reported that *in vitro* exposure of macrophages to crocidolite asbestos fibers resulted in cell death as well as release of oxygen metabolites. This toxicity was prevented by administration of superoxide dismutase, catalase, or deferoxamine. The role of oxygen radicals in asbestos-related inflammation and pulmonary fibrosis has also been assessed using a chronic administration regimen of antioxidants to asbestos-exposed rats (53). The results of these studies suggest a possible role for oxygen radicals (probably derived from inflammatory cells or alveolar macrophages) in asbestos-induced lung injury. In earlier studies, it had been reported that asbestos induces the production of oxygen radicals by AMs *in vitro* and in cell-free reaction mixtures (54,55).

GROWTH FACTORS

Growth factor regulation of the cell cycle with regard to pulmonary cells has been described in several recent reviews (48–51,56,57). Recent studies of fibroblast regulation suggest that the mechanisms of fibroblast proliferation are complex, as macrophage-derived products may both stimulate and/or inhibit cell growth. Growth factors play important roles in the progression of cells through the cell cycle and stimulate quiescent cells to reenter the cell cycle and begin synthesizing deoxyribonucleic acid (DNA). Growth factors that influence early events in G_0/G_1 are labeled *competence* factors. Competence factors such as platelet-derived growth factor (PDGF) and fibronectin stimulate growth-arrested cells to respond to other growth factors, called *progression factors*, which induce cells to initiate DNA synthesis and mitosis. Two progression factors that are considered to be potent stimulators of mesenchymal cell proliferation are interleukin-1 (IL-1), a potent mitogen of human neonatal fibroblasts, and insulin-like growth factor (IGF-1). AMs synthesize and secrete numerous different growth factors for fibroblasts, including IL-1, tumor necrosis factor-α (TNF-α), interleukin-6 (IL-6), fibroblast growth factor (FGF), PDGF, and transforming growth factor-β (TGF-β) (56). Growth factors have been implicated in facilitating the progression of fiber-induced pulmonary fibrosis. Most of the studies linking growth factors and fibrosis have been in association with asbestos exposure. Asbestos fibers were shown to stimulate AMs to produce a PDGF homolog that is mitogenic for rat lung fibroblasts *in vitro* (58). PDGF is considered to be the classic competence factor for fibroblasts (48). In addition, AM-derived PDGF was shown to be chemotactic for fibroblasts *in vitro* (59). In contrast to the experimental data, blood monocytes from asbestotic patients did not express the gene for the β chain of PDGF following culture with the mitogen concanavalin A (Con A); however, monocytes from normal subjects expressed this gene (60). Moreover, unstimulated monocytes from subjects with asbestos exposure released less fibroblast-stimulating activity compared to normal subjects. The authors of this study suggested that peripheral blood monocytes might be immature from patients with asbestos-related disease, implying that lung macrophages are capable of secreting PDGF (60).

Cells recovered by bronchoalveolar lavage are also capable of releasing progression factors for fibroblasts. For example, lavaged AMs from asbestotic patients were found to produce high levels of IGF-1, although only normal levels of IGF-1 messenger ribonucleic acid (mRNA) were measured (61). Asbestos-exposed cells recovered by pulmonary lavage (99% AMs) of rats elaborated a fibroblast growth factor (FGF), also referred to as macrophage-derived growth factor (MDGF), during a period of 1 to 24 weeks following exposure (62). This secretion *in vitro* correlated with the observation of histopathologic changes *in vivo*. However, other studies have not demonstrated such a correlation between *in vitro* fibroblast proliferation and the development of pulmonary fibrosis. Both long and short crocidolite asbestos fibers at similar concentrations induced AMs to secrete fibroblast proliferation factors *in vitro* (63). However, the results of inhalation studies at other laboratories have shown that long asbestos fibers are significantly more pathogenic than short fibers (64). It was surprising to find that fibroblast proliferative activity could not be measured in culture supernatants of cells lavaged from rats instilled with long fibers, despite significant pathologic effects (63). In contrast, short fibers resulted in no significant pathologic pulmonary effects, but significant fibroblast proliferation activity was found in cell culture supernatants from rats exposed to these fibers. The critical target for long crocidolite fibers may have been macrophages within the interstitial compartment, wherein growth factor release could directly stimulate fibroblasts. Short crocidolite fibers may have been phagocytosed and cleared from the lung at a faster rate and thus did not readily reach the interstitium.

In rats instilled with various silicate fibers, it was reported that both MDGF and IL-1 type activity were produced by lavaged macrophages in culture (65). Fibers that produced granulomatous lesions but not pulmonary fibrosis (e.g., attapulgite and short chrysotile 4T30) elicited the production of IL-1 but not MDGF by these cells. These lesions and IL-1 production were decreased over an 8-month postexposure time period. In contrast, exposure to UICC chrysotile B, which produced lung fibrosis, stimulated enhanced production of both IL-1 and MDGF by lavaged cells. The chrysotile B-induced fibrosis was progressive, and MDGF production by cells derived from these animals persisted up to 9 months following the initial exposure (62,65). These results suggest that MDGF production by AMs may play an important role in the progression of fiber-induced pulmonary fibrosis, when compared to IL-1 production, which may serve to influence the nature of the initial inflammatory reaction following exposure to fibers.

Feedback loops are important in the regulation of fibroblast proliferation activity in the lung and indicate that the system is well modulated. It has been reported that IL-1 induces the secretion of prostaglandin E_2 (PGE_2) by fibroblasts, which in turn inhibits growth (66). In addition, PGE_2 may be capable of suppressing the release of fibronectin from AMs (67). Fibronectin has also been associated with the development of pulmonary fibrosis (68). Cultured AMs from patients with idiopathic pulmonary fibrosis released more fibronectin and less PGE_2 than AMs from normal volunteers (67). Stimuli that suppressed fibronectin release by these cells also stimulated PGE_2 release. Studies designed to evaluate the potential alterations of feedback loops in relation to fiber-induced pulmonary fibrosis have not been conducted, although it is likely that the same regulatory pathways are operant.

Progression of fibrotic lung disease also depends on production of connective tissue proteins as well as increased mesenchymal cell proliferation. TGF-β, which induces fibroblast proliferation and is a product of AMs, was also shown to increase elastin production by neonatal rat lung fibroblasts (69). In this regard, it will be important to more fully identify the functions of the different forms of TGF-β and TGF-β receptors on fibroblasts (70,71).

SUMMARY

A current working hypothesis to explain the mechanisms underlying the development of asbestosis in rats proposes that inhaled fibers deposit at alveolar duct bifurcations and recruit macrophages to sites of fiber deposition. Some fibers translocate from airspace to interstitium, wherein they may activate complement in the interstitial compartment, generating chemoattractants to recruit interstitial macrophages. Subsequently, the translocated fibers are phagocytosed by interstitial macrophages and fibroblasts, which produce and/or respond to mitogenic factors, resulting in the synthesis and secretion of connective tissue proteins (collagen). Alternatively, on the alveolar surface, AMs accumulate at sites of fiber deposition, phagocytose fibers, and elaborate cytokines that mediate the growth and proliferation of endothelial, epithelial, and mesenchymal cells. The pattern of asbestos-induced fibrogenesis becomes more complex following chronic exposures. Retention of fibers and consequent accumulation of interstitial fibers combined with sustained inflammatory responses will likely contribute to the development of a diffuse and progressive pattern of pulmonary fibrosis. The studies presented here suggest that immunologic mechanisms are operative in the development of asbestos-related lung disease and, in particular, play a significant role in the AM response to inhaled fibers.

ACKNOWLEDGMENTS

The authors wish to acknowledge Dr. Klara Miller and Dr. Steve Gavett for contributing important insights into the preparation of this chapter.

REFERENCES

1. Advisory Committee Report on Asbestos Cancers to the Director of the International Agency for Research on Cancer. Biological effects of asbestos. *Ann Occup Hyg* 1973;16:9.
2. Kagan E, Solomon A, Cochrane JC, Kuba P, Rocks PH, Webster I. Immunological studies of patients with asbestos. II. Studies of circulating lymphoid numbers and humoral immunity. *Clin Exp Immunol* 1977;28:268.
3. Lange A. An experimental survey of immunological abnormalities in asbestos. I. Nonorgan- and organ-specific autoantibodies. *Environ Res* 1980;22:162.
4. Navatil M, Jezkova Z. Antibodies against pulmonary tissue in individuals with long-term exposure to asbestos dust. *Cas Lek Ces* 1982;121:1608.
5. Turner-Warwick M, Parkes WR. Circulating rheumatoid and anti-nuclear factors in asbestos workers. *Br Med J* 1970;3:492.
6. de Shazo RD, Nordberg J, Baser Y, Bozelka B, Weill H, Salvaggio J. Analysis of depressed cell-mediated immunity in asbestos workers. *J Allergy Clin Immunol* 1983;72:454.
7. Doll NJ, Diem JE, Jones RN, et al. Humoral immunologic abnormalities in workers exposed to asbestos cement dust. *J Allergy Clin Immunol* 1983;72:509.
8. Huuskonen MS, Rasanen YA, Harkonen H, Asp S. Asbestos exposure as a cause of immunological stimulation. *Scand J Respir Dis* 1976;59:326.
9. Kagan E, Solomon A, Cochrane JC, Beissmer EK, Gluckman J, Rocks PH, Webster I. Immunological studies of patients with asbestosis. I. Studies of cell mediated immunity. *Clin Exp Immunol* 1977;28:261.
10. Lange A, Sibinski G, Garncarek D. The follow-up study of skin reactivity to recall antigens and E- and EAC-RFC profiles in blood in asbestos workers. *Immunobiology* 1980;157:1.
11. Miller K, Webster I, Handfield RIM, Skikine MI. Ultrastructure of the lung in the rat following exposure to crocidolite asbestos and quartz. *J Pathol* 1978;124:39.
12. Salvaggio J. Overview of occupational immunologic lung disease. *J Allergy Clin Immunol* 1982;70:5.
13. Miller LG, Sparrow D, Ginns LC. Asbestos circulation correlates with alterations in circulating T-cell subsets. *Clin Exp Immunol* 1983;51:110.
14. Gaumer HR, Doll NJ, Karmal J, Schuyler M, Salvaggio JE. Diminished suppression of cell function in patients with asbestosis. *Clin Exp Immunol* 1981;44:108.
15. Haslem PL, Lukoszek A, Merchant JA, Turner-Warwick M. Lymphocyte responses to phytohaemagglutinin in patients with asbestosis and pleural mesothelioma. *Clin Exp Immunol* 1978; 31:178.
16. Rogol PR, Ryu J, Ginns LC. Reduced natural killer cell activity in asbestos workers. *Am Rev Respir Dis* 1983;127:78.

17. Miller K, Brown RC. The immune system and asbestos-associated disease. In: Dean JH, Luster MI, Munson AE, Amos H, eds. *Immunotoxicology and immunopharmacology*. New York: Raven Press; 1985:429.
18. Gellert AM, Macey MG, Uthayakumor S, Newland AC, Rudd RM. Lymphocyte sub-populations in bronchoalveolar lavage fluid in asbestos workers. *Am Rev Respir Dis* 1985;132:824.
19. Miller K, Weintraub Z, Kagan E. Manifestation of cellular immunity in the rat after prolonged asbestos inhalation. *J Immunol* 1979;123:102.
20. Bekesi G, Roboz J, Fischbein A, Selikoff I. Clinical immunology studies in individuals exposed to environmental chemicals. In: Berlin A, Dean J, Draper MH, Smith EMB, Spreafico F, eds. *Immunotoxicology*. Hingham, MA: Martinus Nijhoff (Commission of the European Communities); 1987:347.
21. WHO. Asbestos and other natural mineral fibres. In: *Environmental health criteria 53, International Programme on Chemical Safety*. Geneva: WHO; 1986:120.
22. Kunkel SL, Fantone JC, Ward PA. Complement mediated inflammatory reactions. *Pathobiol Annu* 1981;11:127.
23. Larsen GL, Henson PM. Mediators of inflammation. *Annu Rev Immunol* 1983;1:335.
24. Snyderman R. Mechanisms of inflammation and leukocyte chemotaxis in rheumatic diseases. *Med Clin North Am* 1986;70:217.
25. Kolb WP, Kolb LM, Wetsel RA, Rogers WR, Shaw JO. Quantitation and stability of the fifth component of complement (C5) in bronchoalveolar lavage fluids obtained from non-human primates. *Am Rev Respir Dis* 1981;123:226.
26. Robertson J, Caldwell JR, Castle JR, Waldman RH. Evidence for the presence of components of the alternative (properdin) pathway of complement activation in respiratory secretions. *J Immunol* 1976;117:900.
27. Joiner KA, Brown EJ, Frank MM. Complement and bacteria: chemistry and biology in host defense. *Annu Rev Immunol* 1984;2:461.
28. Heidbrink PJ, Toews GB, Gross GN, Pierce AK. Mechanisms of complement-mediated clearance of bacteria from the murine lung. *Am Rev Respir Dis* 1982;125:517.
29. Brain JD. Physiology and pathophysiology of pulmonary macrophages. In: Reichard SM, Filkins J, eds. *The reticuloendothelial system*, vol 7B. New York: Plenum Publishing; 1985:315.
30. Warheit DB, Chang LY, Hill LH, Hook GER, Crapo JD, Brody AR. Pulmonary macrophage accumulation and asbestos-induced lesions at sites of fiber deposition. *Am Rev Respir Dis* 1984; 129:301–310.
31. Warheit DB, George G, Hill LH, Snyderman R, Brody AR. Inhaled asbestos activates a complement-dependent chemoattractant for macrophages. *Lab Invest* 1985;52:505–514.
32. Saint-Remy JMR, Cole P. Interactions of chrysotile asbestos fibres with the complement system. *Immunology* 1980;41:431.
33. Wilson MR, Gaumer HR, Salvaggio JR. Activation of the alternative complement pathway and generation of chemotactic factors by asbestos. *J Allergy Clin Immunol* 1977;60:218.
34. Warheit DB, Hill LH, George G, Brody AR. Time course of chemotactic factor generation and the corresponding macrophage response to asbestos inhalation. *Am Rev Respir Dis* 1986;134:128.
35. Warheit DB, Overby LH, George G, Brody AR. Pulmonary macrophages are attracted to inhaled particles through complement activation. *Exp Lung Res* 1988;14:51–66.
36. Warheit DB, Brody AR, Hartsky MA. Predictive value of *in vitro* pulmonary macrophage functional assays to assess *in vivo* clearance of inhaled particles. In: Mossman BT, Begin RO, eds. *Proceedings of the Fourth International Workshop on Effects of Mineral Dusts on Cells*, NATO ASI Series H:Cell Biology vol 30. New York: Springer-Verlag; 1989:347.
37. Warheit DB, Carakostas MC, Bamberger JR, Hartsky MA. Complement facilitates macrophage phagocytosis of inhaled iron particles but has little effect in mediating silica-induced lung inflammatory and clearance responses. *Environ Res* 1991;56:186–203.
38. Pinkerton KE, Pratt PC, Brody AR, Crapo JD. Fiber localization and its relationship to lung reactions in rats after chronic exposure to chrysotile asbestos. *Am J Pathol* 1984;117:484–498.
39. Wagner JC, Berry G, Skidmore JW, Timbrell V. The effects of inhalation of asbestos in rats. *Br J Cancer* 1974;29:252.
40. Bozelka BG, Sestini P, Gaumer HR, Hammad Y, Heather CJ, Salvaggio JE. A murine model of asbestosis. *Am J Pathol* 1983;112:326.
41. Holt PF, Mill J, Young DK. Experimental asbestosis in the guinea pig. *J Pathol Bacteriol* 1966;92:185.

42. Begin R, Rola-Pleszczynski M, Sirois P, et al. Early lung events following low-dose asbestos exposure. *Environ Res* 1981;26:391.
43. Begin R, Rola-Pleszczynski M, Masse S, et al. Asbestos-induced injury in the sheep model: the initial alveolitis. *Environ Res* 1983;30:195.
44. Brody AR, Hill LH, Adkins B Jr, O'Connor RW. Chrysotile asbestos inhalation in rats: deposition pattern and reaction of alveolar epithelium and pulmonary macrophages. *Am Rev Respir Dis* 1981; 123:670–679.
45. Brody AR, Roe MW. Deposition pattern of inorganic particles at the alveolar level in the lungs of rats and mice. *Am Rev Respir Dis* 1983;128:724–729.
46. Brody AR, Hill LH. Interstitial accumulation of inhaled chrysotile asbestos fibers and consequent formation of microcalcifications. *Am J Pathol* 1982;109:107–114.
47. Chang LY, Overby LH, Brody AR, Crapo JD. Progressive lung cell reactions and extracellular matrix production after a brief exposure to asbestos. *Am J Pathol* 1988;131:156–170.
48. Goldstein RH, Fine A. Fibrotic reactions in the lung. The activation of the lung fibroblast. *Exp Lung Res* 1986;11:245–261.
49. King RJ, Jones MB, Minoo P. Regulations of lung cell proliferation by polypeptide growth factors. *Am J Physiol* 1989;257(Lung Cell Mol Physiol)1:L23–L38.
50. Reiser KM, Last JA. Early cellular events in pulmonary fibrosis. *Exp Lung Res* 1986;10:331–355.
51. Crouch E. Pathobiology of pulmonary fibrosis. *Am J Physiol* 1990;259(Lung Cell Mol Physiol 3):L159–L184.
52. Goodglick LA, Kane AB. Cytotoxicity of long and short crocidolite fibers in vitro and in vivo. *Cancer Res* 1990;50:5153–5163.
53. Mossman BT, Marsh JP, Sesko A, et al. Inhibition of lung injury, inflammation, and interstitial pulmonary fibrosis by polyethylene glycol-conjugated catalase in a rapid inhalation model of asbestosis. *Am Rev Respir Dis* 1990;141:1266–1271.
54. Hansen K, Mossman BT. Generation of superoxide (O_2-) from alveolar macrophages exposed to asbestiform and nonfibrous particles. *Cancer Res* 1987;47:1681–1686.
55. Weitzman SA, Graceffa P. Asbestos catalyzes hydroxyl and superoxide radical generation from hydrogen peroxide. *Arch Biochem Biophys* 1984;228:373–376.
56. Kovacs EJ. Fibrogenic cytokines: the role of immune mediators in the development of scar tissue. *Immunol Today* 1991;12:17–23.
57. Rom WM, Travis WD, Brody AR. Cellular and molecular basis of the asbestos-related diseases. *Am Rev Respir Dis* 1991;143:408–422.
58. Kumar RK, Bennett RA, Brody AR. A homologue of platelet-derived growth factor-like molecule produced by human alveolar macrophages *FASEB J* 1988;2:2272–2277.
59. Osornio-Vargas AR, Bonner JC, Badgett A, Brody AR. Rat alveolar macrophage-derived platelet-derived growth factor is chemotactic for rat lung fibroblasts. *Am J Respir Cell Mol Biol* 1990;3:595–602.
60. Schwartz DA, Rosenstock L, Clark JG. Monocyte-derived growth factors in asbestos-induced interstitial fibrosis. *Environ Res* 1989;49:283–294.
61. Rom WM, Basset P, Fells GA, Nukiwa T, Trapnell BC, Crystal RG. Alveolar macrophages release an insulin-like growth factor 1-type molecule. *J Clin Invest* 1988;82:1685–1693.
62. Lemaire I, Beaudoin H, Masse S, Grodin C. Alveolar macrophage stimulation of lung fibroblast growth in asbestos-induced pulmonary fibrosis. *Am J Pathol* 1986;122:205–211.
63. Adamson IYR, Bowden DH. Pulmonary reaction to long and short asbestos fibers is independent of fibroblast growth factor production by alveolar macrophages. *Am J Pathol* 1990;137:523–529.
64. Davis JMG, Addison J, Bolton RE, Donaldson K, Jones AD, Smith T. The pathogenicity of long versus short fibre samples of amostie asbestos administered to rats by inhalation or intraperitoneal injection. *Br J Exp Pathol* 1986;67:415–430.
65. Lemaire I. Selective differences in macrophage populations and monokine production in resolving pulmonary granuloma and fibrosis. *Am J Pathol* 1991;138:487–495.
66. Elias JA, Rossman MD, Zurier RB, Daniele RP. Human alveolar macrophage inhibition of lung fibroblast growth: a prostaglandin-dependent process. *Am Rev Respir Dis* 1985;131:94–99.
67. Ozaki T, Moriguchi H, Nakamura Y, Kamei T, Yasuoka S, Ogura T. Regulatory effect of prostaglandin E_2 on fibronectin release from human alveolar macrophages. *Am Rev Respir Dis* 1990;141:965–969.
68. Fujita J, Rennard SI. Fibronectin in the lung. In: Carsons SE, ed. *Fibronectin in health and disease*. Boca Raton, FL: CRC Press; 1989:215.

69. McGowan SE, McNamer R. Transforming growth factor-β increases elastin production by neonatal rat lung fibroblasts. *Am J Respir Cell Mol Biol* 1990;3:369–376.
70. Kalter VG, Brody AR. Receptors for transforming growth factor-β (TGF-β) on rat lung fibroblasts have higher affinity for TGF-β_1 than for TGF-β_2. *Am J Respir Cell Mol Biol* 1991;4:397–407.
71. Segarini PR. A system of transforming growth factor-β receptors. *Am J Respir Cell Mol Biol* 1991;4:395–396.

Immunotoxicology and Immunopharmacology, Second Edition, edited by J. H. Dean, M. I. Luster, A. E. Munson, and I. Kimber.
Raven Press, Ltd., New York © 1994.

21

Beryllium Lung Disease

The Role of Cell-Mediated Immunity in Pathogenesis

Lee S. Newman

Department of Medicine, Occupational and Environmental Medicine Division and Pulmonary Division, National Jewish Center for Immunology and Respiratory Medicine, University of Colorado School of Medicine, Denver, Colorado 80206

The history of granulomatous lung disease due to beryllium illustrates how the merger of two disciplines, immunology and environmental science, has resulted in both a better understanding of the mechanism of human disease and clinically useful biologic markers of disease. As early as 1949, clinical investigators suggested the possibility of an "immune mechanism" for a newly recognized occupational lung disease occurring among workers exposed to the lightweight metal beryllium (1). In 1951, Sterner and Eisenbud (2) observed an apparent paradox: residents of a community surrounding a beryllium extraction plant were developing beryllium disease at a rate similar to the rate inside the plant, but at lower levels of exposure, seemingly in defiance of the principle of dose–response. They postulated a "hypersensitivity" mechanism despite the primitive understanding of immune mechanisms of the time. This hypothesis steadily garnered support over the next 40 years of clinical and animal research on this disorder. The portrait that emerges is of beryllium, probably interacting with native protein(s), inducing an antigen-specific cell-mediated immune response of pathologic proportion in the pulmonary compartment. In this chapter, we discuss the interrelationships between clinical manifestations of beryllium-related lung disease in humans and the immunopathogenic mechanism, relying where possible on supporting animal and cellular research that helps to inform us about the mechanisms of granulomatous inflammation.

OCCUPATIONAL AND ENVIRONMENTAL EXPOSURES

Interest in beryllium's immunologic and clinical effects stems from the recognition that beryllium presents an ongoing health risk to workers in a variety of industries including aerospace, high-technology ceramics manufacture, dental alloy manufacture, electronics, nuclear reactors, and nuclear weapons, among others. Estimates of the number of beryllium-exposed workers range as high as 800,000, although the actual number is probably lower and remains unknown (3,4). Nonoccupational, environmentally induced beryllium disease occurred in communities around beryllium extraction plants in the 1940s and 1950s due to excessive plant emissions and due to family member contact with beryllium-contaminated clothing (2,5). A recent case of disease in the spouse of a beryllium worker suggests that the risk of such second-hand contact continues in the 1990s (6).

The exposure–response relationship that produces beryllium disease has been the subject of confusion. Most published studies have estimated the rate of disease at 1% to 5% of exposed workers (7,8). When U.S. industry adopted the 1949 Atomic Energy Commission inhalational exposure standard (2 $\mu g/mm^3$ × weighted average for 8-hr day), the acute form of beryllium pneumonitis was virtually eliminated (8). It was believed that adherence to this regulatory standard eliminated chronic beryllium disease as well (7). However, studies conducted in the 1980s demonstrate that chronic disease continues to occur in industry (9,10), possibly at even low levels of exposure (11). It has been commonly, but perhaps incorrectly, believed that beryllium hypersensitivity and disease occur irrespective of the magnitude of exposure. But several recent workplace investigations at a nuclear weapons plant and a beryllium ceramics operation indicate that the risk of disease is related to work task and possibly to the magnitude of past exposure. Our research group observed that although disease prevalence was between 1% and 2% in these two industries, higher rates of disease—up to 16%—were found among workers performing certain work tasks such as machining of metal or of beryllium oxide (12–14). Industry "bystanders" such as secretaries, security guards, and parts inspectors also contract disease, but at a much lower rate. It is not known how small of an exposure can cause beryllium sensitization and disease in humans.

CHRONIC BERYLLIUM DISEASE: THE CLINICAL SPECTRUM

Several recent publications review the clinical features of beryllium-related disease in detail (15–17). The inhalation of beryllium can result in acute pneumonitis, tracheobronchitis, chronic beryllium disease, and increased risk of lung cancer (18,19). Skin contact induces contact dermatitis in some exposed workers. Inoculation of skin with beryllium splinters can produce a local cutaneous granulomatous response. This chapter focuses principally on the chronic granulomatous lung disease, although the skin and lung conditions likely share a common immunopathogenesis.

Patients with chronic beryllium disease gradually develop respiratory symptoms such as shortness of breath and cough, as well as loss of appetite and fatigue over the course of years, with an average latency of approximately 6 to 10 years following first exposure (8). Disease is generally confined to the lungs and to regional

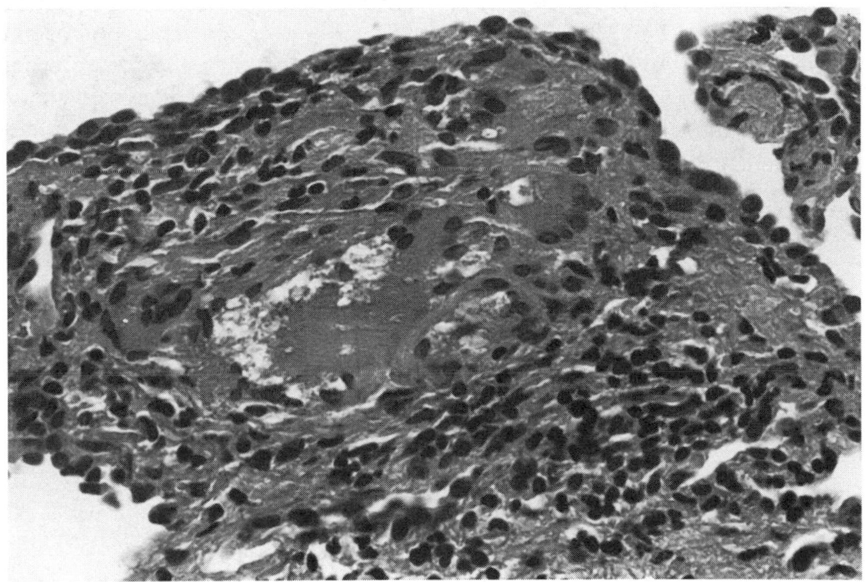

FIG. 1. Lung biopsy from patient with beryllium disease shows noncaseating granulomas with associated giant cells and infiltrates principally consisting of lymphocytes and macrophages. Hematoxylin and eosin stain, ×10.

lymph nodes, although granulomatous involvement of other organs can occur. If not treated with corticosteroids, the disease generally progresses in the lungs, producing secondary effects on the pulmonary circulation and end-stage right heart failure. Pulmonary physiologic effects such as diminution of gas exchange develop as granulomas and mononuclear cells increasingly infiltrate the interstitial space between alveoli and pulmonary capillaries. Chest radiographs, in time, reveal numerous small radiodense opacities scattered throughout the lungs, sometimes associated with obvious mediastinal lymphadenopathy. Lung and lymph node biopsies in these patients typically demonstrate multiple noncaseating granulomas with mononuclear cell (macrophage, lymphocyte, and plasma cell) infiltrates and varying degrees of fibrosis (15,20) (Fig. 1).

None of these clinical findings—symptoms, radiographs, pulmonary physiology, or even pathology—are unique to beryllium disease. A variety of other lung disorders can easily be confused with this diagnosis, including sarcoidosis, hypersensitivity pneumonitis due to inhalation of organic antigens, idiopathic pulmonary fibrosis, granulomatous lung disease due to fungi and mycobacteria, and pneumoconioses, such as silicosis and asbestosis. Not until the advent of immunologic assays of the cellular immune response to beryllium did it become possible to make a highly specific diagnosis, as discussed later.

The clinical course of chronic beryllium disease is variable, but the majority of patients experience a slow, inexorable decline in lung function with respiratory failure occurring in up to 35% of patients (8,21). However, the application of blood tests of the cellular immune response to beryllium now permits the earlier recognition of this disorder, offering an opportunity for earlier treatment that may alter the course of the disease, as discussed later. The mainstay of therapy is daily or alternate day administration of oral corticosteroids in an attempt to suppress the cellular immune response. Such treatment is not curative, but often halts or slows progression. While it is considered medically prudent to remove patients from ongoing exposure, there is little scientific evidence to indicate that cessation of exposure alters the course of disease, with the exception of one study showing that some patients spontaneously improved when they were restricted from their beryllium plant (22). In fact, most patients are first diagnosed long after their last exposure and will continue to decline. Although the majority of beryllium is removed from the lung soon after inhalation, enough beryllium is retained to induce and sustain an ongoing cellular immune response, as suggested by mass absorption data showing beryllium within lung granulomas even in retired workers with the disease (23,24).

IMMUNOPATHOGENESIS OF BERYLLIUM DISEASE

The notion that chronic beryllium disease results from a hypersensitivity response following inhalation of beryllium originated with clinical and epidemiologic evidence that conventional rules of dose–response did not appear to predict who developed disease (1,2). Since that time, we have learned that beryllium disease results from an exhuberant cellular immune response to beryllium (25,26). The observations that lead to this conclusion are summarized in Table 1.

The cardinal histopathologic finding in beryllium disease is the noncaseating granuloma (20) as is typical of antigen-driven cell-mediated immune responses (27). Beryllium is found within the granulomas and within "calcific" inclusion bodies found on some biopsies and is absent from surrounding nonpathologic lung tissue (23).

The first clinical evidence supporting a role for cellular immunity in beryllium disease in humans emerged in 1951 when Curtis (28,29) showed that patients with beryllium disease mounted a delayed-type hypersensitivity response to beryllium salt patch testing and that in some individuals the patch test induced local sarcoid-like granuloma formation at the test site three weeks later (30). Patch testing fell out of favor as a diagnostic tool for beryllium disease, largely because such testing could induce sensitization and anecdotally caused exacerbation of the lung disease in a patch-tested patient (31). Interestingly, recent evidence from the dermatology literature suggests that if a lower concentration (1% solution) of beryllium sulfate is used, patch testing may be safe (32); however, it is not known what impact even this low-dose exposure may have on those individuals with continued workplace exposure.

In a landmark 1970 paper, Hanifin and colleagues (25) examined the *in vitro*

TABLE 1. *Human evidence for a central role of beryllium-specific cellular immunity in the pathogenesis of beryllium disease*

Observation	Reference
Beryllium found in lungs and associated with pathologic lesions	23,24,84
Noncaseating granulomas and mononuclear cell infiltrates found on histologic examination of affected organs	20
Patch testing with beryllium salts induces antigen-specific delayed-type hypersensitivity response, with skin biopsies showing granulomas	28,29
Blood lymphocytes release macrophage migration inhibitory factor, when stimulated by beryllium salts *in vitro*	42
Human macrophages phagocytose beryllium and retain it within vacuoles, producing morphologic changes that correlate with *in vitro* lymphocyte proliferative response	25
Increased mRNA expression for TNF-α and IL-6 by alveolar macrophages, suggesting production of cytokines that may upregulate local immunologic responses	68
Blood lymphocytes proliferate when stimulated by beryllium salts *in vitro*	10,25,33,34,38,39
Lung washing (bronchoalveolar lavage) consists predominantly of CD4+ T lymphocytes	10,36,40
Lung lymphocytes bear "memory" T cell phenotype (CD45 RO+)	43
Lung lymphocytes proliferate when stimulated by beryllium salts *in vitro*	10,36,40
Proliferative response of lung lymphocytes is beryllium specific	43
Proliferative response to beryllium salts is IL-2 dependent	40
Proliferative response to beryllium salts is MHC class II restricted	40
T cell clones that are specific for beryllium salts can be generated from bronchoalveolar lavage and show oligoclonality	40
Individuals who are sensitized to beryllium later develop beryllium disease	44

effects of beryllium salts on monocytes and lymphocytes from patients with beryllium disease, first describing the concentration-dependent *in vitro* lymphocyte proliferative response to beryllium sulfate and to beryllium oxide in a group of seven patients with known patch test reactivity to beryllium sulfate or fluoride. In addition to the lymphocyte transformation, these authors described phenotypic differences in blood monocytes from beryllium-sensitized individuals. They reported that monocytes were larger with more pseudopods and greater cytoplasmic granularity than blood monocytes from normal subjects. These cells developed macrophage morphology within 7 to 9 days *in vitro*, compared with 10 to 14 days for normal subjects' monocytes. Addition of beryllium salts to monocytes did not accelerate the degree or extent of this macrophage morphologic differentiation. Isolated macrophages preincubated with beryllium oxide showed the capacity to phagocytose beryllium, and cells thus "activated" induced autologous lymphocyte thymidine incorporation, even in the absence of added beryllium salts, suggesting a central role for the macrophage in mediating the lymphocyte response (25). Other investigators have verified this *in vitro* cellular immune response to beryllium salts both in the blood and later in lung washing (bronchoalveolar lavage) from patients with this disorder, using morphologic, tritiated thymidine incorporation and macrophage migration inhibition assays (9,10,26,33–42).

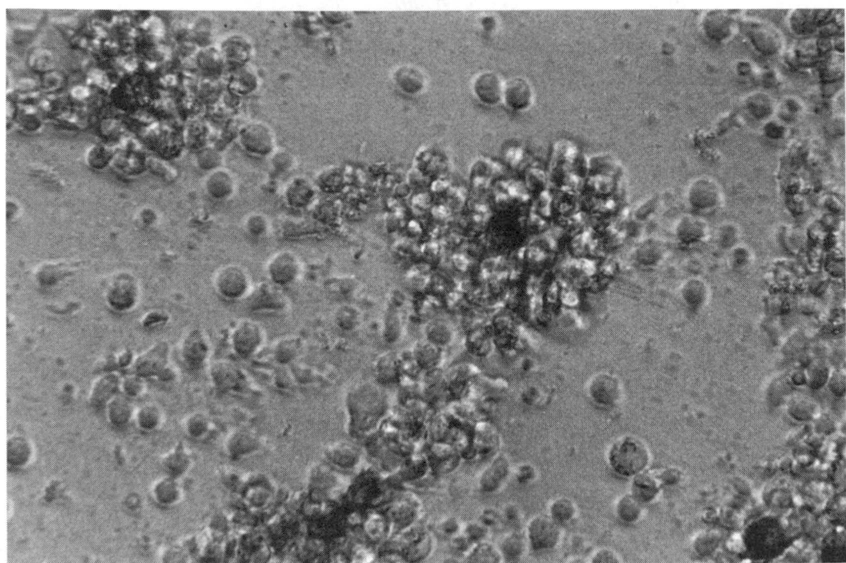

FIG. 2. *In vitro* proliferative response of bronchoalveolar lavage cells from a patient with beryllium disease, following culture with 1×10^{-5} M $BeSO_4$ for 5 days. Majority of cells are T helper lymphocytes. Clusters of blasting T cells can be seen to surround highly granular macrophages.

The lymphocyte response to beryllium salts in chronic beryllium disease is specific for beryllium salts, forming the basis for use of the lymphocyte proliferation assay as a clinical tool, discussed later (Fig. 2). The major lymphocyte populations involved in the beryllium response are T helper cells (CD4+), as suggested by both *in vitro* lymphocyte studies and by the high proportion of lymphocytes within the lungs of patients with this disorder (Fig. 3) (10,37,40). Typically, greater than 80% to 90% of the T lymphocytes in lavage of patients with beryllium disease are CD4+ and mainly of "memory" T cell phenotype (CD45RO+) (43).

Several lines of evidence suggest that these lung cells obey the basic immunologic principles observed in other diseases in which there is a cell-mediated immune response. For example, the T cell response to beryllium is interleukin-2 (IL-2) dependent (40). When Saltini and colleagues (43) blocked IL-2 receptor *in vitro*, they abrogated the beryllium-specific response of T cell lines. Using flow cytometric analysis we have observed increased IL-2 receptor expression on diseased patients' lung lymphocytes stimulated *in vitro* by beryllium sulfate along with increased shedding of soluble IL-2 receptor into the surrounding cell culture supernatant (44). Beryllium-reactive T cell clones expand *in vitro* when augmented by supplemental IL-2. The T cell response to beryllium salts appears to be oligoclonal based on evidence that clones derived from the lungs of patients differ in their antigen receptor β-chain rearrangements (40) and on preliminary data showing a limited oligoclonality based on T cell antigen repertoire assessed by quantitative polymerase

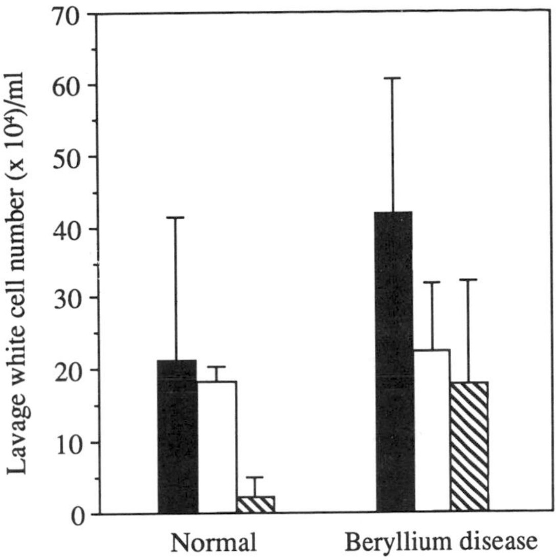

FIG. 3. Bronchoalveolar lavage fluid cellularity in normal subjects ($n = 47$) and beryllium disease patients ($n = 60$). *Bars* indicate total number of white blood cells (■), macrophages (□), and lymphocytes (□) per milliliter of lavage fluid recovered (mean and standard deviation).

chain reaction. Preliminary findings from our laboratory, using flow cytometric analysis with monoclonal antibodies directed against the β subunit of the variable region of the T cell antigen receptor (Vβ), suggest that there probably is a restricted preferential usage of a subpopulation of antigen receptors in beryllium disease.

How do these subpopulations of T cells recognize beryllium? To answer this question, one ultimately must understand the antigen and the mechanisms of antigen presentation. To date, we do not know the nature of the antigen but work on the assumption that it is *not* the beryllium moiety alone [molecular weight (MW) = 9.01] but rather some kind of beryllium–protein complex. Elemental beryllium is an amphoteric alkaline group IIA metal—able to form positive or negative ions in aqueous phase. It forms low-solubility beryllium hydroxide precipitates at neutral pH in physiologic solutions and tissue (45,46). Binding of beryllium to tissue proteins has been demonstrated by several investigators (47–51). Reeves (45) has hypothesized that at physiologic pH electrostatically charged beryllium particles associate with proteins as adsorptive complexes that may serve as the antigen in beryllium disease. However, this remains conjecture. Both exogenous and endogenous nonproteins can bind beryllium. For example, Hall (46) demonstrated that beryllium attaches to naturally occurring sulfated proteoglycans and to polysaccharides such as heparin and chondroitin sulfate; to synthetic, sulfonated, aromatic dyes; and to fixed blood lymphocytes and red blood cells. These beryllium–carrier adducts induced principally a polyclonal B cell lymphoproliferative response in the regional lymph nodes of sheep following subcutaneous injection of the materials

(52) consistent with work from our laboratory in mice showing that beryllium is a B cell but not a T cell mitogen (53).

Despite limited knowledge about the form of the antigen, we and others have begun to examine the cellular immune mechanism using beryllium salts in complete media containing human serum. Work by Saltini et al. (40) demonstrated that antigen recognition of beryllium is major histocompatibility complex (MHC) class II dependent, raising the possibility that beryllium complexes are phagocytosed by antigen-presenting cells, processed and expressed on the cell's surface in the context of MHC class II molecules, and thus presented to T lymphocytes that possess memory for the antigen, triggering lymphocyte proliferation through the appropriate T cell antigen receptor. Other metals that induce a cell-mediated immune response, such as nickel and gold, also appear to require association with MHC class II molecules on the surface of antigen presenting cells (54,55).

The details of MHC restriction and antigen specificity have not been fully investigated in beryllium disease; however, preliminary data suggest that the majority of patients with beryllium disease may share a particular HLA-Dp allele (HLA-Dp Bl) and that this allele might be a genetic marker of the risk for beryllium sensitization in beryllium-exposed populations (56). The incidence of this allele is greater than 20% among normal individuals. Other lines of evidence suggesting a "genetic susceptibility" to beryllium disease derive from the familial occurrence of beryllium disease, occurrence of disease in identical twins (57), and guinea pig and mouse studies showing histocompatibility locus antigen (HLA)-associated strain differences in animal susceptibility to beryllium-induced lung injury (58–62). Much additional research would be needed to unravel the immunogenetics of beryllium disease, especially in regard to (a) the immunologic function of genetic markers; (b) their clinical relevance, as assessed in population-based research of beryllium diseased and beryllium-exposed/nondiseased work forces; and (c) the interaction of genetics with environmental exposure to beryllium.

While a MHC class II/T cell antigen receptor/antigen interaction seems likely to be responsible for the induction of beryllium sensitization, alternative explanations might include (a) direct binding of beryllium to MHC or (b) intracellular triggering of the antigen-presenting cell to generate new antigenic peptides. The later theory gains some very indirect support from work showing histochemical localization of beryllium in the cell nucleus (63), its specific binding to a class of nonhistone nuclear proteins (51), the observed effects of beryllium on cellular enzyme induction and gene transcription (64,65), and as a selective regulator of gene expression (66).

Although it is increasingly clear that beryllium disease develops as a result of a cell-mediated immune response following exposure, it is less clear how or why this response goes awry, resulting in progressive disease. Just as some immunotoxins induce immunosuppression, others such as beryllium result in unabated immunopotentiation. Animal and human studies indicate that the development and maintenance of granulomas in the lungs and other organs depend on the presence of antigen, antigen-presenting cells, memory T lymphocytes, and the synchronous release of key proinflammatory cytokines by effector macrophages and lymphocytes (27,67). After antigen recognition occurs, cells in the lung microenvironment may proliferate locally while others migrate to the site of inflammation along a chemoattractive gradient. As more T cells and activated effector macrophages accumulate in the lung, the granulomatous response becomes amplified through a network of cytokines (67). Preliminary data suggest that this scenario applies to human beryllium disease. Not only do the beryllium-reactive lymphocytes from the lungs of patients with beryllium disease produce IL-2 but alveolar macrophages from these patients also express messenger ribonucleic acid (mRNA) and produce increased quantities of key factors, including tumor necrosis factor-α (TNF-α) and IL-6 (68). These macrophage-derived cytokines are known to potentiate inflammatory and cell-mediated immune responses and, in particular, help upregulate T cell activity (69–74). Hence it is attractive to postulate that a cytokine amplification loop involving macrophages, lymphocytes, and probably other cells in the lung interstitium results in the growth and maintenance of pulmonary granulomas in beryllium disease.

This still does not address squarely the question of why beryllium induces such a sustained inflammatory response. However, a clue to the mechanism underlying granuloma maintenance may come through a better understanding of beryllium's adjuvancy. Beryllium is a known adjuvant (46,52,75–77) capable of increasing expression of immune-associated antigen (Ia) glycoproteins by mouse macrophages in a dose-dependent manner (78), enhancing antigen presentation *in vivo* (76) and inducing slightly increased release of IL-1 (79). Thus it has been hypothesized that the adjuvancy of beryllium, perhaps like that of lipopolysaccharide (LPS), occurs because these compounds initiate or amplify cellular interactions through the induction and release of cytokines (78). In contrast, other investigators have observed lymphocyte proliferation and adjuvant activity due to beryllium unrelated to cytokine production, as measured in the efferent lymphatics of sheep (46). And yet others have demonstrated that beryllium can interact directly with lymphocytes, which when taken in conjunction with the observation that beryllium binds acidic nonhistone nuclear proteins (51) raises the possibility of a direct beryllium–lymphocyte interaction regulating cell division. Clearly, more research is needed to clarify the role of beryllium adjuvancy and the mechanisms that lead to granuloma elicitation and maintenance.

ANIMAL MODELS OF CELL-MEDIATED IMMUNITY TO BERYLLIUM

Although the human was the first "animal model" of beryllium disease, the study of other species has improved our understanding of the role of cell-mediated immunity and of exposure to beryllium. Table 2 summarizes some of the major pathologic and immunologic research on animals exposed to beryllium metal, oxides, and/or salts. The animal models vary widely in the route and schedule of immunization, method and form of beryllium exposure, species, outcome variables measured, and success in inducing sensitization, histologic changes, or both. In several

TABLE 2. *Animal evidence for role of beryllium-specific cellular immunity in the pathogenesis of chronic beryllium disease*

Observation	Reference
Pathologic changes	
Beryllium sulfate inhalation, monkeys, rats, dogs, cats, rabbits, guinea pigs, hamsters, mice	85
Beyllium oxide inhalation, dogs	80,86
Beryllium oxide inhalation, rats	87–89
Beryllium sulfate inhalation, rats	88,90
Beryllium ores (beryl and bertrandite) inhalation, rats and hamsters	88
Beryllium oxide inhalation, nonhuman primates	80
Cell-mediated immune reponse to beryllium	
Guinea pigs	60–62,93
Rats	94,95
Mice	58,82
Sheep	46,52
Dogs	81
Nonhuman primates	80
Cellular effects	
Macrophages	
Instillation of beryllium sulfate induces Ia-positive macrophage exudate	78
Phagocytosis and vacuolization of beryllium	87
Initially decreased phagocytosis, later increased	89
Beryllium acts as adjuvant, directly increasing antigen presentation	75,76
Beryllium increases Ia expression by mouse macrophages	78
Beryllium weakly stimulates release of IL-1	79
Lymphocytes	
Beryllium interacts with lymphocyte membrane	52,91,92
Polyclonal B cell response in sheep *in vivo*	46,52,77
Mitogenic for mouse B cells but not T cells	53

species, the beryllium-specific immunologic response is sometimes, although not always, associated with the development of pulmonary granulomas upon inhalational or intratracheal challenge (see Table 2). The histopathology found in most of the models only vaguely resembles the morphologic appearance of granulomas in humans and usually resolves spontaneously. Nonetheless, the principal conclusions drawn from these animal studies are that (a) beryllium induces a cell-mediated immune response and (b) it can induce granuloma formation.

Recent work in dogs and mice has focused on both immunologic responsiveness and pulmonary pathology (58,80–82). Haley and colleagues (81) exposed dogs to aerosols of beryllium oxide and assessed both lung histology and cellular immune responses over time by performing serial sacrifices. In this study, animals developed patchy granulomatous infiltrates and focal consolidation with lymphocytes, plasma cells, and macrophages, especially in dogs that were exposed to low-fired (500 °C) beryllium oxide. Lesions resolved within 1 year. Lavage cells from dogs that received 50 μg/kg body weight initial lung burden demonstrated a positive lymphocyte proliferative response to beryllium sulfate *in vitro*, confirming sensitization. Newman (82) sensitized mice by a series of subcutaneous injections with beryllium sulfate in incomplete Freund's adjuvant. He demonstrated formation of granulomas within the lungs, but these tended to be poorly formed. Beryllium-specific delayed-type hypersensitivity was confirmed by measuring footpad swelling. Lymphocytes showed a modest proliferative response in sensitized versus control animals (82). Subsequently, Huang and colleagues (58) demonstrated that the quality of the histopathologic and immunologic response to beryllium varies with mouse strain and Ia-associated MHC determinant. Following one of several schedules of preimmunization, animals received intratracheal beryllium sulfate or beryllium oxide. Although bronchoalveolar lavage cells from these mice developed only a low-level lymphocyte proliferative response (two- to fourfold), the lavage and biopsies showed sequential appearance of neutrophils followed by CD4+ lymphocytes and macrophages, forming mature granulomas and some areas of fibrosis. Cutaneous granulomas formed at the site of beryllium exposure.

APPLICATION OF IMMUNOLOGIC MECHANISMS TO DETECTION OF HUMAN DISEASE

Beryllium disease demonstrates how our emerging understanding of immunology can lead to clinical application. Immunologic assessment of beryllium sensitization provides (a) diagnostic information and (b) a useful medical surveillance biomarker that can be used in industry to identify disease at early stages (83).

The use of the beryllium-specific lymphocyte proliferation test (BeLT, also known as the beryllium lymphocyte transformation test or LTT) as a clinical diagnostic tool was suggested by several studies conducted in the 1980s using peripheral blood specimens from patients with disease and from exposed workers (34,35,41). However, the test was felt to be insensitive and poorly reproducible, leading to its abandonment until two events occurred in the 1980s and early 1990s. First, Epstein and colleagues (36) demonstrated that the BeLT could be performed using cells recovered from bronchoalveolar lavage, as an indication of a beryllium-specific cellular immune response occurring within the pulmonary compartment. Second, our group refined the blood BeLT using radiolabeled deoxyribonucleic acid (DNA) precursors as marker of proliferation and then validated the test in field studies of exposed workers. We demonstrated that an improved version of the proliferation assay was reliable and reproducible as an indicator of beryllium sensitization, could identify nearly all the patients that were found to have bronchoalveolar lavage lymphocyte responses to beryllium, and identified patients with disease at a very early stage (9,10,39). Several case series have demonstrated that the BeLT, as an indicator of beryllium-specific cellular immune response, is elevated in patients with beryllium disease, but not elevated in normal subjects, beryllium-exposed normal subjects, beryllium-exposed subjects with other (nongranulomatous) lung diseases, and patients with no beryllium exposure but who have granulomatous diseases such as sarcoidosis and hypersensitivity pneumonitis (36–39) (Fig. 4). Therefore the blood or the lavage BeLT can be used to help diagnose beryllium disease in patients

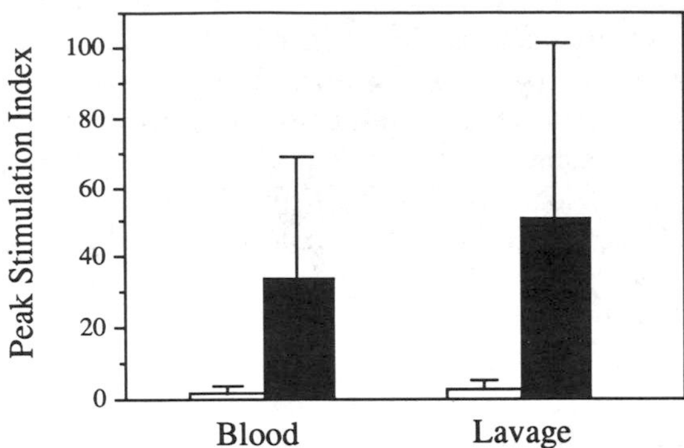

FIG. 4. Peak stimulation index in response to $BeSO_4$ (39) in patients with beryllium disease ($n = 42$), for blood mononuclear cells and bronchoalveolar lavage cells. Shown in *white bars* are blood cell results for 31 normal, nonexposed individuals and lavage cell results for 17 patients who have other forms of granulomatous lung disease *not* due to beryllium (mean and standard deviation).

with compatible lung pathology, helping to differentiate it from similar appearing lung diseases. This assay has now become part of the standard clinical armamentarium in beryllium disease diagnosis. Although the test is performed in only a few centers in the United States, it can be obtained in this country by shipping blood by overnight carrier.

Interestingly, not every individual with an abnormal blood response to beryllium has beryllium disease (9). Some beryllium-sensitized individuals have repeatedly abnormal blood BeLTs but do not have pulmonary pathology, lavage lymphocytosis, or lavage lymphocyte reactivity to beryllium. In our group's experience with 3 years of longitudinal follow-up of beryllium-sensitized/nondiseased individuals, half have progressed, developing granulomas within the lung and accumulating beryllium-reactive T cells in the pulmonary compartment (44). This progress from sensitization to disease occurs even among individuals who have been removed from exposure (44). These data suggest that beryllium sensitization precedes disease. The mode of sensitization and the disease-triggering mechanism are not understood.

Having established the validity of the BeLT in diagnosis, our group turned to the question of whether this assay could be used as a medical surveillance tool for the detection of disease among exposed workers in the beryllium industry (9,12–14). This population-based research using the blood BeLT as a biologic marker of beryllium sensitization was stimulated by the observations that (a) we can identify beryllium-sensitized individuals who have no disease and (b) workers who are found to have disease are often at a subclinical stage (9). They may be asymptomatic, have normal chest radiographs, and normal lung function tests but are found to have both lavage BeLT reactivity and noncaseating granulomas in their lung biopsies. We have observed progression of symptoms, radiographic opacities, and pulmonary physiology in some but not all of these subclinical disease patients, despite removal from exposure (44). In a study of nuclear weapons workers, the blood BeLT was abnormal in 1.9% of exposed workers (9,14). In a study of beryllium-exposed ceramics workers, 1.8% of tested individuals were found to have disease. But interestingly, the prevalence of disease was much higher—as much as 15.8%—in certain jobs in the plant associated with higher dust exposure (13). Compared with other tests used conventionally in medical surveillance, the blood BeLT has proved more sensitive than the patient's report of symptoms, the physician's physical examination, measurement of lung function by spirometry, diffusing capacity, or chest radiograph. In both population-based epidemiologic studies, we observed that the blood BeLT had high positive and negative predictive value for beryllium disease (9,13,14). As a result, the beryllium industry and the Departrnent of Energy initiated broad-based medical screening with this immune biomarker in 1992.

The most useful biomarkers of disease are those that are clearly related to biologic events of pathophysiologic significance (83) as in the case of the BeLT. The BeLT assay specifically measures the relevant T cell proliferative response to beryllium and is highly predictive of disease. The utility of a biomarker of disease depends on the sensitivity of the test: Does it identify disease at early stages? As discussed earlier, the BeLT is superior to any existing clinical screening tool used in beryllium disease detection and identifies preclinical sensitization and subclinical disease. The merit of a biomarker of disease hinges also on whether early detection results in improved outcome for the exposed and/or afflicted individuals. Thus far, it is not known whether those individuals with early disease who are identified through workplace screening with the BeLT have a better prognosis than those who come to clinical attention later in the course of disease. Although it is probable that early diagnosis leads to better patient management, earlier treatment, improved morbidity, and reduced mortality, this warrants further study. Besides such secondary prevention, the blood BeLT could lead to more effective primary prevention. In industries where we have linked the results of blood BeLT testing with exposure data and job histories, we have discovered certain high-risk tasks in the workplace. Equipped with this information, managers, engineers, and industrial hygienists hopefully can make specific modification in work practices and ventilation systems that should reduce the number of new cases of sensitization and disease. It must not be forgotten that beryllium disease only occurs when there has been beryllium exposure. Despite its proven value as a screening tool, the BeLT, like most cell culture-radiolabel incorporation assays, is associated with some intratest, intertest, and interlaboratory variability and provides only a semiquantitative estimate of T cell activity, even when we optimize the methodology (39). Further methodologic refinements may enhance the test's reliability and predictive value.

SUMMARY

Beryllium lung disease occurs when exposure to beryllium results in an exhuberant cell-mediated immune response. Human and animal studies of immunopotentiation due to beryllium have helped us understand the mechanisms underlying metal-induced inflammatory responses within the pulmonary compartment. In turn, such information has provided clinicians and epidemiologists with specific and sensitive biologic markers for use in diagnosis and workplace surveillance efforts.

ACKNOWLEDGMENTS

Research was supported by Physician Scientist Award ES-00173, Grant ES-04843 and SCOR Grant HL-27353 from U.S. Public Health Service, National Institutes of Health. I wish to thank Christine Comment, Beverly Schumacher, Sallie Seay, Margaret Mroz, M.S.P.H., Brian Watson, Cynthia Bobka, Tom Bost, M.D., David Riches, Ph.D., and Kathleen Kreiss, M.D. for their contributions to this work. Special thanks to Nina Eads for her expert secretarial support.

REFERENCES

1. DeNardi JM, Van Ordstrand HS, Carmody MG. Acute dermatitis and pneumonitis in beryllium workers. *Ohio State Med J* 1949;45;567–575.
2. Sterner JH, Eisenbud M. Epidemiology of beryllium intoxication. *Arch Ind Hyg Occup Med* 1951; 4:123–151.
3. National Occupational Health Survey, DHEW Publication No. (NIOSH) 78–114. National Institute for Occupational Safety and Health; 1978.
4. Cullen MR, Cherniack MG, Kominsky JR. Chronic beryllium disease in the United States. *Semin Respir Med* 1986;7:203–209.
5. Lieben J, Metzner F. Epidemiological findings associated with beryllium extraction. *Am Ind Hyg Assoc J* 1959;20:494–499.
6. Newman LS, Kreiss K. Non-occupational chronic beryllium disease masquerading as sarcoidosis: identification by blood lymphocyte proliferative response to beryllium. *Am Rev Respir Dis* 1992; 145:1212–1214.
7. Eisenbud M, Lisson J. Epidemiological aspects of beryllium-induced nonmalignant lung disease: a 30-year update. *J Occup Med* 1983;25:196–202.
8. Kreibel D, Brain JD, Sprince NL. The pulmonary toxicity of beryllium. *Am Rev Respir Dis* 1988; 137:464–473.
9. Kreiss K, Newman LS, Mroz MM, Campbell PA. Screening blood test identifies subclinical berylium disease. *J Occup Med* 1989;31:603–608.
10. Newman LS, Kreiss K, King TE Jr, Seay S, Campbell PA. Pathologic and immunological alterations in early stages of beryllium disease: re-examination of disease definition and natural history. *Am Rev Respir Dis* 1989;139:1479–1486.
11. Cullen MR, Kominsky JR, Rossman MD, et al. Chronic beryllium disease in a precious metal refinery: clinical epidemiologic and immunologic evidence for continuing risk from exposure to low level beryllium fume. *Am Rev Respir Dis* 1987;135:201–208.
12. Kreiss K, Newman LS, Mroz MM, Campbell PA. Screening blood test identifies subclinical beryllium disease. *J Occup Med* 1989;603–608.
13. Kreiss K, Wasserman S, Mroz MM, Newman LS. Beryllium disease screening in the ceramics industry: blood lymphocyte test performance and exposure–disease relations. *J Occup Med* 1993;35:267–274.
14. Kreiss K, Mroz MM, Zhen B, Martyny J, Newman LS. The epidemiology of beryllium sensitization and disease in nuclear workers. *Am Rev Respir Dis* 1993;148:985–991.
15. Rose CS, Newman LS. Hypersensitivity pneumonitis and chronic beryllium disease. In: Schwarz MI, King TE Jr, eds. *Interstitial lung disease*, 2nd ed. St Louis: Mosby Year Book; 1993:231–253.
16. Newman LS. Beryllium. In: Sullivan JB, Krieger GR, eds. *Hazardous materials toxicology*. Baltimore: Williams & Wilkins; 1991:882–890.

17. Kriebel D, Brain JD, Sprince NL, Kazemi H. The pulmonary toxicity of beryllium. *Am Rev Respir Dis* 1988;137:464–474.
18. Ward E, Okun A, Ruder A, Fingerhut M, Steenland K. A mortality study of workers at seven beryllium processing plants. *Am J Ind Med* 1992;22:885–904.
19. Steenland K, Ward E. Lung cancer incidence among patients with beryllium disease: a cohort mortality study. *J Natl Cancer Inst* 1991;83:1380–1385.
20. Freiman DG, Hardy HL. Beryllium disease: the relation of pulmonary pathology to clinical course and prognosis based on a study of 130 cases from the U.S. Beryllium Case Registry. *Hum Pathol* 1970;1:25–44.
21. Kriebel D, Sprince NL, Eisen EA, Greaves IA, Feldman HA, Greene RE. Beryllium exposure and pulmonary functions: a cross-sectional study of beryllium workers. *Br J Ind Med* 1988;45:167–173.
22. Sprince NL, Kanarek DJ, Weber AL, Chamberlin RI, Kazemi H. Reversible respiratory disease in beryllium workers. *Am Rev Respir Dis* 1978;117:1011–1017.
23. Jones Williams W, Kelland D. New aid for diagnosing chronic beryllium disease (CBD): laser ion mass analysis (LIMA). *J Clin Pathol* 1986;39:900–901.
24. Jones Williams W, Wallach ER. Laser microprobe mass spectrometry (LAMMS) analysis of beryllium, sarcoidosis, and other granulomatous diseases. *Sarcoidosis* 1989;6:111–117.
25. Hanifin JM, Epstein WL, Cline MJ. *In vitro* studies of granulomatous hypersensitivity to beryllium. *J Invest Dermatol* 1970;55:284–288.
26. Deodhar SD, Barna B, Van Ordstrand HS. A study of the immunologic aspects of chronic berylliosis. *Chest* 1973;63:309–313.
27. Boros DL. Mechanisms of granuloma formation in the lung. In: Daniele RP, ed. *Immunology and immunologic diseases of the lung*. Boston: Blackwell Scientific Publications; 1988:263–287.
28. Curtis GH. Cutaneous hypersensitivity due to beryllium. *Arch Dermatol Syph* 1951;64:470–482.
29. Curtis GH. The diagnosis of beryllium disease with special reference to the patch test. *Arch Ind Health* 1959;19:150–156.
30. Sneddon IB. Berylliosis case report. *Br Med J* 1955;1:1448–1450.
31. Waksman BH. Discussion of "The diagnosis of beryllium disease with special reference to the patch test" by GH Curtis. *Arch Ind Health* 1959;19:154–156.
32. Haberman AL, Pratt M, Storrs FJ. Contact dermatitis from beryllium in dental alloys. *Contact Dermatitis* 1993;28:157–162.
33. Van Ganse WF, Oleffe J, Van Hove W, Groetenbrie JC. Lymphocyte transformation in chronic berylliosis. *Lancet* 1972;1:1023.
34. Williams WR, Jones Williams WJ. Development of beryllium lymphocyte transformation tests in chronic beryllium disease. *Int Arch Allergy Appl Immunol* 1982;67:175–180.
35. Williams WR, Jones Williams W. Comparison of lymphocyte transformation and macrophage migration inhibition tests in the detection of beryllium hypersensitivity. *J Clin Pathol* 1982;35:684–687.
36. Epstein PE, Dauber JH, Rossman MD, Daniele RP. Bronchoalveolar lavage in a patient with chronic berylliosis: evidence for hypersensitivity pneumonitis. *Ann Intern Med* 1982;97:213–216.
37. Rossman MD, Kern JA, Elias JA, Cullen MR, Epstein PE, Preuss OP, Markham TN, Daniele RP. Proliferative response of bronchoalveolar lymphocytes to beryllium: a test for chronic beryllium disease. *Ann Intern Med* 1988;108:687–693.
38. Bargon J, Kronenberger H, Bergmann L, Buhl R, Meier-Sydow J, Mitrou P. Lymphocyte transformation test in a group of foundry workers exposed to beryllium and non-exposed controls. *Eur J Respir Dis* 1986;69 (Suppl 136):211–215.
39. Mroz MM, Kreiss K, Lezotte DC, Campbell PA, Newman LS. Re-examination of the blood lymphocyte transformation test in the diagnosis of chronic beryllium disease. *J Allergy Clin Immunol* 1991;88:54–60.
40. Saltini C, Winestock K, Kirby M, Pinkston P, Crystal RG. Maintenance of alveolitis in patients with chronic beryllium disease by beryllium-specific helper T cells. *N Engl J Med* 1989;320:1103–1109.
41. Jones William W, Williams WR. Value of beryllium lymphocyte transformation tests in chronic beryllium disease and in potentially exposed workers. *Thorax* 1983;38:41–44.
42. Price CD, Pugh A, Pioli EM, Jones Williams W. Beryllium macrophage migration inhibition test. *Ann NY Acad Sci* 1976;278:204–211.
43. Saltini C, Kirby M, Trapnell BC, Tamura N, Crystal RB. Biased accumulation of T lymphocytes with "memory"-type CD45 leukocyte common antigen gene expression on the epithelial surface of the human lung. *J Exp Med* 1990;171:1123–1140.

44. Newman LS, Mroz MM, Schumacher B, Daniloff E, Kreiss K. Beryllium sensitization precedes chronic beryllium disease. *Am Rev Respir Dis Suppl* 1992;145:A324.
45. Reeves AL. The immunotoxicity of beryllium. In: Gibson GG, Hubbard R, Parke DV, eds. *Immunotoxicity*. London:Academic Press; 1983:261–282.
46. Hall JG. Studies on the adjuvant action of beryllium: effect on individual lymph nodes. *Immunology* 1984;53;105–120.
47. Aldridge WN, Barnes JM, Denz FA. Biochemical changes in acute beryllium poisoning. *Br J Exp Pathol* 1950;31:473–484.
48. Reiner E. Binding of beryllium to proteins. In: Aldridge WN, ed. *Symposium on mechanism of toxicity*. New York: St Martin's Press; 1971:111–125.
49. Vasil'eva EV. Immunologic assessment of a model of experimental berylliosis. *Byull Eksper Biol Med* 1969;III:74–77.
50. Vasil'eva EV. Changes in the antigenic composition of the lungs in experimental berylliosis. *Byull Eksper Biol Med* 1972;II:76–80.
51. Parker VH, Stevens C. Binding of beryllium to nuclear acidic proteins. *Chem Biol Interact* 1979; 26:167–177.
52. Hall JG. Studies on the adjuvant action of beryllium: IV. The preparation of beryllium containing macromolecules that induce immunoblast responses *in vivo*. *Immunology* 1988;64:345–351.
53. Newman LS, Campbell PA. Mitogenic effect of beryllium sulfate on mouse B lymphocytes but not T lymphocytes *in vitro*. *Int Arch Allergy Appl Immunol* 1987;84:223–227.
54. Romagnoli P, Spinas GA, Sinigaglia F. Gold-specific T cells in rheumatoid arthritis patients treated with gold. *J Clin Invest* 1992;89:254–258.
55. Sinigaglia F, Scheidegger D, Garotta G, Scheper R, Pletscher M, Lanzavecchia A. Isolation and characterization of Ni-specific T cell clones from patients with Ni-contact dermatitis. *J Immunol* 1985;135:3929–3932.
56. Richeldi L, Persichini T, Ferrara GB, et al. Chronic beryllium disease association with the HLA-DP 2.1 Allele. *Am Rev Respir Dis Suppl* 1992;145:A324.
57. McConnochie K, Williams WR, Kilpatrick GS, Jones Williams W. Chronic beryllium disease in identical twins. *Br J Dis Chest* 1988;82:431–435.
58. Huang H, Meyer KC, Kubai L, Auerbach R. An immune model of beryllium-induced pulmonary granulomata in mice: histopathology, immune reactivity, and flow-cytometric analysis of bronchoalveolar lavage-derived cells. *Lab Invest* 1992;67:138–146.
59. Turk JL, Polak L. Experimental studies on metal dermatities in guinea pigs. *G Ital Dermatol* 1969; 44:426–430.
60. Barna BP, Chiang T, Pillarisetti SG, Deodhar SD. Immunologic studies of experimental beryllium lung disease in the guinea pig. *Clin Immunol Immunopathol* 1981;20:402.
61. Barna BP, Deodhar SD, Chiang T, Gautam S, Edinger M. Experimental beryllium-induced lung disease: I. Differences in immunologic response to beryllium compounds in strains 2 and 13 guinea pigs. *Int Arch Allergy Appl Immunol* 1984;73:42–48.
62. Barna BP, Deodhar SD, Gautam S, Edinger M, Chiang T, McMahon JT. Experimental beryllium-induced lung disease: II. Analyses of bronchial lavage cells in strains 2 and 13 guinea pigs. *Int Arch Allergy Appl Immunol* 1984;73:49–55.
63. Firket H. Mise en évidence histochimique du béryllium dans des cellules cult. *R Soc Biol (Paris)* 1953;147:167.
64. Witschi HP. Effects of beryllium on deoxyribonucleic acid-synthesizing enzymes in regenerating rat liver. *Biochem J* 1970;120:623–634.
65. Witschi HP, Marchand P. Interference of beryllium with enzyme induction in rat liver. *Toxicol Appl Pharmacol* 1971;20:565–572.
66. Perry ST, Kulkarni SB, Lee K-L, Kenney FT. Selective effect of the metallocarcinogen beryllium on hormonal regulation of gene expression in cultured cells. *Cancer Res* 1982;42:473–476.
67. Kunkel SL, Chensue SW, Strieter RM, Lynch JP, Remick DG. Cellular and molecular aspects of granulomatous inflammation. *Am J Respir Cell Mol Biol* 1989;1:439–447.
68. Bost T, Riches DWH, Carré PC, et al. Alveolar macrophages from patients with beryllium disease and sarcoidosis express increased levels of mRNA for TNF-α and IL-1β but not IL-1β. *Am J Respir Cell Mol Biol* 1994;10:506–513.
69. Garman RD, Jacobs KA, Clark SC, Raulet DH. B-cell-stimulatory factor 2 ($\beta_2$interferon) functions as a second signal for interleukin 2 production by mature murine T cells. *Proc Natl Acad Sci USA* 1987;84:7629–7633.

70. Jayaraman S, Martin CA, Dorf ME. Enhancement of in vivo cell-mediated immune responses by three distinct cytokines. *J Immunol* 1990;144:942–951.
71. Van Snick J. Interleukin-6: an overview. *Annu Rev Immunol* 1990;8:253–278.
72. Houssiau FA, Coulie PG, Olive D, Van Snick J. Synergistic activation of human T cells by interleukin 1 and interleukin 6. *Eur J Immunol* 1988;18:653–656.
73. Cox GW, Melillo G, Chattopadhyay U, Mullet D, Fertel RH, Varesio L. Tumor necrosis factor-α-dependent production of reactive nitrogen intermediates mediates IFN-γ plus IL-2–induced murine macrophage tumoricidal activity. *J Immunol* 1992;149:3290–3296.
74. Bachwich PR, Chensue SW, Larrick JW, Kunkel SL. Tumor necrosis factor stimulated interleukin-1 and prostaglandin E_2 production in resting macrophages. *Biochem Biophys Res Commun* 1986;136:94–101.
75. Salvaggio JE, Flax MH, Leskowitz S. Studies in immunization: III. The use of beryllium as a granuloma-producing agent in Freund's adjuvant. *J Immunol* 1965;95:846–854.
76. Unanue ER, Askonas BA, Allison AC. A role of macrophages in the stimulation of immune responses by adjuvants. *J Immunol* 1969;103:71–78.
77. Denham S, Hall JG. Studies on the adjuvant action of beryllium: III. The activity in the plasma of lymph efferent from nodes stimulated with beryllium. *Immunology* 1988;64:341–344.
78. Behbehani K, Beller DI, Unanue ER. The effects of beryllium and other adjuvants on Ia expression by macrophages. *J Immunol* 1985;134:2047–2049.
79. Unanue ER, Kiely J-M, Calderon J. The modulation of lymphocyte functions by molecules secreted by macrophages: II. Conditions leading to increased secretion. *J Exp Med* 1976;144:155–166.
80. Haley PJ, Finch GL, Hoover MD. The comparative pulmonary toxicity of beryllium metal and oxide in nonhuman primates. *Am Rev Respir Dis Suppl* 1991;143:A219.
81. Haley PJ, Finch GL, Mewhinney JA, Harmsen AG, Hahn FF, Moover MD, Bice DE. A canine model of beryllium-induced granulomatous lung disease. *Lab Invest* 1989;61:219–227.
82. Newman LS. Antigen-specific T cells in a mouse model of beryllium disease. In: Grassi C, Rizzato G, Polli E, eds. *Proceedings of XI World Conference on sarcoidosis and other granulomatous disorders*. Amsterdam: Excerpta Medica; 1988:715–716.
83. Wilcosky TC, Griffith JD. Applications of biological markers. In: Hulka BS, Wilcosky TC, Griffith JD, eds. *Biological markers in epidemiology*. New York: Oxford University Press; 1990:16–27.
84. Schepers GWH. The mineral content of the lung in chronic berylliosis. *J Dis Chest* 1962;42:600–607.
85. Stokinger HE, Sprague GF III, Hall RH, Ashenburg NJ, Scott JK, Steadman LT. Acute inhalation toxicity of beryllium. *Arch Ind Hyg Occup Med* 1950;1:379–397.
86. Robinson FR, Schaffner F, Trachtenberg E. Ultrastructure of the lungs of dogs exposed to beryllium-containing dusts. *Arch Environ Health* 1968;17:193–203.
87. Sanders CL, Cannon WC, Powers GJ, Adee RR, Meier DM. Toxicology of high-fired beryllium oxide inhaled by rodents. 1. Metabolism and early effects. *Arch Environ Health* 1975;30:546–551.
88. Wagner WD, Groth DH, Holtz JL, Madden GE, Stokinger HE. Comparative chronic inhalation toxicity of beryllium ores, bertrandite, and beryl, with production of pulmonary tumors by beryl. *Toxicol Appl Pharmacol* 1969;15:10–29.
89. Hart BA, Harmsen AG, Low RB, Emerson R. Biochemical, cytological, and histological alterations in rat lung following acute beryllium aerosol exposure. *Toxicol Appl Pharrnacol* 1984;75:454–465.
90. Vorwald AJ, Reeves AL, Urban EJ. Experimental beryllium toxicology. In: Stokinger HE, ed. *Beryllium: its industrial hygiene aspects*. New York: Academic Press; 1966;201–234.
91. Skilleter DN, Price RJ, Legg RF. Specific G_1-S phase cell cycle block by beryllium as demonstrated by cytofluorometric analysis. *Biochem J* 1983;216:773–776.
92. Price RJ, Skilleter DN. Stimulatory and cytotoxic effects of beryllium on proliferation of mouse spleen lymphocytes in vitro. *Arch Toxicol* 1985;56:207–211.
93. Reeves AL. Berylliosis as an autoimmune disorder. *Ann Clin Lab Sci* 1976;6:256–262.
94. Votto JJ, Barton RW, Gionfriddo MA, Cole SR, McCormick JR, Thrall RS. A model of pulmonary granulomas induced by beryllium sulfate in the rat. *Sarcoidosis* 1987;4:71–76.
95. Bencko V, Brezina M, Banes B, Cikrt M. Penetration of beryllium through the placenta and its distribution in the mouse. *J Hyg Epidemiol Microbiol Immunol* 1979;23:361–367.

Immunotoxicology and Immunopharmacology, Second Edition, edited by J. H. Dean, M. I. Luster, A. E. Munson, and I. Kimber.
Raven Press, Ltd., New York, 1994.

22

Effects of Gaseous Air Pollutants on Immune Responses and Susceptibility to Infectious and Allergic Disease

MaryJane K. Selgrade and *Matthew I. Gilmour

*Immunotoxicology Branch, Health Effects Research Laboratory, United States Environmental Protection Agency, Research Triangle Park, North Carolina 27711; and *Center for Environmental Medicine and Lung Biology, University of North Carolina, Chapel Hill, North Carolina 27599*

Air pollution has long been considered a risk factor for respiratory infection. Reactive gases, which have been of most concern and hence most extensively studied, are those associated with fossil fuel emissions including ozone (O_3), nitrogen dioxide (NO_2), and sulfur dioxide (SO_2). Epidemiologic studies suggesting a relationship between air pollution and incidence, severity, and duration of symptoms related to respiratory infection span four decades. Lunn et al. (1) reported that chronic upper and lower respiratory tract infections were more prevalent (by approximately 100% and 50%, respectively) in young children living in areas designated as highly polluted (based on smoke and SO_2 emissions) than in relatively "clean" areas of Sheffield, England. Upper respiratory tract infections were recognized by mucopurulent nasal discharge, a history of three or more colds per year, and scarred or perforated eardrums. Lower respiratory tract infections were indicated by persistent or frequent cough, chest cold, or episodes of pneumonia and bronchitis. Excessive acute respiratory disease (primarily sore throat) in children and adults was also found in U.S. communities heavily polluted with SO_2 and suspended sulfates (2). Higher ambient sulfate levels were found to have a positive effect on the incidence of cold or sore throat in children in Chattanooga, Tennessee, but a similar correlation was not found with NO_2 (3). Similarly, Ware et al. (4) found no correlation between respiratory illness and indoor exposure to NO_2 generated by combustion of gas for cooking, and Samet et al. (5) recently reported no association between

The research chapter has been reviewed by the Health Effects Research Laboratory, United States Environmental Protection Agency and approved for publication. Approval does not signify that the contents necessarily reflect the views and policies of the agency, nor does mention of trade names or commercial products constitute endorsement for use.

indoor air exposure to NO_2 and respiratory illness in infants under 2 years old. However, in other studies the incidence of acute respiratory illness was greater in children from households with gas stoves (6) and a 15-ppb increase in household annual NO_2 exposure was associated with an increase of approximately 20% in cumulative incidence of lower respiratory tract symptoms in children (7). More recently, an association was reported between NO_2 exposure and increased incidence of croup in children under 2 years old (8). Finally, exposure to photochemical oxidants (predominantly O_3) has been associated with an increase by as much as 50% in the duration of episodes of coughing, phlegm, and sore throat among nursing students in Los Angeles (9). While the epidemiologic data are sometimes contradictory (particularly with respect to NO_2), several studies suggest that exposure to gaseous air pollutants enhances susceptibility to respiratory infections and, by inference, that these gases may somehow impair host immune defenses in the respiratory tract.

In addition to this evidence that air pollution may have immunosuppressive effects in the respiratory tract, there is now concern that these same pollutants may also exacerbate allergic disease or asthma. Since population studies have shown that both allergens (10,11) and air pollutants, including O_3, NO_2, particulates, SO_2, and mixed pollutants (12–17), appear to enhance asthmatic disease, it is possible that pollutant exposure has effects on immunologic responses to allergens, which may in turn contribute to enhancement of asthma. Because air pollutants themselves provoke nonspecific airway reactivity and alter pulmonary function, it is difficult to test this hypothesis, particularly via epidemiologic studies. Nevertheless, one study did show that individuals living close to a major highway (and hence exposed to higher levels of O_3, NO_2, and other components of automobile exhaust) suffered more frequent and severe allergic reactions to cedar pollen than cohorts living 5 miles from the highway, but with comparable levels of airborne pollen (18).

Because of difficulties inherent in conducting epidemiologic studies, animal models and in some cases human clinical studies have been used to determine the effects of exposure to individual oxidant gases on resistance to challenge with viral, bacterial, or allergenic agents. These studies have also examined effects of pollutants on specific immune responses involved either in host defense against respiratory infection or in mediating allergic reactions. The remainder of this chapter reviews these experimental findings.

DECREASED RESISTANCE TO BACTERIAL INFECTION

One of the most sensitive indicators of air pollutant toxicity is the streptococcus infectivity model developed over 20 years ago (19). In essence, mice are exposed for short periods to single or mixed pollutants before being infected by aerosol with *Streptococcus zooepidemicus* (a group C *Streptococcus*). Mortality is then assessed over a 20-day period and has been shown to increase with increasing concentrations of O_3 (19,20), NO_2 (21,22), phosgene (23), SO_2 (22), and other potentially hazardous substances (reviewed in ref. 24). Significantly enhanced mortality has been demonstrated with this model following 3 hr of exposure to concentrations of O_3 as low as 0.1 ppm (comparable to the current 1-hr national ambient air standard of 0.12 ppm) and at 0.01 ppm phosgene (tenfold below the current threshold limit value). Several investigators have demonstrated that alveolar macrophage (AM) function is impaired following O_3 exposure in mice (25–27), rats (28,29), and rabbits (30,31), as well as in human volunteers (32). NO_2 exposure has also been shown to suppress AM function in rats, rabbits, and humans (33–36). Because AMs are known to be crucial in the inactivation of some gram positive bacteria in the lung (37), it has widely been assumed that enhanced susceptibility to *Streptococcus* following exposure to oxidants was at least in part the result of suppressed AM phagocytic activity.

Recent studies have provided further evidence for the relationship between oxidant-induced suppression of AM phagocytosis and enhancement of susceptibility to *Streptococcus* (38,39) as well as more information on the mechanisms associated with enhanced infection. These studies demonstrated that younger (5-week-old) CD-1 mice are more susceptible to O_3-enhanced streptococcal infection than older (9-week-old) CD-1 mice by a factor of approximately 2 (38) (Fig. 1). Also, C3H/HeJ mice were more susceptible to O_3-enhanced infection than C57BL/6 mice (39). CD-1 mice, the strain that has been historically used for this model, were the most resistant of the three strains tested and differed from the most susceptible strain by a factor of 9 (Fig. 1). These differences in susceptibility were used to explore the mechanisms responsible for O_3 enhancement of bacterial infection.

O_3 suppressed AM phagocytosis of bacteria *in vivo* and impaired clearance of bacteria from the lung in both age groups and strains tested. Strain differences in susceptibility to bacteria were reflected in differences in AM phagocytic activity (Figs. 1 and 2). The data also suggested that other mechanisms, possibly extracellular bacteriostatic components (40) were involved, but suppression of AM phagocytosis appeared to have an important role in O_3 enhancement of streptococcal infection. In young mice, decreased AM activity may have been related to increased prostaglandin E_2 (PGE_2) (38) levels in lavage fluid of O_3-exposed mice since treatment with indomethacin blocked the PGE_2 response and reduced mortality due to infection. Finally, bacteria recovered from O_3-exposed mice expressed a large polysaccharide capsule, which was shown to be antiphagocytic and associated with enhanced virulence relative to the organisms originally deposited in the lung (39). Although this morphologic change was also observed in bacteria isolated from the few air-exposed mice that died, the phenomenon occurred more frequently and rapidly in O_3-exposed mice, suggesting that O_3 predisposed these animals to a more serious infection.

The principal mechanisms currently thought to be responsible for O_3-enhanced susceptibility to streptococcus in mice are shown in Fig. 3. In an air-exposed mouse the scale is tipped in favor of the host, which has fully phagocytic AMs that rapidly inactivate the bacteria from the lung while they are still in an unencapsulated state. It is also likely that other extracellular bacteriostatic factors contribute to the clear-

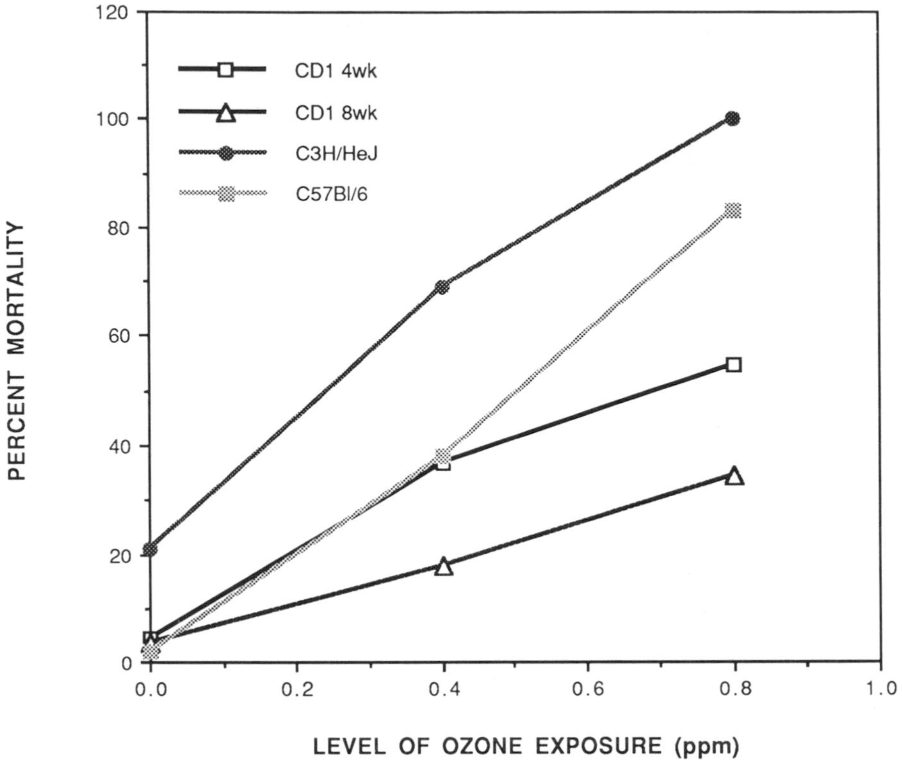

FIG. 1. The effect of a 3-hr O_3 exposure on susceptibility to streptococcal infection in different strains and ages of mice. Intraspecies/age comparisons were derived from data reported by Gilmour et al. (38,39). Concentrations (ppm) at which 40% of mice died, computed for each species from equations derived from the lines in this graph, were as follows: C3H/HeJ = 0.11; C57Bl/6 = 0.39; CD-1 (4 weeks old) = 0.54; CD-1 (8 weeks old) = 0.96.

ance of the bacteria, at least in some strains of mice. In contrast, following O_3 exposure, macrophage phagocytic activity is suppressed. This not only impairs clearance of bacteria but allows time for the expression of an antiphagocytic capsule, which further tips the scale in favor of the bacteria. The same strain differences observed for O_3 enhancement of streptococcal infection were also observed when animals were exposed to NO_2 or phosgene (M.I. Gilmour, *unpublished data*), suggesting that the mechanism of action is the same for all three gases and may also apply to other lower respiratory tract toxicants.

When rats were exposed to O_3 and challenged with streptococci, bacterial clearance from the lung was initially impaired and bacteria isolated from exposed rats exhibited the antiphagocytic capsule, but no mortality was observed (M.I. Gilmour, *unpublished data*). One explanation for the more favorable outcome of infection in the rats may be that polymorphonuclear leukocyte (PMN) infiltration into the lungs of exposed and infected rats peaked on day 1, whereas this peak did not occur in

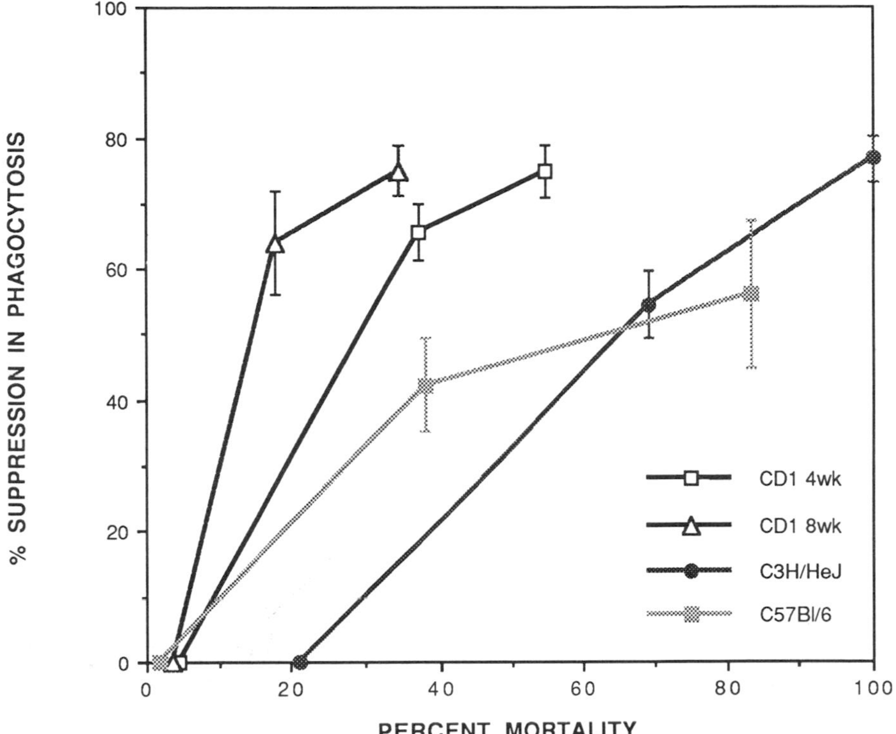

FIG. 2. Relationship between suppression of *in vivo* alveolar macrophage phagocytosis and mortality due to infection. CD-1, 8-week-old mice could tolerate the greatest, and C3H/HeJ mice could tolerate the least, suppression of AM phagocytosis corresponding to their relative susceptibility to O_3-enhanced streptococcal infection shown in Fig. 1. [Graph derived from data reported by Gilmour et al. (38,39).]

mice until day 2 or later (depending on the strain). The hypothesis that this more timely PMN response in the rat is responsible for the resistance of this species to O_3-enhanced infection is supported by the fact that the numbers of bacteria in the lung are markedly increased and infection prolonged in rats treated with antineutrophil serum (M.I. Gilmour, *unpublished data*).

The effects of oxidant air pollutants on several other rodent infectivity models have also been studied. Short-term exposure to 5 or 10 ppm NO_2 decreased intrapulmonary killing of *Mycoplasma pulmonis* and enhanced mortality due to infection (41,42). Again these effects appeared to be related to suppression of AM function (43). Similarly, intrapulmonary inactivation of both *Staphylococcus aureus* and *Pasteurella pneumotropica* was impaired in lungs of mice exposed acutely to O_3 or NO_2. In contrast, similar exposures had no effect or actually enhanced intrapulmonary killing of *Proteus mirabilis* (26,44). In addition to suppression of AM function,

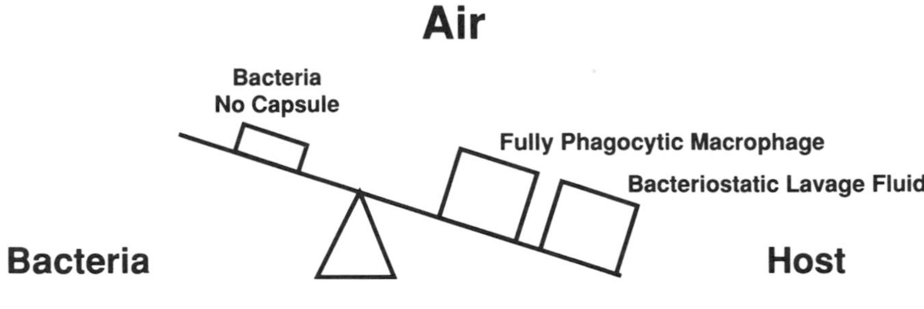

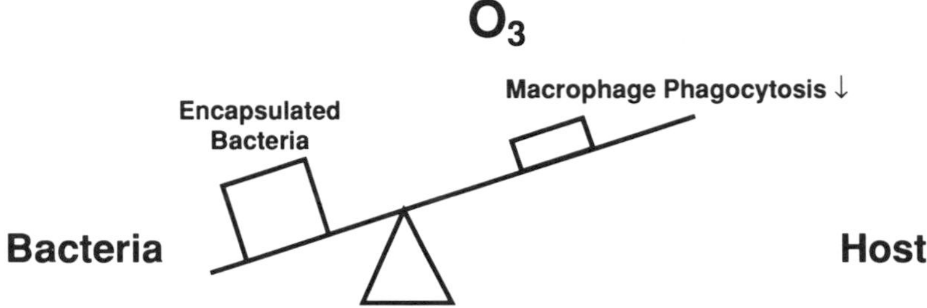

FIG. 3. Summary of mechanisms associated with ozone-enhanced susceptibility to streptococcal infection. Ozone exposure tips the scale in favor of the bacteria by suppressing AM phagocytic activity and allowing bacteria time to form an antiphagocytic capsule.

the authors demonstrated that the dual exposure to both pollutant and the gram-negative organism induced a stronger PMN response than either agent alone, thus augmenting the phagocytic defenses in a synergistic manner, despite AM suppression. Using a *Listeria monocytogenes* infectivity model, O_3 exposure of rats at levels around 1 ppm enhanced mortality due to pulmonary infection, enhanced the severity of lesions in both lung and liver, and impaired clearance of bacteria from the lung (45). Impaired clearance was again attributed to suppressed capacity of macrophages to ingest and kill bacteria in O_3-exposed rats. In addition to direct effects on the macrophage, the authors proposed that impaired macrophage activity might also have been due partly to effects of O_3 on T cell-dependent lymphokine production, which is known to enhance phagocytosis in the *Listeria* model. This latter possibility is supported by the fact that T/B cell ratios in lung and draining lymph nodes, lymphoproliferative responses to *Listeria* antigen in spleen and draining lymph node, and delayed-type hypersensitivity responses to *Listeria* antigen (using a mouse ear swelling test) were all suppressed in mice exposed to O_3. These T cell defects were especially evident if exposure took place during infection. In another study using experimental tuberculosis, an infection similar to *L. monocytogenes* in terms of pertinent host defenses, impaired bacterial clearance was also noted in mice exposed to 1 ppm O_3, 3 hr/d for 3 weeks or more beginning 2 weeks after infection (46).

In summary, it is clear that exposure to oxidant gases enhances susceptibility to several types of bacteria tested in rodent models. O_3 enhancement of these infections (and probably enhancement observed following exposure to other gases) is associated with direct and indirect suppression of AM activity, while PMN responses may in some cases compensate for this deficit. Studies to compare human, rat, and mouse AM and PMN responses to bacteria as well as chemotactic factors in bronchoalveolar lavage fluid are feasible and could provide information that would be useful in terms of extrapolating from animal data to human risk. At present, we know that O_3 suppresses AM function in humans (32), rats (28,29), and mice (38,39) and that *in vitro* exposure of human AMs to O_3 also impairs phagocytic capacity of these cells (47). Also, as in mice, O_3 exposure increases PGE_2 production in human volunteers (48), an effect associated with AM suppression in young mice (38). This suppression of AM activity results in increased susceptibility of mice and rats to certain bacterial infections and suggests that humans exposed to O_3 are likely to be predisposed to bacterial infections in the lower respiratory tract. The seriousness of such infections may depend on how quickly bacteria develop virulence factors and how rapidly PMNs are mobilized to compensate for the deficit in AM function.

EFFECTS ON RESISTANCE TO VIRAL INFECTIONS

In contrast to the extensive literature on the effects of oxidant exposure on susceptibility to bacterial infection, effects of these pollutants on viral infectivity models in experimental animals have been more difficult to demonstrate. This is surprising since 90% of respiratory infections in children and adults up to age 50 appear to be viral rather than bacterial in origin (49). Hence, presumably many of the symptoms described in the epidemiologic studies reviewed in the early part of this chapter were due to viral infections. Of studies describing effects of O_3 exposure on mice infected with influenza virus, two indicated no effect on virus replication in the lung (50,51); two reported reduced severity of infection based on mortality, histopathology, serum albumin levels in lavage fluid, and lung wet/dry weight ratios (52,53); and one indicated increased mortality, pathology, lung wet weight, and alterations in lung function consistent with these effects, but without changes in virus titers in the lung (54). Differences in exposure regimens may account for these discrepancies. In the one instance where influenza infection was enhanced, mice were exposed to 1.0 or 0.5 ppm O_3, 3 hr/d for 5 days and infected after the second exposure. If mice were infected after the fifth exposure, no effects were observed, suggesting that, whatever the effect of O_3, mice adapted very quickly. Since none of the studies demonstrated an increase in virus replication in the lung, there is no evidence that O_3 alters defense mechanisms critical for clearing virus from the lungs of experimentally infected mice. O_3 suppression of certain immunopathologic responses associated with influenza infection may have accounted for the reduced severity of disease in some cases (53), and modulation of immunologic responses might also have been involved in enhanced inflammatory responses seen in other studies. Although O_3 exposure mitigated acute lung injury in mice exposed continuously to 0.5 ppm following infection, chronic lung damage was exacerbated 30 days postinfection. Enhanced postinfluenzal alveolitis and structural changes seen at this time were consistent with fibrogenesis (55).

Similarly, studies of SO_2 exposures as high as 6 ppm showed no effect on influenza virus replication (50,51). However, in several studies there appeared to be additive or synergistic effects on lung inflammatory responses in mice infected with influenza virus and exposed for several days or weeks to SO_2 over a wide range of concentrations (0.1 to 34 ppm) (56–58). Mice exposed to high levels of NO_2 (37 ppm) for 30 days and subsequently challenged with influenza virus actually had a lower incidence of mortality than air-exposed controls (59). However, mice exposed intermittently to 10 ppm NO_2 for 5 days and subsequently infected with influenza virus had increased mortality rates and enhanced interstitial pneumonia (60). As with O_3, differences in exposure regimens may account for differences between studies. Exposure of mice to 5, 10, or 20 ppm NO_2, 4 hr/d for 10 days following infection with Sendai virus (a murine respiratory parainfluenza virus) did not result in increased virus titers in lung but did enhance lung pathology as evidenced by increased lung wet/dry weight ratios and lavage fluid protein and cell counts (61).

In two cases, exposures to toxic gases resulted in increased virus concentrations in the lungs of experimentally infected rodents. Exposure to 5 ppm NO_2, 6 hr/d, for 2 days preceding and 4 days after intratracheal challenge with murine cytomegalovirus (MCMV) resulted in a tenfold increase in lung virus titers and more severe histopathologic changes compared to mice exposed to air (62). Unfortunately, these findings could not be reproduced in another laboratory (63). In another study, rats exposed for 4 hr to a high concentration of phosgene (1 ppm) and challenged 24 hr later with influenza virus exhibited delayed clearance of virus from the lung relative to air controls (64).

Spontaneous pulmonary natural killer (NK) cell activity, thought to be an important host defense against viral infection, was suppressed by phosgene exposure (1.0 ppm for 4 hr) (65) or certain O_3 regimens (1.0 ppm, 23.5 hr/d, for up to 7 days) (66), but enhanced by exposure to lower O_3 concentrations (0.2 and 0.4 ppm for 7 days) (67). Virus-augmented NK cell activity was enhanced in the lung but slightly suppressed in the spleens of mice exposed to 5 ppm NO_2, 3 hr/d for 4 days following MCMV infection (63). Percentages of both T cell populations and NK cells were also lower in the spleens of mice exposed to 0.25 ppm NO_2 for 7 weeks, or 0.35 ppm for 12 weeks (68). Suppressed splenic NK cell activity was reported in rats exposed to a simulated urban profile of NO_2 for 3 weeks (69), but not for more chronic exposures, and no such effects were observed in mice similarly exposed to O_3 (70). From the preceding studies it appears that pulmonary NK cell responses are more likely to be enhanced than suppressed by exposure to reactive gases, whereas some suppression of splenic NK cell responses has been observed on several occasions. A human study appears to be consistent with the animal studies in that a significant increase in NK cell numbers (CD16+) in bronchoalveolar lavage fluid was demonstrated in volunteers exposed to 0.6 ppm NO_2 with moderate exercise, 2 hr/d on 4 days within a 6-day period (71).

Controlled human clinical studies have been no more successful than laboratory animal studies in demonstrating effects of air pollutants on susceptibility to viral infections. No difference in rhinovirus titers or recruitment of neutrophils in nasal secretion, interferon (IFN) levels in lavage fluid, *in vitro* lymphocyte proliferative responses to rhinovirus antigen, or serum-neutralizing antibody levels could be demonstrated between volunteers exposed to 0.3 ppm O_3, 6 hr/d, for 5 days after inoculation of rhinovirus type 39 and those exposed to clean air (72). Similarly, while infection rates (determined by virus-recovery, increased virus-specific antibody in serum or nasal wash, or both) were higher in subjects exposed to 1 or 2 ppm NO_2 (as compared to clean air) 2 hr/d for 3 days and inoculated with influenza virus after the second exposure, the differences were not statistically significant (73). Finally, a single 4-hr exposure of human volunteers to 5 ppm SO_2 prior to challenge with rhinovirus resulted in a reduction in symptoms and lower but more persistent virus shedding (74).

Part of the discrepancy between epidemiologic studies and experimental studies may be related to the parameters used to assess enhancement of infection. Experimental studies tend to view increases in virus titers in the respiratory tract as an indication that pollutant exposure enhances infection, whereas epidemiologic studies rely on symptoms, many of which could be related to enhanced inflammatory or even allergic responses (see later discussion) to the virus in the absence of effects on viral replication. In fact, the above referenced studies suggest that while virus replication does not appear to be particularly vulnerable to pollutant exposure, inflammatory responses to the virus as evidenced by histopathology and lung wet weight do tend to be modulated by pollutant exposure. Also, airway hyperresponsiveness to inhaled methacholine, a cardinal feature of asthma, was demonstrated after exposure of rats to 1 ppm O_3 for 3 hr or in rats infected with influenza virus (75). Airways reactivity (AR) was even further increased when infection and O_3 exposure (either before or after infection) were combined (75). Exposure to 5 ppm NO_2 alone did not enhance AR but when given prior to infection did enhance AR over that observed in air-exposed infected rats. This suggests that pollutants may exacerbate asthmatic-like responses, which sometimes occur as a result of respiratory infection (76). All these data suggest that effects of pollutants on immunologic responses related to inflammation and allergy may provide the most pertinent information on the relationship between immune modulation and susceptibility to viral infection following pollutant exposure.

EFFECT ON ALLERGIC RESPONSES

Unlike the large body of experimental data on the effects of air pollutant exposures on susceptibility to respiratory infections, few studies have investigated the

TABLE 1. *Predominant types of respiratory allergy*

Type	Time to symnptoms	Human example	Animal model	Key immunologic mediators
I	Immediate, 3–15 min	Hay fever	Guinea pig (76), rat (77)	Cytophilic IgE or IgG1; mast cell degranulation
III	Intermediate, 2–6 hr	Farmer's lung	Rabbit (78), guinea pig (79)	IgG or IgM/antigen complexes and complement
IV	Delayed, 6–16 hr	Tuberculosis, berylliosis	Mouse (80)	T cell, monocyte infiltration (DTH response)

interaction between air pollutants and pulmonary allergy. This paucity of data probably stems both from the traditional focus on host–pathogen interaction in pulmonary disease and from difficulties in developing adequate animal models of respiratory allergy. Pulmonary allergy is an inherently complex disease, dependent on a number of host susceptibility factors, and interactions between antigens, immune cells, and mediators. The three most common types of respiratory allergy or hypersensitivity (reviewed in ref. 77 and 78), which might conceivably be modulated by exposure to air pollution, and appropriate animal models are presented in Table 1.

Type I (immediate) hypersensitivity features cytophilic immunoglobulin G1 (IgG1) or IgE antibodies, which bind to the surface of mast cells. Upon reexposure to allergen, antigenic molecules cross-link specific Ig receptor sites, causing mast cell degranulation and the release of vasoactive amines and other mediators responsible for inflammation and bronchoconstriction. In humans, this disease is often manifested as allergy to pollens (hay fever), house dust, and pet dander. These allergens are also regarded as the triggering factor for the majority of asthma attacks (10,11). The most common animal model of type I hypersensitivity is the guinea pig/ovalbumin model (79), where IgG1 is the cytophilic antibody. More recently, IgE-mediated models of disease have now been described in rats (80). Type III (intermediate) hypersensitivity is produced by the interaction of circulating IgG or IgM antibodies with antigen, resulting in immune complex formation and tissue damage from complement components and inflammatory cells. The disease is characterized by alveolar wall thickening, chronic inflammation (mainly PMNs), and granuloma formation. The best known human example of disease is allergic alveolitis or farmer's lung, caused by individuals mounting immune reactions to fungal spores from *Aspergillus* and *Actinomyces* species. This disease has been reproduced by repeated injection and pulmonary challenge regimes using a variety of fungal antigens in rabbits and guinea pigs (81,82). Type IV, delayed-type hypersensitivity (DTH), features a slow T cell-dependent infiltration of monocytes into the lung, granuloma formation, and fibrosis and is most commonly observed in granulomatous diseases such as tuberculosis. Similar models of DTH have been produced in mice using small molecular weight haptens conjugated to large protein carriers

(83). It is generally agreed, however, that hypersensitivity reactions in humans and experimental animal models can incorporate more than one type of response, and thus the above classification, which is less commonly used than in the past, should be used merely as a guideline.

Despite the existence of these allergy models for several years, only a handful of investigators have studied the effect of air pollutant exposure on the development or severity of pulmonary allergy, and all have focused on type I reactions. In 1970, Matsumura (84) reported that guinea pigs exposed to high levels of O_3 (5 to 10 ppm), NO_2 (70 ppm), or SO_2 (330 ppm) for 30 min prior to airway sensitization with ovalbumin antigen had elevated specific antibody titers and increased anaphylactic responses following challenge with aerosolized antigen. In an accompanying study (85) using radiolabeled ovalbumin instilled through the trachea, it was demonstrated that pollutant exposure enhanced dissemination of antigen from the lung to the bloodstream over a 3-hr period. Hence the heightened immunologic responses observed at these high pollutant concentrations were probably due primarily to increased lung permeability resulting in increased flow of antigen to the bloodstream and immune tissue. In a later study using ovalbumin sensitization in the guinea pig (86), daily exposure to lower levels of SO_2 (0.1 to 16.6 ppm) also increased specific antibody levels in serum and bronchoalveolar lavage fluid (BAL) and increased antigen-induced bronchoconstriction.

In a series of studies in mice, Osebold and colleagues (87) demonstrated that continuous exposure to O_3 (0.5 to 0.8 ppm) resulted in elevated levels of albumin, total IgG and IgA antibodies in the BAL fluid of mice, and increased numbers of IgA-containing cells in the lungs. Using a model of ovalbumin induced anaphylaxis in sensitized mice, they also reported that intermittent exposure to O_3 (0.5 to 0.8 ppm) (88), sulfuric acid aerosol (1 mg/m^3), or a combination of both pollutants (89), increased reactivity to subsequent ovalbumin challenge delivered by aerosol. This increased reactivity corresponded to elevated numbers of antigen-specific IgE-producing cells in the lungs (90). Finally, Biagini et al. (91) reported that exposure to 1 ppm O_3 enhanced the development of allergy to inhaled platinum in monkeys.

To date, only two studies have investigated the effect of pollutant exposure on subsequent reactivity to antigen in atopic human volunteers. Molfino et al. (92) reported that exposure to 0.12 ppm O_3 significantly increased bronchial responsiveness to antigen in some individuals. Although they acknowledged weaknesses in design of the experiment and recommended the findings be confirmed, their observations were in accordance with the majority of epidemiologic studies. In contrast, Bascom et al. (93) found no alteration in the acute response to nasal antigen challenge in allergic patients preexposed to O_3 compared to air exposure; however they did report increased upper respiratory tract inflammation following O_3 exposure in those patients in the absence of antigen challenge. Similarly, the bronchial response to inhaled grass pollen was unaffected by prior exposure to 0.1 ppm NO_2 (94).

In addition to studies aimed at identifying the interaction between air pollutants and pulmonary allergy, a number of investigators have reported more general changes in pulmonary immune function during or after exposure to oxidant gases such as O_3 (reviewed in ref. 95). These changes include significant modulation of T lymphocytes in bronchus-associated lymphoid tissue (BALT) and mediastinal lymph nodes (reviewed below), elevation of specific antibody, particularly IgE in some (84,86,87), but not all, cases (96), and suppression of DTH responses (97,98). The relevance of these effects with respect to the hypothesis that air pollution enhances allergic reactions is best understood in the context of the recent discovery of two distinct populations of CD4 T helper (T_H) cells (99). One type (designated T_H1) produces IFN-γ and interleukin-2 (IL-2), which drive DTH reactions and IgG production. T_H2 cells, on the other hand, produce IL-4, which stimulates IgE production, and are therefore key to the initiation of immediate (type I) hypersensitivity reactions. These two populations are antagonistic to each other by virtue of their cytokine profiles, and thus their modulation can influence the types of immune responses that develop. The facts that oxidants enhance some antibody responses, suppress DTH responses, and modulate T cell activity are consistent with the hypothesis that these pollutants disturb the balance between these two cell types in the respiratory tract in a direction that favors type I reactions.

Effects of oxidant exposure on these T cell subpopulations have not been studied; however, Dziedzic and colleagues (100) have reported effects of O_3 on T cells, which suggest that the potential for disturbing the balance of T_H1 and T_H2 in the respiratory tract exists. Exposure to 0.5 ppm O_3, 20 hr/d for 1 to 14 days, caused lymphocyte proliferation in both BALT and mediastinal lymph nodes of rats, which peaked on day 3 of exposure, was still significantly elevated at day 7, and had returned to normal by day 14 (100). Following exposure of mice to 0.7 ppm 20 hr/d for 4 or 14 days, frozen lung sections showed T cell infiltration (Thy 1.2+), but B cells (sIgM+) were virtually nonexistent (101). In mice similarly exposed for 28 days, thymidine uptake in paracortical T cell areas of the mediastinal lymph node was increased during the first 7 days of exposure, and mediastinal lymph node cell responses to concanavalin A were elevated on days 14 to 28 (102). These studies apparently contradict those (reviewed earlier) by Van Loveren et al. (45) in which T/B cell ratios in lung and draining lymph nodes and lymphoproliferative responses to *Listeria* antigen in spleen and draining lymph node were suppressed in infected animals exposed to O_3. Differences in exposure regimens or the presence of an infectious agent in the latter study may account for these discrepancies. In any case, additional work on the effects of pollutant gases on T_H cell populations and related cytokine production are needed to improve our understanding of the immunologic mechanisms associated with potential effects of O_3 on responses to allergens.

SUMMARY

It is clear that oxidant air pollutants modulate immune responses in the lung. The best understood consequence of this modulation is increased susceptibility to a number of bacterial infections in laboratory rodents. Oxidant suppression of AM phagocytic activity appears to have a key role in mediating this effect. Because human studies have shown suppression of AM function as well, it seems likely that increased susceptibility to bacterial infection poses a risk for populations exposed to oxidants. The role that oxidant exposure may have in enhancing viral and allergic disease is much less clear. Effects of air pollutants on viral replication have rarely been demonstrated; however, epidemiologic and experimental studies suggest that these pollutants may modulate allergic or inflammatory responses associated with viral infection. Effects of oxidants on immune responses in the lung, including T cell, antibody, and DTH responses, suggest that these pollutants could potentially enhance allergic type reactions to both viruses and allergens. However, much more work is needed before definitive conclusions can be drawn concerning the effects of air pollutants on viral and allergic disease and associated immune responses. Finally, oxidants are known to elicit inflammatory responses in the lung. The mediators involved have recently been reviewed by Koren et al. (103).

REFERENCES

1. Lunn JE, Knowelden J, Handyside AJ. Patterns of respiratory illness in Sheffield infant schoolchildren. *Br J Prev Soc Med* 1967;21:7–16.
2. French JG, Lowrimore G, Nelson WC, Finklea JF, English T, Hertz M. The effect of sulfur dioxide and suspended sulfates on acute respiratory disease. *Arch Environ Health* 1973;27:129–133.
3. Harrington W, Krupnick AJ. Short-term nitrogen dioxide exposure and acute respiratory disease in children. *J Air Pollut Control Assoc* 1985;35:1061–1067.
4. Ware JH, Dockery DW, Spiro A, Speizer FE, Ferris BG. Passive smoking, gas cooking, and respiratory health of children living in six cities. *Am Rev Respir Dis* 1984;129:366–374.
5. Samet JM, Lambert WE, Skipper BJ, et al. Nitrogen dioxide and respiratory illness in infants. *Am Rev Respir Dis* 1993;148:1258–1265.
6. Speizer FE, Ferris B, Bishop YMM, Spengler J. Respiratory disease rates and pulmonary function in children associated with NO_2 exposure. *Am Rev Respir Dis* 1980:121:3–10.
7. Neas LM, Dockery DD, Ware JH, Spengler JD, Speizer FE, Ferris BG. Association of indoor nitrogen dioxide with respiratory symptoms and pulmonary function in children. *Am J Epidemiol* 1991;134:204–218.
8. Schwartz J, Spix C, Wichmann HE, Malin E. Air pollution and acute respiratory illness in five German communities. *Environ Res* 1991;56:1–14.
9. Schwartz J. Air pollution and the duration of acute respiratory symptoms. *Arch Environ Health* 1992;47:116–122.
10. Burrows B, Martinez FD, Halonen M, Barbee RA, Clines MG. Association of asthma with serum IgE levels and skin-test reactivity to allergens. *N Engl J Med* 1989;320:271–277.
11. Pollart SM, Chapman MD, Fiocco GP, Rose G, Platts-Mills TAE. Epidemiology of acute asthma: IgE antibodies to common inhalant allergens as a risk factor for emergency room visits. *J Allergy Clin Immunol* 1989;83:875–882.
12. Ponka A. Asthma and low level air pollution in Helsinki. *Arch Environ Health* 1991;46:262–270.
13. Shy CM. Health hazards of sulfur oxides: a serious threat in our growing need for electrical power. *Am Lung Assoc Bull* 1977;63:2–8.
14. Phelps HW, Sabel GW, Fischer NE. Air pollution asthma among military personel in Japan. *JAMA* 1961;175:990–993.
15. Levin R, Gilkeson M, McCaldin R. Air pollution and New Orleans asthma. *Public Health Rep* 1962;77:947–954.
16. Bates DV, Sizto R. The Ontario air pollution study: identification of the causative agent. *Environ Health Perspect* 1989;79:69–72.
17. Bresnitz EA, Rest KM. Epidemiological studies of effects of oxidant exposure on human populations. In: Watson AY, Bates R, Kennedy D, eds. *Air pollution, the automobile and public health. Health Effects Institute*. Washington, DC: National Academy Press; 1988:389–413.
18. Ishizaki T, Koizumi K, Ikemori R, et al. Studies of prevalence of Japanese cedar pollinosis among the residents in a densely cultivated area. *Ann Allergy* 1987;58:263–270.

19. Coffin DL, Gardner DE. Interaction of biological agents and chemical air pollutants. *Ann Occup Hyg* 1972;15:219–234.
20. Ehrlich R, Findlay JC, Fenters JD, Gardner DE. Health effects of short-term inhalation of nitrogen dioxide and ozone mixtures. *Environ Res* 1977;4:223–231.
21. Ehrlich R, Henry MC. Chronic toxicity of nitrogen dioxide. I. Effect on resistance to bacterial pneumonia. *Arch Environ Health* 1968;17:860–865.
22. Sherwood RL, Tarkington B, Lippert WE, Goldstein E. Effect of ferrous sulphate aerosols and nitrogen dioxide aerosols on murine pulmonary defense. *Arch Environ Health* 1981;36:130–135.
23. Selgrade MJK, Starnes DM, Illing JW, Daniels MJ, Graham JA. Effects of phosgene exposure on bacterial, viral, and neoplastic lung disease susceptibility in mice. *Inhalation Toxicol* 1989;1:243–259.
24. Gardner DE. Effects of gases and airborne particles on lung infections. In: McGrath JJ, Barnes EB, eds. *Air pollution: physiological effects*. New York: Academic Press; 1982;47–79.
25. Goldstein E, Tyler WS, Hoeprich PD, Eagle C. Ozone and the antibacterial defense mechanisms of the murine lung. *Arch Intern Med* 1971;127:1099–1102.
26. Gilmour MI, Hmieleski RR, Stafford EA, Jakab GJ. Suppression and recovery of the alveolar macrophage phagocytic system during continuous exposure to 0.5 ppm ozone. *Exp Lung Res* 1991; 17:547–558.
27. Canning BJ, Hmieleski RR, Spannhake EW, Jakab GJ. Ozone reduces murine alveolar and peritoneal macrophage phagocytosis: the role of prostanoids. *Am J Physiol* 1991;261(Lung Cell Mol Physiol 5):L227–L282.
28. Oosting RS, Van Golde LMG, Verhoef J, Van Bree L. Species differences in impairment of alveolar macrophage functions following single and repeated ozone exposures. *Toxicol Appl Pharmacol* 1991;110:170–178.
29. Gunnison AF, Finkelstien I, Weidman P, Su W, Sobo M, Schlesinger RB. Age dependent effect of ozone on pulmonary eicosanoid metabolism in rabbits and rats. *Fundam Appl Toxicol* 1990; 15:779–790.
30. Driscoll KE, Vollmuth TA, Schlesinger RB. Acute and subchronic ozone inhalation in the rabbit: response of the alveolar macrophages. *J Toxicol Environ Health* 1987;21:27–43.
31. Zelikoff JT, Kraemer GL, Vogel MC, Schlesinger RB. Immunodulating effects of ozone on macrophage functions important for tumor surveillance and host defense. *J Toxicol Environ Health* 1991;34:449–467.
32. Devlin RB, McDonnell WF, Mann R, Becker S, House DE, Schreinemachers D, Koren H. Exposure of humans to ambient levels of ozone for 6.6 hours causes cellular and biochemical changes in the lung. *Am J Respir Cell Mol Biol* 1991;4:72–81.
33. Suzuki T, Ikeda S, Kanoh T, Mizoguchi I. Decreased phagocytosis and superoxide anion production in alveolar macrophages of rats exposed to nitrogen dioxide. *Arch Environ Contam Toxicol* 1986;15:733–739.
34. Hooftman RN, Kuper CF, Appelman LM. Comparative sensitivity of histopathology and specific lung parameters in the detection of lung injury. *J Appl Toxicol* 1988;8:59–65.
35. Schlesinger RB. Effects of intermittent inhalation exposure to mixed atmosphere of NO_2 and H_2SO_4 on rabbit alveolar macrophages. *J Toxicol Environ Health* 1987;22:301–312.
36. Devlin R, Horstman D, Becker S, Gerrity T, Madden M, Koren H. Inflammatory response in humans exposed to 2.0 ppm NO_2. *Am Rev Respir Dis* 1992;145:A456.
37. Green GM, Kass EH. The role of the alveolar macrophage in the clearance of bacteria from the lungs. *J Exp Med* 1964;119:167–176.
38. Gilmour MI, Park P, Doefler D, Selgrade MJK. Factors which influence the suppression of pulmonary anti-bacterial defenses in mice exposed to ozone. *Exp Lung Res* 1993;19:299–314.
39. Gilmour MI, Park P, Selgrade MJK. O_3-enhanced pulmonary infection with *Streptococcus zooepidemicus* in mice: the role of alveolar macrophage function and capsular virulence factors. *Am Rev Respir Dis* 1993;147:753–760.
40. Coonrod JD, Yoneda K. Detection and partial characterization of antibacterial factor(s) in alveolar lining material of rats. *J Clin Invest* 1983;71:129–141.
41. Parker RF, Davis JK, Cassell GH, et al. Short-term exposure to nitrogen dioxide enhances susceptibility to murine respiratory mycoplasmosis and decreases intrapulmonary killing of *Mycoplasma pulmonis*. *Am Rev Respir Dis* 1989;140:502–512.
42. Nisizawa T, Saito M, Nakayama K, Nishihara T, Imai S, Nakagawa M. Effects of nitrogen dioxide on *Mycoplasma pulmonis* infection and humoral immune responses in mice. *Jpn J Med Sci Biol* 1988;41:175–187.

43. Davis JK, Davidson MK, Schoeb TR, Lindsey JR. Decreased intrapulmonary killing of *Mycoplasma pulmonis* after short-term exposure to NO_2 is associated with damaged alveolar macrophages. *Am Rev Respir Dis* 1992;145:406–411.
44. Jakab GJ. Modulation of pulmonary defense mechanisms by acute exposures to nitrogen dioxide. *Environ Res* 1987;42:215–228.
45. Van Loveren H, Rombout PJA, Wagenaar SS, Walvoort HC, Vos JG. Effects of ozone on the defense to a respiratory *Listeria monocytogenes* infection in the rat. *Toxicol Appl Pharmacol* 1988; 94:374–393.
46. Thomas GB, Fenters JD, Ehrlich R, Gardner DE. Effects of exposure to ozone on susceptibility to experimental tuberculosis. *Toxicol Lett* 1981;9:11–17.
47. Becker S, Madden MC, Newman SL, Devlin RB, Koren HS. Modulation of human alveolar macrophage properties by ozone exposure *in vitro*. *Toxicol Appl Pharmacol* 1991;110:403–415.
48. Madden M, Pape G, Hazucha M, et al. Effects of ibuprofen on lung lavage composition in ozone-exposed subjects. *Am Rev Respir Dis* 1991;143:A699.
49. Evans AS. Epidemiological concepts and methods. In: Evans AS, ed. *Viral infections of humans*. New York: Plenum Press; 1976:1–32.
50. Loosli CG, Buckley RD, Hwang-Kow SY, Hertweck MS, Hardy JD, Serebrin R. Effect of air pollutants on resistance of mice to airborne influenza A virus infection. In: Hass JF, ed. *Airborne transmission and airborne infection*. Utrecht, The Netherlands: Oosthock; 1972:225–231.
51. Fairchild GA. Effects of ozone and sulfur dioxide on virus growth in mice. *Arch Environ Health* 1977;32:28–33.
52. Wolcott JA, Zee YG, Osebold JW. Exposure to ozone reduces influenza disease severity and alters distribution of influenza viral antigens in murine lungs. *Appl Environ Microbiol* 1982;44:723–731.
53. Jakab GJ, Hmieleski RR. Reduction of influenza virus pathogenesis by exposure to 0.5 ppm ozone. *J Toxicol Environ Health* 1988;23:455–472.
54. Selgrade MJK, Illing JW, Starnes DM, Stead AG, Menache MG, Stevens MA. Evaluation of effects of ozone exposure on influenza infection in mice using several indicators of susceptibility. *Fundam Appl Toxicol* 1988;11:169–180.
55. Jakab GJ, Bassett DJ. Influenza virus infection, ozone exposure, and fibrogenesis. *Am Rev Respir Dis* 1990;141:1307–1315.
56. Fairchild GA, Roan J, McCarroll J. Atmospheric pollutants and the pathogenesis of viral respiratory disease. *Arch Environ Health* 1972;25:174–182.
57. Lebowitz MD, Fairchild GA. The effects of sulfur dioxide and A_2 influenza virus on pneumonia and weight reduction in mice: an analysis of stimulus–response relationships. *Chem Biol Interact* 1973;7:317–326.
58. Ukai K. Effects of SO_2 on the pathogenesis of viral upper respiratory infection in mice. *Proc Soc Exp Biol Med* 1977;154:591–596.
59. Buckley RD, Loosli CG. Effects of nitrogen dioxide inhalation on germfree mouse lung. *Arch Environ Health* 1969;18:588–595.
60. Ito K. Effect of nitrogen dioxide inhalation on influenza virus infection in mice. *Jpn J Hyg* 1971; 26:304–314.
61. Jakab GJ. *Modulation of pulmonary defense mechanisms against viral and bacterial infections by acute exposure to nitrogen dioxide*, Res Rep #20. Cambridge, MA: Health Effects Research Institute;1988.
62. Rose RM, Fuglestad JM, Skornik WA, Hammer SM, Wolfthal SF, Beck BD, Brain JD. The pathophysiology of enhanced susceptibility to murine cytomegalovirus respiratory infection during short-term exposure to 5 ppm nitrogen dioxide. *Am Rev Respir Dis* 1988;137:912–917.
63. Selgrade MJK, Daniels MJ, Craig WA, Corsini E, Rosenthal GJ. Effect of NO_2 exposure on virus-augmented natural killer (NK) activity and murine cytomegalovirus infection (MCMV). *Toxicologist* 1992;12:175.
64. Ehrlich JP, Burleson GR. Enhanced and prolonged pulmonary influenza virus infection following phosgene inhalation. *J Toxicol Environ Health* 1991;34:259–273.
65. Burleson GR, Keyes LL. Natural killer activity in Fischer-344 rat lungs as a method to assess pulmonary immunocompetence: immunosuppression by phosgene inhalation. *Immunopharmacol Immunotoxicol* 1989;11:421–443.
66. Burleson GR, Keyes LL, Stutzman JD. Immunosuppression of pulmonary natural killer activity by exposure to ozone. *Immunopharmacol Immunotoxicol* 1989;11:715–735.
67. Van Loveren H, Krajnc EI, Rombout PJA, Blommaert FA, Vos JG. Effects of ozone, hexa-

chlorobenzene, and bis(tri-*n*-butyltin) oxide on natural killer activity in the rat lung. *Toxicol Appl Pharmacol* 1990;102:21–33.
68. Richters A, Damji KS. Changes in T-lymphocyte subpopulations and natural killer cells following exposure to ambient levels of nitrogen dioxide. *J Toxicol Environ Health* 1988;25:247–256.
69. Selgrade MJK, Daniels MJ, Grose EC. Evaluation of immunotoxicity of an urban profile of nitrogen dioxide: acute, subchronic, and chronic studies. *Inhalation Toxicol* 1991;3:389–403.
70. Selgrade MJK, Daniels MJ, Grose EC. Acute, subchronic, and chronic exposure to a simulated urban profile of ozone: effects on extrapulmonary natural killer cell activity and lymphocyte mitogenic responses. *Inhalation Toxicol* 1990;2:375–389.
71. Rubinstein I, Reiss TF, Bigby BG, Stites DP, Boushey HA. Effects of 0.06 ppm nitrogen dioxide on circulating and bronchoalveolar lavage lymphocyte phenotypes in healthy subjects. *Environ Res* 1991;55:18–30.
72. Henderson FW, Dubovi EJ, Harder S, Seal E, Graham D. Experimental rhinovirus infection in human volunteers exposed to ozone. *Am Rev Respir Dis* 1988;137:1124–1128.
73. Goings SA, Kulle TJ, Bascom R, Sauder LR, Green DJ, Hebel JR, Clements ML. Effects of nitrogen dioxide exposure on susceptibility to influenza A virus infection in healthy adults. *Am Rev Respir Dis* 1989;139:1075–1081.
74. Andersen IB, Jensen PL, Reed SE, Craig JW, Proctor DF, Adams GK. Induced rhinovirus infection under controlled exposure to sulfur dioxide. *Arch Environ Health* 1977:32:120–126.
75. Tepper JS, Winsett DW, Dye JA, Burleson GR, Costa DL. Can environmental pollutants exacerbate virus-induced airway hyperresponsiveness. *Toxicologist* 1993;13:A55.
76. Zoratti EM, Busse WW. The role of respiratory infections in airway responsiveness and the pathogenesis of asthma. *Immunol Allergy Clin North Am* 1990;10:449–461.
77. Kaltreider BH. Expression of immune mechanisms in the lung. *Am Rev Respir Dis* 1976;11:347–379.
78. Danielle RP. Introduction: the lung's response to immune injury. In: Danielle RP, ed. *Immunology and immunologic diseases of the lung*. Boston: Blackwell Scientific; 1988:187–191.
79. Andersson P. Antigen-induced bronchial anaphylaxis in actively sensitized guinea pigs. Pattern of response in relation to immunization regime. *Allergy* 1980;35:65–71.
80. Pauwels R. The relationship between airway inflammation and bronchial hyperresponsiveness. *Clin Exp Allergy* 1989;19:395–398.
81. Richerson HB, Cheng FHF, Bauserman SC. Acute experimental hypersensitivity pneumonitis in rabbits. *Am Rev Respir Dis* 1979;104:568–576.
82. Schuyler M, Crooks L. Experimental hypersensitivity pneumonitis: kinetics and dose response. *Am Rev Respir* 1989;139:996–1002.
83. Enander I, Ahlstedt S, Nygren H. Mononuclear cells, mast cells and mucus cells as part of the delayed hypersensitivity response to aerosolized antigen in mice. *Immunology* 1984;51:661–668.
84. Matsumara Y. The effects of ozone, nitrogen dioxide, and sulfur dioxide on the experimentally induced allergic disorder in guinea pigs. I. The effect on sensitization with albumin through the airway. *Am Rev Respir Dis* 1970;102:430–437.
85. Matsumara Y. The effects of ozone, nitrogen dioxide, and sulfur dioxide on the experimentally induced allergic disorder in guinea pigs. I. The effects of ozone on the absorption and the retention of antigen in the lung. *Am Rev Respir Dis* 1970;102:438–443.
86. Reidel F, Kramer M, Scheibenbogen C, Rieger HL. Effects of SO_2 exposure on allergic sensitization in the guinea pig. *J Allergy Clin Immunol* 1988;82:527–534.
87. Osebold JW, Owens SL, Zee YC, Dotson WM, LaBarre DD. Immunological alterations in the lungs of mice following ozone exposure: changes in immunoglobulin levels and antibody containing cells. *Arch Environ Health* 1979;34:258–265.
88. Osebold JW, Zee YC, Gershwin LJ. Enhancement of allergic lung sensitization in mice by ozone inhalation. *Proc Soc Exp Biol Med* 1988;188:259–264.
89. Osebold JW, Gershwin LJ, Zee YC. Studies on the enhancement of allergic lung sensitization by inhalation of ozone and sulfuric and aerosol. *J Environ Pathol Toxicol* 1980;3:221–234.
90. Gershwin LJ, Osebold JW, Zee YC. Immunoglobulin E-containing cells in mouse lung following allergen inhalation and ozone exposure. *Int Arch Allergy Appl Immunol* 1981;65:266–277.
91. Biagini RE, Moorman WJ, Lewis TR, Bernstein IL. Ozone enhancement of platinum asthma in a primate model. *Am Rev Respir Dis* 1986;134:719–725.
92. Molfino NA, Wright SC, Katz I, et al. Effect of low concentrations of ozone on inhaled allergen responses in asthmatic subjects. *Lancet* 1991;338:199–203.

93. Bascom R, Naclerio RM, Fitzgerald TK, Kagey-Sobotka A, Proud D. Effect of ozone inhalation on the response to nasal challenge of allergic subjects. *Am Rev Respir Dis* 1990;142:594–601.
94. Orehek J, Grimaldi F, Muls E, Durand JP, Viala A, Charpin J. Bronchial response to allergens after controlled NO_2 exposure. *Bull Eur Physiopathol Respir* 1981;17:911–915.
95. Jakab GJ, Spannhake EW, Canning BJ, Kleeberger SR, Gilmour MI. The effects of ozone on immune function. *Arch Environ Health [in press]*.
96. Ozawa M, Fujimaki H, Imai T, Honda Y, Watanabe N. Suppression of IgE antibody production after exposure to ozone in mice. *Int Arch Allergy Appl Immunol* 1985;76:16–19.
97. Fujimaki H. Impairment of humoral immune responses in mice exposed to nitrogen dioxide and ozone mixtures. *Environ Res* 1989;48:211–217.
98. Fujimaki H, Shiraishi F, Ashikawa T, Murakami M. Changes in delayed hypersensitivity reaction in mice exposed to O_3. *Environ Res* 1987;43:186–190.
99. Mossman TR, Coffman RL. Heterogeneity of cytokine secretion patterns and functions of T helper cells. *Adv Immunol* 1989;46:111–147.
100. Dziedzic D, Wright ES, Sargent NE. Pulmonary response to ozone: reaction of bronchus-associated lymphoid tissue and lymph node lymphocytes in the rat. *Environ Res* 1990;51:194–208.
101. Bleavins MR, Dziedzic D. An immunofluorescence study of T and B lymphocytes in ozone-induced pulmonary lesions in the mouse. *Toxicol Appl Pharmacol* 1990;105:93–102.
102. Dziedzic D, White HJ. T-cell activation in pulmonary lymph nodes of mice exposed to ozone. *Environ Res* 1986;41:610–622.
103. Koren HS, Devlin RB, Becker S. O_3-induced inflammatory responses in pulmonary cells. In: Shook L, Laskin D, eds. *Xenobiotic induced inflammation: role of cytokines and growth factors*. Orlando, FL: Academic Press; [*in press*].

Immunotoxicology and Immunopharmacology, Second Edition, edited by J. H. Dean, M. I. Luster, A. E. Munson, and I. Kimber.
Raven Press, Ltd., New York © 1994.

23

Effects of Tobacco Smoke on the Immune System

Mohan L. Sopori, *Niranjan S. Goud, and *Alan M. Kaplan

*Department of Immunotoxicology, The Lovelace Institutes, Albuquerque, New Mexico 87108; and *Department of Microbiology and Immunology, University of Kentucky College of Medicine, Lexington, Kentucky 40536*

The lung is an important route of exposure to environmental antigens and pathogens via its airways and systemic exposure to antigens and pathogens via its vascular system. The success or failure of pulmonary defense mechanisms largely determines the manifestation of clinical lung disease. Clearance of particulate antigens from the lung is accomplished by nonspecific and specific defense mechanisms. In the respiratory tract of mammals, nonspecific protection is provided primarily by the mucociliary escalator of the large airways. This process removes the bulk of inhaled foreign matter present in the ambient air (reviewed in refs. 1–3). Protection against particulate material reaching the lung alveoli involves local detoxification via phagocytosis by pulmonary alveolar macrophages (AMs) (4,5). Inhaled substances are also channeled to the regional lymph nodes through interstitial and lymphatic routes (6).

The specific mechanisms of lung defense involve active immunity. Both humoral and cell-mediated immune responses participate in resistance to pulmonary infections (6–13). Microbial neutralizing and opsonizing antibodies and T lymphocytes constitute the pulmonary-specific immune response. Thus any damage to these cells or impairment of their ability to synthesize antibodies, by infectious or toxic agents, may damage pulmonary defense mechanisms, resulting in an increased susceptibility to acute and chronic respiratory tract diseases.

Cigarette smoking has been demonstrated to be a major health risk factor and significantly increases the incidence of cancer of the respiratory tract, upper digestive tract, bladder, kidney, and pancreas (14–17). Epidemiologic studies have also established an association between the use of chewing tobacco and cancer of the oral cavity (18). These inferences have been supported by bioassays in animal models (17–19). Specifically, the application of tobacco smoke condensates and the inhalation of tobacco smoke have been shown to induce cancers in laboratory animals (19–21). Inhalation of cigarette smoke also accelerates the formation of age-related deoxyribonucleic acid (DNA) adducts in the rat lung and nasal mucosa (22).

Long-term exposure to cigarette smoke has been associated with a higher frequency of acute and chronic respiratory tract diseases (23,24), the mechanisms of which have yet to be well delineated. Human smokers have been reported to have an increased incidence of influenza and other respiratory infections and lower titers of antibodies to influenza virus (25–28). It has been postulated that this increased susceptibility reflects cigarette-smoke-induced impairment of the immune system (29). Thus tobacco smoking has been shown to increase leukocyte numbers (30–33), impair granulocyte chemotaxis, increase the release of elastase and superoxide from lung macrophages (34,35), and stimulate degranulation of basophils (36,37). Also, in experimental animals, chronic exposure to tobacco smoke has been reported to significantly decrease lymphocyte proliferation to mitogens, lower antibody production, enhance the growth of tumors, and reduce the size of bronchus-associated lymphoid tissue (BALT) (29,38,39). Exposure to passive or environmental tobacco smoke may also enhance the susceptibility of children to respiratory diseases, but, other than irritation, its effects on the immune system of adults are equivocal (40,41). In the following, we discuss various aspects of cigarette smoking and its biologic consequences including results from experimental animal models designed to study the effects of cigarette smoke on the immune system.

COMPOSITION OF CIGARETTE SMOKE

Tobacco smoke is a complex mixture of particulate and gaseous compounds. It is estimated that cigarette smoke contains over 4000 different chemical constituents, many of which have toxic and/or carcinogenic activity (42–45). The composition of mainstream cigarette smoke (smoke drawn into the mouth during puffs) is quantitatively and, to some extent, qualitatively different from that of sidestream cigarette smoke (smoke formed from a smoldering cigarette between puffing and released into the ambient air) (40,46,47). These differences are due primarily to the lower temperature and limited availability of oxygen inside the burning cone during sidestream smoke formation. While the constituents of mainstream smoke are mainly encountered by the smoker, sidestream cigarette smoke is the major source of environmental or passive tobacco smoke exposure. Although partial pyrolysis products including some toxic, carcinogenic, and cocarcinogenic substances such as nicotine, carbon monoxide (CO), carbon dioxide (CO_2), catechol, benzopyrenes, *N*-nitrosamines [*N*-nitrosodimethylamine, *N*′-nitrosoanabasine, 4-(methylnitrosamino)-1-(3-pyridyl)-1-butanone], and ammonia are enriched in sidestream cigarette smoke, dilution by room air reduces markedly the concentrations passively inhaled by an involuntary smoker (41,48).

Bioassays with cigarette smoke have indicated that the majority of genotoxic and carcinogenic substances as well as nicotine are present in the particulate phase (material from cigarette smoke retained by the Cambridge filter comprising 99.7% of all the particles with diameters of >0.1 μm) of mainstream cigarette smoke (49).

The vapor phase (substances that pass through the Cambridge filter) contains carbon monoxide, carbon dioxide, volatile aldehydes, benzene, ketones, nitrogen oxides, hydrogen cyanide, volatile nitriles, and 400 to 500 minor constituents. Moreover, some components of the vapor phase are known carcinogens in humans and animals (48).

While exposure to the vapor phase alone has not been shown to be tumorigenic in inhalation assays, total smoke induces benign and malignant tumors in the upper respiratory tract of rats and hamsters (45,48). Evidence from studies on contact carcinogenesis suggests that particulates ("tars"), especially the neutral subfraction of the particulate phase, contain the most known tumorigenic and carcinogenic compounds present in cigarette smoke (48). In addition to carcinogens and cocarcinogens, tobacco smoke contains organ-specific carcinogens, supporting the epidemiologic data that cigarette smoke is a risk factor in the etiology of cancer of the esophagus, pancreas, and urinary bladder (17). Nicotine, one of the major constituents of the particulate phase of mainstream cigarette smoke, contributes heavily to the formation of nitrosamines, which are powerful inducers of benign and malignant tumors in the upper respiratory tract and the lung of laboratory animals (50).

IMMUNOLOGIC EFFECTS OF CIGARETTE SMOKE: HUMAN STUDIES

The possibility that increased prevalence of diseases associated with cigarette smoke may in part be due to tobacco smoke-induced changes in immune and inflammatory processes was first recognized in the 1960s (reviewed in ref. 29). A large body of literature now exists regarding the consequences of exposure to cigarette smoke and cigarette smoke extracts on the immune system of both humans and experimental animals and many reports support the hypothesis that cigarette smoking may have significant effects on the immune system (29,38,39). The qualitative and quantitative effects of smoking may depend on the amount and duration of smoke exposure, on the species tested, and, in humans, on the sex and ethnic background of subjects in the study. In the following section we review (a) the immunologic effects of cigarette smoking in humans, (b) effects of exposure to cigarette smoke or smoke extracts on the immune response of experimental animals, and (c) effects of components of cigarette smoke on the immune system.

Although, in humans, cigarette smoking has been demonstrated to be associated with increased susceptibility to numerous infections and a variety of alterations in the humoral and cellular immune system, the degree and extent of these changes vary significantly among studies. Effects of smoking on the following parameters of the immune system have been the subject of most studies.

Cigarette Smoking and Alveolar Macrophages

Cigarette smoking has been implicated as a significant risk factor for acute respiratory tract illnesses (14,23) and chronic obstructive lung disease (24). AMs are the predominant cells recovered from bronchoalveolar lavage (BAL) fluids in normal individuals and cigarette smoking has been documented to induce a variety of changes in these cells (51). In this context, cigarette smoking causes a three- to fivefold increase in the number of AMs (52–55) and a smaller increase in the number of neutrophils (52–57) in the lung. There is good evidence to suggest that the AMs present in smokers are derived from peripheral blood monocytes (58–60).

It appears that AMs from smokers are in a more "active" state than those from nonsmokers. Furthermore, AMs from smokers have alterations in surface membranes (61,62), contain cytoplasmic inclusions (63), and exhibit increased levels of microsomal and lysosomal enzymes (64–66). In addition, smoking also elevates the resting rate of glucose utilization in these cells (67). There is also evidence to suggest that AMs from smokers produced significantly more oxygen radicals and products of myeloperoxidase activity (68,69) and exhibited impaired protein and ribonucleic acid (RNA) synthesis (70–72). Several reports have indicated that cigarette smoking also causes functional alterations in AMs including depression of lymphoproliferative responses to antigens (73,74) and increased migration and chemotactic responsiveness (75,76). Finally, AMs from smokers formed significantly fewer complement-dependent rosettes than from nonsmokers (76,77). However, neutrophil function, assessed by chemotactic, microbicidal, and secretory activities, appeared to be comparable between smokers and nonsmokers (33,34).

Although, smokers' AMs appeared to exist in a more "active" state, comparisons of the phagocytic and bactericidal activities of these cells between smokers and nonsmokers have yielded conflicting results. Some studies with human AMs have detected little difference in the ability of smokers' and nonsmokers' AMs to ingest and kill microorganisms (67,78–81), while others report decreased phagocytosis and/or bactericidal activity of AMs from smokers. Thus Fisher et al. (82) demonstrated that AMs from smokers, compared to nonsmokers, had a lowered ability to ingest carbonized polystyrene latex microspheres. Martin and Warr (61) reported reduced phagocytosis of *Staphylococcus aureus* by smokers' AMs while internalization of *Candida krusei* was the same for smokers and nonsmokers. Green (83) demonstrated that *in vitro* exposure of AMs to cigarette smoke reduced both phagocytic and bactericidal activities for *S. albus* in a dose-dependent manner. King et al. (84) showed that AMs from smokers were able to phagocytose *Listeria monocytogenes* normally but expressed a selective functional deficiency in their ability to kill this facultative intracellular bacteria.

A consistent feature of chronic pulmonary inflammation, caused by cigarette smoking, is that macrophages accumulate in the alveoli and respiratory bronchioli (23,54). Smokers' lungs also have alveolar septal hypercellularity (85). The abundance of AMs in smokers' lungs and their ability to secrete a variety of biologically active substances (86) may play an important role in the pathogenesis of lung tissue. While products of the cyclooxygenase pathway [prostaglandin E_2 (PGE_2), $PGF_{2\alpha}$, leukotriene B_4, and 5-hydroxyeicosatetra enoic acid (5-HETE)] are substantially reduced in AMs by smoking (87–89), increased release of reactive oxygen metabolites and elastase has been reported (35,38,90–95). The latter may contribute to the damage of connective tissue and parenchymal cells of the lung and may therefore play an important role in the pathogenesis of emphysema (35,95–97).

Since cigarette smoking induces recruitment of neutrophils and macrophages from the peripheral blood into the lung, the mechanism by which this accumulation occurs is important for understanding the pathogenesis of smoke-induced lung disease. The CD11/CD18 leukocyte surface adhesion glycoprotein plays an essential role in adhesion-related functions such as migration, chemotaxis, and phagocytosis (98–100). Migration of monocytes from peripheral blood to alveoli would require the binding of CD11/CD18 to its ligand CD54 [intracellular adhesion molecule-1 (ICAM-1)] on endothelial cells within the lung (101). Upon migration into tissues, cells of the mononuclear phagocyte series may undergo maturation and downregulate CD11/CD18 expression (102). Recently, Hoogsteden et al. (103) reported that there is no enrichment of CD11+/CD18+ monocytes in the peripheral blood of smokers and, compared to nonsmokers, the proportion of CD11+/CD18+ AMs is significantly decreased in smokers' BAL fluid. Furthermore, they suggested that increased production of interleukin-1 (IL-1) and other inflammatory cytokines in smokers' AMs resulted in enhanced expression of ICAM-1 (104,105) on endothelial cells within the lung, allowing the migration of monocytes into alveoli (106). In fact, IL-1 production by AMs has been shown to increase in smokers (107).

Other mechanisms proposed for migration of neutrophils and monocytes to alveoli include the presence of chemotactic factors in cigarette smoke (108,109), activation of cells in the lower respiratory tract resulting in the release of chemotactic factors (53,110), and activation of the complement system (111–115). In animal experiments, Kew et al. (113) demonstrated that C5-deficient mice attract significantly fewer neutrophils and AMs to their respiratory tract in response to cigarette smoke than do C5-sufficient mice. Cigarette smoke has been shown to cleave C3, C5, and the alternate complement pathway protein properdin factor B (PFB) *in vitro* (111,112,114,115). Moreover, cigarette smoke can stimulate the epithelial cells lining the airways to release neutrophil chemotactic activity (110). Activation of the complement pathway releases biologically active fragments that may also activate additional mechanisms of leukocyte recruitment. Complement fragments of PFB, C3, and C5 stimulate AMs to release increased amounts of neutrophil chemotactic activity (116–118). There is also evidence that the complement system may direct the influx of neutrophils in other respiratory tract disorders such as bacterial pneumonia (119), adult respiratory distress syndrome (120), and cystic fibrosis (121). Thus it appears likely that more than one mechanism may contribute to the monocyte/neutrophil influx into the lungs of cigarette smokers.

Effects of Cigarette Smoke on Immunoglobulin (Ig) Levels

In spite of some disparity in results, there is general agreement that, excepting IgE, cigarette smoking decreases serum Ig levels (122–129). Several investigators have shown that cigarette smoking causes a significant reduction in the serum levels of IgG, IgA, and IgM (123–125). Anderson et al. (128) reported only a slight decrease in IgM levels and Ferson et al. (122) observed a significant decrease in IgG but not in IgA and IgM levels. Mili et al. (125) reported a negative dose–response correlation between cigarette smoking and the serum IgG levels, while Gulsvik and Fagerhol (126) demonstrated decreased Ig levels in moderate but not heavy smokers.

Unlike the effects on IgG, IgA, and IgM, serum concentrations of IgE are significantly higher in smokers than in nonsmokers (129–140). Although smokers have higher serum IgE levels, a direct proportionality between intensity and duration of smoking to IgE levels is debatable. Zetterstrom et al. (132) and Warren et al. (134) did not find a significant relationship between the amount of smoking and IgE levels, while Bahna et al. (138,139) and Shirakawa et al. (140) observed that IgE levels were highest in mild smokers and decreased with increased cigarette smoking. Levels of IgE increased arithmetically with cigarette smoking in smokers occupationally exposed to hard metals (e.g., cobalt) (140). Cigarette smokers also showed a biphasic response to changes in serum IgD concentrations; light to moderate smoking increased while heavy smoking decreased serum IgD levels (129,141). Finally, autoantibodies, such as antinuclear antibodies and rheumatoid factors, have been found more frequently in smokers than nonsmokers (142).

There appears to be no correlation between cigarette smoking, IgE levels, and skin-test reactivity. In fact, smokers exhibit significantly lower skin-test reactivity for a given value of IgE as compared to nonsmokers (130–134). Eosinophilia frequently observed in smokers is related to IgE levels and skin reactivity in nonsmokers but not in smokers (133). There is some evidence of a relationship between IgE levels and rates of diagnosed asthma, wheeze, and chronic cough and/or sputum in smokers (131). Lehrer et al. (143) demonstrated IgE specific for tobacco antigens in some people, but the frequency was very low and was not significantly increased in smokers. Thus the role of cigarette smoke-induced IgE in the pathogenesis of disease in smokers is not clear.

Effects of Cigarette Smoke on Lymphocytes

One of the well-recognized effects of cigarette smoking in human smokers is leukocytosis (30–33). There is also evidence that smoke-induced leukocytosis is related to the dose of smoking (31). Smokers have significantly increased numbers of all lymphocyte populations (32); however, in light (10 to 19 pack-years) to moderate (20 to 49 pack-years) smokers, there was no difference in the ratios of total T and B lymphocytes between smokers and nonsmokers (32,144,145). In heavy smokers (50 to 120 pack-years) total T cells (CD3+) were increased, but the percentage of CD4+ T cells was decreased and those of CD8+ T cells were increased, leading to a significant decrease in the CD4+/CD8+ ratio (144,145). A decreased CD4+/CD8+ ratio was also reported by Costabel et al. (146,147). On the other hand, Tollerud et al. (57) observed no significant change in the number of

CD3+ cells in smokers from an age- and sex-matched caucasian population with a history of 5 to 50 pack-years, but there was a selective increase in CD4+ T cells resulting in a statistically significant increase in the CD4+/CD8+ ratio. Moreover, the percentage of CD4+ T cells tended to increase as the consumption of cigarettes increased in the population. Increases in the CD4+ T cell population in smokers have also been reported by others (32,125,148,149). Smart et al. (150) found a significant increase in total T cells (CD3+), T cell subsets (CD4+, CD8+, and CD11+), and the CD4+/CD8+ ratio. In contrast to their finding in a caucasian population (57), Tollerud et al. (151) observed a significant dose-related decrease in CD4+ T cells and no change in the CD4+/CD8+ ratio among black smokers, suggesting ethnic background may be an important response modifier.

Results on the effects of cigarette smoke on B cell numbers are generally uniform in that cigarette smoking increases the number of B cells (32,57,125,148,150,152). In contrast, Aizawa et al. (153) found that, compared to nonsmokers, the relative B cell counts were lower among all smokers. However, statistically significant differences were found only between nonsmokers and those who smoked ≤19 years or ≤29 cigarettes/day (153).

The conflict in the above results may reflect variabilities associated with small sample size, race, sex, and age of the population studied. Thus there are significant differences in a number of immunologic parameters between blacks and whites and between men and women of the same race (125,148,151,154).

The relationship between cigarette smoking and lymphocyte function in human smokers is debatable. While lymphocyte function, assessed by phytohemagglutinin (PHA)-induced lymphoproliferation, is elevated in young male smokers (155), the response in older male smokers was significantly decreased in comparison to nonsmokers of the same age group (156). Petersen et al. (157) also found lower mitogen responses in male smokers. Several groups did not find significant differences in lymphocyte responses to PHA and/or concanavalin A (Con A) (32,158–160) or to alloantigens in a mixed lymphocyte reaction (160) between smokers and nonsmokers. However, smokers had significantly decreased *in vitro* suppressor T cell activity on the Ig-secreting response of allogeneic B cells (32).

Since cigarette smoking is associated with an increased incidence of a variety of malignant diseases (16,17,161), several investigators have evaluated the effects of cigarette smoking on natural killer (NK) cell activity in human smokers. Ferson et al. (122) were the first to report that the NK cell activity of peripheral blood leukocytes, against cultured melanoma cells, was significantly lower in smokers than in nonsmokers. Subsequently, these observations were corroborated by others (32,123,162). Hughes et al. (32) found differences in NK but not antibody-dependent cell-mediated cytotoxicity (ADCC) cell activity, whereas Tollerud and coworkers observed that while white smokers exhibited lower NK cell activity (162), black smokers and nonsmokers had comparable NK cell activity (151). Thus effects of cigarette smoke on the NK cell activity may depend on the genetic background of the population studied.

EFFECTS OF CIGARETTE SMOKE ON THE IMMUNE SYSTEM: ANIMAL STUDIES

As in humans, effects of mainstream cigarette smoke exposure in animals have yielded ambiguous results. In experimental animals (mainly rodents), changes in the immune system following exposure to cigarette smoke appear to be dependent on several factors including the level and duration of exposure to cigarette smoke, tar and nicotine content of the smoke, and the species of animal tested. One of the advantages of using experimental animals for these studies is that the investigators can employ inbred strains of animals to control for genetic variability. Animals are exposed to cigarette smoke from a standard reference cigarette so the composition of cigarette smoke is controlled. The University of Kentucky Tobacco and Health Research Institute has developed a number of reference cigarettes of different tar and nicotine content for this purpose (163). Several apparatuses for exposing experimental animals to cigarette smoke have also been developed (164–166). Very rapid changes in chemical composition occur in cigarette smoke after it is generated (49), resulting in potential changes in its biologic activity. Therefore smoking machines are designed to expose laboratory animals to smoke closely resembling human smoking in chemical and mechanical characteristics. A smoking machine, commonly used in the United States for exposing small rodents, was described by Griffith (166) and Griffith and Hancock (167). However, in spite of the well-regulated conditions employed for exposing animals to cigarette smoke, it is impractical to precisely replicate all the parameters of human smoking. Thus, unlike humans who smoke a given quantity of cigarettes over a period of about 16 hr, animals are usually administered their daily dose of cigarette smoke in one to two sessions of 8 to 15 min each. This would significantly reduce the exposure time of these animals to those components of cigarette smoke that have a relatively short *in vivo* half-life. Also, many animal studies involve 5 d/wk exposures, a situation not normally encountered in human smokers. Therefore mainstream cigarette smoke exposures, kinetically comparable to human smokers, may be difficult to accurately replicate in animal models. Nevertheless, results from animal experiments have yielded some promising clues about the mechanism of action of cigarette smoke on the immune system.

Immunologic Effects of Short-Term Smoke Exposure

Esber et al. (168) reported a significant inhibition of humoral antibody (primary and secondary hemagglutinin) responses in mice exposed to very high levels (7 exposures/day) of cigarette smoke or its vapor phase for 7 days before or 2 days after an antigenic challenge. BALB/c mice exposed to cigarette smoke for 3 days or 18 weeks exhibited an altered primary immune response as judged by the splenic architecture (169). Thus smoke-exposed mice, upon antigenic challenge, had less pronounced and/or "short-lived" splenomegaly and reduced expansion of splenic white pulp. In the experiments of Thomas et al. (170), short-term smoke exposure of mice increased the level of serum hemolytic and hemagglutinating antibodies and the numbers of plaque-forming cells (PFCs) in the spleen and lymph nodes. Cigarette smoke inhalation of mice for 10 days (171) and rats for 16 weeks (172) did not lead to a significant alteration of the PFC response. However, Thomas et al. (170), following 5 days of smoke exposure of mice, observed an increased PFC response of spleen but not mediastinal or cervical lymph node cells. Thus it appeared that acute to moderate inhalation of cigarette smoke in rodents did not produce very significant depression of the immune system and, under certain situations, may have enhanced the immunologic response. Inhibition of the antibody response reported by Esber et al. (168) may have reflected the response of animals to acute administration of very high doses of cigarette smoke.

Immunologic Effects of Long-Term Smoke Exposure

Several studies with subchronic (days to months) and chronic exposures (months to years) of smoke inhalation in animals have demonstrated a biphasic effect on immune parameters, producing stimulation of the immune system after subchronic exposure and suppression following chronic exposures. Results from studies on the effects of cigarette smoke on the resistance to challenges with viable tumor cells suggested that C57BL or BALB/c mice exposed to smoke inhalation for 2 to 3 months were more resistant to subcutaneous or intratracheal tumor cell challenges, suggesting enhanced immunity following subchronic smoke exposure (173). However, as exposure time to cigarette smoke was increased, smoke-exposed animals exhibited a progressive decrease in their resistance to these tumors (173). Increased tumor metastases and mortality in chronically smoke-exposed mice were also observed in other experiments (174–177).

The biphasic character of cigarette smoke-induced changes has also been demonstrated for the humoral immune response. The direct and indirect PFC response of the spleen and peripheral lymph nodes to sheep red blood cells (SRBCs) was first enhanced and then depressed by continual exposure to cigarette smoke (170,174, 178–180). Cellular immunity, as assessed by the PHA-induced lymphoproliferative response or development of tumor-specific cytotoxic T cells, was initially increased but continued exposure to cigarette smoke significantly reduced this response (173,174,181,182). Moreover, cigarette smoke containing higher levels of tar and nicotine induced immunologic changes faster than smoke containing lower levels of tar and nicotine (174). A decreased response to the T cell mitogen Con A was observed in monkeys subjected to high doses of chronic smoke inhalation (183).

Chronic exposure of animals to cigarette smoke is associated with increased susceptibility to infectious agents such as murine sarcoma virus (175) and influenza virus (184,185). Using infections with live influenza virus, Mackenzie (184) reported a decreased frequency of seroconversion with chronic smoke inhalation but, conversely, short-term exposure resulted in an enhancement of the immune response. Clearance of *Pseudomonas aeruginosa* from the lungs of 36-week smoke-exposed animals was significantly less efficient than in nonsmoking controls (176). Okazaki et al. (186) observed lower antibody response to *Micropolyspora faeni* in the lungs and spleens of smoke-exposed rabbits. Mackenzie and Flower (185), examining the extent and specificity of the secondary serologic response to influenza virus, observed the production of high titers of less specific (cross-reacting) antibodies in mice exposed to 36 weeks of smoke inhalation.

It has been hypothesized that the effects of chronic cigarette smoke inhalation in animals occur primarily on T cell or T cell-dependent functions; serum antibody responses to T cell-independent (TI) antigens such as polyvinylpyrrolidone (PVP) are generally not inhibited (170,176,177). However, Goud et al. (187) recently reported a significant reduction in the PFC response to PVP in the spleens of smoke-exposed animals. But response to trinitrophenyl (TNP)–Ficoll, another TI antigen, was not affected by smoking. Differences in the method of smoke exposure (5 days versus 7 days) and/or the type of response examined (serum antibody levels versus PFCs) may account for this disparity. Sopori et al. (172) also observed a significant decrease in the PFC response to both T cell-dependent (SRBC) and TI antigens (TNP–*Brucella abortus*) in rats chronically exposed to cigarette smoke. Furthermore, Savage et al. (188) reported that while the numbers of total and antigen-specific B cells in the spleen of smoke-exposed rats were comparable to control, they failed to proliferate in response to antigen, suggesting a smoke-induced B cell defect. In mice, exposed to chronic smoke inhalation, Chang et al. (189) observed a T cell functional defect in lung-associated lymphoid tissue but not in anatomically distant lymph nodes. Thus cigarette smoke may have variable effects on different lymphoid organs. In this regard, while the anti-PVP PFC response in the spleens of smoke-exposed animals was reduced, the response in other lymph nodes was augmented (187). Similarly, rats exposed to cigarette smoke first exhibited a decrease in the PFC response in the lung-associated lymph nodes and, as smoke inhalation was continued, the immune dysfunction subsequently spread to other lymphoid tissues as well (172).

One of the first immune parameters significantly reduced in smoke-exposed animals is the humoral antibody response (172,176,178,187). Chronic cigarette smoke inhalation may inhibit B cell responses in the spleen (172,188). Preliminary experiments in rats, exposed to chronic smoke inhalation, suggested that exposure to smoke impaired the antigen-mediated signal transduction pathway in B cells (190). In addition, cigarette smoke may damage T cell function in the lung-associated lymphoid tissues (189).

Several lines of evidence have suggested that cigarette smoking affects the primary antibody response to an antigen. Thomas et al. (170) found that while the primary PFC response to SRBCs was significantly inhibited in 38-week smoke-exposed mice, the secondary response to this antigen was not affected by cigarette smoking. Mice immunized with sublethal doses of influenza virus, prior to exposure to cigarette smoke, were able to mount a secondary immune response of normal intensity when challenged with the homologous virus strain (185). Thus the immune system of smokers may function normally when responding to an antigen or pathogen encountered prior to smoking.

SMOKELESS CIGARETTES

It is estimated that about 12 million people in the United States use smokeless tobacco (ST) (190–194). Generally, there are two popular methods of ST use—dipping of snuff (finely ground or shredded tobacco) in the oral cavity or chewing coarsely cut tobacco leaves. There is substantial evidence linking the use of ST with oral cancer and a variety of oral conditions such as leukoplakia, dental cavities, discoloration of teeth, gingivitis, localized gum recession, and changes in the soft structure of oral mucosa (195–200). ST has also been found to have systemic effects. For example, chewing of tobacco by pregnant women was found to reduce the birth weight of newborn infants and to increase the incidence of spontaneous abortions and stillbirths in women in India (201,202). In laboratory animals, ST treatment during the gestation period was found to cause weight reduction, delay ossification, and cause an increase in hemorrhages and fetal lethality (203).

Despite the vast amount of data on the toxic effects of ST, the influence of ST on the immune system has not received much attention. In a recent report, it was observed that ST was found to have strong mitogenic potential on murine lymphoid cells in *in vitro* culture (204). In addition to proliferation, an aqueous extract of ST was able to induce a significant increase in polyclonal antibody responses as determined by the PFC assay. This may have been due to the direct effect of ST on B cells. Alternatively, ST may activate macrophages or T cells with the factors secreted by these activated cells inducing the maturation of B cells. In this regard, when the cell-free culture supernatants were analyzed, there was a significant increase of IL-1 activity in spleen cell cultures stimulated with ST extract compared to the control unstimulated cultures as had been previously reported for human leukocytes cultured with tobacco glycoprotein (205). Interestingly, ST extract was also found to induce proliferation of purified splenic T cells but without concomitant induction of IL-2 secretion (204). Similar results have been reported for human T cells where tobacco glycoprotein-induced stimulation was shown to be independent of IL-2 (206). Analysis of intracellular second messengers indicated that stimulation of murine B or T lymphocytes by ST extract did not involve elevation of intracellular Ca^{2+}. Thus it is possible that ST extract was activating lymphocytes by another system of second messengers related to the adenylate cyclase pathway involving cyclic adenosine monophosphate (cAMP). These results were contradictory to those of Lindemann and Park (207), who reported a significant decrease of IL-2- or PHA-induced proliferation of human peripheral blood lymphocytes treated with aqueous extract of ST. The discrepancy in results between these studies may have been due to differences in the concentrations of the tobacco alkaloid nicotine or tobacco glycoprotein in the ST extracts, but these issues will have to be resolved by an analysis of ST extract and more careful evaluation of its constituents.

COMPONENTS OF CIGARETTE SMOKE THAT MAY AFFECT THE IMMUNE SYSTEM

Bioassays with total smoke have indicated that a majority of genotoxic agents reside in the particulate phase (19,45). Cigarette smoke with high tar and nicotine content was shown to be more efficient in inducing immunosuppression (174), suggesting that tar and nicotine may be important immunotoxic components of the cigarette smoke. At the pH of mainstream cigarette smoke, greater than 80% of nicotine is in the particulate fraction (48). Esber et al. (168) observed that acute exposure to cigarette smoke or its vapor phase inhibited the primary and secondary hemagglutinin response. However, the daily dose of cigarette smoke in these experiments was very high. Subsequently, experiments have shown that chronic exposure of rats to the vapor phase of cigarette smoke did not lead to the changes in the immune system observed with whole smoke (208). Water-soluble extracts of tobacco smoke and nicotine are immunosuppressive in animals (209,210). Nicotine was also shown to inhibit the response of rabbit peripheral lymphocytes to Con A and the *in vitro* secondary antibody response of spleen cells to SRBCs (211). Nicotine has been demonstrated to be chemotactic for neutrophils and also enhanced the responsiveness of these cells to chemotactic peptides (109). Thus nicotine, a major component of cigarette smoke, has immunosuppressive potential.

Daily *in vivo* intraperitoneal administration of nicotine for 7 days did not affect the primary antibody response to SRBCs in rats (S. M. Savage et al., *unpublished data*). However, constant exposure of rats to nicotine, via constant-release nicotine pellets, for 3 weeks produced significant depression of the PFC response to SRBCs (208). Thus nicotine in cigarette smoke may contribute to the immunosuppressive properties of cigarette smoke.

CONCLUSIONS

We have attempted to summarize the literature on the effects of cigarette smoking on the immune response. Although controversies abound about the manner and extent to which cigarette smoke influences the immune system, there is a great deal of evidence to suggest that chronic smoking inhibits both humoral and cell-mediated immune responses in humans and experimental animals. In addition, cigarette smoking in humans causes leukocytosis in the lung primarily resulting from the migration of monocytes and neutrophils from the blood. This phenomenon contributes to the bronchitis prevalent in human smokers. There are perhaps several distinct mechanisms, working in concert, that induce the migration of monocytes and neutrophils into the lung. Thus smoke-induced production of chemotactic factors in the serum via the activation of the complement pathway, secretion of chemotactic substances by resident leukocytes in the lung, expression of adhesion molecules on leukocyte membranes, and expression of receptors on endothelial cells at the site of infection all aid the migration and accumulation of leukocytes in smokers' lung.

The mechanism of smoke-induced changes in the active immune response is poorly understood. It is clear, however, that cigarette smoke affects mainly the primary antibody response. Results from animal studies suggest that cigarette smoke may not have tangible effects on the secondary antibody response to an antigen. This also appears to be the case in human smokers (212) and may explain the difficulty in assessing the changes in the immune system of adult human smokers. On the other hand, small children, who have not yet encountered the full repertoire of pathogens, seem more likely to develop susceptibilities to infection due to inhalation of environmental cigarette smoke (213,214).

Animal experiments suggest further that the functional activity of both B and T cells may be compromised by chronic exposure to cigarette smoke. Cigarette smoking does not reduce the number of T or B cells; therefore functional deficits in these populations may reflect either anergy or the presence of suppressor cell-mediated mechanisms.

Cigarette smoke is a very complex mixture of substances and many of these could potentially influence the immune system. Preliminary evidence suggests that nicotine contained in cigarette smoke may affect the B cell membrane signal transduction pathway (208).

Epidemiologic data have established clearly the health risks of cigarette smoking. In contrast, however, cigarette smoking may also decrease the risk of developing some diseases. For example, in spite of the high levels of serum IgE in smokers, environmental allergies are less common in smokers (130,131,133). Similarly, the incidence of pigeon breeders' disease (215), farmers' lung (216), and sarcoidosis (217) are less prevalent in smokers than in nonsmokers. Ulcerative colitis predominantly affects nonsmokers and ex-smokers when compared to smokers (218). The mechanism through which cigarette smoke modifies risk factors to these diseases is presumed to be immunologic in nature. Understanding the cellular and molecular mechanisms through which cigarette smoke affects the system is therefore very important.

ACKNOWLEDGMENTS

This work was supported in part by NIH grant DA04208 and a grant from the Tobacco and Health Research Institute of the University of Kentucky.

REFERENCES

1. Cohen AB, Gold WM. Defense mechanisms of the lung. *Annu Rev Physiol* 1975;37:325–350.
2. Kiburn KH. Clearance mechanisms in the respiratory tract. In: Lee DHK, ed. *Handbook of physiology*. Bethesda, MD: American Physiology Society; 1977:243–262.
3. Wanner A. Clinical aspects of mucociliary transport. *Ann Rev Respir Dis* 1977;116:73–125.
4. Kaltreider HB, Baldwell JL, Adam E. The fate and consequences of an organic particulate antigen instilled into bronchoalveolar spaces of normal canine lungs. *Am Rev Respir Dis* 1977;116:267–280.

5. Green GM, Jakab GJ, Low RB, Davis GS. Defense mechanisms of the respiratory membrane. *Am Rev Respir Dis* 1977;115:479–514.
6. Bice DE, Muggenburg BA. Lung response to antigen. *Semin Respir Med* 1984;5:217–227.
7. Nash DR, Holle B. Local and systemic cellular immune responses in guinea pigs given antigen parenterally or directly into the lower respiratory tract. *Clin Exp Immunol* 1973;13:573–583.
8. Waldman RH, Henney CS. Cell-mediated immunity and antibody responses in the respiratory tract after local and systemic immunization. *J Exp Med* 1991;134:482–494.
9. Thomas WR, Holt PG, Keast D. Local and systemic immune responses of mice after intratracheal and intravenous inoculations of sheep erythrocytes. *Int Arch Allergy Appl Immunol* 1974;46:487–497.
10. Bice DE, Harris DL, Muggenburg BA. Regional immunologic responses following localized deposition of antigen in the lung. *Exp Lung Res* 1980;1:33–40.
11. Abraham E, Freitas AA, Coutinho AA. Purification and characterization of intraparenchymal lung lymphocytes. *J Immunol* 1990;144:2117–2122.
12. Lipcomb MF, Lyons CR, O'Hara RM Jr, Stein-Streilein J. The antigen-induced selective recruitment of specific T lymphocytes to the lung. *J Immunol* 1982;128:111–115.
13. Stein-Streilein J, Bennett M, Mann D, Kumar V. Natural killer cells in mouse lung; surface phenotype, target preference, and response to local influenza virus infection. *J Immunol* 1983; 131: 2699–2704.
14. US Department of Health, Education, and Welfare. A report of the Surgeon General. *Smoking and health*. Washington, DC: US Government Printing Office; 1979.
15. US Department of Health and Human Services. A report of the Surgeon General. *Reducing the health consequences of smoking, 25 years of progress*. Washington, DC: US Government Printing Office; 1989.
16. US Department of Health and Human Services. A report of the Surgeon General. *The health consequences of smoking: cancer*. Washington, DC: US Government Printing Office; 1982.
17. IARC. Monographs on the evaluation of carcinogenic risk of chemicals to humans, vol 38. *Tobacco smoking*. Lyon: IARC; 1986.
18. IARC. Monograph on the evaluation of the carcinogenic risk of chemical to humans, vol 37. *Tobacco habits other than smoking, betel-quid and areca-nut chewing; and some related nitrosamines*. Lyon: IARC; 1985.
19. Hoffmann D, Wynder EL, Rivenson A, Lavoie, EJ, Hecht SS. Skin bioassays in tobacco carcinogenesis. *Prog Exp Tumor Res* 1983;26:43–67.
20. Wynder EL, Wright G. A study of tobacco carcinogenesis. 1. The primary fraction. *Cancer* 1957; 10:255–271.
21. Dalbey WE, Nettesheim P, Griesemer R, Caton JE, Guerin MR. Chronic inhalation of cigarette smoke by F344 rats. *J Natl Cancer Inst* 1980;64:383–390.
22. Gupta RC, Sopori ML, Gairola CG. Formation of cigarette smoke-induced DNA adducts in the rat lung and nasal mucosa. *Cancer Res* 1989;49:1916–1920.
23. Aronson MD, Weiss ST, Ben RL, Komaroff AL. Association between cigarette smoking and acute respiratory tract illness in young adults. *JAMA* 1982;248:181–183.
24. US Department of Health and Human Services. *The health consequences of smoking: chronic obstructive lung disease*. Washington, DC: US Government Printing Office; 1984.
25. Haynes WF, Krstulovic VJ, Loomis AL. Smoking habit and incidence of respiratory tract infections in a group of adolescent males. *Am Rev Respir Dis* 1966;93:730–735.
26. Finklea JF, Sandifer SH, Smith DD. Cigarette smoking and epidemic influenza. *Am J Epidemiol* 1969;90:390–399.
27. Mackenzie JS, Mackenzie IH, Holt PG. The effect of cigarette smoking on susceptibility to epidemic influenza and on serological responses to live attenuated and killed subunit influenza vaccines. *J Hyg (Camb)* 1976;77:409–417.
28. Kark JD, Lebiush M, Rannon L. Cigarette smoke as a risk factor for epidemic A (H^1N^1) influenza in young men. *N Engl J Med* 1982;307:1042–1046.
29. Holt PG, Keast D. Environmentally induced changes in immunological function: acute and chronic effects of inhalation of tobacco smoke and other atmospheric contaminants in man and experimental animals. *Bacteriol Rev* 1977;41:205–214.
30. Corre F, Lellouch J, Schwartz D. Smoking and leukocyte counts. Results of an epidemiological survey. *Lancet* 1971;2:632–634.
31. Friedman CD, Siegelaub AB, Seltzer CC, Feldman R, Colleen MF. Smoking habit and the leukocyte count. *Arch Environ Health* 1973;26:137–143.

32. Hughes DA, Haslam PL, Townsend PJ, Turner-Warwick M. Numerical and functional alteration in circulatory lymphocytes in cigarette smokers. *Clin Exp Immunol* 1985;61:459–466.
33. Noble RC, Penny BB. Comparison of leukocyte count and function in smoking and nonsmoking young men. *Infect Immun* 1975;12:550–555.
34. Abboud RT, Johnson AJ, Richter AM, Elwood RK. Comparison of *in vitro* neutrophil elastase release in nonsmokers and smokers. *Am Rev Respir Dis* 1983;128:507–510.
35. Rodriguez RJ, White RR, Senior RM, Levine EA. Elastase release from human alveolar macrophages: comparison between smokers and nonsmokers. *Science* 1977;198:313–314.
36. Walter S. Blood basophil counts in smokers and nonsmokers. *Indian J Med Res* 1982;76:317–319.
37. Walter S, Walter A. Basophil degranulation induced by cigarette smoking in man. *Thorax* 1982; 37:756–759.
38. Holt PG. Immune and inflammatory function in cigarette smokers. *Thorax* 1987;42:241–249.
39. Johnson JD, Hauchens DP, Kluwe WM, Craig DK, Fisher GL. Effects of mainstream and environmental tobacco smoke on the immune system in animals and humans: a review. *Crit Rev Toxicol* 1990;20:369–395.
40. US Department of Health and Human Services. *The health consequences of involuntary smoking*. Washington, DC: US Government Printing Office; 1986.
41. Samet JM. Environmental tobacco smoke. In: Lippmann M, ed. *Environmental toxicants: human exposures and their health effects*. New York: Van Nostrand Reinhold; 1992:231–265.
42. Stedman RL. The chemical composition of tobacco and tobacco smoke. *Chem Rev* 1968;68:153–207.
43. Schmeltz I, Hoffmann D. Nitrogen-containing compounds in tobacco and tobacco smoke. *Chem Rev* 1977;77:295–311.
44. Gairola C. Genetic effects of fresh cigarette smoke in *Saccharomyces cerevisiae*. *Mutat Res* 1982; 102:123–136.
45. Hoffmann D, Rivenson A, Hecht SS, Hilfrich I, Kobayashi N, Wynder EL. Model studies in tobacco carcinogenesis with Syrian golden hamster. *Prog Exp Tumor Res* 1979;24:370–390.
46. Sterling TD, Kobayashi D. Indoor byproduct level of tobacco smoke: a critical review of literature. *J Air Pollut Control Assoc* 1982;32:250–259.
47. National Research Council Committee on Passive Smoking. *Environmental tobacco smoke: measuring exposures and assessing health effects*. Washington, DC: National Academy Press; 1986.
48. Hoffmann D, Wynder EL. Chemical constituents and bioactivity of tobacco smoke. *IARC Sci Publ* 1986;74:145–165.
49. Dube MF, Green CR. Methods of collection of smoke for analytical purposes. *Recent Adv Tobacco Sci* 1982;8:42–102.
50. Hoffman D, Hecht SS. Perspectives in cancer research: nicotine derived N-nitrosamines and tobacco-related cancer. Current status and future directions. *Cancer Res* 1985;45:935–944.
51. Reynolds HY. Bronchoalveolar lavage. *Am Rev Respir Dis* 1987;135:250–263.
52. Auerback O, Garfunkel L, Hammond EC. Relationship of smoking and age to finding in the lung parenchyma: a microscopic study. *Chest* 1974;65:29–35.
53. Hunninghake GW, Crystal RG. Cigarette smoking and lung destruction. Accumulation of neutrophils in the lung of cigarette smokers. *Am Rev Respir Dis* 1983;128:833–838.
54. Niewoehner DE, Klinerman J, Rice DB. Pathologic changes in the peripheral airways of young cigarette smokers. *N Engl J Med* 1974;291:755–758.
55. Thompson AB, Daughton D, Robbins RA, Ghafouri MA, Oehlerking M, Rennard SI. Intraluminal airway inflammation in chronic bronchitis. Characterization and correlation with clinical parameters. *Am Rev Respir Dis* 1989;840:1527–1537.
56. Ludwig PW, Schwartz BA, Hoidal JR, Niewoehner DE. Cigarette smoking causes accumulation of polymorphonuclear leukocytes in alveolar septum. *Am Rev Respir Dis* 1985;131:828–830.
57. Tollerud DJ, Clark JW, Brown LM, et al. The effects of smoking on T cell subsets: population based survey of healthy caucasians. *Am Rev Respir Dis* 1989;139:1446–1451.
58. Brain J. Free cells in the lungs. *Arch Intern Med* 1970;126:477–483.
59. Blusse Van Oud Alblas A, Van Furth R. Origin, kinetics, and characteristics of pulmonary macrophages in the steady state. *J Exp Med* 1979;149:1504–1518.
60. Bowden D, Adamson I. Role of monocytes and interstitial cells in the generation of alveolar macrophages. I. Kinetic studies of normal mice. *Lab Invest* 1980;42:511–524.
61. Martin RR, Warr GA. Cigarette smoking and human pulmonary macrophages. *Hosp Pract (Off Ed)* 1977;86:97–104.

62. Finch GL, Fisher GL, Hayes TL, Golde DW. Surface morphology and functional studies of human alveolar macrophages from cigarette smokers and nonsmokers. *J Reticuloendoth Soc* 1982;32:1–23.
63. Brody AR, Craighead JE. Cytoplasmic inclusions in pulmonary macrophages of cigarette smokers. *Lab Invest* 1975;32:125–132.
64. Cantrell ET, Warr GA, Busbee DL, Martin RR. Induction of aryl hydrocarbon hydroxylase in human pulmonary alveolar macrophages by cigarette smoking. *J Clin Invest* 1973;52:1881–1884.
65. Harris JO, Olsen GN, Castle JR, Maloney AS. Comparison of proteolytic enzyme activity in pulmonary alveolar macrophages and blood leukocytes in smokers and nonsmokers. *Am Rev Respir Dis* 1975;111:579–586.
66. Martin RR. Altered morphology and increased acid hydrolase content of pulmonary macrophages from cigarette smokers. *Am Rev Respir Dis* 1973;107:596–601.
67. Harris JO, Swenson EW, Johnson JE III. Human alveolar macrophages: comparison of phagocytic ability, glucose utilization, and ultrastructure in smokers and nonsmokers. *J Clin Invest* 1970; 49:2086–2096.
68. Hoidal JR, Fox RB, LeMarbe PA, Perri R, Repine JE. Altered oxidative metabolic responses *in vitro* of alveolar macrophages from asymptomatic cigarette smokers. *Am Rev Respir Dis* 1981; 23:85–87.
69. Ludwig RW, Hoidal JR. Alteration in leukocyte oxidative metabolism in cigarette smokers. *Am Rev Respir Dis* 1982;126:977–980.
70. Low RB. Protein biosynthesis by the pulmonary alveolar macrophages. Conditions of assay and the effects of cigarette smoke extracts. *Am Rev Respir Dis* 1974;110:466–477.
71. Yeager H. Alveolar cells: depressant effect of cigarette smoke on protein synthesis. *Proc Soc Exp Biol* 1969;131:247–250.
72. Ando M, Sugimoto M, Nishi R, et al. Surface morphology and function of human pulmonary alveolar macrophages from smokers and nonsmokers. *Thorax* 1984;39:850–856.
73. Laughter AH, Martin RR, Twomey JJ. Lymphoproliferative responses to antigens mediated by human pulmonary alveolar macrophages. *J Lab Clin Med* 1977;89:1326–1332.
74. Rich EA, Tweardy DJ, Fujiwara H, Ellner JJ. Spectrum of immunoregulatory functions and properties of human alveolar macrophages. *Am Rev Respir Dis* 1987;136:258–265.
75. Warr GA, Martin RR. *In vitro* migration of human alveolar macrophages: effects of cigarette smoking. *Infect Immun* 1973;8:222–227.
76. Warr GA, Martin RR. Chemotactic responsiveness of human alveolar macrophages: effects of cigarette smoking. *Infect Immun* 1974;9:769–771.
77. Reynolds HY, Atkinson JP, Newball HH, Frank MM. Receptors for immunoglobulin and complement on human alveolar macrophages. *J Immunol* 1975;114:1813–1819.
78. Cohen AB, Cline MJ. The human alveolar macrophage: isolation, cultivation *in vitro*, and studies of morphologic and functional characteristics. *J Clin Invest* 1971;50:1390–1398.
79. Jonsson S, Musher DM, Lawrence EC. Phagocytosis and killing of *Haemophilus influenzae* by alveolar macrophages: no difference between smokers and nonsmokers. *Eur J Respir Dis* 1987; 70:309–315.
80. Reynolds HY, Kazmierowski JA, Newball HH. Specificity of opsonic antibodies to enhance phagocytosis of *Pseudomonas aeruginosa* by human alveolar macrophages. *J Clin Invest* 1975;56: 376–385.
81. McLeod R, Mack DG, McLeod EG, Campbell EJ, Estes RG. Alveolar macrophage function and inflammatory stimuli in smokers with and without obstructive lung disease. *Am Rev Respir Dis* 1985;131:377–384.
82. Fisher GL, McNeill KL, Finch GL, Wilson FD, Golde DW. Functional evaluation of lung macrophages from cigarette smokers and nonsmokers. *J Reticuloendoth Soc* 1982;32:311–321.
83. Green GM. Mechanism of tobacco smoke toxicity on pulmonary macrophage cells. *Eur J Respir Dis* 1985;66(Suppl):82–85.
84. King TE Jr, Savici D, Campbell PA. Phagocytosis and killing of *Listeria monocytogenes* by alveolar macrophages: smokers versus nonsmokers. *J Infect Dis* 1988;158:1309–1316.
85. Eidelman D, Saetta MP, Bhezzo H, et al. Cellularity of alveolar walls in smokers and its relation to alveolar destruction. *Am Rev Respir Dis* 1990;141:1547–1552.
86. Unanue ER. Secretory function of mononuclear phagocytes: a review. *Am J Pathol* 1976;83:396–417.
87. Laviolette M, Chang J, Newcombe DS. Human alveolar macrophages: a lesion in arachidonic acid metabolism in cigarette smokers. *Am Rev Respir Dis* 1981;77:397–401.

88. Laviolette M, Coulombe R, Picard S, Braquet P, Borgeat P. Decreased leukotriene B_4 synthesis in smokers' alveolar macrophages *in vitro*. *J Clin Invest* 1986;77:54–60.
89. Wolter NJ, Kunkel SL, Lynch JP, Ward PA. Production of cyclo-oxygenase products by alveolar macrophages in pulmonary sarcoidosis. *Chest* 1983;83:795–815.
90. Hoidal JR, Fox RB, LeMarbe PA, Takiff HE, Repine JE. Oxidative metabolism of alveolar macrophages from young asymptomatic cigarette smokers. *Chest* 1980;77(Suppl):270–271.
91. Joseph M, Tonnel AB, Capron A, Voisin C. Enzyme release and superoxide anion production by human alveolar macrophages stimulated with immunoglobulin E. *Clin Exp Immunol* 1980;40:416–422.
92. Hoidal JR, Niewoehner DE. Lung phagocyte recruitment and metabolic alterations induced by cigarette smoke in humans and in hamsters. *Am Rev Respir Dis* 1982;126:548–552.
93. Greening AP, Lowrie DB. Extracellular release of hydrogen peroxide by human alveolar macrophages: the relationship to cigarette smoking and lower respiratory tract infections. *Clin Sci* 1983; 65:661–664.
94. Razma AB, Lynch JP III, Wilson BS, Ward PA, Kunkel SL. Human alveolar macrophage activation and DR antigen expression in cigarette smokers. *Chest* 1984;85:415–435.
95. McCusker K. Mechanisms of respiratory tissue injury from cigarette smoking. *Am J Med* 1992; 93:18S–21S.
96. Janoff A, Carp H, Laurent P, Raju L. The role of oxidative processes in emphysema. *Am Rev Respir Dis* 1983;127S:31–38.
97. Senior RM, Kuhn C III. The pathogenesis of emphysema. In: Fishman AP, ed. *Pulmonary diseases and disorders*, vol 2, 2nd ed. New York: McGraw-Hill; 1988:1209–1219.
98. Sanchez-Madrid R, Nagy JA, Robbins E, Simon P, Springer TA. A human leukocyte differentiation antigen family with distinct α-subunits and a common β-subunit: the lymphocyte function associated antigen (LFA-1), the C3bi complement receptor (OKM1/Mac-1), and the P150,95 molecules. *J Exp Med* 1983;158:1785–1803.
99. Miller LJ, Schwarting R, Springer TA. Regulated expression of the Mac-1, LFA-1, P150,95 glycoprotein family during leukocyte differentiation. *J Immunol* 1986;137:2891–2900.
100. Springer TA, Anderson DC. The importance of Mac-1, LFA-1 glycoprotein family in monocytes and granulocyte adherence, chemotaxis, and migration into inflammatory sites: insights from an experimental nature. In: *Biochemistry of macrophages*, Ciba Foundation Symposium 118. London: Pitman; 1986:102–126.
101. Wegner CD, Gundel RH, Reily P, Haynes N, Letts LG, Rothlein R. Intracellular adhesion molecule-1 (ICAM-1) in the pathogenesis of asthma. *Science* 1990;247:456–459.
102. Strassmann G, Springer TA, Haskill SJ, Miraglia CC, Lanier LL, Adams DO. Studies on antigen associated with the activation of murine mononuclear phagocytes *in vivo*: differential expression of lymphocyte function-associated antigen in the several stages of development. *Cell Immunol* 1985; 94:265–275.
103. Hoogsteden HC, VanHal PTW, Wijkhuijs JM, Hop W, Verkaik APK, Hilvering C. Expression of the CD11/18 cell surface adhesion glycoprotein family on alveolar macrophages in smokers and nonsmokers. *Chest* 1991;100:1567–1571.
104. Kasama T, Kobayashi K, Fukushima T, et al. Production of interleukin 1-like factor from human peripheral blood monocytes and polymorphonuclear leukocytes by superoxide anion: the role of interleukin 1 and reactive oxygen species in inflamed sites. *Clin Immunol Immunopathol* 1989; 53:439–448.
105. Rothlein R, Czajkowski M, O'Neill MM, Martin SD, Mainolfi E, Merluzzi VJ. Induction of intracellular adhesion molecule 1 on primary and continuous cell lines by proinflammatory cytokines: regulation by pharmacologic agents and neutralizing antibodies. *J Immunol* 1988;141:1665–1669.
106. Bevilacqua MP, Pober JS, Wheeler ME, Cotran RS, Gimbrone MA. Interleukin-1 activation of vascular endothelium. *Am J Pathol* 1985;121:393–403.
107. Ronoux M, Lemarie E, Ronoux G. Interleukin-1 secretion by lipopolysaccharide-stimulated alveolar macrophages. *Respiration* 1989;55:158–168.
108. Bridges RB, Kraal H, Huang JT, Chancellor MB. Effects of tobacco smoke on chemotaxis and glucose metabolism of polymorphonuclear leukocytes. *Infect Immun* 1977;15:115–123.
109. Totti N III, McCusker KT, Campbell EJ, Griffin GL, Senior RM. Nicotine is chemotactic for neutrophils and enhances neutrophil responsiveness to chemotactic peptides. *Science* 1984;223: 169–171.

110. Shoji S, Ertl RF, Rennard SI. Cigarette smoke stimulates release of neutrophil chemotactic activity from cultured bronchial epithelial cells. *Clin Res* 1987;35:539(abst).
111. Kew RR, Ghebrehiwet B, Janoff A. Cigarette smoke can activate the alternate pathway of complement *in vitro* by modifying the third component of complement. *J Clin Invest* 1985;75:1000–1007.
112. Kew RR, Ghebrehiwet B, Janoff A. Characterization of the third component of complement (C3) after activation by cigarette smoke. *Clin Immunol Immunopathol* 1987;44:248–285.
113. Kew RR, Ghebrehiwet B, Janoff A. The fifth component of complement (C5) is necessary for maximum pulmonary leukocytosis in mice chronically exposed to cigarette smoke. *Clin Immunol Immunopathol* 1987;43:73–81.
114. Perricone R, Decarolis C, Desactis G, Fontana L. Complement activation by cigarette smoke condensate and tobacco infusion. *Arch Environ Health* 1983;38:176–179.
115. Robbins RA, Nelson KJ, Gossman GL, Koyama S, Rennard SI. Complement activation by cigarette smoke. *Am J Physiol* 1991;260(Lung Cell Mol Physiol 4):L254–L259.
116. Gadek JE, Hunninghake GW, Zimmerman RL, Crystal RG. Regulation of the release of alveolar macrophage-derived neutrophil chemotactic factor. *Am Rev Respir Dis* 1980;121:723–734.
117. Hensen PM, McCarthy K, Larsen GL, et al. Complement fragment, alveolar macrophages, and alveolitis. *Am J Pathol* 1979;97:93–110.
118. Robbins RA, Justice JM, Rasmussen JK, Russ WD, Thomas KR, Rennard SI. Role of chemotactic factor inactivator in modulating alveolar macrophage-derived neutrophil chemotactic activity. *J Lab Clin Med* 1987;109:164–170.
119. Hopkins H, Stull T, VonEssen SG, Robbins RA, Rennard SI. Neutrophil chemotactic factors in bacterial pneumonia. *Chest* 1989;95:1021–1027.
120. Robbins RA, Russ WD, Rasmussen JK, Clayton MM. Complement activation in the adult respiratory distress syndrome. *Am Rev Respir Dis* 1987;135:651–658.
121. Fick RB, Robbins RA, Squier SU, Schoderbek WE, Russ WD. Complement activation in cystic fibrosis respiratory fluids: *in vivo* and *in vitro* generation of C5a and chemotactic activity. *Pediatr Res* 1986;20:1258–1268.
122. Ferson M, Edwards A, Lind A, Milton GW, Hersey P. Low natural killer-cell activity and immunoglobulin levels associated with smoking in human subjects. *Int J Cancer* 1979;23;603–609.
123. Hersey P, Predergost D, Edwards A. Effects of cigarette smoking on the immune system: follow-up studies in normal subjects after cessation of smoking. *Med J Aust* 1983;2:425–429.
124. Robertson MD, Boyd JE, Collins HPR, Davis JMG. Serum immunoglobulin levels and humoral immune competence in coal workers. *Am J Indus Med* 1984;6:387–393.
125. Mill F, Flanders WD, Boring JR, Annest JL, Destefano AF. The association of race, cigarette smoking, and smoking cessation to measures of the immune system in middle-aged men. *Clin Immunol Immunopathol* 1991;59:187–200.
126. Gulsvik A, Fagerhol MK. Smoking and immunoglobulin levels. *Lancet* 1979;1:449
127. Gerrard JW, Heiner DC, Ko CG, Mink J, Meyers A, Dosman JA. Immunoglobulin levels in smokers and nonsmokers. *Ann Allergy* 1980;44:261–262.
128. Andersen P, Pedersen DF, Bach B, Bonde GJ. Serum antibodies and immunoglobulins in smokers and nonsmokers. *Clin Exp Immunol* 1982;47:467–473.
129. McSharry C, Banham SW, Boyd G. Effect of cigarette smoking on the antibody response to inhaled antigens and the prevalence of extrinsic allergic alveolitis among pigeon breeders. *Clin Allergy* 1985;15:487–492.
130. Burrows B, Halonen M, Barbee RA, Lebowitz MD. The relationship of serum immunoglobulin E to cigarette smoking. *Am Rev Respir Dis* 1981;124:523–525.
131. Burrows B, Halonen M, Lebowitz MD, Knudson RJ, Barbee RA. The relationship of serum immunoglobulin E, allergy skin tests, and smoking to respiratory disorders. *J Allergy Clin Immunol* 1982;70:199–204.
132. Zetterstrom O, Osterman K, Machado L, Johansson SGO. Another smoking hazard: raised serum IgE concentration and increased risk of occupational allergy. *Br Med J* 1981;283:1215–1217.
133. Halonen M, Barbee RA, Lebowitz MD, Burrows B. An epidemiologic study of the interrelationships of total serum IgE, allergy skin test reactivity and eosinophilia. *J Allergy Clin Immunol* 1982;69:221–228.
134. Warren CPW, Holford-Stevens V, Wong C, Manfreda J. The relationship between smoking and total immunoglobulin E levels. *J Allergy Clin Immunol* 1982;69:370–375.
135. Bonini S. Smoking, IgE and occupational allergy. *Br Med J* 1982;284:512–513.

136. Hallgren R, Nou E, Arrendal H, Hiesche K. Smoking and circulating IgE in bronchial carcinoma. *Acta Med Scand* 1982;211:269–273.
137. Stein R, Evans S, Milner R, Rand C, Dolovich J. Isotopic and enzymatic IgE assays in non-allergic subjects. *Allergy* 1983;38:389–398.
138. Bahna SL, Myhre BA, Heiner DC. IgE elevation and suppression by tobacco smoking. *J Allergy Clin Immunol* 1980;65:231–236.
139. Bahna SL, Heiner DC, Myhre BA. Immunoglobulin E pattern in cigarette smokers. *Allergy* 1983; 38:57–64.
140. Shirakawa T, Kusaka Y, Morimoto K. Combined effects of smoking habits and occupational exposure to hard metal on total IgE antibodies. *Chest* 1992;101:1569–1576.
141. Bahna SL, Heiner DC, Myhre BA. Changes in serum IgD in cigarette smokers. *Clin Exp Immunol* 1983;51:624–630.
142. Mathews JD, Hooper BM, Whittingham S, Mackay IR, Stenhouse NS. Association of autoantibodies with smoking, cardiovascular morbidity, and death in a Busselton population. *Lancet* 1993;2:754–758.
143. Lehrer SB, Wilson MR, Karr RM, Salvagio JE. IgE antibody response of smokers, nonsmokers, and "smoke-sensitive" persons to tobacco leaf and smoke antigens. *Am Rev Respir Dis* 1980; 121:168–170.
144. Miller LG, Goldstein G, Murphy M, Ginns LC. Reversible alterations in immunoregulatory T cells in smoking: analysis by monoclonal antibodies and flow cytometry. *Chest* 1982;82:526–529.
145. Ginns LC, Goldenheim PD, Miller LG, et al. T-lymphocyte subsets in smoking and lung cancer: analysis by monoclonal antibodies and flow cytometry. *Am Rev Respir Dis* 1982;126:265–269.
146. Costabel U, Brass KJ, Reuter C, Ruhle K-H, Matthys H. Alteration in immunoregulatory T-cell subsets in cigarette smokers: a phenotypic analysis of bronchoalveolar and blood lymphocytes. *Chest* 1986;90:39–44.
147. Costabel U, Maier K, Teschler H, Wang YM. Local immune components in chronic obstructive pulmonary disease. *Respiration* 1992;59:17–19.
148. Burton RC, Ferguson P, Gary M, Hall J, Hayes M, Smart YC. Effects of age, gender, and cigarette smoking on human immunoregulatory T-cell subsets: establishment of normal ranges and comparison with patients with colorectal cancer and multiple sclerosis. *Diagn Immunol* 1983; 1:216 223.
149. LaVia MF, Hurtubise PE, Parker JW, et al. T-lymphocyte subset phenotypes: a multisite evaluation of normal subjects and patients with AIDS. *Diagn Immunol* 1985;3:75–82.
150. Smart YC, Cox J, Roberts TK, Brinsmead MW, Burton RC. Differential effect of cigarette smoking on recirculating T lymphocyte subsets in pregnant women. *J Immunol* 1986;137:1–3.
151. Tollerud DJ, Brown LM, Blattner WA, Mann DL, Pankiw-Trost L, Hoover RN. T cell subsets in healthy black smokers and nonsmokers. Evidence for ethnic group as an important response modifier. *Am Rev Respir Dis* 1991;144:612–616.
152. Robertson MD, Boyd JE, Fernie JM, Davis DMG. Some immunological studies on coal workers with and without pneumoconiosis. *Am J Ind Med* 1983;4:467–476.
153. Aizawa Y, Takata T, Hashimoto K, Kurihara M, Tominaga M, Miyake H. Lymphocyte subpopulations and lymphocyte reactivity in chronic cigarette smokers. *Jpn J Hyg* 1987;42:747–753.
154. Tollerud DJ, Clark JW, Brown LM, et al. The influence of age, race, and gender on peripheral blood mononuclear cell subset in healthy smokers. *J Clin Immunol* 1989;9:214–222.
155. Silverman NA, Potvin C, Alexander JC Jr, Chretien PB. *In vitro* lymphocyte reactivity and T-cell levels in chronic cigarette smokers. *Clin Exp Immunol* 1975;22:285–292.
156. Vos-Brat LC, Rumke PH. Immunoglobuline concentraties, PHA reacties van lymfocyten *in vitro* en enkele antistof titers van gezonde rokers. *Jaarb Kanker Nederland* 1969;19:49–53.
157. Peterson BH, Steimel LF, Callaghan JT. Suppression of mitogen-induced lymphocyte transformation in cigarette smokers. *Clin Immunol Immunopathol* 1983;27:135–140.
158. Whitehead RH, Hooper BE, Grinshaw DA, Hughes LE. Cellular immune responsiveness in cigarette smokers. *Lancet* 1974;1:1232–1233.
159. Daniele RP, Dauber J, Altose MD, Rawlands DT, Gorenberg DJ. Lymphocyte studies in asymptomatic cigarette smokers. *Am Rev Respir Dis* 1977;116:997–1005.
160. Suciu-Foca N, Molinaro A, Buda J, Rectsma K. Cellular immune responsiveness in cigarette smokers. *Lancet* 1974;1:1062.
161. Doll R, Peto R. Mortality in relation to smoking: 20 years observation on male British doctors. *Br Med J* 1976;2:1525–1536.

162. Tollerud DJ, Clark JW, Brown LM, et al. Association of cigarette smoking with decreased number of circulating natural killer cells. *Am Rev Respir Dis* 1989;139:194–198.
163. Diana JN, Vaught A. *Research cigarettes.* Lexington: The University of Kentucky Printing Services; 1990.
164. Hackney EJ, Weidlich WR, Williams JB. A large capacity cigarette smoking machine. *Tobacco Sci* 1965;161:112–117.
165. Dontenwill W. Experimental investigations on the effect of cigarette smoke inhalation on small laboratory animals. In: *Inhalation carcingenesis,* AEC Symposium Series 18. Oak Ridge, TN: Atomic Energy Commission; 1970:389–412.
166. Griffith RB. A simple machine for smoke analytical studies and total particulate matter collection for biological studies. *Toxicology* 1984;33:33–41.
167. Griffith RB, Hancock R. Simultaneous mainstream–sidestream smoke exposure system I. Equipment and procedures. *Toxicology* 1985;34:123–138.
168. Esber H, Menninger F, Bogden A. Immunological deficiency associated with cigarette smoke inhalation by mice: primary and secondary hemagglutinin response. *Arch Environ Health* 1973; 27:99–104.
169. Ayer DJ, Keast D, Papadimitriou JM. Effects of tobacco smoke on splenic architecture and weight, during the primary immune response of BALB/c mice. *J Pathol* 1981;133:53–59.
170. Thomas WR, Holt PG, Keast D. Humoral immune response of mice with long-term exposure to cigarette smoke. *Arch Environ Health* 1975;30:78–80.
171. Henry CJ, Kouri RE. Smoke inhalation studies in mice. *Final report for the Council of Tobacco Research,* Contract CTR-0030. Bethesda, MD: Microbiological Associates; 1984.
172. Sopori ML, Cherian S, Chilukuri R, Shopp GM. Cigarette smoke causes inhibition of the immune response to intratracheally administered antigens. *Toxicol Appl Pharmacol* 1989;97:489–499.
173. Chalmer J, Holt PG, Keast D. Cell-mediated immune response to transplanted tumors in mice chronically exposed to fresh cigarette smoke. *J Natl Cancer Inst* 1975;52:1129–1134.
174. Holt PG, Chalmer J, Roberts LM, Papadimitriou JM, Thomas WR, Keast D. Low-tar high-tar cigarettes: comparison of effects in mice. *Arch Environ Health* 1976;31:258–265.
175. Thomas WR, Holt PG, Papadimitriou JM, Keast D. The growth of transplanted tumors in mice after chronic inhalation of fresh cigarette smoke. *Br J Cancer* 1974;30:459–462.
176. Holt PG. Cigarette smoking and the immune system: description of an experimental model. In: Clark MA, ed. *Pulmonary disease: defense mechanisms and population at risk.* Lexington: University of Kentucky Printing Services; 1977:214–233.
177. Keast D, Ayre DJ. Effects of chronic tobacco smoke exposure on immune responses in aged mice. *Arch Environ Health* 1981;36:201–207.
178. Thomas WR, Holt PG, Keast D. The development of alteration in the primary immune response of mice by exposure to fresh cigarette smoke. *Int Arch Allergy Appl Immunol* 1974;46:481–486.
179. Thomas WR, Holt PG, Keast D. Antibody production in mice chronically exposed to fresh cigarette smoke. *Experimentia* 1974;30:1469–1470.
180. Thomas WR, Holt PG, Keast D. Effect of cigarette smoking on primary and secondary humoral responses in mice. *Nature* 1973;243:240–241.
181. Thomas WR, Holt PG, Keast D. Cellular immunity in mice chronically exposed to fresh cigarette smoke. *Arch Environ Health* 1973;27:372–375.
182. Holt PG, Chalmer J, Keast D. Development of two manifestations of T lymphocyte reactivity during tumor growth: altered kinetics associated with elevated growth rates. *J Natl Cancer Inst* 1975;55:1135–1142.
183. Sopori ML, Gairola C, DeLucia AJ, Bryant LR, Cherian S. Immune responsiveness of monkeys exposed chronically to cigarette smoke. *Clin Immunol Immunopathol* 1985;36:338–344.
184. Mackenzie JS. The effect of cigarette smoke on influenza virus infection: a murine model system. *Life Sci* 1976;19:409–412.
185. Mackenzie JS, Flower RLP. The effect of long-term exposure to cigarette smoke on the height and specificity of the secondary immune response to influenza virus in a murine model. *J Hyg* 1979; 83:135–141.
186. Okazaki N, Yamaguchi E, Kawakami Y. The effect of long- and short-term exposure of cigarette smoke on hypersensitivity pneumonitis in rabbits. *Am Rev Respir Dis* 1987;135:A158.
187. Goud SN, Kaplan AM, Subbarao B. Effects of cigarette smoke on the antibody response to thymic independent antigens from different lymphoid tissues of mice. *Arch Toxicol* 1992;66:164–169.
188. Savage SM, Donaldson LA, Cherian S, Chilukuri R, White VA, Sopori ML. Effects of cigarette

smoke on the immune response. II. Chronic exposure to cigarette smoke inhibits surface immunoglobulin-mediated responses in B cells. *Toxicol Appl Pharmacol* 1991;111:523–529.
189. Chang JCC, Distler SG, Kaplan AM. Tobacco smoke suppresses T cell but not antigen-presenting cells in the lung-associated lymph nodes. *Toxicol Appl Pharmacol* 1990;102:514–523.
190. Gottlieb A, Pope SK, Rickert VI, Hardin BH. Patterns of smokeless tobacco use by young adolescents. *Pediatrics* 1993;91:75–78.
191. Breurd B. Smokless tobacco use among native American school children. *Public Health Rep* 1990; 105:196–201.
192. Ernster VL, Grady DG, Greene JC, et al. Smokeless tobacco use and health effects among baseball players. *JAMA* 1990;264:218–224.
193. Connolly GN, Winn GM, Hecht SS, Henningfield JE, Walker B, Hoffmann D. The reemergence of smokeless tobacco. *N Engl J Med* 1986;314:1020–1027.
194. Rouse BA. Epidemiology of smokeless tobacco use in the United States: a national study. *Natl Cancer Inst Monogr* 1989;8:29–33.
195. Council on Scientific Affairs. Health effects of smokeless tobacco. *JAMA* 1986;255:1038–1044.
196. Greer RO, Poulson TC. Oral tissue alterations associated with the use of smokeless tobacco by teenagers. *Oral Surg* 1983;56:275–284.
197. Offenbacher S, Weather DR. Effects of smokeless tobacco on the peridontal, mucosal and caries status of adolescent males. *J Oral Pathol* 1985;14:169–181.
198. Surgeon General's Report. The health consequences of using smokeless tobacco: a report of the advisory committee to the Surgeon General. *US Department of Health and Human Services*, publication no 86-2874, 1986.
199. Winn DM, Blot WJ, Shy CL, Pickle LW, Toledo A, Fraumeni JF Jr. Snuff dipping and oral cancer among women in the southern United States. *N Engl J Med* 1981;304:745–749.
200. Wolfe MD, Carlos JP. Oral health effects of smokeless tobacco use in Navajo Indian adolescents. *Community Dent Oral Epidemiol* 1987;15:230–235.
201. Krishna K. Tobacco chewing during pregnancy. *Br J Obstet Gynecol* 1978;85:726–728.
202. Verma RC, Chansoriya M, Kaul KK. Effect of tobacco chewing by mothers on fetal outcome. *Indian Pediatr* 1983;20;105–111.
203. Paulson R, Shanfeld J, Sachs L, Ismail M, Paulson J. Effect of smokeless tobacco on the development of the CD-1 mouse fetus. *Teratogenesis Carcinogen Mutagen* 1988;8:81–93.
204. Goud SN, Zhang L, Kaplan AM. Immunostimulatory potential of smokeless tobacco extract in *in vitro* cultures of murine lymphoid tissues. *Immunopharmacology* 1993;25:95–105.
205. Francus T, Manzo G, Canki M, Thompson LC, Szabo P. Two peaks of interleukin 1 expression in human leukocytes cultured with tobacco glycoprotein. *J Exp Med* 1989;170:327–332.
206. Francus, T, Klein RF, Staiano-Corco L, Becker CG, Siskind GW. Effects of tobacco glycoprotein (TGP) on the immune system. II. TGP stimulates the proliferation of human T cells and the differentiation of human B cells into Ig secreting cells. *J Immunol* 1988;140:1823–1829.
207. Lindemann RA, Park NH. Inhibition of human lymphokine activated killer activity by smokeless tobacco (snuff) extract. *Arch Oral Biol* 1988;33:317–321.
208. Sopori ML, Savage SM, Christner RF, Geng Y-M, Donaldson LA. Cigarette smoke and the immune response: mechanism of nicotine induced immunosuppression. *Adv Biosci* 1993;86:663–672.
209. Roszman TL. Effects of water-soluble products derived from cigarette smoke on the immune response. In: Clark MA, ed. *Pulmonary disease defense mechanisms and population at risk*. Lexington: University of Kentucky Printing Services; 1977:234–249.
210. Jacob CV, Stelzer GT, Wallace JH. The influence of cigarette tobacco smoke products on the immune response. The cellular basis of immunosuppression by a water-soluble condensate of tobacco smoke. *Immunology* 1980;40:621–627.
211. Roszman TL. The effect of nicotine on the immune response. In: *Nicotine and carbon monoxide*. Lexington: University of Kentucky Printing Services; 1975:80–88.
212. Mackenzie JS, Mackenzie IH, Holt PG. The effect of cigarette smoking on susceptibility to epidemic influenza and on serological responses to live attenuated and killed subunit influenza vaccines. *J Hyg* 1976;77:409–417.
213. Hall CB, Hall WJ, Gala CL, MaGill FB, Leddy JP. Long-term prospective study in children after respiratory syncytial virus infection. *J Pediatr* 1984;105:358–364.
214. Tager IB, Segal MR, Munoz A, Weiss ST, Speizer FE. The effect of maternal cigarette smoking on the pulmonary function of children and adolescents. Analyses of data from two populations. *Am Rev Respir Dis* 1987;136:1366–1370.

215. Carrillo T, DeCastro FR, Cuevas M, Diaz F, Cabrera P. Effect of cigarette smoking on the humoral immune response in pigeon fanciers. *Allergy* 1991;46:241–244.
216. Kusaka H, Homma Y, Ogasawara H, et al. Five-year follow-up of *Micropolyspora faeni* antibody in smoking and nonsmoking farmers. *Am Rev Respir Dis* 1989;140:695–699.
217. Harf RA, Ethevenaux C, Gleize J, Perrin-Fayolle M, Guerin JC, Ollagnier C. Reduced prevalence of smokers in sarcoidosis. Results of a case–control study. *Ann NY Acad Sci* 1986;465:625–631.
218. Srivastava ED, Barton JR, O'Mahony S, et al. Smoking, humoral immunity, and ulcerative colitis. *Gut* 1991;32:1016–1019.

Immunotoxicology and Immunopharmacology, Second Edition, edited by J. H. Dean, M. I. Luster, A. E. Munson, and I. Kimber.
Raven Press, Ltd., New York © 1994.

24

Ultraviolet B Radiation and Skin Immunology

Jorge M. Rivas and Stephen E. Ullrich

Department of Immunology, University of Texas, M. D. Anderson Cancer Center, Houston, Texas 77030

The beginning of the 20th century brought with it a wave of intense scientific research and detailed clinical focus into the effects of ultraviolet (UV) radiation on the skin. Early epidemiologic observations by Unna (1) and Dubreuilh (2) on the detrimental effects of UV exposure paved the way to the pioneering empirical studies by Rusch et al. (3) and Blum (4), which clearly demonstrated the cutaneous carcinogenic effect of UV radiation. This spurred a series of investigations that provided insight into the optical nature of the skin and its recognition as the primary target of UV radiation (5). The body of work that eventually evolved from these studies gave rise to the field of photobiology and its more specialized area of photocarcinogenesis. This particular discipline delineated the pathogenic, molecular, and biochemical links between skin cancer and UV radiation. As a separate and independent research endeavor, the immunologic character of the skin was discovered. The observations that T cells selectively localize to the skin, that Langerhans' cells can function as antigen-presenting cells (APCs), and that keratinocytes secrete a wide variety of cytokines once thought to be produced only by cells of the lymphoid lineage supported the existence of skin-associated lymphoid tissues (SALTs) (6).

Studies to determine how UV radiation affects immunologic reactions led to the evolution of a new discipline, photoimmunology. This discipline has brought diverse fields such as immunology, dermatology, and photobiology together into a specialized area of scientific study. To a large extent, photoimmunology developed as a consequence of studies conducted on the immunobiology of UVB-induced skin cancers. In 1974, Kripke (7) observed that the majority of tumors induced in inbred mice following chronic exposure to UVB radiation were unable to grow progressively when transplanted into normal syngeneic recipients. Interestingly, these tumors grew progressively in immunocompromised hosts, suggesting that, unlike chemical carcinogens, UVB exposure induces highly antigenic tumors. How could these highly antigenic tumors develop and grow progressively in the UV-irradiated autochthonous host? The explanation lies in the fact that in addition to being carcinogenic UVB is also immunosuppressive. UVB exposure leads to a selective systemic suppression of tumor immunity in the primary host (8), a state of suppression that is mediated by systemic antigen-specific suppressor T cells (9–13). This chapter focuses on recent studies concerning the mechanisms involved in the suppression of immunity following exposure to UV radiation.

ULTRAVIOLET-INDUCED IMMUNOSUPPRESSION: LOCAL VERSUS SYSTEMIC

The effect of UV radiation on the immune system has generally been divided into local and systemic effects. Local suppression describes a diminished immune response to an antigen or hapten introduced directly at the site of UV irradiation. A UVB-induced defect in Langerhans' cell antigen presentation appears to be essential in the induction of local immunosuppression. Systemic suppression describes a situation where immunologic unresponsiveness is induced following application of the hapten or antigen at a site different and distant from that of irradiation. The induction of systemic immunosuppression is associated with a defect in splenic APC function and appears to be dependent on the release of immunomodulatory cytokines and immunosuppressive substances by UVB-irradiated epidermal cells.

Ultraviolet-Induced Local Immunosuppression

The model of local UV-induced immunosuppression was first described by Toews et al. (14). Mice were exposed to UVB radiation using a dose equivalent to one that produces an erythemal response in normal human skin (approximately 400 J/m^2, per exposure, 4 exposures over a span of 4 consecutive days). Immediately after the last exposure, a contact allergen (dinitrofluorobenzene, DNFB) was applied to the irradiated skin, and 5 days afterward the mice were challenged by applying DNFB to the ears. The induction of contact hypersensitivity (CHS) was assayed 18 to 24 hr later by measuring the resulting ear swelling. Toews and colleagues observed that in comparison to nonirradiated controls, UVB-irradiated animals failed to mount a CHS response. Moreover, the unresponsiveness did not reflect a "null event" because the UV-irradiated mice did not respond to a second application of the same hapten, suggesting the induction of immune suppression. The density of epidermal Langerhans' cells at the site of sensitization appeared to be a critical determinant for the induction of nonresponsiveness. UVB exposure caused a decrease in the number of, and an alteration in the morphology of, epidermal Langerhans' cells. Elmets et al. (15) subsequently demonstrated the presence of suppressor T cells (CD4+, CD8−) in the spleens of mice sensitized through UVB-irradiated skin. The suppressor cells were hapten specific and acted only on the afferent limb of the immune response. The data from these experiments suggested that the introduction of hapten through Langerhans' cell-depleted skin sent a tolerance-inducing signal to the immune system.

A number of recent papers have supported this hypothesis. Cruz et al. (16) obtained a relatively "pure" population of Langerhans' cells by sorting for Ia + epidermal cells with the fluorescence activated cell sorter (FACS). Injecting UVB-irradiated, hapten-conjugated Langerhans' cells into mice prevented the subsequent induction of CHS when the mice were sensitized with hapten. Moreover, it was found that these UV-irradiated cells transmitted a downregulatory immune signal since the animals were unresponsive to a second application of the same hapten. Simon et al. (17) next studied the effects of UVB radiation on the ability of Langerhans' cells to present antigen to different subclasses of CD4 + cells. Two subsets of CD4 + T cells have recently been described in mice (18) and humans (19). These cells are distinguished primarily by their cytokine secretion patterns: T helper 1 (T_H1) cells produce interleukin-2 (IL-2), interferon-γ (IFN-γ), and lymphotoxin (TNF-β) after antigenic stimulation and T helper 2 (T_H2) cells release IL-4, IL-5, IL-6, and IL-10. T_H1 cells help cell-mediated immune reactions such as CHS, whereas T_H2 cells are primarily involved in providing help for antibody production. While Simon et al. (17) observed that FACS "purified" normal Langerhans' cells could present antigen to both T_H1 and T_H2 clones, UVB-irradiated Langerhans' cells were unable to present antigen to T_H1 cells but retained their capacity to present antigen to T_H2 clones. The authors suggest that UVB exposure modulates the costimulatory signals delivered to the T cells, favoring the activation of T_H2 cells. Simon and colleagues (20) subsequently found that when UV-irradiated Langerhans' cells were used as APCs, not only were the CD4 + T_H1 cells nonresponsive, but they became tolerant. The tolerant state was associated with functional inactivation of the T_H1 cells rather than the deletion, hence clonal anergy. Addition of allogeneic splenic adherent cells to cultures of UV-irradiated Langerhans' cells and T_H1 cells prevented the induction of unresponsiveness Thus it appears that UV radiation modulates the expression of, or interferes with the ability of, Langerhans' cells to deliver costimulatory signals [such as the one provided by the B7 molecule (21)] to T cells.

UV exposure also modulates local immune function by activating keratinocytes to produce immunoregulatory cytokines. Yoshikawa and Streilein (22) found that intradermal injection of TNF-α suppressed the induction of CHS, in a manner similar to that seen after UV exposure. Moreover, treatment of UV-irradiated mice with anti-TNF-α antibodies prevented the onset of immunosuppression. Because TNF-α is produced by UV-irradiated keratinocytes (23,24), Yoshikawa and Streilein suggest that locally produced TNF-α interferes with the induction of CHS, perhaps by modulating epidermal Langerhans' cell function.

Further evidence for a role of Langerhans' cells in the induction of local immunosuppression was derived from work conducted in our laboratories by Alcalay et al. (25). In this study, mice were treated topically with either bifunctional psoralens, such as 8-methoxypsoralen, which cross-links complementary strands of deoxyribonucleic acid (DNA) after exposure to UVA, or monofunctional psoralens such as angelicin, which gives rise to intrastrand adducts when exposed to UVA radiation. When mice are treated with 8-methoxypsoralen in conjunction with UVA (PUVA) they exhibit considerable epidermal phototoxicity and a loss of Ia+ Langerhans' cells at the site of irradiation. On the other hand, treatment with angelicin and UVA caused a significant decrease in the number of Ia+ Langerhans' cells, but with no detectable phototoxicity. The application of a contact allergen to the PUVA or angelicin and UVA-treated skin resulted in suppression of CHS, associated with the appearance of suppressor cells in the spleens of the treated animals. These findings suggested that the inflammation and phototoxicity associated with the use of PUVA is not required for the induction of immunosuppression. Furthermore, they suggested that the immunologic unresponsiveness observed was most likely due to the alteration of Langerhans' cells.

The alteration of local immunologic cells at the site of UVB exposure has also been implicated in the suppression of immune function in humans. Human Langerhans' cells are susceptible to the deleterious effects of UVB radiation and UVB exposure does suppress Langerhans' cells APC function (26). Cooper and colleagues (27) confirmed this finding and noted that immediately after UVB exposure the antigen-presenting capacity of CD1+, DR+, Birbeck granule positive, epidermal Langerhans' cells was depressed. Soon after UVB exposure, however, epidermal APC function recovered to values greater than that seen in nonirradiated skin. The enhanced APC function was not due to the reappearance of epidermal Langerhans' cells but rather to the appearance of a CD1−, DR+, Birbeck granule negative, OKM1− OKM5+, melanophage (28). Wavelengths in the UVB region of the spectrum maximally induced the CD1−, DR+ melanophage, with some activity by UVC radiation but no induction following UVA exposure (29). This cell activates suppressor T cells by presenting antigen to a subset of T cells. Human CD4+ T cells can be subdivided into two populations based in the expression of a post-translational modification of CD45 to CD45R. CD45+ cells are found in the subset of CD4+ cells that act as classic helper cells (30,31). CD45R is expressed on CD4+ lymphocytes that provide help for the maturation of CD8+ suppressor cells. (The CD45R+ subpopulation equals the so-called suppressor–inducer subset of CD4 cells.) The UV-induced CD1−, DR+, melanophages preferentially activated CD4+, CD45R+ T cells, suggesting that these melanophages are involved in the induction of suppression (32). This hypothesis was tested by mixing the CD1−, DR+, epidermal cells with autologous peripheral blood T cells. After a 7-day culture, the T cells were isolated. The cells were then added to cultures of pokeweed mitogen (PWM)-stimulated autologous blood mononuclear cells. T lymphocytes isolated from cultures containing CD1−, DR+, UV-irradiated epidermal melanophages suppressed immunoglobulin (Ig) production by the PWM-induced mononuclear cells compared to the levels seen when either unstimulated T cells were added to the mononuclear cells, or when T cells from cultures containing nonirradiated epidermal cells were added (33).

These findings suggest that UVB exposure induces APCs that preferentially activate suppressor T cells. Together with the data generated using experimental animals, it is apparent that UV radiation activates multiple mechanisms at the site of exposure to downregulate the induction of an immune response. UVB exposure modulates Langerhans' cells APC function and not only prevents Langerhans' cells from presenting antigen in a conventional manner but converts the Langerhans' cell into an APC that induces T cell tolerance (17). Moreover, UV-irradiated keratinocytes release immunomodulatory cytokines that may affect local Langerhans' cell function, as suggested by Yoshikawa and Streilein (22). Finally, the recruitment of an APC that presents antigen to suppressor cells, as described by Baadsgaard and Cooper (33) is yet another UVB-activated mechanism that downregulates the induction of a local immune response.

Ultraviolet-Induced Systemic Immunosuppression

The model of UV-induced systemic immunosuppression, as originally described by Jessup and colleagues (34) and Noonan et al. (35), refers to the situation where the UVB radiation is delivered at one site (usually the dorsal skin of mice) and the contact allergen or antigen is applied at a distant nonirradiated site. Hence the alteration of APC function at the site of sensitization is not responsible for the induction of immunosuppression in this model (36,37). Associated with the systemic model of UV-induced immunosuppression is a defect in splenic APC function (38,39) and the induction of antigen-specific suppressor T cells (35). The studies on the UV-induced suppression of contact and delayed-type hypersensitivity (DTH) essentially grew from experiments designed to determine the immunologic profile of tumor-susceptible UV-irradiated mice.

Understanding the mechanism by which UV radiation induces immunosuppression is important for several reasons. Perhaps the major reason is the link between the carcinogenic potential and immunosuppressive effects of UV radiation (40,41). Understanding the mechanisms involved in immunosuppression following UV exposure may provide a rational basis for designing protocols for the prevention and treatment of skin cancer. Similarly, a better understanding of the manner by which UV radiation downregulates the immune response may provide new insights to prevent susceptibility to infectious diseases, since it has been demonstrated that UV radiation can be a predisposing factor for increased immunologic susceptibility to infectious agents (42–46). Finally, the suppression that is induced by UV radiation is unique. UVB radiation suppresses cellular immune reactions in a specific, selective manner without hindering other immune responses such as antibody production (12,47). Thus manipulating the suppressive effects of UV radiation may serve as an innovative strategy for suppressing unwanted immune reactions such as allograft rejection and graft-versus-host disease.

A great deal of information concerning the mechanisms involved in the induction of immunosuppression and suppressor cells by UVB radiation has been generated during the past decade. Sensitization of UV-irradiated mice with contact allergens, protein antigens, foreign erythrocytes, microbial antigens, allogeneic histocompatibility antigens, and hapten-modified self resulted in the induction of suppression and, in most cases tested, antigen-specific suppressor T cells (39,42–46,48–50). Once activated, the UV-induced suppressor T cells (UV-Ts) regulate multiple immunologic pathways: CHS and DTH, T cell proliferation, the generation of cytotoxic T lymphocytes, and antibody formation are all suppressed, in an antigen-specific fashion (48,51–53).

The target of the UV-Ts was determined by taking advantage of the observation that these cells suppressed anti-hapten antibody production (48). UVB-irradiated mice were sensitized with trinitrochlorobenzene (TNCB) to induce trinitrophenyl (TNP)-specific suppressor cells. The UV-Ts were then injected into normal mice, and the recipient animals were immunized with either a T cell-dependent (TNP coupled to erythrocytes) or a T cell-independent (TNP coupled to lipopolysaccharide) antigen. We postulated that if the target of the UV-Ts was T_H cells, they should have no effect on the generation of antibodies in response to TNP–lipopolysaccharide (LPS) but should suppress the antibody response following immunization with TNP–sheep erythrocytes. When UV-Ts were transferred into normal mice, the induction of an anti-hapten antibody response was suppressed when the recipient mice were immunized with T cell-dependent antigens. Conversely, the UV-Ts did not suppress the antibody response to T cell-independent antigens. Because the suppressive effect of UV-Ts was abrogated by the injection of exogenous IL-2, and the production of IL-2 by antigen-activated T cells *in vitro* was suppressed by UV-Ts, we concluded that T_H cell activity was suppressed by UV-Ts (54). Romerdahl and Kripke (55,56) also reported that UV-induced suppressor cells prevent tumor rejection by blocking the generation of T_H cells.

The mechanism employed by UV-induced suppressor cells to downregulate the immune response appears to be through the elaboration of immunosuppressive factors. Steele et al. (57) produced a monoclonal antibody that reacts with suppressive factors produced by a variety of T cells. Injecting this antibody into UV-irradiated mice totally blocked the induction of suppression (58). These findings indicate that although UV irradiation is a unique way to induce suppressor cells, once activated, they use a common mechanism (elaboration of immunosuppressive factors) to downregulate the immune response.

Originally, it was thought that different doses of UV radiation were associated with the induction of local or systemic immunosuppression. Generally, lower doses of UVB radiation (in the range of 1.4 kJ/m^2) were used to induce immunosuppression in the local model, whereas much higher doses (30 to 40 kJ/m^2) were used to induce systemic immunosuppression. Recently, however, Noonan and De Fabo (59) reported the induction of systemic immunosuppression with a relatively small dose (2.2 kJ/m^2) of UVB radiation. They found that the dose of UV needed to suppress the immune response varies according to the strain of mouse tested, and there appears to be no correlation between the dose of UV radiation used and the induction of systemic or local immunosuppression. Others have similarly reported the induction of systemic immunosuppression using relatively low doses of UV radiation (60,61). Therefore using the terms low dose and high dose to describe the effects of UVB radiation on the immune responses appears to be in error and should be discontinued.

Soluble Factors as Mediators of Ultraviolet-Induced Systemic Immunosuppression

Although the phenotype of the UV-induced suppressor cells (CD3+, CD4+, CD8−), their target (T_H cells), and mechanism of suppression (elaboration of suppressive factors) have been discovered over the past few years, what has remained unclear is how splenic antigen-specific suppressor cells are induced following UV exposure. Because the penetrative power of UV radiation affects cells only in the epidermis and very upper layers of the dermis (5), indirect mechanisms have been suggested. Although a variety of hypotheses have been proposed to explain the induction of systemic immunosuppression (39), most of the experimental evidence gathered so far supports the involvement of epidermal-derived suppressive cytokines in the induction of suppression following UVB exposure. These factors include urocanic acid, serum factors from UV-irradiated mice, IL-1, contra-IL-1, contra-CHS, TNF-α, and IL-10.

Urocanic Acid

In 1983, De Fabo and Noonan (62) constructed the action spectrum (wavelength effectiveness) for the UV-induced suppression of CHS and compared it with the known UV-absorbing capability of a variety of epidermal compounds. This analysis identified DNA and urocanic acid (UCA), a deamination product of histidine found naturally in the stratum corneum, as the two best candidates for the UVB-absorbing compound within the skin. Since UCA is only found superficially, the stratum corneum was removed by tape stripping, and the effect this had on the induction of immunosuppression following exposure to UVB radiation was measured. Following tape stripping, UV failed to suppress CHS, suggesting the photoreceptor was located superficially, thus supporting the hypothesis that UCA, and not DNA, is the photoreceptor. Furthermore, De Fabo and Noonan postulated that following UVB exposure trans-UCA is photoisomerized to the cis conformation, and release of cis-UCA induces systemic immunosuppression. Evidence supporting this hypothesis was furnished primarily by studies performed by Ross et al. (63), demonstrating that intravenous injection of cis-UCA into mice depressed their ability to mount a DTH response against herpes simplex virus. Antigen-specific suppressor T cells were found in the spleens of mice injected with cis-UCA. Noonan et al. (64) subsequently focused on the role of cis-UCA in depressing splenic APC function. The ability of splenic dendritic cells isolated from UV-irradiated mice, or mice injected with cis-UCA, to present antigen to immune T cells was examined. The intravenous administration of cis-UCA depressed APC function of splenic dendritic cells in a manner similar to that seen following *in vivo* UV irradiation. Because total-body

UV exposure causes the suppression of DTH, in part through the induction of antigen-specific suppressor T cells, and depresses splenic APC function, these data support a role for cis-UCA in the induction of systemic immunosuppression following UVB irradiation.

Further support for the suppressive effects of cis-UCA comes from the experiments published by Kurimoto and Streilein (65). They report that injecting cis-UCA intradermally into mice before sensitization with a contact allergen impairs the induction of CHS, in a manner similar to that seen following local UVB exposure. The impairment is dependent on the release of TNF-α since the introduction of antibodies to TNF-α abrogates the cis-UCA-induced effect. Furthermore, injecting cis-UCA appears to alter epidermal Langerhans' cell morphology. Kurimoto and Streilein postulate that UVB exposure promotes the release of cis-UCA, which alters Langerhans' cell morphology and activates keratinocytes to release TNF-α. They suggest the net result of local cis-UCA and TNF-α production is to prevent Langerhans' cell migration to the draining lymph nodes, thus preventing sensitization after UV exposure.

Clearly, injecting mice with cis-UCA does induce immunosuppression similar to what is found after total-body UV exposure. There is some question, however, whether UCA is actually the photoreceptor for UV radiation. Morison and Kelly (66) attempted to reproduce the phenomenon described by De Fabo and Noonan and block immunosuppression by removing the stratum corneum prior to UV exposure. While tape stripping was highly effective in removing UCA, it was by itself immunosuppressive. Tape-stripped mice had a 57% reduction in CHS compared to controls. When tape-stripped mice were exposed to UV radiation, Morison and Kelly observed a further reduction in CHS. The suppression observed in tape-stripped UV-irradiated mice was similar to what was found in mice only exposed to UV radiation. Although some residual UCA remained in the tape-stripped mice [tape stripping removed 83% of UCA as measured by high-performance liquid chromatography (HPLC) analysis], these data indicate the UV receptor is not located superficially, suggesting it is not UCA.

Applegate et al. (67) arrived at a similar conclusion using an entirely different experimental system. This study made use of the South American opossum, *Monodelphis domestica*, whose cells contain a photoactivating enzyme that repairs UV-induced pyrimidine dimers. This enzyme repairs pyrimidine dimers after exposure to visible light, cleaving them and restoring the DNA to its original conformation. Applegate et al. observed that CHS was depressed when the marsupials were exposed to UVB radiation. The immunosuppression was abrogated when the animals where exposed to the photoreactivating visible light immediately after UV exposure. The photoreactivating light was not immunosuppressive by itself, nor did it reverse immunosuppression if given prior to UVB exposure. Therefore these findings suggest that DNA and not UCA is the photoreceptor.

A subsequent study by Kripke et al. (68) provided additional data to support the hypothesis that DNA is the UVB photoreceptor in the skin. One of the potential criticisms of the above-mentioned study concerns differences in immune regulation between marsupials and placental mammals (69). Kripke and colleagues therefore devised an alternate method to examine the role of DNA in the induction of UV-induced immunosuppression. This approach made use of liposomes containing the bacterial excision repair enzyme, T4 endonuclease V, an enzyme whose activity is specific for pyrimidine dimers. Upon topical application of these liposomes to murine skin, the liposomes penetrate epidermal cells, destabilize at low pH, and deliver the endonuclease repair enzyme intracellularly, where it initiates pyrimidine dimer repair (70). If the initiating event in UV-induced immunosuppression is the generation of UVB signature mutations (pyrimidine dimers), then the application of these endonuclease-containing liposomes should reverse the induction of immunosuppression. Kripke and colleagues found that treating UV-irradiated mice with liposomes containing the dimer repair enzyme abrogated immunosuppression. Treating UV-irradiated mice with empty liposomes or liposomes containing heat-inactivated enzyme did not abrogate immunosuppression. Because introducing the T4 endonuclease V enzyme into cells repairs pyrimidine dimers *in situ* and reverses UV-induced immunosuppression, Kripke and colleagues suggest the initial event in the induction of suppression by UV radiation is the formation of pyrimidine dimers. Therefore the photoreceptor for UVB must be DNA.

Because of the failure of Morison and Kelly to reproduce the original observation regarding the superficial nature of the UVB photoreceptor, and in light of the studies of Kripke and colleagues demonstrating that reversal of pyrimidine dimer formation abrogates the induction of systemic immunosuppression, we must conclude that DNA and not UCA is the epidermal UVB photoreceptor. It is equally clear, however, that cis-UCA is an immunosuppressive agent and mimics some but not all of the effects of total-body UVB exposure [cis-UCA does not appear to promote the migration of dendritic cells from the skin to the draining lymph nodes in a similar fashion to that described for UVB radiation (71)]. In addition to the studies mentioned above, experiments are currently ongoing to evaluate the potential of using cis-UCA to suppress immune rejection in organ transplantation (72–74). Although cis-UCA holds promise as a novel immunosuppressive agent and may be involved in the induction of immunosuppression following UVB exposure, UCA does not appear to be the UVB photoreceptor in the skin, as originally claimed.

Serum Factors

Transferring serum from UV-irradiated mice into normal recipients suppresses the induction of CHS (75) and DTH (76). Very limited biochemical analysis suggested that this factor had a molecular weight between 1 and 10 kDa; hence it is unlikely to be UCA. In a similar manner, Harriott-Smith and Halliday (77) were able to detect the presence of an immunosuppressive factor(s) in the vascular circulation of animals following UV exposure. This factor suppressed CHS and prevented the adherence inhibition of immunized leukocytes. Little is known about the biochemical characteristics of this factor.

Keratinocyte-Derived Interleukin-1

UV irradiation is capable of inducing IL-1 in the serum of irradiated animals (78) or human volunteers (79). Furthermore, exposing keratinocytes to UVB induces the release of epidermal thymocyte activating factor (ETAF/IL-1) (80). On the basis of these observations, Robertson et al. (81) tested the hypothesis that administration of recombinant IL-1 into normal mice could depress CHS. Intravenous injection of IL-1 did suppress CHS, and suppressor cells were found in the spleens of the IL-1-injected mice. Contrary to the situation seen after UVB exposure, however, these suppressor cells inhibited the elicitation of CHS and not the induction, by preventing the influx of effector cells to the site of challenge. The release of prostaglandins appears to be involved, since prior treatment of these mice with indomethacin, an inhibitor of prostaglandin synthesis, abrogated IL-1-induced suppression. Robertson and colleagues (81) suggest that the suppressive effect of IL-1 reflects a normal feedback mechanism involved in suppressing the effector arm of CHS. Since UVB exposure targets the afferent limb of CHS (82), keratinocyte-derived IL-1 does not appear to play a role in the induction of systemic immunosuppression after UVB exposure.

Contra-CHS and Contra Interleukin-1

Because the skin is the optical barrier against UV radiation, Schwarz and colleagues (83) speculated that UV-irradiated keratinocytes had to secrete suppressive cytokines in addition to the immunostimulating cytokines. To test this hypothesis, Schwarz et al. (83) exposed epidermal cell cultures to UV radiation, waited 24 hr, and injected the supernatants from these cells into mice. Injecting supernatants from UV-irradiated primary epidermal cell cultures, or from UV-irradiated keratinocyte cell lines, into mice suppressed the induction of CHS. No suppression was observed when the mice were injected with supernatants from UV-irradiated fibroblast or monocyte lines. When the supernatants from UV-exposed keratinocyte cultures were fractionated by HPLC, it was found that the suppressive material eluted with an apparent molecular weight between 15 and 50 kDa. Treating the irradiated keratinocytes with indomethacin did not abrogate UV-induced suppression of CHS, indicating keratinocyte synthesis of prostaglandins was not involved.

The supernatants from UV-exposed epidermal cells were subsequently tested for the ability to block IL-1 activity (84). Crude supernatant preparations did not block IL-1 activity; however, when the supernatants were fractionated on HPLC, a suppressive fraction approximately 40 kDa in size, with an isolelectric point of 8.8, was discovered. The activity of this factor was specific for IL-1 since it only blocked IL-1-induced proliferation, without suppressing the proliferative capacity of IL-2- or IL-3-dependent cell lines. Treating the UV-irradiated keratinocytes with cycloheximide depleted all contra-IL-1 activity, indicating a requirement for active protein synthesis.

In order to determine whether the sera of UV-irradiated mice contained contra-

IL-1, Schwarz et al. (85) tested the sera for contra-IL-1 activity. The HPLC analysis revealed a 40-kDa factor whose contra-IL-1 activity peaked 24 hr after UV exposure. The 40-kDa fraction only suppressed IL-1 activity and did not suppress the proliferation of IL-2- or IL-3-dependent cell lines. Neither did this fraction suppress tritiated-thymidine incorporation of EL4 cells, ruling out the possibility of nonspecific DNA synthesis inhibition. These findings indicated that epidermal cells release contra-IL-1 upon exposure to UV radiation. The authors suggest that contra-IL-1 enters the circulation, and this may induce systemic immunosuppression.

Krutmann et al. (86) measured the ability of contra-IL-1 to modulate accessory cell function. Human peripheral blood monocytes served as accessory cells for autologous T cells activated with soluble anti-CD3 antibody. Krutmann and colleagues observed that the addition of contra-IL-1 to CD3-treated monocytes reduced, in a dose-dependent fashion, the proliferative response. Moreover, adding recombinant IL-1α, but not IL-6, restored blastogenesis, also in a dose-dependent manner. These studies demonstrate that contra-IL-1 impairs APC function. Furthermore, they suggest that the well-documented suppression of systemic APC function following UV exposure may be due to the release of keratinocyte-derived contra-IL-1.

Keratinocyte-Derived Interleukin-10

As mentioned earlier, two of the unique characteristics of the systemic immunosuppression induced by UVB exposure are the selective nature of the immunosuppression and the generation of antigen-specific suppression. Because selectivity and specificity are two of the requirements of the "ideal immunosuppressive agent" a focus of our early studies was to determine if UVB exposure could specifically and selectively suppress allograft rejection. During the course of these experiments we observed that UV exposure, coupled with allosensitization, could suppress the immune response to allogeneic histocompatibility antigens and prolong allograft survival in a selective and specific manner (50,87,88). However, the phototoxicity that resulted following UV exposure was an unavoidable consequence and a major drawback in using UVB radiation to suppress allograft rejection. While these studies were in progress, Schwarz and colleagues published their work describing contra-CHS. We immediately modified our system to determine if factors from UVB-irradiated keratinocytes could suppress the immune response to alloantigens in a selective and specific fashion.

Injecting supernatants from UVB-irradiated primary epidermal cell cultures, or UVB-irradiated keratinocyte cell lines, suppressed the induction of DTH to alloantigen. The suppression was associated with the appearance of splenic CD3+, CD4+, and CD8− suppressor T cells, and the suppressor cells were specific for the antigen used to sensitize the factor-injected mice. Treating the keratinocytes with indomethacin did not abrogate the suppressive activity, suggesting that the suppressive factor was not prostaglandin E_2 (PGE_2). Treating the keratinocytes with cycloheximide or treating the supernatants with trypsin did remove all suppressive activity, indicating the factor was a protein. Passing the suppressive material over a concanavalin A (Con A)–agarose column depleted all suppressive activity, indicating the suppressive material is glycosylated (89). Thus injecting the suppressive factor from UV-irradiated keratinocytes mimicked the suppression induced following total-body UVB exposure. Furthermore, the characteristics of the suppressive cytokine resembled contra-CHS as described by Schwarz et al. (83,84).

It was when we began to study the selectivity of the suppression that we first had an indication that we were looking at a cytokine that differed from the one described by Schwarz and colleagues. As mentioned earlier, the immunologic profile of a UV-irradiated animal is unique. While some cellular immune reactions are suppressed (rejection of UVB-induced tumors, CHS, and DTH), humoral immune reactions are normal in these mice. We anticipated that injecting the cytokine from UV-irradiated keratinocytes would yield a similar pattern of immunosuppression. While we could suppress the generation of DTH to hapten-modified self or alloantigen with supernatants from UVB-irradiated keratinocytes, we were unable to suppress CHS (61). At first this finding surprised us because it appeared that our methods were identical to those used by Schwarz and colleagues. Upon closer examination, however, it soon was apparent that the light sources used in our studies differed considerably in their spectral outputs. Schwarz and colleagues used a lamp that produced primarily UVA radiation (68% UVA, 32% UVB), whereas the light source used in our study produced primarily UVB radiation (65% UVB, 35% UVA). Could different wavebands of UV radiation produce unique immunosuppressive factors that had different effects on CHS and DTH? To test this hypothesis we irradiated our keratinocytes with either UVB or pure (>99%) UVA radiation. We found that exposing the keratinocytes to UVB radiation produced a factor that suppressed DTH but not CHS, whereas UVA exposure produced a factor that suppressed CHS but not DTH. Neither factor suppressed antibody formation *in vivo*. Thus it appears that different wavebands of UV radiation activate keratinocytes to produce at least two different immunosuppressive factors, one that suppresses DTH and one that suppresses CHS.

Because the selective nature of UV-induced suppression is very similar to the described biologic activity of cytokine synthesis inhibition factor, or IL-10 (90), we decided to test the hypothesis that UVB radiation stimulates keratinocytes to release IL-10, which is then responsible for inducing systemic immunosuppression. To test this hypothesis we took a number of approaches. First, synthetic oligonucleotides were constructed based on the published cDNA sequence of T cell IL-10. The messenger ribonucleic acid (mRNA) from UV-irradiated keratinocytes was then isolated and analyzed by Northern analysis. At various times after exposure (1, 3, and 6 hr) IL-10 mRNA expression was enhanced. Second, Western blots using IL-10-specific monoclonal antibodies demonstrated that IL-10 was released by UV-irradiated keratinocytes. The keratinocyte-derived IL-10 was biologically active in that it suppressed IFN-γ production by antigen-activated T_H1 cells. Treating the supernatant from the UV-irradiated keratinocytes with neutralizing anti-IL-10 antibody abrogated suppressive activity, indicating that the IL-10 present in the supernatant is responsible for the suppressive activity reported previously (61,89). In addition, IL-10 appears to play an essential role in the induction of suppression following *in vivo* exposure to UVB radiation. Mice were irradiated with 10 to 15 kJ/m^2 of UVB radiation and then injected with either monoclonal rat anti-mouse IL-10 or control normal rat serum. While DTH was significantly suppressed in mice exposed to UVB, or mice exposed to UVB and injected with normal rat serum, injecting UVB-irradiated mice with anti-IL-10 reversed the immunosuppression (91). Thus these findings indicate that keratinocytes synthesize and release IL-10 after UVB exposure and that the secreted IL-10 plays an essential role in the induction of immunosuppression after total-body UV exposure.

The exact mechanism employed by keratinocyte-derived IL-10 to induce systemic immunosuppression remains to be elucidated. We suggest the following scenario (Fig. 1). UVB-induced keratinocyte-derived IL-10 interacts with APCs and impairs their function by downregulating major histocompatibility complex (MHC) class II antigen expression and by blocking the production of monokines (92,93). The impairment of APC function prevents the stimulation of T_H1 clones and DTH is suppressed. The production of IL-10 by UV-irradiated keratinocytes and its effect on the immune system also help to explain the selectivity of the immunosuppression induced by UVB radiation. Because the APCs that present to T_H1 and T_H2 cells appear to differ (94), we propose that, upon the introduction of antigen to UVB-irradiated mice, T_H2 cells are stimulated. Since the cytokines released by these cells (IL-4, IL-5, and IL-6) are essential for B cell activation, proliferation, and differentiation, antibody production is not suppressed. Furthermore, since T_H2 cells also produce IL-10, we suggest that the CD4+ suppressor cells identified in the spleens of UVB-irradiated mice may simply be antigen-activated T_H2 cells. The production of IL-10 by these cells serves to suppress the induction of DTH in the recipient animal, in an antigen-specific manner. A similar mechanism may also be operating in the induction of CD4+ suppressor cells after the application of hapten to UV-irradiated skin (local suppression of immunity). The data of Simon et al. (17) indicate that while UVB-irradiated Langerhans' cells are tolerogenic for T_H1 cells they do stimulate T_H2 cells to proliferate. We suggest that the activated T_H2 clones, by virtue of their IL-10 production, prevent the synthesis of IFN-γ, thus suppressing CHS. These clones are antigen specific and will only secrete IL-10 after being stimulated by the proper antigen. Therefore only the antigen originally used to sensitize the UV-irradiated mouse will trigger these cells, the end result being antigen-specific immunosuppression.

Although keratinocyte IL-10 production is essential for suppressing DTH in UV-irradiated mice, recent studies from this laboratory have suggested that TNF-α production, and not IL-10, is essential for the UVB-induced suppression of CHS. Mice were exposed to 15 kJ/m^2 and then injected with either anti-IL-10, anti-TNF-α, or irrelevant control antibodies. The treated mice were then either sensitized with oxazolone to induce CHS or injected with alloantigen to induce DTH. As described earlier, we found that injecting anti-IL-10 totally reversed the UVB-induced suppression of DTH, whereas injecting these mice with anti-TNF-α did not reverse

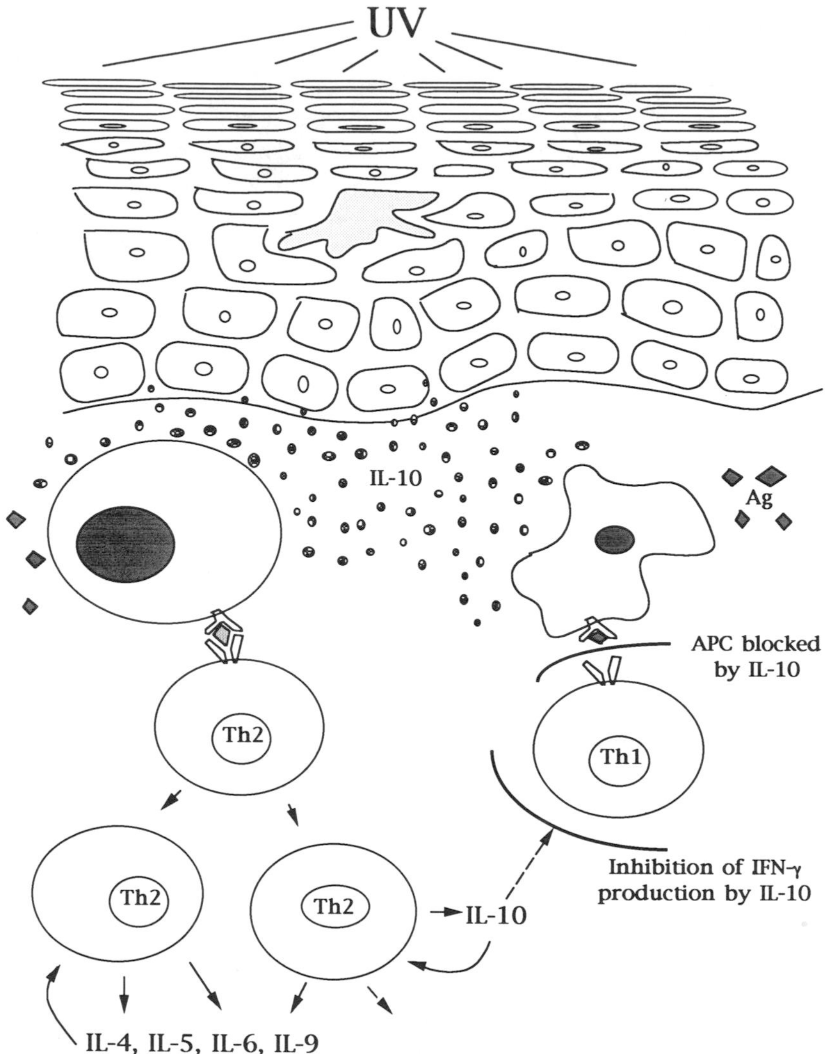

FIG. 1. Working model for the effects of UV-induced keratinocyte-derived IL-10 on systemic immunity. After UV exposure, irradiated keratinocytes produce and release IL-10, which interferes with the presentation of antigen to T_H1 clones and suppresses the induction of DTH. Because T_H1 and T_H2 cells use different APCs, we propose that keratinocyte-derived IL-10 does not affect antigen presentation to T_H2 cells and these cells proliferate. Upon subsequent exposure to antigen these cells are activated to secrete IL-4 and IL-10, thus further limiting DTH. Moreover, we suggest that the adoptive transfer of antigen-specific T_H2 cells from UV-irradiated mice into naive recipients explains the observation that the UV-induced suppressor T cells are antigen-specific CD4+, CD8− T cells.

immunosuppression. On the other hand, injecting anti-IL-10 had no effect on the UVB-induced suppression of CHS, whereas injecting antibodies to TNF-α did reverse the immunosuppression (J. M. Rivas and S. E. Ullrich, *unpublished data*). Thus it appears that different cytokines regulate DTH and CHS following UVB exposure. This information may have important practical applications; for example, the introduction of TNF-α may be useful for suppressing allergic contact dermatitis, whereas IL-10 may be more applicable for suppressing DTH and allograft rejection.

SUMMARY AND CONCLUSIONS

Three facts are readily apparent concerning the effects of UVB radiation on the immune system. First, local events (UV irradiation of the skin) have distant effects. Regardless as to whether the antigen is applied to the irradiated skin or at a distant nonirradiated site, the net result is the induction of systemic immunosuppression, mediated by suppressor T cells. Second, redundant mechanisms have evolved to suppress immunity following UVB exposure. This is most readily apparent when one considers the variety of UV-induced epidermal-derived cytokines that have been shown to suppress the immune response. Third, the depression of APC function appears to be the key to UV-induced immunosuppression. We suggest that the major effect of UVB radiation on the immune system is to modify APC function so that only certain subclasses of T cells, in all probability T_H2 cells, are stimulated. This can happen directly, via mechanisms similar to those described by Simon et al. (20) and Baadsgaard and colleagues (33), or indirectly by the secretion and release of epidermal-derived cytokines, such as cis-UCA (64), contra-IL-1 (86), IL-10 (91), and perhaps TNF-α (65)—cytokines that are known to affect APC function. The net result is that the next time the immune system encounters the antigen, antigen-specific T_H2 cells are activated to secrete cytokines, such as IL-4 and IL-10, that feedback and inhibit the production of IFN-γ by T_H1 cells, thus suppressing cell-mediated immune reactions. This would explain the CD4+ phenotype of the suppressor cells, as well as the selectivity and the specificity of the immunosuppression.

Why did evolution see fit to equip vertebrate animals with multiple mechanisms to suppress the immune system after exposure to an ubiquitous environmental agent? Undoubtedly, the vast mutagenic potential of UVB coupled with the need to maintain homeostasis in the skin resulted in the development of these suppressive mechanisms. One consequence of the interaction between the epidermis and UVB radiation may be the induction of new or altered "skin antigens" that are recognized as foreign by elements of the immune system (95). Perhaps the pressure to prevent anti-skin autoimmune responses selected for the development of UVB-triggered immunosuppression. The suppressive mechanisms described here may all result from the pressure to maintain proper dermatologic function in the face of interaction with carcinogenic and mutagenic environmental agents, such as UVB radiation.

ACKNOWLEDGMENT

Work from this laboratory was supported by grant AR-40824, from the National Institute of Arthritis and Musculoskeletal and Skin Diseases.

REFERENCES

1. Unna PG. *Die Histopathologic der Haukrankheiten*. Berlin: Hirschwald; 1894.
2. Dubreuilh W. Des hyperkeratoses circonscriptes. *Ann Dermatol Syph* (Series 3) 1896;7:1158–1204.
3. Rusch HP, Kline BZ, Bauman CA. Carcinogenesis by UV rays with reference to wavelength and energy. *Arch Pathol* 1941;371:135–146.
4. Blum HF. Ultraviolet radiation and skin cancer: in mice and men. *Photochem Photobiol* 1976; 24:249–254.
5. Everett MA, Yeargers E, Sayre RM, Olson RL. Penetration of epidermis by ultraviolet rays. *Photochem Photobiol* 1966;5:533–542.
6. Streilein JW. Skin associated lymphoid tissue: the next generation. In: Bos D, ed. *Skin immune system*. Boca Raton, FL: CRC Press; 1989:25–48.
7. Kripke ML. Antigenicity of murine skin tumors induced by UV light. *J Natl Cancer Inst* 1974;53: 1333–1336.
8. Fisher MS, Kripke ML. Further studies on the tumor-specific suppressor cells induced by ultraviolet radiation. *J Immunol* 1978;121:1139–1144.
9. Fisher MS, Kripke ML. Systemic alteration induced in mice by ultraviolet light irradiation and its relationship to ultraviolet carcinogenesis. *Proc Natl Acad Sci USA* 1977;74:1688–1692.
10. Daynes RA, Spellman CW. Evidence for the generation of suppressor cells by UV radiation. *Cell Immunol* 1977;31:182–187.
11. Spellman CW, Daynes RA. Modification of immunological potential by ultraviolet radiation. II. Generation of suppressor cells in short-term UV-irradiated mice. *Transplantation* 1977;24:120–126.
12. Spellman CW, Woodward JG, Daynes RA. Modification of immunological potential by ultraviolet radiation. I. Immune status of short-term UV-irradiated mice. *Transplantation* 1977;24:112–119.
13. Ullrich SE, Kripke ML. Mechanisms in the suppression of tumor rejection produced in mice by repeated UV irradiation. *J Immunol* 1984;133:2786–2790.
14. Toews GB, Bergstresser PR, Streilein JW. Epidermal Langerhans' cell density determines whether contact hypersensitivity or unresponsiveness follows skin painting with DNFB. *J Immunol* 1980; 124:445–449.
15. Elmets CA, Bergstresser PR, Tigelaar RE, Wood PJ, Streilein JW. Analysis of the mechanism of unresponsiveness produced by haptens painted on skin to low dose UV radiation. *J Exp Med* 1983; 158:781–794.
16. Cruz PD, Nixon-Fulton J, Tigelaar RE, Bergstresser PR. Disparate effects of in vitro UVB irradiation in intravenous immunization with purified epidermal cell subpopulations for the induction of CHS. *J Invest Dermatol* 1989;92:160–165.
17. Simon JC, Cruz PC, Bergstresser PR, Tigelaar RE. Low dose ultraviolet B-irradiated Langerhans' cells preferentially activate CD4+ cells of the T helper 2 subset. *J Immunol* 1990;145:2087–2091.
18. Mosmann TR, Schumacher JH, Street NF, et al. Diversity of cytokine synthesis and function of mouse CD4+ T cells. *Immunol Rev* 1991;123:209–229.
19. Romagnani S. Human Th1 and Th2 subsets: regulation of differentiation and role in protection and immunopathology. *Int Arch Allergy Immunol* 1992;98:279–285.
20. Simon JC, Tigelaar RE, Bergstresser PR, Edelbaum D, Cruz PD. Ultraviolet B radiation converts Langerhans' cells from immunogenic to tolerogenic antigen-presenting cells: induction of specific clonal anergy in CD4+ T helper 1 cells. *J Immunol* 1991;146:485–491.
21. Razi-Wolf Z, Freeman GJ, Galvin FBB, Nadler L, Reiser H. Expression and function of the murine B7 antigen, the major costimulatory molecule expressed by peritoneal exudate cells. *Proc Natl Acad Sci USA* 1992;89:4210–4214.
22. Yoshikawa T, Streilein JW. Tumor necrosis factor-alpha and ultraviolet light have similar effects on contact hypersensitivity in mice. *Reg Immunol* 1990;3:139–144.

23. Oxholm A, Oxholm P, Staberg B, Bendtzen K. Immunohistological detection of IL-1-like and TNF in human epidermis before and after UVB-irradiation. *Br J Dermatol* 1988;118:369–376.
24. Kock A, Schwarz T, Kirnbauer R, et al. Human keratinocytes are a source for tumor necrosis factor α: evidence for synthesis and release upon stimulation with endotoxin or ultraviolet light. *J Exp Med* 1990;172:1609–1614.
25. Alcalay J, Ullrich SE, Kripke ML. Local suppression of contact hypersensitivity in mice by a monofunctional psoralen plus UVA radiation. *Photochem Photobiol* 1989;50:217–220.
26. Aberer W, Stingl G, Stingl-Gazze LA, Wolff K. Langerhans' cells as stimulator cells in the immune primary epidermal cell lymphocyte reaction: alteration by UVB irradiation. *J Invest Dermatol* 1982; 79:129–135.
27. Cooper KD, Fox P, Neises GR, Katz SI. Effects of UVR on human epidermal cell alloantigen presentation: initial depression of Langerhans' cell dependent function is followed by the appearance of T6-DR+ cells that enhance epidermal alloantigen presentation. *J Immunol* 1985;134:129–137.
28. Cooper KD, Neises GR, Katz SI. Antigen-presenting OKM5+ melanophages appear in human epidermis after ultraviolet radiation. *J Invest Dermatol* 1986;86:363–370.
29. Baadsgaard O, Cooper KD, Lisby S, Wulf HC, Wantzin GL. UVB and UVC, but not UVA, induce the appearance of T6-DR+ antigen-presenting cells in human epidermis. *J Invest Dermatol* 1987; 89:113–118.
30. Morimoto C, Letvin NL, Distaso JA, Aldrich WR, Schlossman SF. The isolation and characterization of human suppressor inducer T cell subset. *J Immunol* 1985;134:1508–1515.
31. Takeuchi T, Schlossman SF, Morimoto C. The 2H4 molecule but not T3-receptor complex is involved in suppressor inducer signals in the AMLR system. *Cell Immunol* 1987;107:107–114.
32. Baadsgaard O, Fox DA, Cooper KD. Human epidermal cells from ultraviolet light-exposed skin preferentially activate autoreactive CD4+2H4+ suppressor–inducer lymphocytes and CD8+ suppressor/cytotoxic lymphocytes. *J Immunol* 1988;140:1738–1744.
33. Baadsgaard O, Salvo B, Mannie A, Dass B, Fox D, Cooper KC. In vivo ultraviolet-exposed human epidermal cells activate T suppressor cell pathways that involve CD4+CD45RA+ suppressor–inducer T cells. *J Immunol* 1990;145:2854–2861.
34. Jessup JM, Hanna N, Palaszynski E, Kripke ML. Mechanisms of depressed reactivity to dinitrochlorobenzene and ultraviolet-induced tumors during ultraviolet carcinogenesis in BALB/c mice. *Cell Immunol* 1978;38:105–115.
35. Noonan FP, De Fabo EC, Kripke ML. Suppression of contact hypersensitivity and its relationship to UV-induced suppression of tumor immunity. *Photochem Photobiol* 1981;34:683–689.
36. Noonan FP, Bucana C, Sauder D, De Fabo EC. Mechanism of systemic immune suppression by UV irradiation in vivo. II. The effects on number and morphology of epidermal Langerhans' cells and the UV-induced suppression of CHS have different wavelength dependencies. *J Immunol* 1984; 132:2408–2413.
37. Morison WL, Bucana C, Kripke ML. Systemic suppression of contact hypersensitivity by UVB radiation is unrelated to the UVB-induced alterations in the morphology and numbers of Langerhans' cells. *Immunology* 1984;52:299–306.
38. Greene MI, Sy MS, Kripke ML, Benacerraf B. Impairment of antigen-presenting cell function by UV radiation. *Proc Natl Acad Sci USA* 1979;76:6591–6595.
39. Noonan FP, De Fabo EC, Kripke ML. Suppression of contact hypersensitivity by ultraviolet radiation: an experimental model. *Springer Semin Immunopathol* 1981;4:293–304.
40. Kripke ML. Immunological mechanisms in ultraviolet radiation carcinogenesis. *Adv Cancer Res* 1981;34:69–106.
41. Yoshikawa T, Rae V, Bruins-Slot W, vand-den-Berg JW, Taylor JR, Streilein JW. Susceptibility to effects of UVB radiation on induction of contact hypersensitivity as a risk factor for skin cancer in humans. *J Invest Dermatol* 1990;95:530–536.
42. Howie SEM, Norval M, Maingay J. Exposure to low dose UVB light suppresses delayed type hypersensitivity to herpes simplex virus in mice by suppressor cell induction. *J Invest Dermatol* 1986;86:125–128.
43. Aurelian L, Yasumoto S, Smith C. Antigen specific immune suppressor factor in herpes simplex type 2 infections of UVB-irradiated mice. *Am Soc Microbiology* 1988;62:2520–2524.
44. Denkins Y, Fidler IJ, Kripke ML. Exposure of mice to UVB radiation suppresses delayed hypersensitivity to *Candida albicans*. *Photochem Photobiol* 1989;49;615–619.
45. Jeevan A, Kripke ML. Effect of a single exposure to ultraviolet radiation on *Mycobacterium bovis* bacillus Calmette–Guerin infection in mice. *J Immunol* 1989;143:2837–2843.

46. Giannini SH. Effects of ultraviolet B irradiation on cutaneous leishmaniasis. *Parasitol Today* 1992; 8:44–48.
47. Norbury KC, Kripke ML, Budman MB. In vitro reactivity of macrophages and lymphocytes from UV-irradiated mice. *J Natl Cancer Inst* 1977;59:1231–1235.
48. Ullrich SE, Yee GK, Kripke ML. Suppressor lymphocytes induced by epicutaneous sensitization of UV-irradiated mice control multiple immunological pathways. *Immunology* 1986;58:185–190.
49. Giannini SH. Suppression of pathogenesis in cutaneous leishmaniasis by UV irradiation. *Infect Immun* 1986;51:838–843.
50. Ullrich SE. Suppression of the immune response to allogeneic histocompatibility antigen by a single exposure to UV radiation. *Transplantation* 1986;42:287–291.
51. Noonan FP, Kripke ML, Pedersen GM, Greene MI. Suppression of contact hypersensitivity by UV radiation is associated with defective antigen presentation. *Immunology* 1981;43:527–533.
52. Ullrich SE. Suppression of lymphoproliferation by hapten-specific suppressor T lymphocytes from mice exposed to UV radiation. *Immunology* 1985;54:343–352.
53. Ullrich SE, Azizi E, Kripke ML. Suppression of the induction of delayed hypersensitivity reactions in mice by a single exposure to UV radiation. *Photochem Photobiol* 1986;43:633–638.
54. Ullrich SE. The effect of ultraviolet radiation-induced suppressor cells on T cell activity. *Immunology* 1987;60:353–360.
55. Romerdahl CA, Kripke ML. Regulation of the immune response against UV-induced skin cancers: specificity of helper cells and their susceptibility to UV-induced suppressor cells. *J Immunol* 1986; 137:3031–3035.
56. Romerdahl CA, Kripke ML. Role of helper T-lymphocytes in rejection of UV-induced murine skin cancers. *Cancer Res* 1988;48:2325–2328.
57. Steele JK, Kawaski H, Kuchroo VK, Minami M, Levy JG, Dorf ME. A monoclonal antibody raised to tumor-specific T cell-derived suppressor factors also recognizes T suppressor inducer factors of the 4-hydroxy-3-nitrophenyl acetyl hapten suppressor network. *J Immunol* 1987;139:2629–2634.
58. Yee GK, Levy JG, Kripke ML, Ullrich SE. The role of suppressor factors in the regulation of the immune response by UV-induced suppressor T lymphocytes. III. Isolation of a suppressor factor with the B16G monoclonal antibody. *Cell Immunol* 1990;126:255–267.
59. Noonan FP, De Fabo EC. Dose response curves for local and systemic immunosuppression are identical. *Photochem Photobiol* 1990;52:801–810.
60. Jeevan A, Kripke ML. Alteration of the immune response to *Mycobacterium bovis* BCG in mice exposed chronically to low dose UV radiation. *Cell Immunol* 1990;130:32–41.
61. Kim T-Y, Kripke ML, Ullrich SE. Immunosuppression by factors released from UV-irradiated epidermal cells: selective effects on the generation of contact and delayed hypersensitivity after exposure to UVA or UVB radiation. *J Invest Dermatol* 1990;94:26–32.
62. De Fabo EC, Noonan FP. Mechanism of immune suppression by ultraviolet irradiation in vivo. I. Evidence for the existence of a unique photoreceptor in skin and its role in photoimmunology. *J Exp Med* 1983;157:84–98.
63. Ross JA, Howie SEM, Maingay J, Simpson TJ. Ultraviolet-irradiated urocanic acid suppresses delayed type hypersensitivity to herpes simplex virus in mice. *J Invest Dermatol* 1986;87:630–633.
64. Noonan FP, De Fabo EC, Morrison H. Cis-urocanic acid, a product formed by UVB irradiation of the skin, initiates an antigen presentation defect in splenic cells in vivo. *J Invest Dermatol* 1988; 90:92–99.
65. Kurimoto I, Streilein JW. Cis-urocanic acid suppression of contact hypersensitivity induction is mediated via tumor necrosis factor-α. *J Immunol* 1992;148:3072–3078.
66. Morison WL, Kelly SP. Urocanic acid may not be the photoreceptor of contact hypersensitivity. *Photodermatology* 1986;3:98–101.
67. Applegate LA, Ley RD, Alcalay J, Kripke ML. Identification of the molecular target for the suppression of contact hypersensitivity by UV radiation. *J Exp Med* 1989;170:1117–1131.
68. Kripke ML, Cox PA, Alas LG, Yarosh DB. Pyrimidine dimers in DNA initiate systemic immunosuppression in UV-irradiated mice. *Proc Natl Acad Sci USA* 1992;89:7516–7520.
69. Infante AJ, Samples NK, Croix DA, Redding TS, VandeBerg JL, Stone WH. Cellular immune response of a marsupial *Monodelphis domestica*. *Dev Comp Immunol* 1991;15:189–199.
70. Yarosh D, Alas LG, Yee V, et al. Pyrimidine dimer removal enhanced by DNA repair liposomes reduces the incidence of UV skin cancer in mice. *Cancer Res* 1992;52:4224–4231.
71. Moodycliffe AM, Kimber I, Norval MA. The effect of ultraviolet B irradiation and urocanic isomers on dendritic cell migration. *Immunology* 1992;77:394–399.

72. Oesterwitz H, Gruner S, Diezel W, Schneider W. Inhibition of rat heart allograft rejection by PUVA treatment of the graft recipient: role of cis-urocanic acid. *Transplant Int* 1990;3:8–11.
73. Gruner S, Diezel W, Stoppe H, Oesterwitz H, Henke W. Inhibition of skin allograft rejection and acute graft-versus-host disease by cis-urocanic acid. *J Invest Dermatol* 1992;98:459–462.
74. Guymer RH, Mandel TE. Urocanic acid as an immunosuppressant in allotransplantation in mice. *Transplantation* 1993;55:36–43.
75. Swartz RP. Role of UVB-induced serum factors in suppression of contact hypersensitivity in mice. *J Invest Dermatol* 1984;83:305–307.
76. Swartz RP. Suppression of DTH to UV radiation induced tumor cells with serum from UVB-irradiated mice. *J Natl Cancer Inst* 1986;76:1181–1184.
77. Harriott-Smith TG, Halliday WJ. Circulating suppressor factors in mice subjected to UV irradiation and contact hypersensitivity. *Immunology* 1986;57:207–211.
78. Gahring LC, Baltz M, Pepys MB, Daynes RA. The effect of UV radiation on the production of ETAF/IL-1 in vivo and in vitro. *Proc Natl Acad Sci USA* 1984;81:1198–1202.
79. Granstein RD, Sauder DN. Whole-body exposure to ultraviolet radiation results in increased serum interleukin-1 activity in humans. *Lymphokine Res* 1987;6:187–191.
80. Sauder DN. Interleukin-1. *Arch Dermatol* 1989;125:679–682.
81. Robertson B, Gahring L, Newton R, Daynes RA. In vivo administration of IL-1 to normal mice decreases their capacity to elicit contact hyper-sensitivity responses: prostaglandins are involved in this modification of the immune response. *J Invest Dermatol* 1987;88:380–387.
82. Kripke ML, Morison WL, Parrish JA. Systemic suppression of contact hypersensitivity in mice by psoralen plus UVA radiation (PUVA). *J Invest Dermatol* 1983;81:87–92.
83. Schwarz T, Urbanska A, Gschnait F, Luger TA. Inhibition of the induction of contact hypersensitivity by a UV-mediated epidermal cytokine. *J Invest Dermatol* 1986;87:289–291.
84. Schwarz T, Urbanska A, Gschnait F, Luger TA. UV-irradiated epidermal cells produce a specific inhibitor of IL-1 activity. *J Immunol* 1987;138:1457–1463.
85. Schwarz TS, Urbanski A, Kirnbauer R, Kock A, Gschnait F, Luger TA. Detection of a specific inhibitor of interleukin-1 in sera of UVB-treated mice. *J Invest Dermatol* 1988;91:536–540.
86. Krutmann J, Schwarz T, Krinbauer R, Urbanska A, Luger TA. Epidermal cell-contra-interleukin 1 inhibits human accessory cell function by specifically blocking interleukin 1 activity. *Photochem Photobiol* 1990;52:738–788.
87. Ullrich SE, Magee MJ. Specific suppression of allograft rejection after treatment of recipient mice with UV radiation and allogeneic spleen cells. *Transplantation* 1988;46:115–119.
88. Magee MJ, Kripke ML, Ullrich SE. Inhibition of the immune response to alloantigen in the rat by exposure to ultraviolet radiation. *Photochem Photobiol* 1989;50:193–200.
89. Ullrich SE, McIntyre BW, Rivas JM. Suppression of the immune response to alloantigen by factors released from ultraviolet-irradiated keratinocytes. *J Immunol* 1990;145:489–498.
90. Mosmann TR. Regulation of immune responses by T cells with different cytokine secretion phenotypes: role of a new cytokine, cytokine synthesis inhibitory factor (IL-10). *Int Arch Allergy Appl Immunol* 1991;94:110–115.
91. Rivas JM, Ullrich SE. Systemic suppression of DTH by supernatants from UV-irradiated keratinocytes: an essential role for interleukin 10. *J Immunol* 1992;149:3865–3871.
92. de Waal Malefyt R, Abrams J, Bennett B, Figdor CG, de Vries JE. Interleukin 10 (IL-10) inhibits cytokine synthesis by human monocytes: an autoregulatory role of IL-10 produced by monocytes. *J Exp Med* 1991;174:1209–1220.
93. Fiorentino DF, Zlotnik A, Vieira P, et al. IL-10 acts on the antigen-presenting cell to inhibit cytokine production by Th1 cells. *J Immunol* 1991;146:3444–3451.
94. Gajewski TF, Joyce J, Fitch FW. Antiproliferative effect of IFN-γ in immune regulation III. Differential selection of Th1 and Th2 murine helper T lymphocyte clones using rIL-2 and rIFN-γ. *J Immunol* 1989;143:15–22.
95. Kripke ML. Immunologic unresponsiveness induced by UV radiation *Immunol Rev* 1984;80:87–102.

Immunotoxicology and Immunopharmacology, Second Edition, edited by J. H. Dean, M. I. Luster, A. E. Munson, and I. Kimber.
Raven Press, Ltd., New York © 1994.

25

Immunotoxicology and Immunopharmacology of the Skin Immune System

*Craig A. Elmets, Uwe Trefzer, and Hasan Mukhtar

*Department of Dermatology, Skin Diseases Research Center, Case Western Reserve University, *University Hospital of Cleveland, Cleveland, Ohio 44106*

As the major interface between an individual and the environment, a principal activity of the skin is to limit access of exogenous pathogens to the internal microenvironment. Originally, this protective function was thought to reside exclusively in the ability of the stratum corneum to act as a physical barrier to these agents and to the less differentiated layers of epidermis to enzymatically modify compounds that were able to evade the permeability barrier. However, recent studies into the biology of cutaneous tissue have demonstrated that the skin is endowed (a) with a distinctive set of cellular elements whose function is immunologic in nature and (b) with a synthetic capacity to secrete a vast array of immunomodulatory cytokines. These components have been termed the skin immune system (1,2). They allow the skin to respond to agents that evade other methods by which it protects other tissues from potentially harmful microbes and chemicals.

Much of the evolutionary driving force that has led to the creation of the skin immune system has come from microbes, which have a specific affinity for cutaneous surfaces. In addition, in today's world, the skin comes in contact with an array of environmental xenobiotics, pharmaceutical agents, and cosmetics. Although many of these agents are removed by other means, some can only be neutralized or eliminated by the skin immune system. In these instances, the interaction of compounds with the skin immune system is appropriate and is clearly beneficial to the host. In other situations, however, the activity of the skin immune system is disproportionate to the potential pathogenicity of the chemical. Such a reaction has been designated as being immunotoxic. Cutaneous immunotoxic reactions may result from either an exaggerated or a diminished immune response to a chemical. Certain chemicals, rather than causing an immunotoxic response, selectively modify the activities of the skin immune system. These immunopharmacologic agents have been used clinically and experimentally as a means of manipulating the skin immune system both to probe its properties and to treat cutaneous diseases that are mediated at least in part by immunologic mechanisms.

This chapter reviews current knowledge regarding the immunotoxicity and immunopharmacology of chemicals that interact with the skin. Strictly speaking, agents capable of causing allergic contact dermatitis and photocontact allergy are also immunotoxic compounds. However, a discussion of these special forms of immunotoxicity is beyond the scope of this chapter. Other chapters within this volume deal specifically with these issues.

COMPONENTS OF THE SKIN IMMUNE SYSTEM

The skin is composed of three separate layers (3). The most superficial layer, called the epidermis, is a continuously renewing, avascular, stratified, keratinizing epithelial tissue. The major cell type, numerically at least, is the keratinocyte, which comprises over 90% of the cells within the epidermis. Keratinocytes undergo progressive differentiation from cuboidal cells (basal cells) attached to the basement membrane to anucleate plate-like cells (cells of the stratum corneum) present at the epidermal–environmental interface. The remainder of the epidermis is comprised of Langerhans' cells, melanocytes, and Merkel's cells. Langerhans' cells and melanocytes each constitute approximately 2% to 4% of all epidermal cells; Merkel's cells are present in somewhat smaller concentrations. Langerhans' cells migrate to the epidermis from the bone marrow, where they reside for long periods of time. As will be discussed later, their function is primarily immunologic in nature. Melanocytes are of neuroectodermal origin and are the pigment-producing cells of the epidermis. Merkel's cells are thought to function as cutaneous mechanoreceptors for touch.

The dermis lies directly beneath the epidermis and is separated from the epidermis by the basement membrane zone. This layer of skin is composed largely of fibroblasts and extracellular matrix proteins such as collagen and elastin. These components of the dermis provide the supporting structure for the skin. The cutaneous microvasculature is found within the dermis. Immunologically relevant cells such as macrophages, dermal Langerhans' cells, and connective tissue mast cells are also present in the dermis. Below the dermis is the subcutaneous tissue, a fatty layer that is also known as the panniculus adiposus.

Initial recognition that the skin might be an active participant in the development of immune responses, rather than a passive participant in such processes, came from observations about the biologic behavior of epidermal Langerhans' cells in cell-mediated immunologic reactions. Lymphocytes were found to preferentially cluster around Langerhans' cells at sites of allergic contact hypersensitivity but not at sites of nonimmunologic irritant reactions within the skin (4). These findings led investigators to postulate that Langerhans' cells are an epidermis-specific antigen-presenting cell (APC), similar to antigen-presenting dendritic cells of the spleen and other tissues. Abundant evidence has accumulated to confirm this hypothesis (1). It is now known that Langerhans' cells are bone marrow derived and that they are the only cells within normal epidermis to express major histocompatibility complex (MHC) class II antigens, the CD1a leukocyte differentiation antigen, receptors for complement (CD11b/CD18), and receptors for the Fc portion of immunoglobulin G (IgG) (CD32) and IgE molecules (FcεRIα) (1). They are able to present haptens (5), soluble proteins (6), alloantigens (7), and tumor antigens (8) to T lymphocytes in *in vitro* proliferation assays. *In vivo* they serve as the primary APC for initiation of allergic contact hypersensitivity to haptens (9,10) and delayed-type hypersensitivity (DTH) to herpes simplex virus (11).

The dynamic role that keratinocytes play in cutaneous cell-mediated immune responses has also attracted special attention. Although they fail to constitutively express MHC class II molecules, cultured keratinocytes upon stimulation with interferon-γ (IFN-γ), express large amounts of these immunologically relevant glycoproteins (12) and also express these determinants *in vivo* in skin diseases associated with a lymphocytic inflammatory infiltrate (13). Furthermore, the low constitutive level of the leukocyte adhesion molecule, intercellular adhesion molecule-1 (ICAM-1), expression on keratinocytes is greatly upregulated *in situ* in a variety of inflammatory skin diseases and on cultured human keratinocytes *in vitro* following treatment with IFN-γ or with tumor necrosis factor-α (TNF-α) (14–17). Keratinocytes also constitutively display the adhesion molecules leukocyte function antigen-3 (LFA-3) (18) and B7/BB-1 on their cell surface (19). The expression of these molecules is important for epidermal T cell trafficking since the ligands for ICAM-1, LFA-3, and B7/BB-1 are leukocyte function antigen-1 (LFA-1), CD2, and CD28, respectively, which are expressed on T lymphocytes. A number of studies have shown that expression of these molecules on the keratinocyte surface increases the binding of T lymphoblasts to monolayers of keratinocytes. Moreover, the presence of ICAM-1 on the keratinocyte cell surface is both spatially and temporally related to the presence of intraepidermal T cells in a variety of cutaneous diseases (14).

Keratinocytes secrete a wide variety of cytokines and growth factors, which play a major role in initiating and/or modulating cell-mediated immunity and inflammation in the skin (20). Table 1 lists several of the mediators synthesized and secreted by the epidermis. For many of these molecules, it is intuitively obvious how they might participate in cutaneous immunologic and inflammatory reactions, although for many the evidence that they actually do so is circumstantial. For example, keratinocyte-derived interleukin-1 (IL-1) is a potent T cell activator, it is a chemoattractant for inflammatory cells, it induces fibroblast proliferation, which may be important for wound healing, and it promotes the activation of epidermal Langerhans' cells (21,22). IL-1 stimulates keratinocytes to secrete other mediators of inflammation including IL-6 and IL-8 (20). TNF-α, another cytokine secreted by keratinocytes (23), increases ICAM-1 and endothelial-leukocyte adhesion molecule-1 (ELAM-1) on keratinocytes and endothelial cells (17,24–26), causes chemotaxis of neutrophils into the skin (27), promotes the survival of epidermal Langerhans' cells

TABLE 1. *Cytokines produced by the epidermis*

Multifunctional cytokines
IL-1α
IL-1β
IL-6
TNF-α
Colony-stimulating factors
GM-CSF
G-CSF
M-CSF
IL-3 (mice)
Growth factors
TGF-α
TGF-β
Basic fibroblast growth factor
Platelet-derived growth factor
Other interleukins
IL-7 (mice)
IL-10

IL, interleukin; GM-CSF, granulocyte–macrophage colony-stimulating factor; G-CSF, granulocyte colony-stimulating factor; M-CSF, macrophage colony-stimulating factor; TGF, transforming growth factor.

(28), and inhibits keratinocyte proliferation (29). Granulocyte–macrophage colony-stimulating factor (GM-CSF), which is also produced by keratinocytes (30), has been shown to be an activating factor for Langerhans' cells (22). Keratinocytes also produce prostaglandin E_2 (PGE_2), which is a negative regulator of inflammatory responses and a growth enhancer of keratinocytes (31,32).

Although the dermis contains a number of cell types of immunologic import, including macrophages, endothelial cells, and Langerhans' cells, investigation into their immunologic properties has, until recently, received little attention. The one exception to this has been the dermal mast cell. Mast cells reside mainly in the perivascular areas of the upper dermis. Their activation by immunologic or nonimmunologic stimuli (e.g., chemical compounds or physical stimuli) results in the release of mediators that are stored in cytoplasmic granules or are synthesized rapidly after mast cell stimulation (33,34). Those mediators include vasoactive substances (e.g., histamine, prostaglandins, leukotrienes), chemotactic factors [e.g., eosinophil factor of anaphylaxis (ECF-A), neutrophil chemotactic factor (NCF), and hydroxy-eicosatetraenoic acid (HETE)], and enzymes (e.g., proteases and acid hydrolases). Mast cells are thought to play an important role in immune and nonimmune inflammation and have an important function in atopic and allergic diseases. They are not only involved in immediate hypersensitivity reactions, mediated by binding of IgE antibodies to receptors on mast cells, but also play a role in DTH reactions of the skin and other tissues (34).

METHODS USED TO ASSESS THE IMMUNOTOXIC AND IMMUNOPHARMACOLOGIC EFFECTS OF DRUGS AND CHEMICALS ON THE SKIN IMMUNE SYSTEM

Assessment of the immunopharmacologic and immunotoxic effects of drugs and chemicals on the skin has made extensive use of three models: (a) allergic contact hypersensitivity in mice and other species of rodents, (b) enumeration of epidermal Langerhans' cell concentrations and antigen-presenting function in humans and mice, and (c) effects on epidermal cytokine production in humans and mice.

Allergic Contact Hypersensitivity

Allergic contact hypersensitivity is a prototypic T lymphocyte-mediated immune response that can be both initiated and elicited in the skin (35). In these assays a hapten is applied topically, which then rapidly conjugates with cutaneous cellular proteins and membranes to form a complete antigen. The complete antigen is "taken up" by Langerhans' cells. Once the Langerhans' cells have taken up antigens, they are internalized, processed, and reexpressed on the Langerhans' cell surface complexed to MHC class II determinants. Langerhans' cells then migrate to regional lymph nodes where they present the antigen to T cells. This results in the clonal expansion of relevant T cell repertoires, which recirculate to sites of antigen application where they create an inflammatory response in an effort to eradicate the antigen administered.

In animals, allergic contact hypersensitivity can be assessed by painting a sensitizing dose of the hapten on the shaved abdominal skin (36). Several days later (typically five) the degree to which sensitization has occurred can be determined by reapplying a smaller dose of the hapten to the ear of each animal. The increment of ear swelling that occurs over subsequent days is used as a quantitative index of the contact hypersensitivity response.

Enumeration of Langerhans' Cell Concentrations

Because the Langerhans' cell is the only cell population in normal epidermis in which the Ca^{2+}/Mg^{2+} adenosine triphosphatase (ATPase) ectoenzyme can be demonstrated by histochemical means and because in normal epidermis it also is the only cell type to express CD1a molecules (in humans) and class II MHC determinants, it has been possible to use these molecules as phenotypic markers to enumerate Langerhans' cell concentrations following treatment with various drugs and chemicals (1). Typically, specimens of epidermis are stained *en face* using indirect immunofluorescence or immunoperoxidase procedures with primary antibodies against MHC class II antigens or against CD1a or using standard histochemical techniques against the ATPase enzyme (37). The number of positively stained cells per square millimeter is then counted and is compared to untreated or vehicle-treated control specimens.

The functional capacity of Langerhans' cells is assessed by using them as APCs in T cell proliferation assays (6,7). In these assays, disaggregated suspensions of epidermal cells are prepared and combined in microtiter plates with (a) purified T lymphocytes that have been rendered devoid of other APC populations and (b) appropriate concentrations of antigen or mitogen. The cells are then cultured for periods of 2 to 6 days, after which the proliferative response of T lymphocytes to Langerhans' cells is assessed by the uptake of tritiated thymidine.

Cutaneous Cytokines

Cytokine production by the epidermis is evaluated by taking cultured keratinocytes and incubating them either with known cytokine inducers or with specific drugs or chemicals that might modulate their production (38). After various periods of time, supernatants from the cultures are removed and placed in standard biologic or immunoassays.

IMMUNOTOXICITY OF CHEMICALS ON THE SKIN

Polyaromatic Hydrocarbons

Many of the studies investigating the immunotoxicity of chemicals on the skin have utilized polyaromatic hydrocarbons as prototypic agents. Because they are the leading cause of chemically induced skin cancer and because they are an important component of crude coal tar, which is applied to the skin as a therapeutic agent in the management of psoriasis and other cutaneous inflammatory disorders, these compounds are of considerable importance to dermatology. Several lines of evidence indicate that these agents interact in a significant way with the skin immune system. At least two of the polyaromatic hydrocarbons—dimethylbenz[*a*]anthracene (DMBA) and benzo[*a*]pyrene (BaP)—when applied topically or injected intradermally, are immunogens capable of initiating and eliciting contact and DTH reactions (39–42). This was first demonstrated in guinea pigs (39–41) but has been shown to occur in inbred strains of mice as well (42). In mice, the development of such a reaction is an acquired phenomenon; it displays immunologic memory, it is antigen specific, and it is transferable to naive syngeneic recipients with lymphocytes from draining lymph nodes, thereby fulfilling all the criteria for classification as an immunologic reaction (42).

With respect to DMBA contact hypersensitivity, at least three genes have been identified that influence the development of the response (43,44). The reaction does not occur in Ah receptor negative strains of mice, implying that metabolism of DMBA is a necessary precondition for immunogenicity and suggesting that, similar to many of the other effects of polyaromatic hydrocarbons, a metabolite rather than

TABLE 2. *Strain variation in the contact hypersensitivity response to dimethylbenz[a]anthracene*

Strain	MHC haplotype	Ah receptor haplotype	Contact hypersensitivity response
DBA/2	d	−	−
SJL/J	s	−	−
RF/J	k	−	−
AKR	k	−	−
C3H	k	+	+
C3H.SW	b	+	−
C57BL/6	b	+	−
C57BL/10	b	+	−
B10.A	a	+	+
B10.D2	d	+	−
B10.S	s	+	−
B10.BR	k	+	+
A/J	a	+	+
A.BY	b	+	−
A.SW	s	+	−
AKR × C57BL/10 F_1	k/b	+	+

the parent compound is responsible for this toxic effect. However, unlike the toxic, mutagenic, and teratogenic effects of DMBA, the magnitude of the contact hypersensitivity response is also influenced by genes within the murine MHC (Table 2). In studies in which strains of mice congenic at the murine MHC were examined for their relative capacity to mount a DMBA contact hypersensitivity response, $H\text{-}2^k$ and $H\text{-}2^a$ haplotype strains developed a much greater response than $H\text{-}2^b$ or $H\text{-}2^d$. There also appears to be a modest impairment in the capacity of C3H/HeJ mice to develop DMBA contact hypersensitivity when compared to C3H/HeN mice. The only known difference between these two strains is at the *Lps* locus, a genetic locus that controls macrophage activation as well as synthesis and release of a number of different cytokines including TNF-α. C3H/HeJ mice have a mutation at the *Lps* locus and, as a result, have a deficit in their capacity to activate macrophages and to synthesize and release cytokines. These animals develop a smaller contact hypersensitivity response to DMBA than do C3H/HeN mice, which are normal at that locus. Thus at least three distinct genetic loci—the Ah receptor locus, the MHC, and *Lps* locus—control induction and expression of contact hypersensitivity to DMBA in inbred strains of mice.

An obvious question to ask has been the extent to which the development of contact hypersensitivity to DMBA influences DMBA carcinogenesis (44). This issue has been addressed by subjecting inbred strains of mice that differ in their capacity to be sensitized to DMBA to the same DMBA cutaneous carcinogenesis protocol. C3H/HeN mice, which have a vigorous contact hypersensitivity response to DMBA, generate substantially fewer tumors than do C3H.SW mice, which do not develop DMBA contact hypersensitivity and which differ from C3H/HeN mice genetically only at the MHC. Moreover, the level of DMBA–deoxyribonucleic acid (DNA) adducts that are formed in C3H/HeN mice is much greater than in C3H.SW mice. These findings are consistent with the hypothesis that the development of contact hypersensitivity to DMBA renders mice resistant to DMBA carcinogenesis and therefore serves a protective role by ameliorating the carcinogenic effects of this agent.

In addition to their ability to initiate immunologic hypersensitivity to themselves, the polyaromatic hydrocarbons have also been shown to suppress the cutaneous cell-mediated immune response to other chemicals. At least for 3-methylcholanthrene (3MC) inhibition occurs only when it is administered to Ah receptor positive strains of mice and does not occur in Ah negative strains that metabolize 3MC poorly (45). This issue has been further investigated with backcross and intercross progeny of C57BL/6 (Ah positive) and DBA/2 (Ah negative) and has been shown to segregate with strains that carry the Ah positive allele (i.e., strains that are able to metabolize the compound). The situation is similar when polyaromatic hydrocarbons are applied topically rather than parenterally. Like intraperitoneal 3MC, topical application of DMBA and BaP inhibits the development of contact hypersensitivity to dinitrofluorobenzene (DNFB) (46,47). However, unlike intraperitoneal 3MC, topical DMBA appears to act locally, at the site of its application, to inhibit cutaneous immunologic function (46). This conclusion is based on the observation that when DMBA is applied at one skin site but DNFB is applied at another skin site, suppression of the DNFB contact hypersensitivity is not observed. There have been no studies examining the effect of noncarcinogenic polyaromatic hydrocarbons on the induction of cutaneous cell-mediated immune responses to other chemicals nor have there been studies investigating whether topically applied polyaromatic hydrocarbons must be metabolized for immunosuppression to occur.

There has been considerable speculation that the polyaromatic hydrocarbons may suppress the induction of immune responses to other chemicals by directly affecting epidermal Langerhans' cells. Because they are potent initiators of cutaneous cell-mediated immune responses and they are located in the epidermis, they represent a logical target for such effects. The data on the effect of polyaromatic hydrocarbons on Langerhans' cell concentrations, however, have yielded conflicting results. On the one hand, repeated weekly applications of DMBA to the skin of mice (48) and to the hamster cheek pouch (49) resulted in a marked reduction in Langerhans' cell densities as detected by ATPase histochemistry and electron microscopy. The decline was present early and persisted for several weeks after the completion of DMBA treatments. On the other hand, epicutaneous application of BaP and catechol produced an increase in the number of identifiable Langerhans' cells (47). Despite the disparity in the effects of these three chemicals on Langerhans' cell densities, all were found to be immunosuppressive (46,47), suggesting either that DMBA inhibits cutaneous cell-mediated immunity differently from BaP and catechol or that mechanisms besides Langerhans' cell depletion operate to inhibit the contact hypersensitivity response when these agents are applied.

Further investigation into the mechanism by which topical application of DMBA inhibits the DNFB contact hypersensitivity response has shown that it is associated with the development of antigen-specific suppressor T lymphocytes, which are able to inhibit the induction of both cellular and humoral immune responses when adoptively transferred to naive syngeneic recipients (46,50). It has also been possible to demonstrate that their activation in this system is due to the direct effects of DMBA on the skin. When the reactive hapten trinitrophenol is conjugated to epidermal cells from DMBA-treated mice and those cells are used to immunize naive syngeneic recipients, suppressor cell induction occurs. However, when regional lymph node cells from skin draining the site of DMBA application are substituted for epidermal cells in these experiments, suppressor cells are not generated (51).

In other experiments, it has been shown that the DMBA-induced reduction in MHC class II determinants in the skin also reduces its immunogenicity for transplantation purposes (52). When allografts are prepared from the skin of mice that have been pretreated with DMBA, prolonged survival of the grafts is observed if they are transplanted to class II disparate recipients. However, if allografts pretreated in this manner are transplanted to mice that differ with respect to MHC class I determinants, no prolongation in graft survival is observed. The findings suggest that enhanced survival of the grafts is a direct consequence of the reduced number of class II molecules that are present on the skin at the time of transplantation.

Although other environmental oncogens such as ultraviolet radiation are known to augment cutaneous production of IL-1 (53), IL-6 (54), IL-10 (55), and TNF-α (23), little is known about the capacity of polyaromatic hydrocarbons to influence cutaneous cytokine synthesis and/or release. Indirect evidence in which strains of mice that differ in their capacity to produce cytokines are treated topically with a tumor-initiating dose of DMBA and are then examined both for differences in epidermal DNA adduct formation and cutaneous tumor formation suggests that DMBA augments cutaneous cytokine production (56). As was mentioned previously, C3H/HeN and C3H/HeJ mice differ only at the *Lps* locus, a gene that controls the biosynthesis and release of IL-1, IL-6, and TNF-α. When subjected to a tumor-initiating dose of DMBA, C3H/HeJ mice that are deficient in their capacity to produce cytokines retain substantially more epidermal DMBA–DNA adducts and develop significantly greater numbers of DMBA-induced tumors than do C3H/HeN mice, which are able to produce normal levels of cytokines. The findings are consistent with the hypothesis that topical application of DMBA leads to the production and release of cytokines that play a protective role in the cutaneous carcinogenesis pathway by reducing the number DMBA-initiated epidermal cells.

Tumor-Promoting Agents

Tumor promoters have also been shown to influence the skin immune system. Tumor promoters refer to a class of compounds that, on repeated application to skin treated with subcarcinogenic doses of carcinogenic chemicals, have the capacity to produce cutaneous tumors (57). Tumor promoters are nonmutagenic and are not tumorigenic when applied to normal skin. Although the mechanism by which tumor promoters, such as the phorbol esters [e.g., 12-*O*-tetradecanoylphorbol 13-acetate (TPA)], ultraviolet radiation, benzoyl peroxide, and anthralin, produce their effects is incompletely understood, all are known to have profound inflammatory effects. Topical application of TPA with as few as four treatments over a 2-week period has been demonstrated to reduce epidermal Langerhans' cell concentrations or to alter their morphology (52,58,59). When TPA-treated mice are evaluated for their capacity to initiate contact hypersensitivity to DNFB, a profound reduction is observed (52,60,61). Inhibition occurred when DNFB was applied at the site of TPA application and when it was painted on a skin site remote from the area to which TPA was applied, implying that TPA has both local and systemic effects (61). This is consistent with the finding that topical application of TPA results in the accumulation of mononuclear phagocytes in the spleen (62). TPA-induced inhibition in the induction of contact hypersensitivity to DNFB is associated with the generation of antigen-specific suppressor T lymphocytes (60).

The immunosuppressive effects of tumor promoters are not restricted to TPA. They are also present when other structurally unrelated classes of tumor promoters are examined for their effect on Langerhans' cells and on the contact hypersensitivity response. Topical application of croton oil and teleocidin both diminish Langerhans' cell concentrations (59,63). *N*-dodecane, ethyl phenylpropriolate, phorbol-12,13-dibenzoate, mezerein, anthralin, butylated hydroxytoluene, hydroperoxide, and benzoyl peroxide all suppress the DNFB contact hypersensitivity response (60,61). In contrast, the non-tumor-promoting agent phorbol and the 4-*O*-methyl TPA analog had no influence on the contact hypersensitivity response (60). Thus there is a rough correlation between the extent of the immunosuppression and the potency of the tumor-promoting activities of each compound.

Other Immunotoxic Chemicals

There is a paucity of data on the immunotoxic effects of other chemicals on the skin immune system. 2,3,7,8-Tetrachlorodibenzo-*p*-dioxin (TCDD) has been shown to increase Langerhans' cell densities in HRS/J +/hr haired mice, but not in their hr/hr hairless littermates (64). Because +/hr mice develop epidermal hyperplasia following topical application of TCDD, whereas hr/hr mice do not, the increase in Langerhans' cell density has been postulated to be due to the production of soluble factors by TCDD-treated epidermis that enhance the accumulation of Langerhans' cells in the skin. In other studies, it has been shown that topically applied urethrane and chrysene do not affect the density of epidermal Langerhans' cells, and that epicutaneous application of urethane does not affect the development of contact hypersensitivity to DNFB (59).

IMMUNOPHARMACOLOGIC AGENTS AND THE SKIN IMMUNE SYSTEM

Because various components of the skin immune system participate in the pathogenesis of many dermatologic diseases, there has been considerable interest in identifying new agents that selectively modify its function and in defining the mechanisms of action of those agents that are now used to alter the activities of the skin immune system.

Corticosteroids

It has been of great interest to examine the effects of topical and systemic corticosteroids on cutaneous immune function because of their extensive use in a variety of inflammatory and immunologic skin disorders. It should be noted that corticosteroids influence several other components of the immune and inflammatory response (65–67). They inhibit T lymphocyte and mononuclear phagocyte activation and mediator release, suppress neutrophil margination to endothelium and decrease their egress out of the vascular space, cause vasoconstriction, and impair eicosanoid synthesis and release. Thus it is not absolutely necessary to invoke a selective effect of corticosteroids on the skin immune system to explain their ameliorative effects on inflammatory dermatologic diseases. Nevertheless, it is quite clear that interactions between corticosteroids and the skin immune system do exist and they influence the cutaneous response to immune and inflammatory stimuli at least to some extent.

In various rodent species and in humans, topical and systemic administration of various corticosteroid preparations produces a profound depletion in the number of Langerhans' cells as identified by a number of cell surface markers with depressed concentrations persisting in some regimens for several weeks (68–71). The magnitude of the reduction is proportional to the dose and to the potency of the steroid employed (71). The capacity of corticosteroid-treated epidermis to present soluble antigens and alloantigens parallels the depressed Langerhans' cell numbers and is not due to an inability of the epidermis to secrete cytokines involved in the antigen presentation process nor is it due to enhanced production of immunosuppressive mediators such as prostaglandins (72). Because the concentration of Langerhans' cells in the epidermis correlates with the capacity of skin to initiate an immune response to contact allergens (9), it is reasonable to speculate that the inhibitory effect of corticosteroids on epidermal Langerhans' cell concentrations is in large part responsible for the inability of corticosteroid-treated skin to sensitize individuals to chemicals capable of causing an allergic contact hypersensitivity reaction (73).

Topical application and systemic administration of corticosteroids are also known to suppress the elicitation of allergic contact hypersensitivity, a finding that provides the rationale for their clinical use in dermatologic diseases. The extent to which a corticosteroid influence on the skin immune system is responsible for these effects, however, is currently unclear.

Less is known about the effects of corticosteroids on epidermal synthesis and secretion of cytokines. Addition of hydrocortisone to keratinocyte cultures results in reduced constitutive and ultraviolet (UV)-induced IL-1 activity in functional assays for that cytokine (74). In addition, it leads to the generation of an inhibitor of IL-1 activity. Physiologic doses of hydrocortisone, prednisolone, and dexamethasone, when added to keratinocyte cultures, have all been shown to inhibit the capacity of cells to synthesize and release IL-6 (54). The effect of corticosteroids on the production of other keratinocyte-derived cytokines has not been examined. *In vitro* administration of corticosteroids does not alter the capacity of IFN-γ or TNF-α to upregulate the expression of ICAM-1 on cultured keratinocytes (75) but does stimulate the production of an inhibitor of keratinocyte human leukocyte antigen (HLA)-DR expression (76).

Within the dermis, prolonged administration of potent topical steroids under occlusion over a 6-week period has been shown to deplete the dermis of mast cells (77). This procedure has been used to reduce the pruritus associated with mastocytosis, a disease in which there are increased numbers of mast cells in the dermis (78). Other studies have shown that corticosteroids inhibit cytokine-stimulated production of IL-6 by human dermal microvascular endothelial cells (79).

Cyclosporine

Cyclosporine is a potent immunosuppressive agent that has been shown to preferentially inhibit the activation of T lymphocytes by impairing the production of IL-2 and other T cell-derived cytokines (80). Although the drug is used primarily to prevent the rejection of transplanted allografts, it is also valuable in the management of a number of other immunologically mediated diseases. Interest in the activity of cyclosporine with respect to the skin immune system is based largely on its efficacy in psoriasis, a cutaneous inflammatory disorder characterized by the development over widespread areas of the body of well-circumscribed, erythematous plaques surmounted by a thick silvery scale (81). Although the pathogenesis of psoriasis remains to be elucidated, increasing evidence indicates that immunologic abnormalities play a critical, but as yet undefined, role. Examination of the effects of cyclosporine on the skin immune system has focused largely on its capacity to inhibit the antigen-presenting function of the skin. Initial studies using murine tissues showed that *in vitro* exposure of freshly prepared normal epidermal cell suspensions containing Langerhans' cells to cyclosporine resulted in a profound inhibition in their capacity to act as APCs in *in vitro* T cell proliferation assays (82). Similar studies have been conducted using human tissue with comparable results (83,84). The inhibition is not due to a decrease in IL-1 production or to a reduction in MHC class II molecule expression, nor is an increase in the synthesis of immunosuppressive prostaglandins a basis for this effect (84).

The extent to which these *in vitro* effects of cyclosporine on Langerhans' cell antigen-presenting function are applicable to the *in vivo* situation is a matter of controversy. The doses of cyclosporine with which epidermal cells were incubated in the *in vitro* studies tend to be higher than normally achieved in the skin *in vivo* (85). In spite of this, when skin has been taken from cyclosporine-treated psoriatic patients, Langerhans' cell antigen-presenting function is markedly reduced (86). The findings suggest either that actual concentrations of drug present in the epidermis are greater than suspected, that Langerhans' cells preferentially accumulate increased amounts of cyclosporine, or that the concentration of cyclosporine required to inhibit the antigen-presenting function of epidermal cells is less *in vivo* than would be predicted from the *in vitro* studies.

Retinoids

The development of retinoids, synthetic derivatives of vitamin A, as pharmaceutical agents has ushered in a new era in therapeutics of epithelial disorders. These drugs have widely been used in the treatment of various dermatoses including acne, psoriasis, keratinizing disorders of the skin, and cutaneous lupus erythematosus (87). Their efficacy in the prevention of skin cancer and their capacity to cause an inflammatory dermatosis (retinoid dermatitis) when administered topically or systemically have provided the impetus to investigate their immunologic activities. Although there are some exceptions, particularly when evaluated in patients with specific disease states (88), most studies have demonstrated that retinoids have an immunopotentiating effect. These include an increase in T lymphocyte proliferation to T cell-dependent mitogens (89), an enhancement in the cytotoxic activity of natural killer (NK) cells (90) and T lymphocytes (91), a simulation of humoral immune responses (92), and an antigen-specific augmentation in tumor immunity (93).

With respect to the skin immune system, systemic administration of retinoids seems to have no appreciable effect on concentrations of Langerhans' cells within the epidermis (90). However, in studies in which suspensions of epidermal cells are incubated with the synthetic retinoid acetretin *in vitro*, a mild inhibition in their ability to act as epidermal APCs in T cell proliferation assays and in the generation of cytotoxic T cells has been observed (94). Treatment of monocytes with similar retinoid doses results in much less of a reduction in their antigen-presenting activities, suggesting that the effect of retinoids is relatively specific for epidermal antigen presentation. The retinoid-induced inhibition in epidermal antigen-presenting function is not reversed by the cyclooxygenase inhibitor indomethacin, indicating that the effect is not prostaglandin mediated.

The effect of retinoic acid on cutaneous immune function *in vivo* has been investigated in experimental animal models and in humans. In mice, dietary supplementation with vitamin A acetate results in an augmented contact hypersensitivity response and in an increase in cell numbers and DNA synthesis in lymph nodes draining the site of primary immunization with optimal and suboptimal doses of the hapten oxazolone (95). An increase in the dinitrochlorobenzene (DNCB) contact hypersensitivity response has also been observed in humans with psoriasis and other cutaneous diseases managed with 13-cis-retinoic acid (96). *In vivo* administration of retinoic acid also accelerates skin allograft rejection in mice, a finding consistent with its immunopotentiating role (97).

Keratinocytes respond to *in vitro* treatment with retinoic acid by increasing their transcription of IL-1α, IL-1β, IL-8, and TGF-α (98,99). For IL-1β, induction by retinoic acid occurs at low concentrations (10^{-10} M) and after short duration in culture (2 to 4 hr), suggesting that retinoic acid must first bind to its intracellular receptor. This does not appear to be the case for IL-8 and TGF-α, since the synthesis of those cytokines is increased by retinoic acid only after prolonged incubation and with rather high retinoic acid concentrations. The retinoid-induced augmentation in IL-1 gene transcription in keratinocytes is accompanied by an increase in protein production that can be found both in cell extracts and in culture supernatants. The various retinoids differ in their capacity to stimulate IL-1 protein with the retinoic acids (retinol and 13-cis-retinoic acid) exerting a greater effect than the monoaromatic retinoids (etretinate and acetretin). Corticosteroids suppress retinoid-induced IL-1 production by keratinocytes.

The *in vivo* influence of retinoids on IL-1 production by the skin appears to be more complex. In rats, acetretin, the major metabolite of etretinate, augments IL-1 concentrations in the epidermis (100), whereas, in humans, topical retinoic acid treatment has no effect on IL-1 concentrations and systemic treatment with aretinoid ethyl ester reduces IL-1a and IL-1β concentrations in psoriatic plaque (101,102).

The synthetic retinoid etretin has been shown to increase the IFN-γ-induced augmentation in ICAM-1 expression on cultured keratinocytes. The capacity of etretin to produce this effect depends on the level of keratinocyte differentiation (75).

REFERENCES

1. Stingl G, Hauser C, Tschachler E, Groh V, Wolff K. Immune functions of epidermal cells. In: Norris DA, ed. *Immune mechanisms in cutaneous disease*. New York: Marcel Dekker; 1989:3–72.
2. Bos JD, Kapsenberg ML. The skin immune sysem (SIS): its cellular constituents and their interactions. *Immunol Today* 1986;7:235–240.
3. Odland GF. Structure of the skin. In: Goldsmith L, ed. *Physiology, biochemistry and molecular biology of the skin*, 2nd ed. New York: Oxford University Press; 1991:3–62.
4. Silberberg I, Baer RL, Rosenthal SA. The role of Langerhans' cells in allergic contact hypersensitivity. A review of findings in man and guinea pigs. *J Invest Dermatol* 1976;66:210–217.
5. Hauser C, Katz SI. Activation and expansion of hapten- and protein-specific T helper cells from nonsensitized mice. *Proc Natl Acad Sci USA* 1988;85:5625–5628.
6. Stingl GL, Gazze-Stingl LA, Aberer W, Wolff K. Antigen presentation by murine epidermal Langerhans' cells and its alteration by ultraviolet light. *J Immunol* 1981;127:1707–1713.
7. Braathen LR, Thorsby E. Studies on human epidermal Langerhans' cells. I. Alloactivating and antigen-presenting capacity. *Scand J Immunol* 1980;11:401–408.

8. Grabbe S, Bruvers S, Gallo RL, Knisely TL, Nazareno R, Granstein RD. Tumor antigen presentation by murine epidermal cells. *J Immunol* 1991;146:3656–3661.
9. Toews GB, Bergstresser PR, Streilein JW. Epidermal Langerhans' cell density determines whether contact hypersensitivity or unresponsiveness follows skin painting with DNFB. *J Immunol* 1980; 124:445–453.
10. Sauder DN, Tamaki K, Moshell AN, Fujiwara H, Katz SI. Induction of tolerance to topically applied TNCB using TNP-conjugated, ultraviolet light-irradiated epidermal cells. *J Immunol* 1981; 127:261–265.
11. Sprecher E, Becker Y. Skin Langerhans' cells play an important role in the defense against HSV-1 infection. *Arch Virol* 1986;91:341–349.
12. Basham TY, Nickoloff BJ, Merigan TC, Morhenn VB. Recombinant gamma interferon differentially regulates class II antigen expression and biosynthesis on cultured normal human keratinocytes. *J Interferon Res* 1985;5:23–32.
13. Auböck J, Romani N, Grubauer G, Fritsch P. HLA-DR expression on keratinocytes is a common feature of diseased skin. *Br J Dermatol* 1986;114:465–472.
14. Boehncke W-H, Kellner I, Konter U, Sterry W. Differential expression of adhesion molecules on infiltrating cells in inflammatory dermatoses. *J Am Acad Dermatol* 1992;26:907–913.
15. Dustin ML, Singer KH, Tuck DT, Springer TA. Adhesion of T lymphoblasts to epidermal keratinocytes is regulated by interferon gamma and is mediated by intercellular adhesion molecule I (ICAM-1). *J Exp Med* 1988;167:1323–1340.
16. Trefzer U, Brockhaus M, Loetscher H, Parlow F, Kapp A, Schopf E, Krutmann J. 55-kd Tumor necrosis factor receptor is expressed by human keratinocytes and plays a pivotal role in regulation of human keratinocyte ICAM-1 expression. *J Invest Dermatol* 1991;97:911–916.
17. Griffiths CE, Voorhees JJ, Nickoloff BJ. Characterization of intercellular adhesion molecule-1 and HLA-DR expression in normal and inflamed skin: modulation by recombinant gamma interferon and tumor necrosis factor. *J Am Acad Dermatol* 1989;20:617.
18. Caughman SW. Adhesion molecules: their roles in cutaneous biology and inflammation. *Prog Dermatol* 1991;25:1–8.
19. Fleming TE, Mirando WS, Elmets CA. Expression of the activation antigen BB-1/B7 on cells of non-hematopoietic origin: keratinocytes from human epidermis. *J Invest Dermatol* 1992;98:577.
20. Schwarz T, Luger TA. Pharmacology of cytokines in the skin. In: Mukhtar H, ed. *Pharmacology of the skin*. Boca Raton, FL: CRC Press; 1992:283–313.
21. Dinarello CA. Interleukin-1 and interleukin-1 antagonism. *Blood* 1991;77:1627–1652.
22. Heufler C, Koch F, Schuler G. Granulocyte/macrophage colony-stimulating factor and interleukin-1 mediate the maturation of murine epidermal Langerhans' cells into potent immunostimulator dendritic cells. *J Exp Med* 1988;167:700–705.
23. Kock A, Schwarz T, Kirnbauer R, Urbanski A, Perry A, Ansel JC, Luger TA. Human keratinocytes are a source for tumor necrosis factor α: evidence for synthesis and release upon stimulation with endotoxin or ultraviolet light. *J Exp Med* 1990;172:1609–1614.
24. Munro JM, Pober JS, Cotran RS. Tumor necrosis factor and interferon γ induce distinct patterns of endothelial activation and associated leukocyte accumulation in skin of *Papio anubis*. *Am J Pathol* 1989;135:121–134.
25. Nickoloff BJ, Griffiths CE, Barker JN. The role of adhesion molecules, chemotactic factors, and cytokines in inflammatory and neoplastic skin disease. *J Invest Dermatol* 1990;94:151S–157S.
26. Barker JN, Sarma V, Mitra R, Dixit VM, Nickoloff BJ. Marked synergism between tumor necrosis factor-alpha and interferon-gamma in regulation of keratinocyte-derived adhesion molecules and chemotactic factors. *J Clin Invest* 1990;85:605–608.
27. Sharpe RJ, Margolis RJ, Askari X, Amento EP, Granstein RD. Induction of dermal and subcutaneous inflammation by recombinant cachectin/tumor necrosis factor (TNF alpha) in the mouse. *J Invest Dermatol* 1988;91:353–357.
28. Koch F, Heufler C, Kampgen E, Schneeweiss D, Bock G, Schuler G. Tumor necrosis factor alpha maintains the variability of murine epidermal Langerhans' cells in culture, but in contrast to granulocyte/macrophage colony-stimulating factor, without inducing their functional maturation. *J Exp Med* 1990;171:159–171.
29. Symington FW. Lymphotoxin, tumor necrosis factor, and gamma interferon are cytostatic for normal human keratinocytes. *J Invest Dermatol* 1989;92:798–865.
30. Kupper TS, Dower S, Birchal N, Clark S, Lee F. Interleukin-1 binds to specific receptors on keratinocytes and induces granulocyte/macrophage colony stimulating factor (GM-CSF)

mRNA and protein, a potential autocrine role of IL-1 in the epidermis. *J Clin Invest* 1988;82:1787–1792.

31. Henke D, Danilowicz R, Eling T. Arachidonic acid metabolism by isolated epidermal basal and differentiated keratinocytes from the hairless mouse. *Biochim Biophys Acta* 1986;876:271–279.
32. Pentland AP, Needleman P. Modulation of keratinocyte proliferation *in vitro* by endogenous prostaglandin synthesis. *J Clin Invest* 1986;77:246–251.
33. Ishisaka K, ed. *Mast cell activation and mediator release*, Progress in Allergy Series, vol 34. Basel: Karger; 1984.
34. Van Loveren H, Teppema JS, Askenase PW. Skin mast cells. In: Bos JD, ed. *Skin immune system (SIS)*. Boca Raton, FL: CRC Press; 1989:171–196.
35. Bergstresser PR. Immune mechanisms in contact allergic dermatitis. *Dermatol Clin* 1990;8:3–11.
36. Phanuphak P, Moorhead JW, Claman HN. Tolerance and contact sensitivity to DNFB in mice. *J Immunol* 1974;112:115–123.
37. Elmets CA, Bergstresser PR, Streilein JW. Differential distributions of Langerhans' cells in organ culture of human skin. *J Invest Dermatol* 1982;79:340–345.
38. Luger TA, Stadler BM, Luger BM, Mathieson BJ, Mage M, Schmidt JA, Oppenheim JJ. Murine epidermal cell derived thymocyte activating factor resembles murine interleukin-1. *J Immunol* 1983;128:2147–2152.
39. Old LJ, Benacerraf F, Carswell E. Contact reactivity to carcinogenic polycyclic hydrocarbons. *Nature* 1963;198:1215–1216.
40. Pomeranz JR. Preliminary studies of tolerance to contact sensitization in carcinogen-fed guinea pigs. *J Natl Cancer Inst* 1972;48:1513–1517.
41. Pomeranz JR, Carney JF, Alarif A. The induction of immunologic tolerance in guinea pigs infused with dimethylbenz[*a*]anthracene. *J Invest Dermatol* 1980;75:488–490.
42. Klemme JC, Mukhtar H, Elmets CA. Induction of contact hypersensitivity to dimethylbenz[*a*]anthracene and benzo[*a*]pyrene in C3H/HeN mice. *Cancer Res* 1987;47:6074–6078.
43. Klemme JC, Mukhtar H, Elmets CA. Strain differences in the development of contact hypersensitivity in mice to a polyaromatic hydrocarbon. *Clin Res* 1988;36:663A.
44. Elmets CA, Athar M, Zaidi SI, Mukhtar H. Contact hypersensitivity of dimethylbenz[*a*]anthracene is influenced by genes within the major histocompatibility complex and at the Ah receptor locus. *Clin Res* 1992;40:309A.
45. Frank DM, Yamashita TS, Blumer JL. Genetic differences in methylcholanthrene-mediated suppression of cutaneous delayed hypersensitivity in mice. *Toxicol Appl Pharmacol* 1982;64:31–41.
46. Halliday GM, Muller HK. Induction of tolerance via skin depleted of Langerhans' cells by a chemical carcinogen. *Cell Immunol* 1986;99:220–227.
47. Ruby JC, Halliday GM, Muller HK. Differential effects of benzo[*a*]pyrene and dimethylbenz[*a*]-anthracene on Langerhans' cell distribution and contact sensitization in murine epidermis. *J Invest Dermatol* 1989;92:150–155.
48. Muller HK, Halliday GM, Knight BA. Carcinogen-induced depletion of cutaneous Langerhans' cells. *Br J Cancer* 1985;52:81–85.
49. Schwartz J, Solt DB, Pappo J, Weichselbaum R. Distribution of Langerhans' cells in normal and carcinogen-treated mucosa of buccal pouches of hamster. *J Dermatol Surg Oncol* 1981;7:1005–1010.
50. Halliday GM, Muller HK. Sensitization through carcinogen-induced Langerhans' cell-deficient skin activates specific long-lived suppressor cells for both cellular and humoral immunity. *Cell Immunol* 1987;109:206–221.
51. Halliday GM, Cavanaugh LL, Muller HK. Antigen presented in the local lymph node by cells from dimethylbenzanthracene-treated murine epidermis activates suppressor cells. *Cell Immunol* 1988;117:289–302.
52. Odling KA, Halliday GM, Muller HK. Enhanced survival of skin grafts depleted of Langerhans' cells by treatment with dimethylbenzanthracene. *Immunology* 1987;62:379–385.
53. Kupper TS, Chua AO, Flood P, McGuire JS, Gubler U. Interleukin 1 gene expression in cultured human keratinocytes is augmented by ultraviolet irradiation. *J Clin Invest* 1987;80:430–436.
54. Kirnbauer R, Köck A, Neuner P, et al. Regulation of epidermal interleukin-6 production by UV light and corticosteroids. *J Invest Dermatol* 1991;96:484–489.
55. Rivas JM, Ullrich S. Systemic suppression of delayed-type hypersensitivity by supernatants from UV-irradiated keratinocytes. An essential role for keratinocyte-derived IL-10. *J Immunol* 1993;149:3865–3871.

56. Elmets CA, Zaidi SI, Bickers DR, Mukhtar H. Immunogenetic influences on the initiation stage of the cutaneous chemical carcinogenesis pathway. *Cancer Res* 1992;52:6106–6109.
57. Agarwal R, Mukhtar H. Cutaneous chemical carcinogenesis. In: Mukhtar H, ed. *Pharmacology of the skin*. Boca Raton, FL: CRC Press; 1992:371–387.
58. Baxter CS, Chalfin K, Andringa A, Miller ML. Qualitative and quantitative effects on epidermal Langerhans' (Ia^+) and Thy-1^+ dendritic cells following topical application of phorbol diesters and mezerein. *Carcinogenesis* 1988;9:1563–1568.
59. Halliday GM, MacCarrick GR, Muller HK. Tumor promoters but not initiators deplete Langerhans' cells from murine epidermis. *Br J Cancer* 1987;56:328–330.
60. Kodari E, Pavone A, Reiners JJ Jr. Induction of suppressor T cells and inhibition of contact hypersensitivity in mice by 12-*O*-tetradecanoylphorbol-13-acetate and its analogs. *J Invest Dermatol* 1991;96:864–870.
61. Kodari E, Pavone A, Reiners JJ Jr. Local- and systemic-mediated suppression of contact hypersensitivity in mice by several structurally unrelated classes of tumor promoters. *Carcinogenesis* 1991;12:1933–1937.
62. Updyke LW, Yoon HL, Chuthaputti A, Pfeifer RW, Yim GKW. Induction of interleukin-1 and tumor necrosis factor by 12-*O*-tetradecanoylphorbol-13-acetate in phorbol ester sensitive (SENCAR) and resistant (B6C3F1) mice. *Carcinogenesis* 1989;10:1107–1111.
63. Lisby S, Baadsgaard O, Cooper KD, Vejlsgaard GL. Decreased number and function of antigen-presenting cells in the skin following application of irritant agents: relevance for skin cancer? *J Invest Dermatol* 1989;92:842–847.
64. Puhvel SM, Sakamoto M, Reisner RM. Effect of TCDD on the density of Langerhans' cells in murine skin. *Toxicol Appl Pharmacol* 1989;99:72–80.
65. Fauci AS, Dale DS, Balow JE. Glucocorticosteroid therapy: mechanisms of action and clinical considerations. *Ann Intern Med* 1976;84:304–315.
66. Katz P, Fauci AS. Immunosuppressives and immunoadjuvants. In: Samter M, Talmage DW, Frank MM, Austen KF, Claman HN, eds. *Immunological diseases*, 4th ed. Boston: Little, Brown; 1988: 675–698.
67. Snyder DS, Unanue ER. Corticosteroids inhibit murine macrophage Ia expression and interleukin 1 production. *J Immunol* 1982;129:1803–1805.
68. Lynch DH, Gurish MF, Daynes RA. Relationship between epidermal Langerhans' cell density, ATPase activity and the induction of contact hypersensitivity. *J Immunol* 1981;126:1892–1897.
69. Belsito DV, Flotte TJ, Lim HW, Baer RL, Thorbecke GJ, Gigli I. Effect of glucocorticosteroids on epidermal Langerhans' cells. *J Exp Med* 1982;155:291–302.
70. Berman B, France DS, Martinelli GP, Hass A. Modulation of expression of epidermal Langerhans' cell properties following *in situ* exposure to glucocorticosteroids. *J Invest Dermatol* 1983;80:168–171.
71. Nordlund JJ, Ackles AE, Lerner AB. The effects of ultraviolet light and certain drugs on Ia-bearing Langerhans' cells in murine epidermis. *Cell Immunol* 1981;60:50–63.
72. Ashworth J, Booker J, Breathnach SM. Effect of topical steroid therapy on Langerhans' cell function in human skin. *Br J Dermatol* 1988;118:457–469.
73. Burrows WM, Stoughton RB. Inhibition of induction of human contact sensitization by topical steroids. *Arch Dermatol* 1976;112:175–178.
74. Kupper TS, McGuire J. Hydrocortisone reduces both constitutive and UV-elicited release of epidermal thymocyte activating factor (ETAF) by cultured keratinocytes. *J Invest Dermatol* 1987; 87:570–573.
75. Kashihara-Sawami M, Norris DA. The state of differentiation of cultured human keratinocytes determines the level of intercellular adhesion molecule-1 (ICAM-1) induction by γ interferon. *J Invest Dermatol* 1992;98:741–747.
76. Smith B, Berman B. Characterization of a glucosteroid-induced inhibitor of interferon-gamma induction of HLA-DR expression. *J Invest Dermatol* 1992;99:35–39.
77. Lavker RM, Schechter NM. Cutaneous mast cell depletion results from topical corticosteroid usage. *J Immunol* 1985;135:2368–2373.
78. Barton J, Lavker RM, Schechter NM, Lazarus GS. Treatment of urticaria pigmentosa with corticosteroids. *Arch Dermatol* 1985;121:1516–1523.
79. Hettmannsperger U, Detmar M, Owsianowski M, Tenorio S, Kammler H-J, Orfanos CE. Cytokine-stimulated human dermal microvascular endothelial cells produce interleukin 6—inhibition by hydrocortisone, dexamethasone, and calcitriol. *J Invest Dermatol* 1992;99:531–536.

80. Shevach EM. The effects of cyclosporine A on the immune system. *Ann Rev Immunol* 1985;3:397–423.
81. Ellis CN, Gorsulowsky DC, Hamilton TA, et al. Cyclosporin A improves psoriasis in a double blind study. *JAMA* 1986;256:3110–3116.
82. Furue M, Katz SI. The effect of cyclosporine on epidermal cells. I. Cyclosporine inhibits accessory cell functions of epidermal Langerhans' cells *in vitro*. *J Immunol* 1988;140:4139–4143.
83. Demidem A, Taylor JR, Grammer SF, Streilein JW. Comparison of effects of transforming growth factor-beta and cyclosporin A on antigen-presenting cells of blood and epidermis. *J Invest Dermatol* 1991;96:401–407.
84. Dupuy P, Bagot M, Michel L, Descourt B, Dubertret L. Cyclosporin A inhibits the antigen-presenting functions of freshly isolated human Langerhans' cells *in vitro*. *J Invest Dermatol* 1991; 96:408–413.
85. Cooper KD, Baadsgaard O, Duell E, Fisher G, Ellis CN, Voorhees JJ. Langerhans' cell sensitivity to *in vitro* versus *in vivo* loading with cyclosporine A. *J Invest Dermatol* 1992;98:259–260.
86. Cooper KD, Baadsgaard O, Ellis CN, Duell E, Voorhees JJ. Mechanisms of cyclosporine A inhibition of antigen-presenting activity in uninvolved and lesional psoriatic epidermis. *J Invest Dermatol* 1992;98:259–260.
87. Dicken CH. Retinoids: a review. *J Am Acad Dermatol* 1984;11:541–545.
88. Soppi A-M, Soppi E, Eskola J, Jansén CT. Cell-mediated immunity in Darier's disease: effect of systemic retinoid therapy. *Br J Dermatol* 1982;106:141–152.
89. Dillehay DL, Li W, Kalin J, Walia AS, Lamon EW. *In vitro* effects of retinoids on murine thymus-dependent and thymus-independent mitogenesis. *Cell Immunol* 1987;107:130–137.
90. McKerrow KJ, Mackie RM, Lesko MJ, Pearson C. The effect of oral retinoid therapy on the normal immune system. *Br J Dermatol* 1988;119:313–320.
91. Dennert G, Lotan R. Effects of retinoic acid on the immune system: stimulation of T killer cell induction. *Eur J Immunol* 1978;8:23–29.
92. Sidell N, Famatiga E, Golub SH. Immunological aspects of retinoids in humans. II. Retinoic acid enhances induction of hemolytic plaque-forming cells. *Cell Immunol* 1984;88:374–381.
93. Malkovsky M, Dore C, Hunt R, Palmer L, Chandler P, Medawar PB. Enhancement of specific antitumor immunity in mice fed a diet enriched in vitamin A acetate. *Proc Natl Acad Sci USA* 1983;80:6322–6326.
94. Dupuy P, Bagot M, Heslan M, Dubertret L. Synthetic retinoids inhibit the antigen presenting properties of epidermal cells *in vitro*. *J Invest Dermatol* 1989;93:455–459.
95. Miller K, Maisey J, Malkovsky M. Enhancement of contact sensitization in mice fed a diet enriched in vitamin A acetate. *Int Arch Allergy Appl Immun* 1984;75:120–125.
96. Fulton RA, Souteyrand P, Thivolet J. Influence of retinoid Ro 10-9359 on cell-mediated immunity *in vivo*. *Dermatologica* 1982;165:568–572.
97. Jurin M, Tannock IF. Influence of vitamin A on immunological response. *Immunology* 1972; 23:283–287.
98. Elder JT, Astrom A, Petterson U, et al. Retinoic acid receptors and binding proteins in human skin. *J Invest Dermatol* 1992;98:36s–41s.
99. Tokura Y, Edelson RL, Gasparro FP. Retinoid augmentation of bioactive interleukin-1 production by murine keratinocytes. *Br J Dermatol* 1992;126:485–495.
100. Schmitt A, Hauser C, Didierjean L, Merot Y, Dayer J-M, Saurat J-H. Systemic administration of etretin increases epidermal interleukin 1 in the rat. *Br J Dermatol* 1987;116:615–622.
101. Gruaz DC, Didierjean L, Grassi J, Frobert Y, Dayer J-M. Interleukin 1 alpha and beta in psoriatic skin. Enzymoimmunoassay, immunoblot studies and effect of systemic retinoids. *Dermatologica* 1989;179:202–206.
102. Gruaz DC, Didierjean L, Gumowski-Sunek D, Saurat J-H. Effect of topical retinoic acid on the interleukin 1α and β immunoreactive pool in normal human epidermis. *Br J Dermatol* 1990; 1123:283–289.

Immunotoxicology and Immunopharmacology, Second Edition, edited by J. H. Dean, M. I. Luster, A. E. Munson, and I. Kimber.
Raven Press, Ltd., New York © 1994.

26

Chemical-Induced Apoptosis in the Immune System

David J. McConkey, *Mikael B. Jondal, and †Sten G. Orrenius

*Department of Cell Biology, University of Texas, M. D. Anderson Cancer Center, Houston, Texas 77030; and *Departments of Microbiology and Tumor Biology, †Institute of Environmental Medicine, Karolinska Institute, S-171 77 Stockholm, Sweden*

In normal tissue physiology, cell death is an important homeostatic mechanism. This is particularly true in the immune system, where it mediates the silencing of autoreactive precursor cells during T and B cell development and eliminates expanded clones at the termination of an immune response. These processes and others are now known to occur via a conserved physiologic mechanism known as apoptosis. Originally defined by morphologic criteria, recent work has identified biochemical and molecular mechanisms that also characterize the process, and it is now clear that its regulation involves signal transduction networks as complex as those regulating cell proliferation and differentiation. Likewise, defects in the control of apoptosis have been linked to various diseases, including cancer, autoimmunity, and acquired immunodeficiency syndrome (AIDS).

Physiologic triggers are not the only ones capable of inducing apoptosis in susceptible target cells, and many immunotoxins exert their effects by stimulating apoptosis by exploiting physiologic control mechanisms. This chapter introduces several of these chemicals and discusses what is known about the mechanisms underlying their actions, particularly with regard to how they relate to known physiologic apoptotic control systems.

DEFINITION OF APOPTOSIS

Apoptosis is a term that was coined by Kerr, Wyllie, and Currie to describe a series of morphologic changes shared by dying cells in various physiologic model systems (1). These include liver atrophy in response to ischemia or low to moderate doses of toxic agents and loss of cells within the adrenal cortex in response to glucocorticoid-induced withdrawal of adrenocorticotropic hormone (ACTH) (1). These alterations were largely detected by electron microscopy and included plasma and nuclear membrane blebbing, organelle relocalization and compaction, chromatin condensation, and production of membrane-enclosed particles containing intracellular material known as *apoptotic bodies*. The changes were easily distinguished from those occurring in cells dying in response to antibody plus complement, high doses of toxic agents, or freezing and thawing—conditions known to induce necrosis, where the morphologic alterations were typified by cellular and organelle swelling and the random spillage of cellular contents into the extracellular milieu. Rather, apoptotic cells display no obvious changes in plasma membrane integrity even while drastic biochemical alterations are underway, and usually apoptotic cells and bodies are specifically recognized and cleared by neighboring cells or phagocytic cells (macrophages) before lysis can occur. Such clearance allows for massive cell turnover without induction of an inflammatory response, another feature of apoptosis that distinguishes the process from necrosis.

Endogenous endonuclease activation, resulting in the cleavage of host chromatin into oligonucleosome-length deoxyribonucleic acid (DNA) fragments (DNA ladders), is the most characteristic biochemical feature of apoptosis (2). Biochemical studies have provided good evidence that a Ca^{2+}/Mg^{2+}-dependent activity is involved. Early work by Hewish and Burgoyne (3) and later by Vanderbilt and colleagues (4) demonstrated the presence of a Ca^{2+}/Mg^{2+}-dependent enzyme activity capable of generating characteristic apoptotic chromatin cleavage patterns, which is present constitutively within nuclei from a variety of cell types. Cohen and Duke (5) implicated this activity in the DNA fragmentation observed in thymocytes undergoing apoptosis, and it has since been linked to DNA fragmentation in other model systems. Candidate Ca^{2+}-dependent endonucleases have been isolated by Gaido and colleagues (6), Arends et al. (7), and Peitsch and co-workers (8), although to date proof that any one is absolutely required for DNA fragmentation in apoptosis is lacking. An alternative enzyme, activated by acidic pH, has been implicated by Barry and Eastman (9) in apoptosis in several cell lines exposed to chemotherapeutic agents. It is possible that redundant mechanisms exist within cells to cleave DNA at the oligonucleosomal linker regions. Evidence has been advanced that DNA fragmentation is directly involved in precipitating cell death during apoptosis (10), further underscoring the importance of the event to the process.

An important feature of apoptosis is that it is often (but not exclusively) dependent on ongoing protein and messenger ribonucleic acid (mRNA) synthesis, as demonstrated by the observation that inhibitors (i.e., cycloheximide and actinomycin D) can prevent the response in many instances (11). These findings have prompted investigators to attempt to isolate and clone potential *lysis genes* to determine the roles they play in regulating the process. For example, Owens and colleagues (12) have isolated a transcript induced in apoptotic cells (RP-8) that encodes a protein containing a zinc finger DNA binding domain, suggesting it may function as a transcriptional regulator. Osborne and co-workers (12a) and Woronicz et al. (12b) have isolated a different transcript (*nur*77) that encodes an orphan member of the steroid hormone receptor superfamily. Independent studies by Askew et al. (13), Evan and colleagues (14), and Shi and co-workers (15) have shown that expression of the oncogene c-myc is often involved in the triggering mechanism. In addition, sustained expression of the c-fos oncogene appears tightly linked to induction of apoptosis *in vivo* (16). However, it should be emphasized that transcription and translation are dispensable for apoptosis in a variety of model systems, including apoptosis induced in target cells by cytotoxic T cells, hyperthermia, or various chemical agents (17,18), as will be discussed later.

Another common characteristic of apoptosis is that it can be blocked by the oncogene Bcl-2 (19) and the adenovirus gene E1B (20). These genes appear to extend the lifespan of cells that would otherwise rapidly undergo apoptosis; they do not immortalize cells. By contrast, the transforming gene of the Abelson virus (v-abl) is capable of blocking apoptosis and immortalizing relevant target cells (21). Apoptosis-inhibiting genes have been conserved through evolution, as evidenced by the recent demonstration that ced-9, a major programmed cell death inhibitor in the nematode *Caenorhabditis elegans* (22), is functionally homologous to Bcl-2 (23). Little is known about the biochemical mechanisms underlying apoptosis inhibition by these gene products, although the demonstration that Bcl-2 (24) and E1B (25) can localize to the nucleus suggests a possible nuclear site of action.

Viral infection, mutation, and DNA damage elicit a physiologic response involving DNA repair systems and induction of the tumor suppressor protein, p53. Recent work has shown that p53 expression can lead to cell cycle arrest and subsequently to induction of apoptosis, apparently depending on the extent of DNA damage (26). Work from Oren's laboratory originally demonstrated that overexpression of p53 by itself is sufficient to induce apoptosis in a myeloid leukemia cell line (27), a result that has been confirmed by Shaw and colleagues (28) in another model system. In addition, independent work from the laboratories of Jacks (29) and Wyllie (30) has demonstrated a p53-dependent pathway of apoptosis in thymocytes that is presumably activated by DNA damage. How DNA damage initiates and how p53 regulates apoptosis are the subjects of intense ongoing investigation.

CHEMICAL-INDUCED APOPTOSIS IN IMMUNE CELLS

A variety of physiologic stimuli, including glucocorticoid hormones, antigen receptor engagement, prostaglandins (PGs), tumor necrosis factor (TNF), and antibodies to the Fas surface antigen, can specifically trigger apoptosis in lymphocytes and other immune cells. Invariably, these responses involve specific receptors and signal transduction systems, and second messengers, including Ca^{2+}, cyclic adenosine monophosphate (cAMP), nitric oxide, and ceramide, have been implicated. The p53-mediated DNA damage response is also an important physiologic apoptosis control mechanism. It appears that toxins that induce apoptosis in their target cells activate the process by exploiting these pathways, either by mimicking receptor-mediated signaling mechanisms or by triggering the DNA damage response (Fig. 1). Some of the more notable of these chemicals are introduced next, along with descriptions of their presumptive modes of action.

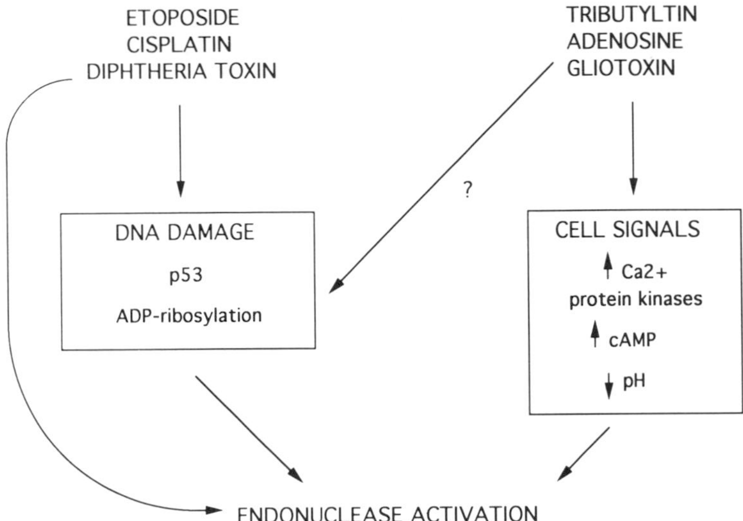

FIG. 1. Physiologic mechanisms underlying chemical-induced apoptosis. Toxic agents that induce DNA damage, such as topoisomerase inhibitors, cisplatin, and diphtheria toxin, are capable of triggering apoptosis in lymphoid target cells via a mechanism involving p53 expression and the cellular DNA damage control response. Alternatively, toxins such as TCDD, tributyltin, adenosine, and gliotoxin appear to exert their actions by interacting with cellular signaling pathways, resulting in inappropriate elevations in the cytosolic Ca^{2+} concentration, protein kinase activation, elevations in cAMP, and/or a decrease in cytosolic pH—events that have been linked to induction of apoptosis.

Dioxin-Induced Thymocyte Apoptosis

The industrial by-product and environmental contaminant 2,3,7,8-tetrachlorodibenzo-*p*-dioxin (TCDD) is the most potent of a group of halogenated, aromatic hydrocarbons that are extremely toxic to laboratory animals. TCDD causes thymic atrophy due to depletion of the immature cortical thymocytes (31), a pattern that is reminiscent of the effects of glucocorticoid hormone treatment. Glucocorticoids and TCDD also have overlapping or indistinguishable effects in other target organs. For example, both are potent inducers of specific isozymes of cytochrome P450 (32), and both suppress B lymphocyte differentiation (33). Moreover, both bind receptors that are closely related members of the steroid hormone receptor superfamily. These receptors are transcriptional regulators that usually induce the expression of specific genetic targets, suggesting that the actions of glucocorticoids and TCDD are mediated by new gene expression.

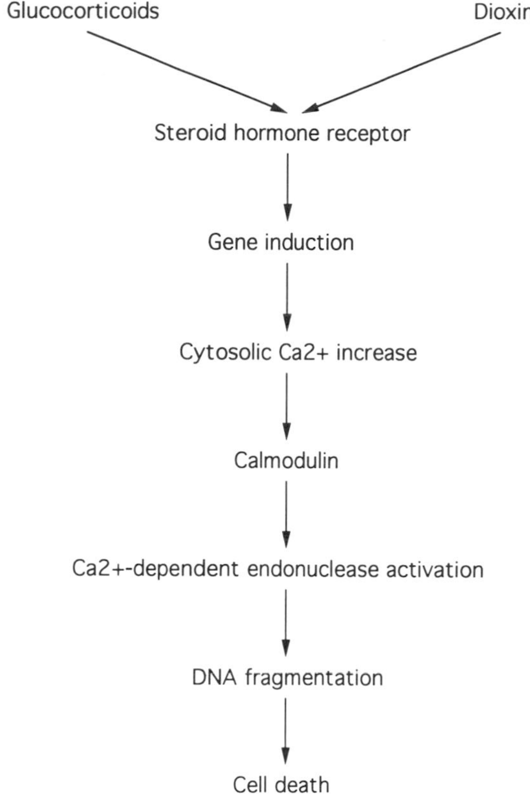

FIG. 2. Shared biochemical events in glucocorticoid- and TCDD-induced thymocyte apoptosis. Previous work has shown that TCDD toxicity is mediated by binding to a cytosolic protein (encoded by the Ah locus) that is a member of the steroid receptor superfamily. Thymocyte apoptosis induced by glucocorticoids or TCDD is preceded by elevations in the cytosolic Ca^{2+} concentration, which are blocked by inhibitors of macromolecular synthesis, suggesting that gene induction mediates the response. Calmodulin antagonists also prevent endonuclease activation. Finally, the endonuclease inhibitor aurintricarboxylic acid can prevent both DNA fragmentation and cell death in apoptotic thymocytes, suggesting that endonuclease activation may be involved in precipitating cell death.

We have presented evidence that TCDD kills immature thymocytes via induction of apoptosis (34). When suspensions of cells are exposed to relatively high doses of the agent, chromatin condensation and DNA fragmentation indistinguishable from that induced by glucocorticoid hormone are observed. Several of the biochemical features of the process are indistinguishable from those evoked during glucocorticoid-induced thymocyte apoptosis, summarized schematically in Fig. 2. For example, the mechanism appears to involve protein synthesis as both DNA fragmentation and cell death can be blocked by the protein synthesis inhibitor cycloheximide. In addition, TCDD stimulates an early, sustained increase in the cytosolic Ca^{2+} concentration due to Ca^{2+} influx that also can be blocked by cycloheximide. In the case of either glucocorticoid- or TCDD-induced thymocyte apoptosis, prevention of the Ca^{2+} increase by treatment with extracellular ethyleneglycol tetraacetic acid (EGTA) or intracellular Ca^{2+}-buffering agents blocks both DNA fragmentation and cell death, indicating that both apoptosis mechanisms are Ca^{2+} dependent. Moreover, calmodulin antagonists block both processes, suggesting the involvement of the important Ca^{2+}-binding protein in the responses. Thus TCDD appears to mimic the glucocorticoid response.

We obtained further evidence for overlap between the mechanisms of glucocorticoid and TCDD action from *in vivo* experiments (35). When young rats are injected with lethal doses of TCDD, thymic atrophy can be detected by 3 days and is complete by about 1 week. We found that loss of glucocorticoid sensitivity perfectly mirrored the time course of TCDD-induced thymic atrophy *in vivo*, indicating that the agents acted on a common target population of cells. Interestingly, at early time points (1 to 2 days postinjection), TCDD exposure actually potentiated the glucocorticoid responsiveness of the cells, an effect that was not observed in response to other stimulators of thymocyte apoptosis (i.e., calcium ionophore treatment). When these cultures were incubated for several hours *in vitro*, spontaneous apoptosis suggestive of *in vivo* priming was observed. Current efforts are aimed at further characterizing the potential synergism between glucocorticoids and TCDD. It is possible that this synergism, and not an independent effect of TCDD alone, is actually responsible for TCDD-induced thymic atrophy *in vivo*.

Organotin Compounds

Organotin compounds are commonly used in plastics production, as pesticides, and in antifoulant paints for water pipes and vessels (36). Tributyltin is the most common form found in the latter, and its tendency to leech into the water supply has caused concern over its toxicity to humans. Previous work has shown that, like dioxin, relatively low doses of tributyltin cause depletion of cortical thymocytes and thymic atrophy in laboratory animals (37). Recent work from one of our laboratories (38) and by Raffray and Cohen (39) has shown that tributyltin stimulates endonuclease activation typical of apoptosis in suspensions of rat thymocytes *in vitro*, suggesting that activation of the physiologic cell death program may underlie its cytotoxicity.

The mechanism of tributyltin-induced apoptosis is particularly unique because of its rapidity. Within 15 min of treatment it is possible to detect a significant increase in DNA cleavage, kinetics that are matched only by rates of DNA fragmentation observed in the targets of cytotoxic T lymphocytes. Endonuclease activation is preceded by and dependent on a sustained increase in the cytosolic Ca^{2+} concentration

(Fig. 1), and treatment with Ca^{2+}-buffering agents or EGTA abrogates both DNA fragmentation and cell death. Inhibitors of protein synthesis have no effect on the response. The Ca^{2+} increase stimulated by tributyltin is mediated by at least three mechanisms, including release from intracellular stores, opening of a membrane ion channel, and inhibition of an adenosine triphosphate (ATP)-dependent plasma membrane Ca^{2+} efflux pathway (40). It is possible that tributyltin opens the same receptor-operated plasma membrane Ca^{2+} channels that mediate Ca^{2+} influx following engagement of antigen receptors on T cells, and that toxicity occurs due to toxin-mediated impairment of cellular Ca^{2+} homeostatic processes.

Gliotoxin-Induced Apoptosis in Macrophages and T Cell Blasts

Gliotoxin is a member of a class of fungal metabolites possessing antimicrobial activity that contain a bridged polysulfide ring (41). The agent also displays antiphagocytic and immunosuppressive activities, effects that may be linked to its ability to inhibit cellular activation functions and trigger apoptosis in macrophages and lymphocytes. Inhibition of activation and induction of apoptosis can be segregated by the dose thresholds required to mediate each response (41), with the former observed at nanomolar and the latter at micromolar concentrations of gliotoxin. The responses in macrophages can also be distinguished by their differential requirements for the epipolythiodioxopiperazine ring: inhibition of macrophage activation exhibits a strict requirement for the structure, whereas induction of apoptosis does not (42).

Gliotoxin-induced apoptosis appears to be mediated by the generation of reactive oxygen species (redox cycling) and subsequent damage to DNA (42,43) (Fig. 1). Incubation of the compound with either plasmid or eukaryotic DNA in the presence of Fe^{3+} results in single- and double-strand breaks detectable on alkaline gels (43). The DNA damage is accompanied by the production of hydrogen peroxide and is abrogated by metal chelators and catalase (43). It would appear that the damage induced in the initial stage of gliotoxin action initiates a secondary response involving endogenous endonuclease activation and DNA laddering (42), effects that are inhibited by the Ca^{2+}/Mg^{2+}-dependent endonuclease antagonist, Zn^{2+} (44). Gliotoxin has also been reported to induce an early increase in the Ca^{2+}-active second messenger inositol triphosphate (44), although whether or not Ca^{2+} plays a role in gliotoxin toxicity remains unclear. These findings are reminiscent, however, of the effects of hydrogen peroxide-induced oxidative stress on renal tubular epithelial cells, where early rises in the cytosolic Ca^{2+} concentration and DNA damage-mediated endonuclease activation have been implicated in the mechanism of cytotoxicity (45).

The actions of gliotoxin do not require ongoing macromolecular synthesis; in fact, gliotoxin itself has been shown to be a potent inhibitor of protein synthesis (44). Moreover, cycloheximide and actinomycin D, commonly used inhibitors of protein and mRNA synthesis, respectively, induce apoptosis in macrophages and activated T cells (44). Therefore the protein machinery involved in the response is present constitutively within the cells and appears only to require a signal for its activation.

Diphtheria Toxin

Diphtheria toxin is a cytotoxic polypeptide that exhibits extreme potency against a variety of eukaryotic cell types. The disulfide-linked active fragment of the toxin is composed of a 20.5-kDa "A" subunit that inhibits protein synthesis by catalyzing the transfer of adenosine 5′-diphosphate (ADP)-ribose to elongation factor 2 (EF-2) and a 40-kDa "B" subunit that serves as the receptor-binding domain. Its ability to inhibit protein synthesis has long been accepted as the basis for the compound's cytotoxicity, although the agent is toxic to some cell types that are not killed by other macromolecular synthesis inhibitors, suggesting the involvement of other biochemical mechanisms as well.

Recent work has indicated that diphtheria toxin induces apoptosis in sensitive target cells, characterized by endonuclease activation leading to the formation of oligonucleosome-length DNA fragments (46,47). A direct correlation exists between translation inhibition and cytolysis (46), and ADP-ribosylation of EF-2 is required (48). Intriguingly, Chang and colleagues (47) have reported that diphtheria toxin possesses intrinsic Ca^{2+} endonuclease activity (Fig. 1); this observation remains somewhat controversial, and it by no means excludes the possibility that host endonuclease is also involved in mediating DNA fragmentation. The finding that diphtheria toxin stimulates ADP-ribosylation may be relevant to its mechanism of action, as activation of poly(ADP-ribose) polymerase in response to DNA damage has been suggested as a trigger for apoptosis (Fig. 1). The latter would fit with the idea that DNA damage control and repair systems are involved in regulating diphtheria toxin-stimulated apoptosis.

Chemotherapeutic Agents

Searle and colleagues (49) demonstrated years ago that chemotherapeutic agents can induce apoptosis in sensitive target cells, although this fact had been overlooked until quite recently. Now work from several independent laboratories has confirmed that antitumor agents are in general quite efficient at inducing apoptosis in their targets (Table 1). Due to years of extensive in-depth investigation, the primary biochemical mechanisms underlying their toxicity are fairly well known; most target DNA, DNA repair enzymes, or metablic processes, the function of which are thought to be more critical for the viability of rapidly dividing tumor cells than for their normal (untransformed) counterparts. One paradox that emerged, however, is that noncycling tumor cells such as the ones that accumulate in chronic lymphocytic leukemia are also effectively targeted by the agents. The finding that apoptosis is the mechanism of cell death underlying their effects resolves the conflict.

TABLE 1. *Chemotherapeutic agents known to induce apoptosis in immune target cells*

Chemical	Site of action	References
Etoposide	Topoisomerase II	17,50,52,56
Novobiocin		50,51
Teniposide		57
Fostriecin		58
Camptothecin	Topoisomerase I	17,50
Cytosine arabinoside	DNA precursor pool	49
1-β-D-arabinofuranosylcytosine (Ara-C)		17,53
2-Chlorodeoxyadenosine		55,59
9-β-D-arabinosyl-2-fluoroadenine (Ara-F)		59
5′-(*N*-Ethyl)carboxamidoadenosine (NECA)		60
Cycloheximide	Protein synthesis inhibitor	17,18,42,49
Puromycin		17
Mitomycin C		49
Actinomycin D	RNA synthesis inhibitor	18,49
Bis-(2-chloroethyl)methylamine	Alkylating agent	54
Ouabain	Na^+/K^+ ATPase	52
Amphidicolin	DNA polymerase	52
Cisplatin	DNA (bifunctional)	52
N-methyl-*N*′-nitro-*N*-nitrosoguanidine	DNA (monofunctional)	52

Two types of apoptosis-inducing chemotherapeutic chemicals that deserve further comment are the topoisomerase inhibitors and the nucleoside analogs used in the treatment of several types of leukemia. The mechanism of action of the topoisomerase inhibitors was originally thought to involve stabilization of enzyme–DNA complexes leading to production of single- or double-strand breaks, which ultimately precipitated cell death. However, the primary damage induced by these agents is often quickly repaired, yet secondary endonuclease-mediated DNA laddering is still induced and cells die by apoptosis. The explanation for this paradox may be found in the observation that induction of apoptosis by topoisomerase inhibitors requires functional p53 (30) and therefore involves the cellular DNA damage control response (Fig. 1). Thus DNA damage likely provides a "signal," which in turn activates the p53-dependent pathway of apoptosis, rather than being directly involved in promoting cell death.

Nucleoside analogs also appear to induce DNA strand breaks, although their mechanisms of action may additionally involve cellular signaling networks (Fig. 1). Illustrating this point, recent work by Robertson and co-workers (59) with chronic lymphocytic leukemia (CLL) cells has shown that apoptosis in response to purine nucleoside analogs can be blocked by treatment with intracellular Ca^{2+} buffering agents and can partially be abrogated by phorbol esters, implicating calcium- and protein kinase C-sensitive signaling pathways in the regulation of the response. Not all populations of CLL cells are killed by the compounds, and the authors demonstrated a strong correlation between the sensitivity of particular CLL samples to spontaneous and induced apoptosis and clinical prognosis, suggesting that apoptosis represents an important mechanism mediating tumor regression in response to treatment. Further evidence for a receptor-mediated signal in adenosine toxicity has been advanced by Kizaki and colleagues (61), who have shown that the response in thymocytes is associated with increases in the cAMP level. It is therefore possible that both DNA damage and cellular signaling are involved in the cytotoxic mechanism.

Macromolecular synthesis is sometimes required for induction of apoptosis in response to chemotherapy. Barry and colleagues (52) reported that both DNA fragmentation and cell killing in Chinese hamster ovary (CHO) cells exposed to cisplatin were blocked by cycloheximide. However, Alnemri and Litwack (51) found that cycloheximide had no effect on novobiocin-induced apoptosis in CEM (acute lymphoblastic leukemic) lymphocytes, and Robertson and co-workers (59) found that macromolecular synthesis inhibitors had no effect on adenosine-induced apoptosis in primary CLL cells in response to purine nucleoside analogs. Indeed, independent reports by Searle and co-workers (49), Kaufmann (17), and Martin et al. (18) have shown that RNA and protein synthesis inhibitors can induce DNA fragmentation and cell death typical of apoptosis in tumor cells *in vivo* and in human promyelocytic leukemic (HL-60) cells *in vitro*. Thus whether or not a macromolecular synthesis requirement is observed may depend on the target cell and the cytotoxic agent in question.

Expression of Bcl-2 may also dictate cellular sensitivity to therapeutic chemicals. Recent work by Tsujimoto (62) and Miyashita and Reed (63) has shown that cells expressing high levels of Bcl-2 are resistant to the cytotoxicity of methotrexate, etoposide, vincristine, cisplatin, cyclophosphamide, and 1-β-D-arabinofuranosylcytosine (Ara-C). The chemicals are still potent growth inhibitors in the cells. However, if the toxins are washed away, cells overexpressing Bcl-2 proliferate much better than control cells. These observations provide further support for the importance of apoptosis in the mechanism of action of antitumor agents and suggest that their effectiveness may in large part be dictated by inherent cellular response mechanisms.

SUMMARY AND CONCLUSIONS

Endogenous endonuclease activation has been implicated in the cytotoxicity of a growing number of immunotoxins. Elevations of the cytosolic Ca^{2+} concentration and DNA damage appear to be common proximal triggers of the response. For the latter, expression of wild-type p53 appears critical, although the biochemical and/or molecular basis for this dependency is unknown. Stimulation of ADP-ribosylation also appears to be involved, and important target substrates, including the endonuclease itself (64) and EF-2, are being identified.

In a clinical context, the observation that apoptosis mediates the cytotoxicity of chemotherapeutic agents is of profound importance to their efficacy. Defining the mechanisms involved in the maintenance of some tumor cell populations in an apoptosis-resistant state (i.e., expression of Bcl-2 and loss of wild-type p53) should allow for the design of strategies to overcome these regulation defects and restore tumor cell responsiveness to treatment. In addition, knowledge of how different physiologic control pathways interact with one another should facilitate the development of synergistic treatment protocols that will improve tumor responsiveness to therapy.

REFERENCES

1. Wyllie AH, Kerr JFR, Currie AR. Cell death: the significance of apoptosis. *Int Rev Cytol* 1980;68: 2251–2305.
2. Wyllie AH. Glucocorticoid-induced thymocyte apoptosis is associated with endogenous endonuclease activation. *Nature* 1980;284:555–556.
3. Hewish DR, Burgoyne LA. Chromatin sub-structure. The digestion of DNA at regularly spaced sites by a nuclear deoxyribonuclease. *Biochem Biophys Res Commun* 1973;52:504–510.
4. Vanderbilt JN, Bloom KS, Anderson JN. Endogenous nuclease: properties and effects on transcribed genes in chromatin. *J Biol Chem* 1982;257:13009–13017.
5. Cohen JJ, Duke RC. Glucocorticoid activation of a calcium-dependent endonuclease in thymocyte nuclei leads to cell death. *J Immunol* 1984;132:38–42.
6. Gaido ML, Cidlowski JA. Identification, purification, and characterization of a calcium-dependent endonuclease (NUC-18) from apoptotic rat thymocytes. *J Biol Chem* 1990;266:18580–18585.
7. Arends MJ, Morris RG, Wyllie AH. Apoptosis: the role of the endonuclease. *Am J Pathol* 1990; 136:593–608.
8. Peitsch MC, Polzar B, Stephan H, Crompton T, MacDonald HR, Mannherz HG, Tschopp J. Characterization of the endogenous deoxyribonuclease involved in nuclear DNA degradation during apoptosis (programmed cell death). *EMBO J* 1993;12:371–377.
9. Barry MA, Eastman A. Identification of deoxyribonuclease II as an endonuclease involved in apoptosis. *Arch Biochem Biophys* 1993;300:440–450.
10. McConkey DJ, Hartzell P, Nicotera P, Orrenius S. Calcium-activated DNA fragmentation kills immature thymocytes. *FASEB J* 1989;3:1843–1849.
11. Raff MC. Social controls on cell survival and cell death. *Nature* 1992;356:397–400.
12. Owens GP, Hahn WE, Cohen JJ. Identification of mRNAs associated with programmed cell death in immature thymocytes. *Mol Cell Biol* 1991;11:4177–4188.

12a. Liu ZG, Smith SW, McLaughlin KA, Schwartz LM, Osborne BA. Apoptotic signals delivered through the T-cell receptor of a T-cell hybrid require the immediate early gene *nur*77. *Nature* 1994;367:281–284.

12b. Woronicz JD, Calnan B, Ngo V, Winoto A. Requirement for the orphan steroid receptor *nur*77 in apoptosis of T-cell hybridomas. *Nature* 1994;367:277–281.

13. Askew DS, Ashmun RA, Simmons BC, Cleveland JL. Constitutive c-myc expression in an IL-3-dependent myeloid cell line suppresses cell cycle arrest and accelerates apoptosis. *Oncogene* 1991; 12:1915–1922.
14. Evan GI, Wyllie AH, Gilbert CS, et al. Induction of apoptosis in fibroblasts by c-myc protein. *Cell* 1992;69:119–128.
15. Shi Y, Glynn JM, Guilbert LJ, Cotter TG, Bissonnette RP, Green DR. Role for c-myc in activation-induced apoptotic cell death in T cell hybridomas. *Science* 1992;257:212–214.
16. Smeyne RJ, Vendrell M, Hayward M, et al. Continuous c-fos expression precedes programmed cell death in vivo. *Nature* 1993;363:166–169.
17. Kaufmann SH. Induction of endonucleolytic DNA cleavage in human acute myelogenous leukemia cells by etoposide, camptothecin, and other cytotoxic anticancer drugs: a cautionary note. *Cancer Res* 1989;49:5870–5878.
18. Martin SJ, Lennon SV, Bonham AM, Cotter TG. Induction of apoptosis (programmed cell death) in human leukemic HL-60 cells by inhibition of RNA or protein synthesis. *J Immunol* 1990;145:1859–1867.
19. Korsmeyer SJ. Bcl-2 initiates a new category of oncogenes: regulators of cell death. *Blood* 1992; 80:879–886.
20. White E, Sabbatini P, Debbas M, Wold WSM, Kusher DI, Gooding LR. The 19-kilodalton adeno-

virus E1B transforming protein inhibits programmed cell death and prevents cytolysis by tumor necrosis factor alpha. *Mol Cell Biol* 1992;12:2570–2580.
21. Evans CA, Owen-Lynch PJ, Whetton AD, Dive C. Activation of the Abelson tyrosine kinase activity is associated with suppression of apoptosis in hemopoietic cells. *Cancer Res* 1993;53:1735–1738.
22. Hengartner MO, Ellis RE, Horvitz HR. *Caenorhabditis elegans* gene ced-9 protects cells from programmed cell death. *Nature* 1992;356:494–499.
23. Vaux DL, Weissman IL, Kim SK. Prevention of programmed cell death in *Caenorhabditis elegans* by human Bcl-2. *Science* 1992;258:1955–1957.
24. Alnemri ES, Robertson NM, Fernandes TF, Croce CM, Litwack G. Overexpression of full-length human Bcl-2 extends the survival of baculovirus-infected Sf9 insect cells. *Proc Natl Acad Sci USA* 1992;89:7295–7299.
25. White E, Blose SH, Stillman BW. Nuclear envelope localization of an adenovirus tumor antigen maintains the integrity of cellular DNA. *Mol Cell Biol* 1984;12:2865–2875.
26. Lane DP. p53, guardian of the genome. *Nature* 1992;358:15–16.
27. Yonish-Rouach E, Resnitzky D, Lotem J, Sachs L, Kimchi A, Oren M. Wild-type p53 induces apoptosis of myeloid leukemic cells that is inhibited by interleukin 6. *Nature* 1991;352:345–347.
28. Shaw P, Bovey R, Tardy S, Sahle R, Sordat B, Costa J. Induction of apoptosis by wild-type p53 in a human colon tumor-derived cell line. *Proc Natl Acad Sci USA* 1992;89:4495–4499.
29. Lowe SW, Schmitt EM, Smith SW, Osborne BA, Jacks T. p53 is required for radiation-induced apoptosis in mouse thymocytes. *Nature* 1993;362:847–849.
30. Clarke AR, Purdie CA, Harrison DJ, Morris RG, Bird CC, Hooper ML, Wyllie AH. Thymocyte apoptosis induced by p53-dependent and independent pathways. *Nature* 1993;362:849–852.
31. McConnell EF, Moore JA, Haseman JK, Harris MW. The comparative toxicity of chlorinated dibenzo-*p*-dioxins in mice and guinea pigs. *Toxicol Appl Pharmacol* 1978;44:335–356.
32. Poland A, Knutson J. 2,3,7,8-Tetrachlorodibenzo-*p*-dioxin and related halogenated aromatic hydrocarbons: examination of the mechanism of toxicity. *Annu Rev Pharmacol Toxicol* 1982;22:517–554.
33. Luster MJ, Germolec DR, Clark G, Wiegand G, Rosenthal GJ. Selective effects of 2,3,7,8-tetrachlorodibenzo-*p*-dioxin and corticosteroid on *in vitro* lymphocyte maturation. *J Immunol* 1988;140:928–935.
34. McConkey DJ, Hartzell P, Duddy SK, Hakansson H, Orrenius S. 2,3,7,8-Tetrachlorodibenzo-*p*-dioxin kills immature thymocytes by Ca^{2+}-mediated endonuclease activation. *Science* 1988;242:256–259.
35. McConkey DJ, Orrenius S. 2,3,7,8-Tetrachlorodibenzo-*p*-dioxin (TCDD) kills glucocorticoid-sensitive thymocytes *in vivo*. *Biochem Biophys Res Commun* 1989;160:1003–1008.
36. Boyer IJ. Toxicity of dibutyl, tributyl, and other organotins to humans and laboratory animals. *Toxicology* 1989;55:253–298.
37. Snoeij NJ, Penninks AH. Seinen W. Dibutyl and tributyltin compounds induce thymus atrophy in rats due to a selective action on thymic lymphoblasts. *Int J Immunopharmacol* 1988;10:891–899.
38. Aw TY, Nicotera P, Manzo L, Orrenius S. Tributyltin stimulates apoptosis in rat thymocytes. *Arch Biochem Biophys* 1990;283:46–50.
39. Raffray M, Cohen GN. Bis(tri-*n*-butyltin)oxide induces programmed cell death (apoptosis) in immature rat thymocytes. *Arch Toxicol* 1991;65:135–139.
40. Chow SC, Kass GEN, McCabe MJ Jr, Orrenius S. Tributyltin increases cytosolic free Ca^{2+} concentration in thymocytes by mobilizing intracellular Ca^{2+}, activating a Ca^{2+} entry pathway, and inhibiting Ca^{2+} efflux. *Arch Biochem Biophys* 1992;298:143–149.
41. Waring P, Eichner RD, Mullbacher A. The chemistry and biology of the immune modulating agent gliotoxin and related epipolythiodioxopiperazines. *Med Res Rev* 1988;4:499–524.
42. Waring P, Eichner RD, Mullbacher A, Sjaarda A. Gliotoxin induces apoptosis in macrophages unrelated to its antiphagocytic properties. *J Biol Chem* 1988;263:18493–18499.
43. Eichner RD, Waring P, Gene AM, Braithwaite AW, Mullbacher A. Gliotoxin causes oxidative damage to plasmid and cellular DNA. *J Biol Chem* 1988;263:3772–3777.
44. Waring P. DNA fragmentation induced in macrophages by gliotoxin does not require protein synthesis and is preceded by raised inositol triphosphate levels. *J Biol Chem* 1990;265:14476–14480.
45. Ueda N, Shah SV. Endonuclease-induced DNA damage and cell death in oxidant injury to renal tubular epithelial cells. *J Clin Invest* 1992;90:2593–2597.
46. Chang MP, Bramhall J, Graves S, Bonavida B, Wisnieski BJ. Internucleosomal DNA cleavage precedes diphtheria toxin-induced cytolysis. *J Biol Chem* 1989;264:15261–15267.

47. Chang MP, Baldwin RL, Bruce C, Wisnieski BJ. Second cytotoxic pathway of diphtheria toxin suggested by nuclease activity. *Science* 1989;246:1165–1168.
48. Morimoto H, Bonavida B. Diphtheria toxin and *Pseudomonas* A toxin-mediated apoptosis. ADP-ribosylation of elongation factor-2 is required for DNA fragmentation and cell lysis and synergy with tumor necrosis factor alpha. *J Immunol* 1992;149:2089–2094.
49. Searle J, Lawson TA, Abbot PJ, Harmon B, Kerr JFR. An electron microscope study of the mode of cell death induced by cancer chemotherapeutic agents in populations of proliferating normal and neoplastic cells. *J Pathol* 1975;116:129–138.
50. Jaxel C, Taudou G, Portemer C, Mirambeau G, Panijel J, Duguet M. Topoisomerase inhibitors induce irreversible fragmentation of replicated DNA in concanavalin A stimulated splenocytes. *Biochemistry* 1988;27:95–99.
51. Alnemri ES, Litwack G. Activation of internucleosomal DNA cleavage in human CEM lymphocytes by glucocorticoid and novobiocin. *J Biol Chem* 1990;265:17323–17333.
52. Barry MA, Behnke CA, Eastman A. Activation of programmed cell death (apoptosis) by cisplatin, other anticancer drugs, toxins, and hyperthermia. *Biochem Pharmacol* 1990;40:2353–2362.
53. Gunji H, Kharbanda S, Kufe D. Induction of internucleosomal DNA fragmentation in human myeloid leukemia cells by 1-beta-D-arabinofuranosylcytosine. *Cancer Res* 1991;51:741–743.
54. O'Connor PM, Wassermann K, Sarang M, Magrath I, Bohr VA, Kohn KW. Relationship between DNA cross-links, cell cycle, and apoptosis in Burkitt's lymphoma cell lines differing in sensitivity to nitrogen mustard. *Cancer Res* 1991;51:6550–6557.
55. Carson DA, Wasson BD, Esparza LM, Carrera CJ, Kipps TJ, Cottam HB. Oral antilymphocyte activity and induction of apoptosis by 2-chloro-2′-arabino-fluoro-2′-deoxyadenosine. *Proc Natl Acad Sci USA* 1992;89:2970–2974.
56. Forbes IJ, Zalewski PD, Giannakis C, Cowled PA. Induction of apoptosis in chronic lymphocytic leukemia cells and its prevention by phorbol ester. *Exp Cell Res* 1992;198:367–372.
57. Roy C, Brown DL, Little JE, et al. The topoisomerase II inhibitor teniposide (VM-26) induces apoptosis in unstimulated mature murine lymphocytes. *Exp Cell Res* 1992;200:416–424.
58. Hotz M, Traganos F, Darzynkiewicz Z. Changes in nuclear chromatin related to apoptosis or necrosis induced by the DNA topoisomerase II inhibitor fostriecin in MOLT-4 and HL-60 cells are revealed by altered DNA sensitivity to denaturation. *Exp Cell Res* 1992;201:184–191.
59. Robertson LE, Chubb S, Meyn RE, Story M, Ford R, Hittelman WN, Plunkett W. Induction of apoptotic cell death in chronic lymphocytic leukemia by 2-chloro-2′-deoxyadenosine and 9-beta-D-arabinosyl-2′-fluoroadenine. *Blood* 1993;81:143–150.
60. Jondal M, Okret S, McConkey DJ. Killing of immature $CD4^+CD8^+$ thymocytes in vivo by anti-CD3 or 5′-(*N*-ethyl) carboxamido-adenosine is blocked by glucocorticoid receptor antagonist RU-486. *Eur J Immunol* 1993;23:1246–1250.
61. Kizaki H, Suzuki K, Tadakuma T, Ishimura Y. Adenosine receptor-mediated accumulation of cyclic AMP-induced T-lymphocyte death through internucleosomal DNA cleavage. *J Biol Chem* 1990; 265:5280–5284.
62. Tsujimoto Y. Stress-resistance conferred by high level of Bcl-2 alpha protein in human B lymphoblastoid cell. *Oncogene* 1989;4:1331–1336.
63. Miyashita T, Reed JC. Bcl-2 oncoprotein blocks chemotherapy-induced apoptosis in a human leukemia cell line. *Blood* 1993;81:151–157.
64. Toshihara K, Tanigawa Y, Burzio L, Koide SS. Evidence for adenosine diphosphate ribosylation of Ca^{2+}, Mg^{2+}-dependent endonuclease. *Proc Natl Acad Sci USA* 1975;72:289–293.

Immunotoxicology and Immunopharmacology, Second Edition, edited by J. H. Dean, M. I. Luster, A. E. Munson, and I. Kimber.
Raven Press, Ltd., New York © 1994.

27

Immune-Mediated Hepatotoxicity

Lesley Helyar and Debra L. Laskin

Department of Pharmacology and Toxicology, Rutgers University, Piscataway, New Jersey 08855

Cells of the immune system and the mediators they release appear to play a key role in the pathogenesis of hepatotoxicity induced by a variety of xenobiotics. Nonparenchymal cells, in particular, those lining the hepatic sinusoids, which include Kupffer cells, endothelial cells, and Ito cells, also participate in this process. Thus following exposure to hepatotoxic agents such as acetaminophen, carbon tetrachloride, galactosamine, or endotoxin, nonparenchymal cells and inflammatory macrophages are activated to release a wide array of proinflammatory and cytotoxic mediators that promote liver damage. In addition, some nonparenchymal cell types also cooperate in specific T lymphocyte-dependent responses induced by hepatotoxins. These findings, together with the discovery that hepatotoxicity can be modified by agents that modulate inflammatory cell and nonparenchymal cell functions, provide evidence that these cells contribute to tissue injury. The cytotoxic process most likely involves mediators such as reactive active oxygen intermediates, reactive nitrogen intermediates, cytokines, hydrolytic enzymes, eicosanoids, and lipid mediators released at the site of tissue injury. Whereas some of the mediators are directly cytotoxic (i.e., hydrogen peroxide, nitric oxide, and peroxynitrite), others degrade the extracellular matrix (i.e., collagenase, and elastase) and/or promote inflammatory cell infiltration and nonparenchymal cell proliferation and activation [i.e., chemotactic factors, colony-stimulating factors (CSFs), interleukin-1 (IL-1), interleukin-6 (IL-6), tumor necrosis factor-α (TNF-α), and platelet activating factor (PAF)]. There is also evidence that activated nonparenchymal cells produce mediators that can modify hepatocyte protein and nucleic acid biosynthesis as well as cytochrome P450-mediated xenobiotic metabolism. This may also contribute to hepatotoxicity. This chapter reviews experimental data implicating nonparenchymal cells and inflammatory macrophages in hepatotoxicity.

IMMUNOLOGIC AND INFLAMMATORY PROPERTIES OF HEPATIC NONPARENCHYMAL CELLS

The majority of the nonparenchymal cells reside within the hepatic sinusoids, positioned between the arterial vasculature and the parenchyma. These cells consist predominantly of Kupffer cells, endothelial cells, and Ito cells. Kupffer cells constitute approximately 80% to 90% of all the macrophages in the body and represent about 29% of the sinusoidal cells in the liver. They are predominantly localized in the lumen of the sinusoids in periportal and central regions of the liver lobule and are anchored to the endothelium by long cytoplasmic processes (1). The major function of Kupffer cells is to clear particulate and foreign materials from the portal circulation, primarily through phagocytosis. Kupffer cells possess both Fc and C3 receptors and are known to phagocytose a wide variety of both opsonized and nonopsonized particles (2). Kupffer cells play a central role in the uptake and detoxification of endotoxin from the portal circulation (3). They also have the capacity to act as antigen-presenting cells (APCs) for the induction of T lymphocyte responses (4). When activated by antigens or inflammatory stimuli, Kupffer cells release superoxide anion, hydrogen peroxide, nitric oxide, hydrolytic enzymes, and eicosanoids that aid in antigen destruction (5,6). Kupffer cells also release a number of different cytokines with immunoregulatory and inflammatory activity including IL-1, IL-6, transforming growth factor-β (TGF-β), PAF, and TNF-α (5,6).

Endothelial cells, which form the walls of the liver sinusoids, represent the major fraction of hepatic nonparenchymal cells (approximately 48%). Endothelial cells function as a selective barrier between the blood and the liver parenchyma. They possess pores or fenestrae that allow direct contact between the plasma and hepatocytes. Endothelial cells also have a well-developed endocytotic capacity as indicated by their unique "bristle-coated" membrane invaginations and vesicles and lysosome-like vacuoles. They can endocytose a variety of particles including glycoproteins, lipoproteins, albumin, lactoferrin, and hyaluronic acid. Endocytosis is accomplished through pinocytotic vesicles and lysosomes, as well as Fc receptors (7,8). Endothelial cells have been reported to display greater levels of phagocytosis than Kupffer cells toward certain types of particles (9,10). In addition, their phagocytic capacity is enhanced when Kupffer cell function is impaired (10). Hepatic endothelial cells can also be activated by inflammatory cytokines to release a variety of mediators that regulate the function of other nonparenchymal cells as well as hepatocytes. These include IL-1, IL-6, IFN, eicosanoids, lysosomal enzymes, nitric oxide and its oxidation products, as well as reactive oxygen intermediates (6,11–13). Thus endothelial cells, like Kupffer cells, appear to be important in immunologic, inflammatory, and regulatory activities in the liver.

Ito cells, also called fat-storing cells, perisinusoidal cells, lipocytes, or stellate cells, represent approximately 20% of the hepatic sinusoidal cells. Ito cells are located between the endothelial cells and hepatocytes or between the hepatocytes. Morphologically, they resemble fibroblasts in that they possess numerous extensions and dilated rough endoplasmic reticulum. Ito cells are the major site in the body for storage of vitamin A, which is localized in intracellular lipid droplets in the form of retinyl esters (14). In addition, they are known to synthesize extracellular matrix proteins, including types I, III, and IV collagen, and there is evidence that they play a role in collagen synthesis in both normal and fibrotic liver (15). Recent studies have suggested that Ito cells may also contribute to inflammatory and immunologic responses in the liver. These cells release a variety of proteins and mediators that have been implicated in tissue injury including nitric oxide, hydrogen peroxide, gelatinase, fibronectin, TGF-β, and CSF-1 (15–17).

ROLE OF MACROPHAGES, ENDOTHELIAL CELLS, AND ITO CELLS IN HEPATOTOXICITY

Treatment of experimental animals with a number of different hepatotoxicants, including acetaminophen, endotoxin, carbon tetrachloride, phenobarbital, allyl alcohol, or galactosamine, is associated with the accumulation of macrophages in the liver (2,18–21). Although the macrophage accumulation is relatively rapid, typically occurring within 48 to 72 hr, the specific location of these cells within the liver varies with the chemical agent. Thus, whereas treatment of rats with acetaminophen or carbon tetrachloride results in accumulation of macrophages in centrilobular regions of the liver, macrophages that accumulate in the liver following lipopolysaccharide (LPS), phenobarbital, carbon tetrachloride, or galactosamine treatment of rats are scattered in clusters throughout the liver lobule (2,18–20,22). These patterns of macrophage localization appear to be correlated with areas of the liver that subsequently exhibit signs of injury (23–25). When macrophages are isolated from livers of hepatotoxicant-treated animals and characterized, they are found to display morphologic and functional properties of activated mononuclear phagocytes. These cells, which consist of resident Kupffer cells and inflammatory macrophages, appear larger and more stellate than cells from untreated rats, are highly vacuolated, and display an increased cytoplasmic/nuclear ratio (2,18,19,26). In addition, macrophages from rats treated with hepatotoxicants such as phenobarbital, acetaminophen, or endotoxin adhere to and spread on culture dishes more rapidly than resident Kupffer cells. These properties are characteristic of morphologically activated macrophages. Macrophages from animals treated with hepatotoxicants also exhibit enhanced phagocytic, chemotactic, cytotoxic, and metabolic activity, as well as increased release of superoxide anion, hydrogen peroxide, nitric oxide and its oxidation products, proteolytic enzymes, IL-1, IL-6, and TNF-α (2,12,18,19,25,27–31). These data suggest that these macrophages are functionally activated. It has been hypothesized that activated Kupffer cells and infiltrating macrophages promote hepatic damage through the release of toxic secretory products (6,31–40). Recent studies from our laboratory have demonstrated that endothelial cells and Ito cells also increase in number and become activated following exposure to hepatotoxicants such as acetaminophen and endotoxin (11–13,16). Like activated hepatic macrophages, these cells are larger and more granular than cells from untreated rats and produce increased amounts of reactive oxygen and nitrogen intermediates, IL-1, and IL-6. The capacity of endothelial cells and Ito cells to produce these mediators may represent an important mechanism by which they participate in inflammatory and immune reactions associated with hepatotoxicity. Vascular endothelial cells have been reported to produce increased amounts of IL-1, IL-6, and IL-8, as well as reactive oxygen and nitrogen intermediates in response to macrophage-derived cytokines (41–45). Similarly, it is possible that cytokines released by nonparenchymal cells and inflammatory macrophages in the liver induce the release of mediators from endothelial cells and Ito cells. These may act in a paracrine and/or autocrine manner to promote cellular proliferation and activation and to induce cytotoxicity. Thus endothelial cells and Ito cells may also participate in the pathogenesis of tissue injury induced by hepatotoxicants.

The precise mechanisms underlying the accumulation and activation of inflammatory macrophages and nonparenchymal cells in the liver following hepatotoxicant exposure are unknown. Damaged tissue and cells release chemotactic and growth-promoting factors for macrophages, endothelial cells, and Ito cells, which may be important in cell migration, proliferation, and activation. A number of factors have been described that induce chemotaxis in phagocytes. Many of these also induce macrophage activation. These include complement fragments, products involved in the kinin and coagulation pathway, collagen and tissue breakdown products, arachidonic acid metabolites, in particular, leukotriene B_4, as well as synthetic peptides related to bacterially derived products (46–49). Recent studies have also characterized several cell-derived chemoattractants for neutrophils and macrophages (50). These belong to a family of phagocyte chemoattractants, which includes macrophage inflammatory proteins, macrophage chemotactic protein, and IL-8, which are thought to participate in early inflammatory responses. Studies from our laboratory have also revealed that hepatocytes treated with acetaminophen or endotoxin *in vitro* or isolated from rats treated with these toxicants produce a factor that attracts and activates Kupffer cells and monocytes (37). We also found that hepatic endothelial cells as well as Kupffer cells produce macrophage chemoattractants and that production of these factors is augmented following hepatotoxicant exposure (51). Thus macrophage accumulation in the liver may be due to release of chemotactic factors from both parenchymal and nonparenchymal cells.

In addition to inducing cellular migration, cytokines produced under inflammatory conditions can promote the growth of inflammatory cells as well as nonparenchymal cells, which may explain, at least in part, the increase in their numbers following hepatotoxicant exposure. For example, our laboratory has discovered that macrophages, endothelial cells, and Ito cells isolated from livers of rats treated with endotoxin display a significantly increased proliferative capacity in response to a number of different inflammatory cytokines including IL-1, CSF-1, and granulocyte–macrophage colony-stimulating factor (GM-CSF). Thus local proliferation and extrahepatic recruitment are likely to contribute to the increased numbers of nonparenchymal cells in the liver following exposure to hepatotoxicants.

Activation of infiltrated macrophages and nonparenchymal cells in the liver also appears to be mediated by inflammatory cytokines and other cell-derived factors produced following hepatotoxicant exposure. For example, our laboratory has discovered that hepatocytes treated with acetaminophen release factors that activate Kupffer cells (37). These factors induce morphologic changes in Kupffer cells that are characteristic of activated macrophages and similar to the morphology of cells isolated from acetaminophen-treated rats (18). Culture medium from hepatocytes treated with acetaminophen, but not acetaminophen itself, also stimulates Kupffer cell phagocytosis, release of superoxide anion, and cytotoxicity (29,37). These data suggest that accumulation and activation of macrophages in the liver following exposure to chemicals like acetaminophen are mediated, at least in part, by factors released from injured hepatocytes.

CYTOTOXIC AND PROINFLAMMATORY MEDIATORS

A variety of mediators are released by activated macrophages and nonparenchymal cells that have been implicated in tissue injury including hydrolytic enzymes, reactive oxygen and nitrogen intermediates, cytokines, and arachidonic acid metabolites. These mediators are likely to act in concert to promote hepatotoxicity.

Reactive Oxygen and Nitrogen Intermediates

One potential mechanism underlying nonparenchymal cell-mediated hepatic injury involves the production of reactive oxygen intermediates such as superoxide anion and hydrogen peroxide. These reactive oxygen intermediates are thought to be primary mediators of macrophage-induced cytotoxicity, of reperfusion and ischemic tissue injury, and of injury associated with both acute and chronic inflammatory diseases (52,53). Following stimulation, activated nonparenchymal cells and inflammatory macrophages release superoxide anion, which reacts with water and other molecules to generate hydroperoxy and hydroxyl radicals. These radicals are even more toxic than superoxide anion and have been linked to membrane, protein, and deoxyribonucleic acid (DNA) damage, lipid peroxidation, and the induction of hepatocyte killing (53–55). Peroxidation of membrane lipids by reactive oxygen intermediates may also induce the formation and release of a number of other vasoactive agents, including prostaglandins, thromboxanes, and leukotrienes. When macrophages are recruited to the liver following hepatotoxicant exposure, they are activated to release hydrogen peroxide and superoxide anion (13,18,19). Stimulation of these cells to produce additional reactive oxygen intermediates has been reported to augment hepatic injury induced by agents such as *Corynebacterium parvum* and galactosamine, whereas administration of antioxidants like superoxide dismutase, allopurinol, or quinone derivatives is hepatoprotective (32,34,39,56–58). These studies support the hypothesis that oxygen-derived free radicals produced by nonparenchymal cells in the liver contribute to the pathogenesis of hepatic injury (6,32,59).

Recent studies have also implicated reactive nitrogen intermediates, in particular, nitric oxide and peroxynitrite, in macrophage-mediated cytotoxicity, in the intracellular destruction of pathogens, and in the regulation of cellular proliferation (60–65). Nitric oxide and its oxidation products, nitrate and nitrite, are produced by activated macrophages, endothelial cells, and Ito cells (12,16). These mediators are thought to contribute to altered hepatic function during sepsis or trauma (66,67). Nitric oxide is also known to react with superoxide anion forming peroxynitrite, a relatively long-lived cytotoxic oxidant that has been implicated in stroke, heart disease, and immune complex-mediated pulmonary edema (68). Peroxynitrite may also initiate lipid peroxidation and can react directly with sulfhydryl groups in cell membranes. Paradoxically, the reaction of superoxide and nitric oxide may also function as a defense against oxidant stress by reducing intracellular levels of these reactive intermediates (68). In this regard, inhibition of nitric oxide synthesis has been reported to augment oxidant-dependent tissue injury induced by *C. parvum* and it has been proposed to play a protective role in the hepatotoxicity of endotoxin (60,69,70). Thus nitric oxide or secondary oxidants generated from nitric oxide may be cytotoxic or hepatoprotective depending on levels of superoxide anion present and the extent to which tissue injury is mediated by reactive oxygen intermediates (68). Nitric oxide may also modulate drug-induced hepatotoxicity by altering cytochrome P450 mixed function oxidase activity. Nitric oxide binds to heme-containing proteins and this may result in either inhibition or activation of enzymes involved in hepatic drug metabolism (63).

Eicosanoids

A variety of eicosanoids are released by activated hepatic macrophages as well as endothelial cells (5,6). The precise role of these reactive species in hepatotoxicity is unknown. Leukotrienes and prostaglandins are generated in acute allergic reactions and it has been shown that these mediators contribute to persistent and late-onset responses to allergens (71). In addition, leukotriene B_4 is known to be a potent polymorphonuclear leukocyte chemoattractant and to induce monocyte IL-1, TNF-α, and hydrogen peroxide production (46,72). Thus release of leukotriene B_4 in the liver may constitute a local control mechanism for the recruitment and activation of inflammatory cells. In this regard, recent studies have demonstrated that administration of lipoxygenase inhibitors or antagonists to mice protected against galactosamine-induced hepatitis (73–76). These data suggest that leukotrienes may be involved in inflammatory liver disease.

Hydrolytic Enzymes

Proteolytic and lysosomal enzymes released from macrophages and endothelial cells such as plasminogen activator, collagenase, elastase, gelatinase, acid phosphatase, and cathepsin D can act directly on hepatocyte membranes, inducing damage. Some of these proteases have been shown to play a role in macrophage-mediated target cell destruction as well as in altered hepatocyte functioning (5,6,40).

Inflammatory Cytokines

Hepatic nonparenchymal cells and inflammatory macrophages are also known to release a number of different cytokines that may contribute to tissue injury (77). These include IL-1, IL-6, and TNF-α, which can act directly on hepatocytes or may indirectly activate other nonparenchymal cells, as well as leukocytes that accumulate in the liver, thus amplifying the inflammatory response (78). IL-1 and IL-6 are low molecular weight proteins that mediate a wide variety of biologic effects (41,45,79). IL-1 induces proliferation and activation of T and B lymphocytes, macrophages, endothelial cells, synovial cells, and epithelial cells (45). IL-1 also augments the cytotoxicity of macrophages and natural killer (NK) cells and, in conjunction with IL-6, induces hepatocyte production of acute-phase proteins (41,45,79). IL-6, also known as hepatocyte stimulating factor-β, stimulates hepatocyte fibronectin and DNA synthesis and glucose and lipid metabolism (41). Both IL-1 and IL-6 depress albumin synthesis and cytochrome P450 activity (41,45,79,80). Recently there have been reports on the synthesis of IL-1 and IL-6 by cells other than macrophages, including hepatic endothelial cells and Ito cells (41,45,79). Like hepatic macrophages, these cells appear to be primed by hepatotoxicants to produce increased amounts of these cytokines (11).

TNF-α is another secretory product of activated macrophages (72,81). It has been implicated not only in the pathogenesis of septic shock and inflammation, but also in the regulation of acute-phase protein gene expression, cytochrome P450 activity, cellular proliferation, and apoptosis (72,81,82). TNF-α also stimulates the release of other immunoregulatory and cytotoxic mediators including IL-1, IL-6, CSF, PAF, prostaglandins, and nitric oxide from inflammatory cells as well as parenchymal and nonparenchymal liver cells (64,72,81). TNF-α may act in concert with these mediators to augment injury in the liver. For example, in endotoxemia associated with alcoholic cirrhosis, TNF-α is thought to be a major mediator of liver damage (83). TNF-α has also been implicated in the hepatotoxicity of acetaminophen, galactosamine, and endotoxin (78,84,85). TNF-α is also known to have deleterious effects on endothelial cells (72). In addition, this mediator sensitizes neutrophils and monocytes to produce reactive oxygen and nitrogen intermediates (64,72,86). The fact that inflammatory cytokines such as IL-1, IL-6, and TNF-α can affect so many different target tissues, and that they are produced by a variety of cell types, suggests that they are major mediators of inflammatory and immune responses.

EFFECTS OF MODIFYING NONPARENCHYMAL CELL FUNCTION ON HEPATOTOXICITY

The best evidence to support the hypothesis that inflammatory macrophages and nonparenchymal cells play a role in liver injury comes from experiments analyzing the effects of agents known to modify the functioning of these cells on hepatotoxicity. Most of these studies have focused on hepatic macrophages. Data from these experiments clearly demonstrate that the degree of hepatic injury induced by a number of different chemicals is directly correlated with macrophage functioning. Thus agents that depress macrophage functioning reduce toxicity, while compounds that augment macrophage activity enhance tissue injury. For example, drugs such as hydrocortisone, certain synthetic steroids, and natural substances that block inflammatory responses protect against liver injury induced by carbon tetrachloride and acetaminophen (87). Similarly, the accumulation of macrophages in the liver and subsequent toxicity of acetaminophen are inhibited by pretreatment of rats with dextran sulfate or gadolinium chloride, compounds also known to depress macrophage activity (88,89). Hepatoprotective effects of gadolinium chloride against allyl alcohol- and carbon tetrachloride-induced injury have also been described (21,90). A number of studies have also demonstrated that activation of hepatic macrophages and/or stimulation of mediator release augments hepatic injury induced by toxic xenobiotics. LPS and poly I:C are potent activators of liver macrophages (2,80). LPS also appears to activate hepatic endothelial cells and Ito cells (13, 16). Studies from our laboratory have demonstrated that treatment of rats with LPS or poly I:C enhances the toxicity of acetaminophen (51). Pretreatment of rats with LPS has also been reported to aggravate injury induced by carbon tetrachloride, galactosamine, and *C. parvum* (91,92). In contrast, animals made tolerant to LPS or treated with the antibiotic polymyxin B, a positively charged detergent that binds to and neutralizes LPS, are protected from hepatotoxicity induced by these agents (92,93). Administration of large doses of vitamin A, which activates Kupffer cells *in vivo* (27,94), has also been reported to augment the hepatotoxicity of carbon tetrachloride as well as allyl alcohol, acetaminophen, and endotoxin (23,95). This is postulated to be due to reactive oxygen intermediates released from vitamin A-activated Kupffer cells. In this regard, methyl palmitate, which blocks Kupffer cell oxidative metabolism, abrogates the enhanced toxicity of carbon tetrachloride induced by vitamin A. Methyl palmitate has also been reported to exert a hepatoprotective effect against galactosamine and 1,2-dichlorobenzene (56,96). Taken together, these observations support the hypothesis that macrophages and the mediators they release contribute to hepatotoxicity.

T CELL-DEPENDENT IMMUNE RESPONSES AND LIVER INJURY

B and T lymphocytes also appear to contribute to tissue injury induced by a number of different hepatotoxicants. The most widely investigated of these agents are the halogenated anesthetics (97,98). Hypersensitivity or autoimmune reactions to these compounds are characterized by the appearance of autoantibodies directed against liver proteins. Metabolites of halothane-type anesthetics are thought to modify hepatocyte proteins to immunogenic forms, which elicit a T cell-mediated immune response. Another immune cell-dependent form of hepatotoxicity induced experimentally by the plant lectin, concanavalin A (Con A), appears to depend on both T lymphocytes and macrophages (99). Administration of Con A to rats results in selective damage to the liver accompanied by increased serum transaminase levels. A role for T lymphocytes in Con A-induced hepatotoxicity is suggested by the presence of infiltrating leukocytes in liver tissue in close association to injured hepatocytes, increased IL-2 in the serum, and the absence of liver injury in mice that lack T and B lymphocytes or are treated with antibodies to deplete these cells. Macrophages, which are known to activate T cells by producing IL-1β, appear to play a critical role in this form of hepatotoxicity as depletion of macrophages by pretreatment with silica particles has been reported to abrogate liver injury.

MODEL OF HEPATOTOXICITY

Based on current experimental data, we have proposed a model of chemically induced hepatotoxicity that includes a role for immune cells and inflammatory mediators (6). According to this model, hepatocytes injured by toxicants release factors that attract Kupffer cells to specific regions of the liver. Additional mononuclear phagocytes are also recruited from blood and bone marrow precursors. Once localized in the injured area, the macrophages become activated by parenchymal and nonparenchymal cell-derived factors and release mediators that induce proliferation and activation of endothelial cells and Ito cells and, in some instances, lymphocytes. Activated macrophages, endothelial cells, and Ito cells also release mediators that contribute to tissue damage. Data from our laboratory and those of other investigators support this model of hepatotoxicity.

CONCLUSION

Hepatotoxicity induced by chemicals is a complex process that involves a variety of cell types and soluble mediators. Although chemicals or their metabolites can directly injure hepatocytes, they may also activate nonparenchymal cells and immune cells and indirectly augment hepatic injury. Reactive mediators produced by inflammatory leukocytes and other nonparenchymal cells in the liver may act as primary mediators of tissue injury and/or they may participate in the inflammatory response by initiating a cascade of additional immunologic reactions that result in tissue damage. Further studies on the nature of mediators released from nonparenchymal cells and their effects on hepatocytes will be particularly relevant for understanding mechanisms of liver injury.

ACKNOWLEDGMENTS

This work was supported by USPHS National Institutes of Health grants GM34310 and ES05022 and an award to L.H. from the New Jersey Commission on Cancer Research.

REFERENCES

1. Bouwens L, Baekeland M, De Zanger R, Wisse E. Quantitation, tissue distribution and proliferation kinetics of Kupffer cells in normal rat liver. *Hepatology* 1986;6:718–722.
2. Pilaro AM, Laskin DL. Accumulation of activated mononuclear phagocytes in the liver following lipopolysaccharide treatment of rats. *J Leukoc Biol* 1986;40:29–41.
3. Mathison JC, Ulevitch RJ. The clearance, tissue distribution, and cellular localization of intravenously injected lipopolysaccharide in rabbits. *J Immunol* 1979:123:2133–2143.
4. Rogoff TM, Lipsky PE. Antigen presentation by isolated guinea pig Kupffer cells. *J Immunol* 1980; 124:1740–1744.
5. Decker K. Biologically active products of stimulated liver macrophages (Kupffer cells). *Eur J Biochem* 1990;192:245–261.
6. Laskin DL. Nonparenchymal cells and hepatotoxicity. *Semin Liver Dis* 1990;10:293–304.
7. Smedstod B, Pertoft H, Eggertsen G, Sundstrom C. Functional and morphological characterization of cultures of Kupffer cells and liver endothelial cell prepared by means of density separation in Percoll, and selective substrate adherence. *Cell Tissue Res* 1985;241:639–649.
8. Steffan AM, Gendrault JL, McCuskey RS, McCuskey PA, Kirn A. Phagocytosis, an unrecognized property of murine endothelial liver cells. *Hepatology* 1986;6:830–836.
9. De Leeuw AM, Praaning-Van Dalen DP, Brouwer A, Knook DL. Endocytosis in liver sinusoidal endothelial cells. In: Wisse E, Knook DL, Decker K, eds. *Cells of the hepatic sinusoid,* vol 2. Amsterdam: Kupffer Cell Foundation; 1989:94–98.
10. Praaning-van Dalen DP, De Leeuw AM, Brouwer A, Knook DL. Rat liver endothelial cells have a greater capacity than Kupffer cells to endocytose N-acetylglucosamine- and mannose-terminated glycoproteins. *Hepatology* 1987;7:672–679.
11. Feder LS, Todaro JA, Laskin DL. Characterization of interleukin-1 and interleukin-6 production by hepatic endothelial cells and macrophages. *J Leukoc Biol* 1993;53:126–132.
12. Gardner CR, Heck DE, Feder LS, McCloskey TW, Laskin JD, Laskin DL. Differential regulation of reactive nitrogen and reactive oxygen intermediate production by hepatic macrophages and endothelial cells. In: Jesaitis AJ, Dratz EA, eds. *The molecular basis of oxidative damage by leukocytes.* Boca Raton, FL: CRC Press; 1992:267–272.
13. McCloskey TW, Todaro JA, Laskin DL. Effects of lipopolysaccharide treatment of rats on hepatic macrophage and endothelial cell antigen expression and oxidative metabolism. *Hepatology* 1992; 16:191–203.
14. Hendriks HFJ, Verhoofstad WAMM, Brower A, Knook DL. Perisinusoidal fat-storing cells are the main vitamin A storage sites in rat liver. *Exp Cell Res* 1985;160:138–149.
15. Ramadori G. The stellate cell (Ito cell, fat storing cell, lipocyte, perisinusoidal cell) of the liver. *Virchows Arch B Cell Pathol* 1991;61:147–158.
16. Helyar L, Bundschuh DS, Laskin JD, Laskin DL. Hepatic fat storing cells produce nitric oxide and hydrogen peroxide in response to bacterially-derived lipopolysaccharide. In: Knook DL, Decker K, eds. *Cells of the hepatic sinusoid,* vol 3. Amsterdam: Kupffer Cell Foundation; 1993;67–69.
17. Pinzani M, Abboud HE, Gesualdo L, Abboud SL. Regulation of macrophage colony-stimulating factor in liver fat-storing cells by peptide growth factors. *Am J Physiol* 1992;262:C876–C881.
18. Laskin DL, Pilaro AM. Potential role of activated macrophages in acetaminophen hepatotoxicity. I. Isolation and characterization of activated macrophages from rat liver. *Toxicol Appl Pharmacol* 1986;86:204–215.
19. Laskin DL, Robertson FM, Pilaro AM, Laskin JD. Activation of liver macrophages following phenobarbital treatment of rats. *Hepatology* 1988;8:1051–1055.
20. MacDonald JR, Beckstead JH, Smuckler EA. An ultrastructural and histochemical study of the prominent inflammatory response in D(+)-galactosamine hepatotoxicity. *Br J Exp Pathol* 1987; 68:189–199.
21. Przybocki J, Reuhl K, Thurman R, Kauffman F. Involvement of nonparenchymal cells in oxygen-dependent hepatic injury by allyl alcohol. *Toxicol Appl Pharmacol* 1992;119:295–301.
22. Thompson WD, Jack AS, Patrick RS. The possible role of macrophages in transient hepatic fibrogenesis induced by acute carbon tetrachloride injury. *J Pathol* 1980;130:65–73.
23. Hendriks HFJ, Horan MA, Durham SK, Earnest DL, Brouwer A, Hollander CF, Knook DL. Endotoxin induced liver injury in aged and subacutely hypervitaminotic rats. *Mech Ageing Dev* 1987; 41:241–249.

24. Jollow DJ, Mitchell JR, Potter WZ, Davis DC, Gillette JR, Brodie BB. Acetaminophen-induced hepatic necrosis. II. Role of covalent binding *in vivo*. *J Pharmacol Exp Ther* 1973;187:195–202.
25. Shiratori Y, Takikawa H, Kawase T, Sugimoto T. Superoxide anion generating capacity and lysosomal enzyme activities of Kupffer cells in galactosamine-induced hepatitis. *Gastroenterology Jpn* 1986;21:135–144.
26. Earnst DL, Brouwer A, Sim W, Horan MA, Hendriks HF, de Leeuw AM, Knook DL. Hypervitaminosis A activates Kupffer cells and lowers the threshold for endotoxin liver injury. In: Kirn A, Knook DL, Wisse E, eds. *Cells of the hepatic sinusoid,* vol 1. Amsterdam: Kupffer Cell Foundation; 1986:277–283.
27. Abril ER, Simm WE, Earnest DL. Kupffer cell secretion of cytotoxic cytokines is enhanced by hypervitaminosis A. In: Wisse E, Knook DL, Decker K, eds. *Cells of the hepatic sinusoid,* vol 2. Amsterdam: Kupffer Cell Foundation; 1989:73–75.
28. Gardner CR, Wasserman AJ, Laskin DL. Differential sensitivity of tumor targets to liver macrophage-mediated cytotoxicity. *Cancer Res* 1987;47:6686–6691.
29. Laskin DL, Pilaro AM. Activation of liver macrophages for killing of hepatocytes following acetaminophen treatment of rats. *Toxicologist* 1988;8:32.
30. Lloyd RS, Triger DR. Studies on hepatic uptake of antigen. III. Studies of liver macrophage function in normal rats and following carbon tetrachloride administration. *Immunology* 1975;29:253–263.
31. Tanner A, Keyhani A, Reiner R, Holdstock G, Wright R. Proteolytic enzymes released by liver macrophages may promote hepatic injury in a rat model of hepatic damage. *Gastroenterology* 1980; 80:647–654.
32. Arthur MJP, Bentley IS, Tanner AR, Saunders PK, Millward-Sadler GM, Wright R. Oxygen-derived free radicals promote hepatic injury in the rat. *Gastroenterology* 1985;89:1114–1122.
33. Chojkier M, Fierer S. D-Galactosamine hepatotoxicity is associated with endotoxin sensitivity and mediated by lymphoreticular cells in mice. *Gastroenterology* 1985;88:115–121.
34. ElSisi AE, Earnest DL, Sipes IG. Vitamin A potentiation of carbon tetrachloride hepatotoxicity: role of liver macrophages and active oxygen species. *Toxicol Appl Pharmacol* 1993;119:295–301.
35. Ferluga J, Allison A. Role of mononuclear infiltrating cells in the pathogenesis of hepatitis. *Lancet* 1978;2:610–611.
36. Freudenberg MA, Keppler D, Galanos C. Requirement for lipopolysaccharide-responsive macrophages in galactosamine-induced sensitization to endotoxin. *Infect Immun* 1986;51:891–895.
37. Laskin DL, Pilaro AM, Ji S. Potential role of activated macrophages in acetaminophen hepatotoxicity. II. Mechanism of macrophage accumulation and activation. *Toxicol Appl Pharmacol* 1986; 86:216–226.
38. Lehman V, Freudenberg MA, Galanos C. Lethal toxicity of lipopolysaccharide and tumor necrosis factor in normal and D-galactosamine-treated mice. *J Exp Med* 1987;165:657–663.
39. Nakae D, Yamamoto K, Yoshiji H, Kinugasa T, Maruyama H, Farber JL, Konishi Y. Liposome-encapsulated superoxide dismutase prevents liver necrosis induced by acetaminophen. *Am J Pathol* 1990;136:787–795.
40. Tanner AR, Deyhani AH, Wright R. The influence of endotoxin *in vitro* on hepatic macrophage lysosomal enzyme release in different models of hepatic injury. *Liver* 1983;3:151–160.
41. Hirano T. Interleukin-6 and its relation to inflammation and disease. *Clin Immunol Immunopathol* 1992;62:S60–S65.
42. Jirik FR, Podor TJ, Hirano T, et al. Bacterial lipopolysaccharide and inflammatory mediators augment IL-6 secretion by human endothelial cells. *J Immunol* 1989;142:144–147.
43. Matsubara T, Ziff M. Increased superoxide anion release from human endothelial cells in response to cytokines. *J Immunol* 1986;137:3295–3298.
44. Ooi BS, MacCarthy EP, Hsu A, Ooi YM. Human mononuclear cell modulation of endothelial cell proliferation. *J Lab Clin Med* 1983;102:428–433.
45. Oppenheim JJ, Kovacs EJ, Matsushima K, Durum SK. There is more than one interleukin 1. *Immunol Today* 1986;7:45–56.
46. Goetzl E, Pickett W. Novel structural determinants of the human neutrophil chemotactic activity of leukotriene B. *J Exp Med* 1981;153:482–487.
47. Laskin DL, Kimura T, Sakakibara S, Riley D, Berg R. Chemotactic activity of collagen-like polypeptides for human peripheral blood neutrophils. *J Leukoc Biol* 1986;39:255–266.
48. Schiffman E, Corcoran B, Wahl S. *N*-formylmethionine peptides as chemoattractants for leukocytes. *Proc Natl Acad Sci USA* 1975;72:1059–1062.

49. Ward PA, Newman LJ. A neutrophil chemotactic factor from C5a. *J Immunol* 1969;102:93–99.
50. Matsushima K, Oppenheim J. Interleukin-8 and MCAF: novel inflammatory cytokines inducible by IL-1 and TNF. *Cytokine* 1989;1:2–13.
51. Laskin DL. Potential role of activated macrophages in chemical and drug induced liver injury. In: Wisse E, Knook DL, Decker K, eds. *Cells of the hepatic sinusoid,* vol 2. Amsterdam: Kupffer Cell Foundation; 1989:284–287.
52. Black HS. Role of reactive oxygen species in inflammatory processes. In: Hensby C, Lowe NJ, eds. *Nonsteroidal anti-inflammatory drugs. Pharmacology and the skin,* vol 2. Basel: Karger; 1989:1–20.
53. DelMaestro RF, Thaw H, Bjork J, Planker M, Arfors KE. Free radicals as mediators of tissue injury. *Acta Physiol Scand Suppl* 1980;492:43–57.
54. Halliwell B, Gutteridge JMC. Oxygen toxicity, oxygen radicals, transition metals and disease. *Biochem J* 1984;219:1–14.
55. Rubin R, Farber JL. Mechanisms of the killing of cultured hepatocytes by hydrogen peroxide. *Arch Biochem Biophys* 1984;228:450–459.
56. Gunawardhana L, Mobley SA, Sipes IG. Modulation of 1,2-dichlorobenzene hepatotoxicity in the Fischer-344 rat by a scavenger of superoxide anions and an inhibitor of Kupffer cells. *Toxicol Appl Pharmacol* 1993;119:205–213.
57. Shiratori Y, Tanaka M, Hai K, Kawase T, Shiina S, Sugimoto T. Role of endotoxin-responsive macrophages in hepatic injury. *Hepatology* 1990;11:183–192.
58. Sugino K, Dohi K, Yamada K, Kawasaki T. Changes in the levels of endogenous antioxidants in the liver of mice with experimental endotoxemia and the protective effects of the antioxidants. *Surgery* 1989;105:200–206.
59. Shiratori Y, Kawase T, Shiina S, et al. Modulation of hepatotoxicity by macrophages in the liver. *Hepatology* 1988;8:815–821.
60. Billiar TR, Curran R, Harbrecht B, Stuehr D, Demetris A, Simmons R. Modulation of nitrogen oxide synthesis in vivo: N^G-monomethyl-L-arginine inhibits endotoxin-induced nitrite/nitrate biosynthesis while promoting hepatic damage. *J Leukoc Biol* 1990;48:565–569.
61. Heck DE, Laskin DL, Gardner CR, Laskin JD. Epidermal growth factor suppresses nitric oxide and hydrogen peroxide production by keratinocytes. Potential role of nitric oxide in the regulation of wound healing. *J Biol Chem* 1992;267:21277–21280.
62. Laskin DL, Heck DE, Punjabi C, Pendino KJ, Laskin JD. Role of nitric oxide in chemically induced tissue injury. *Toxicologist* 1993;13:25.
63. Moncada S, Palmer R, Higgs E. Nitric oxide: physiology, pathophysiology and pharmacology. *Pharmacol Rev* 1991;43:109–142.
64. Punjabi C, Laskin DL, Heck DE, Laskin JD. Production of nitric oxide by bone marrow cells: inverse correlation with proliferation. *J Immunol* 1992;149:2179–2184.
65. Stuehr DJ, Nathan CF. Nitric oxide. A macrophage product responsible for cytostasis and respiratory inhibition in tumor target cells. *J Exp Med* 1989;169:1543–1555.
66. Kilbourn RG, Jubran A, Gross SS, Griffith OW, Levi R, Adams J, Lodato RF. Reversal of endotoxin-mediated shock by N^G-methyl-l-arginine, an inhibitor of nitric oxide synthase. *Biochem Biophys Res Commun* 1990;172:1132–1138.
67. Stark ME, Szurszewski JH. Role of nitric oxide in gastrointestinal and hepatic function and disease. *Gastroenterology* 1992;103:1928–1949.
68. Beckman JS, Crow JP. Pathological implications of nitric oxide, superoxide and peroxynitrite formation. *Biochem Soc Trans* 1993;21:330–334.
69. Frederick J, Hasselgren P, Davis S, Higashiguchi T, Fischer J. Nitric oxide upregulates in vivo hepatic protein synthesis during endotoxemia. *Arch Surg* 1993;128:152–157.
70. Harbrecht B, Billiar T, Stadler J, Demetris A, Ochoa J, Curran R, Simmons R. Inhibition of nitric oxide synthesis during endotoxemia promotes intrahepatic thrombosis and an oxygen radical-mediated hepatic injury. *J Leukoc Biol* 1992;52:390–394.
71. Brain S, Camp R, Greaves M, Jones RR, Woollard PM. The inflammatory responses of human skin to topical application of leukotriene B_4. *Br J Clin Pharmacol* 1984;17:610–611.
72. Beutler B, Cerami A. The biology of cachectin/TNF—a primary mediator of the host response. *Annu Rev Immunol* 1989;7:625–655.
73. Keppler D, Hagmann W, Rapp R, Denzlinger C, Koch HK. The relation of leukotrienes to liver injury. *Hepatology* 1985;5:883–891.

74. Shiratori Y, Tanaka M, Umihara J, Kawase T, Shiina S, Sugimoto T. Leukotriene inhibitors modulate hepatic injury induced by lipopolysaccharide-activated macrophages. *J Hepatol* 1990;10:51–61.
75. Tiegs G, Wendel A. Leukotriene-mediated liver injury. *Biochem Pharmacol* 1988;37:2569–2573.
76. Tiegs G, Wolter M, Wendel A. Tumor necrosis factor is a terminal mediator in galactosamine/endotoxin-induced hepatitis in mice. *Biochem Pharmacol* 1989;38:627–631.
77. Whicher JT, Evans SW. Cytokines in disease. *Clin Chem* 1990;36/37:1269–2181.
78. Shedlofsky SI, McClain CJ. Hepatic dysfunction due to cytokines. In: Kimball ES, ed. *Cytokines and inflammation*. Boca Raton, FL: CRC Press; 1991:235–273.
79. Dinarello CA. Interleukin-1 and its related cytokines. In: Sorg C, ed. *Macrophage-derived cell regulatory factors. Cytokines,* vol 1. Basel: Karger; 1989:105–154.
80. Peterson TC, Renton KW. Kupffer cell factor mediated depression of hepatic parenchymal cell cytochrome P-450. *Biochem Pharmacol* 1986;35:1491–1497.
81. Tracey KJ, Beutler B, Lowry SF, et al. Shock and tissue injury induced by recombinant human cachectin. *Science* 1986;234:470–474.
82. Larrick JW, Wright SC. Cytotoxic mechanism of tumor necrosis factor-α. *FASEB J* 1990;4:3215–3223.
83. Thiele DL. Tumor necrosis factor, the acute phase response and the pathogenesis of alcoholic liver disease. *Hepatology* 1989;9:497–499.
84. Hishinuma I, Nagakawa J, Hirota K, et al. Involvement of tumor necrosis factor-α in development of hepatic injury in galactosamine-sensitized mice. *Hepatology* 1990;12:1187–1191.
85. Laskin DL, Gardner CR, Maurer JK, Driscoll KE. Kupffer cell (KC)-derived tumor necrosis factor-alpha (TNF) as a mediator of hepatotoxicity. *Toxicologist* 1993;13:427.
86. Klebanoff SJ, Vadas MA, Harlan JM, Sparks LH, Gamble JR, Agosti JM, Waltersdorph AM. Stimulation of neutrophils by tumor necrosis factor. *J Immunol* 1986;136:4220–4225.
87. Sudhir S, Budhiraja RD. Comparison of the protective effect of Withaferin-"A" and hydrocortisone against CCl_4 induced hepatotoxicity in rats. *Indian J Physiol Pharmacol* 1992;36:127–129.
88. Husztik E, Lazar G, Parducz A. Electron microscopic study of Kupffer cell phagocytosis blockade induced by gadolinium chloride. *Br J Exp Pathol* 1980;61:624–630.
89. Souhami RL, Bradfield JW. The recovery of hepatic phagocytosis after blockade of Kupffer cells. *J Reticuloendoth Soc* 1981;16:75–86.
90. Edwards MJ, Keller BJ, Kaufman FC, Thurman RG. The involvement of Kupffer cells in carbon tetrachloride toxicity. *Toxicol Appl Pharmacol* 1993;119:275–279.
91. Galanos C, Freudenberg MA, Reuter W. Galactosamine-induced sensitization to the lethal effects of endotoxin. *Proc Natl Acad Sci USA* 1979;76:5939–5943.
92. Nolan JP, Leibowitz AZ. Endotoxin and the liver. III. Modification of acute carbon tetrachloride injury by polymyxin B, an antiendotoxin. *Gastroenterology* 1978;75:445–449.
93. Nolan JP. Endotoxin, reticuloendothelial function and liver injury. *Hepatology* 1981;1:458–465.
94. Sim WW, Abril ER, Earnest DL. Mechanisms of Kupffer cell activation in hypervitaminosis A. In: Wisse E, Knook DL, Decker K, eds. *Cells of the hepatic sinusoid,* vol 2. Amsterdam: Kupffer Cell Foundation; 1989:91–93.
95. ElSisi AE, Hall P, Sim WW, Earnest DL, Sipes IG. Characterization of vitamin A potentiation of carbon tetrachloride-induced liver injury. *Toxicol Appl Pharmacol* 1993;119:280–288.
96. Al-Tuwaijri A, Akdamar K, DiLuzio NR. Modification of galactosamine-induced liver injury in rats by reticuloendothelial system stimulation or depression. *Hepatology* 1981;1:107–113.
97. Gunza JT, Pashayan AG. Postoperative elevation of serum transaminases following isoflurane anesthesia. *J Clin Anesth* 1992;4:336–341.
98. Lind RC, Gandolfi AJ, Hall PM. Subanesthetic halothane is hepatotoxic in the guinea pig. *Anesth Anal* 1992;74:559–563.
99. Tiegs G, Hentschel J, Wendel A. T cell dependent experimental liver injury in mice inducible by concanavalin A. *J Clin Invest* 1992;90:196–203.

Immunotoxicology and Immunopharmacology, Second Edition, edited by J. H. Dean, M. I. Luster, A. E. Munson, and I. Kimber.
Raven Press, Ltd., New York © 1994.

28

Immune-Mediated Downregulation of Cytochrome P450 and Related Drug Biotransformation

Kenneth W. Renton and Steven G. Armstrong

Department of Pharmacology, Dalhousie University, Halifax, Nova Scotia, B3H 4H7, Canada

It is now well established that cytochrome P450-dependent drug biotransformation is compromised during infectious disease or when host defense systems are activated in experimental animals and humans. In the past 15 years there has been remarkable interest in this interaction between the system that protects us from infectious disease and the system that inactivates therapeutic agents and environmental chemicals. In 1976, Renton and Mannering (1) and Leeson et al. (2) demonstrated that interferon (IFN) inducers such as tilorone, quinacrine, polyriboinosinic: polyribocytidylic acid (poly I:C) and *Escherichia coli* endotoxin (lipopolysaccharide, LPS) caused a significant suppression of hepatic microsomal cytochrome P450 content following their administration to rats. The temporal relationship between IFN production and the downregulation of drug metabolism during encephalomyocarditis virus infections or following the administration of immunoactive agents led to the development of the IFN hypothesis that stated "depression of cytochrome P450 is a common property of all interferon-inducing agents including infections" (3). Other immune stimulants can downregulate cytochrome P450 without the involvement of IFN, so that the depression of cytochrome P450 is now thought to occur during the activation of host defense mechanisms in general (3,4).

INTERFERON AND OTHER CYTOKINES

Although it was known that many different IFN-inducing agents decreased drug metabolism (1,2), a casual relationship was not established until we showed that an IFN produced in *E. coli* from cloned genes depressed hepatic microsomal cytochrome P450 (5). This highly purified homogeneous human IFN is a molecular hybrid formed between two of the human leukocyte IFN subtypes. It has been demonstrated to depress hepatic microsomal cytochrome P450, aminopyrine *N*-demethylase, and benzo[*a*]pyrene (BaP) hydroxylase in male mice. This provided the first conclusive direct evidence to support the hypothesis that the production of IFN is a contributing factor in the depression of cytochrome P450 that occurs during infection or following the administration of IFN-inducing agents. Parkinson et al. (6) also observed a significant decrease in hepatic microsomal cytochrome P450 after the administration of IFN-α to female mice. A previous report (7) had shown that a crude preparation of mouse type II IFN (IFN-γ) was capable of causing a depression of cytochrome P450 in hepatic microsomes, and subsequent studies (8,9) with recombinant mouse IFN-γ confirmed that this type of IFN downregulates the levels of cytochrome P450 in the liver. A crude preparation of mouse IFN-β has been shown to have the same effect (5), but to date there have been no reports on the effect of a recombinant IFN-β on cytochrome P450-mediated metabolism. These experiments indicate that all three subtypes of IFN (α, β, and γ) are capable of depressing the cytochrome P450 enzyme system.

An attractive hypothesis is that IFN-inducing agents, infections, or other host defense activators decrease cytochrome P450 only by an IFN-mediated mechanism. However, many of the agents studied as IFN inducers are also more general immune stimulants and have many other effects on host defense activation in addition to their ability to induce the production of IFN. Some immunoactive agents such as the bacteria *Listeria monocytogenes* can cause a decrease in cytochrome P450-mediated metabolism without causing a detectable increase in serum IFN levels (10,11). Endotoxin (LPS), the lipopolysaccharide component of the cell wall of gram-negative organisms, is only a weak inducer of IFN but is one of the more potent immunoactive agents that can depress hepatic drug biotransformation (12). LPS also causes the release of cytokines such as interleukin-1 (IL-1), interleukin-6 (IL-6), and tumor necrosis factor (TNF) (13), all of which are capable of suppressing cytochrome P450 in their own right (14–16).

Human and murine recombinant IL-1α and murine IL-1β have been shown to depress hepatic microsomal cytochrome P450-mediated metabolism after *in vivo* administration to both C3H/HeN and C3H/HeJ mice (9,14,17). Purified IL-1 produced the same effect when incubated directly with mouse or rat hepatocytes (14,18). All these studies with IL-1 suggested that the alterations in hepatic cytochrome P450 observed with endotoxin are consistent with the idea that they may be mediated, at least in part, by this cytokine. Recently, IL-2 has been reported to potentiate the hepatic effects of phenobarbital (19), likely indicating that it too can depress the levels of cytochrome P450 in the liver. Two additional cytokines that have received a great deal of attention are TNF and IL-6, both of which are released by macrophages after endotoxin administration (20). The order of release of various cytokines during sepsis is somewhat controversial but it appears that TNF is released first and in turn results in the release of IL-1 and IL-6 (20). Recombinant human TNF caused a significant depression in the activity of hepatic microsomal cytochrome P450, arylhydrocarbon hydroxylase, and ethoxycoumarin deethylase following administration to mice (16). When human recombinant TNF was incubated with isolated rat hepatocytes, drug metabolism capacity in these cells was unchanged (9,16), suggesting that the effects of TNF are not directly on the parenchymal cells of the liver and that the response requires the release of mediators from other cell types. Such a sequence of events is supported by evidence demonstrating that the supernatants from cultures of human monocytes incubated with recombinant human TNF-α were capable of suppressing ethoxycoumarin deethylase activity in rat hepatocytes (9). Supernatants from TNF-treated monocytes display high IL-1 activity in a thymocyte proliferation assay (21). When the supernatants from the monocyte cultures, stimulated by TNF, were treated with rabbit anti-human IL-1 antiserum, their ability to depress cytochrome P450-mediated metabolism in the hepatocytes was totally blocked. These observations are consistent with the hypothesis that IL-1 released from nonparenchymal cells is the mediator of the effect of TNF on liver cytochrome P450.

IL-6, previously called IFN-β, B cell stimulatory factor-2, and hepatocyte stimulating factor, was originally described in 1980 and is produced by monocytes, macrophages, fibroblasts, and endothelial cells (22). Bacterial endotoxins, TNF, and IL-1 stimulate IL-6 production, and it is probably the ultimate mediator of acute-phase protein synthesis in the liver (22). It is known that LPS can produce an acute-phase response and that cytokines such as IL-1, TNF, and IL-6 are involved in the expression of this response. The acute-phase response causes a myriad of physiologic effects including major changes in the synthesis and secretion of many hepatic proteins (23). As discussed earlier, the cytochrome P450 enzyme system is suppressed after LPS, TNF, and IL-1 administration, and hence there has been interest in determining if IL-6 is a common mediator in the response to these agents. We have shown that IL-6 incubated with isolated mouse hepatocytes for 20 hr results in a significant decrease in total cytochrome P450 content (K. W. Renton and K. Brydon, *unpublished data*), and Williams and co-workers (15) recently demonstrated that recombinant human IL-6 was able to completely block the induction of CYP2B in isolated rat hepatocytes. IL-6 is also capable of downregulating CYP1A1, CYP1A2, and CYP3A3 in hepatoma cells cultured *in vitro* (24). It is generally accepted that IL-6 is a central mediator of acute-phase proteins in the liver and therefore it is possible that the loss of cytochrome P450 activity observed during immune stimulation is simply part of the acute-phase response. Unfortunately, the results obtained on the effects of IL-6 on cytochrome P450 *in vitro* have not been confirmed *in vivo*. Our laboratory and two other groups have shown that although recombinant IL-6 depresses cytochrome P450 forms in isolated hepatocytes, the administration of IL-6 to intact animals has little or no effect (15,25,26; K. W. Renton and K. Brydon, *unpublished data*). In one of these studies (25) IL-6 had a minor effect on some cytochrome P450-dependent pathways and no effect in others, while IL-1, TNF, and LPS had a profound effect on all parameters studied. There is no doubt that the acute-phase response has occurred *in vivo* as measured by a decrease in messenger ribonucleic acid (mRNA) for albumin, which is a well-known negative acute-phase protein. Although the hypothesis resulting from the isolated cell experiments is attractive, the data obtained *in vivo* suggest that the downregulation of cytochrome P450 can occur independently from the production of acute-phase response proteins and this raises serious doubts that IL-6 and the acute-phase response are involved in the chain of events that leads to the loss of cytochrome P450 during host defense activation.

Another situation in which cytochrome P450 is downregulated is during adjuvant-induced arthritis in the rat. Cytochrome P450 and several drug biotransformation pathways are depressed during the inflammatory response in such a model system (27). An example is the decrease in cyclosporin A clearance that occurs during adjuvant-induced arthritis in the rat (28). At the present time no information is available concerning the nature of the cytokines that might be involved in the downregulation of cytochrome P450 caused by the inflammatory response in this model of arthritis.

MECHANISM OF CYTOCHROME P450 DOWNREGULATION

The mechanism involved in the IFN-mediated downregulation of cytochrome P450 is now reasonably well understood. IFN (LeIF-AD) has no effect on cytochrome P450 when incubated directly with hepatic microsomes (6); however, we have observed that a recombinant human IFN-α (IFN-α-CON_1) can decrease total cell cytochrome P450 content when incubated with intact mouse hepatocytes *in vitro* (Moochhala SM and Renton KW *unpublished data*). This suggests that the effect of IFN requires intact cells and that other cell types in the liver are not involved. Non-IFN-inducing agents such as dextran or latex particles that are phagocytosed in the liver can depress cytochrome P450 in parenchymal cells only via an indirect action in the adjacent Kupffer's cells and the release of a factor that acts within the hepatocyte (18,29). The issue of whether or not other cell types are involved in the mechanism causing the downregulation of cytochrome P450 in hepatocytes during host defense activation remains to be completely resolved.

It is now generally accepted that many of the antiviral effects of IFNs are the result of an inhibition of viral protein synthesis (4), and many studies have suggested that the effects of IFN-inducing agents and IFN on cytochrome P450 involve an alteration of apoprotein synthesis or breakdown. The administration of poly I:C for 24 hr along with ^{14}C-labeled amino acids to rats indicated that the incorporation of amino acids into a cytochrome P450 rich fraction of hepatic microsomes is impaired, but their incorporation into other proteins in the liver is unchanged (30). Thus the rate of synthesis of some proteins in the liver was increased by poly I:C while the synthesis of cytochrome P450 appeared to be depressed. This agreed with a previous report indicating that some bands ascribed to cytochrome P450 isoforms on sodium dodecyl sulfate–polyacrylamide gel electrophoresis (SDS–PAGE) were decreased in intensity following the administration of poly I:C, suggesting some degree of isozyme or protein selectivity (31). These two studies were the first to suggest that the loss of cytochrome P450 was due to a selective loss of apoprotein and that the effect was not part of a generalized decrease in the synthesis of all hepatic microsomal proteins. Although Gooderham and Mannering (32) found that the depression in the incorporation of radiolabeled leucine into rough endoplasmic reticulum proteins was also accompanied by an acceleration in the loss of ^{14}C-labeled protein, we were only able to show that the incorporation of labeled methionine into microsomal proteins with molecular weights consistent with those of cytochrome P450 was depressed by a cloned consensus IFN-α-CON$_1$ and that there was no effect on the degradation rate of these same proteins (33). In fact, some experiments indicated that poly I:C treatment resulted in a significant increase in the total incorporation of labeled amino acids into microsomal protein (30). A similar observation was made in studies on the *in vitro* translation of mRNA isolated from animals treated with poly I:C (34). After treatment for 3 days with clofibrate to induce CYP4A1, rats were treated with poly I:C for 24 hr, at which point total hepatic RNA was isolated and translated in an *in vitro* cell-free translation system containing [^{35}S]-methionine. Poly I:C had no effect on the total amount of proteins translated in the liver but the binding of an antibody directed against cytochrome CYP4A1 apoprotein indicated that the translation of this specific protein was depressed by 50%. These data are consistent with the hypothesis that IFN selectively depresses cytochrome P450 levels by decreasing apoprotein synthesis but has little effect on the majority of proteins in the liver.

The first direct evidence indicating that the downregulation of cytochrome P450 by IFN occurred via a depression of apoprotein synthesis was reported independently by three laboratories in 1990 with the demonstration that the downregulation of cytochrome P450 occurs at a pretranslational step in protein synthesis. Renton and colleagues (35,36) provided evidence that IFN decreased cytochrome CYP4A1 mRNA. Total hepatic RNA was isolated from clofibrate-treated rats and a complementary deoxyribonucleic acid (cDNA) probe for cytochrome CYP4A1 mRNA was utilized to identify this specific mRNA. After 6 hr of treatment with poly I:C, cytochrome CYP4A1 mRNA levels were significantly reduced but there was no effect on total hepatic microsomal cytochrome P450 content or lauric acid hydroxylase activity, which is metabolized by cytochrome CYP4A1 (37). After 24 hr of treatment, cytochrome CYP4A1 mRNA levels, total cytochrome P450 content, and lauric acid hydroxylase activities were all significantly reduced. The total amount of mRNA in the liver was unchanged as measured by hybridization to an oligo dT$_{18}$ cDNA probe. Another group reported that the administration of poly I:C to male rats resulted in a significant decrease in total hepatic microsomal cytochrome P450 content and CYP2C11 mRNA and apoprotein levels (38). In a third series of experiments, the administration of recombinant rat IFN-γ to male rats for 24 hr caused a significant decrease in cytochrome CYP3A2 mRNA, specific apoprotein, and CYP3A2-dependent androstenedione 6β-hydroxylase activity; however, this form of cytochrome P450 was unaffected in female rats (39). In all these studies, the loss in mRNA preceded the loss of apoprotein or substrate activity and the magnitude of the suppression of cytochrome P450 mRNA levels observed after the *in vivo* administration of IFN and IFN inducers could entirely account for the loss of apoprotein that was observed, indicating that the decreases in the levels of mRNA were directly responsible for the loss in enzyme and subsequent loss in drug biotransformation capacity. A subsequent study by Morgan (40) demonstrated that poly I:C also caused a significant reduction in the female-specific cytochrome CYP2C12 apoprotein and mRNA levels in female rats; however, in this study the decrease in mRNA levels did not precede the loss of apoprotein, suggesting that there may be differences in the mechanisms by which IFN suppresses different forms of cytochrome P450, or that the mechanisms involved are different in male and female rats. We have since confirmed that an IFN-mediated loss in mRNA also accounts for the downregulation of CYP1A1, CYP1A2, CYP2E1, and CYP3A1 (41,42). The actual mechanism(s) responsible for cytochrome P450 mRNA downregulation by IFN has not been identified, as there have been no reports on the effect of IFN on the transcriptional activity of cytochrome P450 genes or on cytochrome P450 mRNA stability.

As indicated earlier, many immune stimulants are involved in non-IFN-mediated effects on host defense. It is now apparent that endotoxin, TNF, and IL-1 downregulate several forms of cytochrome P450 (CYP1A1, CYP1A2, CYP2C11, CYP2C12, CYP2D, and CYP3A3) in a similar manner to IFN by depressing the levels of mRNA and subsequent apoprotein synthesis (15,26,43,44). IL-6 also decreases the levels of CYP2B1/2 in isolated rat hepatocytes via a loss in the levels of the corresponding mRNA (15). We have recently examined the mechanism involved in the loss of drug metabolism during a bacterial infection (11,45). Initially, we expected that the loss during an active infection would be due to cytochrome P450 destruction by reactive oxygen species, but surprisingly we found that *Listeria* infections caused a downregulation in the synthesis of cytochrome P450 (CYP1A and CYP2D9) in the mouse. This resulted from a profound loss in the levels of mRNA coding for these cytochrome P450 forms. We also found that the loss in CYP1A and its corresponding mRNA, but not for CYP2D9, was preceded by an induction phase early in the infection. It appears now universal that immunoactive agents that can depress drug biotransformation act by a downregulation in the mRNA coding for the various forms of cytochrome P450.

To date, most studies have been in agreement that the loss in cytochrome P450 occurs at a pretranslational step in protein synthesis; however, the exact nature of the step involved remains to be fully elucidated. In a model of inflammation evoked by turpentine or LPS, the rate of transcription for the CYP2C11 gene in male rats was depressed, suggesting that the loss in the corresponding mRNA and protein was mediated by a downregulation in gene expression (46). On the other hand, the expression of the sex-specific CYP2C12 gene in female rats was unaffected, indicating that the loss in this enzyme must be regulated at a post-transcriptional step. Using isolated hepatocytes induced with 2,3,7,8-tetrachlorodibenzo-*p*-dioxin (TCDD), Barker et al. (43) have recently shown that IL-1 or medium conditioned with activated human peripheral monocytes or the U937 monocyte cell line suppresses the transcription rate for CYP1A1 and CYP1A2, indicating that the loss of mRNA and enzymes in these TCDD-induced cells is evoked through an effect of the cytokine on gene expression. This information provides evidence suggesting that a decrease in transcriptional rate could explain the downregulation of at least some forms of cytochrome P450 during the activation of host defense. As this study was confined to *in vitro* experiments with induced hepatocytes, extending this conclusion to the *in vivo* situation should be done with caution as the cytochrome P450 in isolated cell systems often responds differently to immunoactive agents compared to that observed *in vivo*. To date the effect of IFN itself on the transcription rates of cytochrome P450 genes has not been studied and therefore the mechanism involved in the downregulation of cytochrome P450 and its mRNA by IFN remains to be established. It would also be possible to explain the loss of cytochrome P450 at a pretranslational step by a change in mRNA stability that might occur during the activation of host defense processes; however, this possibility has not yet been explored.

In order to explain why so many seemingly different components of host defense downregulate cytochrome P450 in a similar manner by decreasing the levels of mRNA, it has been proposed that a common mediator must be involved in the process. We have shown that IFN action requires the presence of intact cells and the effect in tissues such as the liver may require the involvement of other cell types such as macrophages (6,18,29). It has been established that the effect of IFN in hamsters requires the *de novo* synthesis of an intermediate protein (35,47). Both puromycin and actinomycin D completely blocked the ability of IFN-α-CON_1 to cause a suppression of hepatic cytochrome P450 levels. This finding explains the previous finding of Parkinson et al. (6) that administered IFNs were no longer detectable in serum after 4 hr, while cytochrome P450 levels were still significantly suppressed after 24 hr. The intermediate protein that might mediate the effect of IFN or other immunoactive agents has not been identified.

IFNs that have no antiviral activity in a given species also do not suppress cytochrome P450 in that species (5,6,47,48). Therefore it is possible that the loss in cytochrome P450 is an extension of the establishment of an antiviral state. IFN activates a 2-5A-dependent endonuclease that cleaves viral mRNA (49). IFN also activates a kinase that phosphorylates and inactivates a protein synthesis initiation complex (eIF2) (49). It is generally accepted that the 2-5A-dependent endonuclease cleaves both host and viral RNAs although this issue remains controversial (50). It is therefore possible that 2-5A synthetase is the intermediate protein that is produced by IFN that ultimately leads to a decrease in cytochrome P450. The involvement of this mechanism would result in a change in stability of mRNA—a potential site of action to explain the loss in mRNA that has been widely reported. Xanthine oxidase generates reactive oxygen species that are known to be involved in phagocyte-mediated microbicidal activity. A number of laboratories including our own have produced a large body of evidence correlating the induction of xanthine oxidase and the downregulation of cytochrome P450 (51–53). Although some of the evidence is compelling, the role of xanthine oxidase remains contentious as hepatic xanthine oxidase can be inactivated in animals by tungsten (54) and Mannering et al. (55) demonstrated that tungsten did not prevent the poly I:C-mediated loss in cytochrome P450 in rats. Since growth hormone is a key regulator of CYP2C11 and CYP2C12 expression, it was thought that this hormone may be a mediator of the endotoxin-induced effect; however, recent work by Morgan (56) indicates that the loss of these cytochrome P450 forms occurs independent of the regulatory pathway of the hypothalamic–pituitary axis. The hypothesis that cytochrome P450 is downregulated during the acute-phase response is hard to justify since the key mediator of this response is IL-6. IL-6 downregulates cytochrome P450 only *in vitro* and not *in vivo* despite indications that an acute-phase response had occurred (15,25; K. W. Renton and K. Brydon, *unpublished data*). At present, all data suggest the existence of one or more mediators that are involved in the chain of events that leads to the downregulation of cytochrome P450 during host defense activation. It will be interesting to discover the nature of the modulator(s) that appears to downregulate the expression of the cytochrome P450 enzymes without having general effects on protein synthesis.

CLINICAL IMPLICATIONS OF IMMUNE-MEDIATED CYTOCHROME P450 DOWNREGULATION

The first obstruction that altered drug metabolism may be important in clinical medicine was made by Chang et al. (57), who reported that theophylline clearance was impaired during serologically confirmed upper respiratory tract infections. Renton (58) proposed that these observations could be explained by a loss in cytochrome P450 during the infectious disease and that "in man many other agents which induce the formation of interferon including certain viruses, bacteria and vaccines will alter drug biotransformation and elimination." During an outbreak of influenza in Seattle in 1980, 11 asthmatic children developed a sudden decrease in theophylline clearance and were admitted to hospital with methylxanthine toxicities ranging from headaches to seizures (59). None of the children had experienced problems with theophylline dosage prior to infection. It was postulated that endogenous IFN, known to be released in response to viral infections, played a central role in the drug response of these children. There have been several other documented examples of compromised drug metabolism in infected humans (60–64). Of particular note was the observation of Koren and Greenwald (63) that, during an epidemic of influenza A and parainfluenza 3 in Toronto, there was a significant increase in the number of theophylline levels, which exceeded the therapeutic range. These same authors also described a case of a child with prolonged seizures related to toxic levels of theophylline achieved during a respiratory illness (64). These episodes provide examples of drug-evoked toxicity that can occur during infectious disease.

There have been four reports of altered drug clearance during the clinical use of recombinant IFN-α (65–68). Likewise, hepatic cytochrome P450-dependent metabolism was depressed in microsomes prepared from liver biopsy samples obtained from INF-treated hepatitis patients (69). Similarly, arylhydrocarbon hydroxylase activity is depressed in activated human lymphocytes that are incubated with a recombinant INF-α (70). A review of the literature indicates that IFNs cause a significant depression in the capacity of the liver to metabolize drugs and chemicals in humans and that the magnitude of depression is highly variable. Recent evidence that all members of the cytochrome P450 family of proteins are not depressed equally adds to the complexity and unpredictability of untoward drug responses in infected humans (65,69). These examples serve to illustrate the point that drugs with narrow therapeutic indices should be administered with caution during periods of infectious disease. As the use of IFN and other cytokines in the clinical arena becomes more frequent, there will undoubtedly be an increase in the number of adverse drug reactions due to impaired drug metabolism capacity. A major challenge in clinical practice will be to identify infected patients with susceptibility to drug reactions during episodes of infectious disease.

SIGNIFICANCE AND FUTURE DIRECTIONS

A wide variety of infections impair the metabolism of drugs and chemicals and interfere with their subsequent elimination. It can be predicted that these effects are probably more widespread than has been described and that many infection–drug interactions remain to be detected and reported. These interactions do and will continue to cause problems in drug dosage and toxicity in patients with infectious disease, in vaccinated individuals, in cancer patients receiving IFN or other cytokines, and in any situation in which host defense mechanisms are activated. As the therapeutic use of cytokines and other immunomodulating agents will only increase, it is important to identify the individual products and mechanisms responsible for decreasing the capacity of the liver and other organs to metabolize and subsequently eliminate drugs. A major problem remaining is to identify the reasons causing the huge variability in response in the human population (65,69). Only then will it be possible to identify the patients most at risk and to eliminate these untoward drug responses during the activation of host defense.

Of importance to the research community is the effect of viral infections on drug metabolism in laboratory animals. Although suppliers and institutions take great care in providing highly controlled facilities to prevent infectious disease spread in experimental animals, it must be recognized that outbreaks of infectious disease occur on a regular basis in experimental animals and many colonies of animals carry infectious organisms. Kwong et al. (71) have observed that propranolol clearance and metabolism were augmented during an outbreak of respiratory viral infections (sialodacryoadenitis virus and Kilham virus) in a rat colony. We have previously observed in rats that cytochrome P450 levels were lower than normal and were not responsive to immunostimulants during an outbreak of a respiratory viral illness, suggesting that drug-metabolizing enzymes were already depressed by the operation of host defense mechanisms (3). On the other hand, we did not observe any effect on drug biotransformation during a natural outbreak of mouse hepatitis virus infection in our own facility (72). These reports, along with the large number of studies indicating that infections and/or immunoactive agents depress drug biotransformation in mammalian species, suggest that it remains important to carry out a routine surveillance program in experimental animals used for drug biotransformation studies.

REFERENCES

1. Renton KW, Mannering GJ. Depression of the hepatic cytochrome P-450 monooxygenase system by tilorone (2,7-bis[2-diethylamine ethoxy]fluovene-9-one dihydrochloride. *Drug Metab Dispos* 1976;4:223–231.
2. Leeson GA, Biedenback SA, Chan KY, Gibson JB, Wright GJ. Decrease in the activity of the drug-metabolizing enzymes of rat liver following the administration of tilorone hydrochloride. *Drug Metab Dispos* 1976;4:232–238.
3. Renton KW. Relationships between the enzymes of detoxication and host defense mechanisms. In: Caldwell J, Jacoby WB, eds. *Biological basis of detoxication*. New York: Academic Press; 1983: 307–324.
4. Mannering GJ, Deloria LB. The pharmacology and toxicology of the interferons. An overview. *Annu Rev Pharmacol Toxicol* 1986;26:455–515.
5. Singh G, Renton KW, Stebbing N. Homogenous interferon from *E. coli* depresses hepatic cytochrome P-450 and drug biotransformation. *Biochem Biophys Res Commun* 1982;106:1256–1261.
6. Parkinson A, Lasker J, Kramer MJ, et al. Effects of three recombinant human leukocyte interferons on drug metabolism in mice. *Drug Metab Dispos* 1982;10:579–585.
7. Sonnenfeld G, Harned CL, Thaniyavarn S, Mandel AD, Nerland DE. Type II interferon induction and passive transfer depress the murine cytochrome P450 drug metabolism system. *Antimicrob Agents Chemother* 1980;17:969–972.
8. Franklin MR, Finkle BS. Effect of murine gamma-interferon on the mouse liver and its drug-metabolizing enzymes: comparison with human hybrid alpha-interferon. *J Interferon Res* 1985;5:265–272.
9. Bertini R, Bianchi M, Villa P, Ghezzi P. Depression of liver drug metabolism and increase in plasma fibrinogen by interleukin 1 and tumor necrosis factor: a comparison with lymphotoxin and interferon. *Int J Immunopharmacol* 1988;10:525–530.
10. Azri S, Renton KW. Depression of murine mixed function oxidase during infection with *Listeria monocytogenes*. *J Pharmacol Exp Ther* 1987;243:1089–1094.
11. Azri S, Renton KW. Factor involved in the depression of hepatic mixed function oxidase during infections with *Listeria monocytogenes*. *Int J Immunopharmacol* 1991;13:197–204.
12. Williams JF. Induction of tolerance in mice and rats to the effect of endotoxin to decrease the hepatic microsomal mixed function oxidase system. Evidence for a possible macrophage-derived factor in the endotoxin effect. *Int J Immunopharmacol* 1985;7:501–509.
13. Flohe S, Heinrich PC, Schneider J, Wendel A, Flohe L. Time course of IL-6 and TNF-α release during endotoxin tolerance in rats. *Biochem Pharmacol* 1991;41:1607–1614.
14. Ghezzi P, Saccardo B, Villa P, Rossi V, Bianchi M, Dinarello CA. Role of interleukin-1 in the depression of liver drug metabolism by endotoxin. *Infect Immun* 1986;54:837–840.
15. Williams JF, Bement WJ, Sinclair JF, Sinclair PR. Effects of interleukin-6 on phenobarbital induction of cytochrome P450 IIB in cultured rat hepatocytes. *Biochem Biophys Res Commun* 1991;178: 1049–1055.
16. Ghezzi P, Saccardo B, Bianchi M. Recombinant tumor necrosis factor depresses cytochrome P450-dependent microsomal drug metabolism in mice. *Biochem Biophys Res Commun* 1986;136:316–321.
17. Shedlofski SI, Swim AT, Robinson JM, Gallicchio VS, Cohen DA, McClain CJ. Interleukin-1 depresses cytochrome P450 levels and activities in mice. *Life Sci* 1987;40:233–236.
18. Peterson TC, Renton KW. Kupffer cell factor mediated depression of hepatic parenchymal cell cytochrome P-450. *Biochem Pharmacol* 1986;35:1491–1497.
19. Ansher SS, Puri R, Thompson WC, Habig WH. The effects of interleukin 2 and α-interferon administration on hepatic drug metabolism in mice. *Cancer Res* 1992;52:262–266.
20. Ertel W, Morrison MH, Wang P, Zheng F, Ayala A, Chanddry IH. The complex pattern of cytokines in sepsis. Association between prostaglandins, cachectin and interleukins. *Ann Surg* 1991;214: 141–148.
21. Dinarello CA, Cannon JG, Wolf SM, et al. Tumor necrosis factor (cachectin) is an endogenous pyrogen and induces production of interleukin-1. *J Exp Med* 1986;163:1433–1450.

22. Whicher JT, Evans SW. Cytokines in disease. *Clin Chem* 1990;36:1269–1281.
23. Heinrich PC, Castell JV, Andus T. Interleukin 6 and the acute phase response. *Biochem J* 1990;265: 621–636.
24. Fukuda Y, Ishida N, Noguchi T, Kappas A, Sassa S. Interleukin-6 down regulates the expression of transcripts encoding cytochrome P450 IA1, IA2 and IIIA3 in human hepatoma cells. *Biochem Biophys Res Commun* 1992;184:960–965.
25. Chen YL, Florentin I, Batt AM, Ferrari L, Giroud JP, Chauvelot-Moachon L. Effects of interleukin 6 on cytochrome P450 dependent mixed function oxidases in the rat. *Biochem Pharmacol* 1992;44: 137–148.
26. Wright K, Morgan ET. Regulation of cytochrome P450 IIC12 expression by interleukin-1α, interleukin-6 and dexamethasone. *Mol Pharmacol* 1991;39:468–474.
27. Beck FJ, Whitehouse MW. Effects of adjuvant disease in rats on cyclophosphamide and isophosphamide metabolism. *Biochem Pharmacol* 1973;22:2453–2468.
28. Pollock SH, Mathews HW, D'Souza MJ. Pharmacokinetic analysis of cyclosporin in adjuvant arthritic rats. *Drug Metab Dispos* 1989;17:595–599.
29. Peterson TC, Renton KW. Depressioin of cytochrome P-450-dependent drug biotransformation in hepatocytes after activation of the reticuloendothelial system by dextran sulfate. *J Pharmacol Exp Ther* 1984;229:299–304.
30. Singh G, Renton KW. Inhibition of the synthesis of hepatic cytochrome P-450 by the interferon inducing agent poly rI.rC. *Can J Physiol Pharmacol* 1984;62:379–383.
31. Zerkle TB, Wade AE, Ragland WL. Selective depression of hepatic cytochrome P-450 hemoprotein by interferon inducers. *Biochem Biophys Res Commun* 1980;96:121–127.
32. Gooderham NJ, Mannering GJ. Depression of cytochrome P-450 and alterations of protein metabolism in mice treated with the interferon inducer polyriboinosinic acid.polyribocytidylic acid. *Arch Biochem Biophys* 1986;250:418–425.
33. Moochhala SM, Renton KW. The effect of IFN-α-CON_1 on hepatic cytochrome P-450 and protein synthesis and degradation in hepatic microsomes. *Int J Immunopharmacol* 1991;13:903–912.
34. Renton KW, Moochhhala S, Gibson GG, Makowski R. The interferon mediated loss in cytochrome P-452. In: Benford DJ, et al., eds. *Drug metabolsim—from molecules and man*. London: Taylor and Francis; 1987:448–452.
35. Renton KW, Knickle LC. Regulation of cytochrome P450 during infectious disease. *Can J Physiol Pharmacol* 1990;68:777–781.
36. Knickle LC, Spencer DF, Renton KW. The suppression of hepatic cytochrome P450 mRNA mediated by the interferon inducer polyinosinic acid.polycytidylic acid. *Biochem Pharmacol* 1992;44:604–608.
37. Parker GL, Orton TC. Induction by oxisobutyrates of hepatic and kidney microsomal cytochrome P-450 with specificity towards hydroxylation of fatty acids. In: Gustaffson JA, Carlsted H, Duke J, Mode A, Rafter J, eds. *Biochemistry, biophysics and regulation of cytochrome P-450*. Amsterdam: Elsevier/North-Holland; 1980:373–377.
38. Morgan ET, Norman CA. Pretranslational suppression of cytochrome P450h (IIC11) gene expression in rat liver after administration of interferon inducers. *Drug Metab Dispos* 1990;18:649–653.
39. Craig PI, Mehta I, Murray M, Astrom A, van der Meide PH, Farrell GC. Interferon down regulates the male specific cytochrome P450IIIA2 in rat liver. *Mol Pharmacol* 1990;38:313–318.
40. Morgan ET. Suppression of P450IIC12 gene expression and elevation of active messenger ribonucleic acid levels in the livers of female rats after injection of the interferon inducer poly IC. *Biochem Pharmacol* 1991;42:51–57.
41. Cribb AE, Delaporte E, Kim S, Novak RF, Renton KW. Regulation of cytochrome P-4501A and cytochrome P-4502E induction in the rat during production of interferon-α/β. *J Pharmacol Exp Therap* 1994;268:487–494.
42. Delaporte E, Cribb AE, Renton KW. Modulation of rat hepatic CYP3A1 induction by the interferon inducer poly IC. *Drug Metab Dispos* 1993;21:520–523.
43. Barker CW, Fagan JB, Pascoe DS. Interleukin-1β suppresses the induction of P4501A1 and P4501A2 in isolated hepatocytes. *J Biol Chem* 1992;267:8050–8055.
44. Morgan ET. Suppression of constitutive cytochrome P450 gene expression in livers of rats undergoing an acute phase response to endotoxin. *Mol Pharmacol* 1989;36:699–707.
45. Armstrong S, Renton KW. Mechanism of hepatic cytochrome P450 modulation during *Listeria monocytogenes* infection in mice. *Mol Pharmacol* 1993;43:542–554.
46. Wright K, Morgan ET. Transcriptional and post-transcriptional suppression of P450IIC11 and P450IIC12 by inflammation. *FEBS Lett* 1990;271:59–61.

47. Moochhala SM, Renton KW, Stebbing N. The induction and depression of cytochrome P450 dependent mixed function oxidase by a cloned consensus interferon in the hamster. *Biochem Pharmacol* 1989;38:439–447.
48. Renton KW, Singh G, Stebbing N. Relationship between the antiviral effects of interferons and their abilities to depress cytochrome P-450. *Biochem Pharmacol* 1984;3:3899–3902.
49. Baron SB, Tyring SK, Fleischmann RW, et al. The interferons: mechanism of action and clinical applications. *JAMA* 1991;266:1375–1383.
50. Sen GC. Biochemical pathways in interferon-action. *Pharmacol Ther* 1984;24:235–257.
51. Ghezzi P, Bianchi M, Mantovani A, Spreafico F, Salmona M. Enhanced xanthine oxidase activity in mice treated with interferon and interferon inducers. *Biochem Biophys Res Commun* 1984;119: 144–149.
52. Ghezzi P, Bianchi M, Gianera L, Landolfo S, Salmona M. Role of reactive oxygen intermediates in the interferon-mediated depression of hepatic drug metabolism and protective effect of N-acetylcysteine. *Cancer Res* 1985;45:3444–3447.
53. Moochhala SM, Renton KW. A role for xanthine oxidase in the loss of cytochrome P450 evoked by interferon. *Can J Physiol Pharmacol* 1991;69:944–951.
54. Johnson JL, Rajagopalan KV, Cohen HJ. Molecular basis of the biological function of molybdenum: effect of tungsten on xanthine oxidase and sulfite oxidase in the rat. *J Biol Chem* 1974;249: 859–866.
55. Mannering GJ, Deloria LB, Abbot V. Role of xanthine oxidase in the interferon mediated depression of the hepatic cytochrome P-450 system in mice. *Cancer Res* 1988;48:2107–2112.
56. Morgan ET. Down regulation of multiple cytochrome P450 gene products by inflammatory mediators *in vivo*: independence from hypothalamic–pituitary axis. *Biochem Pharmacol* 1993;45:415–419.
57. Chang KC, Lauer BA, Bell TD, Chai H. Altered theophylline pharmacokinetics during acute respiratory viral illness. *Lancet* 1978;1:1132–1133.
58. Renton KW. Altered theophylline kinetics. *Lancet* 1978;2:160–161.
59. Kraemer MJ, Furukawa C, Koup JP, Shapiro G. Altered theophylline clearance during an influenza outbreak. *Pediatrics* 1982;69:476–480.
60. Fleetham JA, Nakatsu K, Munt PW. Theophylline pharmacokinetics and respiratory infections. *Lancet* 1978;2:898.
61. Clark CJ, Boyd G. Theophylline pharmacokinetics during respiratory viral infection. *Lancet* 1979;1: 492.
62. Forsyth JS, Moreland TA, Ryelance GW. The effect of fever on antipyrine metabolism in children. *Br J Clin Pharmacol* 1982;13:811–815.
63. Koren G, Greenwald M. Decrease in theophylline clearance causing toxicity during viral epidemics. *J Asthma* 1985;22:75–79.
64. Greenwald M, Koren G. Viral induced changes in theophylline handling in children. *Am J Asthma Allergy Pediatr* 1990;3:162.
65. Williams SJ, Farrell GC. Inhibition of antipyrine metabolism by interferon. *Br J Clin Pharmacol* 1986;22:610–612.
66. Williams SJ, Baird-Lambert JA, Farrell GC. Inhibition of theophylline metabolism by interferon. *Lancet* 1987;2:939–941.
67. Jonkman JHG, Nicholson KG, Farrow PR, et al. Effects of α-interferon on theophylline pharmacokinetics and metabolism. *Br J Clin Pharmacol* 1989;27:795–802.
68. Echizen H, Ohta Y, Shirataki H, Tsukamoto K, Umeda N, Ishizaki TJ. Effects of a subchronic treatment with natural human interferons on antipyrine clearance and liver function in patients with chronic hepatitis. *Clin Pharmacol* 1990;30:562–567.
69. Okuno H, Shiozaki Y, Kitao Y, Kunieda K, Seki T, Sameshima Y. Depression of drug metabolizing activity in the human liver by interferon-α. *Eur J Clin Pharmacol* 1990;39:365–367.
70. Moochhala SM, Lee EJD. Effects of recombinant human interferon alpha on arylhydrocarbon hydroxylase activity in cultured human peripheral lymphocytes. *Life Sci* 1991;48:1715–1719.
71. Kwong EC, Laganiere S, Savitch JL, Nelson WL, Shen DD. Alteration in the disposition and metabolism of S(−)propranolol in rats with active respiratory viral infection. *Life Sci* 1988;42: 1245–1252.
72. Armstrong SG, Renton KW. Hepatic cytochrome P450 and related drug biotransformation during an outbreak of mouse hepatitis virus. *Can J Physiol Pharmacol* 1993;71:188–189.

Immunotoxicology and Immunopharmacology, Second Edition, edited by J. H. Dean, M. I. Luster, A. E. Munson, and I. Kimber.
Raven Press, Ltd., New York © 1994.

29

Immunopathogenesis of Autoimmune Diseases

Noel R. Rose

Department of Immunology and Infectious Diseases, Johns Hopkins University School of Hygiene and Public Health, Baltimore, Maryland 21205

The immune response is designed to recognize the myriad of molecules in the world around us. For the purpose of recognizing the nature of these molecules—friend or foe—it employs three types of molecules: immunoglobulins (Igs), T cell receptors (TcRs), and products of the major histocompatibility complex (MHC). In a single individual, the first two of these receptor molecules are expressed clonally on different populations of lymphocytes, whereas the same MHC molecules, belonging to the third type of recognition molecules, are constantly present, to a greater or lesser extent, on the surface of all nucleated cells. The clonal receptors of lymphocytes provide an enormous diversity within a single individual, permitting the immune system to distinguish one molecule from another on the basis of its ability to bind to a particular lymphocyte receptor. MHC gene products are highly polymorphic, thereby characterizing each individual of a species. These receptors enable the immune system to distinguish among different molecules in the external environment, to distinguish self from nonself, and to distinguish one individual from another.

Like other systems of the body, the immune system can go awry. The ability to distinguish self from nonself is relative, not absolute. Many examples of Igs and TcRs reactive with antigens of the host have been demonstrated. Most of these are rendered harmless by the various safeguards of natural immunoregulation. On occasion, however, self-recognition can be the cause of the pathologic phenomenon that we have come to recognize as autoimmune disease.

The present chapter provides a general framework from which an understanding can be obtained of self/nonself discrimination and of its failure, that is, autoimmune disease.

IMMUNOLOGIC RECOGNITION

All lymphocytes arise from a single hematopoietic stem cell located initially in the yolk sac and fetal liver and, later, in the bone marrow. Through a series of steps regulated by peptide messengers, called the colony-stimulating factors, the stem cell differentiates into the precursors of erythrocytes, platelets, macrophages, granulocytes, and lymphocytes. The lymphocyte precursor further differentiates into two principal types of cells: T cells, which mature in the thymus, and B cells, which are derived from the bone marrow precursor without the benefit of subsequent residence in the thymus. Both B cells and T cells acquire the ability of antigen-specific recognition, the B cells through Igs on the cell surface and the T cells through TcRs. After binding their corresponding antigenic determinant, both T cells and B cells are activated and undergo serial replication, producing clones of antigen-specific lymphocytes.

Two major types of B cells are generated. One lineage predominates in embryonic life and subsequently in intestinal mucosa. Most of these B cells express a characteristic marker, CD5. They produce high levels of IgM, much of it reactive as autoantibody. Some circumstantial evidence suggests that these CD5 B cells are the precursors of autoantibody-producing cells in many of the systemic autoimmune diseases, such as lupus erythematosus (1).

Most B cells do not express CD5 but initially express high levels of both IgM and IgD at their cell surfaces. With the cooperation of T cells, they undergo class switching so that, following antigen stimulation, they produce primarily IgG, IgA, or IgE. The predominating Ig class is determined by soluble factors, i.e. cytokines, produced by the cooperating T cells.

The great diversity of Ig-recognition structures depends on the rearrangements of the Ig heavy chains and light chains. A very large (10^6 to 10^7) number of specificities can be produced through these mechanisms. In addition, following the switch to IgG, somatic mutations increase IgG diversity and favor the production of more highly avid antibody molecules.

It is not difficult to detect autoantigen-binding B cells and their Ig products in the normal repertoire. "Natural" autoantibodies are found in the serum of all normal individuals. Most, but not all, of these antibodies are low-affinity IgMs, but IgG antibodies to both internal and cell surface constituents are often found (2). In addition, many monoclonal antibodies produced during malignant transformation of B cells or by *in vitro* hybridization produce autoantibodies (3). Although they react with self-antigens, such antibodies are rarely implicated in autoimmune disease. It has even been suggested that they might have a physiologic function in contributing to the removal of breakdown products produced during normal cell aging and repair (4).

It is therefore likely that B cells have very limited ability to distinguish self from nonself. From the point of view of autoimmune disease, the major question is whether they proceed with the aid of cooperating T cells to produce large quantities of high-affinity autoantibody. When such antibodies are directed against constituents at the cell surface, autoimmune disease may result. Diseases like autoimmune hemolytic anemia and idiopathic thrombocytopenia exemplify disorders in which antibodies are produced to surface constituents of red blood cells and platelets, respectively. Myasthenia gravis results from the production of autoantibodies to the acetylcholine receptor, whereas Graves' disease is caused by production of autoantibodies to the thyrotropin (TSH) receptor on the surface of thyroid epithelial cells.

T cells develop and are programmed in the thymus. The thymus does not generate its own stem cells but acquires the T cell progenitors by immigration of T cell precursors from the yolk sac, from the fetal liver, or, in later life, from the bone marrow. The thymic epithelial cells produce a number of peptide hormones that induce the gene rearrangements needed to form the 10^6 or 10^7 different TcRs. Based on the gene products comprising the TcR, two T cell lineages can be distinguished, those with αβTcR and those with γδTcR. Most mature T cells express the αβTcR, but γδTcR-expressing T cells are dominant on mucosal surfaces (5). Furthermore, αβTcR thymocytes can develop along two major pathways of differentiation. Along one of the pathways, the accessory molecule is CD4, and along the other, it is CD8. TcRs bind antigen with low affinity and require an accessory molecule to trigger cell proliferation. The CD4-bearing population comprises primarily helper and inducer T cells capable of recognizing antigenic peptides in the context of MHC class II molecules and of initiating immune responses. CD8-expressing T cells are mainly cytotoxic lymphocytes, although a population of regulatory T cells may bear the CD8 marker. These cells are capable of recognizing antigenic peptides in the context of MHC class I molecules.

During their development in the thymus, T cells undergo a process of negative and positive selection (6). The vast majority of the αβTcR-expressing thymocytes is fated to die. Thymocytes with an αβTcR that fits self-MHC molecules with high affinity undergo accelerated apoptosis (programmed death), providing negative pressure against such self-reactive T cells. On the other hand, thymocytes with the αβTcR that fit MHC with lower affinity are saved from apoptosis and allowed to differentiate further. T cells with low affinity for self-MHC molecules, which simultaneously recognize a foreign peptide, are subject to positive selection and proliferate in the thymus. They eventually migrate to peripheral lymphoid tissues where they make up the bulk of the MHC-restricted CD4 (inducer) T cells or CD8 (cytotoxic) T cells. Some T cells with lower affinity for self-peptides are not deleted in the thymus. They exit the thymus and are rendered unreactive by entering a state of continued anergy. Tolerance to self at the T cell level therefore depends on the intrathymic deletion or peripheral anergy of T cells with receptors for self-peptides.

Under the conditions of thymic selection, then, many T cells reactive with self-antigens escape thymic deletion and are found in the periphery in an anergic state. Anergic T cells bind their respective peptide but fail to undergo proliferation because they do not receive the necessary nonspecific stimulatory signal (7). This second signal is provided by an antigen-presenting cell (APC) in the form of a soluble cytokine [e.g., interleukin-2 (IL-2)] or a cell surface receptor (B7) that engages its counterpart receptor (CD28) on the T cell. In rare instances, self-reactive T cells can be activated simply by providing a second nonspecific signal. The administration of IL-2 to patients, for example, may induce thyroid autoimmunity (8). In other instances, autoimmunity to self-peptide can be induced by administering autologous antigen together with a potent auxiliary, such as Freund's complete adjuvant. Adjuvants serve both as antigen depots and as stimulators of ILs. Such maneuvers are commonly used to induce experimental autoimmune diseases, such as thyroiditis and encephalomyelitis.

APCs are distinguished by their ability to take up antigenic proteins, to fragment them, and to present the peptide fragments to CD4 T cells. Among the important APCs are macrophages, dendritic cells, and B cells. Antigen processing occurs following uptake of antigen, either by pinocytosis or phagocytosis or, in the case of B cells, by antigen-specific binding and endocytosis. The processed antigen, cleaved by proteolytic enzymes of the lysosomes, appears on the surface of the APC in the form of peptides associated with the products of MHC class II. CD4 T cells recognize antigen only in the form of small peptides bound to MHC class II molecules (9).

Antigens that are synthesized with the cells rather than taken in from the exterior are presented by MHC class I molecules. Transport of the processed peptides of intracellular antigens into the cell's endoplasmic reticulum is mandatory for final assembly of the MHC class I molecules (10). The peptides expressed may be normal or malignant cell products or may result from infection by intracellular pathogens. The complex of protein product plus MHC class I molecule can be recognized by a CD8 T cell with the corresponding TcR.

ABROGATION OF SELF-TOLERANCE

From the basic information described earlier, it is possible to envision several mechanisms by which self-tolerance may be voided and autoimmunity generated. Clonal deletion obviously depends on the presence of self-peptides in the thymus during the development of T cells. Antigens that appear relatively late during fetal development or even after birth may not be represented in the thymus during the earliest stages of T cell development, so that T cells recognizing these antigens may escape from the thymus and take up residence in the periphery. A prime example of such an antigen is myelin basic protein, a major constituent of myelinated central nervous system and peripheral nerves. Other examples are found among late-developing antigens of the reproductive system, including constituents of sperm and zona pellucida.

A second group of self-antigens, unrepresented in the thymus and therefore unavailable for thymic deletion, are organ-specific antigens. Such antigens often reflect the unique function of a particular organ. A prime example is thyroglobulin, the major glycoprotein constituent of the thyroid gland and storage form of the thyroid hormones. This large protein is synthesized by specialized thyroid follicular cells and stored in sac-like follicles in the thyroid. In normal individuals, thyroglobulin circulates in only very low amounts. Substantial tolerance to this antigen therefore fails to develop and it is possible to induce autoimmunity by immunization of thyroglobulin of the same species or even of the same animal, if the injection is accompanied by a powerful adjuvant (11).

Yet another mechanism by which self-tolerance can be terminated is administration of a related protein that shares some determinants with the autologous constituent. T cells are able to recognize the foreign determinants and then cooperate with self-reactive B cells to produce autoantibodies. Thyroglobulin again provides an excellent example of such autoimmune responses, since immunization of rabbits with foreign thyroglobulins can induce the animal to synthesize autoantibodies to rabbit thyroglobulin (12). In recent years, a great deal of attention has been given to molecular mimicry in which sequences of amino acids of pathogenic microorganisms duplicate sequences of autologous antigens. A membrane protein of the β-hemolytic streptococcus, for example, is analogous to certain sequences on cardiac myosin (13). This form of molecular mimicry provides a reasonable explanation for the ability of streptococci to induce rheumatic fever.

Self-reactive T cells not deleted intrathymically are normally held in check in the periphery by anergic mechanisms. Overcoming anergy provides another pathway to autoimmunity. Chronic graft-versus-host (GVH) reactions exemplify such situations. GVH reactions are produced by injecting immunocompetent allogeneic lymphocytes into immunologically unresponsive hosts (14). The injected cells recognize host antigens, proliferate, and liberate cytokines. In appropriately selected genetic combinations, parental spleen cells injected into F1 hybrid recipients induce chronic GVH reactions. The parental cells cannot be rejected by the F1 recipient and react to the alloantigens of the hybrid inherited from the opposite parent. Under these conditions, the recipient produces a number of autoantibodies. The most prominent autoantibodies are directed to erythrocytes and to cell nuclei closely resembling the autoantibodies found in patients with lupus erythematosus. The chronic lymphocyte stimulation of GVH reactions may sometimes lead to lymphoid cell malignancies, associating this form of disease with systemic autoimmunities of the human.

A third device for abrogating self-tolerance is to interfere with normal immunoregulation by specialized populations of T lymphocytes. The existence of immunoregulatory cells, whose function is to prevent autoimmunity, was first inferred from experiments in which neonatal thymectomy was carried out in animals genetically predisposed to certain autoimmune diseases. The obese strain (OS) chicken, for example, is destined to develop a form of autoimmune thyroiditis. The disease is more severe and occurs at an earlier age if the chickens are thymectomized shortly after hatching (15). An alternative strategy to delete immunoregulatory cells is to thymectomize mature rats, accompanying the surgery by irradiation to remove peripheralized regulatory T cells (16). Finally, thymectomy of some strains of mice 2 to 4 days after birth can induce autoimmune responses (17). While the mechanism of this thymectomy-induced autoimmunity is still not completely clear, a reasonable hypothesis is that the procedure removes a population of regulatory T cells that normally restrains self-reactive T cells.

Regulatory T cells can also be found in animals that have recovered spontaneously from autoimmune disease. Rats that have recovered from autoimmune encephalomyelitis, for example, resist reinduction of the disease (18). Spleen cells from these animals can adoptively transfer the unresponsive state to naive recipients. The cell responsible for this unresponsive state, a CD8+ T cell, produces large amounts of transforming growth factor-β, a cytokine known to depress many immunologic responses (19).

EFFECTOR MECHANISMS

The development of autoimmunity is only the first step in the production of autoimmune disease. It is necessary that the corresponding antigen be accessible and that a cytotoxic effector mechanism be active in the body. In the case of autoimmune diseases affecting elements of the blood, antibodies to cell surface antigens can produce disease directly. In autoimmune hemolytic anemia, for example, autoantibodies are most frequently produced to alloantigens of the Rh system (20). Such antibodies attach directly to the blood cell and opsonize it, so that it is taken up by phagocytic cells of the spleen and other organs. In other forms of hemolytic anemias, such as paroxysmal cold hemoglobinuria, antibody binds to the red blood cell at lower temperatures. Upon warming, however, the antibody-coated erythrocytes are lysed by complement. Thus the combination of antibody plus complement can be an effective mediator of autoimmune disease.

In other circumstances, the autoantigen is not available on the cell surface but is released into the bloodstream. Patients with lupus erythematosus commonly produce antibodies to native deoxyribonucleic acid (DNA). This antibody cannot penetrate an intact, viable cell. After cell injury or death, however, the native DNA is released into the bloodstream where it has an opportunity to bind to antigen. These immune complexes tend to localize in capillary beds, particularly in the lung, kidney, and skin. There they may activate complement in these tissues and induce the inflammatory reaction characteristic of this disease (21).

A third mechanism by which antibody can mediate autoimmune disease is to cooperate with leukocytes in producing antibody-dependent cell-mediated cytotoxicity (ADCC). Antibody to thyroglobulin, for example, can attach to cytotoxic leukocytes through receptors for the Fc portion of the antibody molecule (22). In the test tube, these armed leukocytes can lyse tissue cells that bear the corresponding antigen. It is still not known to what extent ADCC reactions occur in the body.

Autoimmune lesions in solid tissues and organs are generally attributed to cell-mediated rather than antibody-mediated immunity. The effector mechanisms involve cytotoxic T cells. In general, cytotoxic T cells are CD8+ cells. Cytotoxic CD4 cells have occasionally been reported. The cytotoxic CD8+ T cell is capable of recognizing its corresponding peptide in conjunction with a matching MHC class I product. The binding of a cytotoxic T cell may directly injure the membrane of the target cell and produce cell lysis. Alternatively, the antigen-binding T cells liberate cytokine products that injure the target cell. Tumor necrosis factor-β, originally termed lymphotoxin, for example, is liberated from antigen-stimulated T cells and kills susceptible tissue cells, especially malignant ones (23). One cytokine produced by T cells, interferon-γ, increases expression of MHC class I, thereby increasing susceptibility to cytotoxic CD8 T cells. MHC class II products may aberrantly be expressed on tissues exposed to interferon-γ, perhaps resulting in cell injury. The increased expression of MHC class II products may initiate additional autoimmune responses, provided that self-antigens are presented in conjunction with the MHC class II molecule and the necessary nonspecific second signals (24). This phenomenon may explain the frequent occurrence of multiple autoimmune responses affecting a single organ, as seen in such autoimmune diseases as atrophic gastritis, chronic thyroiditis, and insulin-dependent diabetes.

Another role of cytokines is to call forth macrophages. These cells are capable of contributing greatly to tissue damage. They are themselves the source of a number of cytokines that may injure cells or interfere with essential metabolic pathways. Macrophages can produce nitric oxide, which may serve as a tissue-damaging agent (25). They are also the source of reactive oxygen derivatives and cytotoxic cytokines, which damage surrounding cells and promote inflammation (26).

Various different effector mechanisms can accompany autoimmune responses. In a certain disease, it is common to find evidence of more than one effector mechanism. In chronic thyroiditis, for example, cytotoxic antibody, immune complex formation, antibody-dependent cytotoxicity, cytotoxic T cells, cytotoxic cytokines, and evidence of superoxide radicals can be found (27). All these factors may contribute to the total picture of autoimmune disease. As one approaches therapy, it is therefore unlikely that blocking a single effector mechanism will be effective in a tissue-localized disease.

HEREDITY AND ENVIRONMENT

In experimental animals, autoimmune disease can be induced by immunization with a self-antigen or a cross-reacting antigen, but a potent adjuvant is generally necessary. In humans, where autoimmune diseases occur without deliberate immunization, a genetic basis of susceptibility to autoimmune disease is apparent. It may be found in the clustering of cases in a particular family or in the sharing of particular genetic traits, particularly the MHC. A well-documented inherited predisposition to the development of autoimmune disease is obvious in human populations (28).

Among genetically identical twins, however, it is rare to find a concordance rate of more than 50%. Two possible explanations can be given for this lack of complete concordance. It may result from stochastic or random variability in genetic expression. On the other hand, essential environmental factors may contribute to autoimmune disease. Several environmental factors are known to provoke autoimmune responses in genetically susceptible humans. Perhaps the most dramatic instance is the occurrence of rheumatic fever in a restricted proportion of patients with β-hemolytic streptococcal pharyngitis, as described previously. The importance of the environmental factor is emphasized by the fact that one can abort the recurrence of rheumatic fever by prophylactic treatment with antibiotics designed to prevent streptococcal infection.

Certain chemicals are also known to induce autoimmune disease in genetically susceptible individuals. D-penicillamine, for example, is responsible for a form of myasthenia gravis in some patients and procainamide is associated with drug-induced lupus erythematosus (29). In all cases of drug-induced autoimmune disease described thus far in the literature, the disease disappeared when the chemical was removed.

The role of environmental pollutants in inducing autoimmune disease has been scantily studied. Some investigations have suggested that silica can induce a form of scleroderma and that mercury salts can be implicated in some cases of autoimmune glomerulonephritis (30,31). Even food additives may prove to be important. Based on studies of the OS chicken, the increasing prevalence of autoimmune thyroid disease observed in the American and West-European populations has been ascribed to increased use of iodized salt (32).

Many mysteries remain to be solved in the realm of immunopathogenesis of autoimmune disease. Clearly, this group of disorders constitutes an important threat to human health and well-being. Moreover, they represent a fascinating problem for the investigator at the interface of immunology and toxicology.

REFERENCES

1. Gadol N, Ault KA. Phenotypic and functional characterization of human Leu 1 (CD5) B cells. *Immunol Rev* 1986;93:23–34.
2. Guilbert B, Dighiero G, Avrameus S. Naturally occurring antibodies against nine common antigens in human sera. *J Immunol* 1982;128:2779–2787.
3. Dighiero G, Lymberi P, Mazie JC, et al. Murine hybridomas secreting natural monoclonal antibodies reacting with self antigens. *J Immunol* 1983;131:2267–2272.
4. Grabar P. Autoantibodies and the physiological role of immunoglobulins. *Immunol Today* 1983; 4:337–340.
5. Goodman T, Lefrancois L. Expression of the gamma-delta T-cell receptor on intestinal CD8+ intraepithelial lymphocytes. *Nature* 1988;333:855–858.
6. Sprent J, Lo D, Gao E-K, Ron Y. T cell selection in the thymus. *Immunol Rev* 1988;101:173–190.
7. Jenkins MK, Schwartz RH. Antigen presentation by chemically modified splenocytes induces antigen-specific T cell unresponsiveness in vitro and in vivo. *J Exp Med* 1987;165:302–319.
8. Rose NR, Metzgar RS, Isaacs E. Studies on organ specificity. VIII. Serologic interrelationships among thyroid extracts of various species revealed by gel-diffusion precipitation techniques. *J Immunol* 1960;84:649–658.
9. Babbitt BP, Allen PM, Matsueda G, Haber E, Unanue ER. Binding of immunogenic peptides to Ia histocompatibility molecules. *Nature* 1985;317:359–361.
10. Yewdell JW, Bennink JR, Hosaka Y. Cells process exogenous proteins for recognition by CTL. *Science* 1988;239:637–640.
11. Witebsky E, Rose NR. Studies on organ specificity. IV. Production of rabbit thyroid antibodies in the rabbit. *J Immunol* 1956;76:408–416.
12. Witebsky E, Rose NR. Studies on organ specificity. VII. Production of antibodies to rabbit thyroid by injection of foreign thyroid extracts. *J Immunol* 1959;83:41–48.
13. Dale JB, Beachey EH. Sequence of myosin-cross-reactive epitopes of streptococcal M proteins. *J Exp Med* 1986;164:1785.
14. Schwartz RS, Beldotti L. Malignant lymphoma following allogeneic disease: transition from an immunological to a neoplastic disorder. *Science* 1965;149:1511–1514.

15. Welch P, Rose NR, Kite JH Jr. Neonatal thymectomy increases spontaneous autoimmune thyroiditis. *J Immunol* 1973;110:575–577.
16. Penhale WJ, Farmer A, McKenna RP, Irvine WJ. Spontaneous thyroiditis in thymectomized and irradiated Wistar rats. *Clin Exp Immunol* 1973;25:225–236.
17. Sakaguchi S, Rose NR. In: Mendelsohn G, ed. *Diagnosis and pathology of endocrine diseases: immune mechanisms in autoimmune disease of endocrine organs*. Philadelphia: Lippincott; 1988: 619–640.
18. Welch AM, Holda JH, Swanborg RH. Regulation of experimental allergic encephalomyelitis. II. Appearance of suppressor cells during the remission phase of the disease. *J Immunol* 1980;125:186–189.
19. Karpus WJ, Swanborg RH. CD4+ suppressor cells inhibit the function of effector cells of experimental autoimmune encephalomyelitis through a mechanism involving transforming growth factor-beta. *J Immunol* 1991;146:1163–1168.
20. Weiner W, Vos GH. *Blood* 1963;22:606–613.
21. Mackworth-Young C, Schwartz RS. Autoantibodies to DNA. *CRC Crit Rev Immunol* 1988;8:147–173.
22. Wasserman J, von Stedingk L-V, Perlmann P, Jonsson J. Antibody-induced *in vitro* lymphocyte cytotoxicity in Hashimoto thyroiditis. *Int Arch Allergy* 1974;47:473–482.
23. Ruddle NH, McGrath K, James T, Schmid DS. Purified lymphotoxin (LT) from class I restricted CTLs and class II restricted cytolytic helpers induce target cell DNA fragmentation. In: Bonavida B, Collier RJ, eds. *Membrane-mediated cytotoxicity*, vol. 45. New York: Alan R Liss; 1987:379.
24. Herskowitz A, Ansari A, Neumann DA, et al. Induction of major histocompatibility complex antigens within the myocardium of patients with active myocarditis: a nonhistologic marker of myocarditis. *J Am Coll Cardiol* 1990;15:624–632.
25. Langrehr JM, Hoffman RA, Lancaster JR Jr, Simmons RL. Nitric oxide—a new endogenous immunomodulator. *Transplantation* 1993;55:1205–1212.
26. Nathan CF, Tsunawaki S. Secretion of toxic oxygen products by macrophages: regulatory cytokines and their effects on the oxidase. In: *Biochemistry of macrophages*, Ciba Foundation Symposium 118. London: Pitman; 1986:211.
27. Rose NR. Pathogenic mechanisms in autoimmune disease. *Clin Immunol Immunopathol* 1989;53 (Suppl):7–16.
28. Nepom GT, Concannon P. Molecular genetics of autoimmunity. In: Rose NR, Mackay IR, eds. *The autoimmune diseases—II*. San Diego: Academic Press; 1992:127–152.
29. Holland K, Spivak JL. Drug-induced immunological disorders of the blood. In: Newcombe DS, Rose NR, Bloom JC, eds. *Clinical immunotoxicology*. New York: Raven Press; 1992:141–153.
30. Uber CL, McReynolds RA. Immunotoxicology of silica. *CRC Crit Rev Toxicol* 1982;10:303–319.
31. Druet P, Pelletier L, Rossort J, Druet E, Hirsch R, Sapin C. In: Kammuller ME, Blocksma N, Seinen W, eds. *Autoimmunity and toxicology; immune dysregulation induced by drugs and chemicals*. Amsterdam: Elsevier; 1989:347–366.
32. Kaplan MH, Sundick RS, Rose NR. Autoimmune diseases. In: Sharma JM, ed. *Avian cellular immunology*. Boca Raton, FL: CRC Press; 1991:183–197.

Immunotoxicology and Immunopharmacology, Second Edition, edited by J. H. Dean, M. I. Luster, A. E. Munson, and I. Kimber.
Raven Press, Ltd., New York © 1994.

30

Chemical-Induced Autoimmunity

Kaye H. Kilburn and *Raphael H. Warshaw

*Department of Medicine, Division of Pulmonary, University of Southern California School of Medicine, Los Angeles, California 90033; and *Working Diseases Detection Services Inc., Claremont, California 91711*

This chapter addresses human autoimmunity associated with chemicals that are not used as drugs and are not metals, thus excluding mercury and arsenic. The major focus is on the evidence for syndromes resembling "collagen disease," which are accompanied by circulating autoantibodies; systemic lupus erythematosus (SLE), scleroderma and dermatomyositis, and nervous system disorders; myasthenia gravis; Guillain–Barré syndrome; and perhaps multiple sclerosis induced by chemicals found in occupational and residential environments.

A 1989 review of immunotoxicology of drugs and environmental chemicals by the Advisory Subgroup in Toxicology of the European Medical Research Councils provided an exceptional departure point for chemical-induced autoimmunity (1). A review of environmentally induced systemic sclerosis disorders was valuable in accessing the German literature in the perspective of silica-induced disease (2), and the possible mechanisms of autoimmune responses to chemicals were thoughtfully reviewed and implications for autoimmune pathogenesis of diseases described by Bigazzi (3).

INTRODUCTORY EXPLANATION AND A CAVEAT

Animal experiments have focused on graft-versus-host disease (GVHD) models or their surrogates emphasizing the popliteal lymph node (PLN) assay in mice to assay chemicals for their potential for autoimmune disorder (1). If the model is accepted, this bioassay can compare autoimmune potential after substituting the side chains and prosthetic groups of molecules like the anticonvulsant hydantoins, succinimides, butyrolactones, and the potential agents of Spanish oil syndrome, the imidazalidinethiones (4,5).

A human cell model system, lymphocyte transformation, may serve as a screening test for chemicals by incubating in the chemical the human lymphocytes from a sensitive individual. This assay is a useful screen but is insufficient to prove an autoimmune pathogenesis. When results are negative, metabolites may be tested after preincubation of hepatic microsomes (P450) with the chemical to convert the chemical to an intermediate that is active *in vivo* (6). Similarly scratch tests may be useful in screening. Besides the PLN assay in mice, other animal models have proved useful. For example, cats develop autoantibodies (antinuclear antibodies, ANAs) and a positive direct antiglobulin test when given 6-propylthiouracil for 4 to 8 weeks (7).

CHEMICALS ASSOCIATED WITH COLLAGEN-LIKE DISEASES

In this section chemicals that have been reported to cause collagen-like diseases are reviewed and compared (Table 1).

Vinyl Chloride (VC)

Vinyl chloride (C_2H_3Cl) was reported in 1974 by Lange et al. (8) to produce a scleroderma-like illness characterized by multisystemic involvement of collagen tissue with pulmonary fibrosis, skin sclerosis, fibrosis of liver and spleen, capillary disturbances, thrombocytopenia, paresthesia, and angiosarcoma of the liver (Table 1). The most extensive study was initiated clinically by Ward et al. (9), who found that 58 (18%) of 320 exposed workers had this scleroderma-like syndrome, 19 were moderately, and 9 were severely disabled. Eight of the latter but none of the moderately disabled group had ANAs. A follow-up by Black et al. (10) of 44 of the 53 available from the 58 workers found 21 had severe and 23 had mild vinyl chloride scleroderma. HLA-DR5 phenotype was of similar frequency in the industrial workers who developed the systemic sclerosis syndrome with vinyl chloride and in 50 classic idiopathic scleroderma patients, but neither anti-centromere nor anti-Scl-70 antibodies were found in the VC group.

Trichloroethylene (TCE) from Occupational Exposure

Scleroderma was described in a 24-year-old woman who used TCE to remove grease from aluminum plates (11). Since 1957, solvents, especially TCE, have shown this association as reported in six of seven patients in Australia (12,13) and in seven of nine patients in Japan (14). Epoxides are formed in the metabolism of TCE, which appear to attack endothelial cells to produce vasculitis. In one fatal case (15), a 19-year-old TCE-exposed dry cleaner died after a few weeks of Raynaud's phenomenon, nail fold hemorrhages, muscle weakness and aching, swollen fingers, and impotence. ANA level was elevated and liver function showed elevated γ-glutyl-transpeptidase and Bromsulphalein retention, but there were no circulating immune complex cells, no lupus erythematosus (LE) cells, and no smooth muscle

TABLE 1. *Possible relationships between human sclerotic and lupus-like diseases and environmental chemical exposures*

Chemical	Reference	Observation
Occupational		
VC	Lange et al. (8) Ward et al. (9) Black et al. (10)	Skin sclerosis Lung fibrosis Nervus system paresthesia Vessels—capillary Inflammation, intimal fibrosis Thrombocytopenia Symptoms—fatigue, cold burning pain, emotional instability, loss of libido, impotence Autoantibodies—not detected
Tetrachloroethylene	Sparrow (70)	19-Year-old male dry cleaner, 4 years, elevated ANA titers, systemic sclerosis
CE	Reinl (11)	24-Year-old woman, degreasing—scleroderma
Solvents	Yamakage and Ishikawa (14)	7/9 Patients in Japan—Raynaud's phenomenon, sclerosis; 6 had lung fibrosis
Solvents, toluene, xylene, white spirit	Walder (12,13)	6/7 Solvent workers in Australia; added 5 in 1983—scleroderma
Carbon tetrachloride and TCE	Saihan et al. (71)	43-Year-old male, neuropathy, Raynaud's phenomenon, sclerosis
Organic solvents	Sverdrup (72)	Scleroderma in 8/9 manufacturing workers
TCE	Lockey et al. (15)	47-Year-old female, fatal scleroderma 6 months after 2.5-hr dermal exposure to TCE
Polymerizing epoxy resins [bis(4-amino-3-methylcyclohexyl methane]	Yamakage et al. (33)	6/233 Workers had skin sclerosis and muscle weakness
Environmental		
TCE and solvents (water exposure)	Byers et al. (17)	ANAs in 10/23 family members of leukemia patients
TCE and solvents	Kilburn and Warshaw (18)	Increased symptoms of SLE and increased ANA titers versus controls
TCE and solvents	Kilburn (*unpublished data*)	Antibodies to smooth muscle and myelin (basic protein)
Spanish oil (syndrome)	Kammuller et al. (4)	PVIZT exposure: pulmonary edema, GVHD, PLN assay
Tryptophan	Silver et al. (22)	9 patients with edema, pruritis, paresthesia, myalgia, scleroderma, eosinophilic fasciitis; 2 with ANA
	Belongia et al. (21)	63 patients with fatigue, muscle tenderness, cramps, arthralgias, rashes, and dyspnea
Hydantoins, succinides, and butyrolactones	Kammuller et al. (4)	Grand mal anticonvulsant PLN assay, petite mal anticonvulsant PLN assay, anticonvulsant PLN assay
Silica	Gunther and Schuchardt (25) Pernis and Paronetto (24) Pearson (23)	25× Increased risk of scleroderma from occupational silica exposure often simultaneous with silicosis; SiO_2 acts as adjuvant

TABLE 1. *Continued.*

Chamical	Reference	Observation
Silicone	Barker et al. (29)	Leakage from gel implants demonstrated *in vitro*
	Van Nunen et al. (32)	SLE classic mixed connective tissue disease—Raynaud's rheumatoid arthritis with Sjögren's syndrome
	Fock et al. (31)	Injected: SLE, scleroderma, idiopathic thrombocytopenic purpura
	Kumagai et al. (28)	Report 18 review 28; of 24 with definite disease, some had been injected with paraffin
	Spiera (30)	4.4% of 113 scleroderma patients had breast implant versus 0.3% of 286 rheumatoid arthritis patients
	Varga et al. (73)	8 patients had progressive systemic sclerosis (PSS), 5 SLE, 6 rheumatoid arthritis, 4 had PSS after silicone gel implants
	Shoaib and Patten (*unpublished data*)	Arthritis in 22, human adjuvant disease or PSS Rh factor in 21, ANA titers increased in 8 after SGI in 17, SG saline in 4, and one silicone injection

or anti-mitochondrial antibodies. The chlorinated alkene solvents resemble VC and are metabolized via epoxides to trichloroacetic acid and trichloroethanol. If this metabolism is intracellular, perinuclear epoxides could adduct to DNA (15). When it occurs near neurofilaments of axons, binding to the neurofilaments interferes with their nutritional function, including transport of protein, causing periodic axonal swelling, an increase in axonal neurofilaments, and secondary demyelination (16).

Environmental Exposure to Trichloroethylene and Solvents

Effects of earlier well-water exposures to TCE, perchloroethylene, and 1,2-trans-dichloroethylene were examined by measuring five autoantibodies in the sera of 23 family members of leukemia patients in Woburn, Massachusetts. Autoantibodies were found in 48% (11/23) of which 10/23 were antinuclear (17). Observations of elevated ANA levels, coupled with increased frequencies of the 11 American Rheumatism Association (ARA) symptoms for SLE in men and women chronically exposed to TCE, 1,1,1-trichloroethene, other volatile organic chemicals (VOCs), and chromium in Tucson, Arizona, strengthened the suggestion that environmental chemical exposure may induce lupus, which resembles the drug-induced lupus (DIL) syndrome (18). Recently, another study that addressed mainly human neurobehavioral effects of environmental chemicals with exposure, again focused on TCE, showed autoantibodies to smooth muscle and immunoglobulin G (IgG) and IgM autoantibodies to myelin basic protein (K. H. Kilburn, *unpublished data*).

Both studies demonstrated impaired neurophysiologic and neuropsychologic performance and affective disturbances shown by elevated Profile of Mood States (POMS) scores and general unwellness with greatly elevated neurologic and respiratory (irritative) complaints.

Spanish Toxic Oil

Spanish toxic oil syndrome was named in 1981 for an epidemic of over 2600 illnesses, including 200 patients with scleroderma, in subjects who had consumed rape seed oil deliberately adulterated with aniline. Over 100 patients died. Important features were fever, respiratory distress with pulmonary edema and pleural effects that were responsible for most deaths, exanthems, flushed cheeks, generalized lymphadenopathy, hepatosplenomegaly, and neurologic signs of cerebral edema (19). ANA titers were elevated in 35% to 80% of patients during the first 8 months of the toxic oil scleroderma-like disease *but dropped after exposure ceased,* so that most were normal after 3 years (20). This temporal sequence resembles the behavior of ANA titers in DIL. A metabolite of phenyl thiourea from Spanish oil, 1-phenyl-5-vinyl-imidazolidinethione (PVIZT), produced a GVHD-like syndrome when experimentally injected in animals and produced a positive popliteal lymph node assay in mice (4,5).

Tryptophan

In 1989 and 1990 a curious syndrome of scleroderma, pruritis, edema, myalgia, and eosinophilic fasciitis was observed in subjects who had taken tryptophan, particularly in Minnesota (21), New Mexico, and South Carolina (22). In nine South Carolina patients, involvement of skin, muscle, nerve, and pulmonary tissue led to skin biopsies, which were typical for scleroderma. Two had ANA titers. Activation of indoleamine-2,3-dioxygenase was postulated together with impairment of the hypothalamic–pituitary–adrenal axis. The 63 Minnesota patients (21) had fatigue, muscle tenderness, cramps, and arthralgias: two-thirds had rashes and one-half were dyspneic and had difficulty climbing stairs. An etiologic link was made to a production product or contaminant, which eluted as a peak during high-pressure liquid chromatography (HPLC) and was associated with reduced powdered carbon in a purification step of the fermentation product by one manufacturer of tryptophan.

Silica, Paraffin, and Silicones

Silica particles have a well-recognized capacity in human subjects and experimental animals to produce adjuvant-like responses or immunostimulation (23,24). A 25-fold increase in scleroderma was seen in German workers with silicosis or silica exposure (25), and 43% of men diagnosed with progressive systemic sclerosis in Pittsburgh had prolonged and heavy silica particle exposure (26). SLE has also been observed in excess (27) in silicosis. Unfortunately, injection of paraffin and silicones and implantation of the latter for breast augmentation provided another wave of iatrogenic connective tissue disease labeled by some as human adjuvant disease (28). Paraffin may behave as an adjuvant, particularly as an emulsion of mineral oil in water stabilized with a surfactant, usually lanolin, to which are added glycoproteins from myobacterial or other microorganisms (23). Adjuvant or immunostimulatory activity has been ascribed not only to Freund's complete adjuvant (23) in an oil vehicle but to silica (24) and to procainamide, hydralazine, D-penicillamine, tienilic acid, and trinitrobenzene sulfonic acid (6).

Scleroderma or human adjuvant illness in women who had breast augmentation, by injection of paraffin or silicones or later silicone gel implants, has been reported repeatedly since 1972 and finally led to Food and Drug Administration (FDA) restrictions on the latter devices in 1992. Their leakage was demonstrated *in vitro* 15 years ago (29).

Silicone Gel Implants

Of 19 implanted women, 5 had SLE, 8 had progressive scleroderma, and 6 had rheumatoid arthritis (30). Of 113 scleroderma patients, 4.4% had breast implants, while, in contrast, only 0.3% of 286 patients with rheumatoid arthritis had breast implants (30). Thrombocytopenic purpura has also been reported (31).

Arthritis followed silicone gel implants or injection, and rheumatoid factor was elevated in 21 of 22 patients and ANA titers in 8 of 22 patients (BO Shoaib and BM Patten, *personal communication*). They also found central nervous system manifestations in many of these 22 patients, including sensory-motor neuropathy in 16, amyotrophic lateral sclerosis (ALS) in 2, multiple sclerosis (MS) in 2, and myositis and myasthenia gravis in one each.

The pathogenesis is unclear but silicone definitely leaks into tissue and free silica particles are found in lymph nodes. Implant gels are composed of polydimethylsiloxane (69%), silica (30%), and catalyst (1%) in a silica elastomere shell. In the United States alone, an estimated 2 million women have received such implants. In light of the known effects of silica and mineral oil adjuvants (23,24), such a large reservoir of silica in the body may induce continual immunostimulation. Fortunately, many patients recover from the connective tissue manifestations after the implants are removed but neurotoxic effects are more lasting (BO Shoaib and BM Patten, *personal communication*) and therapy is difficult (32).

Epoxy Resins

Six of 233 workers using polymerizing epoxy resins had skin sclerosis (33). The active agent is thought to be bis(4-amino-3-methylcyclohexyl methane) entering through the lungs and rapidly producing severe sclerosis of the skin and muscle weakness. This amine is related to amine chemicals used as therapeutic agents: procainamide, D-penicillamine, chlorpromazine, and isoniazid.

Amino Acid-L-Canavanine

A related oddity is the induction of a lupus-like syndrome in cynomolgus monkeys fed L-canavanine, a constituent of alfalfa sprouts, which is characterized by antibodies to nuclear antigens (ANAs), double-stranded DNA, and red blood cells, causing anemia and the deposition of Ig and complement in the kidney and skin (34,35).

Graft Versus Host Disease (GHVD)

Allogenic bone marrow transplantation in human subjects for leukemia has caused severe and incapacitating GVHD. Because of its clinical similarities to VC- and TCE-induced autoimmune disease (36,37), it is included as a foreign chemical disease. GVHD resembles collagen vascular diseases, particularly scleroderma, with dry eyes, pulmonary insufficiency, and wasting (38). Chronic GVHD is characterized by elevated eosinophilia, circulating autoantibodies, hypergammaglobulinemia, and plasmacytosis of lymph nodes and viscera. Malar rashes were common and, after 1 year, thickened hidebound skin and alopecia were characteristic. Eight of 20 patients were reported to have five or more of the ARA criteria for lupus, and 11 of 17 had circulating autoantibodies that were ANAs in eight and mitochrondial in three. Small vessel intimal lesions were common. An *in vitro* active cytotoxic agent against endothelial cells (39) and a non-HLA alloantigen from endothelial cells in scleroderma serum have been implicated in renal allograph rejections (40). Chemical modified membrane determinants on B cells or macrophages plus major histocompatibility complex (MHC) class II molecules are needed to produce GVHD autologous target cells. B cells, hematopoietic cells, or dendritic cells are altered to nonself by chemicals. Then autologous T cells recognize and react against these altered cells (41). In humans the prime candidate chemicals accomplishing this are hydralazine, diphenylhydantoin (DPH), D-penicillamine, nitrofurantoin, mercuric chloride, Epstein–Barr virus, rubella virus, and cytomegalovirus. Models for this sequence typically carry certain major histocompatibility alleles, as an example, nonirradiated F1 mice in which the immunostimulatory or scleroderma pathology may develop. Alternately, the other major pathologic response is suppressive or hypoplastic, manifested by pancytopenia, aplastic anemia, thymic hypoplasia, and hypogammaglobulinemia. GVHD has been modeled by the popliteal lymph node response to injected chemicals in mouse hindlimbs (42).

This GVHD model provides a means to examine chemical induction of scleroderma-like disease as by DPH and similar anticonvulsant drugs (41) as PLN activity. The PLN assay in mice (42) responds to chemical modification of the B cell surface molecule, and MHC class II molecules in mice provide a conceptual framework and an assay system for chemicals that have tied together the once disparate evidence (5).

ORGAN-SPECIFIC AUTOANTIBODIES AND DISEASES

Less evidence has been found thus far of organ-specific autoantibodies induced by chemicals than for syndromes despite acceptance of several important diseases as having an autoimmune pathogenesis (Table 2).

TABLE 2. *Survey of human autoimmune diseases*[a]

Disease	Self-antigens (as defined by the autoantibodies involved)
Autoimmune chronic active hepatitis, virus-negative	Membrane and microsomes of liver cells including cytochrome P450 isoenzymes
Autoimmune hemolytic anemia	Membrane components of erythrocytes
Bullous pemphigoid	Basement membrane of skin
Goodpasture's syndrome (glomerulonephritis and alveolitis with linear Ig deposits along the glomerular and alveolar basement membranes)	Components of the glomerular basement membrane (GBM) and alveolar BM
Guillain–Barré syndrome	Myelin and other components of the sheets of peripheral nerves
Hashimoto's thyroiditis	Cytoplasmic or microsomal thyroid antigen, thyroglobulin
Idiopathic leukocytopenia	Membrane components of leukocytes
Idiopathic thrombocytopenia	Membrane components of platelets
Male infertility (certain cases)	Spermatozoa
Myasthenia gravis	Acetylcholine receptor at the neuromuscular synapsis
Pemphigus vulgaris	Desmosomes linking epithelial cells of the skin
Pernicious anemia	Intrinsic factor (produced by parietal cells for absorption of vitamin B_{12})
Primary Addison's disease	Microsomal antigens in the adrenal cortex
Progressive systemic sclerosis (scleroderma)	Various antigens in cell nuclei, especially nucleoli
SLE	Various nuclear antigens, especially double-stranded DNA; antigens on leukocytes and erythrocytes
Thyrotoxicosis	TSH receptors
Wegener's granulomatosis (inflammatory disease of veins and arteries, especially in the lung and kidneys)	Alkaline phosphatase-like material on endothelial cells and neutrophils (see ref. 50)

Adapted from ref. 1.

[a]Diseases in which pathogenic autoimmune reactions are certain or likely because the self-antigens involved have been relatively well defined.

Hepatitis

Drugs most often associated with autoimmune serologic reactions in 157 cases of hepatitis from five hepatologynists were clometacin, fenofibrate papaverine, and tienilic acid (43). Halothane and tienilic acid (tricryorafen, a uricouria diuretic) produce immunoallergic hepatitis in humans with circulating antibodies against cell organelles. One protein, cytochrome P450-8 from human adult liver microsomes, is recognized in most sera from patients with anti-liver/kidney microsome (anti-LKM_2) antibodies (6). These antibodies specifically inhibit the hydroxylation of tienilic acid by human liver microsomes. This suggests that autoantibodies form when the enzyme (P450-8), present in endoplasmic reticulum, is alkylated by a reactive metabolite and migrates to the surface of the hepatocyte membrane. The modified protein is recognized by the cells reacting to the part of the molecule derived from the reactive metabolite. When this scenario is followed, the strategic borderline between self and nonself, alluded to by Ward (44), has been crossed (1). Thus, autoantibodies formed in hepatitis induced by administering tienilic acid catalyze the metabolic oxidation of the drug. It remains to be demonstrated whether anti-LKM_2 antibodies are responsible for the hepatitis in the 1 affected of 10,000 patients treated with tienilic acid. The recognition of self versus nonself is critical in the pathogenesis of autoimmune disease and the concept of autoimmunity. Therefore, observations that cytochrome P450-8 elicits autoantibodies after conversion by a metabolite that it initiated is important (43).

Renal Disease

Rapidly progressive glomerulonephritis has been seen with and without pulmonary hemorrhage (Goodpasture's syndrome) associated with antibodies to glomerular basement membrane (GBM) both bound and circulating (45). Detailed interviews with 8 patients from a group of 13 with Goodpasture's antiglomerular basement membrane antibody-mediated glomerulonephritis (anti-GBM) (autoimmune glomerulonephritis) found 6 of 8 had extensive exposure to industrial solvents often as a heated vapor or mist (46). Degreasing and painting and paint stripping with heated solvents were frequent. One man fueled jet aircraft. Linearly deposited IgG was demonstrated along GBM by direct immunofluorescent microscopy in five patients and three of four had circulating antibodies. Goodpasture's syndrome has been induced in rabbits by instilling gasoline intratracheally and basement membrane antibodies were found in edematous lungs as well as in the kidneys (47).

Another example is the mercury-induced glomerulopathy in (PVG/C) rats, which is associated with ANAs against nonhistone nucleoprotein and vasculitis (48). Both general T cell reactivity to phytohemagglutinin (PHA) and suppressor cell reactivity to concanavalin A (Con A) were decreased in the mercury-diseased rats, which are comparable to human drug-induced autoimmune disease. It seems logical to extend the search for chemical causes to myasthenia gravis, Guillain–Barré syndrome, and autoimmune thyroiditis (49). The specific autoantibodies to acetylcholine receptor protein and to thyroglobulin are known, methods are well developed, and the frequency of these human diseases provides opportunities to search meticulously for association with chemicals.

Systemic Vasculitis

In some patients with systemic vasculitis, circulating autoantibodies to neutrophil cytoplasmic antigens have been detected using a solid-phase radioimmunoassay and their titers correlated with disease activity (50). Neutrophil alkaline phosphatase has a component inserted in the cell membrane, which might be recognized in systemic vasculitis, and retains its enzymatic activity, which appears to be important in tissue injury.

Neurologic Diseases

Myasthenia gravis is characterized by weak muscles that fatigue quickly in use and is the prototypic antireceptor autoimmune disease with antibodies against the nicotinic acetylcholine receptor (AChR) (51,52) (Table 2). Anti-AChR autoantibodies are controlled by thymic T cells, which arise from impaired self-recognition (52). Levels of anti-AChR above 1.1 U/liter are found in 91% of patients and the thymus is enlarged. D-Penicillamine, a four-carbon fragment of penicillin G with amino and thio groups, is used to treat Wilson's disease because it chelates copper. It has also been used to treat rheumatoid arthritis, where it is thought to modulate T lymphocyte function, immunosuppress the disease, and reduce IgM levels (53). In about 35% of patients with Wilson's disease and rheumatoid arthritis treated with penicillamine, autoimmune diseases develop, including progressive systemic sclerosis, SLE, myasthenia gravis, polymyositis, and membranous glomerulonephritis (54). Between 0.4% and 1% of rheumatoid arthritis patients treated for several months develop myasthenia gravis and antibodies to AChR, frequently with antibodies to striated muscle (53). A mechanism that may induce autoimmune responses in myasthenia gravis is that gold forms a mercaptide with cell surface thiol groups and D-penicillamine forms a mixed disulfide with these same thiol groups (51). In this regard, a possible insight has been provided in lupus psychosis by finding that anti-ribosomal P protein antibodies occur, which are not found in lupus without psychosis, in other psychotics, or in normal controls (55). As central nervous system (CNS) complaints occur in half of lupus patients, this is a promising lead as to the pathogenesis.

ALS is a devastating disease of unknown cause. When the spinal cords and motor cortices of patients with ALS were examined for IgG using immunohistochemical methods, motor neurons showed a granular staining pattern characteristic of binding to rough endoplasmic reticulum. A proportion of pyramidal cells were also stained. No staining was noted in control human tissues. Degenerating horn cells and microglia also stained for HLA-DR (56). Incubation of single mammalian skeletal muscle fibers with IgG from ALS reduced peak Ca^{2+} current in the dehydropyridine-sensitive Ca^{2+} channels. Charge movement and effects were lost when IgG was boiled or absorbed with skeletal tubular membranes (57).

The findings that lupus psychosis was associated with a special antibody, that myasthenia gravis was mediated by an antibody to the acetylcholine receptor, and that ALS showed IgG binding to motor neurons invite speculation that MS, Parkinson–ALS, and dementias of the Alzheimer's disease type may be due to chemical-induced autoimmunity (58). On the one hand, at least three myelin-associated proteins—myelin basic protein, proteolipid protein, and GM-1 ganglioside—elicit autoantibodies. On the other hand, environmental chemicals used in food, cycad fruit in Guam and Japan (59), and ground (chick) peas (60,61) in India, produce characteristic illnesses, chemical-induced neurotoxicity that resembles spontaneous diseases. A Parkinson–ALS disease analog is produced by a cycad-derived amino acid, β-*N*-methylamino-L-alanine (59), and a corticomotor neuronal deficit is produced by the amino acid β-*n*-oxyalylamino-L-alanine from the chick pea (*Lathyrus sativa*) (60,61). Whether immune mechanisms have a role or autoantibodies are present in these models is not known.

Overlap of chemical-induced autoantibody production (ANAs) and chemical neurotoxicity occurred in Tucson residents exposed via well water to TCE and other VOCs plus chromium (18). Although association does not imply a causal link, in a pilot study of Phoenix residents exposed to an even wider assortment of chemicals, especially VOCs, we found neurobehavioral impairments and antimyelin basic protein antibodies—both IgG and IgM (K. H. Kilburn, *unpublished data*).

Perhaps these studies of cohorts exposed to low doses of environmental chemicals who show autoimmune responses (ANAs or anti-SM or anti-myelin antibodies) with LE or scleroderma answer Bigazzi's question: "Are there chemicals whose administration results in irreversible or progressive autoimmune disease?" (3).

Parallel investigation of autoimmunity in the organ-specific disorders could be useful in establishing whether autoantibodies are elicited and, if so, how they are involved in pathogenesis or whether they are simply an epiphenomenon. Epileptic patients treated with diphenylhydantoin have antibodies (ANAs) (37), as do schizophrenic patients treated with chlorpromazine (62), but neither shows additional CNS disease during drug treatment (63). This demonstrates that chemicals may induce autoantibodies without associated disease. However, a proper prospective study of children started on DPH and followed for many years for autoantibodies and associated diseases has not been reported. Thus more data and careful analysis must precede acceptance of each autoantibody-associated disease.

MECHANISMS

VC was postulated to be incorporated by the liver into amino acid synthesis of a structurally abnormal protein, which would be antigenically foreign (9). DNA is a poor immunogen (64) so that a plausible first step is to find a mechanism for increasing its immunogenicity. DNA adducts to epoxides formed during metabolism of chloroalkenes (16). DNA–epoxide adducts may behave similar to formaldehyde–serum albumin conjugates (65), hydralazine (66), hydralazine–human serum albumin conjugates (67), DNA photo-oxidation products (68), and acrylamide and stimulate autoantibodies. If exposure to TCE is chronic, sufficient antigen may be available to form immune complexes. Concomitantly, small chemical molecules, especially epoxides, may attach to B cell surface molecules and thus arouse T cells to react against them as in the Kammuller et al. (4) model.

Two chemicals that cause DIL, procainamide and hydralazine, bind to and alter DNA (66). Hydralazine can complex with soluble nucleoprotein and change its physical properties without changing its antigenicity, while procainamide binds to single-stranded and native DNA (63). Rabbits immunized with hydralazine conjugated to human serum albumin developed rising titers of antibodies to the drug and to single-stranded and native DNA. The importance of the free amine group is shown by studies of *N*-acetylprocainamide, which lacks a free amine group and does not induce ANAs or SLE (63).

GENETIC FACTORS

Just as the linkage of TCE to antinuclear and other autoantibodies and typical lupus symptoms proclaim associations that may have causal significance, the possibility that widely spread environmental contaminants such as polychlorinated biphenyls, especially dioxins, in concert with genetic predisposition, perhaps as manifested by the MHC antigens HLA-DR-5 for scleroderma and HLA-DR-3 for SLE, may explain seemingly peculiar selection and variable disease manifestations within population groups. It is clear that genetic factors influence the risk of chemical-induced SLE or scleroderma acting via the HLA, MHC, acetylation, and cytochrome P450 (43). For example, impaired sulfoxidation of carbocysteine, which is similar to D-penicillamine, was associated with its toxicity in patients with rheumatoid arthritis. In subjects with excessive oxidation, HLA-DR3 was an independent risk factor (69).

Eight mechanisms postulated for autoimmunity due to chemicals, mostly from animal experiments (3), have included complexing with autoantigen (hydralazine); release of autoantigen (gold, cadmium); cross reaction with autoantigen (hydralazine), immunogen, or hapten (penicillamine); inhibition of T suppressor cells (methyldopa, practobol, procainamide, and mercury); stimulation of T helper cells (procainamide, beta blockers, phenytoin, and mercury); stimulation of B cells (mercury, beta-blockers and phenytoin, penicillamine, and iodine); and stimulation of macrophages (penicillamine, propylthiouracil, and iodine).

CONCLUSIONS

Rheumatoid arthritis, LE, and scleroderma can be induced by chemicals that also raise autoantibodies to altered body components (70–73). Rheumatoid arthritis has been induced by silica, paraffin injection, and silicones, and in many instances autoantibodies have been observed (Table 1). Although most of the chemicals that have been reported to induce lupus have been drugs, TCE and other solvents and silicones in breast implants clearly extend and broaden these observations. Scleroderma, in contrast, has been linked more often to industrial chemicals, especially chlorinated and aromatic solvents.

Essentially, we know that (a) mechanisms are diverse; (b) structure–function relationships are not identifiable; (c) chemical-induced delayed-type hypersensitivity has not been explored, but in hepatitis effector T cell reactions are not accompanied by autoantibody production; and (d) genetic predisposition appears to be essential and may be either immunogenic (MHC phenotype) or chemical (acetylator phenotype, sulfoxidizer, or aromatic hydrocarbon receptor).

SPECIFIC DATA GAPS

The need is always for more—*more* cause-directed searches for chemical initiators in patients with autoimmune disease, inclusion of autoantibody measurements in *more* epidemiologic studies of subjects exposed occupationally or environmentally to chemicals, and *more* hypothesis testing of chemical agents in animal models that blend chemical induction against variable genetic endowments. Of further specific importance are explorations on interrelationships between SLE and the sclerosis disorders and CNS disorders building of the elegant models of anti-acetylcholine receptor in myasthenia gravis and Guillain–Barré syndrome, to the dementia and ALS–Parkinson's disease–dementia syndrome. Is there enough evidence for functional CNS impairment in autoimmune CNS disease, particularly in GVHD as in the lupus psychosis anti-ribosomal P protein work, to justify further investigations? If so, it should always be coupled with a diligent, thoughtful search for evidence of chronic exposure to chemicals in each patient's environment.

REFERENCES

1. Gleichmann E, Kimber I, Purchase IFH. Immunotoxicology: suppressive and stimulatory effects of drugs and environmental chemicals on the immune system. *Arch Toxicol* 1989;63:257–273.
2. Haustein UF, Ziegler V. Environmentally induced systemic sclerosis-like disorders. *Int J Dermatol* 1985;24:147–151.
3. Bigazzi PE. Autoimmunity induced by chemicals. *Clin Toxicol* 1988;26:125–156.
4. Kammuller ME, Penninks AH, deBakker JM, et al. An experimental approach to chemically induced systemic (auto)-immune alterations. The Spanish toxic oil syndrome as an example. In: Fowler BA, ed. *Mechanism of cell injury: implications for human health*. New York: Wiley; 1987: 175–192.
5. Kammuller ME, Bloksma N, Seinen W. Chemical-induced autoimmune reactions and Spanish toxic oil syndrome: focus on hydantoins and related compounds. *Clin Toxicol* 1988;26:157–174.
6. Beaune PH, Dansette PM, Mansuy D, et al. Human anti-endoplasmic reticulum autoantibodies appearing in a drug-induced hepatitis are direct against a human liver cytochrome P-450 that hydroxylates the drug. *Proc Natl Acad Sci USA* 1987;84:551–555.

7. Aucoin DP, Peterson ME, Hurvitz AI, et al. Propylthiouracil-induced immune-mediated disease in the cat. *J Pharmacol Exp Ther* 1985;234:13–18.
8. Lange CE, Juhe S, Veltman G. Uber das auftreten von angiosarkomen der leber bei zwei arbeitern der PVC-herstellenden industrie. *Dtsch Med Wochenschr* 1974;99:1598–1599.
9. Ward AM, Udnoon S, Watkins J, Walker AE, Darke CS. Immunological mechanisms in the pathogenesis of vinyl chloride disease. *Br Med J* 1976;1:936–938.
10. Black CM, Welsh KI, Walker AE, et al. Genetic susceptibility to scleroderma-like syndrome induced by vinyl chloride. *Lancet* 1983;1:53–55.
11. Reinl W. Sklerodermic durch trichlorethylen-einworking? *Zentralbl Archeitamed Arteitsschutz* 1957;7:58–60.
12. Walder BK. Solvents and scleroderma. *Lancet* 1965;2:436.
13. Walder BK. Do solvents cause scleroderma? *Int J Dermatol* 1983;22:157–158.
14. Yamakage A, Ishikawa H. Generalized morphea-like scleroderma occurring in people exposed to organic solvents. *Dermatologica* 1982;165:186–193.
15. Lockey JE, Kelly CR, Cannon GW, et al. Progressive systemic sclerosis associated with exposure to trichloroethylene. *J Occup Med* 1987;29:493–496.
16. Savolainen H. Some aspects of the mechanisms by which industrial solvents produce neurotoxic effects. *Chem Biol Interact* 1977;18:1–10.
17. Byers VS, Levin AS, Ozonoff DM, Baldwin RW. Association between clinical symptoms and lymphocyte abnormalities in a population with chronic domestic exposure to industrial solvent-contaminated domestic water supply and a high incidence of leukaemia. *Cancer Immunol Immunother* 1988;27:77–81.
18. Kilburn KH, Warshaw RH. Prevalence of symptoms of systemic lupus erythematosus (SLE) and of fluorescent antinuclear antibodies associated with chronic exposure to trichloroethylene and other chemicals in well water. *Environ Res* 1992;57:1–9.
19. Tabuenca JM. Toxic-allergic syndrome caused by ingestion of rapeseed oil denatured with aniline. *Lancet* 1981;2:567–568.
20. Alonso-Ruiz A, Zea-Mendoze AC, Salazar-Vallinas JM, Rocamora-Ripoll A, Beltran-Gutierrez J. Toxic oil syndrome: a syndrome with features overlapping those of various forms of scleroderma. *Semin Arthritis Rheum* 1986;15:200–212.
21. Belongia EA, Hedberg CN, Gleich GJ, et al. An investigation of the cause of eosinophilia–myalgia syndrome associated with tryptophan use. *N Engl J Med* 1990;323:357–365.
22. Silver RM, Heyes MP, Maize JC, Quearry B, Vionnet-Fausset M, Sternberg EM. Scleroderma, fasciitis and eosinophilia associated with the ingestion of tryptophan. *N Engl J Med* 1990;322:874–881.
23. Pearson CM. Development of arthritis, periarthritis, periostitis in rats given adjuvants. *Proc Soc Exp Biol Med* 1973;143:95–99.
24. Pernis B, Paronetto F. Adjuvant effect of silica (tridymite) on antibody production. *Proc Soc Exp Biol Med* 1962;110:390–392.
25. Gunther G, Schuchardt E. Silikose und progressive. *Sklerodermie Dtsch Med Wochenschr* 1970;95: 467–468.
26. Rodnan GP, Benedek TG, Medsger TA, Gammarata RJ. The association of progressive systemic sclerosis (scleroderma) with coal miners' pneumoconiosis and other forms of silicosis. *Ann Intern Med* 1967;66:323–334.
27. Ziskind M, Jones RN, Weill H. Silicosis. *ARRD* 1967;113:643–664.
28. Kumagai Y, Shiokawa Y, Medsger TA, Rodnan GP. Clinical spectrum of connective tissue disease after cosmetic surgery. *Arthritis Rheum* 1984;27:1–12.
29. Barker DE, Retsky MI, Schultz S. Bleeding of silicone from bag-gel breast implants, and its clinical relation to fibrous capsule reaction. *Plast Reconstr Surg* 1978;61:836–841.
30. Spiera H. Scleroderma after silicone augmentation mammoplasty. *JAMA* 1988;260:236–238.
31. Fock KM, Feng PH, Tey BH. Autoimmune disease developing after augmentation mammoplasty: report of 3 cases. *J Rheumatol* 1984;11:98–100.
32. Van Nunen SA, Gatenby PA, Basten A. Post-mammoplasty connective tissue disease. *Arthritis Rheum* 1982;25:694–696.
33. Yamakage A, Ishikawa H, Saito Y, Hattori A. Occupational scleroderma-like disorder occurring in men engaged in the polymerization of epoxy resins. *Dermatologica* 1980;161:33–44.
34. Malinow MR, Bardana EJ, Pirofsky B, Craig S. Systemic lupus erythematosus-like syndrome in monkeys fed alfalfa sprouts: role of a nonprotein amino acid. *Science* 1982;216:415–417.

35. Bardana EJ, Malinow MR, Houghton DC, et al. Diet-induced systemic lupus erythematosus (SLE) in primates. *Am J Kidney Dis* 1982;1:345–351.
36. Gleichmann E, Gleichmann H. Graft-versus-host reaction: a pathogenetic principle for the development of drug allergy, autoimmunity and malignant lymphoma in non-chimeric individuals. Hypothesis. *Z Krebsforsch* 1976;85:91–109.
37. Gleichmann E, Pals ST, Rolink AG, Radaszkiewicz T, Gleichmann H. Graft-versus-host reactions: clues to the etiopathology of a spectrum of immunological diseases. *Immunol Today* 1984;5:324–332.
38. Shulman HM, Sullivan KM, Weiden PL, et al. Chronic graft-versus-host syndrome in man. *Am J Med* 1980;69:204–216.
39. Kahaleh MB, Sherer GK, LeRoy EC. Endothelial injury in scleroderma. *J Exp Med* 1979;149:1326–1339.
40. Moraes JR, Stastny P. A new antigen system expressed in human endothelial cells. *J Clin Invest* 1977;60:449–454.
41. Gleichmann H, Pals ST, Radaszkiewicz T. T cell-dependent B-cell proliferation and activation induced by the drug diphenylhydantoin in mice. *Hematol Oncol* 1983;1:165–176.
42. Ford WL, Burr W, Simonson M. A lymph node weight assay for the graft-versus-host activity of rat lymph cells. *Transplantation* 1970;10:258–266.
43. Homberg JC, Andre C, Abuaf N. A new anti-liver-kidney microsome antibody (anti-LKM2) in tienilic acid induced nephritis. *Clin Exp Immunol* 1984;55:561–570.
44. Ward AM. Evidence of an immune complex disorder in vinyl chloride workers. *Proc R Soc Med* 1976;69:289–291.
45. Lerner RA, Glassock RJ, Dixon FJ. The role of anti-glomerular basement membrane antibody in the pathogenesis of human glomerulonephritis. *J Exp Med* 1967;126:989–1004.
46. Beirne GJ, Brennan JT. Glomerulonephritis associated with hydrocarbon solvents. *Arch Environ Health* 1972;25:365–369.
47. Yamamoto T, Wilson CB. Binding of anti-basement membrane antibody to alveolar basement membrane after intratracheal gasoline instillation in rats. *Am J Pathol* 1987:126:497–505.
48. Weening JJ, Hoedemaeker J, Bakker WW. Immunoregulation and anti-nuclear antibodies in mercury-induced glomerulopathy in the rat. *Clin Exp Immunol* 1981;45:64–71.
49. Patterson PY, Day ED. Neuroimmunologic disease: experimental and clinical aspects. In: Dixon FJ, Fisher DW, eds. *The biology of immunologic disease*. Sunderland, MA: Sinauer Associates; 1983.
50. Lockwood CM, Bakes D, Jones S, et al. Association of alkaline phosphatase with an autoantigen recognised by circulating anti-neutrophil antibodies in systemic vasculitis. *Lancet* 1987;1:716–720.
51. Smiley JD, Moore SE. Southwestern internal medicine conference: molecular mechanisms of autoimmunity. *Am J Med Sci* 1988;295:478–496.
52. Stobo JD. Autoimmune antireceptor diseases. In: Dixon FJ, Fisher DW, eds. *The biology of immunologic disease*. Sunderland, MA: Sinauer Associates; 1983.
53. Jaffe IA. Penicillamine treatment of rheumatoid arthritis: rationale, pattern of clinical response, and clinical pharmacology and toxicology. *NY Acad Med* 1976;354:11–24.
54. Bacon PA, Tribe CR, MacKenzie JC, Verrier Jones J, Cumming RH, Amer B. Penicillamine nephropathy in rheumatoid arthritis. *Q J Med* 1976;180:661–684.
55. Bonfa E, Glombek SJ, Kaufman LD, Skelly S, Weissbach H, Brot N, Elkon KB. Association between lupus psychosis and antiribosomal P protein antibodies. *N Engl J Med* 1987;317:265–271.
56. Engelhardt JI, Appel SH. IgG reactivity in the spinal cord and motor cortex in amyotrophic lateral sclerosis. *Arch Neurol* 1990;47:1210–1216.
57. Delbono O, Garcia J, Appel SH, Stefani E. IgG from amyotrophic lateral sclerosis affects tubular calcium channels of skeletal muscle. *Am J Physiol* 1991;260:C1347–C1351.
58. Benzing WC, Jufson EJ, Jennes L, Armstrong DM. Reduction of neurotensin immunoreactivity in the amygdala in Alzheimer's disease. *Brain Res* 1990;537:298–302.
59. Spencer PS, Nunn PB, Hugo J, et al. Guam amyotrophic lateral sclerosis–Parkinson–dementia linked to a plant excitant neurotoxin. *Science* 1987;237:517–522.
60. Kissler A. Lathyismus monatschrift. *Psychiatr Una Neurol* 1947;113:345–375.
61. Ludolph AC, Hugon J, Dwivedi MP, Schaumburg HH, Spencer PS. Studies on the aetiology and pathogenesis of motor neuron diseases. *Brain* 1987;110:149–165.
62. Schoen RJ, Trentham DE. Drug-induced lupus: an adjuvant disease? *Am J Med* 1981;71:5–8.
63. Weinstein A. Drug-induced systemic lupus erythematosus. *Prog Clin Immunol* 1980;4:1–21.
64. Friou GJ. Double-stranded DNA: an antigen of unique significance. *J Lab Clin Med* 1978;91:545–549.

65. Patterson R, Dykewicz MS, Evans R, et al. IgG antibody against formaldehyde human serum proteins: a comparison with other IgG antibodies against inhalant proteins and reactive chemicals. *J Allergy Clin Immunol* 1989;84:359–366.
66. Eldredge NT, Robertson WVB, Miller JJM. The interaction of lupus-inducing drugs with deoxyribonucleic acid. *Clin Immunol Immunopathol* 1974;3:263–271.
67. Yamauchi Y, Litwin A, Adams L, Zimmer H, Hess EV. Induction of antibodies to nuclear antigens in rabbits by immunization with hydralazine–human serum albumin conjugates. *J Clin Invest* 1975; 56:958–969.
68. Blomgren SE, Vaughan JH. The immunogenicity of photo-oxidized DNA and of the photoproduct of DNA and procainamide hydrochloride. *Arthritis Rheum* 1968;11:470.
69. Emery P, Panayi GS, Huston G, et al. D-Penicillamine induced toxicity in rheumatoid arthritis: the role of sulphoxidation status and HLA-DR3. *J Rheumatol* 1984;11:626–632.
70. Sparrow GP. A connective tissue disorder similar to vinyl chloride disease in a patient exposed to perchloroethylene. *Clin Exp Dermatol* 1977;2:17–22.
71. Saihan EM, Burton JL, Heaton KW. A new syndrome with pigmentation, scleroderma, gynaecomastia, Raynaud's phenomenon and peripheral neuropathy. *Br J Dermatol* 1978,99.437–440.
72. Sverdrup B. Do workers in the manufacturing industry run an increased risk of getting scleroderma (letter)? *Int J Dermatol* 1984;23:629.
73. Varga J, Schumacher HR, Jimenez SA. Systemic sclerosis after augmentation mammoplasty with silicone implants. *Ann Intern Med* 1989;111:377–383.

Immunotoxicology and Immunopharmacology, Second Edition, edited by J. H. Dean, M. I. Luster, A. E. Munson, and I. Kimber.
Raven Press, Ltd., New York © 1994.

31

Mercury and Autoimmunity

Lucette Pelletier, Maria Castedo, Blanche Bellon, and *Philippe Druet

*INSERM U28, Hospital Broussais, 75674 Paris Cedex, France; *Department of Nephrology, INSERM U28, Hospital Broussais, University of Paris, 75674 Paris Cedex, France*

Mercury (Hg) has been used for thousands of years, such as in mirror making or the felt hat industry. Hg compounds were also used as antiseptic agents, laxatives, vaginal contraceptive agents, or diuretics, but now their therapeutic usage is quite limited (reviewed in refs. 1 and 2). However, even today, Hg is still used in the manufacture of thermometers, fluorescent light tubes, batteries, and chlorine (2,3). In some countries, metallic Hg, used to refine gold, causes a serious problem of public health (4). In addition, Hg in dental amalgam could have deleterious effects due to Hg release (5). Finally, although illicit, Hg is also present in skin lightening creams (6), still used in some countries.

Hg compounds exist either as inorganic mercury or organomercurials in which Hg is covalently bound to carbon such as methylmercury. Hg is mainly inhaled and is oxidized from Hg^0 to Hg^{2+} in erythrocytes, a process that requires catalase and hydrogen peroxide and is antagonized by glutathione peroxidase (2,8). Individual variations in the ability to oxidize Hg^0, depending on genetic background and environmental factors, would condition susceptibility to toxic effects. Methylmercury, present in fish, is mainly absorbed through the gastrointestinal tract and undergoes partial biotransformation to inorganic Hg by demethylation (7,8).

Acute exposure to high concentrations of Hg vapor induces an erosive bronchitis (9) and an interstitial pneumonitis, while chronic exposure to toxic amounts of Hg targets the central nervous system and induces a dysfunction of renal tubular epithelial cells (2). Besides the toxic effects on tubular cells, an immunologically mediated glomerulopathy can occur (1). Clinical presentation is initially that of a heavy proteinuria or a nephrotic syndrome with normal renal function and normal blood pressure. Histologically, this glomerulopathy can be a membranous glomerulopathy with granular immunoglobulin G (IgG) deposits evidenced by immunofluorescence or a minimal glomerular change disease thought to be mediated by T lymphocytes. In some cases, Igs were found linearly deposited along the glomerular basement membrane and were or were not associated with granular IgG deposits (10). This suggests that, in some patients, anti-glomerular basement membrane antibodies may be produced. An increased prevalence of anti-laminin antibodies (laminin is a component of glomerular basement membrane) was reported in workers exposed to Hg vapor (11) but this study was not confirmed in a later study (12).

Development of experimental models of Hg-induced autoimmunity argue that Hg can be deleterious by acting on the immune system. In the chapter, we describe these models because they can be useful for understanding human situations and because they represent potent tools to understand mechanisms of autoimmunity and thereby those supporting tolerance.

First, we describe the models of drug-induced autoimmunity and then we discuss mechanisms that could be at play in the induction phase of the disease and in the spontaneous regulation phase of the disease in susceptible strains of rats. Next, the effects of $HgCl_2$ in the Lewis (LEW) strain of rats are discussed.

EXPERIMENTAL MODELS OF MERCURY-INDUCED AUTOIMMUNITY

$HgCl_2$-Induced Autoimmunity in Rats

Brown Norway (BN) rats injected with nontoxic amounts of $HgCl_2$ (100 μg/100 g body weight three times a week) develop an immunologically mediated disease (13–23) characterized by a T cell-dependent B cell polyclonal activation, which is responsible for the impressive increase in serum IgE concentration (from less than 10 μg/ml up to 5 mg/ml), for the production of many antibodies directed against exogenous elements [e.g., trinitrophenyl (TNP) and red blood cells] and autoantibodies [e.g., deoxyribonucleic acid (DNA), laminin, and other elements of glomerular basement membrane (GBM) antibodies such as collagen IV, entactin, thyroglobulin, and myeloperoxidase]. The disease is characterized by a glomerulopathy evolving in two phases: first, linear anti-GBM antibody deposition along the glomerular capillary pattern, and second, a change in the pattern of immunofluorescence with the appearance of granular glomerular IgG deposits. This second phase corresponds to what is found in patients with Hg-induced membranous glomerulopathy. Clinically, rats exhibit an abnormal proteinuria frequently associated with a nephrotic syndrome but there is no renal failure (14,15). Rats also develop a mucositis, Sjögren's syndrome (19), and a vasculitis in the gut (23) that is associated with anti-myeloperoxidase antibodies (22). The B cell polyclonal activation does not affect all B cell clones, because, for example, anti-myelin basic protein antibodies are not found during the Hg disease. The role for T cells in targeting autoimmunity has been well demonstrated; thus BN rats deprived of T cells either genetically or after adult thymectomy, lethal irradiation, and reconstitution with fetal liver cells are completely protected from Hg-induced autoimmunity (24). In addition, transfer of T cells from diseased BN rats into naive syngeneic BN rats induced a mild form of autoimmunity. If recipients are depleted also of CD8+ suppressor/cytotoxic cells with an anti-CD8 monoclonal antibody, the disease is marked with an increase in serum IgE concentration to around 700 μg/ml, circulating and kidney-bound anti-GBM antibodies, as well as a significant proteinuria (25). This shows that (a) T cells from Hg-exposed animals were responsible for autoimmunity, that (b) they may cooperate with normal syngeneic B cells for antibody production, and (c) they initiate a regulatory circuit implying CD8+ suppressor cells.

Several points are of interest:

1. The genetic control of susceptibility to Hg-induced autoimmunity.
2. The influence of route, of dosage, and of the chemical form of Hg compounds in the occurrence of the disease.
3. The way by which this disease can be modulated since this disease resembles by some features anti-GBM antibody-mediated glomerulonephritis in humans.

Genetic Control

The susceptibility to Hg-induced autoimmunity is genetically controlled (Table 1) (26–28) and some strains such as LEW rats are completely resistant even when rats are injected with high doses (400 μg/100 g body weight instead of 100). Some strains such as BN (26,28) or MAXX (29) rats develop linear IgG deposits along the glomerular capillary wall, while others such as DZB rats only develop a membranous glomerulopathy. It is interesting to note that $HgCl_2$ induces a B cell polyclonal activation in both BN (15–18) and DZB rats (30), though these two strains exhibit two different types of glomerulopathies. In addition, in the two strains, there is a tremendous increase in serum IgE concentration. Susceptibility depends on three or four genes, depending on the parameter looked for, one of which is major histocompatibility complex (MHC)-linked. The development of histologic lesions is inherited as a dominant trait, while it is suggested that the development of proteinuria in rats that possess genes for Hg-induced susceptibility requires homo-

TABLE 1. *Genetic control of susceptibility to mercury-induced autoimmunity*

Strain	RT1 haplotype	Autoimmune nephritis
BN, MAXX	n	Anti-GBM GN, ICGN
DZB	u	ICGN
LEW, AS, BS, ...	l	None
(BN × LEW)F1	n/l	Anti-GBM GN, ICGN
BN.1L	n	None
LEW.1N	l	None
(BN.1L × LEW.1N)F1	l/n	Anti-GBM GN, ICGN
LOU, WAG	u	None
Wistar Furth	u	ICGN
AUG	c	ICGN

Anti-GBM GN, anti-glomerular basement membrane antibody-mediated glomerulonephritis; ICGN, immune complex type glomerulonephritis.

TABLE 2. *Genetic control of mercury-induced glomerulopathy*

Strain	RT1 genes	Non-RT1 genes	Anti-GBM Ab response	Type of GN	Abnormal proteinuria
BN	n	B	+ + +	Anti-GBM/ICGN	+ + +
LEW	l	L	–	—	–
(BN × LEW) F1	n/l	B/L	+ +	Anti-GBM/ICGN	–
(BN.1L × LEW.1N) F1	n/l	B/L	+ +	Anti-GBM/ICGN	–
(BN × LEW.1N) F1	n	B/L	+ + +	Anti-GBM/ICGN	+ + +
(BN × BN.1L) F1	n/l	B	+ + +	Anti-GBM/ICGN	+ + +
(LEW × LEW.1N) F1	n/l	L	–	—	–
MAXX	n	B + L	+ + +	Anti-GBM/ICGN	+ +
AO	u	A	–	ICGN	–
(AO × BN) F1	u/n	A/B	+ +	Anti-GBM/ICGN	+ +
DZB	u	A + B	+ +	ICGN	+ +

Non-RT1 genes from BN (B), LEW (L), or AO (A) rats. Anti-GBM, anti-glomerular basement membrane antibody-mediated glomerulonephritis (GN); ICGN, immune complex type GN.

zygosity for one gene of the RT1 complex and at least one gene of the non-RT1 background (Table 2) (28). The development of $HgCl_2$-induced immune complex type glomerulonephritis in the absence of linear deposition of anti-GBM antibodies is also genetically determined and one gene is linked to MHC class II molecules (28). Thus AO strain (RT1-u) is susceptible while AO.1P congenic rats differing from the former at the RT1B and RT1D loci (l) are resistant. The fact that $HgCl_2$-injected DZB rats (RT1-u) develop a significant proteinuria while AO rats do not could be related to the presence of non-RT1 genes of BN origin in the former strain.

Mode of Administration

$HgCl_2$ given intravenously, orally, or intratracheally induces the disease in a similar way (31). Exposure to Hg vapor also induces the autoimmune disease in BN rats (32). Methylmercury or pharmaceutical ointments and solutions containing organic Hg are effective even when these products were applied on wounds or on normal skin (33).

In the susceptible strain, the effects of $HgCl_2$ depend on dosage (14; Pelletier L. *unpublished data*). Thus the increase in serum IgE concentration is positively correlated with the dosage and this parameter is less well regulated for low doses (Fig. 1). Serum IgE concentrations of rats injected with low doses (5 or 10 μg/100 g body weight thrice a week) exhibit kinetics with multiple waves (Fig. 1).

Modulation of the Disease

$HgCl_2$-induced autoimmunity in BN rats is easily prevented and cured by immunosuppressive agents such as cyclosporin A (34,35) and cyclophosphamide (36,37) even administered for a short period (days 0 to 10) after initiating $HgCl_2$ injections.

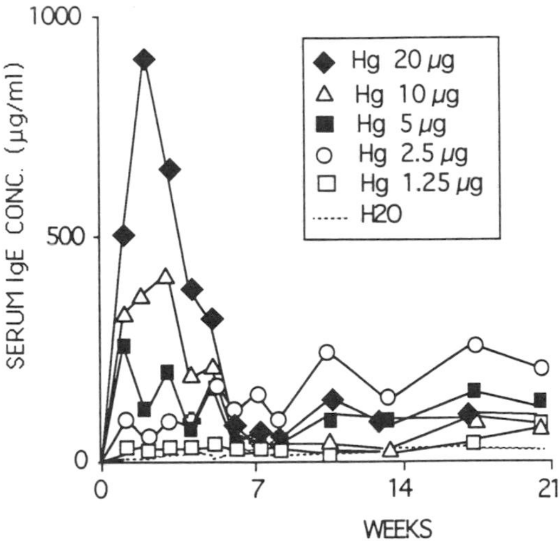

FIG. 1. Kinetics of serum IgE concentration in BN rats injected with various doses of $HgCl_2$ (from 20 to 1.25 μg/100 g body weight thrice weekly) or control solution (H_2O).

In addition, cyclosporin A-pretreated rats become unresponsive to $HgCl_2$ for more than 5 weeks (35); lymphoid cells cannot transfer the protective effect and unresponsiveness is broken by injection of naive syngeneic lymphoid cells. This suggests that protection against the disease is associated with a functional inactivation of pathogenic T cells. Transplantation of a spleen from BN rats injected with $HgCl_2$ for 15 days into naive recipients completely prevents the appearance of the disease when $HgCl_2$ injections are begun 2 months later (38), suggesting that in these models, as in other models of autoimmunity (39–44), it is possible to vaccinate against the disease by injecting "attenuated" autoreactive T cells.

$HgCl_2$-Induced Autoimmunity in Other Species

Hg-induced nephritis has been described also in mice and rabbits (45–48). Thus Roman-Franco et al. (48) have described in rabbits a disease resembling that described in BN rats with an anti-GBM-mediated glomerulopathy. In mice, it has been shown that Hg is not present in the glomeruli (47) and these findings are in agreement with recent data (Pelletier L. *unpublished data*) in BN rats injected with $HgCl_2$ obtained by staining kidney sections with an anti-Hg monoclonal antibody (49). Some strains of mice given $HgCl_2$ produce antinuclear antibodies (50–52); MHC-linked genes play an important role in this response and H-2^s mice are particularly susceptible. H-2^s mice also develop a polyclonal B cell activation with an increase in serum IgG and IgE concentrations (53). Some strains develop a glomerulopathy; BALB/c mice develop mesangial IgG deposits (45–47) and antinuclear antibodies have been recovered from the kidneys (47). Other authors have shown that $HgCl_2$-injected BALB/c mice present subepithelial deposits, produce anti-gp-330 antibodies and are proteinuric (54).

Nature and Specificity of T Cells Involved in Mercury-Induced Autoimmunity

Autoreactive CD4+ cells are detected in BN rats as early as days 4 to 6. T cells from $HgCl_2$-injected BN rats proliferate in the presence of B cells exposed to the toxin or of B cells from normal BN rats, and in both cases the proliferation is blocked when stimulator cells are preincubated with an anti-class II monoclonal antibody (55,56). Thus native as well as $HgCl_2$-modified class II molecules can stimulate T cells. It is possible that there is only one autoreactive T cell population. In this case, even if induced *in vivo* by a modification of class II molecules, these anti-class II T cells recognize and are activated by cells whether they express native or "modified" class II molecules. Alternatively, it cannot be excluded that specific anti-Hg T cells and autoreactive anti-class II T cells are present together. Indeed, it has been suggested that $HgCl_2$ may induce the former cells in mice (57).

At this time, we do not know if these autoreactive T cells recognize empty MHC class II molecules or, as is more likely, a self-peptide in the groove of the MHC class II molecule. Indeed, empty class II molecules would not be stable enough to persist at the cell membrane while the association of a peptide with a class II molecule would allow it. It has been shown functionally or even chemically that self-peptides are constitutively expressed in self-class II molecules (58,59) such as peptides derived from class II molecules themselves (59,60). It has recently been reported that an autoreactive T cell clone recognizes a DR1-derived peptide expressed by DR1 molecules (60); thus it cannot be excluded that $HgCl_2$–induced anti-class II T cells recognize a peptide from MHC class II molecules presented by the intact class II molecule.

In mice, humans, and probably rats, CD4+ T cells can be divided into two subsets of T helper (T_H) cells: T_H1 and T_H2 cells (61,62). T_H1 cells produce interleukin-2 (IL-2), interferon-γ (IFN-γ), and tumor necrosis factor-β (TNF-β) and use IL-2 as a growth factor; they are responsible mainly for delayed-type hypersensitivity reactions and can cooperate with B cells for antibodies of the IgG2a isotype in mice. T_H2 cells produce IL-4, IL-5, IL-6, and IL-10 and can use IL-2 or IL-4 as growth factors; they are mainly involved in B cell help and particularly in antibodies of the IgA, IgG1, and IgE isotypes. Each subset downregulates the other one. $HgCl_2$ activates preferentially T_H2 cells in BN rats (63). Indeed, $HgCl_2$ induces an increase in the expression of MHC class II molecules on B cells (64) and messenger ribonucleic acid (mRNA) for IL-4 has been detected in lymphocytes from BN rats injected with $HgCl_2$ (Sanedi A *unpublished data*). In addition, in mice susceptible to Hg-induced autoimmunity, treatment with an anti-IL-4 monoclonal antibody partially prevents the disease (65). One reason that could explain the preferential activation of T_H2 cells to the detriment of T_H1 cells is that $HgCl_2$ depletes cells of free cysteine and of the reduced form of gluthathione, groups that play an important role in the production and the responsiveness to IL-2 by T cells (66). Thus T_H2 cells that can be IL-2 independent would be favored. Interestingly, the effects of depletion in reduced glutathione are much less important in LEW rats as judged by the capacity of lymphocytes from $HgCl_2$-injected LEW rats to produce IFN-γ in response to a T cell mitogen.

How Are Anti-Class II T Cells Induced?

In the normal situation, it is admitted that autoreactive clones are deleted and/or anergized (67–73). However, at least potential autoreactive clones persist at the periphery but their affinity is low and they do not induce B cell activation (67,68). $HgCl_2$ could increase this affinity by binding to class II molecules or to the T cell receptor or both (Fig. 2). $HgCl_2$ could also increase gene expression of molecules involved in the presentation of self-peptides, or in T or B cell activation/differentiation. This could explain the increase in the expression of class II molecules on B cells induced by $HgCl_2$ (64,74). In any case, the increase in the affinity of the autoreactive anti-class II T cells for B cells could lead to activation, proliferation, and differentiation of B cells. The fact that these autoreactive cells are probably T_H2 would also favor their role in B cell differentiation. T cell lines from BN rats injected with $HgCl_2$ have recently been derived that will allow researchers to dissect the part of autoreactive T cells in B cell activation and in the disease.

Mercury-Induced Glomerulopathy

Antinuclear antibodies have been found in PVG/c rats injected with $HgCl_2$ (75,76) and have been eluted from kidneys (76); similar results have been obtained in BALB/c mice injected with $HgCl_2$. In BN (77,78) and in DZB (30) rats, anti-laminin antibodies are probably responsible for the glomerulopathy (Table 3). In BN rats, it has recently been strongly suggested that anti-laminin antibodies are responsible for both the linear and the granular pattern in immunofluorescence (38). It has been proposed that autoantibodies to GBM components may bind transiently in a linear pattern to the interface of GBM with epithelial cells, which would be followed by redistribution of these complexes (77,79), perhaps because deposition of antibodies causes a hyperproduction of the GBM component. The modification of the interaction between GBM and epithelial cells would lead to a loss of functional integrity of the filtration barrier and proteinuria.

Mercury-Induced Autoregulation

Multiple factors are probably involved in Hg-induced autoregulation and it is possible that only one of them being present is sufficient to achieve it (Table 4).

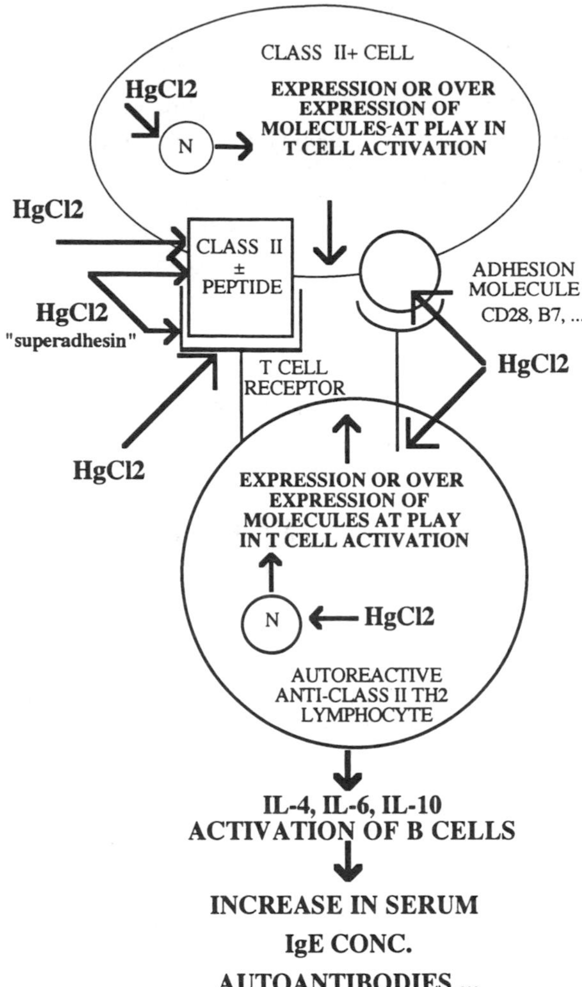

FIG. 2. Putative mechanisms that may activate normally silent autoreactive anti-MHC self-class II T cells in BN rats. $HgCl_2$ increases the affinity of the T cell receptor (Ψ) of an autoreactive anti-class II for the self-class II MHC molecule or a self-peptide associated with the MHC class II molecule (□). It could act directly by binding at least one of these molecules. It could also act by binding adhesion molecules (Ψ, ○) that would lead to the delivery of a costimulatory signal. Finally, it cannot be excluded that $HgCl_2$ acts by increasing expression of a gene implicated in cell activation/proliferation and/or differentiation.

CD8+ suppressor cells able to inhibit autoreactive cells have been described concomitantly with improvement of rats (56,80) but depletion of CD8+ cells does not prevent regulation (81,82). However, such a treatment renders convalescent rats more susceptible to rechallenge with $HgCl_2$ (82), showing that suppressor cells play an important role in acquired resistance to $HgCl_2$-induced autoimmunity. Anti-id-

TABLE 3. *Possible explanations for an anti-laminin antibody-mediated glomerulopathy in $HgCl_2$-injected BN rats*

A low threshold of activation of anti-laminin autoreactive B cells in BN rats favors anti-laminin antibody production.
$HgCl_2$ increases the metabolism of laminin and of other components of extracellular matrix (metalloproteinases?) that favors activation of anti-laminin lymphocytes.
Activated T cells and/or macrophages release cytokines modifying vascular permeability and favoring the development of glomerulopathy.

iotypic antibodies have also been demonstrated (83,84) but their role has not been proved. The decrease in the frequency of autoreactive T cells (56) could be due either to death or functional inactivation of cells. Finally, it has recently been shown that there is a change in the balance of T_H1/T_H2 at the time of recovery with emergence of T_H1 cells. Indeed, this phase is associated with the production of INF-γ (J. Aten, *personal communication*) and a better capacity to produce IL-2 in response to various stimuli than normal BN rats (L. Pelletier, *unpublished data*). Moreover, treatment of BN rats with an anti-IL-2 receptor monoclonal antibody, that impairs preferentially T_H1 cells, delays the return of serum IgE concentration to normal values (85).

EFFECTS OF $HgCl_2$ IN LEW RATS

LEW rats injected with $HgCl_2$ do not exhibit autoimmunity and develop a non-antigen-specific immunosuppression (86). This immunosuppression is mediated by non-antigen-specific suppressor T cells responsible for a depression of T cell functions and a protection against organ-specific autoimmune diseases such as Heymann's nephritis (87) or experimental autoimmune encephalomyelitis (EAE) (88). In the latter case, it has been shown that suppressor cells are CD8+ since treatment of $HgCl_2$-injected LEW rats immunized with myelin and treated with an anti-CD8 monoclonal antibody (mAb) completely abrogates protection (89). As demonstrated by limiting dilution analysis in this model, non-antigen-specific suppressor cells are very frequent (around 1/1000 lymphocytes) when compared to the frequency of autoreactive anti-myelin T cells (around 1/10,000) (90). This shows that, in LEW rats, $HgCl_2$ does not affect activation of myelin-specific autoreactive cells but acts

TABLE 4. *Spontaneous regulation of mercury-induced autoimmunity*

Suppressor cells: resistance to rechallenge
Idiotypic network: anti-idiotypic antibodies and/or T cells
Decrease in the frequency of autoreactive T cells
Change in the balance of T_H1/T_H2 autoreactive T cells

thereafter. Curiously, in spite of a high frequency of suppressor cells, 20% of rats injected with $HgCl_2$ and immunized with myelin are not protected; this is probably due to the emergence of contrasuppressor cells that allow some autoreactive cells to escape suppression (their frequency is around 1/10,000 lymphocytes) (90). It is tempting to speculate that these contrasuppressor cells represent a homeostatic response to an increase in the frequence of suppressor cells.

Resistance of LEW rats to Hg-induced autoimmunity is neither due to CD8+ suppressor cells since treatment with an anti-CD8 mAb does not trigger autoimmunity (81) nor due to an absence of autoreactive T cells since $HgCl_2$ triggers autoreactive anti-self-class II T cells as frequently as in BN rats (91). It could be due to a difference in the nature of the autoreactive T cells between the two strains: they could belong to the T_H1 subtype in LEW rats and to the T_H2 subtype in BN rats. We have derived a CD4+ anti-self-class II T cell line from $HgCl_2$-injected LEW rats that is probably of the T_H1 subtype and that acts as a suppressor/inducer line since it protects from active EAE by the bias of suppressor CD8+ cells (91). These suppressor cells resemble the so-called anti-ergotypic suppressor cells (92) that recognize a marker of activation of T cells and that have been described in models of T cell vaccination. It remains to be determined if these cells suppress via a direct interaction with the cell to be suppressed or if cytokines such as transforming growth factor-β (TGF-β) (93) are at play. Development of suppressor lines would permit an answer. In any case, $HgCl_2$-induced suppressor cells could represent an exacerbation of a physiologic process in which such suppressor cells generated after any immunization would limit the immune response.

CONCLUSIONS

Experimental models of drug-induced immune dysregulation have allowed an understanding of the mechanisms that underlie some toxin-induced nephropathies in humans. In these models, it has been shown that $HgCl_2$ and some other toxins may break down tolerance to anti-MHC class II autoreactive T cells. More interestingly, depending on the strain, anti-class II T cell-mediated autoreactivity will result in an autoimmune disease or in an immunosuppression and this is probably due to the fact that, in the first case, these T cells would be of the T_H2 subtype while in the second case, they would be of the T_H1 subtype.

REFERENCES

1. Fillastre JP, Druet P, Méry JP. Proteinuria associated with drugs and substances of abuse. In: Cameron JS, Glassock RJ, eds. *The nephrotic syndrome*. New York: Marcel Dekker; 1988:697–744.
2. Berlin M. Mercury. In: Friberg L, Nordberg GF, Vouk VB, eds. *Handbook on the toxicology of metals*. Amsterdam: Elsevier; 1986:387–445.
3. Clarkson TW, Hursh JB, Sager PR, Syversen TLM. Mercury. In: Clarkson TW, Friberg L, Nordberg GF, Sager PR, eds. *Biological monitoring of toxic metals*. New York: Plenum Press; 1988: 199–246.

4. Byrne L. Brazil' s mercury poisoning disaster. *Br Med J* 1992;304:1397–1399.
5. Weiner JA, Nylander M, Berglund F. Does mercury from amalgam restorations constitute a health hazard? *Sci Total Environ* 1990;99:1–22.
6. Kibukamusoke JW, Davies DE, Hutt MSR. Membranous nephropathy due to skin lightening cream. *Br Med J* 1974;2:646–647.
7. Halbach S, Ballatori N, Clarkson TW. Mercury vapor uptake and hydrogen peroxide detoxification in human and mouse red blood cells. *Toxicol Appl Pharmacol* 1988;96:517–524.
8. Lind B, Friberg L, Nylander M. Preliminary studies on methylmercury biotransformation and clearance in the brain of primates: II Demethylation of mercury in brain. *J Trace Elem Exp* 1988;1:49–56.
9. Levin M, Jacobs J, Polos PG. Acute mercury poisoning and mercurial pneumonitis from gold ore purification. *Chest* 1988;94:554–556.
10. Lindqvist KY, Makene WJ, Shaba JK, Nantulya V. Immunofluorescence and electron microscopic studies of kidney biopsies from patients with nephrotic syndrome possibly induced by skin lightening creams containing mercury. *East Afr Med J* 1974;51:168–169.
11. Lauwerys R, Bernard A, Roels H, Buchet JP, Gennart JP, Mahieu P, Foidart JM. Anti-laminin antibodies in workers exposed to mercury vapour. *Toxicol Lett* 1983;17:113–116.
12. Bernard AM, Roels HR, Foidart JM, Lauwerys RL. Search for anti-laminin antibodies in the serum of workers exposed to cadmium, mercury vapour or lead. *Int Arch Occup Environ Health* 1987; 59:303–309.
13. Sapin C, Druet E, Druet P. Induction of anti-glomerular basement membrane antibodies in the Brown-Norway rat by mercuric chloride. *Clin Exp Immunol* 1977;28:173–178.
14. Druet P, Druet E, Potdevin F, Sapin C. Immune type glomerulonephritis induced by $HgCl_2$ in the Brown-Norway rat. *Ann Immunol (Inst Pasteur)* 1978;129C:777–792.
15. Bellon B, Capron M, Druet E, et al. Mercuric chloride-induced autoimmunity in Brown Norway rats: sequential search for anti-basement membrane antibodies. *Eur J Clin Invest* 1982;12:127–133.
16. Prouvgst-Danon A, Abadie A, Sapin C, Bazin H, Druet P. Induction of IgE synthesis and potentiation of anti-ovalbumin IgE response by $HgCl_2$ in the rat. *J Immunol* 1981;126:699–702.
17. Hirsch F, Couderc J, Sapin C, Fournie G, Druet P. Polyclonal effect of $HgCl_2$ in the rat, its possible role in an experimental autoimmune disease. *Eur J Immunol* 1982;12:620–625.
18. Pelletier L, Pasquier R, Guettier C, et al. $HgCl_2$ induces T and B cells to proliferate and differentiate in BN rats. *Clin Exp Immunol* 1988;71:336–342.
19. Aten J, Bosman CB, Rozing J, Stjnen T, Hoedemaeker PJ, Weening JJ. Mercuric chloride-induced autoimmunity in the Brown Norway rat. Cellular kinetics and major histocompatibility complex antigen expression. *Am J Pathol* 1988;133:127–138.
20. Pusey CD, Bowman C, Morgan A, Weetman AP, Hartley B, Lockwood CM. Kinetics and pathogenicity of autoantibodies induced by mercuric chloride in the Brown Norway rat. *Clin Exp Med* 1990;81:76–82.
21. Prummel B, Aten J, Bosman C, Van der Wal AM, Hoedemaeker PJ, Weening JJ. Modulation by cyclosporin A (Cy A) of toxin-induced autoimmune reactions and glomerulonephritis in the Brown-Norway rat (BN). *Kidney Int* 1985;28:696.
22. Esnault VLM, Mathieson PW, Thiru S, Oliveira DBG, Lockwood CM. Autoantibodies to myeloperoxidase in Brown Norway rats treated with mercuric chloride. *Lab Invest* 1992;67:114–120.
23. Mathieson PW, Thiru S, Oliveira DBG. Mercuric chloride-treated Brown-Norway rats develop widespread tissue injury including necrotizing vasculitis. *Lab Invest* 1992;67:121–129.
24. Pelletier L, Pasquier R, Vial MC, Mandet C, Moutier R, Salomon JC, Druet P. Mercury-induced autoimmune glomerulonephritis. Requirement for T cells. *Nephrol Dial Transplant* 1987;1:211–218.
25. Pelletier L, Pasquier R, Rossert J, Vial MC, Mandet C, Druet, P. Autoreactive T cells in mercury disease. Ability to induce the autoimmune disease. *J Immunol* 1988;140:750–754.
26. Druet E, Sapin C, Günther E, Feingold N, Druet P. Mercuric chloride induced anti-glomerular basement membrane antibodies in the rat. Genetic control. *Eur J Immunol* 1977;7:348–351.
27. Sapin C, Mandet C, Druet E, Günther E, Druet P. Immune complex type disease induced by $HgCl_2$ in the Brown-Norway rat. Genetic control of susceptibility. *Clin Exp Immunol* 1982;48:700–702.
28. Aten J, Veninga A, de Heer E, Rozing J, Nieuwenhuis P, Hodemaeker P, Weening JJ. Susceptibility to the induction of either autoimmunity or immunosuppression by mercuric chloride is related to the MHC haplotype. *Eur J Immunol* 1991;21:611–616.
29. Henry GA, Jarnot BM, Steinhoff MM, Bigazzi PE. Mercury-induced renal autoimmunity in the MAXX rat. *Clin Immunol Immunopathol* 1992;49:187–203.

30. Aten J, Veninga A, Bruijn JA, Prins FA, De Heer E, Weening JJ. Antigenic specificities of glomerular-bound autoantibodies in membranous glomerulopathy induced by mercuric chloride. *Clin Immunol Immunopathol* 1992;63:89–102.
31. Bernaudin JF, Druet E, Druet P, Masse P. Inhalation or ingestion of organic or inorganic mercurials produces autoimmune disease in rats. *Clin Immunol Immunopathol* 1981;20:129–135.
32. Hua J, Pelletier L, Berlin M, Druet P. Autoimmune glomerulonephritis induced by mercury vapour exposure in the Brown-Norway rat. *Toxicology* 1993;79:119–129.
33. Druet P, Teychenne P, Mandet C, Bascou C, Druet P. Immune type glomerulonephritis induced in the Brown-Norway rat with mercury containing pharmaceutical products. *Nephron* 1981;28:145–148.
34. Baran D, Vendeville B, Vial MC, Bascou C, Cosson C, Teychenne P, Druet P. Effect of cyclosporin A on mercury-induced autoimmune glomerulonephritis in the Brown-Norway rat. *Clin Nephrol* 1986;25:S175–S180.
35. Aten J, Bosman CB, De Heer E, Hoedemaeker PJ, Weening JJ. Cyclosporin A induces long-term unresponsiveness in mercuric chloride induced autoimmune glomerulonephritis. *Clin Exp Immunol* 1988;73:307–311.
36. Pusey CD, Bowman C, Peters DK, Lockwood CM. Effects of cyclophosphamide on autoantibody synthesis in the Brown Norway rat. *Clin Exp Immunol* 1983;54:697–704.
37. Pelletier L, Pasquier R, Vial MC, Mandet C, Hirsch F, Druet P. Effect of methylprednisolone and cyclophosphamide in mercury-induced autoimmune glomerulonephritis. *Nephrol Dial Transplant* 1987;2:2–9.
38. Icard P, Pelletier L, Vial MC, Mandet C, Pasquier R, Michel A, Druet P. Evidence for a role of antilaminin-producing B cell clones that escape tolerance in the pathogenesis of $HgCl_2$-induced membranous glomerulopathy. *Nephrol Dial Transplant* 1993;8:122–127.
39. Cohen IR. Regulation of autoimmune disease. Physiological and therapeutic. *Immunol Rev* 1986; 94:5–36.
40. Lider O, Karin N, Shinitzky M, Cohen IR. Therapeutic vaccination against adjuvant arthritis using autoimmune T cells treated with hydrostatic pressure. *Proc Natl Acad Sci USA* 1987;84:4577–4580.
41. Lider O, Reshef T, Beraud E, Ben-Nun AA, Cohen IR. Anti-idiotypic network induced by T cell vaccination against experimental autoimmune encephalomyelitis. *Science* 1988;239:181–183.
42. Sun D, Ben-Nun A, Wekerle H. Regulatory circuits in autoimmunity: recruitment of counterregulatory CD8+ T cells by encephalitogenic CD4+ T cell line cells. *Eur J Immunol* 1988;18:193–199.
43. Jingwu Z, Schreurs M, Medaer R, Raus JCM. Regulation of myelin basic-protein-specific helper T cells in multiple sclerosis: generation of suppressor T cell lines. *Cell Immunol* 1992;139:118–130.
44. Lohse AW, Mor E, Reshef T, Meyer zum Büschenfelde KH, Cohen IR. Inhibition of mixed lymphocyte reaction by T cell vaccination. *Eur J Immunol* 1990;20:2521–2524.
45. Eneström S, Hultman P. Immune-mediated glomerulonephritis induced by mercuric chloride in mice. *Experientia* 1984;40:1234–1240.
46. Hultman P, Eneström S. The induction of immune complex deposits in mice by peroral and parenteral administration of mercuric chloride: strain dependent susceptibility. *Clin Exp Immunol* 1987; 67:283–292.
47. Hultman P, Eneström S. Mercury-induced antinuclear antibodies in mice: characterization and correlation with renal immune complex deposits. *Clin Exp Immunol* 1988;71:269–274.
48. Roman-Franco AA, Turiello M, Albini B, Ossi E, Milgrom F, Andres GA. Anti-basement membrane antibodies and antigen–antibody complex in rabbits injected with mercuric chloride. *Clin Immunol Immunopathol* 1978;9:464–481.
49. Wylie DE, Lu D, Carlson LD, Carlson R, Babacan KF, Schuster SM, Wagner FW. Monoclonal antibodies specific for mercuric ions. *Proc Natl Acad Sci USA* 1992;89:4104–4108.
50. Robinson CJG, Abraham AA, Balazs T. Induction of anti-nuclear antibodies by mercuric chloride in mice. *Clin Exp Immunol* 1984;58:300–306.
51. Robinson CJG, Balazs T, Egorov IK. Mercuric chloride, gold sodium thiomalate, and D-penicillamine-induced anti-nuclear antibodies in mice. *Toxicol Appl Pharmacol* 1986;86:156–169.
52. Mirtcheva J, Pfeiffer C, Bruijn JA, Jaquesmart F, Gleichmann E. Immunological alterations induced by mercury compounds. III. H-2A acts as an immune response and H-2E as an immune "suppression" locus for $HgCl_2$-induced anti-nucleolar autoantibodies. *Eur J Immunol* 1989;19: 2257–2261.
53. Pietsch P, Vohr HW, Degitz K, Gleichmann E. Immunopathological signs inducible by mercury compounds. II. $HgCl_2$ and gold sodium thiomalate enhance serum IgE and IgG concentrations in susceptible mouse strains. *Int Arch Allergy Appl Immunol* 1989;90:47–53.

54. Fleuren GJ, de Heer E, Van Burgers J, Osnabrugge C, Hoedemaeker PJ. Mercuric chloride-induced glomerulopathy in Balb/c mice. *Kidney Int* 1985;28:702.
55. Pelletier L, Pasquier R, Hirsch F, Sapin C, Druet P. Autoreactive T cells in mercury-induced autoimmune disease: in vitro demonstration. *J Immunol* 1986;137:2548–2554.
56. Rossert J, Pelletier L, Pasquier R, Druet P. Autoreactive T cells in mercury-induced autoimmune disease. Demonstration by limiting dilution analysis. *Eur J Immunol* 1988;18:1761–1766.
57. Gleichmann E, Vohr HW, Stringer C, Nuyens J, Gleichmann H. Testing the sensitization of T cells to chemicals. From murine graft-versus-host (GVH) reactions to chemical-induced GVH-like immunological diseases. In: Kammüller ME, Bloksma N, Seinen W, eds. *Autoimmunity and toxicology*. Amsterdam: Elsevier; 1989:363–390.
58. Lorenz RG, Allen PM. Direct evidence for functional self-protein/Ia molecule complexes in vivo. *Proc Natl Acad Sci USA* 1988;85:5220–5223.
59. Rudensky AY, Preston-Hurlbut P, Hong S-C, Barlow A, Janeway CA Jr. Sequence analysis of peptides bound to MHC class II molecules. *Nature* 1991;353:622–627.
60. Liu Z, Sun Y-K, Xi Y-P, Harris P, Suciu Foca N. T cell recognition of self-human histocompatibility leukocyte antigens (HLA)-DR molecules. *J Exp Med* 1992;175:1663–1668.
61. Mosmann TR, Cherwinski H, Bond MW, Giedlin MA, Coffman RL. Two types of murine helper T cell clones I. Definition according to profiles of lymphokine activities and secreted proteins. *J Immunol* 1986;136:2348–2357.
62. Mosmann TR, Coffman RL. Heterogeneity of cytokine suppression patterns and functions of helper T cells. *Adv Immunol* 1989;46:111–147.
63. Dubey C, Bellon B, Druet P. TH1 and TH2 dependent cytokines in experimental autoimmunity and immune reactions induced by chemicals. *Eur Cytokine Netw* 1991;2:147–152.
64. Dubey C, Bellon B, Hirsch F, Kuhn J, Vial MC, Goldman M, Druet P. Increased expression of class II major histocompatibility complex molecules on B cells in rats susceptible or resistant to $HgCl_2$-induced autoimmunity. *Clin Exp Immunol* 1991;86:118–123.
65. Ochel M, Vohr HW, Pfeiffer C, Gleichmann E. IL-4 is required for the IgE and IgG1 increase and IgG1 autoantibody formation in mice treated with mercuric chloride. *J Immunol* 1991;146:3006–3011.
66. Van der Meide PH, de Labie MCDC, Botman CAD, van Bennekom WP, Olsson T, Aten J, Weening JJ. Mercuric chloride downregulates T cell interferon-gamma production in Brown Norway but not in Lewis rats; role of glutathione. *Eur J Immunol* 1993;23:675–681.
67. Nossal GJV. Immunologic tolerance: collaboration between antigen and lymphokines. *Science* 1989;245:147–153.
68. Gill RG, Haskins K. Molecular mechanisms underlying diabetes and other autoimmune diseases. *Immunol Today* 1993;14:49–51.
69. Kappler JW, Roehm N, Marrack P. T cell tolerance by clonal elimination in the thymus. *Cell* 1987;49:273–280.
70. Ramsdell F, Lantz T, Fowlkes BJ. A nondeletional mechanism of thymic self tolerance. *Science* 1989;246:1038–1041.
71. Jones LA, Chin LT, Longo DL, Kruisbeek AM. Peripheral clonal elimination of functional T cells. *Science* 1990;250:1726–1729.
72. Lo D, Freedman J, Hesse S, Brinster RL, Sherman L. Peripheral tolerance in transgenic mice: tolerance to class II MHC and non-MHC transgene antigens. *Immunol Rev* 1991;122:87–102.
73. Jenkins MK. The role of division in the induction of clonal anergy. *Immunol Today* 1992;13:69–73.
74. McCabe M, Lawrence DA. The heavy metal lead exhibits B cell-stimulatory factor by enhancing B cell Ia expression and differentiation. *J Immunol* 1990;145:671–677.
75. Weening JJ, Fleuren GJ, Hoedemaeker PJ. I. Demonstration of anti-nuclear antibodies in mercury-induced glomerulopathy in the rat. *Lab Invest* 1978;39:405–411.
76. Weening JJ, Hoedemaeker PJ, Bakker WW. Immunoregulation and anti-nuclear antibodies in mercury-induced glomerulopathy in the rat. *Clin Exp Immunol* 1981;45:64–71.
77. Fukatsu A, Brentjens JR, Killen PD, Kleinman HK, Martin GR, Andres GA. Studies on the formation of glomerular immune deposits in rats injected with mercuric chloride. *Clin Immunol Immunopathol* 1987;45:35–47.
78. Makker SP, Kanalas JJ. Renal antigens in mercuric chloride induced anti-GBM autoantibody glomerular disease. *Kidney Int* 1990;37:64–71.
79. Bruijn JA, Hoedemaeker PJ, Fleuren GJ. Biology of disease. Pathogenesis of anti-basement membrane glomerulopathy and immune-complex glomerulonephritis: dichotomy dissolved. *Lab Invest* 1989;61:480–488.

80. Bowman C, Mason DW, Pusey CD, Lockwood CM. Autoregulation of autoantibody synthesis in mercuric chloride in the Brown Norway rat I. A role for T suppressor cells. *Eur J Immunol* 1984; 14:464–470.
81. Pelletier L, Rossert J, Pasquier R, Vial MC, Druet P. Role of CD8+ T cells in mercury-induced autoimmunity or immunosuppression in the rat. *Scand J Immunol* 1990;30:65–74.
82. Mathieson PW, Stapleton K, Oliveira DBG, Lockwood CM. Immunoregulation of mercuric chloride-induced autoimmunity in Brown Norway rats: a role for CD8+ T cells revealed by in vivo depletion studies. *Eur J Immunol* 1991;21:2105–2109.
83. Chalopin JM, Lockwood CM. Autoregulation of autoantibody synthesis in mercuric chloride in the Brown Norway rat. II. Presence of antigen augmentable plaque forming cells in the spleen is associated with humoral factors behaving as auto-antiidiotypic antibodies. *Eur J Immunol* 1984;14:470–475.
84. Guéry JC, Druet P. A spontaneous hybridoma producing autoanti-idiotypic antibodies that recognize a V_κ-associated idiotope in mercury-induced autoimmunity. *Eur J Immunol* 1990;20:1027–1031.
85. Dubey C, Kuhn J, Vial MC, Druet P, Bellon B. Anti-interleukin 2 receptor monoclonal antibody therapy supports a role for TH1-like cells in $HgCl_2$-induced autoimmunity in rats. *Scand J Immunol* 1993;37:406–412.
86. Pelletier L, Pasquier R, Rossert J, Druet P. $HgCl_2$ induces nonspecific immunosuppression in LEW rats. *Eur J Immunol* 1987;17:49–54.
87. Pelletier L, Galceran M, Pasquier R, Ronco P, Verroust P, Bariety J, Druet P. Down-modulation of Heymann's nephritis by mercuric chloride. *Kidney Int* 1987;32:227–232.
88. Pelletier L, Rossert J, Pasquier R, et al. Effect of $HgCl_2$ on experimental allergic encephalomyelitis in Lewis rats. $HgCl_2$-induced down-modulation of the disease. *Eur J Immunol* 1988;18:243–247.
89. Rossert J, Pelletier L, Pasquier R, Villarroya H, Oriol R, Druet P. $HgCl_2$-induced perturbation of the T cell network in experimental allergic encephalomyelitis. I. Characterization of T cells involved. *Cell Immunol* 1991;137:367–378.
90. Pelletier L, Rossert J, Pasquier R, Villarroya H, Oriol R, Druet P. $HgCl_2$-induced perturbation of the T cell network in experimental allergic encephalomyelitis. II. In vivo demonstration of the role of T suppressor and contrasuppressor cells. *Cell Immunol* 1991;137:379–388.
91. Castedo M, Pelletier L, Rossert J, Pasquier R, Villarroya H, Druet P. Mercury-induced autoreactive anti class II T cell line protects from experimental autoimmune encephalomyelitis by the bias of antiergotypic cells in Lewis rats. *J Exp Med* 1993;177:881–889.
92. Lhose AW, Mor F, Karin N, Cohen IR. Control of experimental autoimmune encephalomyelitis by T cells responding to activated T cells. *Science* 1989;244:820–822.
93. Karpus WJ, Swanborg RH. CD4+ suppressor cells inhibit the function of effector cells of experimental autoimmune encephalomyelitis through a mechanism involving transforming growth factor-β. *J Immunol* 1991;146:1163–1168.

Immunotoxicology and Immunopharmacology, Second Edition, edited by J. H. Dean, M. I. Luster, A. E. Munson, and I. Kimber.
Raven Press, Ltd., New York © 1994.

32

Autoallergic Responses to Drugs

Mechanistic Aspects

John W. Coleman and *Edith Sim

*Department of Pharmacology and Therapeutics, University of Liverpool, Liverpool L69 3BX, United Kingdom; and *Department of Pharmacology, Oxford University, Oxford OX1 3QT, United Kingdom*

DRUG AUTOALLERGY IN PERSPECTIVE

The mechanisms underlying the majority of adverse drug reactions are reasonably well understood in terms of the known pharmacology or toxicology of the causative agent. We have a sound grasp, for example, of how paracetamol overdose causes liver damage, how aspirin and related drugs cause gut damage, and how corticosteroids induce metabolic disturbance. In addition, there are well-documented examples of drugs that interfere with the actions, metabolism, or clearance of another, and of individuals who may be predisposed to an "idiosyncratic" reaction due to abnormal receptor expression or genetic deficiency of a metabolizing enzyme (1). Other drugs (e.g., thalidomide) are toxic to the growing fetus. On the other side of the coin, a substantial minority of adverse drug reactions cannot be explained rationally from pharmacologic or toxicologic principles. Many of these, in terms of clinical symptoms and laboratory test results, appear to be mediated by or involve disruption of the immune system and are therefore loosely classified as "allergic." An allergic etiology is implicated in as many as 10% to 25% of all adverse drug reactions (2). With the possible exception of some immunoglobulin E (IgE) antibody-mediated reactions, we have a poor understanding of the mechanistic basis of allergic compared to direct toxic drug reactions. This reflects the additional layer of complexity introduced when having to consider the role of the immune system as an intermediary factor.

A distinction can be made between immunologically mediated adverse drug reactions that represent true *drug hypersensitivity* reactions and those that are *autoallergic* in nature. In drug hypersensitivity the adverse reaction occurs as a consequence of an immune response directed against the drug. Examples include immediate anaphylactic reactions mediated by IgE antibody directed against penicillins (3) or muscle relaxant anesthetics (4), or cell-mediated delayed skin reactions to topically applied medications (5). Drug hypersensitivity reactions and their underlying mechanisms have been reviewed extensively elsewhere (6–8) and are not covered here. In drug autoallergy, on the other hand, which is the subject of this chapter, the adverse reaction results from an immune response directed against the body's own tissue, cell, or plasma constituents. The autoallergic reaction may be either tissue specific, in which a particular tissue or cell type becomes the target for antibody-mediated toxicity, or tissue nonspecific, in which a universal subcellular (e.g., microsomal protein) or nuclear [e.g., deoxyribonucleic acid (DNA) or histone] constituent is targeted. This disease often resembles idiopathic systemic lupus erythematosus (SLE). Examples of tissue-specific reactions, which are discussed in more detail later, include quinidine-induced thrombocytopenia, penicillin- or methyldopa-induced hemolytic anemia, and severe halothane-induced hepatitis. Examples of tissue nonspecific reactions include SLE-like disorders induced by procainamide, hydralazine, phenytoin, methimazole, succinimides, carbamazapine, chlorpromazine, sulfonamides, and D-penicillamine (9).

With our current state of knowledge, it is not possible to predict which individuals are at risk of autoallergic reactions to which compounds. It is clear that there are likely to be many predisposing genetic factors and unidentified environmental factors in addition to the known environmental exposure to the drug itself. However, now that the mechanism of antigen processing and presentation is beginning to be unraveled, and effector mechanisms of immune clearance are better understood at the molecular level, these advances should provide an ideal springboard for defining how drugs interact with these processes to stimulate production of an autoallergic response. In this chapter we review the major types of autoallergic drug reactions from a mechanistic point of view, with reference to experimental and clinical evidence and specific drug examples.

CONCEPTS OF IMMUNOLOGIC TOLERANCE AND DRUG-INDUCED BREAKDOWN OF TOLERANCE

It is a central tenet of immunology that the immune system is able to recognize and mount a concerted and highly directed attack against foreign material but is tolerant toward the body's own constituents. However, immunologic tolerance to self is not absolute. Autoantibodies can be induced experimentally in animals and are seen in a number of human autoimmune diseases such as rheumatoid arthritis, SLE, and myasthenia gravis. Thus it is clear that mammals retain the capacity to mount an antibody response to self, but this response is suppressed in healthy individuals. The cellular basis of tolerance is that B lymphocytes with the capacity to produce autoantibodies are rendered nonfunctional through lack of an appropriate population of T helper (T_H) lymphocytes. Corecognition of chemically linked antigenic determinants by T and B cells is essential for T–B cell cooperation that leads to antibody synthesis (10,11). The unavailability of the anti-self T_H cell is believed to result from clonal deletion (12).

There is little evidence to suggest that drugs that cause autoallergy do so by acting directly on B cells (the antibody-producing lymphocytes) since nonspecific B cell activation has not been described. It is therefore considered more likely that drugs induce autoantibody production indirectly by activation of T cells (the B cell regulating lymphocytes). Activation of T cells could occur either by drug conjugation to self-proteins to induce new antigenic determinants, or by modification of T cells such that they are induced to respond to self. Several theoretical models implicating T cells as central to drug-induced autoallergy, together with supporting experimental and clinical evidence, are discussed later. A further concept, which we consider in some detail, is that drugs that cause systemic autoimmune disease, typified by SLE, might do so by inhibiting the clearance of immune complexes (that may occur naturally at low levels or may be partly drug-induced) by impairing the function of the complement system. This mechanism is considered as an adjunct rather than as an alternative to theories that implicate T cells as central to drug-induced autoallergy.

It should be borne in mind that the classes of drugs that can cause autoallergic reactions are chemically and pharmacologically extremely heterogeneous, and the types of autoantibodies that are induced are not uniform in their specificity. Therefore it is unlikely that a single unifying concept of drug-induced autoallergy would encompass this diversity. More probably, a variety of mechanisms are involved, and in some instances these may operate in conjunction with one another.

DRUG-INDUCED ANTIBODY RESPONSES TO MODIFIED SELF

In this section we consider autoallergic responses in which the drug-induced antibodies recognize drug-modified self. In such reactions the drug or a metabolite conjugates to self and forms an integral component of the determinant that is recognized by the antibody. In laboratory assays, the test antigen comprises a self-protein or cell or tissue extract that has been modified by treatment with the drug or a metabolite. The antibody recognizes the drug-modified but not the native form of the protein.

To understand how drugs might induce antibody to modified self, we need to consider how antigen is recognized by T and B cells, and how these cells cooperate in the immune response. In classic experiments, Mitchison (10) showed that in the antibody response to a chemical hapten in mice there is a requirement for a population of lymphocytes (T_H cells) that recognize a "carrier" determinant on a foreign protein that is chemically linked to the hapten. Our understanding of T–B cell cooperation was furthered by the experiments of Lanzavecchia (11), who showed that B cells can process and present antigen to T cells to induce expansion of an antigen-specific population of T_H cells. B cells capture antigen via cell surface immunoglobulin (Ig), accumulate it intracellularly, and process and present it in conjunction with self major histocompatibility complex (MHC) class II molecules to T cells (11). The expanded population of T cells that recognize the appropriately presented antigen provides help to the B cell by production of soluble protein molecules [interleukin-4 (IL-4), IL-5, and IL-6]. This mechanism satisfies the requirement for chemical linkage between T and B cell determinants (10) but differs from earlier models in that there is no longer a requirement for simultaneous recognition of the two determinants: T cells can provide help to any B cell that presents the appropriate antigen. In this model a bridge between the T and B cell is provided by the interaction between the antigen receptor on the T cell and the antigenic determinant presented in conjunction with the MHC molecule on the B cell. A scheme showing how T and B cells may cooperate in the antibody response to drug-modified self is illustrated in Fig. 1.

According to our understanding of how T and B cells cooperate, as outlined earlier, to induce an antibody response against drug-modified self, the drug or a metabolite must generate separate but chemically linked determinants that can be recognized by both T and B cells (Fig. 1). Although antigenic determinants (haptens) generated by small chemicals such as trinitrophenol and drugs such as penicillamine or penicillins are readily recognized by both T cells (13–15) and B cells (10,16), the limiting factor in hapten generation is the chemical reactivity of the compound. Some drugs such as penicillin (16,17), captopril (18), and D-penicillamine (19,20) are inherently chemically reactive and readily generate antigenic determinants on cells and proteins (reviewed in ref. 21). Other drugs that cause autoallergy, including phenytoin, mianserin, and sulfanilamide, have been shown to conjugate covalently to liver microsomal proteins *in vitro* by the action of reduced nicotinamide adenine dinucleotide phosphate (NADPH)-dependent enzymes

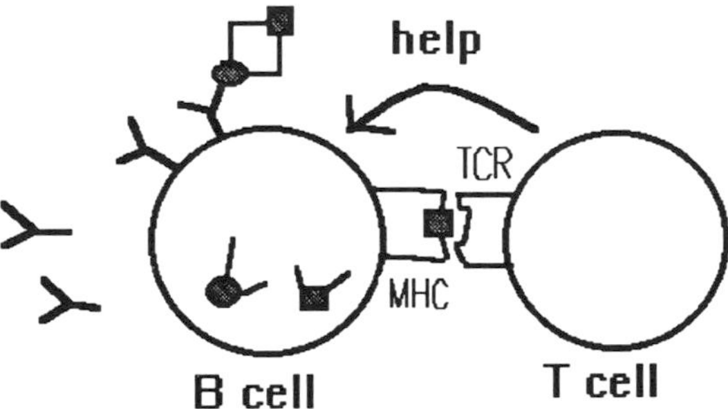

FIG. 1. Schematic representation showing how a drug might induce an antibody response to drug-modified self. The *small filled circles* represent the drug-derived determinant that is recognized by Ig receptors on B cells: in this model these determinants incorporate components of self. The *small filled squares* represent drug-derived determinants that are recognized by T cells: these may or may not incorporate components of self. The B cell internalizes the conjugate incorporating the drug-derived determinants and processes it to a form that is presented in conjunction with a MHC class II molecule to the appropriate drug-specific T cell. As a consequence of this cognate recognition of the antigen, the T cell provides help to the B cell that is than induced to synthesize and export antibodies that recognize the drug-modified self molecule. MHC, class II MHC molecule; TCR, T cell receptor for antigen. Based on ideas from ref. 11.

(22). With the proviso that such conjugation reactions have not been reported *in vivo*, it is conceivable that drug–protein conjugates generated in the liver might find their way to lymphoid tissues to induce an immune response. It seems less likely that a reactive metabolite generated in the liver might be able to reach remote target cells and tissues in a form that retains sufficient reactivity to enter into conjugation reactions. In the case of halothane-induced severe hepatitis (23), this difficulty does not arise since a halothane-derived liver antigen is generated *in vivo*, presumably via metabolism in the liver, and the liver subsequently becomes the target for antibody-mediated toxicity. However, when the tissue or cell target is remote from the liver, it might be more realistic to expect that a reactive metabolite is generated in the target tissue. It has been shown that activated neutrophils or isolated myeloperoxidase can generate reactive metabolites from several drugs including hydralazine, propylthiouracil and phenytoin (24), and procainamide (25). Such a process provides an attractive mechanism for generation of drug-derived antigens on peripheral blood cells that might then become the target for immune attack.

Selected drugs, namely, penicillin, quinidine, halothane, and tienilic acid (ticrynafen), which are good examples of compounds that can induce antibody responses to drug-modified self, and which have attracted much research interest, are discussed in further detail below.

Blood Dyscrasias

Penicillin binds to proteins via a covalent bond and the penicilloyl moiety has been detected on red blood cells of all patients receiving more than 10^7 units of the antibiotic daily—a high dose (26). Even though binding of penicillin to red blood cells occurs commonly, only a small proportion of patients develop high-affinity IgG antibodies specific for the penicilloyl group on erythrocytes (27). These patients develop immune hemolytic anemia (28).

Drug-dependent antibodies have also been associated with other blood disorders and there has been a great interest in thrombocytopenia due to quinidine-dependent development of antibodies (29). Early reports indicated that antibodies that were produced in response to treatment with quinidine would only react with platelets if the drug were present during the reaction. The antibodies appear to be low-affinity antibodies and the proteins on the platelet surface to which the antibodies bind have been determined through observing the effects of aggregation of normal and genetically defective Bernard–Soulier platelets, which lack the platelet glycoprotein known as Ib (30). These studies have been extended to show that it is the complex between glycoprotein Ib and X that is recognized by the antisera and there is also a common reactivity with another platelet surface glycoprotein complex, IIb/IIIa (31). Subsequently, it has been possible to further define the reactivities present in the antisera from patients with quinidine-induced thrombocytopenia and the earlier reports of the ascendency of the immunogenicity of the Ib/IX have been confirmed. It has been possible to identify particular proteolytic peptide fragments on which the antigenic sites reside by competition with monoclonal antibodies against the native proteins (32,33).

It is unclear why particular patients develop these antibodies. A further intriguing observation is that the degree of thrombocytopenia does not appear to be related to the antibody titer in the serum (34), which may indicate that it is due to a difference in the platelets of different individuals. There has been interest in investigating polymorphism in metabolism of quinidine but it has not been possible to correlate with polymorphism in sparteine or debrisoquine metabolism (35). A distinct polymorphism is involved in quinidine oxidation.

Hepatitis

As well as causing blood dyscrasias, antibodies recognizing a combination of drug and self antigen have also been associated with hepatitis. There are rare indications that quinidine can cause autoimmune hepatotoxicity but the best investigated drugs implicated in autoimmune hepatitis are halothane and tienilic acid.

Halothane ($CF_3CHClBr$) is an inhalation anesthetic with widespread use. It induces hepatotoxicity in around 20% of individuals. There is a mild form, which is the most common and which is unlikely to have an immune basis (23). The other adverse reaction to halothane is rare, occurring only in 1 in 20,000 uses of the drug. The resulting hepatitis is severe and is a result of an autoallergic reaction. This severe idiosyncratic adverse reaction has been thoroughly investigated at the molecular level. Patients who develop this adverse reaction have in their serum antibodies that recognize a limited number of specific liver proteins (36). The proteins that were recognized by these antibodies could be demonstrated after sodium dodecyl sulfate–polyacrylamide gel electrophoresis (SDS–PAGE) and immunoblotting. A similar spectrum of proteins reactive with halothane-induced antibodies could be observed in livers from patients anesthetized with halothane who died of heart failure shortly after surgery and livers of rabbits and rats treated with halothane (37). The proteins in livers of patients and animals not treated with halothane did not react with the specific antisera, thus demonstrating that the antigens incorporate a drug-induced determinant. The patients whose livers were investigated were extremely unlikely to have halothane-induced hepatitis and these experiments clearly suggested that halothane was bound covalently to liver proteins but that the binding of halothane alone was not a sufficient stimulus for the development of severe autoimmune hepatitis. From *in vitro* experiments with rat liver microsomes, it is known that before halothane binds covalently to protein, the anesthetic has to be oxidized via a cytochrome P450-dependent mechanism to the trifluoroacetylhalide (38). There are up to five different polypeptides recognized by antibodies from all the individuals with autoallergic hepatitis due to halothane who have been investigated. The reactivity with the protein is not due to recognition of the trifluoroacetic acid (TFA)–halide haptenic group only because it cannot be inhibited completely with TFA–lysine. There must also be a protein component to the antigenic site. It would seem that the binding of halothane occurs in all or most animals exposed to the drug. In order to identify the nature of the proteins to which TFA binds, painstaking protein purification studies have been carried out using as starting material livers from rats treated with halothane (37). The nature of the antigens include microsomal carboxylesterase and sulfide isomerase. These are abundant proteins found within the lumen of the endoplasmic reticulum (ER) and are not involved in halothane metabolism. It is proposed that the oxidized metabolite is generated on the cytoplasmic face of the ER via cytochrome P450 and then is transported via an unknown mechanism across the ER where a nonspecific reaction occurs with adjacent proteins. It may be that the TFA–halide causes disruption of the integrity of the ER membrane, allowing access to the lumen. It is unclear how the covalent binding of these proteins to the halothane metabolite leads to sensitization. In affected individuals there must be additional predisposing factors. It has been postulated that these antigens are exposed at the surface of hepatic cells during membrane recycling and that this may be necessary for the autoallergic liver damage to occur. However, in the idiopathic condition primary biliary cirrhosis, there are antibodies that are specific for components of the mitochondrial enzyme pyruvate dehydrogenase (39), and with antibodies against intracellular components, it is difficult to dissociate whether these antibodies have been generated as a result of cell damage or whether they initiate cell damage.

Hepatitis with an autoimmune etiology has also been observed as a result of treatment with the diuretic tienilic acid. The drug is metabolized by a specific hepatic cytochrome P450. It has been observed that patients with allergic hepatitis as a result of therapy with tienilic acid have antibodies that recognize the specific P450 (40). The drug is not used frequently.

DRUG-INDUCED ANTIBODY RESPONSES TO UNMODIFIED SELF

We turn now to those autoallergic reactions in which the drug-induced autoantibodies recognize self-proteins in their native form. These reactions include those of the tissue-specific and non-tissue-specific types. In laboratory assays for antibody, the test antigen is unmodified blood cells or plasma or tissue protein. These reactions are true autoimmune responses since the determinant that is recognized by antibody, and therefore by the B cells that synthesize it, does not incorporate a drug-derived determinant. However, the determinant that is recognized by the T_H cells that promote the B cell response may be drug-derived.

Several theories, stemming largely from experimental work in rodents, have been put forward that attempt to explain the induction of autoantibodies to unmodified self. In the first of these, Allison and colleagues (41,42) suggested that drugs might break tolerance by binding to self-macromolecules so as to generate a new determinant that could be recognized by T cells. T cells recognizing this new determinant would clonally expand and go on to provide help for B cells that recognized adjacent autoantigens (unmodified self) on the same drug–self conjugate. These in turn

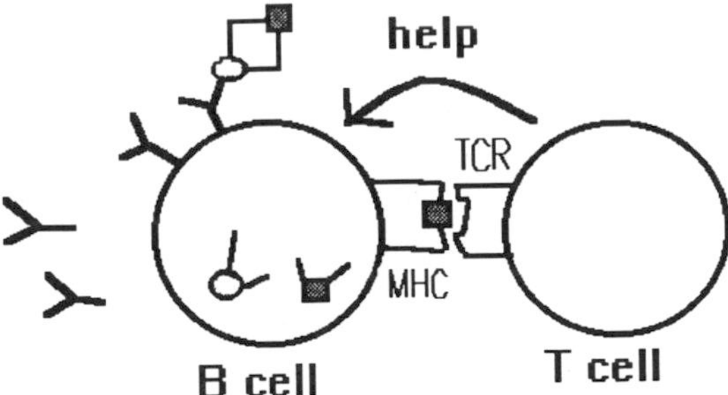

FIG. 2. A scheme showing how a drug might induce a response to unmodified self. The *small open circles* represent self while the *small filled squares* represent the drug-induced determinant to be recognized by the T cell. Otherwise the scheme is identical to that shown in Fig. 1. Based on ideas from refs. 41 and 42.

would clonally expand and differentiate into autoantibody-producing plasma cells (Fig. 2). In this way the normal process of suppression that operates through either clonal or functional deletion of T_H cells is effectively bypassed.

A considerable body of experimental evidence, largely from work with mice, supported Allison's concept. Administration of arsenilic acid-conjugated autologous thyroglobulin or dinitrophenylated autologous Ig to mice led to breakdown of tolerance and elicitation or autoantibodies to these self-proteins (43,44). Along similar lines, mice sensitized to *p*-aminobenzoic acid (PAB) and then administered PAB-conjugated isologous red blood cells developed a T cell-dependent antibody response to their own red blood cells, with consequent hemolytic anemia (45). These studies show clearly that autoimmunity can be induced experimentally by administration of modified self and provide a mechanistic model of drug-induced autoimmune reactions, particularly of the tissue- or protein-specific type.

A second theory of drug-induced autoimmunity was arrived at by Gleichmann and colleagues (46) by analogy with graft-versus-host (GVH) disease. In experimentally induced GVH disease in mice, in which grafted T lymphocytes mount a response against allogeneic histocompatibility antigens of the host, a spectrum of immunologically mediated pathologic changes is seen. In most cases, when the donor and grafted cells differ at both MHC class I and II molecules, a T_H cell response to class II predominates, leading to excessive antibody production, including autoantibodies to nuclear antigens, double-stranded DNA, erythrocytes, and thymocytes (46–49). A severe immune complex glomerulonephritis is also seen in which antibodies to nuclear antigens are implicated (50). Cognate interaction between expanded clones of donor T_H cells and host B cells carrying "foreign" MHC class II leads to polyclonal B cell activation and uncontrolled antibody production. The close similarity between the immunopathologic and autoimmune changes seen in experimental GVH disease and those seen in autoimmune diseases in general, particularly those of the tissue nonspecific type such as SLE, led Gleichmann et al. (46) to postulate that a mechanism analogous to that of stimulatory GVH disease,

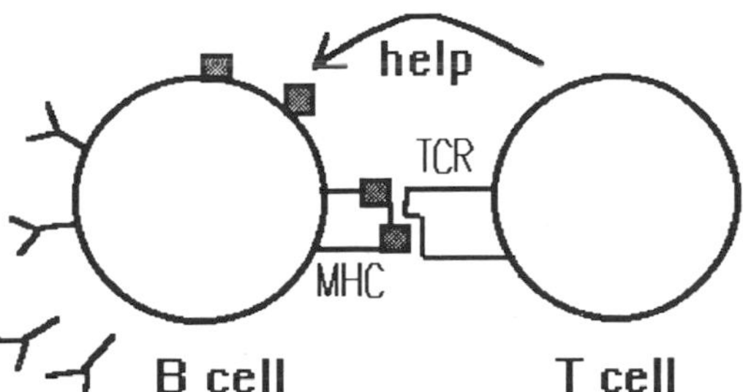

FIG. 3. A representation of how a drug might bind to a self-MHC molecule so as to make it appear foreign to a T cell. As a result of the cognate recognition of altered MHC, the T cell provides help indiscriminately to any B cell that carries drug-altered MHC molecule, resulting in polyclonal antibody synthesis. Based on ref. 46.

that is, indiscriminate activation of B cells by T cells, might underlie autoimmune disease. To explain drug-induced autoimmunity, they postulated that a drug or metabolite might interact chemically with self-MHC molecules on antigen-presenting cells (macrophages and B cells) in such a way as to make them appear as nonself to T cells. These T cells, following clonal expansion, would then provide help indiscriminately to all B cells carrying the drug-modified self-MHC molecule (46). Assuming that the drug modifies MHC molecules without regard for the antigen specificity of the B cell, the resulting cognate T–B cell interaction would lead to polyclonal B cell activation and induction of synthesis of antibodies of multiple, including anti-self, specificities (Fig. 3).

Studies in rodents support the analogy drawn by Gleichmann and colleagues between GVH-induced and chemical-induced autoimmunity. Repeated injections of low doses of mercuric chloride (51,52), D-penicillamine (53), or gold salts (54) into the susceptible Brown Norway (BN) strain of rats lead to multiple immune disruptive changes resembling those seen in mice with GVH disease. These changes include elevation of circulating Igs, particularly IgE, and induction of autoantibodies to the glomerular basement membrane (with associated glomerulopathy), DNA, IgG, and collagen and nuclear and nucleolar proteins (55). The disease is accompanied by increased numbers of B cells—CD4+ (helper type) T cells—and expression of MHC class II molecules on a number of cell types is elevated (55). It is T cell dependent, since it is not seen in T cell-depleted animals and can be transferred by T cells to syngeneic recipients (55). The elevations in IgE and IgG1 in mercury-treated susceptible mice and raised levels of IL-4 mRNA in CD4+ T cells implicate the T_H2 subset of T_H cells in this response (55). Of further interest is the finding that autoantibodies of shared idiotype can be detected in BN rats in which autoimmunity was induced either by GVH reactions or by drugs (D-penicillamine or gold) or mercuric chloride (56). This finding suggests that the same B cell clones are activated in chemical and GVH-induced disease—supporting the concept that both forms of autoimmunity have a common underlying etiology (46).

It is much more difficult to obtain direct or even indirect evidence that autoallergic reactions to drugs are mediated in human patients via activation of T cells that respond to drug-derived determinants, as would be predicted by the theories of Allison and Gleichmann. Antibodies directed against self or drug-modified self are reported in many tissue-specific and systemic autoallergic reactions, but there are few reports of drug-sensitized T cells and their association with autoallergic disease. Detection of sensitized T cells in preparations of human blood mononuclear cells by proliferation assays is notoriously difficult, even to conventional antigens. In the case of drug-induced antigens the difficulty is compounded by the fact that often we are ignorant of the chemical nature of the antigen, whether it is a plasma protein or cellular site, and how it is generated. Hence the appropriate form of the antigen may not be available for use in tests. Nonetheless, there have been a limited number of reports of T cell responsiveness to drugs that can cause autoallergic reactions, including captopril (57), penicillin (58), carbamazepine (59), and gold salts (60). However, in each of the above studies the T cell sensitivity was not associated primarily with autoallergy but with drug-induced skin reactions, probably caused by a classic cell-mediated type IV hypersensitivity reaction. Likewise, in humans with contact sensitivity to nickel, CD4+ T cells can be cloned, which show specificity for autologous nickel-treated MHC class II positive cells, and these cloned T cells can activate autologous B cells in the presence of nickel (61). Again, however, this irritation is not accompanied by systemic autoimmunity, although this may be due to the fact that the nickel is applied topically rather than systemically.

A third theory of drug-induced autoimmunity is that of Druet and colleagues who suggest that certain drugs and chemicals might induce, or protect from suppression (derepress), populations of T cells that recognize unmodified self-MHC (62,63). The consequences of induction of T cells reactive to unmodified self-MHC would be entirely analogous to those seen in GVH disease, and predicted in the Gleichmann model, namely, indiscriminate activation of B cells, accompanied by polyclonal antibody production (46,64). The difference is that the chemical's effect is targeted at the T cell rather than the B cell (shown schematically in Fig. 4). In the BN rat model of D-penicillamine, gold-, and mercury-induced autoimmunity, T

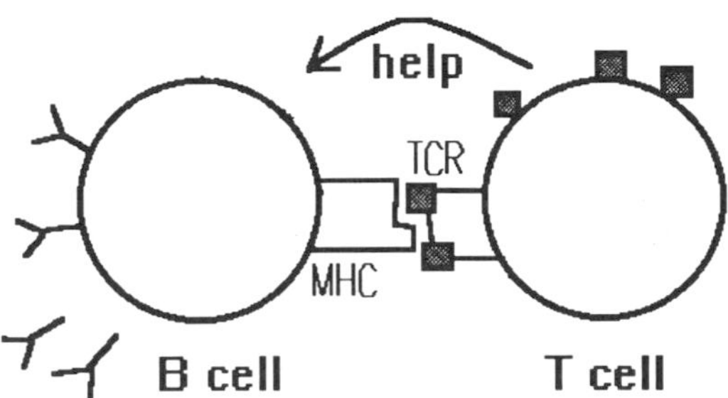

FIG. 4. A representation of how a drug might target a T cell receptor (TCR) such that it can no longer distinguish self from nonself. The consequence of the T–B cell interaction is as for the model depicted in Fig. 3. Based on refs. 62–64.

cells that recognize unmodified self-MHC class II molecules on normal B cells have been reported, rather than T cells that recognize chemically modified self (62–66). This finding supports the concept that mercury and other drugs and chemicals might induce autoreactivity by modifying T cells (Fig. 4) rather than B cells (Fig. 3). Certain drugs, including 5-azacytidine, hydralazine, and procainamide, induce DNA methylation and autoimmunity, leading to the suggestion that they might induce a population of T cells with anti-self reactivity by derepressing gene activation (67,68).

Antibodies that recognize self-determinants have been described on treatment of patients with certain aromatic anticonvulsants and also methyldopa. While drug-specific T cells or T cells with altered recognition of self-MHC have not been identified in these cases, nevertheless, the antibody reactivity is with unmodified self-determinants and is induced by exposure to the drug and almost certainly is induced via drug-mediated disruption of T cell-dependent immune regulation. Recent advances in our understanding of autoallergic responses induced by these kinds of drugs are discussed further below.

Aromatic Anticonvulsants

Antibodies recognizing cytochromes P450 have been detected in the sera of individuals with hypersensitivity reactions to phenytoin, phenobarbital, and carbamazepine, which included hepatitis in two out of the nine patients described (69). The antibodies appeared to recognize the cytochromes both in rat microsomes and the purified rat proteins. There was also a cross-reactivity detected with a human liver microsomal protein of 53,000 molecular weight, although this could not be identified unequivocally as cytochrome P450. The interesting point raised by these studies is that it did not appear necessary that the antigen had been exposed to drug prior to reacting with antibodies in the patient's serum nor does the presence of antibodies allow a profile of the autoimmune reactivity to be predicted. Although the numbers are small (five cases), no sign of antibodies was detected in patients on chronic anticonvulsant therapy with no toxicity. Again it is difficult to dissociate the pathologic cause-and-effect nature of the presence of these antibodies but their presence indicates strongly that an autoallergic response is involved.

These drugs have also been associated with development of antibodies against a range of other subcellular components, including ribonuclear protein, and with a condition resembling SLE in which deposits of subcellular antigens and antibodies are found at inappropriate tissue sites.

Methyldopa

Thrombocytopenia associated with the antihypertensive drug methyldopa has been repeatedly described (70) and the antibodies that have been detected react with platelets in the absence of the drug. However, autoimmune hemolytic anemia is a more prevalent adverse reaction with methyldopa. The development of antibodies against red blood cells occurs in greater than 10% of patients who take the drug, as detected by the ability to agglutinate erythrocytes using anti-human Ig. Although it has not been investigated exhaustively (71), methyldopa does not appear to bind to erythrocytes to act as a hapten. The majority of these individuals with antibodies on the red blood cell surface will not develop hemolytic anemia, although the clearance of the antibody-coated erythrocytes via the reticuloendothelial system is impaired (72). Only 1% of individuals who take methyldopa will develop hemolytic anemia and it seems that there is no impairment of reticuloendothelial cell function, measured *in vivo* in these patients (72,73). The specificity of anti-erythrocyte antibodies after treatment with methyldopa is directed against the Rhesus antigens (73) but a thorough analysis has not been carried out at the molecular level. From serologic studies, it appears that there is no difference in the pattern of reactivity of antibodies of those who do and those who do not develop the autoimmune hemolytic anemia, nor is there any difference in the distribution of Ig subclasses. It may be that the polymorphism resides in the erythrocytes themselves. Erythrocyte stability has clearly been demonstrated to be subject to polymorphism: individuals who develop paroxysmal nocturnal hemoglobinuria have been found to have a defect in the ability to synthesize the glycophosphatidylinositol lipid anchor of several erythrocyte antigens including acetylcholinesterase and decay accelerating factor (DAF) (74). The mechanism by which antibodies are induced in response to methyldopa is unclear. However, it has been demonstrated *in vitro* that monocytes from patients with antibodies but no hemolytic anemia did not ingest the antibody-coated erythrocytes (75). The impairment of phagocytic function may be related to the development of autoantibodies but much more work is required before firm hypotheses can be proposed.

DRUG-DEPENDENT IMPAIRMENT OF COMPLEMENT ACTIVITY

In this section drugs are considered that have been shown to inhibit a key reaction in activation of the classical pathway of complement (76). The drugs considered fall into two categories:

1. Those that themselves inhibit the classical pathway of complement, for example, the antihypertensive hydralazine and the antiarthritic drug D-penicillamine.
2. Drugs whose metabolites are classical pathway inhibitors, for example, the antiarrhythmic agent procainamide.

These drugs induce SLE-like symptoms in which antibody–antigen complexes become deposited in tissues (e.g., vascular epithelium) and stimulate tissue inflammatory responses (77). The antibodies found in patients treated with these drugs are specific for subcellular components. Although, as has been described above for methyldopa and penicillin-induced hemolytic anemia, not all patients who develop antibodies eventually have autoallergy (78). It has been observed that procainamide patients with a particular antibody specificity profile recognizing histones 2A and

2B are at greatest risk of developing SLE (79). While the previous discussion on the role of T cells in stimulation of autoantibody production is pertinent to this group of drugs, the role of specific T cell activation by these drugs or their metabolites has not been determined in patients.

The complement system is a multipurpose defense and removal system and is best known historically for its role in lysis of bacterial and eukaryotic cells. It is now becoming clear that the complement system also has an important direct role in removal of subcellular debris from damaged tissue (80) since DNA and mitochondria can bind to C1q of the classic pathway and activate the cascade (81). The third part complement plays is in removal of immune complexes of antibody and antigen (82,83). The specificities of the antibodies that are found in immune complex disease associated with hydralazine, penicillamine, and procainamide are against subcellular components (77). Therefore in order to approach understanding of development of the autoimmune conditions it is important to understand the effects of these drugs on complement activation. Any event that inhibits activation of the classic pathway of complement will interfere with both clearance of subcellular debris and clearance of immune complexes. The role of complement activation in clearance of cellular debris and immune complexes is through promoting opsonization and phagocytosis. Thus any inhibition of complement activation may well decrease phagocytosis of cell debris and of immune complexes. In the case of cell debris, it is proposed that this increases the likelihood that antibodies against subcellular components will be generated. For immune complexes, complement activation through the classic pathway inhibits precipitation of antibody–antigen complexes (82). So inhibition of the classic complement pathway both inhibits phagocytosis and promotes formation of large complexes. Thus inhibition of the classic pathway of complement is likely to induce inappropriate deposition of immune complexes in tissues such as vascular epithelium (77), where they are found in SLE. Individuals who are lacking the classic complement components C1, C2, and C4 are at increased risk of idiopathic SLE (83), which strongly supports a physiologic role for the cascade in immune complex clearance.

A central event following complement activation is the coating of the activating surface with C3, which leads to ingestion of material and/or solubilization, if the complement-activating surface is an immune complex. When this occurs through the classic pathway, an essential preliminary step is the binding of the protein C4. C4 is polymorphic and is encoded at two loci within the MHC, and there have been many studies showing that lack of the functional activity of the C4 component is one predisposing factor in idiopathic SLE (84,85). The mechanism of activation of complement components C3 and C4, both of which are homologous and become bound covalently to the site of complement activation, has been established (86). Within these molecules there is an internal thiol ester group, which becomes exposed and can, for less than 1 msec, bind covalently to the complement activating surface via an ester or an amide bond (Fig. 5). Other nucleophilic groups in the fluid phase can compete with this binding reaction and become covalently bound to the activated thiol ester site (87). We have shown that hydralazine (88) and penicillamine (89)

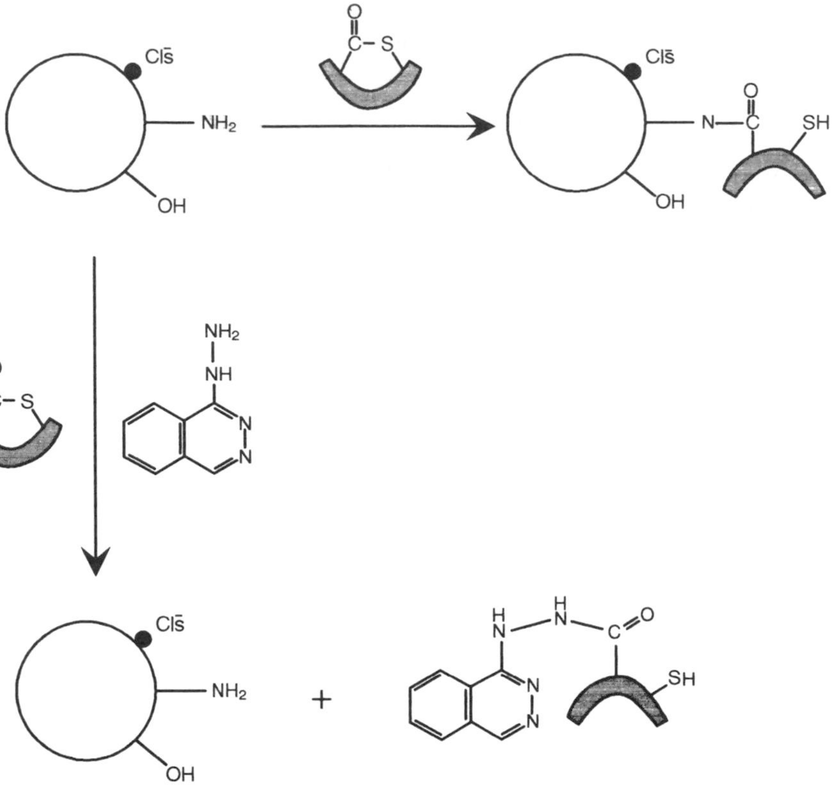

FIG. 5. Mechanism of inhibition of covalent binding of complement component C4. The *open circle* represents the complement-activating surface, either an immune complex or subcellular component with surface hydroxyl and amino groups. The complement-activating surface binds and activates the first component of complement and the subcomponent C1$\bar{s}$ is shown. C1$\bar{s}$ activates C4 (*filled shape*) by proteolytic cleavage at a single site. When C4 is activated, the thiol ester that is buried in C4 becomes exposed and for less than 1 msec can bind covalently to adjacent hydroxyl groups via ester formation or through adjacent amino groups, as illustrated. C4 then becomes covalently bound to the complement-activating surface by an amide linkage. The particle with C4 attached is the focus for further complement activation and C3 binding. This promotes phagocytosis and, in the case of immune complexes, regulates their size. Nucleophilic compounds in solution, including hydralazine as illustrated, can compete with the complement-activating surface for binding to activated C4. The result is that hydralazine (or other nucleophile) becomes covalently bound to C4. This C4 remains in solution and cannot act as a focus for further complement activation on the surface of either an immune complex or a subcellular particle (see refs. 89, 97, and 103 for further details). Ninety percent of the C4 that is activated will react with water, and only up to 10% will react with either the activating surface or other competing nucleophiles such as hydralazine, as illustrated. The sizes of the particles and molecules are not to scale. C1$\bar{s}$ is 83,000 kDa; C4 is 200,000 kDa.

will each compete with the thiol ester site in C4 and inhibit the covalent binding of C4 to an activating surface if the drug is present *during* activation of C4. These drugs become bound to the thiol ester site in C4, which is the mechanism whereby they inhibit C4 binding to a complement-activating surface (90).

Procainamide itself is not inhibitory, but an oxidative metabolite of procainamide, the hydroxylamine form, does inhibit the covalent binding reaction of C4 to a complement-activating surface (91). It has been observed that procainamide is oxidized both by liver microsomes (92,93) and by activated phagocytes via myeloperoxidase (25,94,95). Therefore when phagocytes are ingesting immune complexes, the local generation of the hydroxylamine metabolite of procainamide could become of considerable importance in inhibiting the covalent binding of C4 to immune complexes in the vicinity.

The inhibition of covalent binding of C4 by hydralazine, the hydroxylamine metabolite of procainamide and penicillamine, to a complement-activating surface is clearly effective *in vitro*. The short-lived nature of the active site of C4 on activation means that the drug must be present during C4 activation for inhibition to be observed. Once C4 is activated in plasma, C4 with hydralazine or penicillamine covalently bound would be rapidly degraded to the C4d fragment, which accounts for only 1% to 2% of the total C4 in plasma (96). Of all the C4d that is present in plasma (10 μg/ml), the maximum amount that would be expected to have a molecule of drug bound is 1 μg/ml (87). This may explain why antibodies against hydralazine or penicillamine as a hapten have rarely been found. There has been controversy over the therapeutic concentration of hydralazine, but penicillamine inhibits the covalent binding reaction of C4 within the therapeutic range of the drug (89,97) and *in vivo* penicillamine causes a reduction in the deposition of C3 in rheumatic joints (98), which indicates that inhibition of the covalent binding reaction *in vivo* is effective.

Inhibition of C4 covalent binding and consequently of C3 covalent binding, initially to subcellular debris and also to immune complexes of antibody and subcellular antigens, will reduce phagocytosis of these complexes and is also likely to promote tissue deposition of complexes of antibodies and subcellular antigens as are found in SLE. However, the roles of complement inhibition and cellular mechanisms in drug-induced-allergy are not mutually exclusive. They are both likely to contribute to the final clinical picture observed.

Polymorphism is also likely to be important in determining which individual develops an adverse reaction. The C4 type of an individual contributes to susceptibility to idiopathic SLE: particularly a null allele at the C4A locus (84,85,99). Nonfunctioning (null) C4 alleles have also been associated with hydralazine- (100), procainamide- (101), and penicillamine-induced (102) autoimmune adverse effects.

In vitro studies with C4A and C4B, which are gene products of different gene loci, have demonstrated that the C4A isotype is inhibited to a greater extent by hydralazine (103) and also particularly by penicillamine (97). The C4A isotype is inhibited eight to ten times more effectively than the C4B isotype by penicillamine. A partial deficiency of C4A has been described in penicillamine-induced autoimmunity (102), which again is compatible with the *in vitro* preference of penicillamine inhibition of C4A. Individuals with a lower concentration of C4A would be likely to be more susceptible to further inhibition of this particular C4 isotype. The C4A isotype is thought to have an important role in immune complex clearance (86).

An additional major contributing factor in determining susceptibility to drug-induced SLE is the ability to metabolize the drug. There is clear evidence that this is the case with hydralazine (104) and procainamide (105). Hydralazine, a hydrazine, and procainamide, an arylamine, are both metabolized by the polymorphic arylamine *N*-acetyltransferase (106). The induction of an allergic autoimmune reaction to each of these drugs is correlated with the slow acetylator phenotype (104,105). The association with slow acetylation is a direct functional association and is not due to the linkage of the slow acetylation to a more direct genetic marker, since penicillamine, which is not metabolized by arylamine *N*-acetyltransferase, does not show a correlation with *N*-acetyltransferase genotype (107). A correlation has been made between penicillamine-induced toxicity and sulfoxidation (108) but the molecular genetic basis of penicillamine sulfoxidation has not been established.

CONCLUSIONS

Induction of drug-induced autoallergy is likely due to a range of factors. These may differ depending on the drug and the physiologic state and genetic makeup of the individual. It is clear in many of the examples cited above that only a subgroup of patients who develop drug-induced antibodies either against drug conjugates or against self-components then experience a recognized autoallergic reaction. This is not understood. It is likely that the ability to metabolize drugs and the type of complement components as well as the T cell and cytokine responses of individuals are important contributory factors.

ACKNOWLEDGMENTS

J.W.C. is supported by the Wellcome Trust and the Commission of the European Communities; E.S. is supported by the Wellcome Trust and the Arthritis and Rheumatism Council.

REFERENCES

1. Park BK, Pirmohamed M, Kitteringham NR. Idiosyncratic drug reactions: a mechanistic evaluation of risk factors. *Br J Clin Pharmacol* 1992;34:377–395.
2. De Weck AL. Immunopathological mechanisms and clinical aspects of allergic reactions. In: De Weck AL, Bundgaard H, eds. *Allergic reactions to drugs*. Berlin: Springer-Verlag; 1983:75–133.

3. Ahlstedt S, Kristofferson A. Immune mechanisms for induction of penicillin allergy. *Prog Allergy* 1982;30:67–134.
4. Assem E-SK, ed. *Allergic reactions to anaesthetics*, vol 30 of Monographs in allergy. Basel: Karger; 1992.
5. Cronin E. *Contact dermatitis*. London: Churchill Livingstone; 1980.
6. Park BK, Coleman JW, Kitteringham NR. Drug disposition and drug hypersensitivity. *Biochem Pharmacol* 1987;36:581–590.
7. Pohl LR, Satoh H, Christ DD, Kenna JG. Immunologic and metabolic basis of drug hypersensitivities. *Annu Rev Pharmacol* 1988;28:367–387.
8. Park BK, Kitteringham NR. Drug–protein conjugation and its immunological consequences. *Drug Metab Rev* 1990;22:87–144.
9. Kammuller ME, Bloksma N, Seinen W, eds. *Autoimmunity and toxicology*. Amsterdam: Elsevier; 1989.
10. Mitchison NA. The carrier effects in the secondary response to hapten–protein conjugates II. Cellular cooperation. *Eur J Immunol* 1971;1:18–27.
11. Lanzavecchia T. Antigen-specific interaction between T and B cells. *Nature* 1985;314:537–539.
12. Kappler JW, Roehm N, Marrack P. T-cell tolerance by clonal elimination in the thymus. *Cell* 1987;49:273–280.
13. Martinez-Alonso C, Coutinho A, Bernabe RR, Augustin A, Haas W, Pohlit H. Hapten-specific helper T cells. I. Collaboration with B cells to which the hapten has been directly conjugated. *Eur J Immunol* 1980;10:403–410.
14. Nagata N, Hurtenbach U, Gleichmann E. Specific sensitization of Lyt-1$^+$2 T cells to spleen cells modified by the drug D-penicillamine or a stereoisomer. *J Immunol* 1986;136:136–142.
15. O'Donnell CA, Coleman JW. A T-cell response to the anti-arthritic drug penicillamine in the mouse: requirements for generation of the drug-derived antigen. *Immunology* 1992;76:604–609.
16. Christie G, Coleman JW, Park BK. Drug–protein conjugates XVII. The effect of storage on the antigenicity and immunogenicity of benzylpenicillin in the rat. *Biochem Pharmacol* 1988;37:4121–4128.
17. Kitteringham NR, Christie G, Coleman JW, Yeung JHK, Park BK. Drug–protein conjugates XII. A study of the disposition, irreversible binding and immunogenicity of penicillin in the rat. *Biochem Pharmacol* 1987;36:601–608.
18. Park BK, Grabowsksi PS, Yeung JHK, Breckenridge AM. Drug–protein conjugates I. A study of the covalent binding of [^{14}C]captopril to plasma proteins in the rat. *Biochem Pharmacol* 1982; 31:1755–1760.
19. Coleman JW, Foster AL, Yeung JHK, Park BK. Drug–protein conjugates XV. A study of the disposition of D-penicillamine in the rat and its relationship to immunogenicity. *Biochem Pharmacol* 1988;37:737–742.
20. O'Donnell CA, Foster AL, Coleman JW. Penicillamine and penicillin can generate antigenic determinants on rat peritoneal cells *in vitro*. *Immunology* 1991;72:571–576.
21. Coleman JW. Allergic reactions to drugs: current concepts and problems. *Clin Exp Allergy* 1990; 20:79–85.
22. Kitteringham NR, Lambert C, Maggs JL, Colbert J, Park BK. A comparative study of the formation of chemically reactive drug metabolites by human liver microsomes. *Br J Clin Pharmacol* 1988;26:13–21.
23. Neuberger J, Williams R. Immunology of drug and alcohol-induced liver disease. *Balliere's Clin Gastroenterol* 1987;1:707–722.
24. Uetrecht JP. Idiosyncratic drug reactions: possible role of reactive metabolites generated by leukocytes. *Pharmacol Res* 1989;6:265–273.
25. Rubin RL, Curnutte JT. Metabolism of procainamide to the cytotoxic hydroxylamine by neutrophils activated in vitro. *J Clin Invest* 1989;83:1336–1343.
26. Levine B, Redmond A. Immunochemical mechanisms of penicillin-induced Coombs positivity and haemolytic anaemia in man. *Int Arch Allergy Appl Immunol* 1967;31:594–606.
27. Petz LD, Branch DR. Drug-induced haemolytic anaemia. In: Chaplin D, ed. *Immune heamolytic anaemias*, vol 12 of Methods in haematology. New York: Churchill Livingstone; 1973:47–94.
28. Worlledge SM. Immune drug-induced hemolytic anemias. *Semin Hematol* 1973;10:327–344.
29. Kelton JG, Huang AT, Mold N, Logue G, Rosse WF. The use of in vitro techniques to study drug-induced pancytopenia. *N Engl J Med* 1979;301:621–629.
30. Lerner W, Carusa R, Faig D, Kaspatkin S. Drug-dependent and non drug-dependent antibodies in drug-induced thrombocytopenia purpura. *Blood* 1985;66:306–311.

31. Pfueller SL, Bilston RA, Logan D, Gibson JM, Firkin BG. Quinine and quinidine induced thrombocytopenia. *Blood* 1988;72:1155–1162.
32. Vistentin GP, Newman PJ, Aster RH. Characteristics of quinine- and quinidine-induced antibodies specific for platelet glycoproteins IIb and IIIa. *Blood* 1991;77:2668–2675.
33. Chong BH, Xiaping D, Berndt MC, Horn S, Chesterman CN. Characterization of the binding domains on platelet glycoproteins Ib-Ix and IIb-IIIa for the quinine/quinidine-dependent antibodies. *Blood* 1991;77:2190–2199.
34. Saleh MN, Dhodophar N, Allen K, LoBuglio AF. Quinidine-induced thrombocytopenia. *Henry Ford Hosp Med J* 1989;37:28–32.
35. Brosen K, Davidsen F, Gram LF. Quinidine kinetics after a single oral dose in relation to the sparteine oxidation polymorphism in man. *Br J Clin Pharmacol* 1990;29:248–253.
36. Kenna JG, Neuberger J, Williams R. Identification by immunoblotting of three halothane-induced liver microsomal polypeptide antigens recognised by antibodies in sera from patients with halothane-associated hepatitis. *J Pharmacol Exp Ther* 1987;242:733–740.
37. Kenna GJ. The molecular basis of halothane-induced hepatitis. *Biochem Soc Trans* 1991;19:191–195.
38. Gandalfi AJ, White RD, Sipes IG, Pohl LR. Bioactivation and covalent binding of halothane in vitro: studies with [^{3}H]- and [^{14}C]-halothane. *J Pharm Exp Ther* 1980;214:721–725.
39. Yeaman SJ, Fussey SPM, Danner DJ, James OFW, Mutimer DJ, Bassendine MF. Primary biliary cirrhosis: identification of two major M2 mitochondrial autoantigens. *Lancet* 1988;1:1067–1070.
40. Beaune PH, Dansette PM, Mansuy D. Human anti-endoplasmic reticulum antibodies appearing in a drug-induced hepatitis are directed against a human liver cytochrome P-450 that hydroxylates the drug. *Proc Natl Acad Sci USA* 1987;84:551–555.
41. Allison AC, Denman AM, Barnes RD. Co-operating and controlling functions of thymus-derived lymphocytes in relation to autoimmunity. *Lancet* 1971;2:135–140.
42. Allison AC. Theories of self tolerance and autoimmunity. In: Kammuller ME, Bloksma N, Seinen W, eds. *Autoimmunity and toxicology*. Amsterdam: Elsevier; 1989:67–115.
43. Weigle WO. The production of thyroiditis and antibody following injection of unaltered thyroglobulin into rabbits previously stimulated with altered thyroglobulin. *J Exp Med* 1965;122:1049–1062.
44. Iverson GM. Ability of CBA mice to produce anti-idiotypic sera to 5563 myeloma protein. *Nature* 1970;227:273–274.
45. Yamashita U, Takami T, Hamasaka T, Kitigawa M. The role of hapten-reactive T-lymphocytes in the induction of autoimmunity in mice. II. Termination of self tolerance to erythrocytes by immunization with hapten-isologous erythrocytes. *Cell Immunol* 1976;25:32–40.
46. Gleichmann E, Pals ST, Rolink AG, Radaszkiewicz, Gleichmann H. Graft-versus-host reactions: clues to the etiopathology of a spectrum of immunological diseases. *Immunol Today* 1984;5:324–332.
47. van Rappard-van der Veen FM, Rolink AG, Gleichmann E. Diseases caused by reactions of T lymphocytes towards incompatible structures of the MHC. VI. Autoantibodies characteristic of SLE induced by abnormal T-B cell cooperation across I-E. *J Exp Med* 1982;155:1555–1560.
48. Rolink AG, Pals ST, Gleichmann E. Allosuppressor and allohelper T cells in acute and chronic GVH disease. II. F_1 recipients carrying mutations at H-2K and/or IA. *J Exp Med* 1983;157:755–771.
49. Rolink AG, Gleichmann E. Allosuppressor and allohelper T cells in acute and chronic graft v host disease. *J Exp Med* 1983;158:546–558.
50. Rolink AG, Gleichmann H, Gleichmann E. Diseases caused by reactions of T lymphocytes to incompatible structures of the major histocompatibility complex in immune complex glomerulonephritis. *J Immunol* 1983;130:209–215.
51. Druet P, Druet E, Potdevin F, Sapin C. Immune type glomerulonephritis induced by $HgCl_2$ in the Brown Norway rat. *Ann Immunol (Inst Pasteur)* 1978;129C:777–792.
52. Hirsch F, Couderc J, Sapin C, Fournie G, Druet P. Polyclonal effect of $HgCl_2$ in the rat, its possible role in an experimental autoimmune disease. *Eur J Immunol* 1982;12:620–625.
53. Tournade H, Pelletier L, Pasquier R, Vial M-C, Mandet C, Druet P. D-Penicillamine-induced autoimmunity in Brown-Norway rats. Similarities with $HgCl_2$-induced autoimmunity. *J Immunol* 1990;144:2985–2991.
54. Schuhmann D, Kubicka-Muranyi M, Mirtschewa J, Gunther J, Kind P, Gleichmann E. Adverse immune reactions to gold. I. Chronic treatment with a Au(I) drug sensitizes mouse T cells not to Au(I) but to Au(III) and induces autoantibody formation. *J Immunol* 1990;145:2132–2139.

55. Goldman M, Druet P, Gleichmann E. T_H2 cell in systemic autoimmunity: insights from allogeneic diseases and chemically induced autoimmunity. *Immunol Today* 1991;12:223–227.
56. Guery JC, Tournade H, Pelletier L, Druet E, Druet P. Rat anti-glomerular basement membrane antibodies in toxin-induced autoimmunity and in chronic GVH reactions share recurrent idiotypes. *Eur J Immunol* 1990;20:101–105.
57. Smit AJ, Van der Laan S, De Monchy J, Kallenberg CGM, Donker AJM. Cutaneous reactions to captopril. Predictive value of skin tests. *Clin Allergy* 1984;14:413–419.
58. Bell SJD, Pichler WJ. Penicillin-allergic patients react to penicillin-modified "self." *Allergy* 1989; 44:199–203.
59. Zakrzewska JM, Ivanyi L. In vitro lymphocyte proliferation by carbamazepine, carbamazepine-10,11-epoxide, and oxcarbamazepine in the diagnosis of drug-induced hypersensitivity. *J Allergy Clin Immunol* 1988;82:110–115.
60. Verwilghen J, Kingsley GH, Gambling L, Panayi GS. Activation of gold-reactive lymphocytes in rheumatoid arthritis patients treated with gold. *Arthritis Rheum* 1992;35:1413–1418.
61. Sinigaglia F, Scheidegger D, Garotta G, Scheper R, Pletscher M, Lanvavecchia A. Isolation and characterisation of Ni-specific T cell clones from patients with Ni-contact dermatitis. *J Immunol* 1985;135;3929–3932.
62. Pelletier L, Pasquier R, Hirsch F, Sapin C, Druet P. Autoreactive T cells in mercury-induced autoimmune disease: In vitro demonstration. *J Immunol* 1986;137:2548–2554.
63. Rossert J, Pelletier L, Pasquier R, Druet P. Autoreactive T cells in mercury-induced autoimmune disease: demonstration by limiting dilution analysis. *Eur J Immunol* 1988;18:1761–1766.
64. Pelletier L, Bellon B, Tournade H, et al. Chemical-induced autoimmunity. *Immunol Ser* 1991; 55:315–353.
65. Chalopin JM, Lockwood CM. Autoregulation of autoantibody synthesis in mercuric chloride nephritis in the Brown Norway rat II. Presence of antigen-augmentable plaque-forming cells in the spleen is associated with humoral factors behaving as auto-anti-idiotype antibodies. *Eur J Immunol* 1984;14:470–475.
66. Pelletier L, Pasquier R, Rossert J, Vial MC, Druet P. Autoreactive T cells in mercury-induced autoimmunity. *J Immunol* 1988;140:750–754.
67. Richardson B. Effect of an inhibitor of DNA methylation on T cells. II. 5-Azacytidine induces self reactivity in antigen-specific T4+ cells. *Hum Immunol* 1986;17:456–470.
68. Cornacchia E, Golbus J, Maybaum J, Strahler J, Hanash S, Richardson B. Hydralazine and procainamide inhibit T cell DNA methylation and induce autoreactivity. *J Immunol* 1988;140:2197–2200.
69. Leeder SJ, Riley RJ, Cook VA, Spielberg SP. Human anti-cytochrome P450 antibodies in aromatic anti-convulsant-induced hypersensitivity reactions. *J Pharmacol Exp Ther* 1992;263:360–367.
70. Shalev O, Brezis M. Methyldopa induced thrombocytopenia in chronic lymphatic leukemia. *N Engl J Med* 1977;297:471.
71. Lo Buglio AF, Jandl JH. The nature of alpha-methyldopa antibody. *N Engl J Med* 1967;276:658–665.
72. Kelton JG. Impaired reticuloendothelial function in patients treated with methyldopa. *N Engl J Med* 1985;313:596–600.
73. Murphy WG, Kelton JG. Immune haemolytic anaemia and thrombocytopaenia with drugs and antibodies. *Biochem Soc Trans* 1991;19:183–186.
74. Lubin DM, Atkinson JP. Decay accelerating factor, biochemistry, molecular biology and function. *Annu Rev Immunol* 1989;7:35–58.
75. Branch DR, Gallagher MT, Shulman IA, Mison AP, Sysiokian AL, Petz LD. Reticuloendothelial cell function in alpha methyldopa induced hemolytic anemia. *Vox Sang* 1983;45:278–287.
76. Sim E. Drug-induced immune complex disease. *Biochem Soc Trans* 1991;19:164–170.
77. Mongey A-B, Hess EV. Drug-related lupus. *Curr Opin Rheumatol* 1989;1:353–359.
78. Woosley RL, Drayer DE, Reidenberg MM, Neis AS, Carr K, Oates JA. Effect of acetylator phenotype on the rate at which procainamide induces antinuclear antibodies and the lupus syndrome. *N Engl J Med* 1978;298:1157–1159.
79. Totoritis MC, Tan EM, McNally EM, Rubin RL. Association of antibody to histone complex H2A-H2B with symptomatic procainamide-induced lupus. *N Engl J Med* 1988;318:1431–1436.
80. Weisman HF, Bartow T, Leppo MK, et al. Soluble CR1 in vivo inhibitor of complement-suppressed post-ischaemic myocardial inflammation and necrosis. *Science* 1990;249:146–151.
81. Giclas PC, Pinkard RN, Olson MS. In vivo activation of complement by isolated human heart subcellular membranes. *J Immunol* 1979;122:146–151.

82. Schifferli J, Bartolotti SR, Peters DK. Inhibition of immune precipitation by complement. *Clin Exp Immunol* 1980;42:387–392.
83. Whaley K, Lemercier C. In: Sim E, ed. *Natural immunity-humoral factors*. Oxford: Oxford University Press; 1993:121–150.
84. Batchelor JR, McMichael AJ. Progress in understanding HLA and disease associations. *Br Med Bull* 1987;43:156–183.
85. Dunckley H, Gatenby PA, Hawkins B, Naito S, Serjeantson SW. Deficiency of C4 is a genetic determinant of systemic lupus erythematosus in three ethnic groups. *J Immunogenetics* 1987;14: 219–229.
86. Campbell RD, Law SK, Reid KBM, Sim RB. Structure, organisation and regulation of the complement genes. *Ann Rev Immunol* 1988;6:161–195.
87. Sim RB, Twose T, Paterson D, Sim E. The covalent binding reaction of complement component C3. *Biochem J* 1981;193:115–127.
88. Sim E, Gill EW, Sim RB. Drugs that induce systemic lupus erythematosus. *Lancet* 1984;2:422–424.
89. Sim E, Dodds AW, Goldin A. Inhibition of the covalent binding of complement component C4 by penicillamine, an anti-rheumatic drug. *Biochem J* 1989;259:415–419.
90. Sim E. Drug-induced immune complex disease. *Complement Inflamm* 1989;6:119–126.
91. Sim E, Stanley L, Gill EW, Jones A. Metabolites of procainamide and practolol inhibit complement components C3 and C4. *Biochem J* 1988;251:323–326.
92. Uetrecht JP. Reactivity and possible significance of hydroxylamine and nitroso metabolites of procainamide. *J Pharmacol Exp Ther* 1985;232:420–425.
93. Budinsky RA, Roberts RM, Coats EA, Adams L, Hess EV. The formation of procainamide hydroxylamine by rat and human liver microsomes. *Drug Metab Dispos* 1987;15:37–43.
94. Uetrecht JP. Mechanism of drug-induced lupus. *Chem Res Toxicol* 1988;1:133–143.
95. Rubin RL, Burlingame RW. Drug-induced autoimmunity: a disorder at the interface between metabolism and immunity. *Biochem Soc Trans* 1991;19:153–159.
96. Folkerson J, Teisner B, Petersen NE, et al. Preparation of antibodies against C4 and for quantification of C4d. *J Clin Lab Immunol* 1985;16:163–167.
97. Edmonds SD, Gibb A, Sim E. Effect of thiol compounds on human complement component C4. *Biochem J* 1993;289:801–805.
98. Mellbye OJ, Munthe E. Effect of penicillamine on complement *in vivo* and *in vitro*. *Ann Rheum Dis* 1977;36:453–458.
99. Batchelor JR, Fielder AHL, Walport MJ, et al. Family study of the major histocompatibility complex in HLA DR3 negative patients with systemic lupus erythematosus. *Clin Exp Immunol* 1987;70:364–371.
100. Spiers CN, Fielder AHL, Chapel HM, Batchelor JR. Hydralazine-induced systemic lupus erythematosus. *Lancet* 1989;1:922–924.
101. Mongey A-B, Balakrishnan K, Ball E, Brand R, Hess EV, Sim E, Adams L. HLA types in procainamide-induced SLE. *55th Annual Meeting of American College of Rheumatology* 1991; abst no 1071.
102. Clarkson RWE, Sanders PA, Grennan DM. Complement C4 null alleles as a marker of gold or D-penicillamine toxicity in the treatment of rheumatoid arthritis. *Br J Rheumatol* 1992;31:53–54.
103. Sim E, Law SKA. Hydralazine binds covalently to complement component C4. Different reactivity of C4A and C4B gene products. *FEBS Lett* 1985;184:323–327.
104. Perry HM, Tan EM, Carmody S, Sakamoto A. Relationship of acetyltransferase activity to antinuclear antibodies and toxic symptoms in hypertensive patients treated with hydralazine. *J Lab Clin Med* 1970;76:114–125.
105. Reidenberg MM. Chemical induction of systemic lupus erythematosus and lupus like illnesses. *Arthritis Rheum* 1981;24:1004–1008.
106. Sim E, Hickman D, Coroneos E, Kelly SL. Arylamine N-acetyl-transferase. *Biochem Soc Trans* 1992;20:304–309.
107. Hickman D, Risch A, Camilleri J, Sim E. Genotyping human polymorphic arylamine N-acetyltransferase: identification of new slow allotypic variants. *Pharmacogenetics* 1992;2:217–226.
108. Madhok R, Zoma A, Torley HI, Capell HA, Waring R, Hunter JA. The relationship of sulfoxidation status to efficacy and toxicity of penicillamine in the treatment of rheumatoid arthritis. *Arthritis Rheum* 1990;33:574–577.

Immunotoxicology and Immunopharmacology, Second Edition, edited by J. H. Dean, M. I. Luster, A. E. Munson, and I. Kimber.
Raven Press, Ltd., New York © 1994.

33

Drug-Induced Autoimmunity

Michael E. Kammüller and *Nanne Bloksma

*Department of Drug Safety and Toxicology, Sandoz Pharma Ltd., CH-4002 Basel, Switzerland; and *Research Institute of Toxicology, Section of Immunotoxicology, Utrecht University, NL 3508 TD Utrecht, The Netherlands*

The phenomenon of drug-induced autoimmune diseases has frequently been reviewed since the first sulfadiazine-induced case of systemic lupus erythematosus (SLE) was recognized by Hoffman in 1945 (see refs. 1–5 and references cited therein). At first, the reports were sporadic, but gradually specific (groups of) drugs with the potential to induce SLE emerged (4,6). Besides SLE—approximately 1% to 12% of all the diagnosed cases of SLE have been attributed to drugs (4,6–8)—other, more cell-specific, forms of drug-induced autoimmune disorders, such as immune-mediated granulocytopenia (3), hemolytic anemia (9), and thrombocytopenia (10) have been documented as well. The variety of mechanisms that may be at play in drug-induced autoimmune disorders have been listed and discussed elsewhere (3,5,11–13). In trying to analyze drug-induced autoimmune reactions from a toxicologic point of view, the following questions need to be addressed: (a) Are there particular chemical or pharmacologic properties that endow some low molecular weight (LMW) compounds with the potential to provoke autoimmune reactions? (b) Can drug-induced autoimmune disorders be reproduced in animals? (c) Which methods or parameters allow hazard identification? (d) Do drugs actually induce autoimmune disorders *de novo* or by activation of a predisposition, or do they act by a combination of mechanisms, and if so, what makes some individuals more susceptible to the development of these disorders than others?

CHEMICAL AND PHARMACOLOGICAL ASPECTS

A large variety of drugs, with a molecular weight of less than 1000 daltons, have been associated with induction of autoimmune disorders in susceptible individuals (2,3). These drugs belong to different chemical classes and include among others derivatives of *aromatic amines* (procainamide, practolol), *hydrazines* (hydralazine), *hydantoins* (phenytoin, mephenytoin, ethotoin, nitrofurantoin), *thioureylenes* (methimazole, propylthiouracil), *oxazolidinediones* (trimethadione, paramethadione), *succinimides* (ethosuximide, methsuximide, phensuximide), *dibenzazepines* (carbamazepine), *phenothiazines* (chlorpromazine), *sulfonamides* (sulfasalazine, sulfadiazine), *pyrazolones* (phenylbutazone), *amino acids* (D-penicillamine, captopril, methyldopa), *allyl amines* such as zimeldine, and, furthermore, halothane, mercuric chloride, and gold preparations. With few exceptions, these compounds are heterocyclic and many contain at least one aromatic group, suggesting that particular chemical entities may favor induction of immune disregulation.

From a pharmacologic point of view, the majority of drugs that induce autoimmune disease can be ranked among β-adrenergic-receptor-blocking compounds. drugs acting at the central nervous system (CNS), antithyroidal agents, and anti-infectious agents. While there is no conclusive evidence of the involvement of their pharmacologic mode of action in adverse immune effects, this may be expected on the basis of circumstantial evidence. There is, for example, a functional connectivity between immune, nervous, and endocrine systems, which is, at least partially, affected by shared receptors and mediators among the systems (14,15). It is therefore not unlikely that CNS drugs modulate immune responses by acting at these receptors or inducing common mediators. Such a mode of action might also explain the observation that chemically different CNS drugs cause similar immune side effects, since CNS drugs from different chemical classes have been shown to share a common molecular topography (16).

ANIMAL MODELS OF DRUG-INDUCED AUTOIMMUNE REACTIONS

Most attempts to induce autoimmune disorders with drugs in experimental animals have been unsuccessful (2), and presently only few reproducible models of drug-induced autoimmune disease are available. Among these glomerulonephritis induced by mercuric chloride- and gold-containing compounds and by D-penicillamine in inbred Brown Norway rats and B10.S mice have been best studied (17).

Within the scope of this chapter we aim to address several issues concerning drug-induced autoimmune reactions from a toxicologic perspective. No attempt is made to give a comprehensive overview of the various possible mechanisms of drug-induced autoimmune reactions (see refs. 3, 5, and 11–13). Discussions will focus on selected aspects of diphenylhydantoin (DPH) activities (e.g., phenytoin, Dilantin, and Epanutin) as an example, since many properties of this drug have been studied in great detail, both in the laboratory and in the clinic.

DIPHENYLHYDANTOIN CAN INDUCE IMMUNODEFICIENCY, LYMPHOPROLIFERATION, AND AUTOIMMUNITY

The discovery of the anticonvulsant activity of DPH by Merritt and Putnam in 1938 (18) represented a milestone in the treatment of convulsive disorders. Today,

DPH is a widely used anticonvulsant drug. The compound exerts a stabilizing effect on excitable neurons and cardiac myocytes (among others) by decreasing resting Na^+ fluxes or Na^+ currents that flow during action potentials. In this respect its action resembles that of local anesthetics (19). Thus, at therapeutically relevant concentrations (below 10 μM), DPH suppresses episodes of repetitive neuronal firing (19). Based on its molecular structure, DPH is believed to interact with particular receptor sites in the CNS (16). The pharmacokinetic properties of DPH are markedly influenced by its limited aqueous solubility and by dose-dependent elimination. DPH is bound by about 90% to plasma proteins, in particular, to albumin (19).

Adverse effects of DPH are relatively common and have been well documented for the CNS, endocrine, gastrointestinal, hematopoietic, and immune systems (20). Whereas some adverse side effects (e.g., CNS effects) of DPH are dose-related and thus predictable, others, specifically DPH-induced allergic and autoimmune disorders, seem to be unpredictable. Fortunately, serious adverse immunologic effects are rare, but in those cases the drug needs to be withdrawn (19,21). Other untoward immune side effects are less rare and have been amply documented and studied in humans and experimental animals.

In humans, the effects of DPH on the immune system diverge widely. Notably, immunoglobulin A (IgA) deficiency and impairment of delayed-type hypersensitivity, T cell mitogen responsiveness, and T helper cell function point to the immunosuppressive action of DPH (22–24). In fact, based on the immunosuppressive properties, DPH has been considered as a valuable drug in the treatment of rheumatoid arthritis (25,26). Other side effects reveal the capacity of DPH to elicit a spectrum of lymphoproliferative disorders at low incidence, including lymphoma, lymphadenopathy, and autoimmune diseases such as SLE, scleroderma, and vasculitis (6,20).

Animal experiments have confirmed some of the immunosuppressive actions of DPH in humans. In mice, in particular, suppression of antibody formation (24, 27,28), natural killer (NK) cell activity, and cytotoxic T lymphocyte function (29) have been found.

Krueger et al. (30,31) have shown that DPH can cause atrophy of lymphoid organs as well as lymphoproliferation in mice. They exposed three strains of female mice differing in spontaneous lymphoma incidence—that is, C3Hf mice ($H\text{-}2^k$; resistant), C57BL mice ($H\text{-}2^b$; low spontaneous incidence), and SJL mice ($H\text{-}2^S$; high spontaneous incidence)—to DPH (approximately 40 mg DPH/kg/d) via liquid diet starting at week 8 to 12 of age. Autopsies were done every 8 weeks starting 2 months after the start of treatment. C3Hf mice revealed only mild lymph node and thymus enlargement and moderate to marked splenomegaly after 6 months of treatment, which was reflected histologically in the lymph nodes by diffuse histiocytosis and in the spleen by red pulp as well as a moderate follicular hyperplasia. After 8 months cortical and paracortical atrophy in lymph nodes with a diffuse increase of reticulum cells and histiocytes was recognized. No lymphoma development was noted in C3Hf mice after 10 months of treatment (32). C57BL mice showed a transient enlargement of lymphoid organs at about 6 to 8 weeks and atrophy of the thymic cortex and of the T cell-harboring paracortex of lymph nodes after about 4 months of DPH administration. The lymph node atrophy was still present at 8 months of treatment when thymic hyperplastic cortical nodules became manifest. This resulted in thymic lymphoma in 12% of the animals at 12 months of treatment, a clear increase compared to the observed spontaneous lymphoma incidence of 4% by 18 months of age. Thymus and lymph node atrophy observed in C57BL mice was also seen in the susceptible SJL mice. But already at 4 to 8 months of treatment 25% of the mice showed lymphomatous enlargement of thymus and lymph nodes, and 75% of the mice had B cell lymphomas in spleen and lymph nodes at 6 to 8 months. In untreated SJL mice a similar incidence of spontaneous B cell lymphoma is only observed by 8 to 12 months (30). The mechanisms underlying the DPH-induced acceleration of lymphoma development in SJL and C57BL mice is unknown. Susceptibility or resistance is probably dependent on the genetic makeup or the presence or absence of endogenous lymphomatogenous retroviruses that can be activated by DPH. A similar explanation may be given for the lack of effects of DPH in Fischer 344 rats that showed no higher incidence of lymphoma or signs of autoimmune disease during oral exposure to DPH up to 23 mg/kg/d for 2 years compared to controls (33). In mice a relation between lymphoma induction and pharmacokinetics of DPH is not very likely, since Atlas et al. (34) have demonstrated that C57BL/6 and C3H mice are fast metabolizers of DPH, and SJL mice are slow metabolizers.

The ability of DPH to cause thymus cortex atrophy has recently been confirmed by Hirai and Ichikawa (35) in ICR mice given up to 60 mg DPH/kg/d from 3 weeks of age. The atrophy was dose-dependent, already apparent after 3 days of treatment, and persisted over 30 days in treated animals. Since DPH caused a dose-dependent two- to fourfold increase of serum glucocorticoid levels in these mice, thymus effects have been attributed to the thymolytic effect of this hormone. The ability of DPH to elevate glucocorticoid levels in mice (35) or to mediate itself glucocorticoid-like effects via the glucocorticoid receptor (36) has also been suggested by Bloksma et al. (37) to explain the beneficial effects of DPH in C57BL/6-*lpr*/*lpr* mice that develop lymphoproliferative disease and SLE-like symptoms. In this study DPH was administered to 6-week-old mice via the drinking water (approximately 65 mg/kg/d) for 6 months. It was found that DPH significantly reduced the lymphadenopathy as well as autoantibody levels. This effect seems rather unique, since various treatments, like irradiation (38), androgens (39), cyclosporin A (CsA) (40), prostaglandin E_1 (41), and calorie restriction (42), were found to reduce only one of both parameters in MRL-*lpr*/*lpr* mice. Since glucocorticoids were reported to exert both effects (43), the above-described properties of DPH were suggested to be involved. Immunosuppression as a consequence of a direct or indirect glucocorticoid action of DPH may also explain why DPH fails to induce autoimmune disease in rodents. Moreover, it possibly permits proliferative expansion of certain lymphoid cell populations and lymphoma development in susceptible strains.

Kohler et al. (44) obtained evidence that the developing immune system is more susceptible to DPH than that of adults. They treated adult female C3H mice twice a day by gavage with 25 mg/kg DPH from the day of copulation until delivery and sacrificed mothers and neonates 5 days thereafter (44). While thymuses and spleens of the mothers were apparently normal, neonatal thymuses showed a reduction of the thymic cortex accompanied by an apparent enlargement of the reticuloepithelial tissue. In the spleens an enlargement of the white pulp associated with lymphocyte accumulation in the periarteriolar lymphocyte sheaths was seen. Furthermore, prenatal DPH exposure affected postnatal immune system function, as reported by Chapman and Roberts (45). The offspring of BALB/c mice that were dosed daily by gavage on gestation days 9 through 18 with 0, 20, 40, or 60 mg/kg/d showed a dose-related reduction of antibody formation against type III pneumococcal polysaccharide at 25 days but not at 15 weeks of age. According to Chapman and Roberts (45), the humoral defect is likely to be related to the development of purulent eye exudates in the offspring observed on day 12 of age, because its incidence and persistence were dependent on the DPH dose as well. Moreover, the degree of DPH-induced humoral immunosuppression appeared higher in offspring born with an open eye defect than in the physically normal offspring. Therefore it was suggested that effects of DPH on humoral immune function and physical development were related. Cell-mediated immunity as assessed by the delayed-type hypersensitivity response to the contact allergen oxazolone, however, was not affected in these mice (45).

Thus animal studies enable recognition of the immunosuppressive and lymphoproliferative activities of DPH as observed in humans but fail to demonstrate the autoimmunizing potential of DPH.

ARE IMMUNODEFICIENCY, LYMPHOPROLIFERATION, AND AUTOIMMUNITY RELATED?

Patients with primary immunodeficiency, especially various B cell deficiencies, are known to have a high incidence of autoimmune disease (46). For example, selective IgA deficiency is associated with systemic autoimmune diseases, such as SLE (46,47). Moreover, drugs with a documented ability to cause systemic autoimmune disorders, that is, DPH (48) and D-penicillamine (49), have been shown to reduce secretory and/or serum IgA levels. However, the relationship between IgA deficiency and susceptibility to autoimmune disease is not known. It most likely is influenced by other factors, since the prevalence of selective IgA deficiency in a normal population is much higher (1 in 700) than the prevalence of systemic autoimmune disease.

In contrast to B cell immunodeficiencies, profound, inherited T cell deficiencies are apparently not associated with autoimmune disorders (46). However, the association between development of immunodeficiency, benign or neoplastic lymphoproliferation, and autoimmune diseases, particularly in the context of thymic abnormalities, is well known (50). It has been observed upon immunosuppressive treatment, among others with cyclophosphamide and CsA. The reversibility of lymphoproliferative lesions upon withdrawal of the immunosuppressive drug therapy suggests a causal relationship (51). Recent studies in rodents have provided more solid evidence of the relationship between the development of autoimmune disease and induced disturbance of thymus function (52,53). Notably, CsA, which is successfully used in the prevention of transplant rejection and treatment of various autoimmune diseases in humans, has been shown to interfere with the deletion of T cells recognizing autoantigens in the thymic medulla and to cause organ-specific and systemic autoimmune disease under specific conditions. This occurs when CsA is given to neonates (52), but not older animals (54), and to bone marrow transplant recipients that received a high dose of irradiation prior to transplantation (54,55). The development of autoimmune disease under these conditions has been attributed to the absence of an established regulatory peripheral T cell repertoire. Because CsA may interfere at different levels of immunologic tolerance, autoreactive T cells leaving the thymus as a consequence of CsA treatment may not be functionally inactivated in the periphery (56). However, a recent study using the bone marrow transplant model in different mouse strains suggested the involvement of other mechanisms, because effects of CsA on T cell deletion did not correlate with development of autoimmune effects (57). The study suggests a polyfactorial etiology of CsA-induced autoimmune disease and may explain why autoimmune side effects have been observed only rarely in CsA-treated human bone marrow transplant patients (58).

Both CsA and DPH have immunosuppressive activities and affect the thymus. Although some neonatal exposure experiments with DPH have been performed (44,45), autoimmune side effects were not reported. This may be related to the different intrathymic targets of both compounds. CsA is thought to disturb thymocyte differentiation by affecting interdigitating and epithelial cells (59), while DPH affects the more immature cortical thymocytes probably by a glucocorticoid-mediated effect (see above). As pointed out by Schuurman et al. (59) such differences in intrathymic targets may have different consequences for immune function ranging from immunodeficiency to autoimmune disorders. It illustrates the complex relationship between immunodeficiency, lymphoproliferation, and autoimmune effects and the difficulty of immunotoxicologic hazard identification and risk assessment at this point.

HAZARD IDENTIFICATION IN TOXICOLOGIC TESTING: DETECTION OF IMMUNE DISREGULATION

Currently, there are no predictive assays developed and validated to identify the potential of drugs to induce systemic hypersensitivity or autoimmune responses in the early phases of drug development. These side effects usually become manifest only during advanced clinical development. As indicated earlier (60), the conditions used in routine preclinical toxicologic screening are obviously not optimal for the detection of the immune-disregulating potential of drugs and chemicals (e.g., small animal number, use of outbred animal strains, dynamics of disease development versus snapshot determinations, and lack of predictive parameters). An economically and practically relevant question concerning screening studies is whether actual evidence of an agent's ability to induce manifest hypersensitivity or autoimmune disease should be and can be obtained, or whether (preferably short-term) assays not measuring the actual clinical endpoints can be sufficiently predictive in this respect. As it has become clear that T cells are primary players in the initiation and perpetuation of spontaneous (41,61) as well as induced systemic autoimmune disorders (17,62), an important aspect to study in toxicology is whether a drug's ability to cause more or less persistent T cell activation is predictive of its ability to cause allergic and/or autoimmune side effects.

In Vivo Parameters

In addition to morphologic examinations in routine toxicologic studies (63), measurements of some immunologically relevant serum parameters can provide important information about antibody-mediated responses. Parameters may comprise levels of total immunoglobulins and of various immunoglobulin (sub)classes, immune complexes, and some commonly observed autoantibodies, for example, antinuclear (ANAs), anti-histone, and anti-single-stranded deoxyribonucleic acid (denatured; ssDNA) autoantibodies. Some of these autoantibodies proved to be useful in the diagnosis of procainamide-induced SLE in humans as shown by Rubin (64). Measurement of these parameters at suitably chosen intervals, especially during subchronic and chronic exposition, may obviate the snapshot nature of the histopathologic examinations and will give a reflection of cellular and humoral immune function in time. With regard to autoantibody measurements it is important to measure both total immunoglobulin classes and subclasses. This can be illustrated by murine models of spontaneous SLE in which a switch from IgM to IgG autoantibodies could be associated with development of overt disease (41,65). Also, data on drug-induced SLE in humans point in this direction. ANAs in patients with procainamide-induced SLE appeared to be of the IgG class (in particular IgG1 and IgG3), whereas IgM ANAs are predominant in asymptomatic users of the drug (64). Furthermore, the relatively low incidence of chlorpromazine-induced SLE has been related to its preferential induction of IgM ANAs (66).

Noninvasive routine methods for monitoring and predicting cell-mediated autoimmune reactions in toxicity studies are virtually lacking. Although levels of serum and urinary neopterin were shown to be a nonspecific but useful biochemical parameter to monitor T cell activation in humans (67), experiments in mice have shown that the murine analog, biopterin, is not a useful marker as judged by the only marginal changes observed in various induced and spontaneous autoimmune models (37,68). A more recently introduced parameter to monitor human T cell activation nonspecifically is the soluble interleukin-2 receptor (sIL-2R: p55 chain) (69,70). Although both T cells and macrophages shed sIL-2R upon activation, its levels in serum and to a lesser extent in urine paralleled various kinds of T cell-mediated immune processes in humans (71). Since sIL-2R can be measured by enzyme-linked immunoadsorbent assay (ELISA), it could fit very well into routine toxicologic procedures, but its relevance in animal models has still to be assessed. This is not the case for sIL-6R in serum and urine, which has been measured in various mouse strains with genetically defined autoimmune disease and was found to correlate very well with manifestation and severity of the disease as shown by Suzuki et al. (72).

It remains to be established whether cytokine profile measurements will become useful tools in drug safety studies. Various cytokines are involved in the induction and development of autoimmune diseases. This indicates that T helper (T_H1 or T_H2) cells may be the dominant mediators in a particular disease (17,70). While such studies provide valuable insight in the etiology of the different diseases, it is to be questioned whether such detailed data need to be obtained in routine toxicity studies. For instance, there is evidence that the quite opposite effects of mercuric chloride observed in different strains of rats and mice are mediated by preferential T_H1 or T_H2 cell activation (17). An additional problem is that levels of many cytokines in the circulation as well as lymphoid organs are low or undetectable, even when symptoms are clearly manifest (73). A clear exception is IL-6, which is profoundly elevated in serum and/or tissue in many inflammatory conditions (73,74). Therefore it may function as a marker of inflammatory action of chemicals in early screening, thus selecting the compounds to be tested in various other assays to assess the cause of the inflammatory action.

Short-Term Assays

Based on the hypothesis that chemicals may elicit autoimmune disorders by a mechanism resembling graft-versus-host (GVH) reactions, Gleichmann et al. (11,75) have adopted an existing GVH assay, the popliteal lymph node assay (PLNA), to study chemical-induced immune reactions. In the adopted assay a chemical (without adjuvant) instead of a lymphoid cell suspension is subcutaneously injected into the footpad of mice, and the reaction of the draining PLN is assessed by measuring weight or cell number. Whereas the classical GVH reaction is caused by donor T cell reactions against genetically foreign major histocompatibility complex (MHC) molecules of the recipient, the chemical-induced PLN reaction is caused by recipient T cell reactions against chemically altered self-protein/peptides, including self-MHC molecules. Using the PLNA, many drugs known to occasionally induce immune-mediated systemic side effects in humans were shown to trigger significant reactions in mice and rats (75–88). Injection of DPH and D-penicillamine without adjuvant into the footpad of mice induced a T cell-dependent weight increase that could be characterized morphologically by early T cell activation followed by proliferation and maturation of B cells (77,83). Maturation was confirmed by the demonstration of increased numbers of IgM- and, especially, IgG-producing cells (77,89) and of increased secretion of these immunoglobulins (84–86). Effects observed were very similar to those induced during a local GVH reaction in the PLN (83). Study of the kinetics and morphology of DPH- and nitrofurantoin-induced PLN reactions has verified the resemblance with a local GVH reaction and showed that the PLN reactions could clearly be distinguished from those induced by sheep red blood cells, a T cell-dependent antigen, lipopolysaccharide (LPS), a B cell mitogen, and the contact sensitizer dinitrochlorobenzene (83). Immunogenetic studies in mice with DPH (89) and D-penicillamine (78) have indicated that the extent of PLN enlargement is controlled by MHC (H-2) as well as non-MHC genes. Complete nonresponder strains were not found. Furthermore, the PLNA was able to discriminate between structurally closely related compounds, as shown for chemical congeners of D-penicillamine (78), DPH (80), and zimeldine (84–86). For zimeldine also a distinction between the immunologic and pharmacologic activity could be made (86).

The virtual elimination of pharmacokinetic factors inherent to the assay and/or the limited possibility for local metabolic conversion may account for the false-negative results, such as in the case of procainamide (81). As shown in a recent study, the deficit may be overcome by the use of an *in vitro* drug-metabolizing system (90). Thus the PLNA seems to be a versatile tool to recognize T cell-activating drugs and chemicals, including autoimmunogenic chemicals. However, further mechanistic studies and interlaboratory validation are required, before the assay can be recommended for routine use in preclinical toxicity screening.

MULTIFACTORIAL ETIOLOGY: DIFFICULTIES FOR RISK ASSESSMENT

The spectrum of factors associated with autoimmune diseases have been reviewed extensively (2,91,92) and appropriately termed "The Mosaic of Autoimmunity" (91). The concerted action of individual factors and the chemical appear to somehow determine whether or not autoimmune disease will develop (2,91). For example, there is ample circumstantial evidence that only minor environmental triggers suffice to evoke SLE in individuals with a strong genetic predisposition to the disease, while stronger environmental stimuli are needed to trigger disease in individuals with less of a genetic predisposition (20,91). This was elegantly evidenced by Hang et al. (65) in different mouse strains. They showed that the relative contribution of endogenous and exogenous factors to the induction of disease can vary and that the factors probably complement each other.

Risk assessment ideally requires knowledge of all endogenous as well as exogenous factors that influence susceptibility to drug-induced untoward immune reactions. In practice this will be impossible, since there are numerous factors, most of which are ill-defined or unknown, and since these will differ between drugs or groups of drugs under investigation. However, factors having major influence on immune reactions are becoming more and more defined.

Immunogenetics

Ample data have shown that polymorphisms of MHC genes play a crucial role in the initiation and regulation of specific immune responses. Therefore it is not surprising that several associations between the genetic makeup of the MHC and autoimmune diseases have been found (93). Less data are available on chemical-induced autoimmune diseases, but firm evidence of the role of the MHC in the induction of autoantibody formation and glomerulonephritis by mercuric chloride has been obtained in inbred rats (62,94) as well as in mice (95).

Metabolism

Metabolic polymorphisms also might define susceptibility. Notably, individuals that are slow acetylators of procainamide and hydralazine (64,96) and poor sulfoxidizers of D-penicillamine (97) and sulfonamides (98) have an increased chance to develop adverse systemic immunologic disorders. These observations have led to the suggestion that particular reactive metabolites may be implicated in the pathogenesis. Polymorphisms of drug metabolism may result not only in a different rate of elimination of the parent compound or its metabolites but also in formation of particular metabolites due to stereoselective metabolism (99). For example, the extent of formation of 5-ethyl-5-phenylhydantoin from mephenytoin was found to be determined by a stereoselective metabolism of the *R*- and *S*-enantiomers (99). Because 5-ethyl-5-phenylhydantoin (Nirvanol), used at the beginning of this century for the treatment of chorea, caused a high incidence of mild to severe immunologic disorders in children and adults (100), this particular metabolite may be implicated in the immunotoxic effects of mephenytoin.

Stress Responses

Glucocorticoids released from the adrenal glands in response to stress have profound effects on the immune system, and genetic variation in the magnitude of such a response can determine the susceptibility to autoimmune disease. For example, the low stress-responsive Lewis rat is highly susceptible to induction of cell-mediated autoimmune diseases, for example, experimental allergic encephalomyelitis. In contrast, the high stress-responsive PVG rat is resistant to the disease but becomes highly susceptible upon adrenalectomy and when given glucocorticoid replacement at only basal levels (101). There is as yet no indication that high-stress responders, which tend to produce more vigorous humoral immunity than cell-mediated immunity, are more susceptible to antibody-mediated autoimmune disorders. Regarding the influence of the stress genotype on immune reactions, it should be noted that various drugs themselves can influence the production or action of glucocorticoids as a side effect and so inhibit, potentiate, or modulate immune reactions elicited by themselves.

Confounding and Conditional Factors

Although a drug's potential to cause autoimmune disease may reflect its intrinsic chemical or pharmacologic characteristics, the underlying disease necessitating treatment may be at play as well. For instance, epileptic seizures can be an initial symptom of SLE in some patients and precede other features of the syndrome by years (20,102). Therefore antiepileptic drugs given to treat the convulsions may be mistakenly considered as causative agents of the autoimmune disease. On the other hand, the relatively high frequency of epileptic seizures and the low incidence of autoimmune disease among the general population (103) suggest that other host and environmental factors are likely to be more important in provoking SLE.

Another example concerns drugs used to treat bacterial infections, like penicillins, sulfonamides, and nitrofurantoin. These are relatively frequent inducers of immunologic side effects. Since infectious agents themselves have been implicated in the etiology of autoimmune diseases, this may lead to a biased implication of these drugs in the diseases. On the other hand, it is not unlikely that sensitization of T cells to the drugs is stimulated by infection, for instance, as a consequence of the adjuvant action of cytokines generated during infection. Likewise, the suggestion by Bryson et al. (57) is interesting in this connection: T cells, which contribute to the normal or drug-induced autoreactive T cell pool, can be activated by microbial superantigens produced as a result of microbial growth after drug-induced immunosuppression, resulting in the induction or exacerbation of autoimmune reactions.

CONCLUSIONS

Hazard identification of the autoimmune disease-inducing potential of a given compound in routine toxicology, as currently practiced, will remain difficult in the near future. Because drugs may interact with the immune system at different levels, it is unlikely that one assay or methodology will be able to predict the autoimmunizing potential of the various classes of drugs. Nevertheless, the association between development of immunodeficiency, benign or neoplastic lymphoproliferation, and autoimmune diseases, particularly in the context of thymic abnormalities, should be investigated further. New approaches like the PLNA may provide a promising short-term indicator of a drug's potential to induce T cell activation. In the absence of any other useful assay system in this context, further mechanistic and validation studies with the PLNA should be encouraged.

To establish adequate parameters that allow hazard identification, further research into the mechanisms of drug-induced autoimmune reactions is required. A major challenge for the development of predictive toxicity testing methods and risk assessment represents the analysis of the contribution of individual factors to the development of disease.

ACKNOWLEDGMENTS

We wish to thank Drs. H. J. Schuurman and R. Bechter for critically reviewing the manuscript for this chapter.

REFERENCES

1. Adams LE, Hess EV. Drug-related lupus. Incidence, mechanisms and clinical implications. *Drug Safety* 1991;6:431–449.
2. Kammüller ME, Bloksma N, Seinen W. Autoimmunity and toxicology. Immune disregulation induced by drugs and chemicals. In: Kammüller ME, Bloksma N, Seinen W, eds. *Autoimmunity and toxicology*. Amsterdam: Elsevier Science Publishers; 1989:3–34.
3. Uetrecht JP. The role of leukocyte-generated reactive metabolites in the pathogenesis of idiosyncratic drug reactions. *Drug Metab Rev* 1992;24:299–366.
4. Dubois EL, Wallace DJ. Drugs that exacerbate and induce systemic lupus erythematosus. In: Wallace DJ, Dubois EL, eds. *Dubois' lupus erythematosus*, 3rd ed. Philadelphia: Lea & Febiger; 1987:450–469.
5. Bigazzi PE. Autoimmunity induced by chemicals. *Clin Toxicol* 1988;26:125–156.
6. Zürcher K, Krebs A. *Cutaneous side effects of systemic drugs. A commentated synopsis of today's drugs*. Basel: Karger; 1980.
7. Siegel M, Lee SL, Peress NS. The epidemiology of drug-induced systemic lupus erythematosus. *Arthritis Rheum* 1967;10:407–415.
8. Michet CL, McKenna CH, Elveback LR, Kaslow RA, Kurland LT. Epidemiology of systemic lupus erythematosus and other connective tissue diseases in Rochester, Minnesota, 1950 through 1979. *Mayo Clin Proc* 1985;60:105–113.
9. Packman CH, Leddy JP. Drug-related immunologic injury of erythrocytes. In: Williams WJ, Beutler E, Erslev AJ, Lichtman MA, eds. *Hematology*, 4th ed. New York: McGraw-Hill; 1990: 681–686.
10. Aster RH. George JN. Thrombocytopenia due to enhanced platelet destruction by immunologic mechanisms. In: Williams WJ, Beutler E, Erslev AJ, Lichtman MA, eds. *Hematology*, 4th ed. New York: McGraw-Hill; 1990:1370–1398.
11. Gleichmann E, Pals ST, Rolink AG, Radaszkiewicz T, Gleichmann H. Graft-versus-host reactions: clues to the etiopathology of a spectrum of immunological diseases. *Immunol Today* 1984; 5:324–332.
12. Allison AC. Theories of self tolerance and autoimmunity. In: Kammüller ME, Bloksma N, Seinen W, eds. *Autoimmunity and toxicology*. Amsterdam: Elsevier Science Publishers; 1989:67–115.
13. Duggan MAK, Court JB. A proposed mechanism of production of the autoimmune and lymphoproliferative side-effects of β-adrenergic-site-blocking drugs and hydantoin anticonvulsants. *Ann Clin Res* 1981;13:406–418.
14. Blalock JE. A molecular basis for bidirectional communication between the immune and neuroendocrine systems. *Physiol Rev* 1989;69:1–32.
15. Moingeon P, Bidart JM, Albemici GF, Bohuon C. Characterization of a peripheral-type benzodiazepine binding site on human circulating lymphocytes. *Eur J Pharmacol* 1983;92:147–149.
16. Lloyd EJ, Andrews PR. A common structural model for central nervous system drugs and their receptors. *J Med Chem* 1986;29:453–462.
17. Goldman M, Druet P, Gleichmann E. T_H2 cells in systemic autoimmunity: insights from allogeneic diseases and chemically-induced autoimmunity. *Immunol Today* 1991;12:223–227.
18. Merritt HH, Putnam TJ. Sodium diphenylhydantoinate in treatment of convulsive disorders. *JAMA* 1938;111:1068–1073.
19. Rall TW, Schleifer LS. Drugs effective in the therapy of the epilepsies. In: Goodman Gilman A,

Rall TW, Nies AS, Taylor P, eds. *Goodman and Gilman's the pharmacological basis of therapeutics*, 8th ed. New York: Pergamon Press; 1990:436–462.

20. Alarcon-Segovia D, Alarcon-Riquelme M. Autoimmune reactions induced by diphenylhydantoin and nitrofurantoin. In: Kammüller ME, Bloksma N, Seinen W, eds. *Autoimmunity and toxicology*. Amsterdam: Elsevier Science Publishers; 1989:151–166.
21. Scherokman B, Jabbari B. The risks and benefits of withdrawing antiepileptic therapy. *Drug Safety* 1993;8:399–403.
22. Sorrell TC, Forbes IJ. Depression of immune competence by phenytoin and carbamazepine. *Clin Exp Immunol* 1975;20:273–285.
23. Bluming A, Homer S, Khiroya R. Selective diphenylhydantoin-induced suppression of lymphocyte reactivity *in vitro*. *J Lab Clin Med* 1976;88:417–422.
24. Margaretten NC, Warren RP. Effect of phenytoin on antibody production: use of a murine model. *Epilepsia* 1987;28:77–80.
25. MacFarlane DG, Clark B, Panayi GS. Pilot study of phenytoin in rheumatoid arthritis. *Ann Rheum Dis* 1986;45:954–956.
26. Richards IM, Fraser SM, Hinter JA, Capell HA. Comparison of phenytoin and gold as second line drugs in rheumatoid arthritis. *Ann Rheum Dis* 1987;46:667–669.
27. Seager J, Coovadia HM, Soothill JF. Reduced immunoglobulin concentration and impaired macrophage function in mice duc to diphenylhydantoin. *Clin Exp Immun* 1978;33:437–440.
28. Tucker AN, Hong L, Boorman GA, Pung O, Luster MI. Alteration of bone marrow cell cycle kinetics by diphenylhydantoin: relationship to folate utilization and immune function. *J Pharmacol Exp Ther* 1985;234:57–62
29. Okamoto Y, Shimizu K, Tamura K, et al. Effects of phenytoin on cell-mediated immunity. *Cancer Immun Immunother* 1988;26:176–179.
30. Krueger GRF. The pathology of diphenylhydantoin-induced lymphoproliferative reactions in animals. In: Kammüller ME, Bloksma N, Seinen W, eds. *Autoimmunity and toxicology*. Amsterdam: Elsevier Science Publishers; 1989:391–413.
31. Krueger GRF, Bedoya VA. Hydantoin-induced lymphadenopathies and lymphomas: experimental studies in mice. *Recent Results Cancer Res* 1978;64:265–270.
32. Krueger G, Harris D, Sussman E. Effect of dilantin in mice. II. Lymphoreticular tissue atypia and neoplasia after chronic exposure. *Z Krebsforsch* 1972;78:290–302.
33. Jang JJ. Takahashi M, Furukawa F, Toyoda K, Hasegawa R, Sato H, Hayashi Y. Long-term *in vivo* carcinogenicity study of phenytoin (5,5-diphenylhydantoin) in F344 rats. *Food Chem Toxicol* 1987;25:697–702.
34. Atlas SA, Zweier JL Nebert DW. Genetic differences in phenytoin pharmacokinetics. *In vivo* clearance and *in vitro* metabolism among inbred strains of mice. *Dev Pharmacol Ther* 1980;1:281–304.
35. Hirai M, Ichikawa M. Changes in serum glucocorticoid levels and thymic atrophy induced by phenytoin administration in mice. *Toxicol Lett* 1991;56:1–6.
36. Katsumata M, Gupta C, Baker MK, Sussdorf CE, Goldman AS. Diphenylhydantoin: an alternative ligand of a glucocorticoid receptor affecting prostaglandin generation in A/J mice. *Science* 1982;218:1313–1315.
37. Bloksma N, De Bakker JM, van Rooijen HJM, Punt P, Seinen W, Kammüller ME. Long-term treatment with 5,5–diphenylhydantoin reduces lymphadenopathy and anti-ssDNA autoantibodies in C57BL/6-*lpr*/*lpr* mice. *Int J Immunopharmacol* 1994;16:261–268.
38. Theofilopoulos AN, Balderas R, Shawler DL, Izui S, Kotzin BL, Strober S, Dixon FJ. Inhibition of T cell proliferation and SLE-like syndrome of MRL/I mice by whole body or total lymphoid irradiation. *J Immunol* 1980;125:2137–2142.
39. Steinberg AD, Roths JB, Murphy ED, Steinberg RT, Raveche ES. Effects of thymectomy or androgen administration upon the autoimmune disease of MRL/Mp-*lpr*/*lpr* mice. *J Immunol* 1980; 125:871–873.
40. Mountz JD, Smith HR, Wilder RL, Reeves JP, Steinberg AD. Cs-A therapy in MRL-*lpr*/*lpr* mice: amelioration of immunopathology despite autoantibody production. *J Immunol* 1987;138:157–163.
41. Theofilopoulos AN, Dixon FJ. Murine models of systemic lupus erythematosus. *Adv Immunol* 1985;37:269–390.
42. Kubo C, Day NK, Good RA. Influence of early or late dietary restriction on life span and immunological parameters in MRL/Mp-*lpr*/*lpr*. *Proc Natl Acad Sci USA* 1984;81:5831–5835.

43. Koizumi T, Nakao Y, Matsui T. Effects of corticosteroids and 1,24R-dihydroxy-vitamin D3 administration on lymphoproliferation and autoimmune disease in MRL/MP-*lpr*/*lpr* mice. *Int Arch Allergy Appl Immunol* 1985;77:396–404.
44. Kohler C, Jeanvoine G, Pierrez J, Olive D, Gerard H. Modifications of the thymus and splenic thymic dependent zones after in utero exposure to phenytoin: qualitative and quantitative analysis in C3H mice. *Dev Pharmacol Ther* 1987;10:405–412.
45. Chapman JR, Roberts DW. Humoral immune dysfunction as a result of prenatal exposure to diphenylhydantoin: correlation with the occurrence of physical defects. *Teratology* 1984;30:107–117.
46. Rosen FS. Autoimmunity and immunodefiency disease. In: Evered D, Whelan J, eds. *Autoimmunity and autoimmune disease*, Ciba Foundation Symposium 129. Chichester: Wiley; 1987:135–148.
47. Cleland LG, Bell DA. The occurrence of systemic lupus erythematosus in two kindreds in association with severe selective IgA deficiency. *J Rheumatol* 1978;5:288–293.
48. Seager J, Jamison DL, Wilson J, Hayward AR, Soothill JF. IgA deficiency, epilepsy, and phenytoin treatment. *Lancet* 1975;2:632–635.
49. Hjalmarson O, Hanson LÅ, Nilsson LÅ. IgA deficiency during D-penicillamine treatment. *Br Med J* 1977;1:549.
50. Fudenberg HH. Immunological deficiency, autoimmune disease, and lymphoma: observations, implications, and speculations. *Arthritis Rheum* 1966;9:464–472.
51. Starzl TE, Nalesnik MA, Porter KA, et al. Reversibility of lymphomas and lymphoproliferative lesions developing under cyclosporin-steroid therapy. *Lancet* 1984;1:583–587.
52. Sakaguchi S, Sakaguchi N. Organ-specific autoimmune disease induced in mice by elimination of T cell subsets. V. Neonatal administration of cyclosporine A causes autoimmune disease. *J Immunol* 1989;142:471–480.
53. Sakaguchi S, Sakaguchi N. Thymus and autoimmunity: capacity of the normal thymus to produce pathogenic self-reactive T cells and conditions required for their induction of autoimmune disease. *J Exp Med* 1990;172:537–545.
54. Hess AD, Fischer AC. Immune mechanisms in cyclosporine-induced syngeneic graft-versus-host disease. *Transplantation* 1989;48:895–900.
55. Glazier A, Tutschka PJ, Farmer ER, Santos GW. Graft-versus-host disease in cyclosporine A-treated rats after syngeneic and autologous bone marrow reconstitution. *J Exp Med* 1983;158:1–8.
56. Prud'Homme GJ, Parfrey NA, Vanier LE. Cyclosporine-induced autoimmunity and immune hyperreactivity. *Autoimmunity* 1991;9:345–356.
57. Bryson JS, Caywood BE, Kaplan AM. Relationship of cyclosporine A-mediated inhibition of clonal deletion and development of syngeneic graft-versus-host disease. *J Immunol* 1991;147:391–397.
58. Jones RJ, Vogelsang GB, Hess AD, et al. Induction of graft-versus-host disease after autologous bone marrow transplantation. *Lancet* 1989;1:754–757.
59. Schuurman H-J, Van Loveren H, Rozing J, Vos JG. Chemicals trophic for the thymus: risk for immunodeficiency and autoimmunity. *Int J Immunopharmacol* 1992;14:369–375.
60. Kammüller ME, Bloksma N, Seinen W. Toxicological considerations on immune disregulation induced by drugs and chemicals. In: Kammüller ME, Bloksma N, Seinen W, eds. *Autoimmunity and toxicology*. Amsterdam: Elsevier Science Publishers; 1989:443–457.
61. Singer PA, Theofilopoulos AN. T-cell receptor Vβ repertoire expression in murine models of SLE. *Immunol Rev* 1990;118:103–127.
62. Druet P, Pelletier L, Rossert J, Druet E, Hirsch F, Sapin C. Autoimmune reactions induced by metals. In: Kammüller ME, Bloksma N, Seinen W, eds. *Autoimmunity and toxicology*. Amsterdam: Elsevier Science Publishers; 1989:347–361.
63. Kuper CF, Beems RB, Bruijntjes JP, Schuurman H-J, Vos JG. Normal development, growth, and aging of the thymus. In: Mohr U, Dungworth DL, Capen CC, eds. *Pathobiology of the aging rat. Volume 1: Blood and lymphoid, respiratory, urinary, cardiovascular, and reproductive systems*. Washington, DC: ILSI Press; 1992:25–48.
64. Rubin RL. Autoimmune reactions induced by procainamide and hydralazine. In: Kammüller ME, Bloksma N, Seinen W, eds. *Autoimmunity and toxicology*. Amsterdam: Elsevier Science Publishers; 1989:119–150.
65. Hang L, Aguado MT, Dixon FJ, Theofilopoulos AN. Induction of severe autoimmune disease in normal mice by simultaneous action of multiple immunostimulators. *J Exp Med* 1985;161:423–428.

66. Canoso RT, De Oliveira RM. Characterization and antigenic specificity of chlorpromazine-induced antinuclear antibodies. *J Lab Clin Med* 1986;108:213–216.
67. Fuchs D, Hausen A, Reibnegger G, Werner ER, Dierich MP, Wachter H. Neopterin a marker for activated cell-mediated immunity: application in HIV infection. *Immunol Today* 1988;9:150–155.
68. Kammüller ME, van Rooijen HJM, Seinen W, Bloksma N. Urinary biopterin levels in mice during graft-versus-host reactions and during exposure to 5,5-diphenylhydantoin. *Int J Immunopharmacal* 1991;13:463–473.
69. Balderas RS, Josimovic-Alasevic O, Diamantstein T, Dixon FJ, Theofilopoulos AN. Elevated titers of cell-free interleukin 2 receptor in serum of lupus mice. *J Immunol* 1987;139:1496–1500.
70. Kroemer G, Andreu JL Gonzalo JA, Gutierrez-Ramos JC, Martinez-A C. Interleukin-2, autotolerance, and autoimmunity. *Adv Immunol* 1991;50:147–235.
71. Colvin RB, Preffer FI, Fuller TC, Brown MC, Ip SH, Kung PC, Cosimi AB. A critical analysis of serum and urine interleukin-2 receptor assays in renal allograft recipients. *Transplantation* 1989; 48:800–805.
72. Suzuki H, Yasukawa K, Saito T, Narazaki M, Hasegawa A, Taga T, Kishimoto T. Serum soluble interleukin-6 receptor in MRL/*lpr* mice is elevated with age and mediates the interleukin-6 signal. *Eur J Immunol* 1993;23:1078–1082.
73. Troutt AB, Kelso A. Lymphokine synthesis *in vivo* in an acute murine graft-versus-host reaction: mRNA and protein measurements *in vivo* and *in vitro* reveal marked differences between actual and potential lymphokine production levels. *Int Immunol* 1993;5:399–407.
74. Bauer J, Hermann F. Interleukin-6 in clinical medicine. *Ann Hematol* 1991;62:203–210.
75. Gleichmann E, Vohr H-W, Stringer C, Nuyens J, Gleichmann H. Testing the sensitization of T cells to chemicals. From murine graft-versus-host (GVH) reactions to chemical-induced GVH-like immunological diseases. In: Kammüller ME, Bloksma N, Seinen W, eds. *Autoimmunity and toxicology*. Amsterdam: Elsevier Science Publishers; 1989:363–390.
76. Gleichmann H. Studies on the mechanism of drug sensitization: T-cell-dependent popliteal lymph node reaction to diphenylhydantoin. *Clin Immunol Immunopathol* 1981;18:203–211.
77. Gleichmann HIK, Pals ST, Radaszkiewicz T. T-cell-dependent B-cell proliferation and activation induced by administration of the drug diphenylhydantoin to mice. *Hematol Oncol* 1983;1:165–176.
78. Hurtenbach U, Gleichmann H, Nagata N, Gleichmann E. Immunity to D-penicillamine: genetic, cellular, and chemical requirements for induction of popliteal lymph node enlargement in the mouse. *J Immunol* 1987;139:411–416.
79. Stiller-Winkler R, Radaszkiewicz T, Gleichmann E. Immunopathological signs in mice treated with mercury compounds—I. Identification by the popliteal lymph node assay of responder and non-responder strains. *Int J Immunopharmacol* 1988;10:475–484.
80. Kammüller ME, Seinen W. Structural requirements for hydantoins and 2-thiohydantoins to induce lymphoproliferative popliteal lymph node reactions in the mouse. *Int J Immunopharmacol* 1988; 10:997–1010.
81. Kammüller ME, Thomas C, De Bakker JM, Bloksma N, Seinen W. The popliteal lymph node assay in mice to screen for the immune disregulating potential of chemicals—a preliminary study. *Int J Immunopharmacol* 1989;11:293–300.
82. Thomas C, Groten J, Kammüller ME, De Bakker JM, Seinen W, Bloksma N. Popliteal lymph node reactions in mice induced by the drug zimeldine. *Int J Immunopharmacol* 1989;11:693–702.
83. De Bakker JM, Kammüller ME, Muller ESM, Lam AW, Seinen W, Bloksma N. Kinetics and morphology of chemically induced popliteal lymph node reactions compared with antigen-, mitogen-, and graft-versus-host-reaction-induced responses. *Virchows Arch B Cell Pathol* 1990;58: 279–287.
84. Thomas C, Punt P, Warringa R, Högberg T, Seinen W, Bloksma N. Popliteal lymph node enlargement and antibody production in the mouse by zimeldine and related compounds with varying side chains. *Int J Immunopharmacol* 1990;12:561–568.
85. Thomas C, Lippe W, Högberg T, Seinen W, Bloksma N. Induction of popliteal lymph node enlargement and antibody production in the mouse pyridylallylamines related to zimeldine. *Int J Immunopharmacol* 1990;12:569–576.
86. Thomas C, Lippe W, Seinen W, Bloksma N. Popliteal lymph node enlargement and antibody production in the mouse induced by drugs affecting monoamine levels in the brain. *Int J Immunopharmacol* 1991;13:621–629.
87. Krzystyniak K, Brouland J-P, Panaye G, Patriarca C, Verdier F, Descotes J, Revillard J-P. Activa-

tion of $CD4^+$ and $CD8^+$ lymphocyte subsets by streptozotocin in murine popliteal lymph node (PLN) test. *J Autoimmun* 1992;5:183–197.
88. Verdier F, Virat M, Descotes J. Applicability of the popliteal lymph node assay in the Brown-Norway rat. *Immunopharmacol Immunotoxicol* 1990;12:669–677.
89. Bloksma N, Kammüller ME, Punt P, Seinen W. Strain-dependence of primary popliteal lymph node reactions to subcutaneous injection of diphenylhydantoin in mice. In: Kammüller ME. *A toxicolological approach to chemical-induced autoimmunity*. Utrecht: PhD Thesis; 1988:79–92.
90. Katsutani N, Shionoya H. Popliteal lymph node enlargement induced by procainamide. *Int J Immunopharmacol* 1992;14:681–686.
91. Shoenfeld Y, Isenberg D. The mosaic of autoimmunity. The factors associated with autoimmune disease. In: *Research monographs in immunology*, vol. 12. Amsterdam: Elsevier Science Publishers; 1989.
92. Mackay IR, Rose NR. Autoimmunity: horizons. In: Rose NR, Mackay IR, eds. *The autoimmune diseases II*. San Diego: Academic Press; 1992:409–430.
93. Welsh KI, Black CM. Genetic aspects of the acquired connective tissue diseases. *Semin Dermatol* 1985;4:152–163.
94. Aten J, Veninga A, De Heer E, Rozing J, Nieuwenhuis P, Hoedemaeker PJ, Weening JJ. Susceptibility to the induction of either autoimmunity or immunosuppression by mercuric chloride is related to the major histocompatibility complex class II haplotype. *Eur J Immunol* 1991;21:611–616.
95. Mirtcheva J, Pfeiffer C, de Bruijn J, Jacquesmart F, Gleichmann E. Immunological alterations inducible by mercury compounds: III. H-2A acts as an immune response and H-2E as an immune "suppression" locus for $HgCl_2$-induced antinucleolar autoantibodies. *Eur J Immunol* 1989;19: 2257–2261.
96. Hein DW, Weber WW. Metabolism of procainamide, hydralazine, and isoniazid in relation to autoimmune(-like) reactions. In: Kammüller ME, Bloksma N, Seinen W, eds. *Autoimmunity and toxicology*. Amsterdam: Elsevier Science Publishers; 1989:239–265.
97. Emery P, Panayi GS, Huston G, et al. D-Penicillamine-induced toxicity in rheumatoid arthritis. The role of sulphoxidation status and HLA-DR3. *J Rheumatol* 1984;11:626–632.
98. Sheer NH, Spielberg SP, Grant DM, Tang BK, Kalow W. Differences in metabolism of sulfonamides, predisposing to idiosyncratic toxicity. *Ann Intern Med* 1986;105:179–184.
99. Wedlund PJ, Aslanian WS, Jacqz E, McAllister CB, Branch RA, Wilkinson GR. Phenotype differences in mephenytoin pharmacokinetics in normal subjects. *J Pharmacol Exp Ther* 1985;234:662–669.
100. Pilcher JD, Gerstenberger HJ. Treatment of chorea with phenylethyl-hydantoin. *Am J Dis Child* 1930;40:1239–1249.
101. Mason D. Genetic variation in the stress response: susceptibility to experimental allergic encephalomyelitis and implications for human inflammatory disease. *Immunol Today* 1991;12:57–60.
102. Dubois EL, Wallace DJ. Clinical and laboratory manifestations of systemic lupus erythematosus. In: Wallace DJ, Dubois EL, eds. *Dubois' lupus erythematosus*, 3rd ed. Philadelphia: Lea & Febiger; 1987:317–449.
103. Janz D. Epilepsy: seizures and syndromes. In: Frey H-H, Janz D, eds. *Antiepileptic drugs*. Berlin: Springer-Verlag; 1985:3–34.

Immunotoxicology and Immunopharmacology, Second Edition, edited by J. H. Dean, M. I. Luster, A. E. Munson, and I. Kimber.
Raven Press, Ltd., New York © 1994.

34

Clinical Aspects of Allergic Contact Dermatitis

Peter S. Friedmann

Department of Medicine, University of Liverpool, Royal Liverpool University Hospital, Liverpool L69 3BX, United Kingdom

Situated at the interface between the *milieu interieur* and the external world, the skin is exposed to a wide variety of physical, chemical, and microbial assaults. The skin has to perform a number of functions related to its interface position. It provides a physical barrier and maintains that barrier through the capacity to repair physical breaches caused by injury. The stratum corneum or horny layer provides not only a formidable physical barrier to penetration by microbes, but it also forms the vitally important permeability barrier that limits passage of water, electrolytes, and many chemical substances. An additional function of skin, important in defense against invasion from without, is the capacity to respond to physical and chemical perturbation by recruitment of inflammatory processes. A component of this inflammatory response is the skin's function as an immune organ. The immune function of skin presumably evolved to deal with microbes including viruses, fungi, and parasites, such as the scabies mite, that succeed in breaching the outer physical barrier to penetrate the epidermis. When the skin responds to chemical perturbation by substances that are "antigenic," no distinction is made between antigens that are of microbial origin and others that may be derived from the environment. Therefore the antimicrobial immune response in skin is closely reflected by the allergic contact hypersensitivity response. This is a delayed hypersensitivity response characterized by the infiltration of CD4+ T lymphocytes into both dermis and epidermis. The contact hypersensitivity system has been used to study mechanisms involved in the immune response. In examining the immune responses activated in skin, a number of aspects must be considered. These include factors involved in the induction of responses—the afferent limb—and also important determinants affecting expression of established immune reactivity—the efferent limb.

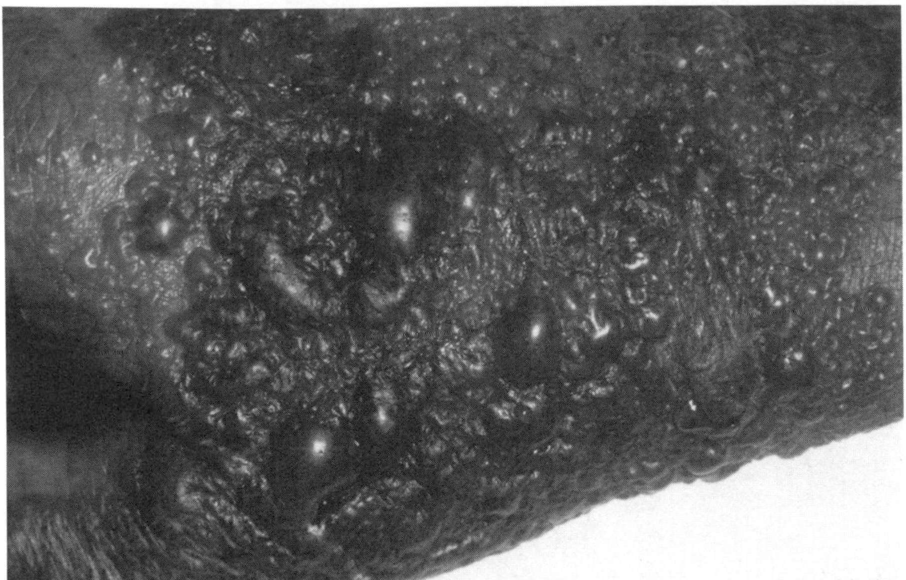

FIG. 1. Acute allergic contact dermatitis reaction to a topical antiseptic applied to the back of the hand. Note characteristic multilocular blisters.

CONTACT HYPERSENSITIVITY AS A CLINICAL PROBLEM

Immune responses to fungi or parasites that penetrate into the viable layers of epidermis are recognized clinically as *eczema*. The immune/allergic response to environmental antigens results in the inflammatory reaction of allergic contact eczema or dermatitis. This often happens as an unwanted consequence of exposure to substances in the work or domestic environment. Contact with the causal substance results in a characteristic pattern of inflammation. The vascular response comprises vasodilation, resulting in redness (erythema), and increased permeability with edema formation, causing swelling and induration. In addition, edema forms within the epidermis, separating epidermal cells (spongiosis), and collections of fluid form blisters (vesicles) that, when large, can be seen to be multilocular because of fusion of small vesicles (Fig. 1). There is perivascular inflammatory infiltration of lymphomononuclear cells in the dermis. The most important immunologic component is probably CD4+ T cells, which are also found in the epidermis (for more details see later discussion). The clinical recognition of allergic contact dermatitis is based on the anatomic distribution of lesions in areas matching physical contact with likely provoking agents in the environment. The picture can become confused because many chemical substances in the environment can provoke inflammatory reactions in the skin, which are not mediated by specific immune mechanisms; these reactions are referred to as irritant reactions. Reactions to irritants are usually categorized as acute, when they follow a single exposure to the substance, or chronic, when they result from repeated or cumulative exposure to the compounds. Responses to irritants must be mentioned here because, as will be seen later, certain mechanisms are common to both the non-immune- and immune-mediated processes. The presence of specific cell-mediated immune hypersensitivity (CMI) is demonstrated formally by epicutaneous patch test challenge with the relevant substance. The inflammation develops over 24 to 48 hr and may last 4 to 6 days. The crucial aspect of the technique is that concentrations of antigen must be used that are nonirritant and hence will not elicit a nonspecific inflammatory response.

Incidence and Prevalence of Allergic Contact Dermatitis

Estimation of incidence and prevalence of contact dermatitis in a whole population is very difficult. A number of surveys have been performed and most have been cross-sectional; that is, they have looked at a population sample that is presumed to represent the general population with no selection in relation to exposure or disease status. Most studies have used questionnaires, asking for the presence of skin troubles on the hands, and most followed up with clinical examination to confirm responses to the questionnaires. These surveys have mainly given estimates for the occurrence of eczema without distinction between irritant or allergic contact dermatitis. Figures for the prevalence of hand dermatitis include 1.7% in Sweden (1), 6.3% in Sweden (2), 2% in the United States (3), and 6.1% in London (4). For a detailed summary of these surveys see Coenraads and Smit (5).

In the working population of the Western world, occupational skin disease accounts for about one-third of all chronic occupational diseases. Eczema and contact dermatitis are responsible for 85% to 95% of all causes of occupational skin diseases (6,7).

Exposure to sensitizing substances is obviously a prerequisite for the formation of allergic contact sensitivity, but, given comparable exposure, there are a number of factors that contribute to whether and how sensitivity is manifested.

STUDIES OF SUSCEPTIBILITY TO CONTACT SENSITIZATION

The immune response to contact allergens comprises two distinct components: the initiation of sensitization (the afferent limb) and the expression of the sensitivity once it is established (the efferent limb). Both these components of the response are influenced by systemic factors, including genetic constitution, age, and sex, as well as local factors, including regional differences in skin thickness, barrier function, and vasculature. Many attempts have been made to examine the importance of these in determining immune responsiveness.

What determines whether an individual will develop an immune/hypersensitivity response to a substance? Antigenic strength or potency is still not well understood, but some substances such as dinitrochlorobenzene (DNCB), diphenylcyclopropenone (DPCP), oxazolone, and urushiol (poison ivy) are highly potent and appear able to induce sensitization in all normal people. Substances such as metallic salts of nickel, cobalt, and chromium and an extensive range of organic compounds are weak antigens and appear only to sensitize some subjects. It is not known whether every individual has the capacity to respond to weak sensitizers. The concentration of antigen is critical and local factors such as occlusion or coincident inflammation, which potentiate percutaneous absorption, may augment the sensitizing potency of a substance.

Once a substance penetrates the outer barrier of the stratum corneum, the induction of sensitization is mediated by special antigen-presenting cells—Langerhans' cells. In summary, upon contact with a chemical, Langerhans' cells in the epidermis descend into the dermis and migrate via the afferent lymphatics to the regional lymph node. Here, they enter the paracortical areas, the home of T lymphocytes (8–10). If the substance is an antigen it appears to provoke this migration. Also, the Langerhans' cell expresses the substance on its surface in combination with the class II molecules of the major histocompatibility complex (MHC), HLA-DR in humans. This complex of HLA-DR-associated antigen is recognized by a T lymphocyte expressing the appropriate, specific T cell receptor. The specific, receptor-mediated binding with the antigen-bearing Langerhans' cell causes activation of the T cell, which results in proliferation and expansion of the clone to establish a population of CD4+ effector T cells. These processes are dealt with in detail elsewhere in this book.

Once some degree of clonal expansion has occurred, immunologic "memory" is established, which allows a quicker response upon reencounter with the antigen. If the clonal expansion continues, at some point some of the daughter cells will leave the node to enter the circulation. Once in the circulation they are available to participate in immune surveillance and to traffic through the tissues. Their presence is manifested by the inflammatory response of contact allergic eczema that develops at sites of encounter with their specific antigen. The regulation of many steps in these events is not yet understood. For instance, it is unknown what determines how many initial T cells are encountered by the antigen-bearing Langerhans' cells, how many divisions the expanding T cell clone undergoes, what signals some T cells to leave the node, or what contributes to the generation of the inflammatory response in the efferent stage. It is the variability in these steps that probably accounts for the heterogeneity of immune responsiveness seen in human beings. However, despite the many steps that are involved in the generation of an immune response, the human immune system, like other physiologic systems, exhibits generally predictable dose–response relationships. Using experimental sensitization with DNCB, analysis of these dose–response relationships has given a physiologic perspective to many of the static and qualitative phenomena observed experimentally.

EXPERIMENTAL SENSITIZATION WITH DNCB

DNCB is a highly potent contact sensitizer and has been used for many studies of human immune responses (11–16). The author and colleagues examined the effects

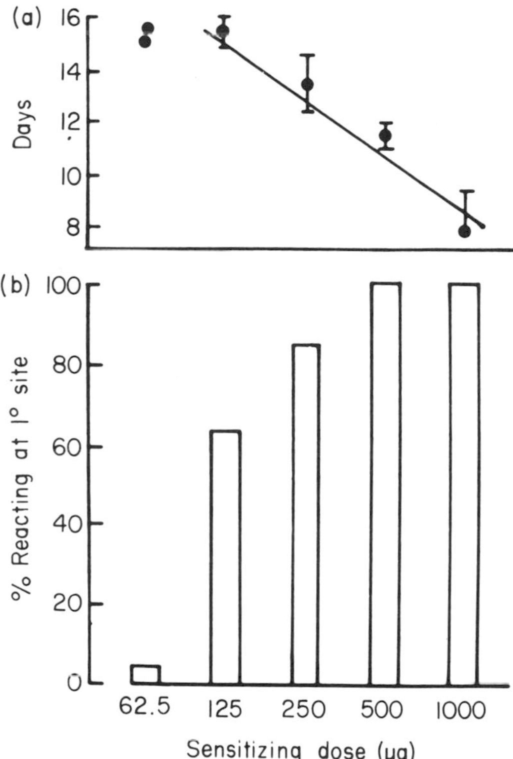

FIG. 2. "Late" flare reaction at site of primary sensitization with DNCB. **A:** Proportion of subjects developing such reactions with different sensitizing doses **B:** Time of appearance of reaction. (Reproduced from ref. 36, with permission.)

of varying the sensitizing dose of DNCB on contact sensitization, and also the dose–response relationships of the elicitation reaction (16–18). Five groups of normal subjects with no history of contact sensitivity or inflammatory skin disease received sensitizing doses of 62.5, 125, 250, 500, or 1000 μg of DNCB in acetone. The sensitizing dose was applied to the flexor aspect of the forearm on a standard, 3-cm diameter area, followed by occlusion for 48 hr. Some DNCB remains bound in the skin for several weeks and hence is available to act as a continuous challenge. As soon as the DNCB-specific T cells enter the circulation, they can respond to this challenge, generating inflammation at the site—a reaction that has been called the "delayed flare" by earlier workers. It was observed that the time of onset of this reaction was inversely related to sensitizing dose (Fig. 2). This implied that the clonal expansion had been quicker, which suggests that a greater number of cells had been activated at the outset.

Four weeks after induction of sensitization, a graded series of challenges (3.125, 6.25, 12.5, and 25 μg) were applied to the other forearm on standard 1-cm patch

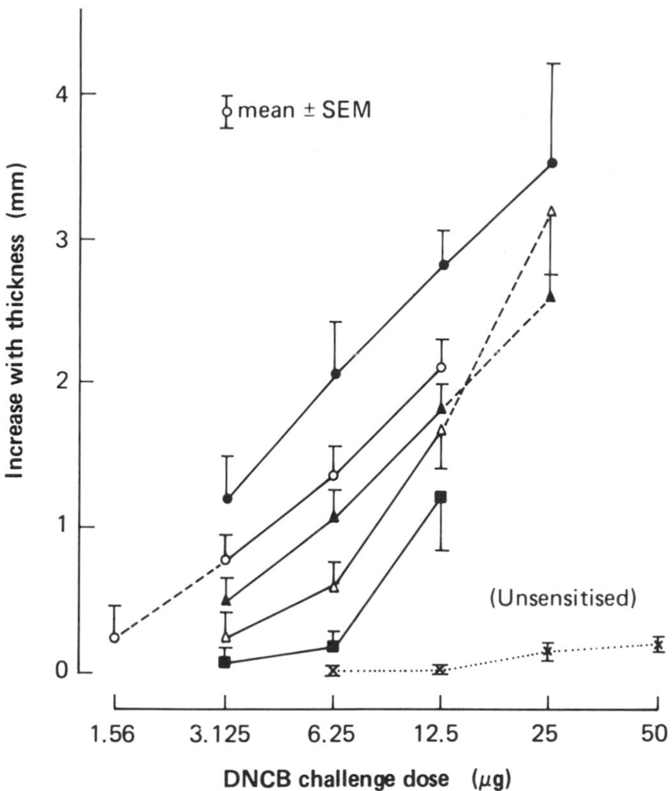

FIG. 3. Response to challenge with DNCB in subjects challenged with different doses of DNCB. ●, Sensitizing dose (SD) 1000 μg; ○, SD 500 μg; ▲, SD 250 μg; Δ, SD 125 μg; ■, SD 62.5 μg; X, unsensitized controls to show irritant effect. Responses measured with calipers as skin fold thickness. (Reproduced from ref. 16, with permission.)

test felts (Al-test) for 24 hr. Forty-eight hours after application, the responses were measured with Harpenden calipers as increases in skin fold thickness (16).

DNCB is an irritant, so in order to interpret challenge responses the irritant effect was first examined in unsensitized normal subjects. The irritant reaction was mainly one of erythema and not edema (Fig. 3). Within the range of challenge doses studied, the threshold for irritance was at 25 μg and there was little further increase in thickness at higher challenge doses. Hence the small degree of thickness change due to irritance was assumed to be constant and not to contribute significantly to the specific immune reaction. Because of the problem of detecting a degree of reactivity so low, it could only be elicited by challenge doses above the threshold for irritance, subjects with no response below this 25-μg dose were regarded, arbitrarily, as unsensitized. Using the clinical assessment of an indurated (edematous) response to challenge with 12.5 μg to indicate that sensitivity was detectable, it was found that the proportions of subjects sensitized showed a sigmoid relationship with the log of

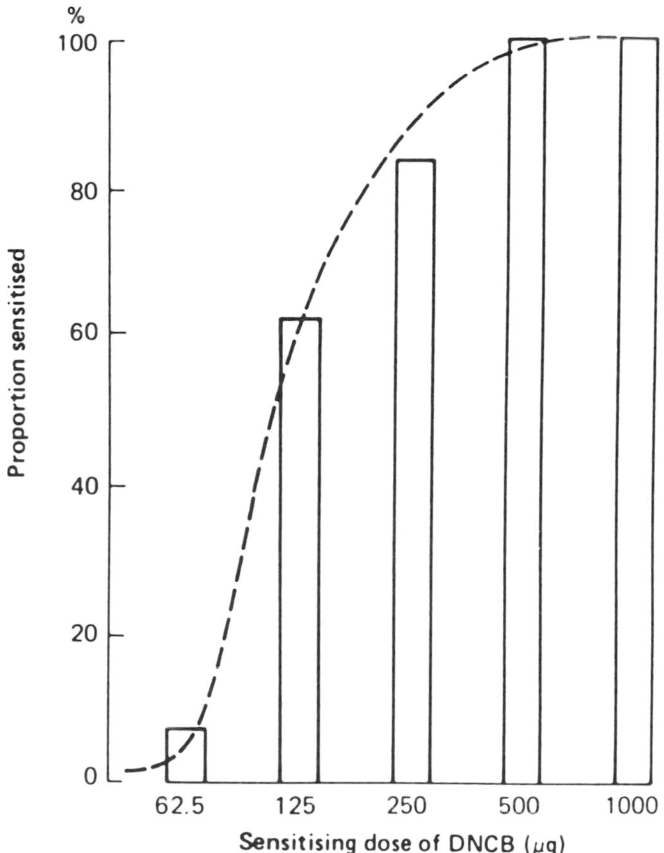

FIG. 4. Proportion of normal subjects sensitized by different doses of DNCB. (Reproduced from ref. 16, with permission.)

sensitizing dose (Fig. 4). Thus 100% of people were sensitized by an initial application of 500 μg of DNCB. When the sigmoid log dose–response curve was linearized by logit transformation, the dose required to sensitize 50% of subjects (ED_{50}) was estimated as 116 μg. This was subsequently tested and indeed 13 of 26 subjects were sensitized (19).

The next observation was that as sensitizing dose increased, not only were more people made clinically sensitive, but they were sensitized to a greater degree. Challenge of these five groups produced a family of dose–response curves that appear to be the lower portions of sigmoid curves (Fig. 3). The tops of the curves were not reached within the range of doses used. Analysis of the linear portions confirmed they were parallel and the calculated slopes are shown in Fig. 5. It can be seen that as sensitizing dose increases, the challenge dose–response curve is shifted progressively to the left, indicating greater reactivity.

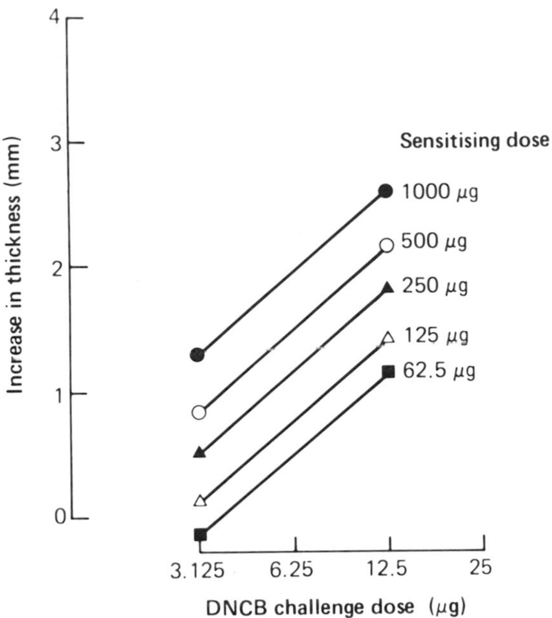

FIG. 5. Responses to challenge with DNCB in normal subjects sensitized 4 weeks previously. The calculated slopes of the linear portions of dose—response curves are shown. (Reproduced from ref. 17, with permission.)

It is an informative observation that the position of the dose–response curve, but not its slope, is altered by changing the strength of the sensitizing stimulus. Thus the slope of the curve seems likely to be determined by the local inflammatory response, the increments of change being proportional to the log of the eliciting stimulus. The position of the challenge dose–response curve reflects the "degree of sensitivity" of an individual or group of subjects. Since the curves are parallel, they can be represented by the responses at any chosen challenge dose. So if, for example, the response at the 12.5-μg challenge dose for each group of subjects is plotted against the sensitizing dose, a curve is obtained which shows that as sensitizing stimulus increases so there is a uniform, linear augmentation of degree of sensitivity (Fig. 6). This probably reflects the proliferative expansion of a clone or clones of antigen-specific effector T cells or, conceivably, of both T effector and T suppressor cells. However, in the latter case their net contribution would have to increase uniformly. The slope of the curve in Fig. 6, which reflects increase in sensitivity with increasing sensitizing dose, reflects the contribution of regulatory factors, augmenting or "helper" factors being likely to increase the slope, while inhibitory or "suppressor" factors being likely to depress it. The slope of this curve therefore represents the "susceptibility" to contact sensitization by DNCB in normal subjects. The slope of the curve would be expected to alter with disease or treatment that modifies susceptibility.

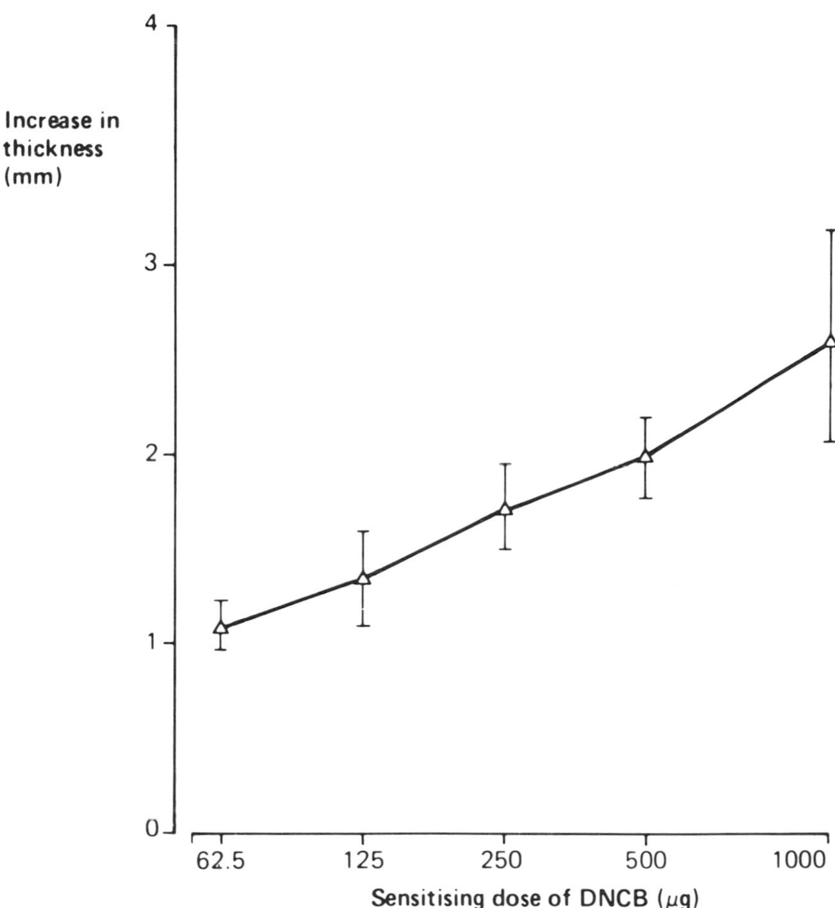

FIG. 6. Relationship between degree of sensitization and sensitizing dose. The skin fold thickness responses to challenge with 12.5 μg of DNCB from each group of subjects are plotted against sensitizing doses. Data from five groups of healthy subjects shown in Fig. 5. *Bars* are standard error of mean (SEM). (Reproduced from ref. 17, with permission.)

Variation in Susceptibility to Contact Sensitization

There is considerable variation in susceptibility to contact sensitization even among people who appear "normal" in every sense. Thus at any sensitizing dose below the 100% effective dose—for example, 250 μg—a proportion of people appeared not to be sensitized at all. These will be discussed further below. Of those who gave clinically "positive" reactions to the challenges, there was a very wide range of responses that appeared normally distributed. It is also a clinical observation that some individuals appear to form contact sensitivities readily to a wide range of environmental substances. This group was studied to see whether they

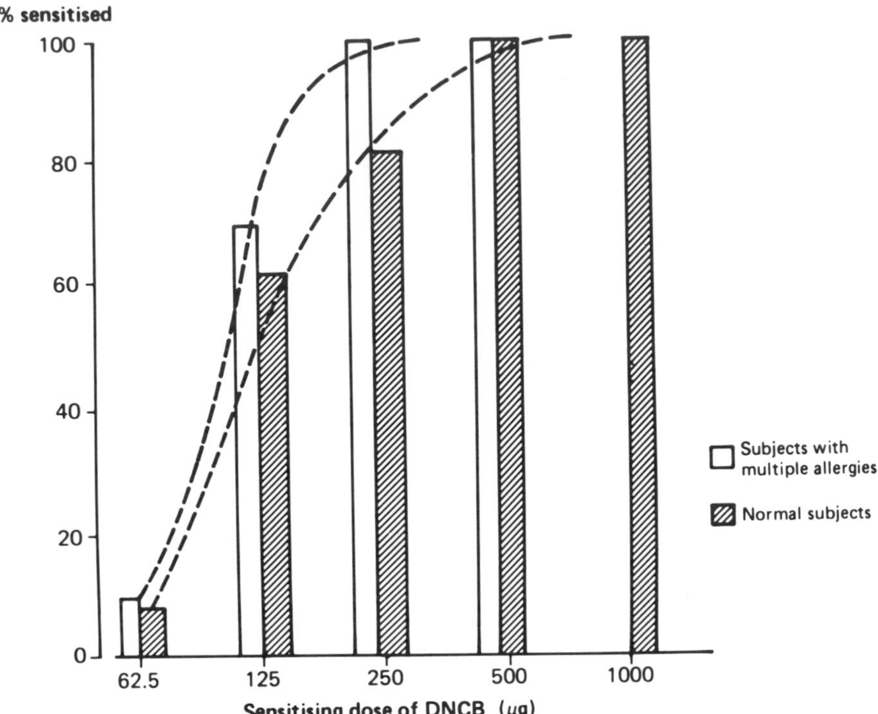

FIG. 7. Proportions sensitized by different doses of DNCB. Comparison of normal subjects, as in Fig. 4, with four groups of individuals with multiple contact allergies to environmental sensitizers. (Reproduced from ref. 18, with permission.)

were different in their capacity to respond to DNCB. Subjects with sensitivity to three or more antigens in the European standard patch test battery were identified from the diagnostic patch test clinic; patients with active eczema were excluded. The protocol for sensitization with DNCB was as described except that the 1000-μg sensitizing dose was not used. It was found that at each sensitizing dose proportionally more subjects could be sensitized (Fig. 7) and the 100% sensitizing dose was 250 μg. The sensitized subjects were more responsive than "normal" subjects (Fig. 8), with the challenge dose–response curves being displaced upward compared with those of the normal subjects (16,19). Very interestingly, the slopes of the curves were parallel, indicating the increased contact sensitivity was not simply due to an increased capacity to generate inflammatory reactions in skin.

When the curve is plotted showing the relationship between degree of sensitization and sensitizing dose for this group of people with multiple contact sensitivities, it has a much greater slope than that for people without such allergies (Fig. 9) (18). In other words, there is a greater augmentation of sensitivity produced by any increase in sensitizing dose.

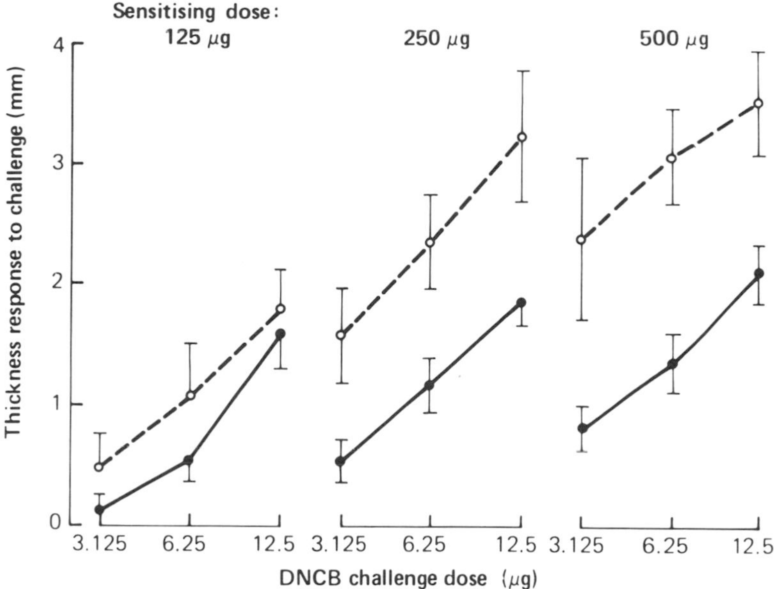

FIG. 8. Responses to challenge with DNCB in subjects with multiple contact sensitivities (○) compared with those from normal subjects (●). Data from three groups are shown, sensitized with 125, 250, and 500 μg DNCB, respectively.

One question that arises is whether the acquisition of one contact sensitivity increases susceptibility to further sensitization by other antigens. However, the studies by Moss et al. (20) included some subjects with multiple contact sensitivities following occupational exposure. These subjects did not differ in their reactivity to DNCB, suggesting that previous contact sensitivity does not enhance subsequent susceptibility to sensitization.

The subjects with multiple contact sensitivities might be a qualitatively different subgroup or they might be at one tail of the normal distribution. When people who had only a single contact sensitivity to nickel were tested with the same protocol, the slope of the curve for increasing sensitization with sensitizing dose was intermediate (20). This supports the idea that there is a normal distribution for susceptibility to contact sensitivities—"high responders" lying at one tail of the normal distribution and the other tail presumably being the "low responders."

Subclinical Sensitization

The previous discussion concerning the range of susceptibility to contact sensitization touched on the point that, at submaximal sensitizing doses of DNCB, a proportion of people appeared not to have become sensitized. The question that arises from this is what has happened immunologically in these unresponsive subjects?

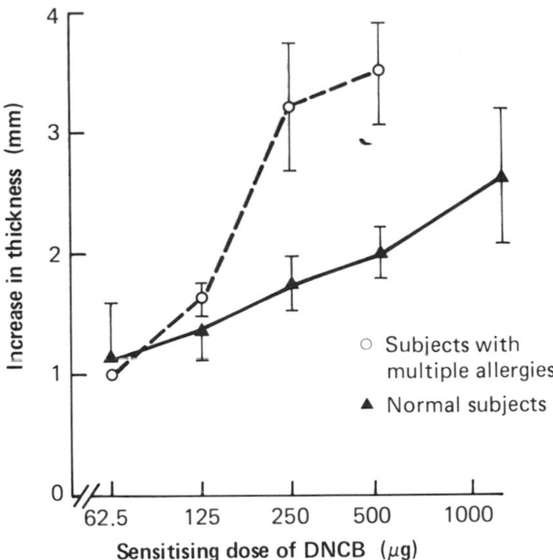

FIG. 9. Augmentation of sensitivity with increasing sensitizing dose of DNCB. Degree of sensitization, obtained from response at 12.5-μg challenge dose, is plotted against sensitizing dose for normal subjects and those with multiple allergies. (Reproduced from ref. 18, with permission.)

Was it a complete failure of response or has their immune system responded to the stimulus at a subclinical level? If this were the case, it would be expected that the initial sensitizing dose has in fact primed the system, initiating expansion of the specifically committed clone(s) to establish some degree of immunologic memory. From this it might be predicted that a second sensitizing stimulus would induce an augmented or boosted response. This is in fact the case as shown by the following observations. The approach used to test the possibility made use of the fact that the challenge regimen of four DNCB doses (3.125, 6.25, 12.5, and 25 μg; total 46.9 μg) is itself a moderately potent sensitizing stimulus. Thus the degree of reactivity of control subjects sensitized by application of the challenge regimen alone could be determined with a second, elicitation challenge 4 weeks after the first sensitizing exposure (Fig. 10). Responses could be compared with those from subjects given the same regimen but who had first received a low-potency sensitizing stimulus. Therefore a group of normal people received 116 μg DNCB on a 3-cm circle of forearm skin as initial sensitizing stimulus. This had previously been shown to be the 50% effective sensitizing dose (19). When challenged 4 weeks later, half the subjects showed no clinically detectable response. These unresponsive subjects were challenged a second time after 4 more weeks (Fig. 10). They gave greatly augmented responses compared with the control subjects who 4 weeks previously had received the challenge regimen alone as a sensitizing stimulus (Fig. 11). This showed clearly that the two sensitizing stimuli had interacted positively, the first subclinical stimulus having established immunologic memory, which greatly aug-

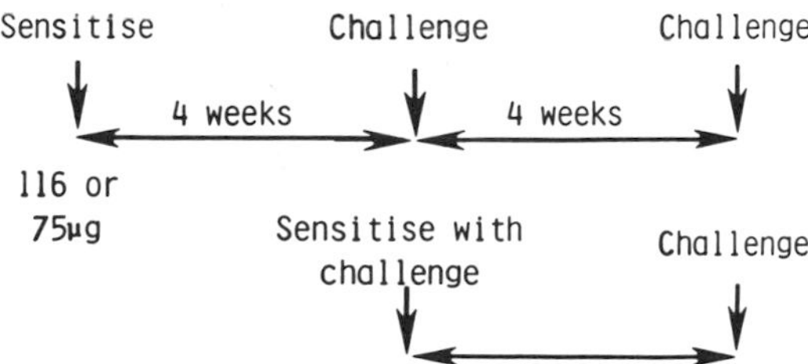

FIG. 10. Protocol for sensitization and challenge to assess subclinical sensitization. Experimental subjects received an initial dose of 116 or 75 μg of DNCB. Four weeks later they were challenged and subjects who were unresponsive received a further challenge after 4 more weeks. Control subjects received the challenge regimen to induce sensitization and their degree of reactivity was determined 4 weeks later with an eliciting challenge. (Reproduced from ref. 19, with permission.)

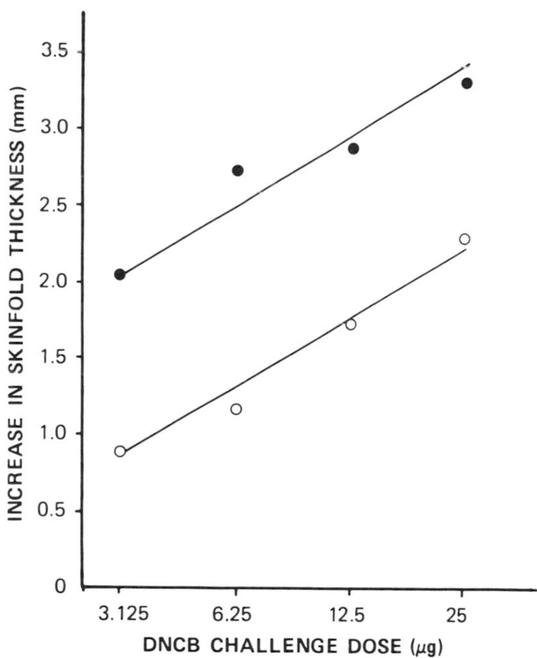

FIG. 11. Augmentation of responsiveness by subclinical sensitization. After an initial dose of 116 μg of DNCB, subjects were challenged 4 weeks later. Unresponsive subjects received a second challenge to determine their degree of reactivity (●). Control subjects were sensitized by application of the challenge regimen (○). (Reproduced from ref. 19, with permission.)

mented the response to the second sensitizing stimulus. This experiment was repeated using the 25% effective sensitizing dose (75 μg DNCB) as the subclinical priming dose (19). Again, the subjects who were unresponsive to the first elicitation challenge were given a second challenge after a further 4 weeks. These people were significantly more responsive than the controls and hence had clearly been sensitized at a subclinical level by the primary sensitizing dose (19).

Thus it is clear that a state of subclinical sensitization can be established by exposure to low doses of antigen. This indicates therefore that the quantitative dose relationship of contact sensitization by DNCB extends down into the subclinical range. This fits with the clonal expansion of antigen-specific T lymphocytes but supports the idea that, below certain levels of proliferation, these cells remain within the lymph nodes and cannot participate in cutaneous challenge responses.

FACTORS INFLUENCING SUSCEPTIBILITY TO CONTACT SENSITIZATION

A number of studies have been performed to examine the basis of susceptibility to contact sensitivity.

Age

The ability to become sensitized to contact antigens such as DNCB is very little altered with age (16,21). Analysis of the relationship between sensitizability and age showed no simple relationship (16), although there is a complex interaction between age and sex. Thus greatest responses were seen in young females, while lowest responses were obtained from old males (16). Also, sensitizability is found to decline slightly after the age of 70.

A more important factor in relation to clinical problems from contact hypersensitivity is that with increasing age there is a greater chance of exposure to environmental allergens. Thus the frequency of clinical problem of contact sensitization and positive patch tests increases with age at least up to the sixth decade.

Genetic Factors

Work in experimental animals provides many examples showing that genetic factors can be of major importance. Thus inbred guinea pigs of strain II can be sensitized with chromate and beryllium but not mercury, whereas animals of strain XIII can be sensitized with mercury but not with chromate or beryllium (22). In humans, observations have been made on naturally occurring sensitivity, such as that to nickel, and also on results of deliberate experimental sensitization with chemicals. Walker et al. (23) used two experimental sensitizers—DNCB and *p*-nitrosodimethylaniline (NDMA)—to investigate responsiveness in families. It was found that if both parents could be sensitized by both agents then their children were more likely to be sensitized than children whose parents failed to sensitize. However, it was not established whether this was simply quantitative in that they were less responsive but could have been sensitized by a bigger dose of antigen, or whether it was qualitative in that nonresponders could not be sensitized at all. Work by the present author and colleagues suggests these would only be quantitative differences—that some humans are more susceptible to forming contact allergies (19,24) (see later discussion). Menné and Holm (25,26) studied female twins. They found that among 30 pairs of monozygotic and 41 pairs of dizygotic twins, with proven nickel allergy in one member of the pair, the frequency of hand eczema was 41% in both groups. In monozygotic twins with one of the pair having nickel sensitivity, the chance of the other developing nickel sensitivity was comparable to the background population level—rather strong evidence against genetic control of susceptibility.

A number of studies have examined whether susceptibility to contact sensitivity is linked to a human leukocyte antigen (HLA) phenotype. In people with nickel sensitivity, HLA-DRw6 was found to be increased up to twofold (37.7% compared to 15.6% in control subjects) (27). White et al. (28) examined 67 patients with multiple (three or more) independent contact allergies and found no overall HLA association with high susceptibility status. There was a slight but nonsignificant increase in frequency of HLA-DR4 in subjects whose allergies included nickel, and of HLA-DR6 in those sensitized to rubber accelerators. Overall, apart from the report by Walker et al. (23), there is very little to suggest that human susceptibility to contact hypersensitivity is under genetic control. One caveat, however, is that all studies of HLA sensitization reviewed by the author have used control populations that were not screened to exclude the presence of contact sensitivity. Therefore small differences may in fact be larger. Also, if human susceptibility to contact sensitivity is normally distributed, as indicated by the experimental studies with DNCB, then it is not surprising that there is no obvious link with HLA or other genetic factors.

Sex

The main factor that appears to be a determinant in susceptibility to contact hypersensitivity is femaleness. Thus it is well-known that autoimmune diseases are more common in women. Also, more women than men present with problems relating to contact hypersensitivity. In Newcastle upon Tyne (United Kingdom), analysis of results of patch tests with the European standard battery of antigens, performed over 5 years in nearly 2200 consecutive patients with eczema, showed the ratio of women to men with at least one positive patch test was greater than 3:1 (29). However, this might reflect either a fundamental sex difference or differences in exposure to environmental antigens.

Several authors have examined susceptibility to contact hypersensitivity formally. Most have used experimental sensitization in different ways and have used response to challenge to make the qualitative decision that an individual is sensitized or not. Walker et al. (23) used DNCB, while Leyden and Kligman (30) and Jordan and King (31) used repetitive exposure to panels of several antigens; all found small increases in the proportion of females becoming sensitized. Rees (32) used experimental sensitization with DNCB but quantified responses to challenge by measurement of edema as skin fold thickness. It was shown that, at the particular sensitizing dose used, the proportion of females sensitized was slightly greater—80% of males compared to 100% of females. However, the females gave much greater responses at each challenge dose and the slope of the dose–response curve was steeper (32). This shows that proper quantification can be much more powerful for such comparisons. It also illustrates the point that this methodology gives information about the whole immune response—afferent and efferent components together. In particular, the influence of systemic factors such as heredity, genetics, or sex cannot be examined separately on the afferent or efferent limbs of the response. Therefore, in the future, it may be that *in vitro* techniques such as limiting dilution analysis, which allows direct enumeration of the number of cells specifically sensitized to a particular antigen, will allow cleaner analysis of the afferent phase. On the other hand, factors that can be applied locally can be analyzed with great discrimination in either the afferent or the local, efferent responses to challenge.

Local Factors in Induction of Contact Sensitivity

As mentioned, systemic factors are likely to affect both afferent and efferent components of the immune response. However, local factors can have an important influence on either the afferent or efferent limbs of the response. As seen from the experiments using different sensitizing doses of DNCB, the concentration of antigen is a major determinant of degree of sensitization. In those observations, the concentration of antigen was varied on a fixed area of 3-cm diameter. Therefore the dose per unit area was being changed. The effect of this variable was explored by changing the area of application and total dose applied while maintaining a constant dose per unit area. As seen from Table 1 a total dose of 62.5 μg applied to a 3-cm diameter circle of area 7.1 cm^2 caused clinical sensitivity in only 2 of 24 (8%) subjects. When the same dose of 62.5 μg was applied to a circle 1.5 cm in diameter (1.8 cm^2), six of seven subjects (89%) were sensitized (33). When the sensitizing stimuli are expressed as concentration per unit area, they are 8.8 μg/cm^2 and 35.4 μg/cm^2, respectively, a fourfold difference. A 250-μg dose applied to a 3-cm diameter circle gives a concentration of 35.4 μg/cm^2, that is, the same as that for 62.5 μg applied to a 1.5-cm circle (Table 1). Although the total doses differ by a factor of 4, they have the same sensitizing potency, causing sensitization in 81% and 89% of subjects, respectively (Table 1). Moreover, the degree of reactivity shown by the sensitized subjects in the two groups was found to be identical (33) (Fig. 12). These observations were extended by choosing another concentration—16.4 μg/cm^2 of DNCB. Three groups were sensitized at this concentration but the area and total dose applied were varied (Table 1). Thus one group received 232 μg on a 4.25-cm circle, one group received 116 μg on a 3-cm diameter circle, and one group re-

TABLE 1. *Relationship between proportions sensitized, area of application, and sensitizing dose of DNCB*

	Application site		Sensitizing dose			
Row	Diameter (cm)	Area (cm^2)	Total (μg)	Concentration (μg/cm^2)	Number of subjects	Percentage sensitized
1	3	7.1	1000	142	24	100
2	3	7.1	500	71	40	100
3	3	7.1	250	35.4	30	83
4	3	7.1	125	17.7	30	63
5	3	7.1	62.5	8.8	24	8
6	1.5	1.8	62.5	35.4	7	86
7	2.1	3.5	58	16.4	22	55
8	3	7.1	116	16.4	34	50
9	4.25	14.2	232	16.4	15	66
10	1 cm felt	0.8	30	38	28	93
11	3 mm felt	0.08	3	38	15	26

Data are from several studies with DNCB. The first five rows are the normal subjects from Figs. 3 and 4. Row 6 gives the same dose per unit area as row 3. In rows 7 to 9 the areas were half and double the standard 7.1 cm^2 but the dose per unit area was constant.

Reproduced from ref. 24, with permission.

ceived 58 μg on a 2.1-cm diameter circle. Again, the proportions sensitized were not significantly different—55%, 50%, and 66%, respectively ($P<0.5$) (33). Also, the degree of reactivity elicited by challenge was not significantly different between the three groups (33). From these results it might be predicted that there would be no reduction of sensitization if the area of application were reduced to an infinitesimal size. To test this prediction a group of people were sensitized using the smallest practicable area. To achieve this, a dose of 30 μg of DNCB in acetone was applied to a standard 1-cm Al-test disk to give a concentration of 38 μg/cm^2. This stimulus (0.8 cm^2) sensitized 90% of the normal subjects. Disks 3 mm in diameter (0.08 cm^2) were cut out with a biopsy punch and applied as sensitizing stimulus (Table 1). The concentration was still 38 μg/cm^2 but this area of application was one-tenth that of the 1-cm patch. This induced clinical sensitization in only 26% and their degree of responsiveness was reduced in proportion (34).

Altogether, these observations indicate that for a given concentration of DNCB per unit area there is a plateau above which increases in area, and hence of total dose, cause very little increase in sensitizing effect. Below that plateau, change in area and total dose exhibit a dose–response relationship as might be expected. These findings can be interpreted in terms of the relationship between the numbers of Langerhans' cells and the numbers of antigen molecules per cell. Hence for a fixed number of Langerhans' cells within a given area, varying the number of antigen molecules per cell causes potent changes in the induction stimulus. By contrast, at any given number of molecules per Langerhans' cell—constant concentration per unit area—altering the number of antigen-bearing Langerhans' cells above a particular plateau level makes only a small difference to sensitivity. Below this plateau, however, changing the number of Langerhans' cells has a strong influence on sensi-

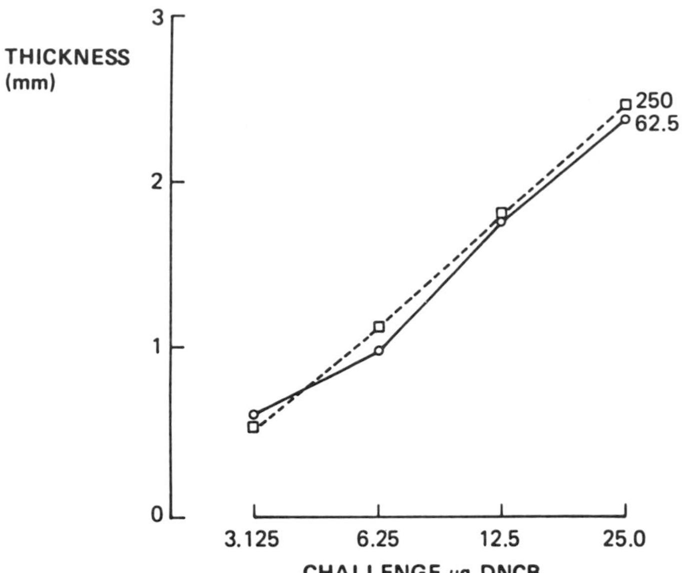

FIG. 12. Responses to challenge with DNCB in groups of subjects sensitized with the same dose per unit area, 35.4 μg/cm^2 of DNCB. □, Subjects successfully sensitized with 250 μg on a 3-cm diameter circle; ○, subjects sensitized with 62.5 μg on a 1.5-cm diameter circle. (Reproduced from ref. 33, with permission.)

tization (35,36). This interpretation is supported by the observations of Macatonia et al. (8). They showed that, in mice, increasing the concentration of sensitizing antigen resulted in dose-related increases in the numbers of antigen-bearing Langerhans' cells in the regional lymph nodes. Moreover, there was a dose-related increase in the amount of antigen per Langerhans' cell.

Local Factors in Expression of Contact Sensitivity

Inflammatory reactivity of skin varies considerably with anatomic site. This has been demonstrated most clearly with irritant substances. Thus reactivity to the irritant dimethylsulfoxide (DMSO) is greatest on the forehead with progressively reduced reactivity on the upper back, antecubital fossa, forearm, lower leg, and wrist (37,38). Similar variations were found in response to benzalkonium chloride (39). Also, Lawrence et al. (40) showed that, on the forearm, there were consistent site-related variations in the responses to anthralin, another irritant. Thus responsiveness was greater proximally and laterally.

Local factors are also important in the expression of immune responses in skin and these will have an important effect on the clinical manifestations of contact sensitivity as well as the responses to formal challenge. Magnusson and Hersle (39) performed simultaneous patch tests on several body sites of people known to be sensitized to the test antigen. Upper back was most reactive, followed by lower back, forearm, upper arm, and thigh. In the previous account of normal responses to DNCB, it was argued that the slope of dose–response curves for response measured as change of skin thickness reflected local cutaneous inflammatory factors. This also appears to apply for the slope of the dose–response curve when measured as erythema with a reflectance instrument. The experimental confirmation of this was obtained by quantification of responses to serial dilutions of nickel sulfate in petrolatum applied to the back and forearm of nickel-sensitive patients (41). Fourfold dilutions of nickel sulfate from 5% downwards were applied on Finn chambers for 48 hr. The responses were graded clinically as "positive" when there was palpable erythema and quantified with a reflectance instrument by measurement of increase in erythema over baseline. The back was much more reactive in that the threshold concentration required to produce a positive response was one-quarter to one-eighth of the threshold on the forearm. Also, the slope of the erythema dose–response curve was much steeper (Fig. 13).

These local differences in reactivity may result in clinical problems from certain substances such as cosmetics occurring on one area, for instance, the face, but not on other areas such as the hands.

POTENTIATION OF ALLERGIC RESPONSES

A clinical problem is seen when a person appears to become allergic to something such as a cosmetic, but patch test challenge with the separate ingredients applied in the standard concentrations fails to detect the contact sensitivity. This apparent methodologic weakness of patch testing can be explained by results from an interesting study by McClelland and Shuster (42). Since allergic contact hypersensitivity responses are dose related, it is clear that doubling the concentration of an antigen will increase the strength of the response. If the concentration of antigen is below the threshold level, then, if doubled, it may come above the threshold and so elicit a "positive" response. McClelland and Shuster showed this in people who were sensitive to two different contact allergens. They were challenged with a doubling dilution series of each antigen separately and also combined at each dilution. There was a complete summation so, at any concentration, the response to the two antigens combined was about the same as the sum of the individual responses at that concentration. Moreover, mixtures of antigens at subclinical levels indeed crossed the threshold and elicited clinically detectable responses.

A similar phenomenon was shown when an irritant was substituted for one of the antigens (43). The method was slightly different, but when sites challenged with a subthreshold dose of antigen for 24 hr were given the additional irritant challenge for the second 24 hr, then significant clinically positive responses were obtained. A similar but less well-quantified study was performed by Sonnex and Ryan (44). They showed that pretreatment of skin with thurfyl nicotinate cream, a rubefacient,

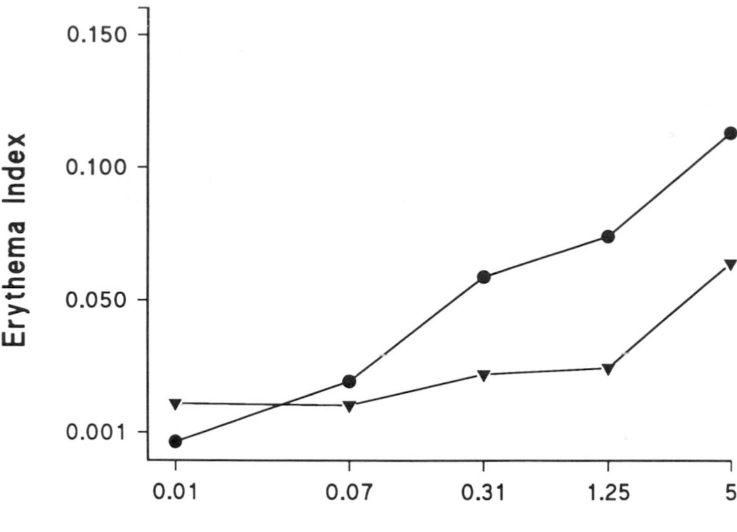

FIG. 13. Erythemal dose–response to challenge with serial dilutions of nickel sulfate in yellow soft paraffin on the back (●) and forearm (▼). Data are from seven nickel-sensitive volunteers. Erythema was quantified by means of a reflectance instrument (Diastron).

followed by patch testing with 20 substances causes a significant increase in the number of positive patch test reactions.

It is clear that an irritant may augment absorption of antigen, raising its effective concentration. Also, as will be seen later, irritants like antigens activate processes in the skin aimed at recruitment of immune surveillance mechanisms. The two stimuli for these mechanisms can clearly summate to increase the likelihood of antigen-specific effector T cells entering the tissues to encounter the low dose of antigen.

"Angry Back" and "Excited Skin Syndrome"

These terms must be mentioned because they are often alluded to in the clinical practice of diagnostic patch testing . The term "angry back" was coined by Mitchell in relation to the phenomenon of multiple positive patch test reactions occurring on the same individual (45,46). He showed that if substances giving weak (+) reactions were retested singly at a later time, a significant proportion, 42%, were negative. He presumed this meant they were in fact, false positives and did not represent genuine sensitization. Bruynzeel et al. (47) performed a similar study and arrived at a similar conclusion. By contrast, Bandman and Agathos (48) found only 8.6% of such so-called false-positive responses became negative upon retesting. The difference has been explained on the basis of different methodology, including retesting strong reactions as well as weak ones. Maibach (49) broadened the term to "excited skin syndrome" to indicate that a generalized hyperirritability could occur in skin. The central tenet of the idea is that one strong patch test reaction creates the hyperreactive state. Evidence that this is not so was presented by Kligman and Gollhausen (50). They first challenged a range of volunteers with irritants or sensitizers to which they were sensitive, to obtain baseline responses. Then they generated strong responses with sensitizers such as DNCB, nickel, or rhus oleoresin of poison ivy. They placed the challenges at the corners of a square on the backs of subjects sensitized to these agents. Then various challenges, either irritants or sensitizers, were placed within the squares. No augmentation was seen of any response compared with the baseline. The present author has made similar but less comprehensive observations (*unpublished data*). This would seem to cast serious doubt on the concept that a general phenomenon exists in which a strong local patch test or irritant response can induce hyperreactivity. However, Magnusson and Hellgren (51) observed that when test subjects developed a reaction due to the adhesive tape used to apply patch tests, a much greater frequency of positive responses was seen. Also, Bruynzeel et al. (52) showed that guinea pigs pretreated with Freund's complete adjuvant became hyperreactive both to allergens and irritants. These two observations add the perspective, which is, in fact, present in slightly loose form in the literature and is perhaps highlighted by Bjornberg (53), that hyperirritability is seen when there is active dermatitis present.

There is still much work to be done to define the conditions under which such hyperreactivity occurs. However, it is conceivable that the prerequisite is for the presence of active skin inflammation that is accompanied by increased levels of circulating cytokines. These could have the effect of priming the skin vasculature in the same way as local, subthreshold applications of irritant or allergen. The question that preoccupies clinicians of whether reactions on an angry back are genuine or false positives may be resolved by *in vitro* techniques such as analysis of the antigenic specificities of reacting lymphocytes.

RECRUITMENT OF IMMUNE AND INFLAMMATORY MECHANISMS IN SKIN

As mentioned in the early part of this chapter, a vital function of skin is defense against invasion by microbes. Since the skin is under continuous assault by chemical substances in the environment, it seems probable that efficient mechanisms must be present to activate or recruit immune surveillance to "inspect" any substance that penetrates the outer barrier. The critical event in a cell-mediated immune response to an antigen is the specific interaction between the relevant T cell receptor on the surface of a CD4+ T lymphocyte and the antigen, presented in association with MHC class II determinants, on the surface of an antigen-presenting cell. After this interaction, the T cell responds by releasing cytokines, of which interferon-γ (IFN-γ) appears most important, to augment the recruitment of other lymphomononuclear cells (54). When an antigen enters the skin, the statistical likelihood is very low of a chance encounter between the antigen and a specifically committed T cell trafficking through the tissues in its performance of immune surveillance. This jeopardizes the protective efficiency of the response and it is becoming clear that the skin plays an active role to increase the efficiency of immune surveillance.

It could be predicted that, following chemical or even physical perturbation, mechanisms would be activated to increase trafficking of T cells through the tissues. Furthermore, such recruitment mechanisms must be nonspecific in that they cannot distinguish whether or not the provoking substance is microbial in origin. Moreover, these mechanisms must operate independently of whether or not the host has been previously sensitized, and, in addition, they must become activated rapidly.

A number of studies have found evidence of these mechanisms by examining skin after application of various chemical provoking substances including irritants and antigens to which mice (55) or humans (56–59) were known to be specifically sensitive or nonsensitive. The main changes detected relate, on the one hand, to expression of cell adhesion molecules on dermal microvascular endothelium and, in some circumstances, also on epidermal keratinocytes, and on the other hand, to increased numbers of putative antigen-presenting cells in the superficial dermis.

In prechallenge resting skin some dermal vessels express intercellular adhesion molecule-1 (ICAM-1) but generally endothelial cell leukocyte adhesion molecule-1 (ELAM-1) and vascular cell adhesion molecule-1 (VCAM-1) are not detectable. The scanty population of immune cells is mainly perivascular and comprises CD3+ T cells, CD14+ macrophages, and occasional CD1a+ Langerhans' cells. In the epidermis, although CD1a+ Langerhans' cells are present, there is no expression of ICAM-1 and, depending on the antibody used, some staining of basal cells for tumor necrosis factor-α (TNF-α) and interleukin-1α (IL-1α) can be detected (59). After challenge with irritants or sensitizers such as nickel, *p*-phenylenediamine, urushiol, or DNCB, and regardless of whether individuals are sensitive or not, there are similar changes seen up to 8 hr.

Changes in Adhesion Molecules

Increased expression in ICAM-1, ELAM-1, and VCAM-1 was first detectable after only 2 hr and increased in intensity to reach a maximum at 24 hr (Fig. 14) (59). Interestingly, in people known to be sensitive to the challenge substance and also at sites challenged with irritants, the numbers of vessels expressing ICAM-1 also showed a significant increase at 8 hr (Fig. 15) (59). Some authors have also found that ICAM-1 is expressed in focal patches on basal keratinocytes. Griffiths and coworkers (56,57) found this at 4 hr with progressive increase with time, while others have found it only by 24 hr after challenge (58).

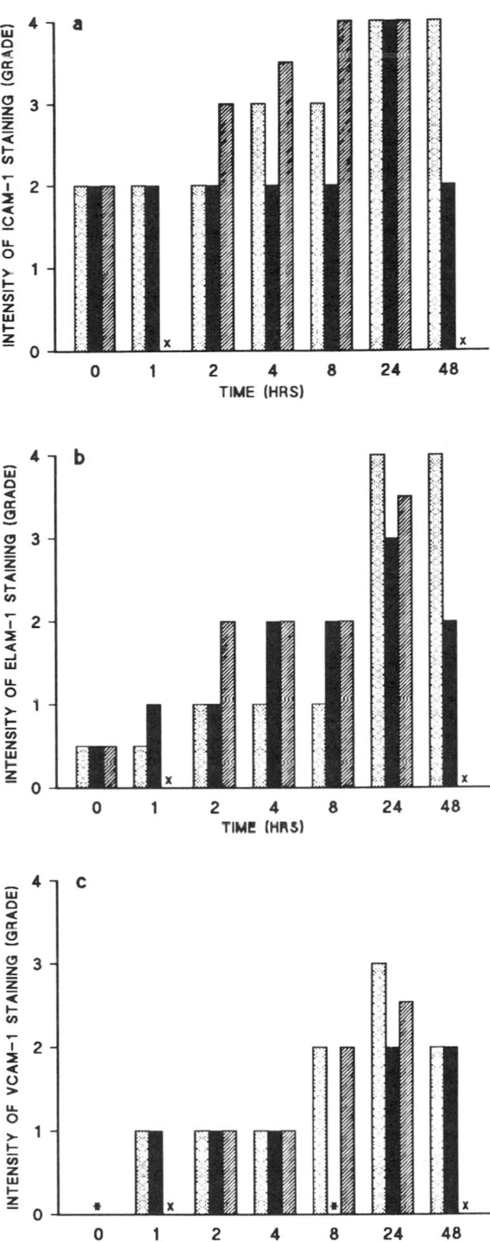

FIG. 14. Intensity of staining of adhesion molecules at various times after challenge. ▨, Reaction in individuals known to be sensitive to the challenge; ■, reaction in individuals known to be nonsensitized to the challenge; □, irritant reactions. Panels (a) ICAM-1, (b) ELAM-1, (c) VCAM-1. *, No staining observed; X, no biopsies at these time points. (Reproduced from ref. 59, with permission.)

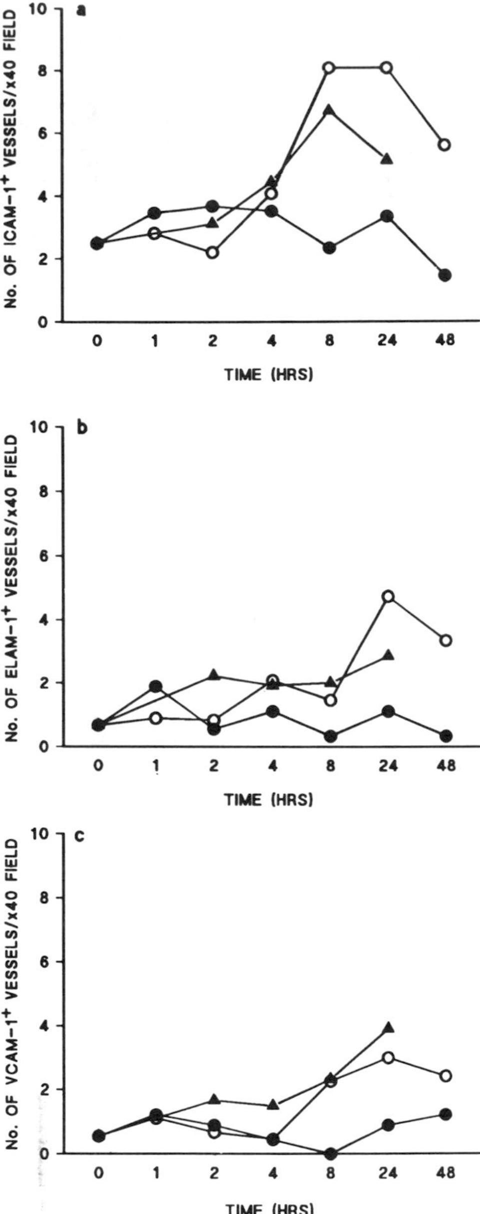

FIG. 15. Adhesion molecule expression by dermal microvascular endothelial cells at various times after epicutaneous challenge. ○, Reaction in individuals known to be sensitive to provoking stimulus; ●, reaction in subjects known to be nonsensitive to provoking stimulus; ▲, irritant reactions. Panels (a) ICAM-1, (b) ELAM-1, (c) VCAM-1. Points are numbers of vessels per 40 × high power field. (Reproduced from ref. 59, with permission.)

Immune Cells

By 2 to 4 hr after challenge there is an increase in the numbers of CD1a+ Langerhans' cells in the superficial dermis. This change appears proportional to the "strength" of the provoking agent, occurring most with irritants such as anthralin or highly potent sensitizers such as DNCB (59). However, it is even seen at 24 hr with innocuous chemical mixtures such as white soft paraffin (58). No changes are detected in the dermal mononuclear cell infiltrate up to 8 hr. However, by 24 hr skin biopsies from subjects sensitized to the provoking substance show a significant mononuclear cell infiltrate comprised mainly of T cells of phenotypes CD3+, CD4+, and CD45RO+, which represents memory T cells. Among the T cells, occasional cells were observed that expressed CD25, the p55 chain of the IL-2 receptor. This marker is thought to be expressed by T cells that have been activated following binding of the T cell receptor with its homologous antigen/MHC class II complex (60). A few CD4+ T cells are seen in the epidermis, while deeper in the dermis CD14+ monocytes/macrophages are increased.

In sensitized individuals generating positive responses to antigen challenge, the T cell infiltrate continues to increase to 48 hr, at which time many CD1b+ dermal dendrocytes are seen adjacent to superficial dermal capillaries. Interestingly, these cells are strongly stained by anti-VCAM-1 antibodies (59). In the fully developed reaction, IL-8 expression is seen on keratinocytes too (57).

In summary, these observations indicate the following sequence of events. Chemical perturbation induces rapid expression of adhesion molecules by dermal microvascular endothelium. This appears to be a direct effect since it is seen with cultured endothelial cells too (61). There may also be expression of ICAM-1 by keratinocytes, although this is not detected by most workers. Moreover, keratinocytes exposed to urushiol *in vitro*, express ICAM-1 by 48 hr (56,62). There is also a rapid (2 hr) increase in the number of dermal Langerhans' cells that have been shown to carry antigens (63). Thus the conditions are established to recruit T cells to perform immune surveillance. Activated memory T cells are particularly rich in lymphocyte function associated antigen-1 (LFA-1) and cutaneous lymphocyte antigen (CLA), the ligands for ICAM-1 and ELAM-1, respectively (64–66). Therefore the initial expression of ELAM-1 and ICAM-1 by endothelial cells is probably sufficient to allow attachment of T cells to the endothelium. After attachment, the T cells must express β_1-integrins including VLA-3, -5 and -6, which are ligands for collagen, fibronectin, and laminin, which will be required for emigration into the tissues (67). If no T cell recognizes its target antigen, the whole reaction subsides over a few hours. However, once a specifically committed T cell recognizes its target antigen on the surface of a Langerhans' cell, it becomes activated, expressing CD25 and releasing cytokines including IFN-γ and TNF-α. These will upregulate adhesion molecule expression further and recruit other T cells into the area to participate in the inflammatory reaction recognized clinically as allergic contact eczema.

These observations made in humans demonstrate no qualitative differences between the early effects of substances that are sensitizers or irritants, while the distinctive consequences of activation of sensitized T cells only develop from 8 hr at the earliest. Similar findings were made in mice by Malorny et al. (55). However, a study by Enk and Katz (68) used sensitive molecular biologic techniques to detect messenger ribonucleic acid (mRNA) for various cytokines after mice were treated with irritant (sodium lauryl sulfate), haptens, and also tolerogens. They observed certain differences in the early, 4-hr, profile of cytokines. Although TNF-α, IFN-γ, and granulocyte–macrophage colony-stimulating factor (GM-CSF) were increased in the epidermis by all compounds, only the contact sensitizers upregulated IL-1α, IL-1β, and macrophage inflammatory protein-2 (MIP-2). It remains to be seen whether human skin will also show these qualitative differences in response to exposure to different types of provoking chemical.

The recognition that contact with chemicals activates this complex response, which is independent of the immune status of the host, will allow explanation of many phenomena observed clinically. For instance, it shows why subthreshold concentrations of antigens and/or irritants can summate to generate clinically detectable responses. If the nonspecific recruitment mechanisms are activated to a greater extent, the chance of an antigen-specific T cell entering the tissues to find its antigen will be increased in proportion.

REFERENCES

1. Agrup G. Hand eczema and other dermatoses in South Sweden. *Acta Derm Venereol Suppl (Stockh)* 1969;49:61.
2. Meding BE, Swafbeck G. Prevalence of hand eczema in an industrial city. *Br J Dermatol* 1987; 116:627–634.
3. Johnson MLT, Roberts J. Skin conditions and related need for medical care among persons 1–74 years. *Vital Health Stat* 1978;11.
4. Rea JN, Newhouse ML, Halil T. Skin diseases in Lambeth. A community study of prevalence and use of medical care. *Br J Prev Soc Med* 1976;30:107–114.
5. Coenraads P-J, Smit J. Epidemiology. In: Rycroft RJG, Menné T, Frosch PJ, Benezra C, eds. *Textbook of contact dermatitis*. Berlin: Springer-Verlag; 1992.
6. Mathias CGT. The cost of occupational disease. *Arch Dermatol* 1985;121:332–334.
7. Emmet EA. The skin and occupational disease. *Arch Environ Health* 1984;39:144–149.
8. Macatonia SE, Edwards AJ, Knight SC. Dendritic cells and the initiation of contact sensitivity to fluorescein isothiocyanate. *Immunology* 1986;59:509–514.
9. Kinnaird A, Peters SW, Foster JR, Kimber I. Dendritic cell accumulation in draining lymph nodes during the induction phase of contact allergy in mice. *Int Arch Allergy Appl Immunol* 1989;89:202–210.
10. Okamoto H, Kripke ML. Effector and suppressor circuits of the immune response are activated *in vivo* by different mechanisms. *Proc Natl Acad Sci USA* 1987;84:3841–3845.
11. Rostenberg A, Kanof NM. Studies in eczematous sensitizations. *J Invest Dermatol* 1941;4:505–513.
12. Epstein WL, Maibach HI. Immunologic competence of patients with psoriasis receiving cytotoxic drug therapy. *Arch Dermatol* 1965;91:599–606.
13. Eilber FR, Morton DL. Impaired immunologic reactivity and recurrence following cancer surgery. *Cancer* 1970;25:362–367.
14. Catalona WJ, Taylor PY, Rabson AS, Chretien PB. A method for dinitrochlorobenzene contact sensitization. *N Engl J Med* 1972;286:362–367.
15. Bleumink E, Nater JP, Koops S, The TH. A standard method for DNCB sensitization testing in patients with neoplasms. *Cancer* 1974;33:911–915.

16. Friedmann PS, Moss C, Shuster S, Simpson JM. Quantitative relationships between sensitising dose of DNCB and reactivity in normal subjects. *Clin Exp Immunol* 1983;53:709–711.
17. Friedmann PS, Moss C. Quantification of contact hypersensitivity in man. In: Maibach HI, Lowe NJ, eds. *Models in dermatology*, vol 2. Basel: Karger; 1985:275–281.
18. Friedmann PS. Immune functions of skin. In: Thody AJ, Friedmann PS, eds. *Scientific basis of dermatology. A physiological approach*. Edinburgh: Churchill Livingstone; 1986:58–73.
19. Friedmann PS, Rees J, Matthews JNS. Low dose exposure to antigen induces subclinical sensitisation. *Clin Exp Immunol* 1990;81:507–509.
20. Moss C, Friedmann PS, Shuster S, Simpson JM. Susceptibility and amplification of sensitivity in contact dermatitis. *Clin Exp Immunol* 1985;61:232–241.
21. Schwartz M. Eczematous sensitisation in various age groups. *J Allergy* 1953;24:143–148.
22. Polak L, Barnes JM, Turk JL. The genetic control of contact sensitisation to inorganic metal compounds in guinea pigs. *Immunology* 1968;14:707–711.
23. Walker FB, Smith PO, Maibach HI. Genetic factors in human allergic contact dermatitis. *Int Arch Allergy Appl Immunol* 1967;32:453–462.
24. Friedmann PS. The immunology of allergic contact dermatitis: the DNCB story. In: Dahl MV, ed. *Advances in dermatology*, Vol. 5. Chicago: Year Book Medical Publishers; 1989:175–195.
25. Menné T, Holm NV. Hand eczema in nickel-sensitive female twins. *Contact Dermatitis* 1983;9: 289–296.
26. Menné T, Holm NV. Genetic susceptibility in human allergic contact sensitisation. *Semin Dermatol* 1986;5:301–306.
27. Mozzanica N, Rizzolo L, Veneroni G, Diotti R, Hepeisen S, Finzi AF. HLA-A, B, C and DR antigens in nickel contact sensitivity. *Br J Dermatol* 1990;122:309–313.
28. White SI, Friedmann PS, Stratton A. HLA antigens and Langerhans' cell density in contact dermatitis. *Br T Dermatol* 1986;115:447–452.
29. Moss C. *Studies of cutaneous sensitisation to dinitrochlorobenzene in man* [DM thesis]. Oxford: Oxford University, 1983.
30. Leyden JJ, Kligman AM. Allergic contact dermatitis: sex differences. *Contact Dermatitis* 1977;3: 333–336.
31. Jordan WP, King SE. Delayed hypersensitivity in females. *Contact Dermatitis* 1977;3:19–26.
32. Rees JL, Friedmann PS, Matthews JNS. Sex differences in susceptibility to development of contact hypersensitivity to dinitrochlorobenzene. *Br J Dermatol* 1989;120:371–374.
33. White SI, Friedmann PS, Moss C, Simpson JM. The effect of altering area of application and dose per unit area on sensitization by DNCB. *Br J Dermatol* 1986;115:663–668.
34. Rees JL, Friedmann PS. Area of application does affect strength of sensitisation by DNCB. *J Invest Dermatol* 1988;91:404.
35. Friedmann PS. Contact hypersensitivity. *Curr Opin Immunol* 1989;1:690–693.
36. Friedmann PS. Graded continuity or all or none—studies of the human immune response. *Clin Exp Dermatol* 1991;16:79–84.
37. Vandervalk PGM, Maibach HI. Potential for irritation increases from the wrist to the cubital fossa. *Br J Dermatol* 1989;121:709–712.
38. Frosch PJ. Cutaneous irritation. In: Rycroft RJG, Menne T, Frosch PJ, Benezra C, eds. *Textbook of contact dermatitis*. Berlin: Springer-Verlag; 1992:33–35.
39. Magnusson B, Hersle K. Patch test methods II. Regional variations of patch test responses. *Acta Derm Venereol* 1965;45:257–261.
40. Lawrence CM, Howel D, Shuster S. Site variation in anthralin inflammation on forearm skin. *Br J Dermatol* 1986;114:609–613.
41. Memon AA, Friedmann PS. Studies on the reproducibility of the contact hypersensitivity response. *Br J Dermatol* [*submitted*].
42. McClelland J, Shuster S. Contact dermatitis with negative patch tests: the additive effect of allergens in combination. *Br J Dermatol* 1990;122:623–630.
43. McClelland J, Shuster S, Matthews JNS. "Irritants" increase the response to an allergen in allergic contact dermatitis. *Arch Dermatol* 1991;127:1016–1019.
44. Sonnex TS, Ryan TJ. An investigation of the angry back syndrome using Trafuril. *Br J Dermatol* 1987;116:361–370.
45. Mitchell JC. The angry back syndrome: eczema creates eczema. *Contact Dermatitis* 1975;1:193–194.
46. Mitchell JC, Maibach HI. The angry back syndrome: the excited skin syndrome. *Semin Dermatol* 1982;1:9–13.

47. Brunyzeel DP, von Blomberg-van der Flier BME, Van Ketel WG, et al. Depression or enhancement of skin reactivity by inflammatory processes in the guinea pig. *Int Arch Allergy Appl Immunol* 1983;72:67–70.
48. Bandman H-J, Agathos M. New results and some remarks to the "angry back syndrome." *Contact Dermatitis* 1981;7:23–26.
49. Maibach HI. The ESS: excited skin syndrome. In Ring J, Burg G, eds. *New trends in allergy*. New York: Springer-Verlag; 1981:208–221.
50. Kligman A, Gollhausen R. The "angry back": a new concept or old confusion? *Br J Dermatol* 1986;115(suppl 31):93–100.
51. Magnusson B, Helgren L. Skin irritating and adhesive characteristics of some different tapes. *Acta Derm Venereol* 1962;42:463–472.
52. Brunyzeel DP, van Ketel WG, von Blomberg-van der Flier BME, Scheper RJ. Angry back or the excited skin syndrome. *J Am Acad Dermatol* 1983;8:392–397.
53. Bjornberg A. *Skin reaction to primary irritance in patients with eczema* [PhD dissertation]. Göteborg: Göteborg University, 1968.
54. Issekutz TB, Stoltz JM, van der Meide P. Lymphocyte recruitment in delayed-type hypersensitivity: the role of IFN-γ. *J Immunol* 1988;140:2989–2993.
55. Malorny U, Knop J, Burmeister G, Sorg C. Immunohistochemical demonstration of migration inhibitory factor (MIF) in experimental allergic contact dermatitis. *Clin Exp Immunol* 1988;71:164–170.
56. Griffiths CEM, Nickoloff BJ. Keratinocyte adhesion molecule-1 (ICAM-1) expression precedes dermal T lymphocytic infiltration in allergic contact dermatitis (rhus dermatitis). *Am J Pathol* 1989; 135:1045–1053.
57. Griffiths CEM, Barker JNWN, Kunkel S, Nickoloff BJ. Modulation of leucocyte adhesion molecules, a T-cell chemotaxin (IL-8) and a regulatory cytokine (TNF-α) in allergic contact dermatitis (rhus dermatitis). *Br J Dermatol* 1991;124:519–526.
58. Sterry W, Kunne N, Weber-Matthiesen K, Brasch J, Mielke V. Cell trafficking in positive and negative patch-test reactions: demonstration of a stereotypic migration pathway. *J Invest Dermatol* 1991;96:459–462.
59. Friedmann PS, Strickland I, Memon AA, Johnson PM. Early time-course of recruitment of immune surveillance in human skin after chemical provocation. *Clin Exp Immunol* 1993;91:351–356.
60. Meuer SC, Hussey RE, Cantrell D, Hodgdon IC, Schlossman SF, Smith KA, Reinherz EL. Triggering of the T3-Ti antigen receptor complex results in clonal T-cell proliferation through an interleukin-2 dependent autocrine pathway. *Proc Natl Acad Sci USA* 1984;81:1509–1513.
61. Meinardus-Hager G, Goebeler M, Gutwald J, Sorg C. The allergen nickel chloride directly induces distinct expression patterns of leucocyte adhesion molecules on human endothelial cells. *J Invest Dermatol* 1992;98:539.
62. Barker JNWN, Mitra RS, Griffiths CEM, et al. Keratinocytes as initiators of inflammation. *Lancet* 1991;337:211–215.
63. Carr MM, Botham PA, Gawkroger DJ, McVittie EM, Ross JA, Stewart IC, Hunter JAA. Early cellular reactions induced by dinitrochlorobenzene in sensitized human skin. *Br J Dermatol* 1984; 110:637–641.
64. Shimizu Y, Shaw S, Graber N, Gopal TV, Horgan KJ, Van Seventer GA, Newman W. Activation-independent binding of human memory T cells to adhesion molecule ELAM-1. *Nature* 1991;349: 799–781.
65. Picker LJ, Kishimoto TK, Smith CW, Warnock RA, Butcher EC. ELAM-1 is an adhesion molecule for skin homing T cells. *Nature* 1991;349:796–799.
66. Berg EL, Yoshino T, Rott LS, et al. The cutaneous lymphocyte antigen is a skin lymphocyte homing receptor for the vascular lectin endothelial cell–leucocyte adhesion molecule 1. *J Exp Med* 1991; 174:1461–1466.
67. Butcher EC. Leucocyte–endothelial cell recognition: three (or more) steps to specificity and diversity. *Cell* 1991;67:1033–1036.
68. Enk AH, Katz SI. Early molecular events in the induction phase of contact sensitivity. *Proc Natl Acad Sci USA* 1992;89:1398–1402.

Immunotoxicology and Immunopharmacology, Second Edition, edited by J. H. Dean, M. I. Luster, A. E. Munson, and I. Kimber.
Raven Press, Ltd., New York © 1994.

35

Clinical Aspects of Respiratory Hypersensitivity to Chemicals

Jonathan A. Bernstein and I. Leonard Bernstein

Department of Internal Medicine, Division of Immunology and Allergy, University of Cincinnati Medical Center, Cincinnati, Ohio 45267

Hypersensitivity reactions occur in the lung as the result of direct immunologic effects on the lung parenchyma by toxins, chemicals, drugs, or infectious agents. A spectrum of respiratory disorders has been described in individuals exposed to systemic or inhaled xenobiotics including asthma, hypersensitivity pneumonitis, pulmonary fibrosis, and pulmonary infiltrates with eosinophilia (PIE) (1). The increased recognition of asthma and other pulmonary hypersensitivity disorders has been most pronounced in the workplace, presenting a formidable health problem for the worker and employer that can no longer be ignored. The most commonly diagnosed respiratory hypersensitivity disorder induced by chemicals is occupational asthma (OA), which accounts for 2% to 15% of all new cases of asthma (2). The actual prevalence of this disease may be higher as many symptomatic workers leave their jobs prior to a definitive diagnosis of OA. Since currently available OA prevalence statistics are derived from cross-sectional surveys conducted in specific industries in different countries, it is not possible to accurately estimate the true prevalence of OA for the entire industrial workforce (2,3).

The progressive rise in the number of occupational respiratory hypersensitivity cases is partially attributable to innovative industrial technology, which led to the introduction of many new chemicals into the work environment. As a result, there are now over 200 chemicals in the workplace known to cause respiratory hypersensitivity disorders (2,3). Low molecular weight (LMW) chemical agents (MW< 1000 daltons) are unique as they require linkage with an endogenous protein carrier to form a complex multivalent hapten–protein conjugate, which results in new epitopes capable of eliciting an immune response (2). Synthesis of these conjugates has facilitated *in vitro* and *in vivo* investigation of the LMW chemical agents known to cause respiratory hypersensitivity disorders with particular attention to polyisocyanates, acid anhydrides, organic acids, and metallic salts. Because of the unique properties of LMW chemical antigens and their ubiquitous presence in industry, it is appropriate to review the progress made in our understanding of respiratory hypersensitivity reactions encountered in the work environment. This chapter reviews the immunopathogenic mechanisms responsible for the clinical manifestations of these reactions observed in workers exposed to LMW chemical agents, focusing on OA. Other hypersensitivity respiratory syndromes such as hypersensitivity pneumonitis and drug-induced pneumonitis are discussed as they pertain to individual groups of LMW chemicals including drugs.

MECHANISMS OF RESPIRATORY HYPERSENSITIVITY REACTIONS

Immunosurveillance of large workforces exposed to LMW chemical agents has been the major source of information for defining the underlying immune responses responsible for respiratory hypersensitivity reactions. For many of these LMW chemicals, one or more of the immune responses described by the Gell–Coombs classification have been invoked to explain the clinical syndromes manifested by sensitized workers. For example, type I immune responses, which require host sensitization and induction of specific immunoglobulin E (IgE) antibodies to a chemical ligand, have been described for acid anhydrides, polyisocyanates, and other reactive chemical agents (1,4,5). Type II or cytotoxic immune responses, which occur when IgM and IgG antibodies activate the complement pathway after adhering to specific tissue antigens, have been postulated as the causes of a Goodpasture-like syndrome presenting with hemorrhagic pulmonary lesions and hemolytic anemia in workers exposed to high concentrations of trimellitic anhydride (TMA) (6). Type III immune complex-mediated reactions, which cause tissue destruction associated with deposition of antibody–antigen complexes and complement activation, may be implicated in the pathogenesis of drug- and chemical-induced pulmonary lesions (1,7). Finally, there is accumulating evidence that supports the involvement of type IV cell-mediated responses in respiratory hypersensitivity reactions after exposure to several LMW chemicals such as toluene diisocyanate and plicatic acid (1,8). These reactions are initiated when T lymphocyte receptors interact with antigenic determinants contained within type I or type II major histocompatibility complex (MHC) molecules expressed on the surfaces of antigen-presenting cells (APCs) (8).

Proposed mechanisms for OA induced by LMW chemicals have been divided into nonimmunologic and immunologic categories summarized in Table 1 (3). Several examples of LMW antigens causing OA through nonimmunologic mechanisms have been recognized. Direct injury to the bronchial epithelial cells by the chemical's toxic effects has been described for acid anhydrides and plicatic acid, the organic acid of interest in western red cedar, or by environmental irritants such as ozone or sulfur dioxide (9–11). Damaged bronchial epithelial cells (BECs) are believed to permit easier access of xenobiotics into the underlying lamina propria where they may exert direct effects on inflammatory cells and the bronchial microvasculature. Stimulation of sensory vagal afferents in and beneath the epithelium

TABLE 1. *Classification of mechanisms of occupational asthma* (3)

Nonimmunologic mechanisms
Reflex bronchoconstriction
Irritant bronchoconstriction (i.e., reactive airways dysfunction syndrome)
Pharmacologically induced bronchoconstriction
Immunologic mechanisms
Immediate hypersensitivity response (IgE mediated)
High molecular weight allergens
Low molecular weight allergens
Mixed (immunologic and nonimmunologic) allergens
IgG antibody and/or immune (antigen–antibody) complex response
Complement pathway activation
Cell-mediated response

may result in reflex bronchoconstriction and increased nonspecific bronchial hyperresponsiveness (NSBHR). BECs also release cytokines and bioactive mediators with chemotactic, inflammatory, and other potent physiologic properties that contribute to the increase and persistence of bronchial hyperresponsiveness (BHR) (1,12).

Shepherd et al. (13) have proposed a neurophysiologic mechanism for OA using a guinea pig model. Exposure of afferent nerve endings to toluene diisocyanate (TDI) is known to cause the release of tachykinins, substance P, and neurokinin A, resulting in airway hyperresponsiveness that is further potentiated by TDI's ability to inhibit neutral endopeptidase, the ectoenzyme responsible for tachykinin degradation (13). TDI also stimulates local release of substance P and calcitonin gene-related peptide (CGRP) from efferent nerve endings, a route of neurogenic inflammation that completely bypasses the central nervous system (14).

Some LMW chemical antigens, such as plicatic acid derived from western red cedar, have been demonstrated to activate either the classic or alternative complement pathways, resulting in production of anaphylatoxins capable of activating mast cells to release bioactive mediators (9). The clinical relevance of this *in vitro* pathway has not been demonstrated. Nonimmunologic "pharmacologic" mechanisms have also been described for organophosphate insecticides with anticholinesterase activity, resulting in hypercholinergic BHR (1). Immunologic mechanisms have been described for many of the reactive LMW chemical agents known to induce OA. Anhydrides, for example, have been reported to cause OA by IgE-mediated, cytotoxic, immune complex-, and cell-mediated immune mechanisms (4,6). IgE-mediated mechanisms have similarly been described for polyisocyanates, plicatic acid, azo dyes, and some metallic salts (5,15,16). Many individuals sensitized by these substances also manifest elevated IgG antibody levels but the role of the IgG isotype in the pathogenesis of OA is still unknown (17,18).

LMW chemicals have been speculated to interact cognitively with T lymphocytes, causing activation and release of lymphokines necessary for initiation of the inflammatory cascade, which leads to asthma (1). Definitive involvement of T lymphocytes in OA was first demonstrated by Gallagher et al. (19), who described a relatively specific delayed hypersensitivity response—leukocyte inhibitory factor activity—in a majority of TDI-exposed subjects. This activity disappeared after cessation of exposure (19). Several years later an increase of circulating peripheral CD8 + cells and eosinophils was noted after TDI-specific inhalational challenges of workers diagnosed with OA (20). More recently, T lymphocyte involvement has been documented to occur in OA induced by nickel and cobalt metal salts (21,22). Taken together, these findings strongly support a role for cellular immunity in OA.

The involvement of a cell-mediated immune mechanism in OA has been further enhanced by experimental data recognizing the importance of T helper (T_H) lymphocyte functional heterogeneity. Mosmann et al. (23,24), using a murine model, identified two T_H cell subsets (T_H1 and T_H2) by their differential production of cytokines. Both T_H cell subsets produced interleukin-3 (IL-3) and granulocyte–macrophage colony-stimulating factor (GM-CSF), which are pleuripotent cell growth factors. However, T_H1 cells secreted primarily IL-2, interferon-γ (IFN-γ), and tumor necrosis factor-β (TNF-β), whereas T_H2 cells preferably secreted IL-4, IL-5, IL-6, IL-10 and IL-13 (23–24a). Expression of IgE-mediated immune responses was found to correspond to a predominance of T_H2 cells and cell-mediated immune responses were found to correspond to a predominance of T_H1 cells. In a murine OA model, similar evidence for T_H cell heterogeneity was shown by a preferential activation of T_H2 cells by phthalic and trimellitic anhydrides (PA and TMA) and diphenylmethylene diisocyanate. Animals sensitized by these chemicals demonstrated IgE synthesis and respiratory sensitization, whereas 2,4–dinitrochlorobenzene (DNCB), a potent contact sensitizing chemical, favored activation and cytokine release by T_H1 cells (25–27). Evidence supporting a similar model of T_H cell heterogeneity in humans has been presented and may eventually explain some aspects of the complex immunopathogenic role of cellular immunity in OA (28). More recently, a subset of human T_H cells (T_H0), which has not yet differentiated into T_H1 and T_H2 varieties and produces a mixture of cytokines found in both T_H1 and T_H2 subsets, has been reported (29).

PATHOPHYSIOLOGY

Specific bronchoprovocation studies performed on workers with OA induced by LMW chemicals such as diisocyanates have been helpful in characterizing the physiologic changes occurring in the bronchial airways. These studies have usually correlated well with the occupational history and histopathologic changes demonstrated by bronchoalveolar lavage (BAL) and transbronchial biopsy (TBBx) (30–32). Chronic BHR has been shown to correspond to the migration of inflammatory cells into the airways (31). However, LMW chemical agents characteristically induce different patterns of bronchospastic reactions. Results of specific bronchoprovocation studies with various chemicals have demonstrated that 10% to 20% of these bronchial reactions are early asthmatic reactions (EARs), 30% to 50% are late asthmatic reactions (LARs), and 30% to 50% are dual asthmatic reactions (DARs) (2).

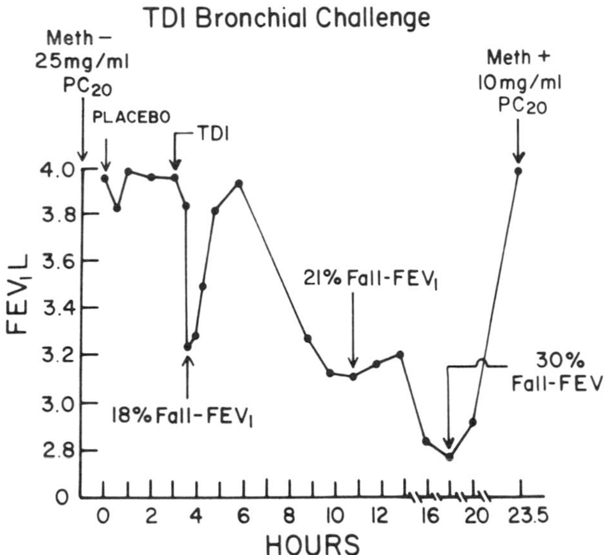

FIG. 1. Dual-phase airway response in polyisocyanate-exposed workers (2).

Isolated EARs are more commonly seen with high molecular weight (HMW) antigens such as animal and plant proteins, whereas isolated LARs are characteristically seen in OA induced by LMW chemicals. DARs are frequently seen in IgE-mediated OA induced by either HMW or LMW agents (2). LARs occur approximately 4 to 12 hr after exposure to the LMW antigen and are associated with influx of inflammatory cells into the airways (2). Contrary to what had previously been reported, studies have demonstrated that an increase in BHR may precede cellular infiltrates as early as 2 hr postchallenge with antigen (33,34). Figure 1 illustrates a characteristic DAR bronchoprovocation response after challenge with TDI and the increased NSBHR, which frequently persists after exposure (2). It should be mentioned that these asthmatic reactions may vary depending on the bronchial challenge method utilized and the chemical properties of the LMW antigen.

The immunopathogenic basis of inflammation for OA closely resembles the findings for NOA, illustrated in Fig. 2 (28). Common pathologic features of acute OA and NOA include airway smooth muscle contraction, edema, and fluid accumulation with the loss of lung parenchymal support (35,36). Airway obstruction results from the influx of inflammatory cells, which cause increased edema and mucus production, smooth muscle hypertrophy, and subepithelial fibrosis secondary to collagen deposition (35,36). These changes lead to chronic airway inflammation, which correlates with persistent BHR, a hallmark feature of asthma.

Because of OA's pathogenic similarity to NOA, OA has served as a convenient epidemiologic model for studying mechanisms of airway inflammation in asthma. Bronchoscopy has facilitated this process by permitting an easy access for the col-

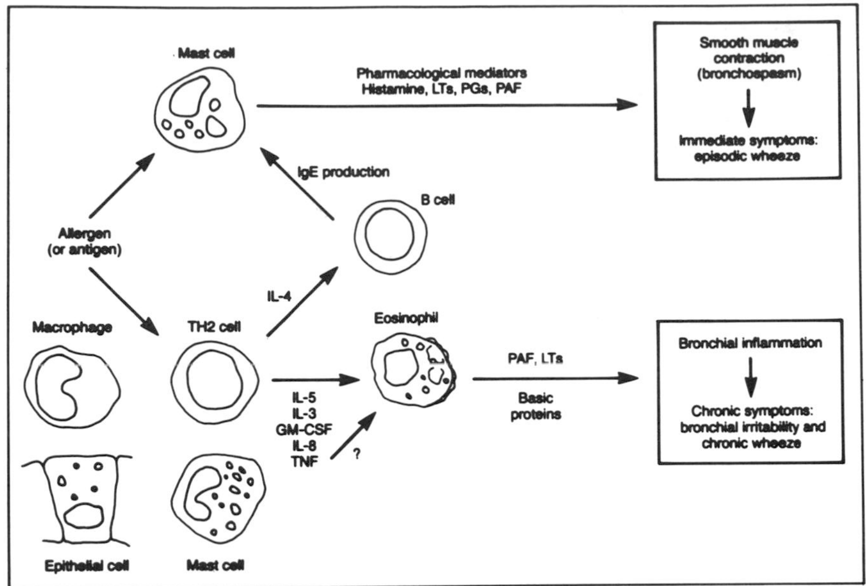

FIG. 2. Immunopathogenesis of asthma (28).

lection of tissue samples by TBBx and airway washings using BAL. BAL fluids obtained from normal, NOA and OA subjects have similar cell count distributions (90% to 95% alveolar macrophages, 5% to 10% lymphocytes, and the remainder leukocytes and epithelial cells) (31). The number and distribution of inflammatory cells remain unchanged in asymptomatic OA subjects but rise in individuals with persistent BHR or active OA (10). Saetta et al. (37) have examined TBBx's from workers diagnosed with TDI OA and found increased numbers of inflammatory cells compared to normal nonasthmatic subjects. Activated eosinophils and lymphocytes were observed in the mucosal and submucosal layers while activated mast cells were identified only in the epithelium (37). The biopsies also revealed thickening of the reticular basement membrane layer secondary to deposition of collagen produced by myofibroblasts (types 1 to 3) and widened spaces between the basal epithelial cells (37,38). This latter finding was thought to contribute to a loss in cellular adhesion between the basilar epithelial and columnar cells, resulting in epithelial cell desquamation and subsequent loss of intercellular adhesion molecules, which regulate the traffic of inflammatory cells into the airways of patients with NOA (39). The importance of adhesion molecules in the pathogenesis of OA has not yet been investigated.

Lung biopsies from patients with OA have revealed increased numbers of activated T cells and eosinophils (37,38). Eosinophilia has correlated with elevations of IL-5, the cytokine responsible for growth, differentiation, and activation of eosinophils (37). T cells that release IL-5 modulate eosinophil adherence, chemotaxis, cellular activation, and release of their cationic and other toxic proteins (40). Patients with OA have increased numbers of activated T lymphocytes, eosinophils, and mast cells similar to what is found in NOA, suggesting that a T lymphocyte–eosinophil interaction is important in OA (37,38).

The inflammatory cells recruited into the airways release bioactive mediators that are responsible for the physiologic changes seen in asthma. BAL has been useful for identifying the presence of these mediators during EARs and LARs induced by occupational agents. For example, the lipoxygenase metabolite, LTB_4, has been detected shortly after a TDI challenge whereas LTE_4 presents early on in the EAR induced by plicatic acid (41,42). LTE_4 is also found in the urine during the EAR induced by many LMW chemicals including TDI but disappears during the LAR (43). Many other mediators such as histamine, platelet-activating factor (PAF), and prostaglandins have been detected in BAL fluids obtained from subjects with OA (42).

Finally, BAL fluids obtained during LARs induced by diisocyanates and plicatic acid contain increased amounts of albumin as a result of microvascular leakage and mucosal edema. The presence of albumin in BAL fluid has been used as a reliable marker for detecting active asthma (44).

SPECIFIC CHEMICAL AGENTS CAUSING RESPIRATORY HYPERSENSITIVITY

Polyisocyanates

Polyisocyanates are responsible for more cases of occupationally related lung disease today than any other class of LMW chemical. An estimated 5% to 10% of workers exposed to polyisocyanates develop OA (2). These compounds have reactive N=C=O side chains that are useful for the production of polyurethane foams, elastomers, adhesives, coatings, and paint hardeners used in the automotive, building, and spray paint industries (45). The polyisocyanate compounds, hexamethylene diisocyanate (HDI), 4,4′-diphenylmethylene diisocyanate (MDI), and toluene diisocyanate (TDI) (Fig. 3) are the most commonly used agents commercially and therefore have been responsible for most of the cases of occupational lung disease reported around the world (5,45). Even though the chemical properties of these polyisocyanate compounds vary, exposed symptomatic workers demonstrate significant cross reactivity between these chemicals, which makes them easier to study as a group (45,46). For instance, TDI and HDI are volatile at room temperature whereas MDI requires heating above 60°C before emitting vapor fumes, but all these polyisocyanates clinically affect the respiratory system. Table 2 summarizes the chemical properties of polyisocyanates (45).

Polyisocyanates are irritating to the mucous membranes of the eyes, nose, and lung. Respiratory disorders induced by polyisocyanates include bronchiolitis obliterans, hypersensitivity pneumonitis, and OA (5). The natural course of polyisocyanate-induced OA is variable and may persist for years even after cessation of expo-

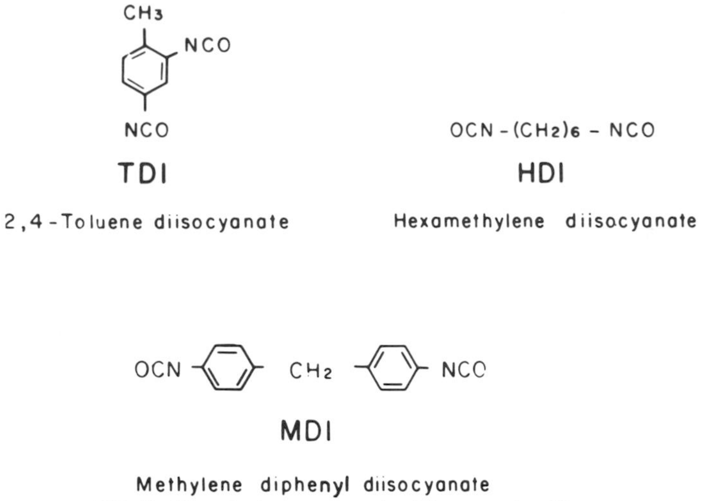

CH3
NCO
NCO
TDI
2,4-Toluene diisocyanate

OCN-(CH2)6 - NCO
HDI
Hexamethylene diisocyanate

OCN CH2 NCO
MDI
Methylene diphenyl diisocyanate

FIG. 3. Chemical structures of polyisocyanates (5).

TABLE 2. *Chemical properties of polyisocyanates* (45)

Property	HDI	TDI	MDI
Partial listing of uses	As cross-linking agent in preparations of materials, contact lenses, and medical absorbents, and production of polyurethane and spray paints	Polyurethane coatings in floor and wood finishes and sealers; paints; elastomers in coated fabrics and clay pipe seals; in adhesives; cross-linking agent for nylon 6; manufacture of polyurethane foam	Bonding rubber to rayon and nylon; in two-component polyurethane coating systems; to produce polyurethane lacquer coatings; production of thermoplastic polyurethane resins, millable gums, and spandex fibers
Commercial formulations	Mononer; trimer (biuret)	2,4-TDI; 2,6-TDI mixtures of 80:20 and 65:35	
Boiling point	127°C at 9.8 mm Hg	251°C at 760 mm Hg	196°C at 5 mm Hg
Melting point	−67°C	19.5–21.5°C	37°C
Molecular weight	168.22	174.15	250.27
TLV	8-hr TWA = 0.005 ppm (0.034 mg/m^3) (1988)	8-hr TWA = 0.005 ppm (0.036 mg/m^3); STEL = 0.02 ppm (0.14 mg/m^3) (1988)	8-hr TWA = 0.005 ppm (0.51 mg/m^3) (1988)

TLV, threshold limit value; TWA, time-weighted average; STEL, short-term exposure limit.

sure (47,48). No identifiable risk factors for developing OA such as atopy, smoking, preexisting asthma, or gender have been identified (49). The amount of polyisocyanate exposure required to induce asthma or other upper airway symptoms is unknown but has been demonstrated to occur below the accepted threshold limit value (TLV) of 20 ppb (45). Animal studies have demonstrated physiologic, histologic, and immunologic changes after exposure to TDI as low as 1 ppb (50). In humans, most reports of polyisocyanate-induced OA have resulted from large exposures such as accidental chemical spills. Once these individuals become sensitized their symptoms can be reproduced with exposure to polyisocyanate concentrations as low as 1 ppb (51).

Rats and guinea pigs have been used to study the uptake and distribution of polyisocyanates into the respiratory tract using ^{14}C radioactive tracers (52). In these animal models the majority of polyisocyanate uptake occurred in upper and lower airways, while the alveoli were spared (45,52).

Most of the early *in vitro* investigation of polyisocyanates in animals and humans has involved conjugation of these LMW chemicals to autogenous albumin proteins (53). Although the chemical characterization of these isocyanate–albumin conjugates has been well described, it is still unknown whether these experimental conjugates reflect the immunopathogenic events in the respiratory tract after polyisocyanate exposure and sensitization (46,53). Recently, a 70,000-kDa molecular weight protein, identified as laminin, has been identified as the endogenous protein carrier that TDI conjugates with in the airways (54,55).

Polyisocyanates induce a spectrum of immune responses (Gell–Coombs 1 to 4) in addition to toxic and neuroreflex effects in the lung. Cell-mediated immune responses have been identified using lymphocyte blast transformation and leukocyte inhibitory factor assays (1). More recently, CD8+ lymphocytes have been found to increase in the peripheral circulation after specific TDI bronchoprovocation (20,56). Markers of IgE-mediated immune responses such as immediate cutaneous reactivity and specific serum IgE antibody to monoisocyanate–protein conjugates have been demonstrated in a minority of TDI-exposed workers (19,46,50). Although specific IgE and IgG antibodies are found more frequently in symptomatic workers with positive polyisocyanate inhalational challenges, they can also be found in workers with a negative challenge and therefore do not directly correlate with the presence of airway disease (48). A heterogeneous isotypic antibody response has been observed for the various polyisocyanates (19,46). For instance, HDI-exposed subjects are more likely to produce specific IgE and IgG antibodies compared to MDI workers, who may produce IgE, IgG, or IgM, or TDI workers who seldom elicit an antibody response (19,57–59). Serologic assays using polyisocyanate–albumin conjugates yield positive results more frequently than skin testing. However, reliable accuracy of both of these tests depends on using conjugates that have been carefully characterized to avoid ligand oversubstitution of the protein carrier, which could give rise to false-positive results (53).

Polyisocyanate-induced OA is associated more frequently with an LAR, which corresponds to the infiltration of inflammatory cells (polymorphonuclear cells and eosinophils) into the airways, resulting in chronic asthma with persistent BHR (60). This observation is supported by the inhibition of the LAR, BHR, and influx of inflammatory cells into the airways after pretreatment with corticosteroids (60). Initiation of these airway inflammatory events may be the result of the chemicals' toxic or immunologic effects on epithelial and alveolar macrophage cells, resulting in the release of bioactive chemotactic mediators (e.g., leukotriene B_4, IL-5, or IL-8) (61–63). Because there is significant overlap between inflammatory cells and the mediators they release, it is extremely difficult to determine the specific role of each cell leading to airway inflammation. However, the inflammatory cascade of events that occur with TDI-induced OA results in severe pathologic changes (e.g., mucus plugging, airway edema, smooth muscle hypertrophy, and basement membrane thickening with collagen deposition) that can lead to death if not recognized and treated. Even when the worker is removed from exposure, airway inflammation and BHR can persist for long periods of time. Thus there is a need for industries to develop environmental surveillance and monitoring programs in order to minimize the worker's exposure and risk for developing occupational lung disease (64).

Acid Anhydrides

Acid anhydrides are a group of reactive organic compounds that are constituents of alkyd and epoxy resins (Fig. 4) (65,66). Alkyl resins, which usually contain phthalic anhydride (PA) and maleic anhydride (MA), are used in paints, varnishes, and plastics, whereas epoxy resins, made from epichlorhydrin and bisphenol A, require curing with acid anhydrides for use in adhesive, casting, coating, and sealant materials (65,66). Trimellitic acid anhydride (TMA) has greater thermal stability than the other anhydride compounds and therefore is used as a plasticizer for the production of wire and cable coatings (66). TMA has also been used in the paint, textile, and paper industries (66). Anhydrides cause reactions in humans through their direct toxic effects primarily affecting the eyes, nose, skin, and lungs. In addition to their toxic effects, anhydrides are known to cause a spectrum of hypersensitivity reactions, which have been classified according to their clinical presentation as IgE, cytotoxic, immune complex-, or cell-mediated mechanisms (4,6,65, 66). Several animal models have been developed to study the effects of anhydrides. Rats exposed to TMA by inhalation develop pathologic lung features of interstitial pneumonitis with hemorrhagic foci (67). These changes begin to occur after 6 days of exposure but, after 10 days, reveal dramatic intra-alveolar hemorrhage, macrophage infiltration, and epithelial and endothelial cell injury (68,69). BAL fluid from these rat lungs contained higher antibody levels compared to the serum levels (70). This model corresponds to TMA-induced pulmonary hemorrhage and pneumonitis in some exposed workers (71).

The rhesus monkey has been used to study TMA-induced antibody immune responses using TMA haptenized erythrocytes (72). IgG, IgA, and IgM were found in the serum in response to this conjugate whereas only IgA and IgM were found in

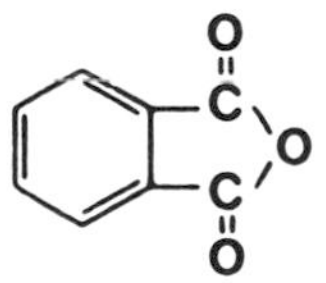

Phthalic (PA)

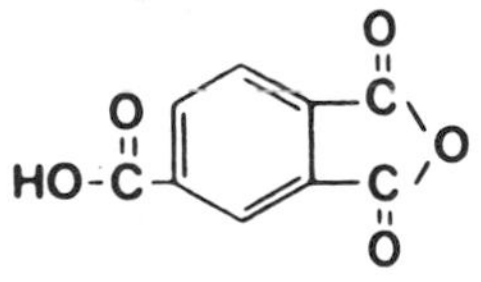

Trimellitic (TMA)

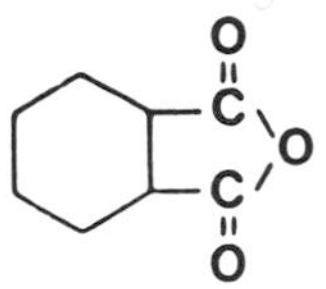

Hexahydrophthalic (HHPA)

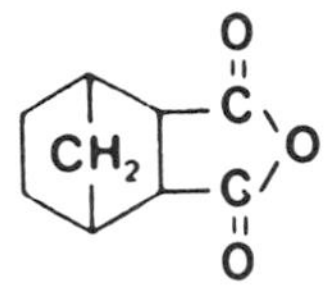

Himic (HA)

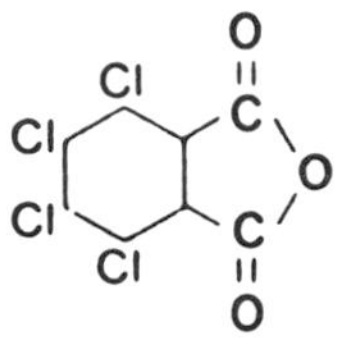

Tetrachlorophthalic (TCPA)

FIG. 4. Chemical structures of acid anhydrides (65).

BAL fluids (72). Although specific IgE antibodies were not demonstrated, subsequent experiments were successful in passively transferring human TMA-specific reaginic-like antibodies into the monkey's airways, which resulted in BHR (73). This model has been used to explain the IgE-mediated reactions manifested by a subset of TMA-exposed workers (73).

Other anhydride compounds have been demonstrated to induce occupation-related lung disorders in exposed workers. Wernfors et al. (74) and Bernstein and coworkers (75,76) studied immune responses in workers exposed to PA, himic anhydride (HA), and hexahydrophthalic anhydride (HHPA) and found heterogeneous reactions among them. IgE-mediated reactions were demonstrated against the hapten and newly formed antigenic determinants when the anhydrides were conjugated to the protein carrier molecule (65,74–76). Increased IgG levels have also been reported in these patients and in one study elevated IgG4 levels were thought to be involved in the immunopathogenesis of OA (17).

The late respiratory systemic syndrome (LRSS) resembles hypersensitivity pneumonitis in that symptoms begin 4 to 12 hr after TMA exposure and are associated with a productive cough in addition to systemic symptoms of fever, chills, and arthralgias/myalgias (6,77). This syndrome develops after a latency period of exposure (6,77). IgG and IgA antibodies have been demonstrated in response to TMA–

human serum albumin (HSA) conjugates (4). The pulmonary disease–anemia syndrome has been described in workers after very high exposure to TMA fumes (4,6,77). This syndrome also has a latency period with symptoms ranging from dyspnea, hemoptysis, anemia, and pulmonary infiltrates, which can result in restrictive lung disease (4,6,77). Elevated total antibody levels to TMA–protein conjugates have been demonstrated in these patients (77). Antibodies found in response to TMA–HSA in both of these syndromes are directed toward the new antigenic determinants that are formed as the result of TMA binding to protein (4). Antibody specificity has been shown for TMA, PA, and tetrachlorophthalic anhydride (TCPA) (78,79).

Prospective epidemiologic studies evaluating work exposure to TMA have found that TMA-induced immunologic lung disease is sporadic and uncommon (80,81). Latency periods are highly variable. Asthma and rhinitis followed by LRSS were most commonly diagnosed in these workers (81). A large epidemiologic study of TCPA workers found TCPA-specific IgE antibody in 12% of atopic workers and 6% of nonatopic workers (82). Furthermore, a strong correlation between TCPA specific IgE antibodies and smoking was found (79). Although the IgE levels decreased after 1 year, skin test reactivity persisted up to 4 years (83). In a survey of PA-exposed workers in four different plants, 24% were found to have rhinitis, 11% had bronchitis, and 2.8% had OA (74). A small group of workers exposed to HHPA have also been evaluated. Specific IgE antibody to HHPA–HSA was increased in 12 patients and 4 of these workers were diagnosed with OA (76). Several of these workers also had nasal and eye symptoms (76). Two out of 20 HA-exposed workers were found to have OA with increased specific IgE to HA–HSA (75). Additional longitudinal epidemiologic studies are necessary to learn more about the immunopathogenesis of respiratory hypersensitivity reactions induced by anhydrides.

Wood Dusts

Wood dusts are responsible for several occupationally related lung disorders including hypersensitivity pneumonitis, organic dust toxic syndrome, asthma, chronic bronchitis, and a mucous membrane irritation syndrome (84). Although individuals have typically developed symptoms in their occupational setting, hobbyists working with wood are also at risk for these pulmonary reactions. Western red cedar (*Thuja plicata*) has been the most extensively investigated of the wood dusts (85). This wood is harvested in the Pacific Northwest region of Canada and the United States and has been used to make pools, shingles, and lumber for building construction purposes. Western red cedar wood dust contains a variety of chemicals including tannin, dyes, pitch, resins, and gums (85). These chemicals can be extracted from the cedar wood by steam distillation to form volatile and nonvolatile components. Volatile components contain tropolones, natural fungicides that protect the wood from decay, and nezucone, an aromatic compound that can induce asthma in susceptible individuals (86,87). Most of the nonvolatile residue consists primarily of plicatic acid (MW = 440 daltons), which has subsequently been found to be responsible for most of the wood dust-induced OA in exposed workers (85). Red cedar dust TLVs range between 2.5 and 5 mg/mm^3 but workers have developed OA at levels below 2 mg/mm^3 (85). Red cedar OA typically presents after a latency exposure period of 6 weeks to 3 years with symptoms of cough, chest tightness, and wheezing (85,88). Symptoms may present as an upper respiratory infection or common cold with rhinorrhea and usually manifest as nocturnal coughing and wheezing that progressively worsens over time (85,88). Large groups of workers with red cedar OA have been studied. Preexisting atopy and NSBHR are not risk factors for developing symptoms in these individuals (88). Interestingly, nonsmokers or ex-smokers had a higher incidence of red cedar OA compared to active smokers (88). Specific bronchial challenges to plicatic acid in workers with severe red cedar OA reveal biphasic asthmatic reactions (EARs and LARs) associated with increased BHR (89,90). Immediate skin testing and serum IgE antibodies have not been diagnostically useful in these individuals. Bronchial challenges, initially using very low concentrations of plicatic acid, are often necessary to make a diagnosis (89).

Several nonimmunologic and immunologic mechanisms have been postulated to cause plicatic acid-induced OA (9). In high concentrations, plicatic acid has been demonstrated to activate the classical complement pathway, leading to the generation of the anaphylatoxins C3a and C5a, which are both capable of activating basophils and mast cells to release bioactive mediators (9). Plicatic acid is also toxic to the bronchial epithelium (91). Several features of plicatic acid-induced OA support an IgE-mediated mechanism, including the low prevalence of red cedar asthma in the exposed work population, the small amount of wood dust required to trigger asthma, and the characteristic latency period prior to the onset of symptoms (92). IgE antibody has been demonstrated *in vitro* or *in vivo* in many of these patients (85). *In vitro* assays using plicatic acid conjugated to HSA found specific IgE antibodies in 30% of patients whose diagnosis with red cedar OA was confirmed by specific inhalational challenges, but this serologic response did not correlate with cutaneous reactivity in these patients (16). It had previously been speculated that the LAR observed in patients with red cedar OA represented a type III immune response, but this theory has been supplanted by more recent work suggesting that the LAR is the result of late inflammatory changes secondary to the type I IgE-mediated response (44).

BAL fluids sampled during the LAR in these individuals have revealed eosinophils and bronchial epithelial cells (44). Bronchial biopsies performed on these patients demonstrated thickening of the basement membrane with infiltration of eosinophils into the bronchial epithelium and submucosa similar to what is found with NOA (44). Increased CD4+ cells have also been found in the BAL fluids 48 hr after specific bronchial challenge in individuals manifesting a LAR to plicatic acid with a concomitant decrease in peripheral blood CD4+ cells (31,93). The exact role of CD4+ lymphocytes in red ceder OA or in OA in general is still unclear.

Follow-up studies of OA worker populations who left their jobs have found that

40% recovered whereas 60% continued to experience asthma exacerbations. Many of these latter individuals required treatment with inhaled or systemic corticosteroids (88). Individuals who have continued working in the wood dust environment, despite wearing respiratory devices, have had progression of their disease manifested as a decrease in the ratio of 1-sec forced expiratory volume to vital capacity (FEV_1/VC) and increase in BHR (88).

Other wood dusts have been recognized as causing OA including abirncana, African maple wood, African zebrawood, kejaat wood, mahogany, and quillaja bark (31,94–97). Many of these individuals have demonstrated cutaneous reactivity and specific IgE-mediated antibodies to these wood dusts (31,94–97). Other wood dusts, such as California redwood, cedar of Lebanon, Central American walnut, cocabolla, eastern white cedar, and iroko, have not been associated with immediate cutaneous reactivity or serum-specific IgE antibodies (98–104).

Wood dusts are known to cause several hypersensitivity pneumonitis disorders including maple bark disease, sequoiosis, suberosis, and wood pulp workers disease (105–109). These diseases are caused by sensitization to fungi, including *Cryptostroma corticale* (maple bark), *Alternaria, Aspergillus,* and *Thermoactinomyces vulgaris,* contaminating the wood dust or bark of the tree (105–109). Several of these syndromes have been associated with IgG-precipitating antibodies to a specific antigenic determinant of the fungus (105–109).

The organic dust toxic syndrome, a systemic syndrome consisting of fever, rigors, nonproductive cough, and generalized malaise, is occasionally experienced by wood dust workers (110). Chronic bronchitis, consisting of a chronic productive cough, has also been described in these workers (111). Finally, wood dusts can induce other nonrespiratory symptoms including allergic conjunctivitis, rhinitis, dermatitis, and adenocarcinoma of the nasopharynx (112,113).

Metallic Salts

Metallic salts are responsible for a variety of pulmonary reactions. Because of their solubility in aqueous media, they can be readily dissociated and transported as metal ions into the lungs, where they can cause tissue destruction or sensitization (114). The fumes or dusts of metallic salts, once inhaled, can result in chemical pneumonitis, bronchitis, pulmonary emphysema, and adult respiratory distress syndrome (ARDS). Table 3 lists the metals that have most commonly been implicated with causing pulmonary immunologic and nonimmunologic disorders (114–116).

Immunologic Mechanisms

Platinum is used in the mining and metallurgical industries, as a catalyst in the chemical industry, and in catalytic converters used to reduce automobile exhaust emissions (114,115). Chloroplatinate salts are highly allergenic compared to the other metallic salts but platinum salt skin testing does not correlate well with the

TABLE 3. *Examples of inhaled metallic salts known to cause pulmonary reactions* (114–116)

Metal salt	Sources of exposure	Injury produced
Aluminum	Aluminum smelting	Potroom asthma
Antimony trichloride, antimony pentachloride	Steel industry, organic catalysts	Pulmonary edema
Cadmium	Electroplating, paint and pesticide manufacturing, cutting plated metals	Diffuse airway and lung injury; renal injury; lung carcinogen, pulmonary fibrosis
Cobalt sulfate/chloride	Metal alloy manufacture, especially tungsten carbide catalyst	Acute inhalation can cause pulmonary edema; chronic exposure may cause interstitial fibrosis, asthma
Copper sulfate	Vineyard sprayers	Patchy pneumonitis
Manganese dioxide	Chemical, battery manufacturing	Parenchymal injury
Nickel carbonyl/sulfate	Metal alloys, electroplating, welding	Pulmonary edema, asthma
Chloroplatinum	Mining and metallurgical industries, as a catalyst in the chemical industry, in catalytic converters	Asthma
Selenium hydrochloride	Metal industry, paints, glass production	Airway injury
Titanium tetrachloride	Dyes, pigments, sky writing	Upper airway injury
Vanadium pentoxide	Catalyst in chemical and petroleum industries	Asthma, tracheitis, and bronchitis
Zinc oxide	Steel, pavement and pesticide industries	Asthma

incidence of OA (117). However, workers with positive platinum skin tests have a higher incidence of allergic rhinitis and asthma compared to exposed workers with negative skin tests (118). Workers with platinum-induced OA demonstrate prick test reactivity to concentrations of platinum salts as low as 10^{-9} mg/ml and the skin test has therefore been used as a method for surveillance and early recognition of sensitized workers (118). Cigarette smoking has been implicated as a significant risk factor for platinum sensitization (117). The immunologic pathogenesis of platinum salt-induced OA has been shown to be type I IgE-mediated, which may also involve reaginic IgG4, supported by skin testing, radioallergosorbent test (RAST) inhibition, and specific IgE radioimmunoassays (117,118). Chronic platinum salt exposure may also result in nonspecific immunopotentiation of the IgE antibody response (117,118).

Nickel is widely used in mining, milling, smelting, and refinishing processes. Some nickel salts are extremely toxic to the central nervous system and the lung and therefore have restricted TLVs (15 $\mu g/mm^3$). Nickel-induced asthma, however, is rare (119,120). Individual case reports have found reactive hemagglutinating antibodies to nickel and, more recently, nickel-specific IgE antibodies using a nickel–HSA conjugate (15).

Chromium is widely used in electroplating processes and as a metal alloy in pigments, leather tanning, cement, and for the production of chromate salts (121). Hexavalent chromium compounds, such as chromium trioxide and mono- and bichromates are believed to be more allergenic because their solubility allows them easier access into body tissues (121). Chromates are prevalent in the work environment. They have been divided into carcinogenic and noncarcinogenic groups. The monochromates and bichromates are noncarcinogenic and have been occasionally implicated as causes of OA (121). Although prick skin tests to chromate salts have been negative in the reported cases of OA, one individual was demonstrated to have immediate bronchial hyperreactivity after a chromate-specific challenge and IgE-specific antibodies (15). Cell-mediated immune mechanisms have been postulated to induce pulmonary disease as one patient experienced an isolated late asthmatic reaction after a chromate bronchial challenge (122).

Cobalt salts are used to produce alloys for electrical, automobile, and aircraft industries. Cobalt is found in safety razor blades, surgical instruments, high-speed diamond polishing disks, glass, and enamel (123). Five percent of cobalt-exposed workers develop OA that needs to be distinguished from hard metal disease, which causes interstitial pneumonia and pulmonary fibrosis (124,125). Workers with cobalt-induced OA produce specific IgE antibodies and exhibit lymphocyte proliferation in response to free cobalt or cobalt–HSA. These findings suggest that specific IgE antibodies and cobalt-sensitized lymphocytes are involved in the immunopathogenesis of cobalt-induced asthma (125).

Nonimmunologic Mechanisms

Vanadium pentoxide has been used as a catalyst in the chemical and petroleum industries (126). Inhalational exposure to this metallic salt is very irritating to the upper respiratory tract. Acute tracheitis and bronchitis resulting in persistent bronchial hyperresponsiveness have been described after exposure (126). "Boilermaker's bronchitis" refers to vanadium-induced asthma that occurs in workers who clean oil tanks (126).

Zinc is used as an alloy for making steel and is important in the pavement and pesticide industries (114). Metal fume fever refers to a constellation of systemic symptoms including coughing, shortness of breath, and generalized myalgias and arthralgias occurring 4 to 12 hr after exposure to zinc oxide fumes, which can last 1 to 2 days (127). OA has also been reported to occur after zinc oxide exposure (128). At high doses zinc chloride, used in taxidermy, oil refining, and galvanizing iron, causes lung injury that can result in pulmonary edema (116).

Cadmium has not been associated with OA. However, inhalational exposure can result in impaired respiratory function and diffusing capacity with radiologic signs of emphysema that may be complicated by pulmonary fibrosis (114,115).

Aluminum is used in potrooms of the aluminum smelting process (129). Several gases and particulate matter commonly found in the potroom may induce asthma.

TABLE 4. *Miscellaneous low molecular weight chemicals inducing asthma*

Azobisformamide
Azodicarbonamide
Colophony
Other soldering fluxes
Formaldehyde
Chloramine-T
Persulfates
Diazonium salts (azo dyes)
1°, 2°, 3°, 4° Amines

These include dust containing cryolite, alumina, sulfur dioxide, carbon oxides, fluorides, and particulate organic matter. The causes and immune mechanisms of potroom asthma are unknown (129). Subjects with potroom asthma develop shortness of breath, wheezing, chest tightness, and cough, which occur hours after exposure. These symptoms become more frequent and severe with reexposure. Prognosis of potroom asthma is variable as 40% of workers have persistent asthma after leaving their work environment (129).

Additional Chemical and Pharmaceutical Agents

A number of other LMW chemicals have been associated with respiratory hypersensitivity disorders (Table 4). Azobisformamide and azodicarbonamide, used in the plastic industry to introduce gas into plastic, induce asthma in some exposed workers (130,131). An IgE-mediated immune response has not been demonstrated. Primary, secondary, tertiary, and quaternary amines have been reported to cause OA (132–135a). These chemicals are used in the rubber, cosmetic, photographic, paint, and pharmaceutical industries (132–135a). Investigators have described cutaneous and respiratory sensitivity symptoms to piperazine, which is an antihelminthic drug (135). Prolonged exposure to amines correlates well with the development of respiratory symptoms manifested as chronic bronchitis. The mechanisms responsible for amine-induced OA have not been clearly established (132–135a). Colophony, a pine tree resin containing abietic and pumaric acids, is commonly used as a soldering flux to prevent erosion in the electronics industry (136). Colophony inhalation challenges may induce an isolated early, isolated late, or dual asthmatic response in susceptible individuals (136). Atopy is a weak, predisposing factor for colophony-induced OA, but smoking is not a risk factor for developing BHR. The immunologic mechanism for colophony-induced lung disease is unknown and specific antibodies have not been demonstrated (137). It is worth noting that other soldering fluxes that contain zinc chloride, ammonium chloride and polyether, an alcohol–polypropylene glycol, or ethanolamine have also been reported to cause OA (138,139).

The safety of small amounts of airborne formaldehyde constitutes a concern to the general public. Formaldehyde is commonly used in hospitals, by furniture manufacturers, and in the textile industry (140,141). At high concentrations, formaldehyde causes well-recognized irritant side effects involving the nasal and conjunctival mucosa (140,141). Bronchial constriction with obstructive lung disease has been noted to occur in normal subjects exposed to 3 ppm of formaldehyde during exercise (140,141). Investigators have repeatedly found reduced expiratory flow rates in the small airways of formaldehyde-exposed workers. However, the overall incidence of formaldehyde-induced occupational lung disease is very low (140,141). A few case reports have demonstrated formaldehyde-specific antibodies in the sera of exposed workers that correlates to their lung disease. However, an immunologic basis for this disorder is uncommon (140,141).

Chloramine-T, a sterilizing agent commonly used in the food and beverage industry, may cause OA (142,143). An IgE-mediated mechanism for chloramine-T-induced OA has been proved based on immediate skin tests and serum specific IgE antibodies to a *p*-toluenesulfonyl side group (144). Persulfates (ammonium persulfate), which are commonly used by hair dressers in their hair styling preparations, have been linked to causing a number of OA cases after exposure (145). Diazonium salts, used in photocopying processes, produce an azo dye after exposure with light. LARs have been observed to occur in exposed workers undergoing a specific azo dye bronchial challenge (146). Increased levels of specific IgE antibodies to a diazonium tetrafluoroborate–HSA conjugate have been found in workers in the polymer industry (147). OA also occurs in workers exposed to reactive dyes used in the textile industry (148). An IgE-mediated mechanism has been confirmed for these dyes by immediate skin test reactivity and serum-specific IgE antibodies (148).

Respiratory hypersensitivity reactions to pharmaceutical agents have frequently been reported (Table 5) (1,149,150). Several antibiotics cause OA confirmed by specific inhalation tests. An IgE-mediated immune mechanism has been postulated to be responsible for several of these reactions based on the demonstration of specific immediate cutaneous reactivity and inhalational challenges (1,149,150).

Drug-induced pulmonary infiltrates may result from anaphylactic or anaphylactoid reactions, acute or chronic pneumonitis involving the alveoli or interstitium, lupus-like reactions, or fibrosis (149,150). The immunopathogenesis for most of these reactions is not completely understood. Drug-induced pulmonary infiltrates may be associated with peripheral and tissue eosinophilia (PIE syndromes) (1). Nitrofurantoin, a sulfonamide analog, causes pulmonary infiltrates that can lead to irreversible fibrosis if not recognized and discontinued (1,150). These reactions may occur due to the host's decreased catabolism of the drug's cytotoxic metabolites combined with a secondary immune response to the metabolite(s). Drug-induced lupus, most commonly seen with the antiarrythmic agent procainamide, is believed to represent an autoimmune response to the drug's reactive metabolites formed by oxidation of the primary aromatic amine (1,150). Metabolism of procainamide's primary arylamine may also lead to the production of procainamide hydroxylamine, which, after oxidation to a nitroso metabolite, may bind to histones or other proteins to form multivalent conjugates capable of inducing autoantibody

TABLE 5. *Drugs causing hypersensitivity lung disease* (150)

Cytotoxic drugs	Noncytotoxic drugs
Bleomycin	Nitrofurantoin
Methotrexate	Sulfasalazine
Procarbazine	Sulfadimethoxine
	Diphenylhydantoin
	Carbamazepine
	Chlorpropamide
	Imipramine
	Isoniazid
	Para-aminosalicylic acid
	Penicillin
	Cromolyn
	Dantrolene
	Methylphenidate
	Mephenesin carbamate
	Hydralazine
	Mecamylamine
	Ampicillin

formation (1). A number of chemotherapeutic agents have been reported to cause pulmonary interstitial or pleural fibrosis (e.g., bleomycin, cyclophosphamide, and busulfan). However, an immunologic basis for these drug reactions has not been established (149,150).

Pyrolysis fumes of polyvinyl chloride (PVC) are responsible for causing "meat wrapper's asthma" (151). This has been described in workers in meat packing plants exposed to the thermal degradation products of the plastic meat packing material (151). Specific inhalation tests to PVC and the price label adhesive fumes have confirmed these findings (152,153). Other chemicals known to cause respiratory reactions include the acrylates, organophosphate insecticides, freon, hexachlorophene (a topical disinfectant), furan (used to produce molds in foundries), styrene in plastic workers, machining fluids, and several noxious acids (154–162). Underlying immunologic mechanisms for PVC and other chemically induced pulmonary reactions have not been demonstrated (154–162).

Miscellaneous Syndromes

The multiple chemical sensitivity syndrome is a term that has been used to describe a constellation of nonspecific systemic symptoms occurring after exposure to a wide variety of irritating agents (163). Patients present with headaches, food intolerance, fatigue, lack of concentration, and depression, which they attribute to their work environments (163). The heterogeneous spectrum of their symptoms has made it very difficult to perform scientifically well-designed epidemiologic investigations of these individuals. Immunologic evaluation is usually normal. Search for environmental factors at work and home that aggravate their symptoms have been unsuccessful in identifying specific causes. In many instances, these individuals have been found to suffer from depression (163).

Reactive airways dysfunction syndrome (RADS) refers to the onset of bronchial hyperresponsiveness after a single exposure to high levels of irritant vapors, fumes, gas, or smoke (164). The histopathology of this disorder is very similar to asthma. The underlying mechanism(s) for this syndrome has not been proved. A high irritant exposure resulting in massive airway injury is believed to cause epithelium desquamation, resulting in exposure of irritant nerve fibers that can induce neurogenic inflammation (164,165). Diagnosis of this disorder requires a careful medical and occupational history with pulmonary function testing to confirm BHR. RADS is treated similarly to asthma (164,165).

CONCLUSIONS

Human respiratory hypersensitivity reactions to chemicals have emerged as important determinants of pulmonary immunotoxicology. Because of advancing industrial technology, a greater number of chemicals continue to be introduced into the work environment. The unique physical properties of LMW chemicals partially explains their capacities to sensitize exposed individuals. The current immunotoxicologic uncertainties about many of these chemicals can only be answered through further epidemiologic studies that monitor adverse drug reactions and large worker populations exposed to these chemicals. Such studies should be directed toward identifying risk factors, the natural course, and prognosis for these respiratory hypersensitivity disorders. Immunosurveillance programs designed and implemented by some industries to monitor workers exposed to specific chemicals have already been successful in decreasing the incidence of these respiratory disorders (166).

REFERENCES

1. Bernstein IL. Pulmonary hypersensitivity disorders. In: Newcombe DS, Rose NR, Bloom JC, eds. *Pulmonary hypersensitivity disozders*. New York: Raven Press; 1992;191–202.
2. Bernstein DI. Occupational asthma. *Clin Allergy* 1992;76:917–934.
3. Bernstein JA. Occupational asthma. *Postgrad Med* 1992;92:109–118.
4. Patterson R, Zeiss CR, Pruzansky JJ. Immunology and immunopathology of trimellitic anhydride pulmonary reactions. *Allergy Clin Immunol* 1982;70:19–23.
5. Bernstein IL. Isocyanate-induced pulmonary diseases: a current perspective. *J Allergy Clin Immunol* 1982;70:24–31.
6. Zeiss CR, Wolkonsky P, Pruzansky JJ, Patterson R. Clinical and immunologic evaluation of trimellitic anhydride workers in multiple industrial settings. *J Allergy Clin Immunol* 1982;70:15–18.
7. Patterson R, Grammer LC. Methods of analysis of occupational lung disease. *J Allergy Clin Immunol* 1986;78:1063–1066.
8. Solway P, Fish S, Passmore H, Gefter M, Coffee R, Manser T. Regulation of the immune response to peptide antigens: differential induction of immediate-type hypersensitivity and T cell proliferation due to changes in either peptide structure or major histocompatibility complex haplotype. *J Exp Med* 1991;174:847–858.
9. Chan-Yeung M. Immunologic and nonimmunologic mechanisms in asthma due to western red cedar (*Thuja plicata*). *J Allergy Clin Immunol* 1982;70:32–37.

10. Harkonen H, Nordman H, Korhonen O. Long-term effects of exposure to sulfur dioxide. *Am Rev Respir Dis* 1983;128:890–893.
11. Horstman DH, Folinsbee LJ, Ives PJ, Aabdul-Salaam S, McDonnell WF. Ozone concentration and pulmonary response relationships for 6.6-hour exposures with five hours of moderate exercise to 0.08, 0.10 and 0.12 ppm. *Am Rev Respir Dis* 1990;142:1158–1163.
12. Sheppard D. Airway hyperresponsiveness mechanisms in experimental models. *Chest* 1989;96: 1165–1168.
13. Sheppard D, Thompson JE, Scypinski L, Dusser D, Nadel JA, Borson DB. Toluene diisocyanate increases airway responsiveness to substance P and decreases airway neutral endopeptidase. *J Clin Invest* 1988;81:1111–1115.
14. Thompson JE, Scypinsky LA, Gordon T, Sheppard D. Tachykinins mediate the acute increase in airway responsiveness caused by toluene diisocyanate in guinea pigs. *Am Rev Respir Dis* 1987;136:43–49.
15. Novey HS, Habib M, Wells ID. Asthma and IgE antibodies induced by chromium and nickel salts. *J Allergy Clin Immunol* 1983;72:407–412.
16. Tse KS, Chan H, Chan-Yeung M. Specific IgE antibodies in patients with occupational asthma due to western red cedar (*Thuja plicata*). *Clin Allergy* 1982;12:249–258.
17. Nielsen J, Welinder H, Schutz A, Skerfring S. Specific serum antibodies against phthalic anhydride in occupationally exposed subjects. *J Allergy Clin Immunol* 1988;82:126–133.
18. Butcher BT, Bernstein IL, Schwartz HJ. Guidelines for the clinical evaluation of occupational asthma due to small molecular weight chemicals. *J Allergy Clin Immunol* 1989;84:834–838.
19. Gallagher JS, Tse CST, Brooks SM, Bernstein IL. Diverse profiles of immunoreactivity in toluene diisocyanate (TDI) asthma. *J Occup Med* 1981;23:610–616.
20. Finotto S, Fabbri LM, Rado V, Mapp CE, Maestrelli P. Increase in numbers of CD8 positive lymphocytes and eosinophils in peripheral blood of subjects with late asthmatic reactions induced by toluene diisocyanate. *Br J Ind Med* 1991;48:116–121.
21. Herzog CH, Villiger B, Braun P. Nickel-specific T cell clones in asthma—preferential use of V-beta 14 in T cell receptor beta chain. *Eur Respir Rev* 1991;4:4255.
22. Kusaka Y, Nakona Y, Shirakawa T, Morimoto K. Lymphocyte transformation with cobalt in hard metal asthma. *Ind Health* 1989;27:155–163.
23. Mosmann TR, Coffman RL. Heterogeneity of cytokine secretion patterns and functions of helper T cells. *Adv Immunol* 1989;46:111–147.
24. Mosmann TR, Schumacher JH, Street NF, et al. Diversity of cytokine synthesis and function of mouse CD4+ T cells. *Immunol Rev* 1991;123:209–229.
24a. Zurawski G, deVries JE, Interleukin 13, an interleukin 4-like cytokine that acts on monocytes and B cells, but not on T cells. *Immunol Today* 1994;5:19–26.
25. Dearman RJ, Kimber I. Differential stimulation of immune function by respiratory and contact chemical allergens. *Immunology* 1991;72:563–570.
26. Dearman RJ, Kimber I. Divergent immune responses to respiratory and contact chemical allergens: antibody elicited by phthalic anhydride and oxazolone. *Clin Exp Allergy* 1992;22:241–250.
27. Dearman RJ, Spence LM, Kimber I. Characterization of murine immune responses to allergenic diisocyanates. *Toxicol Appl Pharmacol* 1992;112:190–197.
28. Corrigan CJ, Kay AB. T cells and eosinophils in the pathogenesis of asthma. *Immunol Today* 1992;13:501–506.
29. Parronchi P, De Carli M, Manetti R, et al. IL-4 and IFN (α and γ) exert opposite regulatory effects on the development of cytolytic potential by Th1 and Th2 human T cell clones. *J Immunol* 1992; 149:2977–2983.
30. De Monchy GR, Kauffman HF, Venge P, et al. Bronchoalveolar eosinophils following allergen-induced late-phase asthmatic reactions. *Am Rev Respir Dis* 1985:131:373–376.
31. Chan-Yeung M, Leriche J, McLean L, Lam S. Comparison of cellular and protein changes in bronchial lavage fluid of symptomatic and asymptomatic patients with red cedar asthma on follow-up examination. *Clin Allergy* 1988;18:359–365.
32. Summary and recommendations of a workshop on the investigative use of fiberoptic bronchoscopy and bronchoalveolar lavage in asthmatics. *Am Rev Respir Dis* 1985;132:180–182.
33. Durham SR, Graneck BJ, Hawkins R, Newman-Taylor AJ. The temporal relationship between increases in airway responsiveness to histamine and late asthmatic responses induced by occupational agents. *J Allergy Clin Immunol* 1987;79:398–406.
34. Steinberg DR, Bernstein DI, Bernstein IL, Murlas CG. Bronchial reactivity increases early in both immediate and dual phase responders to allergen. *J Allergy Clin Immunol* 1987;79:249.

35. Roche WR, Beasley R, Williams JH, Holgate ST. Subepithelial fibrosis in the bronchi of asthmatics. *Lancet* 1989;1:520–524.
36. Beasley R, Roche WR, Roberts JA, Holgate ST. Cellular events in the bronchi in mild asthma and after bronchial provocation. *Am Rev Respir Dis* 1989;139:806–817.
37. Saetta M, Di Stefano A, Maestrelli P, et al. Airway mucosal inflammation in occupational asthma induced by toluene diisocyanate. *Am Rev Respir Dis* 1992;145:160–168.
38. Saetta M, Maestrelli P, De Stefano A, et al. Effect of cessation of exposure to toluene diisocyanate (TDI) on bronchial mucosa of subjects with TDI-induced asthma. *Am Rev Respir Dis* 1992;145:169–174.
39. Wagner CD, Gundel RH, Reilly P, et al. Intercellular adhesion molecule-1 (ICAM-1) in the pathogenesis of asthma. *Science* 1990;247:456–459.
40. Hamid Q, Azzawi M, Ying S, et al. Expression of mRNA for interleukin-5 in mucosal bronchial biopsies from asthma. *J Clin Invest* 1991;87:1541–1546.
41. Zocca E, Fabbri LM, Boschetto P, et al. Leukotriene B4 and late asthmatic reactions induced by toluene diisocyanate. *J Appl Physiol* 1990;68:1576–1589.
42. Chan-Yeung M, Chan H, Tse KS, Salari H, Lam, S. Histamine and leukotrienes release in bronchoalveolar lavage fluid during plicatic acid induced bronchoconstriction. *J Allergy Clin Immunol* 1989;84:762–768.
43. Manning PJ, Rokach J, Malo J, et al. Urinary leukotriene E_4 levels during early and late asthmatic responses. *J Allergy Clin Immunol* 1990;86:211–220.
44. Lam S, LeRiche J, Phillips D, Chan-Yeung M. Cellular and protein changes in bronchoalveolar lavage fluid after late asthmatic reactions in patients with red cedar asthma. *J Allergy Clin Immunol* 1987;80:44–50.
45. Kennedy AL, Brown WE. Isocyanates and lung disease: experimental approaches to molecular mechanisms. *Occup Med* 1992;7:301–329.
46. Baur X. Immunologic cross-reactivity between different albumin-bound isocyanates. *J Allergy Clin Immunol* 1983;71:197–205.
47. Luo JC, Nelsen KG, Fischbein A. Persistent reactive airway dysfunction syndrome after exposure to toluene diisocyanate. *Br J Ind Med* 1990;47:239–241.
48. Butcher BT, O'Neil CE, Reed MA, Salvaggio JE, Weill H. Development and loss of toluene diisocyanate (TDI) reactivity: immunologic, pharmacologic and provocative inhalation challenge studies. *J Allergy Clin Immunol* 1982;70:231.
49. Mapp CE, Boschetto P, Dal Vecchio L, Maestrelli P, Fabbri LM. Occupational asthma due to isocyanate. *Eur Respir J* 1988;1:273–279.
50. Karol MN. Respiratory effects of inhaled isocyanates. *CRC Crit Rev Toxicol* 1986;16:349–379.
51. Butcher BT, Karr RM, O'Neil CE, et al. Inhalation challenge and pharmacologic studies of TDI sensitive workers. *J Allergy Clin Immunol* 1979;64:146.
52. Kennedy AL, Stock MF, Alarie Y, Brown WE. *Uptake and distribution of ^{14}C during and following inhalation exposure to radioactive toluene diisocyanate*. New York: Academic Press; 1989:280–285.
53. Tse CST, Pesce AJ. Chemical characterization of isocyanate–protein conjugates. *Toxicol Appl Pharmacol* 1979:51:39–46.
54. Kennedy AL, Brown WE. Modification of airway proteins and induction of secondary responses by inhalation exposure to isocyanates. *Am Rev Respir Dis* 1989;139:387A.
55. Kennedy AL, Wilson TR, Brown WE. Analysis of function alterations of laminin modified by isocyanates *in vivo* and *in vitro*. *Am Rev Respir Dis* 1990;141:A706.
56. Bentley AM, Maestrelli P, Saetta M, et al. Activated T-lymphocytes and eosinophils in the bronchial mucosa in isocyanate-induced asthma. *J Allergy Clin Immunol* 1992;89:821–829.
57. Grammer LC, Eggum P, Silverstein M, Shaughnessy MA, Liotta JL, Patterson R. Prospective immunologic and clinical study of a population exposed to hexamethylene diisocyanate. *J Allergy Clin Immunol* 1988;82:627–633.
58. Liss GM, Bernstein DI, Moller DR, Gallagher JS, Stephenson RL, Bernstein IL. Pulmonary and immunologic evaluation of foundry workers exposed to methylene diphenyldiisocyanate (MDI). *J Allergy Clin Immunol* 1990;85:1076–1082.
59. Lushniak BD, Reh CM, Gallagher JS, et al. Indirect assessment of exposure to MDI by evaluation of specific immune responses to MDI-HSA in foam workers. *J Allergy Clin Immunol* 1990;85:251.
60. Fabbri LM, Maestrelli P, Saetta M, Mapp CE. Bronchial hyperreactivity: mechanisms and physiologic evaluation airway inflammation during late asthmatic reactions induced by toluene diisocyanate. *Am Rev Respir Dis* 1991;143:537–538.

61. Fabbri LM, Boschetto P, Zocca E, et al. Bronchoalveolar neutrophilia during late asthmatic reactions induced by toluene diisocyanate (TDI). *Am Rev Respir Dis* 1987;136:36–42.
62. Mattoli S, Miante S, Calabro F, Mezzett M, Fasoli A, Allegra L. Bronchial epithelial cells exposed to isocyanates potentiate activation and proliferation of T cells. *Am Physiol Soc* 1990;259:L320–L326.
63. Mattoli S, Masiero M, Calabro F, et al. Eicosanoid release from human bronchial epithelial cells upon exposure to toluene diisocyanate *in vitro*. *J Cell Physiol* 1990;142:379–385.
64. Paggiaro P, Bacci E, Paoletti P, et al. Bronchoalveolar lavage and morphology of the airways after cessation of exposure in asthmatic subjects sensitized to toluene diisocyanate. *Chest* 1990;98:536–542.
65. Bernstein DI, Gallagher JS, D'Souza L, Bernstein IL. Heterogeneity of specific-IgE responses in workers sensitized to acid anhydride compounds. *J Allergy Clin Immunol* 1984;74:794–801.
66. Venables K. Low molecular weight chemicals, hypersensitivity, and direct toxicity: the acid anhydrides. *Br J Ind Med* 1989;46:222–232.
67. Leach CL, Hatoum NS, Ratjczak HV, Zeiss CR, Roger JC, Garvin PJ. The pathologic and immunologic response to inhaled trimellitic anhydride in rats. *Toxicol Appl Pharmacol* 1987;87:67–80.
68. Ledbetter AD, Leach CL, Hatoum NS, Roger JC. The generation and detection of particulate aerosol of trimellitic anhydride and trimellitic acid for inhalation exposures. *Am Ind Hyg Assoc J* 1987;48:35–40.
69. Zeiss CR, Leach CL, Smith LJ, et al. A serial immunologic and histopathologic study of lung injury induced by trimellitic anhydride. *Am Rev Respir Dis* 1988;137:191–196.
70. Chandler MJ, Zeiss CR, Leach CL, et al. Levels and specificity of antibody in bronchoalveolar lavage (BAL) and serum in an animal model of trimellitic anhydride-induced lung injury. *J Allergy Clin Immunol* 1987;80:223–229.
71. Leach CL, Hatoum NS, Ratacjak HV, Zeiss CR, Garvin PJ. Evidence of immunologic control of lung injury induced by trimellitic anhydride. *Am Rev Respir Dis* 1988;137:186–190.
72. Patterson R, Roberts M, Harris KE, Levitz D, Zeiss CR. Pulmonary and systemic immune responses in rhesus monkeys to intrabronchial administration of trimellitic anhydride. *Clin Immunol Immunopathol* 1980;15:357–366.
73. Dykewicz MS, Patterson R, Harris KE. Induction of antigen-specific bronchial reactivity to trimellityl–human serum albumin by passive transfer of serum from human to rhesus monkeys. *J Lab Clin Med* 1988;111:459–465.
74. Wernfors M, Nielsen J, Schutz A, Zkerfring S. Phthalic anhydride-induced occupational asthma. *Int Arch Allergy Appl Immunol* 1986;79:77–82.
75. Rosenman KD, Bernstein DI, O'Leary K, Gallagher JS, D'Souza L, Bernstein IL. Occupational asthma caused by himic anhydride. *Scand J Work Environ Health* 1987;13:150–154.
76. Moller DR, Gallagher JS, Bernstein DI, Wilcox TG, Burroughs HE, Bernstein IL. Detection of IgE-mediated respiratory sensitization in workers exposed to hexahydrophthalic anhydride. *J Allergy Clin Immunol* 1985;75:663–672.
77. Zeiss CR, Patterson R, Pruzansky JJ, Miller MM, Rosenberg M, Levitz D. Trimellitic anhydride-induced airway syndromes: clinical and immunologic studies. *J Allergy Clin Immunol* 1987;60:96–103.
78. Maccia CA, Bernstein IL, Emmett EA, Brooks SM. *In vitro* demonstration of specific IgE in phthalic anhydride hypersensitivity. *Am Rev Respir Dis* 1976;113:701–704.
79. Howe W, Venables KM, Topping MD, et al. Tetrachlorophthalic anhydride asthma: evidence for specific IgE antibody. *J Allergy Clin Immunol* 1983;71:5–11.
80. Zeiss CR, Mitchell JH, Van Peenen PFD, et al. A twelve year clinical and immunologic evaluation of workers involved in the manufacture of trimellitic anhydride (TMA). *Allergy Proc* 1990;11:71–77.
81. Zeiss CR, Wolkonsky P, Chacon R, et al. Syndromes in workers exposed to trimellitic anhydride. A longitudinal clinical and immunologic study. *Ann Intern Med* 1983;98:18–24.
82. Venables K, Topping MD, Howe W, Lucznska CM, Hawkins R, Newman-Taylor AJ. Interaction of smoking and atopy in producing specific IgE antibody against a hapten protein conjugate. *Br Med J* 1985;290:201–204.
83. Venables KM, Topping MD, Nunn AJ, Howe W, Newan-Taylor AJ. Immunological and functional consequences of clinical tetrachlorophthalic anhydride induced asthma after four years of avoidance of exposure. *J Allergy Clin Immunol* 1987;80:212–218.
84. Enarson DA, Chan-Yeung M. Characterization of health effects of wood dust exposures. *Am J Ind Med* 1990;17:33–38.
85. Chan-Yeung M, Barton G, MacLean L, Grzybowski S. Occupational asthma and rhinitis due to western red cedar (*Thuja plicata*). *Am Rev Respir Dis* 1973;108:1094–1102.

86. Belleau B, Burba J. Occupancy of adrenergic receptors and inhibition of catechol *o*-methyl transferase by tropolones. *J Med Chem* 1986;6:755–759.
87. Shida T, Mimaki K, Sasaki N, Nakagama Y, Hattovi O. Western red cedar asthma: occurrence in Oume City, Tokyo and results of inhalation test using "nezucone" aromatic substance of western red cedar. *Arerugi* 1971;20:915–921.
88. Chan-Yeung M, MacLean L, Paggiaro PL. Follow-up study of 232 patients with occupational asthma caused by western red cedar (*Thuja plicata*). *J Allergy Clin Immunol* 1987;79:792–796.
89. Paggiaro PL, Chan-Yeung M. Pattern of specific airway response in asthma due to western red cedar (*Thuja plicata*): relationship with length of exposure and lung function measurements. *Clin Allergy* 1987;17:333–339.
90. Cockcroft DW, Cotton DJ, Mink JT. Nonspecific bronchial hyperreactivity after exposure to western red cedar. *Am Rev Respir Dis* 1979;119:505–510.
91. Ayars GH, Altman LC, Frazier CE, Chi EY. The toxicity of constituents of cedar and pine woods to pulmonary epithelium. *J Allergy Clin Immunol* 1989;83:610–618.
92. Chan-Yeung M, Kennedy S, Vedal S. A longitudinal study of red cedar sawmill workers. *Am Rev Respir Dis* 1990;141:A80.
93. Gerblich AA, Campbell A, Schuyler M. Changes in T-lymphocyte subpopulations after antigenic bronchial provocation in asthma. *N Engl J Med* 1984;310:1349.
94. Hinojosa M, Moneo I, Domingues J, Delgrado E, Losado E, Alcover R. Asthma caused by African maple (*Triplochiton scheroxylon*) wood dust. *J Allergy Clin Immunol* 1984;74:782–786.
95. Ordman D. Wood dust as an inhalant allergen: bronchial asthma caused by kejaat wood (*Pterocarpus angolensis*). *S Afr Med J* 1949;23:973–975.
96. Bush RK, Yunginger JW, Reed C. Asthma due to African zebrawood (*Microberlinia*) dust. *Am Rev Respir Dis* 1978;227:601–604.
97. Raghuprasad PD, Brooks SM, Litwin A, Edwards JJ, Bernstein IL, Gallagher J. Quillaja bark (scrap bark) induced asthma. *J Allergy Clin Immunol* 1980;65:285–287.
98. Chan-Yeung M, Abboud R. Occupational asthma due to California redwood (*Sequois sempervirens*) dusts. *Am Rev Respir Dis* 1976;114:1027–1031.
99. Greenberg M. Respiratory symptoms following brief exposure to cedar of Lebanon (*Cedra Libani*) dust. *Clin Allergy* 1972;2:219–224.
100. Bush RK, Clayton D. Asthma due to Central American walnut (*Juglans olanchana*) dust. *Clin Allergy* 1983;13:389–394.
101. Eaton KK. Respiratory allergy to exotic wood dust. *Clin Allergy* 1973;3:307–310.
102. Cartier A, Chan H, Malo JL, Pineau L, Tse KS, Chan-Yeung M. Occupational asthma caused by eastern white cedar (*Thuja occidentalis*) with demonstration that plicatic acid is present in this wood and is the causative agent. *J Allergy Clin Immunol* 1986;77:639–645.
103. Azofra J, Olaquibel JM. Occupational asthma caused by iroko wood. *Allergy* 1989;44:156–158.
104. Pickering CAC, Batten JL, Pepys J. Asthma due to inhaled wood dusts—western red cedar and iroko. *Clin Allergy* 1972;2:213–218.
105. Emanuel DA, Wenzel FJ, Lawton BR. Pneumonitis due to *Cryptostroma corticale* (maple-bark disease). *N Engl J Med* 1966;274:1413–1418.
106. Cohen HI, Merigan TC, Kosek JC, Eldridge F. Sequoiosos. A granulomatous pneumonitis associated with redwood sawdust inhalation. *Am J Med* 1967;43:785–794.
107. Avila R, Villar TG. Suberosis. Respiratory disease in cork workers. *Lancet* 1968;1:620–621.
108. Schlueter DP, Fink JN, Hensley GT. Wood-pulp workers' disease: a hypersensitivity pneumonitis caused by *Alternaria*. *Ann Intern Med* 1972;77:907–914.
109. Malmberg P, Palmgren U, Rask-Anderson A. Relationship between symptoms and exposure to moldy dust in Swedish farmers. *Am J Ind Med* 1986;10:316–317.
110. doPico GA, Reddan W, Flaherty D, et al. Respiratory abnormalities among grain handlers: a clinical, physiologic and immunologic study. *Am Rev Respir Dis* 1977;115:915–927.
111. Chan-Yeung M, Vedal S, Kus J, MacLean L, Enarson D, Tse KS. Symptoms, pulmonary function and bronchial hyperreactivity in western red cedar workers compared with those in office workers. *Am Rev Respir Dis* 1984;130:1038–1041.
112. Mitchell J, Chan-Yeung M. Contact allergy from *Frullania* and respiratory allergy from *Thuja*. *Can Med Assoc J* 1974;110:653–657.
113. Acheson ED, Cowdell RH, Hadfield E, Macbeth RG. Nasal cancer in woodworkers in the furniture industry. *Br Med J* 1968;2:587–597.
114. Nemery B. Metal toxicity and the respiratory tract. *Eur Respir J* 1990:3:202–219.

115. Metals and the lung. Editorial. *Lancet* 1984; Oct 20.
116. Sheppard D. Chemical agents. In: Murray JF, Nadel JA, eds. *Textbook of respiratory medicine*. Philadelphia: Saunders; 1988:1631–1645.
117. Brooks SM, Baker DB, Gann PH, et al. Cold air challenge and platinum skin reactivity in platinum refinery workers. *Chest* 1990;97:1401–1407.
118. Biagini RE, Bernstein IL, Gallagher JS, Moorman WJ, Brooks S, Gann PH. The diversity of reaginic immune responses to platinum and palladium metallic salts. *J Allergy Clin Immunol* 1985; 76:794–802.
119. Malo JL, Cartier A, Gagnon G, Evans S, Dolovich J. Isolated late asthmatic reaction due to nickel sulfate without antibodies to nickel. *Clin Allergy* 1985;15:95–99.
120. Malo JL, Cartier A, Doepner M, Nieboer E, Evans S, Dolovich J. Occupational asthma caused by nickel sulfate. *J Allergy Clin Immunol* 1982;69:55–59.
121. Burrows D. The dichromate problem. *Int J Dermatol* 1984;23:215–220.
122. Moller DR, Brooks SM, Bernstein DI, Cassedy K, Enrione M, Bernstein IL. Delayed anaphylactoid reaction in a worker exposed to chromium. *J Allergy Clin Immunol* 1986;77:451–456.
123. Gheysens B, Auwerx J, Van den Eeckkhout A, Demedts M. Cobalt-induced bronchial asthma in diamond polishers. *Chest* 1985;88:740–744.
124. Shirakawa T, Kusaka Y, Fukimura N, et al. Occupational asthma from cobalt sensitivity in workers exposed to hard metal dust. *Chest* 1989;95:29–37.
125. Shirakawa T, Kusaka Y, Fujimura N, Goto S, Morimoto K. The existence of specific antibodies to cobalt in hard metal asthma. *Clin Allergy* 1988;18:451–460.
126. Musk AW, Tees JG. Asthma caused by occupational exposure to vanadium compounds. *Med J Aust* 1982;1:183–184.
127. Malo JL, Cartier A. Occupational asthma due to fumes of galvanized metal. *Chest* 1987;92:375–377.
128. Kawane H, Soejima R, Umeki S, Niki Y. Metal fume and asthma. *Chest* 1988;93:1116–1117.
129. Chan-Yeung M, Wong R, MacLean L, et al. Epidemiologic health study of workers in an aluminum smelter in British Columbia. *Am Rev Respir Dis* 1983;127:465–469.
130. Malo JL, Pineau L, Cartier A. Occupational asthma due to azobisformamide. *Clin Allergy* 1985;15:261–264.
131. Norand JC, Grange F, Hernandez C, et al. Occupational asthma after exposure to azodicarbonamide: report of four cases. *Br J Ind Med* 1989;46:60–62.
132. Belin L, Wass U, Audnusson G, Mathiasson L. Amines: possible causative agents in the development of bronchial hyperreactivity in workers manufacturing polyurethanes from isocyanates. *Br J Ind Med* 1983;40:251–257.
133. Vallieres M, Cockcroft DW, Taylor DM, Dolovich J, Hargreave FE. Dimethyl ethanolamine-induced asthma. *Am Rev Respir Dis* 1977;115:867–871.
134. Lam S, Chan-Yeung M. Ethylenediamine-induced asthma. *Am Rev Respir Dis* 1980:121:151–155.
135. Hagmar L, Bellander T, Bergoo B, Simonsson BG. Piperazine-induced occupational asthma. *J Occup Med* 1982;24:193–197.
135a. Bernstein JA, Stauder T, Bernstein DI, et al. A combined respiratory and cutaneous hypersensitivity syndrome induced by work exposure to quaternary amines. *J Allergy Clin Immunol* 1994 [in press].
136. Burge PS, Harries MG, O'Brien IM, et al. Respiratory disease in workers exposed to solder flux fumes containing colophony (pine resin). *Clin Allergy* 1978;8:1–14.
137. Burge PS. Occupational asthma due to soft soldering fluxes containing colophony (rosin, pine resin). *Eur J Respir Dis* 1982;63:65–67.
138. Weir DC, Robertson AS, Jones S, et al. Occupational asthma due to soft corrosive soldering fluxes containing zinc chloride and ammonium chloride. *Thorax* 1989;44:220–223.
139. Stevens JJ. Asthma due to soldering flux: a polyether alcohol-polypropylene glycol mixture. *Ann Allergy* 1976;36:419–422.
140. Thrasher JD, Wojdani A, Cheung G, Heuser G. Evidence for formaldehyde antibodies and altered cellular immunity in subjects exposed to formaldehyde in mobile homes. *Arch Environ Health* 1987;42:347–350.
141. Imbus HR. Clinical evaluation of patients with complaints related to formaldehyde exposure. *J Allergy Clin Immunol* 1985;76:831–840.
142. Dijkman JG, Vooren PH, Kramps JA. Occupational asthma due to inhalation of chloramine-T. 1. Clinical observations and inhalation-provocation studies. *Int Arch Allergy Appl Immunol* 1981; 64:422–427.

143. Kramps JA, van Toorenenbergen AW, Vooren PH, et al. Occupational asthma due to inhalation of chloramine-T. II. Demonstration of specific IgE antibodies. *Int Arch Allergy Appl Immunol* 1981; 64:428–438.
144. Wass U, Belin L, Eriksson NE. Immunological specificity of chloramine-T-induced IgE antibodies in serum from a sensitized worker. *Clin Allergy* 1989;19:463–471.
145. Blainey AD, Ollier S, Cundell D, et al. Occupational asthma in a hairdressing salon. *Thorax* 1986;41:42–50.
146. Graham V, Coe MJS, Davies RJ. Occupational asthma after exposure to a diazonium salt. *Thorax* 1981;36:950–951.
147. Luczynska CM, Hutchcroft BJ, Harrison MA, et al. Occupational asthma and specific IgE to diazonium salt intermediate used in the polymer industry. *J Allergy Clin Immunol* 1990;85:1076–1082.
148. Alanko K, Keskinen H, Byorksten F, et al. Immediate-type hypersensitivity to reactive dyes. *Clin Allergy* 1978;8:25–31.
149. Cooper JAD Jr, White DA, Matthay RA. Drug-induced pulmonary disease. Part 1: cytotoxic drugs. *Am Rev Respir Dis* 1986;133:321–340.
150. Cooper JAD Jr, White DA, Matthay RA. Drug-induced pulmonary disease. Part 2: noncytotoxic drugs. *Am Rev Respir Dis* 1986;133:488–506.
151. Pauli G, Bessot JC, Kopferschitt MC, et al. Meat wrapper's asthma: identification of the causal agent. *Clin Allergy* 1980;10:263–269.
152. Vandervort R, Brooks SM. Polyvinyl chloride film thermal decomposition products as an occupational illness. *J Occup Med* 1977;19:188–191.
153. Brooks SM, Vandervort R. Polyvinyl chloride film thermal decomposition products as an occupational illness. *J Occup Med* 1977;19:192–196.
154. Nakazawa T. Occupational asthma due to alkyl cyanoacrylate. *J Occup Med* 1990;32:709–710.
155. Bryant DH. Asthma due to insecticide sensitivity. *Aust N Z J Med* 1985:15:66–68.
156. Malo JL, Gagnon G, Cartier A. Occupational asthma due to heated freon. *Thorax* 1984;39:628–629.
157. Nagy L, Orosz M. Occupational asthma due to hexachlorophene. *Thorax* 1984;39:630–631.
158. Cockcroft DW, Cartier A, Jones G, et al. Asthma caused by occupational exposure to a furan-based binder system. *J Allergy Clin Immunol* 1980;66:458–463.
159. Tarlo SM, Wong L, Roos J, et al. Occupational asthma caused by latex in a surgical glove manufacturing plant. *J Allergy Clin Immunol* 1990;85:626–631.
160. Spaner D, Dolovich J, Tarlo S, et al. Hypersensitivity to natural latex. *J Allergy Clin Immunol* 1989;83:1135–1137.
161. Moscato G, Biscaldi G, Cottica D, et al. Occupational asthma due to styrene: two case reports. *J Occup Med* 1987;29:957–960.
162. Kennedy SM, Greaves IA, Kriebel D, Eisen EA, Smith TJ, Woskie SR. Acute pulmonary responses among automobile workers exposed to aerosols of machining fluids. *Am J Ind Med* 1989; 15:627–641.
163. Black DW, Rathe A. Total environmental allergy: 20th century disease or deception? *Res Staff Physician* 1990;34:47–54.
164. Brooks SM, Weiss MA, Bernstein IL. Reactive airways dysfunction syndrome (RADS). *Chest* 1985;88:376–384.
165. Boulet LP. Increases in airway responsiveness following acute exposure to respiratory irritants. *Chest* 1988;94:476–480.
166. Bernstein DI, Korbee L, Stauder T, et al. The low prevalence of occupational asthma and IgE mediated sensitization to diphenylmethane diisocyanate (MDI) in a plant engineered for minimal exposure to diisocyanates. *J Allergy Clin Immunol* 1993;92:387–396.

Immunotoxicology and Immunopharmacology, Second Edition, edited by J. H. Dean, M. I. Luster, A. E. Munson, and I. Kimber.
Raven Press, Ltd., New York © 1994.

36

Immune-Mediated Side Effects of Antirheumatic Drug Therapy

Johanna J. Verwilghen and *Gabriel S. Panayi

*Department of Rheumatology, Northwestern Memorial Hospital, Chicago, Illinois 60611; and *Rheumatology Unit, Guy's Hospital, London SE1 9RT, United Kingdom*

In this chapter we do not intend to provide an exhaustive list of immune effects associated with all the various agents used in the treatment of rheumatoid arthritis. Instead, we have elected to focus on a selected number of therapeutic agents. Particular emphasis is placed on recent advances in our understanding of the immune-mediated side effects of gold and D-penicillamine treatment. This is an exciting and rapidly evolving field. Indeed, more is known concerning immunopathogenetic mechanisms of gold- and D-penicillamine-induced side effects than concerning immunologic effects associated with any of the other so-called disease-modifying agents. Furthermore, studies of the immunologic disturbances caused by gold have, as a valuable spin-off, cast considerable light on the mechanisms of action of this agent in the treatment of patients with rheumatoid arthritis.

GOLD SALTS

Gold salts have been used in the treatment of rheumatoid arthritis for almost 70 years. However, there is no clear understanding of the mechanisms of action of these slow-acting, second-line agents (1). *In vitro* studies have shown that gold has potent immunosuppressive effects, and this may explain its disease-modulating effects (2). However, treatment with gold salts is associated with a high frequency of adverse reactions. Indeed, after several months of treatment, at the time when the disease-ameliorating effect becomes apparent, side effects necessitate discontinuation of gold therapy in up to one-third of patients (3). Furthermore, it is of particular interest that the very patients who respond best to gold treatment are the ones most likely to develop adverse reactions (4). A number of recent studies, discussed later, have reported interesting observations that may provide an explanation for the clinical picture of the toxic manifestations as well as the temporal coincidence between the onset of these side effects and clinical benefit from gold therapy (5–7).

TABLE 1. *Comparison of clinical manifestations of gold-induced side effects and graft-versus-host disease*

System or organ	Gold-induced pathology	GVH disease
Skin	Maculopapular rash, erythroderma, lichen planus, alopecia	Maculopapular rash, total body erythema, lichen planus, alopecia, onychodysplasia, scleroderma
Gastrointestinal tract	Nausea, diarrhea, abdominal pain, stomatitis, mouth ulcers, colitis	Anorexia, nausea, diarrhea, abdominal pain, paralytic ileus, mucositis, sicca syndrome
Liver	Cholestatic jaundice, hepatitis	Cholestatic jaundice, hepatitis, hepatic failure
Immune system	Lymphadenopathy, IgA[a] deficiency	Lymphadenopathy, immunodeficiency
Hematopoietic system	Thrombocytopenia, aplastic anemia, leukopenia, agranulocytosis, eosinophilia	Thrombocytopenia, aplastic anemia, pancytopenia
Kidney	Immune complex nephritis	
Lung	Alveolitis, pneumonitis, pulmonary fibrosis	Bronchiolitis obliterans

[a]IgA, immunoglobulin A.

Clinical and Immunologic Manifestations Induced by Gold Salts

A variety of immune-mediated side effects can follow treatment of patients having rheumatoid arthritis with gold salts (Table 1). Of interest are the striking similarities between the clinical features of gold-induced side effects and graft-versus-host (GVH) disease (Table 1). In addition, gold salts can induce abnormalities of the immune system. These include antigen-specific T lymphocyte dysfunction, B cell hyperactivity leading to hypergammaglobulinemia, and the production of autoreactive antibodies (2).

Pathogenesis of Gold-Induced Side Effects

The pathogenetic mechanisms responsible for gold-induced side effects remain unclear. An increased risk of adverse immune reactions to gold salts is associated with human leukocyte antigen (HLA)-B35, HLA-DR2, and HLA-DR3, as well as the non-HLA linked slow sulfoxidation status (1,8). The immunopathologic appearances of the adverse cutaneous immune reactions to gold salts, which may resemble lichen planus (9) and are characterized by the accumulation of CD4+ (helper) T cells, and the association of these side effects with HLAs both suggest that T lymphocytes and antigen-presenting cells play a central role in the pathogenesis (1). Since rheumatoid arthritis is characterized by a chronic cell-mediated immune response in the synovium, most likely mediated by the persistent presentation of unknown antigenic peptides, presented on the HLA molecules, to disease-causing T cells (10), a common mechanism might explain both the toxic and disease-ameliorative effects of gold salts. Recently, Sinigaglia and colleagues (7) presented data indicating that gold salts can bind directly to and structurally modify the major histocompatibility complex (MHC) class II molecules. These authors reported that gold salts specifically alter that region of the MHC class II molecule that interacts with a given T cell receptor (7). A functional equivalent of an allogeneic MHC molecule is thus generated and this could result in T lymphocyte activation. Indeed, we (5) and others (6) reported that patients with gold-induced dermatitis have T lymphocytes that are activated by gold salts, and this T cell activation is MHC restricted.

Conclusions

As gold salts alter the structure of the MHC class II molecules on antigen-presenting cells, thereby creating a functional equivalent of an allogeneic molecule, gold salts alter the immunogenicity of potentially stimulating cells bearing MHC class II molecules. This may lead to the development of side effects in a GVH-like pattern (11), which may explain the striking clinical similarities between gold-related pathology and GVH disease. In addition, one could hypothesize that gold salts, by altering the molecular configuration of the binary complex of HLA class II/rheumatoid antigenic peptide, could suppress rheumatoid synovitis by preventing activation of disease-causing T cells (12). Further studies analyzing the exact alterations of the MHC class II molecules induced by gold salts as well as determining the nature of the T cell receptor of gold-responsive T cells, by cloning techniques, may lead to the development of specific monoclonal antibodies against the T cell receptor of these cells. Such antibodies could then be used in the prevention or treatment of gold-induced dermatitis, which severely limits the use of what is otherwise an effective antirheumatic drug.

D-PENICILLAMINE

D-Penicillamine was introduced in 1963 for the treatment of rheumatoid arthritis (13). As with the gold salts, the rationale for use of this agent was based on theoretical assumptions that soon turned out to be incorrect. Indeed, even now, there is no clear understanding of the mechanisms of action of this second-line agent. *In vitro* studies have shown that D-penicillamine has potent immunosuppressive effects, and this may partly explain its disease-modulating effects (14–16). However, as with gold salts, use of D-penicillamine is associated with a high frequency of adverse reactions. Here, we focus only on the immune-mediated side effects and do not discuss those side effects resulting from the copper- or cysteine-depleting capacity of D-penicillamine. Similarly, clinical effects resulting from the collagen-damaging effect of D-penicillamine are not discussed.

TABLE 2. *Clinical manifestations of penicillamine- and antimalarial-induced side effects*

System or organ	D-Penicillamine	Antimalarial drugs
Nervous system	Myasthenia gravis, polymyositis, dermatomyositis	Myasthenic reactions, myopathy, polyneuropathy
Skin	Alopecia, maculopapular rash, exanthema, lichenoid lesions, pemphigus	Alopecia, maculopapular rash, lichenoid lesions, urticarial and exfoliative rashes
Gastrointestinal tract	Stomatitis, oral ulcers, anorexia, nausea, colitis	Anorexia, nausea, diarrhea
Liver	Cholestatic jaundice	
Immune system	Lupus erythematosus-like disease, IgA deficiency	
Hematopoietic system	Thrombocytopenia, leukopenia, agranulocytosis, pure red blood cell aplasia, eosinophilia	Leukopenia, agranulocytosis, aplastic anemia, leukemia
Kidney	Goodpasture's syndrome, immune complex membranous glomerulonephritis, lupus nephritis, renal vasculitis	
Endocrine system	Graves' disease, autoimmune insulin syndrome	
Lung	Interstitial fibrosis, obliterative bronchiolitis	

Clinical and Immunologic Manifestations Induced by D-Penicillamine

Treatment with D-penicillamine creates disturbances of the immunologic system, as evidenced by the appearance of autoantibodies as well as of symptoms and signs compatible with an autoimmune disease process. All such autoimmune manifestations, including autoantibodies, disappear slowly after stopping the drug. Table 2 shows the various immune-mediated syndromes that have been associated with D-penicillamine. Despite major structural, metabolic, and pharmacologic differences, the time course of efficacy and the spectrum of toxicity of penicillamine are similar to those observed with gold salts (Table 1). Moreover, patients who develop adverse reactions while on gold appear to have an increased risk for the development of similar reactions to D-penicillamine (17,18).

Pathogenesis of Penicillamine-Induced Side Effects

The pathogenetic mechanisms responsible for penicillamine-induced side effects remain unclear. However, the observation that an increased risk of side effects with penicillamine treatment is associated with the HLA-B8/DR3 and HLA-DR4 haplotypes suggests a role for immune-mediated mechanisms (19,20). The molecular basis for the induction of D-penicillamine-induced autoimmunity has been studied in considerable detail in animal models (21,22). Gleichmann and colleagues have suggested that D-penicillamine may induce side effects by one of three different mechanisms. As D-penicillamine is characterized by reactivity with thiol groups, this agent may react with membrane proteins. Alternatively (or additionally), they may affect intracytoplasmic and intranuclear compartments or may alter protein trafficking and processing in immunocompetent cells (22). The authors propose three mechanisms of actions, none of which are necessarily mutually exclusive (22). First, penicillamine may modify the structure of MHC class II molecules, or self-peptides, at the surface of antigen-presenting cells. The modified epitopes would then be recognized as foreign by the T cells and thus induce a GVH disease-like syndrome, similar to that induced by gold salts (21,22). Second, the agent may alter the structure or the specificity of the T cell receptor, either by direct binding at the T cell surface or by acting at the gene level. Third, by reacting with other membrane proteins, such as adhesion molecules, penicillamine might amplify T cell–B cell interactions—independent of the specificity of the T cells—and so function as a "superadhesin" (22).

Conclusions

If D-penicillamine in humans can alter the immunogenicity of HLA-DR molecules and, as a consequence, induce a GVH disease-like syndrome, the striking similarity between the side effects induced by gold salts and D-penicillamine becomes understandable. However, to date, there is no clear proof that any of the proposed pathogenic mechanisms of D-penicillamine occur in humans and further studies examining the molecular mechanisms of D-penicillamine-induced side effects are clearly needed.

SULFASALAZINE

Sulfasalazine is an acid azo compound of 5-aminosalicylic acid and sulfapyridine that was synthesized in the late 1930s. At the time, rheumatoid arthritis was thought to be a chronic granulomatous disease with a probable infectious cause. Accordingly, it was hypothesized that a compound containing both salicylate and a sulfonamide would be a potentially useful therapeutic agent. However, it was not until a report by McConkey and colleagues (23), published in 1978, that its efficacy in the treatment of rheumatoid arthritis was appreciated. The mode of action of sulfasalazine remains unknown. Interest has focused on the effects other than antibacterial in the hope that these may provide clues to the mechanism(s) of action of sulfasalazine in patients with rheumatoid arthritis. *In vitro* studies have shown that sulfasalazine inhibits T cell (24) and B cell function (25), as well as natural killer (NK) cells (26). However, most of these studies reported the immunosuppressive effect at concentrations higher than those attained in the serum of patients receiving therapeutic doses of the drug. Some authors have suggested that the higher concentration of the drug in the gastrointestinal tract (twice the serum levels) suppresses the activity of gut-associated lymphoid tissue, thus asserting its immunomodulatory effect (27).

During treatment with sulfasalazine, approximately one in four patients stop taking the drug because of side effects. The most common side effects (nausea, vomiting, dizziness, and abdominal pain) as well as less frequently observed side effects (bone marrow suppression and hepatitis) are seen in patients with the slow acetylator phenotype and do not appear to be immunologically mediated. However, despite its immunosuppressive effect, treatment with sulfasalazine is associated with immune-mediated side effects. Systemic lupus-type syndromes occur rarely and, not surprisingly, are more frequently seen in patients with a preexisting positive antinuclear antibody test (28). More common immunologic side effects are mucocutaneous reactions (exfoliative dermatitis, bullous erythema multiforme, and epidermal necrolysis). Desensitization to sulfasalazine, which can be done in an outpatient setting, enables the majority of patients developing these cutaneous reactions to continue treatment (29). Pulmonary complications due to sulfasalazine have been reported anecdotally. Symptoms occurred within the first few months of treatment and were accompanied by infiltrations in chest radiographic films, fever, and peripheral blood eosinophilia (30). These symptoms and signs, suggesting an allergic reaction, resolve after discontinuation of sulfasalazine.

ANTIMALARIALS

Antimalarials have been used to treat rheumatoid arthritis since 1951, when the remission-inducing effect of quinocrine was reported (31). However, although multiple antimalarial compounds have been developed and used for connective tissue disease, the compounds currently used are the 4-aminoquinoline derivatives chloroquine and hydroxychloroquine. These antimalarial medications have gained favor because they offer the best ratio of efficacy to toxicity. However, even with these compounds, potential toxicity limits their use. The mechanisms by which antimalarial drugs act to alleviate rheumatoid arthritis have not been determined. Two possible mechanisms of action are (a) inhibition of enzyme activity and (b) interference of cell activities in compartments that function in an acid cell environment, such as lysosomes. These basic drug actions may subsequently affect pathways, such as the immune cascade, that more directly lead to joint lesions. Antimalarial suppression of the immune system may be mediated by inhibition of interleukin-1 production by monocytes (32). Concentrations of chloroquine as low as 1 μg/ml suppress *in vitro* lymphocyte proliferation (32). Indeed, we have shown that peripheral blood lymphocytes from patients treated with chloroquine and aspirin have a decreased responsiveness to phytohemagglutinin stimulation when compared with cells from patients treated with aspirin alone (33).

The somewhat weaker antirheumatic activity of antimalarial drugs when compared with other second-line agents is offset by a superior safety profile. The benefit applies to both drug tolerance and serious toxicity. Potential ocular toxicity is a particular concern as loss of vision caused by retinopathy has been reported. However, it is now apparent that, with low daily dosage and regular ophthalmologic examination, visual loss almost never occurs. Other reported side effects of antimalarial drugs are similar to those of gold salts and penicillamine and are shown in Table 2. The pathogenetic mechanisms of these adverse reactions remain unknown. Future studies will be needed to determine whether any of these side effects are immune mediated.

REFERENCES

1. Panayi GS. Immunological and immune-mediated toxic effects of gold compounds used in the treatment of rheumatoid arthritis. In: Dayan AD, ed. *Immunotoxicity of metals and immunotoxicology*. New York: Plenum Press; 1990:155–158.
2. Lipsky PE. Immunomodulatory effect of gold compounds. In: Nuki G, Gumpel JM, eds. *Myocrisin, 50 years experience*. London: Medi-Cine Communications International Ltd; 1985:39–48.
3. Lockie LM, Smith DM. Forty-seven years experience with gold therapy in 1,019 rheumatoid arthritis patients. *Semin Arthritis Rheum* 1985;14:238–246.
4. Caspi D, Tishler M, Yaron M. Association between gold induced skin rash and remission in patients with rheumatoid arthritis. *Ann Rheum Dis* 1989;48:730–732.
5. Verwilghen J, Kingsley GH, Gambling L, Panayi GS. Activation of gold-reactive T lymphocytes in rheumatoid arthritis patients treated with gold. *Arthritis Rheum* 1992;35:1413–1418.
6. Romagnoli P, Spinas GA, Sinigaglia F. Gold specific T cells in rheumatoid arthritis patients treated with gold. *J Clin Invest* 1992;89:254–258.
7. Sinigaglia F, Takacs B, Romagnoli P. Immunologically relevant interactions between metals and peptide complexes. Presented at the 8th International Congress of Immunology, Budapest, 1992.
8. Panayi GS, Wooley PH, Batchelor JR. Genetic basis of rheumatoid disease: HLA antigen, disease manifestations and toxic reactions to drugs. *Br Med J* 1978;2:1326–1328.
9. Wooley PH, Griffin J, Panayi GS, Batchelor JR, Welsh KI, Gibson TJ. HLA-DR antigens and toxic reaction to sodium aurothiomalate and D-penicillamine in patients with rheumatoid arthritis. *N Engl J Med* 1980;303:300–302.
10. Penneys NS, Ackerman AB, Gottlieb NL. Gold dermatitis: a clinical and histopathological study. *Arch Dermatol* 1974;109:372–376.
11. Verwilghen J, Panayi GS. Side effects induced by gold salts: a graft-versus-host like disease. *J Lab Clin Med* 1994;123:777–780.
12. Kingsley G, Pitzalis C, Panayi GS. Immunogenetic and cellular immune mechanisms in rheumatoid arthritis: relevance to new therapeutic strategies. *Br J Rheumatol* 1990;29:58–64.
13. Jaffe IA. Comparison of the effect of plasmapheresis and penicillamine on the level of circulating rheumatoid factor. *Ann Rheum Dis* 1963;22:71–73.
14. Kosha A. Effects of oral administration of D-penicillamine on T and B lymphocytes in peripheral blood of rheumatoid patients. *Tokohu J Exp Med* 1979;129:233–238.
15. Olsen NJ, Jasin HE. Decreased pokeweed mitogen-induced IgM and IgM rheumatoid factor synthesis in rheumatoid arthritis patients treated with gold sodium thiomalate or penicillamine. *Arthritis Rheum* 1984;27:985–994.
16. Riestra JL, Harth M, Rodrigues A, Larrea CL. Effects of D-penicillamine on mononuclear cells in vitro. *Rheumatol Int* 1988;8:119–124.
17. Webley M, Coomes EN. Is penicillamine therapy influenced by previous gold? *Br Med J* 1978;2:91.
18. Halla JT, Cassidy J, Hardin JG. Sequential gold and penicillamine therapy in rheumatoid arthritis. Comparative study of effectiveness and toxicity and review of the literature. *Am J Med* 1982;72: 423–426.
19. Bernelot Moens HJ, Ament HJW, Feltkamp TEW, van der Korst JK. Long term follow-up of treatment with D-penicillamine for rheumatoid arthritis: efficacy and toxicity in relation to HLA antigens. *J Rheumatol* 1987;14:1115–1119.
20. Gladman DD, Anhorn KAB. HLA and disease manifestations in rheumatoid arthritis. *J Rheumatol* 1986;13:274–276.

21. Gleichmann E, Pals ST, Rolink AG, Radaszkiewickz T, Gleichmann H. Graft-versus-host reactions: clues to the etiopathology of a spectrum of immunological diseases. *Immunol Today* 1984;5: 324–332.
22. Goldman M, Druet P, Gleichmann E. TH2 cells in autoimmunity: insights from allogeneic diseases and chemically induced autoimmunity. *Immunol Today* 1991;12:223–227.
23. McConkey B, Amos RS, Butler EP. Salazopyrin in rheumatoid arthritis. *Agents Actions* 1978;8: 438–441.
24. Symmons DPM, Salmon M, Farr M, Bacon PA. Sulphasalazine treatment and lymphocyte function in patients with rheumatoid arthritis. *J Rheumatol* 1988;15:575–579.
25. Comer SS, Jasin HE. In vitro immunomodulatory effects of sulphasalazine and its metabolites. *J Rheumatol* 1988;15:580–586.
26. Gibson PR, Jewell DP. Sulphasalazine and derivates, natural killer activity and rheumatoid arthritis. *Clin Sci* 1985;69:177–184.
27. Sheldon PJ, Welsh C, Grindulis KA. Sulphasalazine in rheumatoid arthritis: pointers to a gut-mediated immune effect. *Br J Rheumatol* 1988;17:344–349.
28. Farr M, Scott DGI, Bacon A. Side effect profile of 200 patients with inflammatory arthritis treated with sulphasalazine. *Drugs Suppl* 1986;32:49–53.
29. Bax DE, Amos RS. Sulphasalazine in rheumatoid arthritis: desensitizing the patient with a skin rash. *Ann Rheum Dis* 1986;45:139–140.
30. Jones GR, Malone DN. Sulphasalazine induced lung disease. *Thorax* 1972;27:713–717.
31. Freedman A, Bach F. Mepacrine and rheumatoid arthritis. *Lancet* 1951;2:231–232.
32. Salmeron G, Lipsky PE. Immunosuppressive activity of chloroquine: inhibition of human monocyte function. *Arthritis Rheum* 1982;25:S132.
33. Panayi GS, Neill WA, Duthie JJR, McCormick JN. Action of chloroquine phosphate in rheumatoid arthritis. I. Immunosuppressive effect. *Ann Rheum Dis* 1973;32:316–321.

Immunotoxicology and Immunopharmacology, Second Edition, edited by J. H. Dean, M. I. Luster, A. E. Munson, and I. Kimber.
Raven Press, Ltd., New York © 1994.

37

Allergy to Laboratory Animals

Philip A. Botham and *Eric L. Teasdale

*ZENECA Central Toxicology Laboratory, Alderley Park, Macclesfield, Cheshire SK10 4TJ, United Kingdom; and *Department of Safety, Health, and Environment, ZENECA Pharmaceuticals, Alderley Park, Macclesfield, Cheshire SK10 4TF, United Kingdom*

The interest of the scientific, clinical, and clinico-legal communities in the syndrome known as allergy to laboratory animals (ALA) has been generated only with the last 20 years. Since 1970, there has been a rapidly increasing number of publications on the subject, in the form of both scientific research papers and reviews and advisory and guidance documents from various industry associations and governments. ALA is not a new disease, however. There is considerable, albeit mainly anecdotal, evidence that ALA has been a major occupational health problem for many years and has resulted in significant morbidity among scientists and technicians working with laboratory animals.

It was not until the 1970s, however, that the scale of the problem could be quantified. Now, a large number of epidemiologic investigations have confirmed that ALA is probably the greatest occupational risk to the health of individuals working with animals. As a consequence of this, several countries have recognized that legislation designed to protect employees from the development of occupational disease should include ALA and that employees who develop asthma due to exposure to laboratory animals should qualify for appropriate compensation payments.

Although many of the allergenic proteins responsible for ALA have been characterized and can be measured, there is still very little known about the level and type of exposure to animals that result in ALA. Neither is there a very clear understanding of why certain types of individuals appear to be more susceptible to the development of the problem or why, once sensitized, some are more "allergic" than others. This lack of knowledge has also made the prevention and treatment of ALA very difficult.

This chapter reviews the recent scientific progress that has been made in this area, but it also highlights where there are still deficiencies in our understanding and where further research is required.

IMMUNOLOGIC MECHANISMS OF ALLERGY TO LABORATORY ANIMALS

In common with other "atopic diseases" such as hay fever and house dust allergy, ALA is an immunoglobulin E (IgE)-mediated syndrome (1). Specific IgE antibodies are produced in genetically susceptible individuals in response to exposure to allergens derived from the urine, dander, serum, and saliva of laboratory animals (see later discussion). However, it is not always possible to detect these antibodies using the standard diagnostic techniques of skin prick testing and radioallergosorbent testing (RAST), even in individuals with confirmed exposure-related symptoms. Hunskaar and Fosse (2) recently reviewed the results of 17 published studies of ALA and found that, on average, only 57% of people with clinical allergy associated with exposure to rats or mice were skin test positive to extracts derived from rat and mouse urine, dander, and serum. This probably reflects a number of problems, the most important being that the extracts used were generally crude preparations derived by a variety of methods from these tissues and with little or no characterization or quality control. Other explanations are possible, however, including the presence in patients' sera of only low levels of antibodies, undetectable with the standard diagnostic methods, a lack of the causative allergen in the extracts used for the tests, and incorrect clinical diagnosis. It may also be possible that the symptoms of some individuals are mediated by other mechanisms, immunologic or nonimmunologic.

LABORATORY ANIMAL ALLERGENS

Although many, even recent, epidemiologic studies of ALA have used crude extracts of urine, dander, serum, or saliva as diagnostic reagents, methods have been available for several years to purify and characterize the allergenic components. Thus, for example, in rat urine there are two major allergens: Rat n IB (also known as α-2u-globin) and Rat n IA (prealbumin). The former (which has a molecular weight of 16,000 to 17,000 kDa with pI values of 5.4, 5.6, and 5.8) is present in higher quantities than the latter (which has a molecular weight of 20,000 to 21,000 kDa with pI values of 4.5 and 4.6) (3). In mouse urine, the major allergen is Ag1 (also known as prealbumin), which has a molecular weight of 17,000 to 20,000 kDa with pI values in the range of 4.2 to 4.9. Another major allergen is found in mouse dander and has been named Ag3 (4). Major allergens are normally defined as those for which the sera of 50% or more of clinically allergic subjects show binding of IgE (by techniques such as crossed radioimmunoelectrophoresis) and for which at least 25% show strong specific binding (5).

A few studies have investigated cross-reactivity between species and even between strains (6). It has also been suggested that male rats may have more Rat n IA allergen in their dander, urine, and saliva than females (7). However, these important issues (particularly in terms of the management of ALA) have received little attention and it is recommended that further studies of species cross-reactivity and sex differences are conducted using purified and well-characterized allergens. It is also recommended that diagnostic testing in ALA should be conducted using purified allergens and that a commercially available supply of these materials should be made available.

DIAGNOSIS OF ALLERGY TO LABORATORY ANIMALS

The most common symptoms of ALA are rhinitis and irritation and watering of the eyes. Skin rashes are also common and take the form of urticaria (nettle rash) or papula or vesicular erythema (8). Wheals may develop on the skin around bites or scratches especially if the area is contaminated with urine or saliva from the animal (6). The clinically more serious condition, allergic asthma, may occur on its own or more usually in association with other symptoms and may present as an immediate or as a delayed reaction (9).

The diagnosis of allergy to laboratory animals is mainly clinical; taking a proper history will identify both the allergic state and the connection with work. It is also important to make use of both preemployment and follow-up questionnaires. The former is obviously designed to help in the screening out of those likely to be allergic—particularly if they suffer from asthma. The follow-up questionnaire should be used in a well-designed health surveillance program. It should include questions designed to determine the periods of contact with animals, the duties performed (e.g., feeding, cleaning, weighing), the symptoms experienced when exposed to animals, the use of specific respiratory protection, and any possible development of symptoms.

The use of immunologic tests (skin tests and RASTs) may support any diagnosis. However, ALA is an allergic syndrome that shares with the common atopic diseases—hay fever and house dust mite allergy—a similar clinical picture and an IgE-mediated pathogenesis. It has been estimated that there are over 200 agents and specific biologic materials in use in the workplace that can trigger an allergic response. There are many more substances that can do likewise outside the work environment. As mentioned earlier, immunologic studies have shown that only 57% of individuals who develop ALA have IgE antibodies specific for laboratory animal-derived allergens (2). Therefore clinical history should always be the major basis on which a diagnosis is made.

A secondary problem with immunologic tests is that there is currently a lack of good quality diagnostic reagents. As they now come under the control of the regulatory authorities, companies previously involved in their manufacture have found the process of authorization too time consuming, expensive, and laborious.

It is often said that even in organizations that maintain an effective health surveillance program, there is a great deal of underreporting of ALA. Highly trained biologists may fear that admitting to symptoms of allergy, with possible subsequent confirmation, could threaten their career or limit work in their chosen speciality. It is important to educate employees at the time of commencing work with laboratory animals. There should be an ongoing program to continue the education process to ensure full understanding of the ways in which it is possible to reduce the risk of developing the disease and of reducing the frequency and severity of symptoms in allergic individuals. The importance of early reporting of symptoms should be encouraged so that modifications to working practices and to the type of respiratory protective equipment issued can, if possible, be made.

PREVALENCE AND INCIDENCE OF ALLERGY TO LABORATORY ANIMALS

The prevalence of ALA, that is, the number of cases of the disease present in a population at a specified time, expressed as a percentage of the total population, has been estimated using a variety of epidemiologic techniques in studies over the last 20 years. Hunskaar and Fosse (2) have found that in 19 studies, published between 1972 and 1988, the prevalence of ALA was in some cases as low as 11% to 15%, but in others it was over 30%. When the data were pooled, giving a total exposed population of 4988, the overall prevalence was 21%. Subsequently, several other studies have confirmed this picture (see refs. 10 and 11), the most notable being that of Aoyama et al. (12), who studied 5641 workers in Japanese laboratory animal facilities and found a prevalence rate of 23%. In all these studies, the data are predominantly concerned with exposure to rats, mice, guinea pigs, and rabbits.

The heterogeneity of the methods used in these studies makes it very difficult to compare individual studies; some used only self-administered questionnaires, whereas others required a thorough clinical history and a range of diagnostic testing. The definition of "exposed to laboratory animals" also varied, with some studies excluding individuals with relatively infrequent exposure and others including people who were probably never exposed to animal allergens. Reported prevalences may be low because allergic individuals have left employment due to their medical condition. Conversely, prevalence studies may overestimate the problem if no account is taken of previous exposure to laboratory animals, either in past employment or from household pets.

Further analysis of the data from these studies, for example, to look for the effect of exposure on the development of ALA or to investigate the relative allergenicity of different species, is therefore of doubtful value. What is clear, however, is that ALA affects at least one-fifth of people who work with laboratory rodents and rabbits. It is perhaps worth speculating what the response of regulatory authorities would be if this sort of prevalence rate were seen with occupational allergy caused by exposure to a synthetic chemical. While there is no doubt that ALA is now recognized by several authorities as an important occupational disease, its association with exposure to "natural products" (i.e., animals) means that it is still associated more with hay fever and house dust allergy—a nuisance rather than a major health problem—than with allergy caused by exposure to, say, an isocyanate.

There have been far fewer studies of the incidence of ALA. Incidence is defined as the number of cases of the disease occurring in a population during a specified period of time, expressed as a percentage of the total population. We have conducted three major prospective studies of ALA. In the first (13), 15% or 148 individuals studied developed ALA during their first year of employment with the company. The symptoms were generally mild and restricted to rhinitis, conjunctivitis, and urticaria, but there was a 2% incidence of asthma. This contrasted with a retrospective study, which was conducted concurrently, where 13 of 24 subjects with ALA who had worked with animals for up to 16 years were suffering from asthma. This suggested that most individuals who become allergic to laboratory animals develop the condition in a mild form, perhaps during their first year of employment, but that some then progress to more severe forms of the disease with further exposure.

This study was followed by a larger prospective investigation of 383 individuals (14), in which it was found that the "first year incidence" of ALA fell from 37% in 1980 and 1981 to 12% by 1984. This reduction coincided with the introduction of a site order and code of practice for working with animals, which were designed to reduce potential exposure to allergens (e.g., by mandatory use of personal protective equipment and by extensive use of educational programs). Some individuals in each yearly cohort were also monitored for a further 2 years, but, although additional subjects developed ALA during this time, there was no evidence for an increase in the intensity of the symptoms and the overall incidence of asthma was again only 2%. Two-thirds of those individuals who developed ALA during their first 3 years of employment did so during the first year. A third study (P. A. Botham et al., *unpublished data*) has shown that the reduction in "first year incidence" has been maintained at around 10% up to 1990. Kibby et al. (10) found a similar incidence of ALA (13%) in the first 2 years of exposure of 69 animal-exposed workers in a U.S. government research facility.

These studies suggest that ALA tends to develop in a mild form during the first few years of occupational exposure to animals, and that its incidence, and perhaps its severity, can be controlled by the introduction of appropriate management controls. However, none of the studies reported to date have considered the effect of previous exposure to animals and there has been no attempt made to measure actual or potential exposure to allergens. Further prospective studies are needed to address these issues so that the effects of management controls on incidence and severity can be better assessed and their cost effectiveness established.

PREDISPOSING FACTORS

Many of the prevalence and incidence studies referred to earlier have also tackled the vexing question of predisposing factors in the development of ALA. However, as the majority of the studies were cross-sectional, it is difficult to determine the significance of some of the findings. A similar picture is seen with the whole area of occupational asthma. Thus, although underlying nonspecific airways hyperreactivity, atopic diathesis, and cigarette smoking are believed to be important factors in asthma due to high molecular weight allergens, they have not usually been measured immediately before employment (reviewed in ref. 15).

The prospective studies of ALA (13,14) studied the influence of preexisting atopy on the development of ALA. Atopy was defined as a positive skin prick test (greater than 3-mm wheal) to grass pollen allergens and/or house dust mite allergen at the preemployment medical check. A significantly greater proportion of atopic individuals became symptomatic than nonatopics (19% to 43% compared with 3% to 6%) during the first year of exposure, but this discrepancy was not maintained, as more nonatopics developed ALA in the second and third years of exposure. The prospective study of Kibby et al. (10) looked at a number of historic findings as possible predictors of ALA. The best predictor was the presence of at least three historic atopic indicators. Five such indicators were assessed: history of hay fever, of childhood skin rashes, of other allergies, and of asthma and a family history of allergy. However, the relative risk was only 2.5.

All these studies concluded that the exclusion of atopics from working with animals could not be justified because for every case of ALA that would theoretically be prevented, at least three individuals who would never develop the problem would also be denied employment.

Das et al. (15) attempted to study the effect of smoking history and the results of preemployment skin tests and measurements of nonspecific airways reactivity on the development of ALA in trainee animal health technicians. Unfortunately, interpretation of the data was complicated by the findings that precareer selection bias had already occurred due to previous exposure to animals.

All these findings indicate that further studies of predisposing factors in ALA must focus on people as they begin work with laboratory animals and particularly on those who have no past occupational exposure. Failure to control these factors will lead to the same difficulties of interpretation that have accompanied every study of ALA to date.

EXPOSURE TO ALLERGENS AND THE DEVELOPMENT OF ALLERGY TO LABORATORY ANIMALS

The measurement of airborne allergens was first described by Agarwal et al. (16). They captured allergenic particles greater than 0.3 μm in diameter on a filter through which constant air flow was maintained. The filters were then eluted with buffer and allergen was measured using a RAST inhibition technique. This was subsequently adapted for use with mouse allergens (17). Several groups have since used similar approaches to estimate exposure to a number of laboratory animal allergens (reviewed in ref. 18).

Interpretation and comparison of results from these studies are again very difficult, however, because the elution techniques and assay procedures have varied sufficiently to give rise to large (and probably artifactual) variations in measured allergen concentrations. A number of common findings can be highlighted though. Allergen load is related to stocking density, air circulation, and humidity, and measurements of room allergen levels can significantly underestimate the levels generated locally, for example, during the handling of an animal, and hence underestimate potential exposure.

Although it has been suggested that the most heavily exposed individuals are the most likely to develop ALA (10), prospective studies are needed to better define the relation between exposure levels (and patterns of exposure) and the incidence of the disease. Only then will it be possible to focus on the most appropriate management and engineering controls required to minimize the development of ALA.

TREATMENT, MANAGEMENT, AND PREVENTION OF ALLERGY TO LABORATORY ANIMALS

The symptoms of allergy have been noted previously: congested nose and sneezing, skin rashes, or the more serious allergic asthma. All may be reduced in intensity by removal of the individual from exposure to the allergens. Orally administered antihistamines are the drugs of choice for symptomatic management of urticaria. However, it is the symptoms affecting the chest that may require more urgent attention to resolve discomfort. The β_2-agonists have become the most frequently prescribed drugs for asthma. The β-agonists, such as salbutamol, are bronchodilator drugs and are regarded as "symptomatic" treatment, in contrast to "anti-inflammatory" or "prophylactic" treatment such as inhaled corticosteroids or sodium cromoglycate. The management of asthma in ALA should therefore consist of prevention with anti-inflammatory agents and relief of breakthrough symptoms with β-agonists (19).

There is also a chance that anaphylaxis could occur—perhaps following a bite (20). Clorpheniramine maleate should be administered and salbutamol by inhaler if the patient is conscious but wheezy. In a case of collapse, hydrocortisone should be administered and, if there is no response, epinephrine should be given.

However, the mainstay of management of staff working with laboratory animals is minimizing exposure to animal allergens by appropriate engineering or procedural controls or, if these are not practical, by the provision of suitable personal protective equipment (desensitization is not a feasible option because the success rate is small and the inherent risks are too great).

PREEMPLOYMENT SELECTION AND SCREENING

In the United Kingdom, an employer is free not to employ staff on the basis of a medical recommendation with regard to likely susceptibility to ALA. Therefore all candidates who are to work with laboratory animals should be medically assessed as part of the preemployment selection process. The medical assessment should always include a detailed occupational history (with dates) plus a questionnaire on medical history, including details of any allergic conditions with the time of occurrence, results of investigations, and treatment past and present.

Consideration should be given to recommending to management rejection of a candidate where there is a history of ALA or of chronic skin disease, asthma, or other cardiorespiratory disorders likely to make the candidate more susceptible to the induction or the consequences of ALA (21,22). Investigations such as lung function tests and skin prick tests may usefully contribute to the preemployment medical assessment. Atopics identified by skin prick testing should be warned of their increased chance of developing the disease early in their work with animals but, as mentioned earlier, should not be excluded simply on the basis of their atopic status.

PROTECTION AGAINST EXPOSURE TO ALLERGENS

Exposure to laboratory animal-derived allergens may be minimized by implementing engineering control systems. These have recently been reviewed by Hunskaar and Fosse (23). The most effective control is by containing animals within enclosures such as isolators or cage boxes with filtered tops. If this is not practical, adequate ventilation should be installed. Experimental work has shown that general room ventilation without directed laminar flow is not effective in controlling exposures in people carrying out specific operations involving allergens but will lower the general background level in the area. This can be assisted by adjusting the humidity but this must be compatible with the needs of the animals and the comfort of operators. Effective control of specific operations can only be maintained by the use of laminar flows in the order of 0.5 $msec^{-1}$. This level of air flow is necessary to overcome eddies and other air currents and thermals and movement within the area. It is usually not practical to provide this level of air flow over the whole area of an animal room because of the high costs involved, but an alternative is the provision of local workstations. These are segregated areas in part of the animal accommodation or adjacent to it. They should be designed to be large enough for the operations to be carried out but not over large to minimize the quantity of air required for adequate control.

While it should be policy to control the exposure of individuals to hazardous materials by engineering methods, there are occasions where the only practical means of control of atmospheric contaminants is by the use of respiratory protective equipment. This should be of a type designated for use with toxic dusts, for example, one of those listed in Part 6 of the (U.K.) HSE Certificate of Approval (Respiratory Protective Equipment). In practice, it is found that disposable masks (e.g., 3M 8800 or 8810) are the most comfortable to wear and are acceptable to the workforce. Alternatively, high-efficiency ventilated visors and helmets can be recommended. These have been found to be readily accepted and very effective in practice, even with sensitized personnel (24). It must be said, however, that these can give a sensation of isolation and make communication with colleagues difficult—particularly if worn for long periods.

Piecemeal modification of existing facilities is unlikely to be efficient or cost effective in reducing the incidence of allergy to laboratory animals and therefore ventilation control, the principle of segregation of working areas from animal housing areas, and personal protective measures must be considered together.

ARE THERE "SAFE" LEVELS OF LABORATORY ANIMAL ALLERGENS?

Experiments were conducted to determine whether there are levels of allergen below which sensitized people can work without experiencing symptoms. This was indeed found to be the case (*unpublished data*); however, the volunteers merely sat in the room where animals were housed while the levels of allergen were estimated. While this work has provided evidence to support the efforts made to provide engineering solutions to the problem of ALA, in practice, sudden high levels of allergen may be sufficient to trigger symptoms in those sensitized. Such peaks have been found when animals are lifted to face height for inspection and palpation. Any release of allergen (e.g., when the animal urinates) will lead to a high local level of allergen, in the breathing zone of the scientist.

The exposure levels required to induce sensitization in healthy (unsensitized) individuals have not been formally demonstrated. In fact, it may be ethically unjustified to conduct trials to determine the dose of allergen that produces symptoms in those who are not already sensitized. Not only could this seriously interfere with the lives of individuals so exposed, but it could also prove life-threatening.

LEGISLATION AFFECTING ALLERGY TO LABORATORY ANIMALS

The United States, Canada, Japan, and most countries in Europe have laws regarding general aspects of health and safety at work. In the United Kingdom, the Health and Safety at Work Act of 1974 details the responsibility of employers and employees in general terms. Under common law, an employer has a duty to take reasonable care of employees' health and safety and to conduct the business in such a way as not to expose employees to an unnecessary risk. The fact that an employee contracts a condition or disease that is prescribed by regulations as due to the nature of one's employment does not automatically make the employer liable under common law for the injury. The employee must still prove that the employer was negligent in exposing the employee to the risk of contracting such injury, and proof of negligence will depend on considerations such as whether the employer maintained a safe system of work. The general practice of the company or laboratory will be relevant to judgment in these matters. In addition to one's duty under common law, an employer has to observe a number of statutory provisions relating to the safety, health, and welfare of employees, the breach of which makes the employer liable to prosecution under the Health and Safety at Work Act of 1974 as well as to an action for damages.

Occupational asthma following exposure to laboratory animals is a condition that, in many countries, attracts compensation or industrial injury benefit. It is often referred to as one of the "prescribed" diseases. This makes it advisable for companies to prepare a general policy statement on this subject. Such a policy should include a statement of the company attitude to preemployment selection and medical screening, medical surveillance during employment, relocation, and dismissal.

An employer also has a duty to consider removing an employee who has developed ALA to a safer job or even to terminate the employment if the risk caused by the condition is too great. If relocation is sought, the company should seek to make all reasonable endeavors to achieve this aim in full and proper consultation with the employee. In the event of an employee refusing to cooperate, a reasonable employer cannot permit the employee to remain exposed to the hazard.

SUMMARY

A great many institutions, companies, and other organizations are involved in work using laboratory animals. ALA is probably one of the most important occupational health problems in the majority of these institutions. The prevention of ALA by screening out every susceptible individual is not yet possible. Therefore it is important to minimize the chances of the disease developing by ensuring that effective engineering controls and personal protective equipment are in place and to have a strategy for managing the adverse effects of ALA should they occur. These initiatives should not be viewed in isolation, however, but rather as part of an integrated approach to managing a high-quality operation.

REFERENCES

1. Gross NJ. Allergy to laboratory animals: epidemiologic, clinical and physiologic aspects, and a trial of cromolyn in its management. *J Allergy Clin Immunol* 1980;66:158–165.
2. Hunskaar, Fosse RT. Allergy to laboratory mice and rats: a review of the pathophysiology, epidemiology and clinical aspects. *Lab Anim* 1990;24:358–374.
3. Eggleston PA, Newill CA, Ansari AA, et al. Task-related variation in airborne concentrations of laboratory animal allergens: studies with Rat nI. *J Allergy Clin Immunol* 1989;84:347–352.
4. Price JA, Longbottom JL. Allergy to mice. I. Identification of two major mouse allergens (Ag1 and Ag3) and investigations of their possible origin. *Clin Allergy* 1987;17:43–53.
5. Lowenstein H. Quantitative immunoelectrophoretic methods as a tool for the analysis and isolation of allergens. *Prog Allergy* 1978;25:1–62.
6. Longbottom J. Occupational allergy due to animal allergens. *Clin Immunol Allergy* 1984;4:19–36.
7. Walls AF, Longbottom JL. Quantitative immunoelectrophoretic analysis of rat allergen abstracts. I. Antigenic characterisation of fur, urine, saliva and other rat-derived materials. *Allergy* 1983;38: 501–512.
8. Agrup G, Belin L, Sjostedt L, Skerfving S. Allergy to laboratory animals in laboratory technicians and animal keepers. *Br J Ind Med* 1986;43:192–198.
9. Lutsky I. Occupational asthma in laboratory animal workers. In: Frazier CA, ed. *Occupational asthma*. New York: Van Nostrand Reinhold; 1980:193–208.

10. Kibby T, Powell G, Cromer J. Allergy to laboratory animals: a prospective and cross-sectional study. *J Occup Med* 1989;31:842–846.
11. Sjostedt L, Willers S. Predisposing factors in laboratory animal allergy: a study of atopy and environmental factors. *Am J Ind Med* 1989;16:199–208.
12. Aoyama K, Ueda A, Manda F, Matsushita T, Ueda T, Yamauchi C. Allergy to laboratory animals: an epidemiological study. *Br J Ind Med* 1992;49:41–47.
13. Davies GE, Thompson AV, Niewola Z, et al. Allergy to laboratory animals: a retrospective and a prospective study. *Br J Ind Med* 1983;40:442–449.
14. Botham PA, Davies GE, Teasdale EL. Allergy to laboratory animals: a prospective study of its incidence and of the influence of atopy on its development. *Br J Ind Med* 1987;44:627–632.
15. Das R, Tager IB, Gamsky T, Schenker MB, Royce S, Balmes JR. Atopy and airways reactivity in animal health technicians. A pilot study. *J Occup Med* 1992;34:53–60.
16. Agarwal MK, Yunginger JW, Swanson MC, Reed CE. An immunochemical method to measure atmospheric allergens. *J Allergy Clin Immunol* 1981;68:194.
17. Twiggs JT, Agarwal MK, Dahlberg MJE, Yunginger JW. Immunochemical measurement of airborne mouse allergens in a laboratory animal facility. *J Allergy Clin Immunol* 1982;69:522–526.
18. Gordon S, Tee RD, Lowson D, Wallace J, Newman Taylor AJ. Reduction of airborne allergenic urinary proteins from laboratory rats. *Br J Ind Med* 1992;49:416–420.
19. Chung KF. The current debate concerning β-agonists in asthma: a review. *J R Soc Med* 1993;86:96–100.
20. Teasdale EL, Davies GE, Slovak AJM. Anaphylaxis following bites by rodents. *Br Med J* 1983; 286:1480.
21. Lutsky I, Kalbfleisch JH, Fink JN. Occupational allergy to laboratory animals: employer practices. *J Occup Med* 1983;25:372–376.
22. Newill CA, Evans R, Khoury MJ. Pre-employment screening for allergy to laboratory animals—an epidemiological evaluation of its potential usefulness. *J Occup Med* 1986;28:1158–1164.
23. Hunskaar S, Fosse RT. Allergy to laboratory mice and rats: a review of its prevention, management and treatment. *Lab Anim* 1993;27:206–221.
24. Slovak AJM, Orr RG, Teasdale EL. Efficacy of the helmet respirator in occupational asthma due to laboratory animal allergy (LAA). *Am Ind Hyg Assoc J* 1985;46:411–415.

Immunotoxicology and Immunopharmacology, Second Edition, edited by J. H. Dean, M. I. Luster, A. E. Munson, and I. Kimber.
Raven Press, Ltd., New York © 1994.

38

Immune Responses to Contact and Respiratory Allergens

Ian Kimber and Rebecca J. Dearman

Immunology Group, Research Toxicology Section, ZENECA Central Toxicology Laboratory, Alderley Park, Macclesfield, Cheshire SK10 4TJ, United Kingdom

Chemical allergy describes the adverse health effects that result from the provocation in susceptible individuals of specific immune responses to the inducing material. Such responses are manifestations of a functionally intact and normally operating immune system and do not differ substantially from the protective immune responses that provide host defense against pathogenic microorganisms and malignant disease. Simplistically, the recognition of and response to chemicals by the immune system can be considered to be a case of mistaken identity. Such does not imply, however, that the immune responses required for the induction and elicitation of chemical allergic disease are themselves simple. Immune responses directed against chemicals exhibit some unique characteristics in terms of both the routes via which exposure usually occurs and the way in which antigen is handled by the immune system. Furthermore, probably as a consequence of the limited array of epitopes displayed by chemical allergens, genetic and acquired variations in responsiveness are more apparent and assume greater importance clinically.

The two types of chemical allergic reaction that are of most significance to the immunotoxicologist and occupational health physician are contact hypersensitivity (allergic contact dermatitis) and respiratory allergy.

CONTACT HYPERSENSITIVITY

Contact allergy is an example of a delayed-type hypersensitivity reaction and as such is dependent on the action of T lymphocytes and cell-mediated immune responses. By definition, exposure to contact sensitizing chemicals occurs via the skin, which in susceptible individuals results in a primary immune response and the activation and clonal expansion of T lymphocytes (1,2).

Induction of Skin Sensitization

Following encounter with a skin-sensitizing chemical, a primary immune response is induced in the lymph nodes draining the site of exposure. Such responses are characterized initially by lymphocyte activation and hyperplasia in the paracortical region of the lymph node (3–5). Sensitization fails to develop in animals deprived of, or congenitally deficient in, mature T lymphocytes (6–8). The initiation phase of contact sensitization can be considered to be complete when clonal expansion of responsive T lymphocytes has occurred and, as a consequence, there are available systemically increased numbers of allergen-reactive cells capable of mounting an accelerated and more aggressive response to the inducing chemical following subsequent exposure. The vigor of the T lymphocyte proliferative response induced in draining lymph nodes correlates closely with the extent to which sensitization develops and the severity of cutaneous allergic reactions that will be elicited following challenge (9). Perhaps not unexpectedly, T lymphocyte activation and proliferation in response to topically applied chemical allergens appear to be subject to homeostatic control mechanisms (10–12). Although contact sensitization can be transferred successfully to naive recipients with T lymphocytes alone, the available evidence indicates that the majority of contact allergens also induce humoral immune responses and hapten-specific antibodies. The relevance of antibodies for the initiation and expression of contact sensitivity is unclear, although they, or the anti-idiotypic antibodies they provoke, may serve an immunoregulatory function (13,14).

Antigen Processing and Presentation

The effective induction of contact sensitization demands that the chemical allergen reaches the draining lymph nodes in sufficient quantity and in an appropriate form to stimulate T lymphocyte activation. The role of Langerhans' cells is of central importance here (15,16). Langerhans' cells (LCs), which are bone marrow derived, display a dendritic morphology with a large surface area to volume ratio and form a contiguous network in the epidermis where they provide a trap for cutaneous antigen (17). In response to skin sensitization a proportion of the LCs at the site of exposure, many of which bear high levels of antigen, are induced to migrate from the epidermis, via the afferent lymphatics, to the draining lymph nodes (18–22). The movement of LCs from the skin is associated with both phenotypic and functional changes. Resident epidermal LCs are relatively inefficient antigen-presenting cells and fail to stimulate primary responses by naive T lymphocytes (23,24). However, while in transit to the lymph nodes, LCs acquire the characteristics of mature immunostimulatory dendritic cells (DCs). The antigen-bearing DCs that arrive in the lymph nodes exhibit, in comparison with the LCs from which they derive, a substantial increase in the membrane expression of both intercellular adhesion molecule-1 (ICAM-1) and major histocompatibility complex (MHC) class

II (Ia) antigen—determinants that facilitate, respectively, interaction with, and presentation of antigen to, T lymphocytes (25,26).

As a consequence, antigen-bearing DCs are, unlike LCs, able to form stable clusters with T cells (27). Interestingly, the changes to which LCs are subject during migration *in vivo* mirror those found to result from the culture of LCs in the presence of keratinocytes or keratinocyte-conditioned medium (23,28,29). By analogy with *in vitro* studies, it would appear that although the LCs found within the epidermis are ineffective antigen-presenting cells for naive T lymphocytes, they are able to process efficiently protein antigens and to produce immunogenic peptide fragments that will associate with Ia molecules (30,31). During culture this function is exchanged for immunostimulatory activity and the ability to provoke responses by T lymphocytes (30,31). There is little doubt that naive and memory T cells exhibit different requirements for antigen presentation (24,32)—a higher stimulation threshold being necessary for activation of the former (33). While LCs are unable to stimulate responses by naive T lymphocytes, it is probable that resident LCs play an important role in the local activation of primed or memory T cells during the elicitation phase of contact hypersensitivity (16).

The need for active processing of chemical allergens, as it is understood in the context of protein antigens, is unclear. Certainly the intimate association of chemical with host protein to form an immunogenic complex will be necessary. It is not known, however, whether hapten conjugates formed with skin proteins are internalized, digested, and presented in the conventional way, or whether chemical allergens can associate directly and productively with membrane Ia determinants. In theory, either or both processes could occur; what happens in practice has still to be determined. It is now apparent that the changes that influence LC function and that are necessary for the initiation of contact sensitization are dependent on the local availability of cytokines.

Epidermal Cytokines

The development of the LC/DC lineage from multipotent progenitors within the stem cell compartment of the bone marrow or cord blood has been shown recently to be driven by cytokines and, in particular, granulocyte–macrophage colony-stimulating factor (GM-CSF) and tumor necrosis factor-α (TNF-α) (34–37). This is of some interest as it is these cytokines that appear to exert the greatest influence on the further development and functional activity of epidermal LCs.

Until recently, keratinocytes were considered to be immunologically inert. It is now known, however, that these cells can produce constitutively, or can be induced to produce, a wide variety of cytokines including interleukin-1α (IL-1α), IL-6, IL-8, and IL-10, transforming growth factors α and β (TGF-α and TGF-β), monocyte chemotaxis and activating factor (MCAF), interferon-induced protein-10 (IP-10), macrophage inflammatory protein-2 (MIP-2), GM-CSF, and TNF-α (38–40). In addition, LCs themselves are considered to be an important, major, or even exclusive source of some epidermal cytokines such as IL-1β, MIP-1α, and IL-6 (39,41–43).

The increased immunostimulatory activity of LCs that results from culture is dependent on the presence of keratinocyte-derived products, in particular, GM-CSF and possibly IL-1 (44–46). It is likely therefore that the functional maturation characterizing the passage of LCs to the draining lymph nodes is effected by these and possibly other cytokines produced locally by keratinocytes in response to chemical exposure. Epidermal cytokines also provide the stimulus for LCs to leave the skin. Recent studies have shown that TNF-α will cause the movement away from the epidermis of LCs and the accumulation in draining nodes of DCs (47,48; Cumberbatch and Kimber *unpublished data*). Moreover, a reduced availability of TNF-α has been shown to impair markedly the arrival of DCs in draining nodes following skin sensitization or local irradiation with ultraviolet B light (49; *unpublished data*). The migration and maturation of LCs during the induction phase of skin sensitization and the effective transport and presentation of chemical allergen therefore require the sequential and/or concerted action of epidermal cytokines. TNF-α provides a signal, and probably the sole signal, for LC migration and GM-CSF acting together with IL-1, and possibly other cytokines, effects the functional maturation necessary for stimulation of primary T lymphocyte responses (Fig. 1). It is likely, of course, that local stimuli other than those resulting from skin sensitization are able to provoke or augment the production of epidermal cytokines. As a consequence, cutaneous trauma may serve to modulate the efficiency of skin sensitization secondary to cytokine-induced changes in the activity of LCs (50).

Elicitation Reactions

As the result of sensitization there exists a pool of allergen-reactive memory T lymphocytes that will be triggered to effect the cutaneous inflammatory reaction following subsequent exposure to the same chemical. Such effector cells are primarily of the CD4+ phenotype, although there is evidence that CD8+ cells and lymphocytes expressing the γδ T cell receptor may also play a role (51,52).

It is possible to distinguish phenotypically between naive and memory/effector CD4+ cells as a function of differential expression of the CD45 common leukocyte antigen. Naive T lymphocytes are characterized by possession of the high molecular weight isoform of this determinant, designated CD45RA. In contrast, memory/effector cells express a truncated form of the molecule, CD45RO (53,54). It has been found that in contact allergic reactions and in a variety of other skin lesions it is CD45RO+ cells that predominate within the inflammatory site (55–57). It is assumed that the predominance of memory/effector cells over naive T lymphocytes is due to the preferential immigration of CD45RO+ cells from the circulation into areas of cutaneous inflammation and that this, in turn, results from the selective expression of relevant adhesion molecules (58). It has been shown that at sites of allergic contact dermatitis there is an elevated expression on vascular endothelial

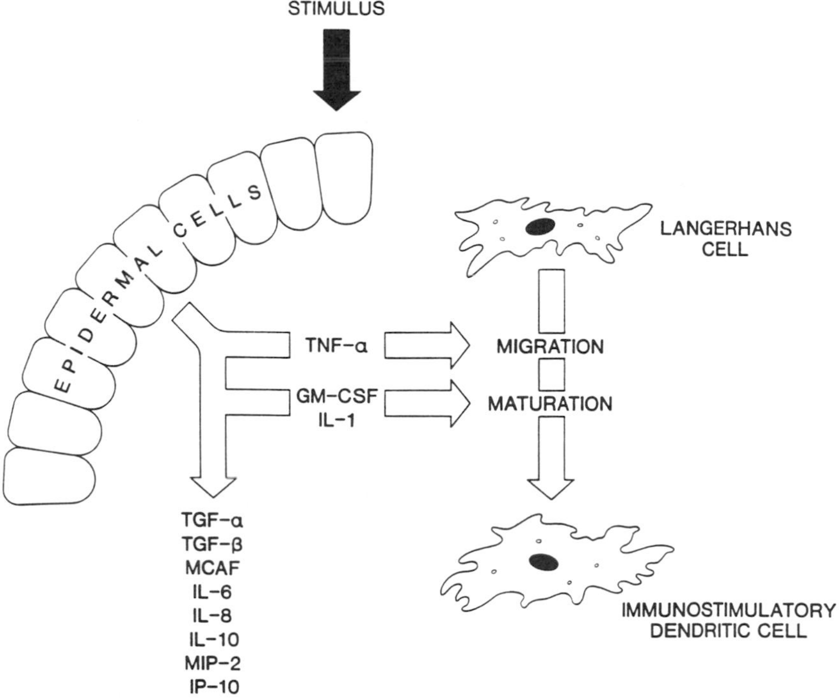

FIG. 1. The production by epidermal cells of cytokines following local trauma and the influence of cytokines on Langerhans cell migration and maturation. Tumor necrosis factor α (TNF-α), granulocyte/macrophage colony-stimulating factor (GM-CSF), interleukins 1, 6, 8, and 10 (IL-1, IL-6, IL-8, and IL-10), transforming growth factors α and β (TGF-α and TGF-β), monocyte chemotaxis and activating factor (MCAF), macrophage inflammatory protein 2 (MIP-2), and interferon-induced protein 10 (IP-10).

cells of several inducible adhesion molecules [ICAM-1, vascular cell adhesion molecule-1 (VCAM-1), and endothelial–leukocyte adhesion molecule-1 (ELAM-1)], which are known to influence T cell migration (59). Superimposed on changes that may allow the selective recruitment of memory cells is the existence of receptor–ligand interactions, which facilitate the anatomic homing of T lymphocytes. Such tissue-selective homing, in theory, enhances the efficiency of immune reactions by targeting effector cells to tissues similar to those where the inducing antigen was encountered initially and local to where the primary immune response was provoked. In this respect it is ELAM-1, recently renamed E-selectin, that is of particular relevance to cutaneous immune function. E-selectin has affinity for an antigen designated CLA (cutaneous lymphocyte-associated antigen), which is found on the majority of T lymphocytes infiltrating inflammatory skin sites, but on only a small proportion of T cells in extracutaneous tissue or in peripheral blood (60–62). The expression by primed T lymphocytes of leukocyte-function associated antigen-1 (LFA-1), a member of the β_2-integrin family, and of CLA ligands, respectively, for

ICAM-1 and E-selectin, facilitates attachment to endothelial cells. Further progress may then require the expression by T lymphocytes of additional integrins with affinity for components of the tissue matrix. After recruitment from the blood, the migration of such cells from the perivascular areas of the dermis toward the epidermis may be directed by chemotactic gradients. Tissue fluid derived from contact hypersensitivity lesions, but not from normal skin, contains a chemotactic factor for T lymphocytes (63). Furthermore, IL-8 has been shown to act as a T cell chemoattractant (64) and interferon-γ (IFN-γ) to be a potent mediator of lymphocyte recruitment into delayed-type hypersensitivity skin reactions (65).

It has been suggested also that an early event during the elicitation phase of contact hypersensitivity is the local release of vasoactive amines, which facilitate the subsequent entry of effector cells (66). A mandatory role for vasoactive amines in contact allergic reactions remains controversial, however.

Following the recruitment of memory T lymphocytes it is possible that they recognize and respond to antigen displayed by LCs. Alternatively, keratinocytes may acquire the ability to serve as antigen-presenting cells. In immune and inflammatory skin reactions, characterized by the infiltration and accumulation of T lymphocytes, keratinocytes are induced to express both ICAM-1 and Ia antigen—the important signals being IFN-γ and TNF-α (67–69). Whatever the relevance of keratinocytes in the context of active antigen presentation, it has been proposed that, secondary to the induction of ICAM-1 expression, these cells will assist in the retention of effector T lymphocytes displaying LFA-1, which have arrived at the inflammatory site.

It is clear therefore that, in addition to an important role during the induction phase of skin sensitization, cytokines produced either by epidermal cells or by cells infiltrating the epidermis influence the development of contact allergic reactions. Keratinocyte-derived cytokines effect changes in the dermal vascular endothelium (TNF-α and IL-1) and serve as chemoattractants for T lymphocytes (IL-8). IFN-γ, produced presumably by activated T lymphocytes, serves to enhance further the infiltration of T cells and also acts in concert with TNF-α to induce the expression by keratinocytes of ICAM-1, which in turn encourages the retention of T lymphocytes. The accumulation and activation of T cells and the subsequent release of cytokines and other mediators provoke in skin the inflammatory reaction recognized clinically as allergic contact dermatitis.

RESPIRATORY HYPERSENSITIVITY

The ability of proteins to cause respiratory allergic disease is well established. Implicated also in the induction of occupational allergic respiratory hypersensitivity are chemicals including, for example, certain diisocyanates, acid anhydrides, reactive dyes, and platinum salts (70–73). Allergy of the respiratory tract may take a variety of forms. Attention here will focus, however, on those allergic responses that are characterized by asthma and/or rhinitis and that are considered usually to be examples of type I (immediate-type) hypersensitivity reactions. Immediate-type allergic reactions are defined classically as being effected by homocytotropic antibody, the most important class of which is immunoglobulin E (IgE). There is no doubt that, in immediate-onset respiratory hypersensitivity induced in susceptible individuals by exposure to protein allergens, specific IgE antibody provides a clear correlate of sensitization and is the key element in initiation of acute allergic reactions. There is an increasing awareness, however, that the pathogenesis of asthma itself and, in particular, development of the chronic symptoms of bronchial inflammation and irritation require the involvement of T lymphocytes and cellular immune processes (74,75). In chemical respiratory allergy the case for a universal association of IgE with immunologic sensitization appears less compelling. Although in human studies IgE antibody specific for all chemical respiratory allergens has been found, in some instances (notably with the isocyanates), respiratory hypersensitivity in the absence of detectable specific IgE antibody has been claimed (76). Such findings may reflect simply a technical problem and the failure to use appropriate or sufficiently sensitive detection methods. Alternatively, it is possible in some cases that chemicals are able to provoke respiratory symptoms characteristic of type I hypersensitivity reactions in the absence of IgE antibody. It is nevertheless true that the induction of specific IgE antibody is likely usually to be a central event in the development of respiratory sensitization.

T Cells, Cytokines, and Immunoglobulin E Antibody

T helper (T_H) cells, as defined by possession of the membrane determinant CD4, exhibit functional heterogeneity (77,78). In 1986 Mosmann and colleagues (79) identified two types of cloned murine T_H cell, designated T_H1 and T_H2. The most remarkable distinguishing feature of these functional subpopulations of T_H cells is that, following activation, they produce different spectra of cytokines. Both produce GM-CSF and IL-3. However, only T_H1 cells secrete IFN-γ, IL-2, and TNF-β (lymphotoxin) and only T_H2 cells secrete IL-4, IL-5, IL-6, and IL-10 (77,78). It has been found more recently that a similar heterogeneity among human T_H cells exists also (80,81). A clear division of CD4+ cells into T_H1 and T_H2 phenotypes is undoubtedly an oversimplification. Other T_H populations have been described including T_H0 cells, which produce cytokines of both T_H1 and T_H2 type (78,82). It is probable that T_H1 and T_H2 cells represent in functional terms the most differentiated forms of CD4+ T lymphocytes and develop from common precursors (such as T_H0 cells) during the evolution of an immune response (Fig. 2). The drive toward a more differentiated function and the appearance of CD4+ cells with a phenotype of selective cytokine production will be dictated by conditions prevailing in the local microenvironment. Cytokines themselves appear to play an important role in directing the development of T_H populations. IL-4 facilitates and may be essential for the generation of T_H2 cells. In contrast, IFN-γ favors the development of T_H1 cells (83–86). The fact that cytokines produced by CD4+ cells have the ability to regulate reciprocally their own development and differentiation suggests that any perturbation in the balance between T_H1- and T_H2-type responses induced during immune activation will be sustained and amplified as the response progresses. The cellular

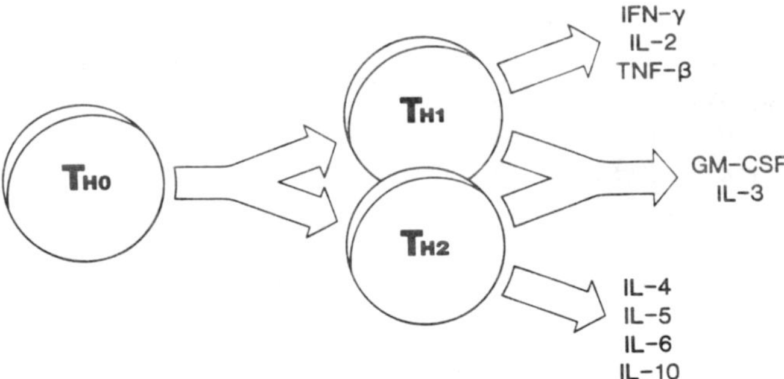

FIG. 2. The functional diversity of T_H cells. T_H1 and T_H2 cells derive from common precursors (including T_H0 cells). Both T_H1 and T_H2 cells produce IL-3 and GM-CSF. However, only T_H1 cells secrete IFN-γ, IL-2, and TNF-β (lymphotoxin) and only T_H2 cells secrete IL-4, IL-5, IL 6, and IL-10.

source of the cytokines that initially provide the signals necessary for T_H cell differentiation is of interest and it has been suggested recently that elements of the nonadaptive immune system are important in this respect. It is hypothesized that IFN-γ derived from natural killer (NK) cells will favor the development of T_H1 cells, while mast cell-derived IL-4 will promote T_H2-type responses (87). In addition to the relative availability of cytokines, the nature and dose of the inducing antigen, the conditions under which it is presented, and the characteristics of the antigen-presenting cell itself are likely to be critical determinants of the selective development of T_H responses. It has been found in experimental systems that the allelic forms of MHC class II molecules in the context of which the antigen is displayed, the density of the Ia/antigen ligand complex, the source of antigen-presenting cells, and the availability of the costimulatory cytokine IL-1 all influence the balance between induced T_H1 and T_H2 subpopulations (88–91).

The relevance of T_H cell heterogeneity to the development of allergy is that the soluble products of CD4+ cells have a decisive influence on the induction of IgE antibody responses. Studies in mice have shown that IL-4, a product of T_H2 cells, is necessary for the induction and maintenance of IgE antibody production (92). The critical role of this cytokine in IgE responses has recently been emphasized further by studies of mice homozygous for a mutation that inactivates the gene for IL-4. Such animals lack detectable IgE and fail to mount IgE responses (93). Conversely, mice that possess a transgene for this cytokine and that constitutively produce IL-4 exhibit high levels of serum IgE (94,95). In contrast, IFN-γ serves to inhibit IgE antibody production (96). These cytokines also regulate reciprocally the synthesis of human IgE (97,98).

The induction of IgE responses and the development of immediate-type hypersensitivity will be favored therefore by allergens, or conditions of exposure to allergens, which result in preferential activation of T_H2 cells. The selective stimulation of T_H1-type responses will normally be nonpermissive for the induction of IgE antibody. T_H1 cell activation by chemical allergens is, however, consistent with the induction of contact sensitization. It is known that T_H1 cells effect delayed-type hypersensitivity reactions and that IFN-γ plays an important role in this process (99–101). It has been found recently that topical exposure of mice to chemicals known to cause occupational respiratory hypersensitivity in humans results in the induction of immune responses characteristic of preferential T_H2 cell activation. Conversely, chemical contact allergens known or suspected not to induce respiratory sensitization were shown to provoke qualitatively different immune responses indicative of the selective activation of T_H1 cells (102–108). It may be therefore that the physicochemical properties of the inducing allergen and/or the conditions under which it is handled, processed, and presented by the immune system will dictate the quality of response that is provoked preferentially and the type of allergic reaction or reactions that will be manifest following subsequent exposure. On the basis of available evidence it appears that the majority of chemical respiratory allergens have at least some potential to cause contact sensitization in experimental systems. Such is not necessarily incompatible with the induction by such chemicals of preferential T_H2-type responses. One can speculate that, although the balance of immune activation induced by respiratory allergens is biased toward activation of T_H2 cells and that as a consequence the stimulatory effect of IL-4 on IgE production outweighs the inhibitory influence of IFN-γ, there are still sufficient allergen-reactive T_H effector lymphocytes to elicit a dermal hypersensitivity reaction following challenge. Alternatively, such observations may reflect the tempo of qualitative changes in the immune response following initial stimulation and the time necessary to achieve a situation where the influence of T_H2 cells predominates.

The differential stimulation of T_H cells by chemical allergens has consequences other than for the regulation of IgE antibody production. The preferential induction of T_H2-type responses will influence the elicitation of immediate-type hypersensitivity reactions. IL-3, IL-4, and IL-10 are all mast cell growth factors or cofactors (109,110) and IL-5 is a growth and differentiation factor for eosinophils (111). Moreover, it has been found recently that IL-4 is capable of augmenting the secretory potential of mast cells and will enhance the release of serotonin following stimulation (112,113). Here again reciprocal antagonistic effects of cytokines may be important. IFN-γ not only depresses mast cell secretory function (112–114) but also inhibits the antigen-induced infiltration of eosinophils into the respiratory tract of sensitized mice (115). In contrast, IL-4 has been shown to reduce significantly the severity of contact allergic reactions in mice (116).

There is increasing evidence that divergent T_H cell responses also characterize allergic disease in humans. Virtually all allergen-specific T cell clones derived from the peripheral blood of nickel-sensitive donors have been found to secrete high levels of IFN-γ but low or undetectable levels of IL-4 and IL-5 (117,118). However, T cell clones specific for *Dermatophagoides pteronyssimus* (house dust mite) and grass pollen (aeroallergens that induce in susceptible individuals IgE-mediated hypersensitivity reactions) were found to produce T_H2-type cytokines but not IFN-γ (119). Similarly, CD4+ cell clones prepared from lesional skin biopsies of house dust mite-allergic atopic dermatitis patients were shown to be of T_H2 phenotype on the basis of cytokine production (120). A predominance of T_H2-type cells in the sites of cutaneous reactions in atopic individuals has been demonstrated also by *in situ* hybridization. The cells infiltrating lesional skin expressed messenger ribonucleic acid (mRNA) for IL-3, IL-4, IL-5, and GM-CSF but not for IFN-γ (121).

It should be emphasized that in addition to the quality of immune response provoked in the context of selective T_H cell development, other factors may serve to influence the production of IgE antibody. Thus, for example, prostaglandin E_2 has been found to promote murine IgE responses (122,123) and there exist soluble IgE binding factors that regulate the production of human IgE (124).

The selective stimulation of T_H2 cell responses and IL-4 production will be determined at least in part by the nature and concentration of the inducing antigen and probably by the route of exposure and the immunologic environment in which antigen is first encountered (102–104,125,126). It is likely also that extrinsic factors are important. Several studies have shown that tobacco smoking is associated with increased plasma levels of IgE antibody (127,128). Furthermore, there is evidence available from experimental systems that diesel exhaust particulates and sulfur dioxide augment the production of IgE antibody and allergic sensitization in response to ovalbumin (129–131). There is a growing appreciation from epidemiologic studies that atmospheric pollution may aggravate asthma (132). The extent to which this is in turn attributable to adjuvant-like effects of air pollutants for IgE production is as yet unclear. Superimposed on immunologic and environmental factors is the existence of genetic variation in terms of both IgE antibody production and susceptibility to the development of allergic disease. Only a proportion of the exposed population displays symptoms of chemical respiratory allergy. The variables that influence the quality of the provoked immune response, the vigor of IgE antibody production, and susceptibility to the development of allergic disease are summarized in Fig. 3.

Elicitation Reactions

Occupational asthma has the characteristic features of airway smooth muscle contraction, edema, and fluid accumulation—changes initiated presumably by the degranulation of local mast cells and the release of inflammatory mediators such as histamine and leukotrienes. It has been suggested recently that cell-mediated immune processes may act in concert with, or independently of, IgE antibody in the elicitation of respiratory chemical allergic reactions (75). Chronic inflammation plays an important role in asthma and is associated with an accumulation in the bronchial mucosa of leukocytes, mucus production, the destruction and sloughing of airway epithelial cells, and subepithelial fibrosis secondary to collagen deposition (133,134). Central to the development of chronic bronchial inflammation and injury are eosinophils acting together with infiltrating T lymphocytes (75,135,136). While the exact role of eosinophils in the development of pulmonary hypersen-

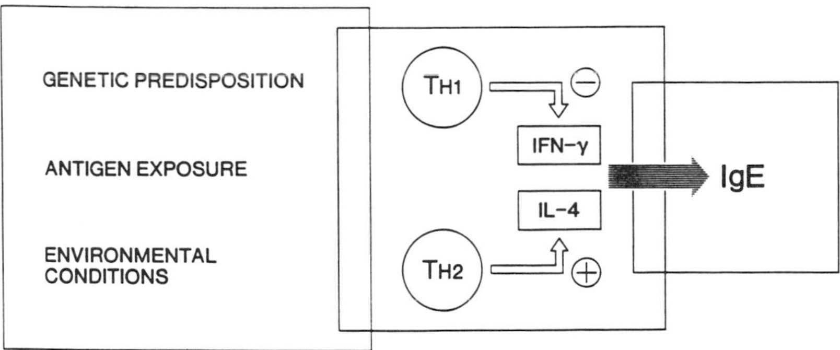

FIG. 3. Factors that influence the induction of IgE responses. The production of IgE is controlled pivotally by the reciprocal effects of the cytokines IFN-γ and IL-4, products, respectively, of activated T_H1 and T_H2 cells. The preferential activation of T_H cell responses will be determined by the nature of the inducing antigen and the way in which it is handled by the immune system. In addition, the vigor of IgE responses will be influenced by environmental conditions and inherent genetic susceptibility.

sitivity has yet to be elucidated fully, it is clear that the initiation of local eosinophilia at the site of allergen-induced respiratory reactions is controlled by IL-5, derived presumably from T_H2 cells (137–139). One view is that asthma is invariably associated with the activity of T lymphocytes and eosinophils and that in those cases where asthma results from allergic sensitization an important initiating event is IgE-mediated mast cell degranulation, which triggers the accumulation of inflammatory cells. Alternatively, it remains a possibility that in some cases allergic respiratory hypersensitivity induced by chemicals can be elicited in the absence of IgE antibody. Although the uniform involvement of IgE in the pathogenesis of chemical respiratory allergy needs to be explored further, it is apparent that the induction of T_H2 cell-type responses is of central importance.

REFERENCES

1. Kimber I. Contact sensitivity. In: Miller K, Turk J, Nicklin S, eds. *Principles and practice of immunotoxicology*. Oxford: Blackwell Scientific Publications; 1992:104–124.
2. Scheper RJ, von Blomberg BME. In: Rycroft RJG, Menne T, Frosch PJ, Benezra C, eds. *Textbook of contact dermatitis*. Berlin: Springer-Verlag; 1992:11–27.
3. Oort J, Turk JL. A histological and autoradiographic study of lymph nodes during the development of contact sensitivity in guinea pigs. *Br J Exp Pathol* 1965;46:147–154.
4. Turk JL. Cytology of the induction of hypersensitivity. *Br Med Bull* 1967;23:3–8.
5. Parrott DMV, de Sousa MAB. Changes in the thymus-dependent areas of lymph nodes after immunological stimulation. *Nature* 1966;212:1316–1317.
6. Davies AJS, Carter RL, Leuchars E, Wallis V. The morphology of immune reactions in normal, thymectomized and reconstituted mice. II. The response to oxazolone. *Immunology* 1969;17:111–126.
7. de Sousa MAB, Parrott DMV. Induction and recall in contact sensitivity. Changes in the skin and draining lymph nodes of intact and thymectomized mice. *J Exp Med* 1969;130:671–684.

8. Pritchard H, Micklem HS. Immune responses in congenitally thymusless mice. I. Absence of response to oxazolone. *Clin Exp Immunol* 1972;10:151–161.
9. Kimber I, Dearman RJ. Investigation of lymph node cell proliferation as a possible immunological correlate of contact sensitizing potential. *Food Chem Toxicol* 1991;29:125–129.
10. Kimber I, Shepherd CJ, Mitchell JA, Turk JL, Baker D. Regulation of lymphocyte proliferation in contact sensitivity: homeostatic mechanisms and a possible explanation of antigenic competition. *Immunology* 1989;66:577–582.
11. Kimber I, Foster JR, Baker D, Turk JL. Selective impairment of T lymphocyte activation following contact sensitization with oxazolone. *Int Arch Allergy Appl Immunol* 1991;95:142–148.
12. Baker D, Kimber I, Ahmed K, Turk JL. Antigen-specific and nonspecific depression of proliferative responses induced during contact sensitivity in mice. *Int J Exp Pathol* 1991;72:55–65.
13. Sy M-S, Moorhead JW, Claman HN. Regulation of cell-mediated immunity by antibodies: possible role of anti-receptor antibodies in the regulation of sensitivity to DNFB in mice. *J Immunol* 1979;123:2593–2598.
14. Moorhead JW. Antigen receptors on murine T lymphocytes in contact sensitivity. III. Mechanisms of negative feedback regulation by autoanti-idiotypic antibody. *J Exp Med* 1982;155:820–830.
15. Breathnach SM. The Langerhans cell. Centenary review. *Br J Dermatol* 1988;119:463–469.
16. Kimber I, Cumberbatch M. Dendritic cells and cutaneous immune responses to chemical allergens. *Toxicol Appl Pharmacol* 1992;117:137–146.
17. Shelley WB, Juhlin L. Langerhans cells form a reticuloepithelial trap for external contact allergens. *Nature* 1976;261:46–47.
18. Silberberg-Sinakin I, Thorbecke GJ, Baer RL, Rosenthal SA, Berezowsky V. Antigen-bearing Langerhans cells in skin, dermal lymphatics and in lymph nodes. *Cell Immunol* 1976;25:137–151.
19. Knight SC, Krejci J, Malkovsky M, Colizzi V, Gautam A, Asherson GL. The role of dendritic cells in the initiation of immune responses to contact sensitizers. I. In vivo exposure to antigen. *Cell Immunol* 1985;94:427–434.
20. Mactonia SE, Edwards AJ, Knight SC. Dendritic cells and the initiation of contact sensitivity to fluorescein isothiocyanate. *Immunology* 1986;59:509–514.
21. Kinnaird A, Peters SW, Foster JR, Kimber I. Dendritic cell accumulation in draining lymph nodes during the induction phase of contact allergy in mice. *Int Arch Allergy Appl Immunol* 1989;89:202–210.
22. Cumberbatch M, Kimber I. Phenotypic characteristics of antigen-bearing cells in the draining lymph nodes of contact sensitized mice. *Immunology* 1990:71:404–410.
23. Schuler G, Steinman RM. Murine epidermal Langerhans cells mature into potent immunostimulatory dendritic cells in vitro. *J Exp Med* 1985;161:526–546.
24. Inaba K, Schuler G, Witmer MD, Valinsky J, Atassi B, Steinman RM. Immunologic properties of purified epidermal Langerhans cells. Distinct requirements for stimulation of unprimed and sensitized T lymphocytes. *J Exp Med* 1986;164:605–613.
25. Cumberbatch M, Gould SJ, Peters SW, Kimber I. MHC class II expression by Langerhans cells and lymph node dendritic cells: Possible evidence for maturation of Langerhans cells following contact sensitization. *Immunology* 1991;74:414–419.
26. Cumberbatch M, Peters SW, Gould SJ, Kimber I. Intercellular adhesion molecule-1 (ICAM-1) expression by lymph node dendritic cells: comparison with epidermal Langerhans cells. *Immunol Lett* 1992;32:105–110.
27. Cumberbatch M, Illingworth I, Kimber I. Antigen-bearing dendritic cells in the draining lymph nodes of contact sensitized mice: cluster formation with lymphocytes. *Immunology* 1991;74:139–145.
28. Shimada S, Caughman SW, Sharrow SO, Stephany D, Katz SI. Enhanced antigen-presenting capacity of cultured Langerhans cells is associated with markedly increased expression of Ia antigen. *J Immunol* 1987;139:2551–2555.
29. Tang A, Udey MC. Inhibition of epidermal Langerhans cell function by low dose ultraviolet B radiation. Ultraviolet B radiation selectively modulates ICAM-1 (CD54) expression by murine Langerhans cells. *J Immunol* 1991;146:3347–3355.
30. Streilein JW, Grammer SF. In vitro evidence that Langerhans cells can adopt two functionally distinct forms capable of antigen presentation to T lymphocytes. *J Immunol* 1989;143:3925–3933.
31. Streilein JW, Grammer SF, Yoshikawa T, Demidem A, Vermeer M. Functional dichotomy between Langerhans cells that present antigen to naive and memory/effector T lymphocytes. *Immunol Rev* 1990;117:159–183.

32. Inaba K, Steinman RM. Resting and sensitized T lymphocytes exhibit distinct (antigen presenting cell) requirements for growth and lymphokine release. *J Exp Med* 1984;160:1717–1735.
33. Gajewski TF, Schell SR, Nau G, Fitch FW. Regulation of T cell activation. Differences among T-cell subsets. *Immunol Rev* 1989;111:79–110.
34. Caux C, Dezutter-Dambuyant C, Schmitt D, Banchereau J. GM-CSF and TNF-α cooperate in the generation of dendritic Langerhans cells. *Nature* 1992;360:258–261.
35. Reid CDL, Stackpoole A, Meager A, Tikerpae J. Interactions of tumor necrosis factor with granulocyte–macrophage colony-stimulating factor and other cytokines in the regulation of dendritic cell growth in vitro from early bipotent CD34$^+$ progenitors in human bone marrow. *J Immunol* 1992;149:2681–2688.
36. Inaba K, Inaba M, Romani N, et al. Generation of large numbers of dendritic cells from mouse bone marrow cultures supplemented with granulocyte/macrophage colony-stimulating factor. *J Exp Med* 1992;176:1693–1702.
37. Santiago-Schwarz F, Belilos E, Diamond B, Carsons SE. TNF in combination with GM-CSF enhances the differentiation of neonatal cord blood stem cells into dendritic cells and macrophages. *J Leukoc Biol* 1992;52:274–281.
38. Barker JNWN. Role of keratinocytes in allergic contact dermatitis. *Contact Dermatitis* 1992;26: 145–148.
39. Enk AH, Katz SI. Early molecular events in the induction phase of contact sensitivity. *Proc Natl Acad Sci USA* 1992;89:1398–1402.
40. Enk AH, Katz SI. Identification and induction of keratinocyte-derived IL-10. *J Immunol* 1992; 149:92–95.
41. Matsue H, Cruz PD Jr, Bergstresser PR, Takashima A. Langerhans cells are the major source of mRNA for IL-1β and MIP-1α among unstimulated mouse epidermal cells. *J Invest Dermatol* 1992;99:537–541.
42. Heufler C, Topar G, Koch F, Trockenbacher B, Kampgen E, Romani N, Schuler G. Cytokine gene expression in murine epidermal cell suspensions: interleukin 1β and macrophage inflammatory protein 1α are selectively expressed in Langerhans cells but are differentially regulated in culture. *J Exp Med* 1992;176:1221–1226.
43. Schreiber S, Kilgus O, Payer E, Kutil R, Elbe A, Mueller C, Stingl G. Cytokine pattern of Langerhans cells isolated from murine epidermal cell cultures. *J Immunol* 1992;149:3525–3534.
44. Witmer-Pack MD, Olivier W, Valinsky J, Schuler G, Steinman RM. Granulocyte/macrophage colony-stimulating factor is essential for the viability and function of cultured murine epidermal Langerhans cells. *J Exp Med* 1987;166:1484–1498.
45. Heufler C, Koch F, Schuler G. Granulocyte/macrophage colony-stimulating factor and interleukin 1 mediate the maturation of murine epidermal Langerhans cells into potent immunostimulatory dendritic cells. *J Exp Med* 1988;167:700–705.
46. Picut CA, Lee CS, Dougherty EP, Anderson KL, Lewis RM. Immunostimulatory capabilities of highly enriched Langerhans cells in vitro. *J Invest Dermatol* 1988;90:201–206.
47. Cumberbatch M, Kimber I. Dermal tumour necrosis factor-α induces dendritic cell migration to draining lymph nodes and possibly provides one stimulus for Langerhans cell migration. *Immunology* 1992;75:257–263.
48. Kimber I, Cumberbatch M. Stimulation of Langerhans cell migration by tumor necrosis factor α (TNF-α). *J Invest Dermatol* 1992;99:48S–50S.
49. Moodycliffe AM, Kimber I, Norval M. The effect of ultraviolet B irradiation and urocanic acid isomers on dendritic cell migration. *Immunology* 1992;77:394–399.
50. Cumberbatch M, Scott RC, Basketter DA, Scholes EW, Hilton J, Dearman RJ, Kimber I. Influence of sodium lauryl sulphate on 2,4-dinitrochlorobenzene-induced lymph node activation. *Toxicology* 1993;77:181–191.
51. Gocinski BL, Tigelaar RE. Roles of CD4$^+$ and CD8$^+$ T cells in murine contact sensitivity revealed by in vivo monoclonal antibody depletion. *J Immunol* 1990;144:4121–4128.
52. Ptak W, Askenase PW. γδ T cells assist αβ T cells in adoptive transfer of contact sensitivity. *J Immunol* 1992;149:3503–3508.
53. Akbar AN, Terry L, Timms A, Beverley PCL, Janossy G. Loss of CD45R and gain of UCHL1 reactivity is a feature of primed T cells. *J Immunol* 1988;140:2171–2178.
54. Clement LT, Yamashita N, Machin AM. The functionally distinct subpopulations of human CD4 helper/inducer T lymphocytes defined by anti-CD45R antibodies derive sequentially from a pathway that is regulated by activation-dependent post-thymic differentiation. *J Immunol* 1988;141: 1464–1470.

55. Silvennoinen-Kassinen S, Ikaheimo I, Karvonen J, Kauppinen M, Kallioinen M. Mononuclear cell subsets in the nickel allergic reaction in vitro and in vivo. *J Allergy Clin Immunol* 1992;89:794–800.
56. Markey AC, Allen MH, Pitzalis C, Macdonald DM. T-cell inducer populations in cutaneous inflammation: a predominance of T-helper-inducer lymphocytes in the infiltrate of inflammatory dermatoses. *Br J Dermatol* 1990;122:325–332.
57. Frew AJ, Kay AB. UCHL1$^+$ (CD45RO$^+$) "memory" T-cells predominate in the CD4$^+$ cellular infiltrate associated with allergen-induced late-phase skin reactions in atopic subjects. *Clin Exp Immunol* 1991;84:270–274.
58. Sterry W, Bruhn S, Kunne N, Lichtenberg B, Weber-Mattheisen K, Brusch J, Mielke V. Dominance of memory over naive T cells in contact dermatitis is due to differential tissue immigration. *Br J Dermatol* 1990;123:59–64.
59. Griffiths CEM, Barker JNWN, Kunkel S, Nickoloff BJ. Modulation of leukocyte adhesion molecules, a T-cell chemotaxin (IL-8) and a regulatory cytokine (TNF-alpha) in allergic contact dermatitis (rhus dermatitis). *Br J Dermatol* 1991;124:519–526.
60. Picker LJ, Kishimoto TK, Smith CW, Warnock RA, Butcher EC. ELAM-1 is an adhesion molecule for skin-homing T cells. *Nature* 1991;349:796–799.
61. Picker LJ, Treer JR, Ferguson-Darnell B, Collins PA, Bergstresser PR, Terstappen LWMM. Control of lymphocyte recirculation in man. II. Differential regulation of the cutaneous lymphocyte-associated antigen, a tissue-selective homing receptor for skin-homing T cells. *J Immunol* 1993; 150:1122–1136.
62. Bos JD, Kapsenberg ML. The skin immune system: progress in cutaneous biology. *Immunol Today* 1993;14:75–78.
63. Larsen CG, Ternowitz T, Larsen FG, Thestrup-Pedersen K. Epidermis and lymphocyte interactions during an allergic patch test reaction. Increased activity of ETAF/IL-1 epidermal derived lymphocyte chemotactic factor and mixed lymphocyte reactivity in persons with type IV allergy. *J Invest Dermatol* 1988;90:230–233.
64. Barker JNWN, Jones ML, Mitra RS, Fantone JC, Kunkel SL, Dixit VM, Nickoloff BJ. Modulation of keratinocyte-derived interleukin-8 which is chemotactic for neutrophils and T lymphocytes. *Am J Pathol* 1991;139:869–876.
65. Issekutz TB, Stoltz JM, Meide P. Lymphocyte recruitment in delayed-type hypersensitivity. The role of IFN-γ. *J Immunol* 1988;140:2989–2993.
66. Van Loveren H, Askenase PW. Delayed hypersensitivity is mediated by a sequence of two different T cell activities. *J Immunol* 1984;133:2397–2401.
67. Basham TY, Nickoloff BJ, Merigan TC, Morhenn VB. Recombinant gamma interferon induces HLA-DR on cultured human keratinocytes. *J Invest Dermatol* 1984;83:88–92.
68. Dustin ML, Singer KH, Tuck DT, Springer TA. Adhesion of T lymphocytes to epidermal keratinocytes is regulated by interferon-gamma and is mediated by intercellular adhesion molecule-1 (ICAM-1). *J Exp Med* 1988;167:1323–1340.
69. Griffiths CEM, Voorhees JJ, Nickoloff BJ. Characterization of intercellular adhesion molecule-1 and HLA-DR in normal and inflamed skin: modulation by interferon-gamma and tumor necrosis factor. *J Am Acad Dermatol* 1989;20:617–629.
70. Salvaggio JE, Butcher BT, O'Neil CE. Occupational asthma due to chemical agents. *J Allergy Clin Immunol* 1986;78:1053–1057.
71. Salvaggio JE. The impact of allergy and immunology on our expanding industrial environment. *J Allergy Clin Immunol* 1990;85:689–699.
72. Karol MH. Occupational asthma and allergic reactions to inhaled compounds. In: Miller K, Turk J, Nicklin S, eds. *Principles and practice of immunotoxicology*. Oxford: Blackwell Scientific Publications; 1992:228–241.
73. Grammer LC. Occupational immunologic lung disease. In: Patterson R, Grammer LC, Greenberger PA, Zeiss CR, eds. *Allergic diseases. Diagnosis and management*. Philadelphia: Lippincott; 1993:745–762.
74. Corrigan CJ. Allergy of the respiratory tract. *Curr Opin Immunol* 1992;4:798–804.
75. Corrigan CJ, Kay AB. T cells and eosinophils in the pathogenesis of asthma. *Immunol Today* 1992;13:501–507.
76. Newman Taylor AJ. Clinical and epidemiological methods in investigating occupational asthma. *Clin Immunol Allergy* 1984;4:3–21.
77. Mosmann TR, Coffman RL. Heterogeneity of cytokine secretion patterns and functions of helper T cells. *Adv Immunol* 1989;46:111–147.

78. Mosmann TR, Schumacher JH, Street NF, et al. Diversity of cytokine synthesis and function of mouse $CD4^+$ T cells. *Immunol Rev* 1991;123:209–229.
79. Mosmann TR, Cherwinski H, Bond MW, Giedlin MA, Coffman RL. Two types of murine helper T cell clone. I. Definition according to profiles of lymphokine activities and secreted proteins. *J Immunol* 1986;136:2348–2357.
80. Romagnani S. Human T_H1 and T_H2 subsets: doubt no more. *Immunol Today* 1991;12:256–257.
81. Romagnani S, Del Prete G, Maggi E, et al. Human T_H1 and T_H2 subsets. *Int Arch Allergy Immunol* 1992;99:242–245.
82. Bendelac A, Schwartz RH. T_h0 cells in the thymus. The question of T-helper lineages. *Immunol Rev* 1991;123:169–188.
83. Swain SL, Bradley LM, Croft M, et al. Helper T-cell subsets: phenotype, function and the role of lymphokines in regulating their development. *Immunol Rev* 1991;123:115–144.
84. Coffman RL, Varkila K, Scott P, Chatelain R. Role of cytokines in the differentiation of $CD4^+$ T-cell subsets in vivo. *Immunol Rev* 1991;123:189–207.
85. Abehsira-Amar O, Gibert M, Joliy M, Theze J, Jankovic DL. IL-4 plays a dominant role in the differential development of T_H0 into T_H1 and T_H2 cells. *J Immunol* 1992;148:3820–3829.
86. Hsieh C-S, Heimberger AB, Gold JS, O'Garra A, Murphy KM. Differential regulation of T helper phenotype development by interleukins 4 and 10 in an αβ T-cell-receptor transgenic system. *Proc Natl Acad Sci USA* 1992;89:6065–6069.
87. Romagnani S. Induction of T_H1 and T_H2 responses: a key role for the "natural" immune response? *Immunol Today* 1992;13:379–381.
88. Weaver CT, Hawrylowicz CM, Unanue ER. T helper cell subsets require the expression of distinct costimulatory signals by antigen-presenting cells. *Proc Natl Acad Sci USA* 1988;85:8181–8185.
89. Chang T-L, Shea CM, Urioste S, Thompson RC, Boom WH, Abbas AK. Heterogeneity of helper/inducer T lymphocytes. III. Responses of IL-2- and IL-4-producing (T_H1 and T_H2) clones to antigens presented by different accessory cells. *J Immunol* 1990;145:2803–2808.
90. Gajewski TF, Pinnas M, Wong T, Fitch FW. Murine T_H1 and T_H2 clones proliferate optimally in response to distinct antigen-presenting cell populations. *J Immunol* 1991;146:1750–1758.
91. Pfeiffer C, Murray J, Madri J, Bottomly K. Selective activation of T_H1- and T_H2-like cells in vivo. Response to human collagen IV. *Immunol Rev* 1991;123:65–84.
92. Finkelman FD, Katona IM, Urban JF Jr, et al. IL-4 is required to generate and sustain in vivo IgE responses. *J Immunol* 1988;141:2335–2341.
93. Kuhn R, Rajewsky K, Muller W. Generation and analysis of interleukin-4 deficient mice. *Science* 1991;254:707–710.
94. Tepper RI, Levinson DA, Stanger BZ, Campos-Torres J, Abbas AK, Leder P. IL-4 induces allergic-like inflammatory disease and alters T cell development in transgenic mice. *Cell* 1990;62:457–467.
95. Burstein HJ, Tepper RI, Leder P, Abbas AK. Humoral immune functions in IL-4 transgenic mice. *J Immunol* 1991;147:2950–2956.
96. Finkelman FD, Katona IM, Mosmann TR, Coffman RL. IFN-γ regulates the isotypes of Ig secreted during in vivo humoral immune responses. *J Immunol* 1988;140:1022–1027.
97. Del Prete G, Maggi E, Parronchi P, et al. IL-4 is an essential factor for the IgE synthesis induced in vitro by human T cell clones and their supernatants. *J Immunol* 1988;140:4193–4198.
98. Pene J, Rousset F, Briere F, et al. IgE production by normal human B cells induced by alloreactive T cell clones is mediated by IL-4 and suppressed by IFN-γ. *J Immunol* 1988;141:1218–1224.
99. Cher DJ, Mosmann TR. Two types of murine helper T cell clones. II. Delayed type hypersensitivity is mediated by T_H1 clones. *J Immunol* 1987;138:3688–3694.
100. Fong TAT, Mosmann TR. The role of IFN-γ in delayed-type hypersensitivity mediated by T_h1 clones. *J Immunol* 1989;143:2887–2893.
101. Diamanstein T, Eckert R, Volk H-D, Kupier-Weglinski J-W. Reversal by interferon-γ of inhibition of delayed-type hypersensitivity induction by anti-CD4 or anti-interleukin 2 receptor (CD25) monoclonal antibodies. Evidence for the physiological role of the $CD4^+$ T_h1^+ subset in mice. *Eur J Immunol* 1988;18:2101–2103.
102. Dearman RJ, Kimber I. Differential stimulation of immune function by respiratory and contact chemical allergens. *Immunology* 1991;72:563–570.
103. Dearman RJ, Kimber I. Divergent immune responses to respiratory and contact chemical allergens: antibody elicited by phthalic anhydride and oxazolone. *Clin Exp Allergy* 1992;22:241–250.
104. Dearman RJ, Spence LM, Kimber I. Characterization of murine immune responses to allergenic diisocyanates. *Toxicol Appl Pharmacol* 1992;112:190–197.

105. Dearman RJ, Mitchell JA, Basketter DA, Kimber I. Differential ability of occupational chemical contact and respiratory allergens to cause immediate and delayed dermal hypersensitivity reactions in mice. *Int Arch Allergy Immunol* 1992;97:315–321.
106. Dearman RJ, Basketter DA, Kimber I. Variable effects of chemical allergens on serum IgE concentration in mice. Preliminary evaluation of a novel approach to the identification of respiratory sensitizers. *J Appl Toxicol* 1992;12:317–323.
107. Dearman RJ, Basketter DA, Coleman JW, Kimber I. The cellular and molecular basis for divergent allergic responses to chemicals. *Chem Biol Interact* 1992;84:1–10.
108. Kimber I, Dearman RJ. The mechanisms and evaluation of chemically-induced allergy. *Toxicol Lett* 1992;64/65:79–84.
109. Smith CA, Rennick DM. Characterization of a murine lymphokine distinct from interleukin 3 (IL-3) possessing a T-cell growth factor activity and a mast cell growth factor activity that synergizes with IL-3. *Proc Natl Acad Sci USA* 1986;83:1857–1861.
110. Thompson-Snipes L, Dhar V, Bond MW, Mosmann TR, Moore KW, Rennick DM. Interleukin-10: a novel stimulatory factor for mast cells and their progenitors. *J Exp Med* 1991;173: 507–510.
111. Yokota T, Coffman RL, Hagiwara H, et al. Isolation and characterization of lymphokine cDNA clones encoding mouse and human IgA-enhancing and eosinophil-colony stimulating factor activities. Relationship to interleukin 5. *Proc Natl Acad Sci USA* 1987;84:7388–7392.
112. Coleman JW, Holliday MR, Buckley MG. Regulation of the secretory function of mouse peritoneal mast cells by IL-3, IL-4 and IFN-γ. *Int Arch Allergy Immunol* 1992;99:408–410.
113. Coleman JW, Holliday MR, Kimber I, Zsebo KM, Galli SJ. Regulation of mouse peritoneal mast cell secretory function by stem cell factor, IL-3 or IL-4. *J Immunol* 1993;150:556–562.
114. Coleman JW, Buckley MG, Holliday MR, Morris AG. Interferon-γ inhibits serotonin release from mouse peritoneal mast cells. *Eur J Immunol* 1991;21:2559–2564.
115. Iwamoto I, Nakajima H, Endo H, Yoshida S. Interferon γ regulates antigen-induced eosinophil recruitment into the mouse airways by inhibiting the infiltration of $CD4^+$ T cells. *J Exp Med* 1993; 177:573–576.
116. Gautam SC, Chikkala NF, Hamilton TA. Anti-inflammatory action of IL-4. Negative regulation of contact sensitivity to trinitrochlorobenzene. *J Immunol* 1992;148:1411–1415.
117. Kapsenberg ML, Wierenga EA, Stiekma FEM, Tiggelman AMBC, Bos JD. T_H1 lymphokine production profiles of nickel-specific $CD4^+$ T lymphocyte clones from nickel contact allergic and non-allergic individuals. *J Invest Dermatol* 1992;98:59–63.
118. Kapsenberg ML, Wierenga EA, Bos JD, Jansen HM. Functional subsets of allergen-reactive human $CD4^+$ T cells. *Immunol Today* 1991;12:392–395.
119. Parronchi P, Macchia D, Piccinni M-P, et al. Allergen and bacterial antigen-specific T-cell clones established from atopic donors show a different profile of cytokine production. *Proc Natl Acad Sci USA* 1991;88:4538–4542.
120. van der Heijden FL, Wierenga EA, Bos JD, Kapsenberg ML. High frequency of IL-4-producing $CD4^+$ allergen-specific T lymphocytes in atopic dermatitis lesional skin. *J Invest Dermatol* 1991; 97:389–394.
121. Kay AB, Ying S, Varney V, et al. Messenger RNA expression of the cytokine gene cluster, interleukin 3 (IL-3), IL-4, IL-5 and granulocyte/macrophage colony stimulating factor, in allergen-induced late phase cutaneous reactions in atopic subjects. *J Exp Med* 1991;173:775–778.
122. Ohmori H, Hikida M, Takai T. Prostaglandin E_2 as a selective stimulator of antigen-specific IgE response in murine lymphocytes. *Eur J Immunol* 1990;20:2499–2503.
123. Roper RL, Phipps RP. Prostaglandin E_2 and cAMP inhibit B lymphocyte activation and simultaneously promote IgE and IgG1 synthesis. *J Immunol* 1992;149:2984–2991.
124. Pene J. Regulatory role of cytokines and CD23 in the human IgE antibody synthesis. *Int Arch Allergy Appl Immunol* 1989;90:32–40.
125. Snapper CM, Pecanha LMT, Levine AD, Mond JL. IgE class switching is critically dependent upon the nature of the B cell activator, in addition to the presence of IL-4. *J Immunol* 1991;147: 1163–1170.
126. Marcelletti JF, Katz DH. Antigen concentration determines helper T cell subset participation in IgE antibody responses. *Cell Immunol* 1992;143:405–419.
127. Zetterstrom O, Osterman K, Machado L, Johansson SG. Another smoking hazard: raised serum IgE concentration and increased risk of occupational allergy. *Br Med J* 1981;283:1215–1217.

128. Venables KM, Topping MD, Howe W, Luczynska CM, Hawkins R, Newman Taylor AJ. Interaction of smoking and atopy in producing specific IgE antibody against a hapten protein conjugate. *Br Med J* 1985;290:201–204.
129. Muranaka M, Suzuki S, Koizumi K, Takafuji S, Miyamoto T, Ikemori R, Tokiwa H. Adjuvant activity of diesel-exhaust particulates for the production of IgE antibody in mice. *J Allergy Clin Immunol* 1986;77:616–623.
130. Takafuji S, Suzuki S, Koizumi K, Tadokoro K, Miyamoto M, Ikemori R, Muranaka M. Diesel-exhaust particulates inoculated by the intranasal route have an adjuvant activity for IgE production in mice. *J Allergy Clin Immunol* 1987;79:639–645.
131. Riedel F, Kramer M, Scherbenbugen C, Rieger CHL. Effects of SO_2 exposure on allergic sensitization in the guinea pig. *J Allergy Clin Immunol* 1988;82:527–534.
132. Wardlaw AJ. The role of air pollution in asthma. *Clin Exp Allergy* 1993;23:81–96.
133. Roche WR, Beasley R, Williams JH, Holgate ST. Subepithelial fibrosis in the bronchi of asthmatics. *Lancet* 1989;1:520–524.
134. Beasley R, Roche WR, Roberts JA, Holgate ST. Cellular events in the bronchi in mild asthma and after bronchial provocation. *Am Rev Respir Dis* 1989;139:806–817.
135. Gleich GJ. The eosinophil and bronchial asthma: current understanding. *J Allergy Clin Immunol* 1990;85:422–436.
136. Bentley AM, Maestrelli P, Saetta M, et al. Activated T-lymphocytes and eosinophils in the bronchial mucosa in isocyanate-induced asthma. *J Allergy Clin Immunol* 1992;89:821–829.
137. Chand N, Harrison JE, Rooney S, et al. Anti-IL-5 monoclonal antibody inhibits allergic late phase bronchial eosinophilia in guinea pigs: a therapeutic approach. *Eur J Pharmacol* 1992;211:121–123.
138. Iwami T, Nagai H, Suda H, Tsuruoka N, Koda A. Effect of murine recombinant interleukin-5 on the cell population in the guinea-pig airways. *Br J Pharmacol* 1992;105:19–22.
139. Iwami T, Nagai H, Tsuruoka N, Koda A. Effect of murine recombinant interleukin-5 on bronchial reactivity in guinea-pigs. *Clin Exp Allergy* 1993;23:32–38.

Immunotoxicology and Immunopharmacology, Second Edition, edited by J. H. Dean, M. I. Luster, A. E. Munson, and I. Kimber.
Raven Press, Ltd., New York © 1994.

39

Predictive Models for Assessment of Contact Photoallergy

G. Frank Gerberick

Human Safety Division, Procter & Gamble, Cincinnati, Ohio 45239

Contact photoallergy (CPA) is a cell-mediated immunologic reaction to chemicals that histologically and mechanistically resembles allergic contact hypersensitivity (1,2). The critical factor differentiating these reactions is that the chemicals that produce CPA reactions require activation by ultraviolet (UV) radiation in order to induce and elicit the response (Fig. 1). Although photoallergens absorb energy over a wide energy spectrum, predominantly the UVA (320 to 400 nm) range is associated with CPA. Two mechanisms have been postulated to explain formation of the photoproducts responsible for the induction of photosensitization responses (3–6). In the first mechanism, a photoallergen in its excited state reacts with proteins to form an antigen. In the second, the excited state of the photoallergen is converted into a simple contact allergen that binds to protein. Following formation via either pathway, it is believed that the photoallergen is processed by epidermal Langerhans' cells (LCs), which transport the processed antigenic determinant (photohapten) to regional lymph nodes. Therein, antigen-specific T helper cells recognize LC-bound antigen [in conjunction with major histocompatibility complex (MHC) class II antigen] and are triggered to proliferate and promote the dissemination of effector and memory T cells that are able to elicit a cutaneous response upon subsequent encounter with the inducing antigen.

To gain a better understanding of the mechanism of contact photoallergy, investigators have used mouse models to examine the immunologic aspects of CPA (7–10). Takigawa and Miyachi (7) demonstrated that CPA to tetrachlorosalicylanilide (TCSA), a known human contact photoallergen, could be transferred with TCSA-sensitized lymph node cells to naive recipients that were genetically identical at the MHC, whereas attempts were unsuccessful using histoincompatible strains, immune sera, or polymorphonuclear cells. Moreover, treatment of lymph node cells with anti-Thy-1.2 monoclonal antibody and complement abrogated the response, demonstrating that T lymphocytes were required for CPA. More recently, Tokura et al. (9) reported that subcutaneous inoculation of TCSA photohapten-modified

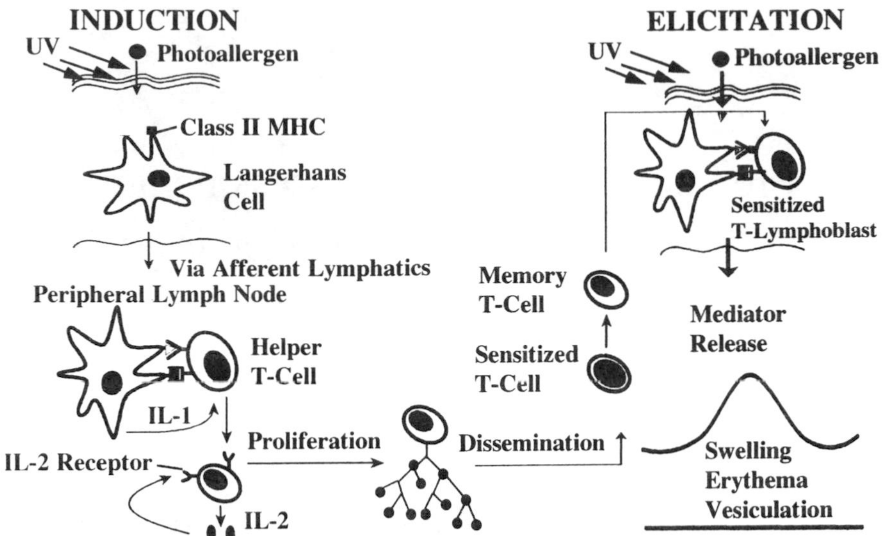

FIG. 1. Immunologic mechanism of contact photoallergy.

spleen cells into syngeneic mice induced a highly specific CPA response detected by ear swelling upon epicutaneous challenge with TCSA painting plus UVA irradiation. Cell-transfer experiments indicated that Thy-1+, L3T4+, Lyt-2− (CD4+) immune lymph node cells were responsible for transfer of the sensitivity. These studies demonstrate that CPA to TCSA in inbred mice is a specific delayed-contact hypersensitivity reaction, requiring T cells, and restricted by gene products of the MHC. In our laboratory, we have demonstrated that mice treated with TCSA+UVA demonstrate an increase both in local lymph node dendritic cell number and in lymphocyte proliferation (11). Moreover, we have shown that LC-enriched epidermal cells photohapten-modified with TCSA+UVA are capable of stimulating a significant lymphocyte-blastogenesis response when cultured with TCSA-sensitized lymphocytes, but not with naive or musk ambrette photosensitized lymphocytes (12). The results of these investigative studies further substantiate the delayed hypersensitivity nature of a CPA response.

CPA clinical responses characteristically range from a simple erythema to a severe vesiculobullous eruption. Histologically, the response is characterized by epidermal edema and vesicle formation and a dense perivascular infiltrate. Clinically, CPA reactions do not occur as frequently as contact allergic dermatitis reactions; however, the number of reports of chemicals eliciting possible photoallergic responses has increased (13–16). In general, removal of the offending photoallergen will eliminate the problem once the eruption has subsided. However, a small percentage of patients with CPA develop a sensitivity to light itself, presumably without further contact with the offending agents or related structures. This condition is referred to as persistent light reactivity (17). Phototesting often reveals abnormal reactivity of the normal untreated skin to UVB or to both UVB and UVA wavelengths. The mechanisms are not known, but the wavelengths for the reaction include UVB and perhaps result in autosensitization induced through photoautooxidation of histidine in epidermal proteins (18).

In 1939, Epstein (19,20) first differentiated photoallergy from phototoxicity for the drug sulfanilamide. The most notable CPA human data were compiled much later, between 1960 and 1970, on eruptions induced by the halogenated salicylanilides and related antibacterial compounds (5). Wilkinson (21) reported 53 cases of CPA to TCSA, an antimicrobial agent incorporated into soaps to reduce bacterial colonization. Phenolic compounds introduced to replace TCSA were also associated with causing CPA, including bithionol, hexachlorophene dichlorophene, the carbanilides, fentichlor, Jadit, and chloro-2-phenylphenol (1). In addition to the halogenated salicylanilides, other materials of various classes have been associated with causing CPA (Table 1). For example, two fragrance materials have been associated with contact photodermatitis, 6-methylcoumarin (22,23) and musk ambrette (6,24). In addition, musk ambrette has been reported to be responsible for the induction of a persistent light reaction similar to that noted with the halogenated salicylanilides (6).

Unfortunately, few studies have been conducted involving investigation of the wavelengths required for elicitation of photocontact allergic dermatitis in sensitized humans. As stated, UVA is usually sufficient for elicitation of photoallergic re-

TABLE 1. *Substances reported to produce photoallergic contact dermatitis in humans: classes and compounds*

Antimicrobial agents
3,3′,4′,5-Tetrachlorosalicylanilide (TCSA)
3,4′,5-Tribromosalicylanilide (TBS)
3,4,4′,-Tribromocarbanilide (TCC)
Hexachlorophene
Bithionol
Fentichlor
Fragrances
Musk ambrette
6-Methylcoumarin
Plant derivatives
Balsam of Peru
Wood mixture
Lichen mixture
Sunscreens
p-Aminobenzoic acid (PABA)
Octyl dimethyl PABA
Oxybenzones
Butyl methoxydibenzoylmethane
Drugs
Sulfanilamide
Chlorpromazine
Promethazine

sponses. Freeman and Knox (25) and Cripps and Enta (26), using narrow wave bands, showed that responses to the halogenated salicylanilides in pretreated skin could be elicited over a relatively wide portion of the UVA spectrum. Similar findings were obtained with 6-methylcoumarin (27). In contrast, Emmett (28) demonstrated that photoallergy was only provoked by UVB wavelengths when using diphenhydramine. Action spectrum studies for evaluating the wavelengths needed for the induction phase of CPA are also rare. Kaidbey and Kligman (27,29) have identified the photoallergic potential of various coumarin derivatives, including 6-methylcoumarin, using a human maximization protocol. In humans, Kaidbey (29) has shown that simulated solar radiation, which includes UVB and UVA radiation, was more effective than UVA radiation alone in inducing CPA to 6-methylcoumarin. When simulated solar radiation (UVB plus UVA) was used for induction and UVA alone for challenge, 15 of 25 subjects were sensitized; whereas when UVB radiation was omitted during the induction phase, only 4 of 24 subjects were sensitized. It was proposed that shorter UV wavelengths are more efficient for the activation of 6-methylcoumarin.

CLINICAL CONTACT PHOTOALLERGY TESTING

Diagnostic Patch Testing

The diagnosis of photocontact dermatitis is suspected by the clinical picture, including the character and distribution of the eruption (e.g., eruption is most notably in sun-exposed areas such as face and hands). Similar to the identification of a contact allergen, the contact photoallergen is identified by photopatch testing, which is accomplished by patch testing with a nonirritating concentration of the potential offending agent. Basically, the material is patched at two sites for 24 hr, after which time one site is irradiated, generally with UVA radiation (320 to 400 nm) only. The amount of UVA radiation required for photopatch testing is considerably less than the amount that is directly phototoxic. Twenty-four hours after irradiation, the nonirradiated and irradiated sites are evaluated. A positive response in a UVA-treated site alone represents a photoallergic reaction; whereas a positive response in both irradiated and nonirradiated sites represents contact allergic dermatitis at least, and, on occasion, both simultaneously. In addition, a positive reaction is one that reproduces the clinical lesions morphologically and, in some instances, histologically (2). Of course, as is the case with diagnostic patch testing for contact allergy, it is critical that the clinician determine whether or not the photoallergy is relevant to the photodermatitis, either as a primary cause or as an aggravating factor.

A number of different groups exist that perform photopatch testing including the Scandinavian Photo Dermatology Research Group, North American Contact Dermatitis Group, and Germany, Austria, and Switzerland Photopatch Test Group. From 1980 to 1985, the Scandinavian group showed that musk ambrette and *p*-aminobenzoic acid were the leading photosensitizers (30). Other less common photosensitizers included fentichlor, balsam of Peru, and tetrachlorosalicylanilide. The Germany, Austria and Switzerland Photopatch Test Group conducted a photopatch study between 1985 and 1990 (31) and found the most frequent photoallergens to include tiaprofenic acid, fentichlor, and carprofen. In 1988, Menz et al. (32) published results of a 6-year experience at the Mayo Clinic that showed the most frequent positive reactions were due to chlorpromazine, musk ambrette, and promethazine. Most recently, DeLeo et al. (33) published results of photopatch testing in New York from 1985 to 1990. Ten of the responses were due to fragrance ingredients (musk ambrette and 6-methylcoumarin) and 18 were due to sunscreen agents (nine to *p*-aminobenzoic acid and esters, nine to oxybenzone). Interestingly, the authors report that the incidence of photoallergy due to fragrances is declining, while reactions to sunscreen agents are increasing.

Predictive Photoallergy Testing

Kaidbey and Kligman (29,34) developed a photomaximization procedure to identify potential contact photoallergens. As mentioned previously, CPA is similar to contact allergy insofar as it comprises both an induction and elicitation phase. In most studies, 25 healthy volunteers are evaluated with the test material. The test material is applied to the skin and is occluded; 24 hr later the site is uncovered and irradiated with three minimal erythema doses (MED) of solar simulated radiation [UVB (290 to 320 nm) + UVA (320 to 400 nm)]. Generally, the UV source is a 150-W xenon arc solar simulator, which characteristically has an emission spectrum that is continuous, extending from 290 to 410 nm. The induction process is performed twice weekly for 3 weeks, using the same skin area. The test subjects are challenged 10 to 14 days after the last photoinduction routine. The test material is applied to normal skin under occlusion at a site different from the induction site, and 24 hr later the area is irradiated with UVA (4 J/cm^2). Control sites receive UVA only or test material without UVA. All sites are evaluated clinically 2 or 3 days later for inflammation. Kaidbey and Kligman (29,34) successfully photosensitized normal human volunteers to various known photoallergens, including TCSA, 3,5-dibromosalicylanilide, bithionol, 6-methylcoumarin, chlorpromazine, and sodium omadine. However, negative results were obtained with *p*-aminobenzoic acid and musk ambrette, which have produced photoallergic reactions clinically.

PRECLINICAL CONTACT PHOTOALLERGY TESTING

Guinea Pig Photoallergy Testing

The classic studies of Landsteiner and Chase (35) established the guinea pig as the model laboratory animal for investigating allergic contact dermatitis to simple chemicals. Therefore the guinea pig has been the species of choice for CPA studies.

TABLE 2. *Guinea pig contact photoallergy methods*

Reference	Potentiation method	Induction radiation[a] source/dose	Number of inductions	Challenge radiation source/dose
Vinson and Borselli (62)	—	FSL/15 min	5	FSL/15 min
Harber et al. (37)	Tape stripping	FSL/1 J/cm^2 FBL/30 J/cm^2	3	FBL/9 J/cm^2
Morikawa et al. (63)	—	FSL + FBL/11.8 J/cm^2	10	FBL/11.2 J/cm^2
Maurer (36)	Freund's adjuvant	Xenon/10 min	12	Xenon/3 or 10 min
Ichikawa et al. (40)	Freund's adjuvant + tape stripping	FSL/6.6 J/cm^2 FBL/10.2 J/cm^2	5	FBL/10.2 J/cm^2
Jordan (39)	Mechanical irritation	FSL/50–90m J/cm^2 FBL/30 J/cm^2	15	FBL/20 J/cm^2
Gerberick and Ryan (41)	Freund's adjuvant	FBL/10 J/cm^2	6	FBL/10 J/cm^2

[a]FSL, fluorescent sun lamps; FBL, fluorescent black lights.

Guinea pig tests developed for CPA testing are summarized in Table 2 and have been reviewed previously by Mauer (36). The methods summarized in Table 2 involve an induction phase and challenge phase. During the induction phase, guinea pigs are treated by repeated epidermal application of test compound followed by UV radiation. A combination of UVB plus UVA or UVA alone is used. After a rest period of 7 to 14 days, the animals are challenged with subirritant doses of test compound followed by UVA irradiation. Appropriate controls for photoallergy testing include induction with test material plus UVA followed by challenge with test material alone (contact sensitization), sham treatment during induction and challenge with test material and UVA (phototoxicity), and, finally, sham treatment for induction and challenge with test material alone (irritation).

The early models developed could readily detect photoallergens such as TCSA, tribromosalicylanilide, and chlorpromazine. By contrast, other known human photoallergens such as musk ambrette and 6-methylcoumarin went undetected when tested in conventional guinea pig models. Therefore investigators modified the guinea pig methods to enhance the sensitivity of the tests. Agents used to enhance the responses of the guinea pigs included combinations of UVA and UVB irradiation, sodium lauryl sulfate, cellophane tape stripping, skin abrasion, and Freund's complete adjuvant (36–40). With the exception of the latter, these techniques were designed to compromise the stratum corneum barrier and thus enhance cutaneous penetration of photosensitizers. Ichikawa et al. (40) modified a model developed by Harber et al. (37) to demonstrate that the use of Freund's complete adjuvant and cellophane tape stripping allowed for the detection of two human photoallergens, musk ambrette and 6-methylcoumarin. Since these known human photoallergens can be detected successfully in guinea pigs, Ichikawa's modified Harber technique is a model generally considered appropriate for photoallergy testing. Moreover, we have shown that this method is also capable of detecting the known sunscreen photoallergen, *p*-aminobenzoic acid (41).

Mouse Photoallergy Testing

In addition to the guinea pig photoallergy models, mouse models (Table 3) have been developed for investigating CPA (8,42–45). We have used a mouse ear swelling (MES) model for CPA testing that is a modification of previously reported methods (8,42,43). Specifically, the modifications included the addition of a third induction and the expansion of the irradiation spectrum to include both UVB and UVA radiation during the induction and elicitation phases of the response. In addition, we have used the model to investigate the effect of time between test material application and irradiation for the induction phase and to examine the coexistence of CPA and contact allergy.

As mentioned, we have incorporated UVA and UVB for both the induction and elicitation of CPA (46). Investigators have demonstrated the need for both UVA and UVB radiation during induction, but not elicitation, to successfully detect various photoallergens (29,47,48). For example, Maguire (48) demonstrated, using a mouse model, that photosensitization to bisphenol A requires UVB radiation. He showed that only mice photosensitized with UVB plus UVA during induction and UVA at challenge showed positive photoallergic reactions. Similarly, Giudici and Maguire (47) demonstrated in the mouse that UVA radiation alone fails to induce photoallergy to sulfanilamide and chlorpromazine when systemically administered. However, when UVA and UVB radiation was used during the induction phase and

TABLE 3. *Mouse contact photoallergy models*

Reference	Potentiation method	Induction radiation[b] source/dose	Number of inductions	Challenge radiation source/dose
Maguire and Kaidbey (42)	CY[a]	FSL/0.1 J/cm^2 FBL/5 J/cm^2	2	FBL/5 J/cm^2
Granstein et al. (8)	CY	FSL/0.3 J/cm^2 FBL/4 J/cm^2	2	FBL/4 J/cm^2
Miyachi and Takigawa (43)	CY	FSL/2.5 hr	2	FBL/2.5 hr
Wirestrand and Ljunggren (44)	CY	FSL/0.1 J/cm^2 FBL/5 J/cm^2	2[c]	FBL/5 J/cm^2
Gerberick and Ryan (45)	CY	FSL/30 mJ/cm^2 FBL/10 J/cm^2	3	FSL/30 mJ/cm^2 FBL/10 J/cm^2

[a]CY, cyclophosphamide.
[b]FSL, fluorescent sun lamps; FBL, fluorescent black lights.
[c]Mice are induced and challenged by intraperitoneal administration of the test material followed by UV irradiation.

TABLE 4. *Detection of known human photoallergens using a mouse ear swelling photoallergy model*

Chemical	Mouse[a] ear swelling model	Human[b] photomaximization method
3,3′,4′,5-Tetrachlorosalicylanilide	+	+
Bithionol	+	+
Musk ambrette	+	−
6-Methylcoumarin	+	+
Fentichlor	+	nd[c]
Bisphenol A	+	nd
Chlorpromazine	+	−
p-Aminobenzoic acid	+	−
Sodium omadine	+	+
Sulfanilamide	+	−
Coumarin	−	nd
Homosalate	−	nd

[a]See ref. 45.
[b]See ref. 29.
[c]nd, not determined.

UVA radiation alone was used for the challenge phase, photoallergy to systemically administered sulfanilamide and chlorpromazine in the mouse was detected. We found that the use of UVB plus UVA radiation for both induction and challenge significantly increased the photoallergic response to 6-methylcoumarin, but not TCSA or musk ambrette (46). Thus it may be appropriate to use both UVB and UVA radiation during both the induction and challenge phases when performing predictive photoallergy testing.

Employing a mouse photoallergy model, we successfully detected ten known human photoallergens representing various classes of materials, including antimicrobials, antifungals, drugs, fragrances, and sunscreens (Table 4). Included in the list are five clinically relevant photoallergens (TCSA, bithionol, 6-methylcoumarin, chlorpromazine, and sodium omadine), which have been detected in humans using a photomaximization protocol (29,34). In addition, and more importantly, three additional clinically relevant human photoallergens—sulfanilamide, musk ambrette, and *p*-aminobenzoic acid (16,49,50), which have been tested but not detected with the human protocol (29,34)—were shown to be photoallergens using the mouse model. These three compounds were also detected as photoallergens in the guinea pig (36,41,51). Fentichlor and bisphenol A, two compounds not tested in humans but reported as human contact photoallergens (52–54), were also detected in the mouse. Coumarin and homosalate, two chemicals that are not typically categorized as photoallergens (16,29,36,55), were unable to induce photoallergy in the mouse.

These results extend the initial findings of Miyachi and Takigawa (43) and Maguire and Kaidbey (42) that the mouse is a useful model for investigative as well as for predictive photoallergy testing. The mouse models are more quantitative than guinea pig models in that they use an objective assay to measure elicitation of CPA in previously sensitized animals. Moreover, the mouse photoallergy models are less time consuming, require fewer animals per test material, and are less costly than currently employed guinea pig models.

Alternative Photoallergy Testing Methods

Lowell (56) has proposed the use of an *in vitro* tier approach for assessing photoallergic potential of chemicals. The first step of this scheme involves examination of the absorption spectrum of the substance. If sunlight wavelengths are absorbed, then photobinding to protein is studied. Lowell also measures photooxidation of histidine as a test for photoirritation and to aid interpretation of the photobinding results. Lowell states that if photobinding is negative, then a potential for photoallergy is not expected and further testing is not required. Animal testing would be required to address the issue of photoallergen potency. Lowell proposes that photoallergens, following absorption of light energy, produce reactive species that bind chemically to protein to generate a complete antigen. In support, Pendlington and Barratt (57) have reported that a number of photoallergens exhibit photobinding to protein and the correlation of the *in vitro* experiments with *in vivo* findings appear to be excellent. Other investigators have also demonstrated the photobinding of photoallergens to proteins. Much of the work has been summarized by Lowell (56). In future studies, it would be interesting to use mammalian cells (e.g., LCs) as the target since photobinding of a substance to cell surface proteins is involved in photoallergy, not binding to serum proteins.

Scholes et al. (58) have evaluated the murine local lymph node assay (MLLNA) for use as a predictive model for assessing the contact photoallergenicity of chemicals. The MLLNA has been developed recently as an alternative method for the identification of skin-sensitizing chemicals (59,60). The results demonstrated that the photo-MLLNA was capable of identifying moderate photoallergic potential. Two known weak photoallergens, musk ambrette and 6-methylcoumarin, went undetected, suggesting that the assay, as designed, was insufficiently sensitive to identify weak photoallergic potential. Moreover, two known photoirritants, acridine and anthracene, were positive in the photo-MLLNA. The authors propose that the positive responses may be due to the ability of these chemicals to modify skin protein, thereby leading to the generation of modified skin proteins that are antigenic.

FUTURE NEEDS FOR PREDICTIVE PHOTOALLERGY TESTING

Dermatitis caused by contact photoallergens is rare compared to that caused by irritants and contact allergens. For this reason, less effort has been directed toward the development, validation, and standardization of predictive methods for the assessment of photoallergic potential. As new methods are developed, however, the robustness and predictability of the methods need to be determined by conducting interlaboratory validation studies as has been the case for the recently developed alternative methods for skin irritation and skin allergy testing. For the validation of new alternative CPA methods, investigators will need to use known weak photoallergens such as musk ambrette and 6-methylcoumarin for validation of their methods as well as the use of structurally similar chemicals that are known not to be photoallergenic.

Since the early days of developing models for photoallergy testing, much experience has been gained in our understanding of how to administer UV wavelengths necessary for initiating a photoallergic response. In any phototesting, it is critical that investigators know the output of the radiation source and the spectral response of the radiation detector. In the future, it would be beneficial to use solar simulators and spectrum radiometers for photoallergy testing. Solar simulators can be equipped with appropriate filters, so they can deliver radiation that simulates sunlight. In some cases, investigators are using FS40 bulbs, which are known to inappropriately deliver UVC radiation in addition to UVB (61). Spectrum radiometers would allow for the exact determination of the radiation source spectral output and intensity. For those investigators that use broad-spectrum radiometer detectors to determine their radiation dose, they need to be keenly aware that measurements obtained are directly dependent on the spectral response of the radiometer detector.

Finally, more studies are needed to determine the wavelengths required for elicitation of CPA responses in humans and animals. As previously stated, UVA radiation is usually sufficient for elicitation of photoallergic responses. With appropriate radiation sources, it should be possible to investigate further action spectra, which will aid understanding of which wavelengths are responsible for the induction and elicitation of CPA by comparison to the absorption spectrum of the test chemical. In addition, further studies are needed to evaluate the issue of metabolism and photosensitization. It has been suggested that metabolism is not an issue for photoallergy testing and that one only needs to look at the absorption spectrum of an unknown chemical (56). Action spectrum studies will also indirectly address the issue of metabolism and its role in CPA.

REFERENCES

1. Stephens TJ, Bergstresser PR. Fundamental concepts in photoimmunology and photoallergy. *J Toxicol Cutan Ocular Toxicol* 1985;4:193–218.
2. Epstein JH. Photocontact allergy in humans. In: Marzulli FN, Maibach HI, eds. *Dermatotoxicology*. Washington, DC: Hemisphere Publishing; 1987:441–456.
3. Willis I, Kligman AM. The mechanism of the persistent light reactor. *J Invest Dermatol* 1968; 51:385–394.
4. Harber LC, Baer RL. Pathogenic mechanisms of drug-induced photosensitivity. *J Invest Dermatol* 1972;58:327–332.
5. Herman PS, Sams WM Jr. Cellular reactions in contact photoallergy. *Int Arch Allergy Appl Immunol* 1971;41:551–558.
6. Giovinazzo VJ, Harber LC, Armstrong RB, Kochevar IE. Photoallergic contact dermatitis to musk ambrette. Clinical report of two patients with persistent light reactor patterns. *J Am Acad Dermatol* 1980;3:384–393.

7. Takigawa M, Miyachi Y. Mechanisms of contact photosensitivity in mice: I. T cell regulation of contact photosensitivity to tetrachlorosalicylanilide under the genetic restrictions of the major histocompatibility complex. *J Invest Dermatol* 1982;79:108–115.
8. Granstein RD, Morison WL, Kripke ML. The role of UVB radiation in the induction and elicitation of photocontact hypersensitivity to TCSA in the mouse. *J Invest Dermatol* 1983;80:158–162.
9. Tokura Y, Takigawa M, Yamada M. Induction of contact photosensitivity to TCSA using photohapten-modified syngeneic spleen cells. *Arch Dermatol Res* 1988;280:207–213.
10. Miyachi Y, Takigawa M. Mechanisms of contact photosensitivity in mice: II. Langerhans cells are required for successful induction of contact photosensitivity to TCSA. *J Invest Dermatol* 1982;78:363–365.
11. Gerberick GF, Ryan CA, Fletcher ER, Howard AD, Robinson MK. Increased number of dendritic cells in draining lymph nodes accompanies the generation of contact photosensitivity. *J Invest Dermatol* 1991;96:355–361.
12. Gerberick GF, Ryan CA, Von Bargen EC, Stuard SB, Ridder GM. Examination of tetrachlorosalicylanilide (TCSA) photoallergy using in vitro photohapten-modified Langerhans cell-enriched epidermal cells. *J Invest Dermatol* 1991;97:210–218.
13. de Groot AC, van der Walle HB, Jagtman BA, Weyland JW. Contact allergy to 4-isopropyl-dibenzoylmethane and 3-(4′-methylbenzylidene) camphor in the sunscreen Eusolex 8021. *Contact Dermatitis* 1987;16:249–254.
14. Knobler E, Almeida L, Ruzkowski AM, Held J, Harber LC, DeLeo VA. Photoallergy to benzophenone. *Arch Dermatol* 1989;125:801–804.
15. Thune P, Eeg-Larsen T. Contact and photocontact allergy in persistent light reactivity. *Contact Dermatitis* 1984;11:98–107.
16. Wennersten G, Thune P, Jansen CT, Brodthagen H. Photocontact dermatitis: current status with emphasis on allergic contact photosensitivity occurrence, allergens, and practical phototesting. *Semin Dermatol* 1986;5:277–289.
17. Vandermaesen J, Roelandts R, Degreef H. Light on the persistent light reaction–photosensitivity dermatitis–actinic reticuloid syndrome. *J Am Acad Dermatol* 1986;15:685–692.
18. Kochevar IE. Photoallergic responses to chemicals. *Photochem Photobiol* 1979;30:437–442.
19. Epstein S. Photoallergy and primary phototoxicity to sulfanilamide. *J Invest Dermatol* 1939;2:243–247.
20. Epstein S. Phototoallergy and primary photosensitivity to sulfanilamide. *Dermatologica* 1941;83: 63–66.
21. Wilkinson DS. Photodermatitis due to tetrachlorosalicylamide. *Br J Dermatol* 1969;73:123–127.
22. Kaidbey KH, Kligman AM. Contact photoallergy to 6-methylcoumarin in proprietary sunscreens. *Arch Dermatol* 1978;114:1709–1710.
23. Jackson RT, Nesbitt LT Jr, DeLeo VA. 6-Methylcoumarin photocontact dermatitis. *J Am Acad Dermatol* 1980;2:124–127.
24. Raugi GJ, Storrs FJ. Photosensitivity from men's colognes (letter). *Arch Dermatol* 1979;115:106.
25. Freeman RG, Knox JM. The action spectrum of photocontact dermatitis. *Arch Dermatol* 1968;97: 130–136.
26. Cripps DJ, Enta T. Absorption and action spectra studies on bithionol and halogenated salicylanilide photosensitivity. *Br J Dermatol* 1970;82:230–242.
27. Kaidbey KH, Kligman AM. Photosensitization by coumarin derivatives; structure–activity relationships. *Arch Dermatol* 1981;117:258–263.
28. Emmett EA. Diphenhydramine photoallergy. *Arch Dermatol* 1974;110:249–252.
29. Kaidbey K. The evaluation of photoallergic contact sensitizers in humans. In: Marzulli FN, Maibach HI, eds. *Dermatotoxicology*. Washington, DC: Hemisphere Publishing; 1987:457–468.
30. Thune P, Jansen C, Wennersten G, Rystedt I, Brodthagen H, McFadden N. The Scandinavian multicenter photopatch study 1980–1985: final report. *Photodermatology* 1988;5:261–269.
31. Hölzie E, Neumann N, Hausen B, et al. Photopatch testing: the 5-year experience of the German, Austrian, and Swiss Photopatch Test Group. *J Am Acad Dermatol* 1991;25:59–68.
32. Menz J, Muller SA, Connolly SM. Photopatch testing: a six-year experience. *J Am Acad Dermatol* 1988;18:1044–1047.
33. DeLeo VA, Suarez SM, Maso MJ. Photoallergic contact dermatitis: results of photopatch testing in New York, 1985 to 1990. *Arch Dermatol* 1992;128:1513–1518.
34. Kaidbey KH, Kligman AM. Photomaximization test for identifying photoallergic contact sensitizers. *Contact Dermatitis* 1980;6:161–169.
35. Landsteiner K, Chase MW. Experiments on transfer of cutaneous sensitivity to simple compounds. *Proc Soc Exp Biol Med* 1942;49:688.

36. Maurer T. Experimental contact photoallergenicity: guinea pig models. *Photodermatology* 1984;1: 221–231.
37. Harber LC, Targovnik SE, Baer RL. Contact photosensitivity patterns to halogenated salicylanilides in man and guinea pigs. *Arch Dermatol* 1967;96:646–656.
38. Horio T. The induction of photocontact sensitivity in guinea pigs without UVB radiation. *J Invest Dermatol* 1976;67:591–593.
39. Jordan WP Jr. The guinea pig as a model for predicting photoallergic contact dermatitis. *Contact Dermatitis* 1982;8:109–116.
40. Ichikawa H, Armstrong RB, Harber LC. Photoallergic contact dermatitis in guinea pigs: improved induction technique using Freund's complete adjuvant. *J Invest Dermatol* 1981;76:498–501.
41. Gerberick GF, Ryan CA. Contact photoallergy testing of sunscreens in guinea pigs. *Contact Dermatitis* 1989;20:251–259.
42. Maguire HC Jr, Kaidbey K. Experimental photoallergic contact dermatitis: a mouse model. *J Invest Dermatol* 1982;79:147–152.
43. Miyachi Y, Takigawa M. Mechanisms of contact photosensitivity in mice. III. Predictive testing of chemicals with photoallergenic potential in mice. *Arch Dermatol* 1983;119:736–739.
44. Wirestrand LE, Ljunggren B. Photoallergy to systemic quinidine in the mouse: dose–response studies. *Photodermatology* 1988;5:201–205.
45. Gerberick GF, Ryan CA. A predictive mouse ear-swelling model for investigating topical photoallergy. *Food Chem Toxicol* 1990;28:361–368.
46. Gerberick GF, Ryan CA. The use of UVB and UVA to induce and elicit contact photoallergy in the mouse. *Photodermatol Photoimmunol Photomed* 1990;7:13–19.
47. Giudici PA, Maguire HC Jr. Experimental photoallergy to systemic drugs. *J Invest Dermatol* 1985;85:207–211.
48. Maguire HC Jr. Experimental photoallergic contact dermatitis to bisphenol A. *Acta Derm Venereol (Stockh)* 1988;68:408–412.
49. Giovinazzo W, Harber LC, Bickers DR, Armstrong RB, Silvers DN. Photoallergic contact dermatitis to musk ambrette. Histopathologic features of photobiologic reactions observed in a persistent light reactor. *Arch Dermatol* 1981;117:344–348.
50. Horio T, Higuchi T. Photocontact dermatitis from *p*-aminobenzoic acid. *Dermatologia* 1988;156: 124–128.
51. Harber LC, Armstrong RB, Ichikawa H. Current status of predictive animal models for drug photoallergy and their correlation with drug photoallergy in humans. *J Natl Cancer Inst* 1982;69:237–244.
52. Burry JN. Photoallergies to fentichlor and multifungin. *Arch Dermatol* 1967;95:287–290.
53. Allen H, Kaidbey K. Persistent photosensitivity following occupational exposure to epoxy resin. *Arch Dermatol* 1979;115:1307–1310.
54. Ramsay CA. Skin responses to ultraviolet radiation in contact photodermatitis due to fentichlor. *J Invest Dermatol* 1979;72:99–102.
55. Cronin E. *Contact dermatitis*. Edinburgh: Churchill Livingstone; 1980:414–460.
56. Lowell WW. A scheme for in vitro screening of substances for photoallergic potential. *Toxic in Vitro* 1993;7:95–102.
57. Pendlington RU, Barratt MD. Photochemical binding of photoallergens to human serum albumin: a simple in vitro method for screening potential photoallergens. *Toxicol Lett* 1985;24:1–6.
58. Scholes EW, Basketter DA, Lovell WW, Sarll AE, Pendlington RU. The identification of photoallergic potential in the local lymph node assay. *Photodermatol Photoimmunol Photomed* 1991;8:249–254.
59. Kimber I, Weisenberger C. A murine local lymph node assay for the identification of contact allergens. *Arch Toxicol* 1989;63:274–282.
60. Kimber I, Hilton J, Weisenberger C. The murine local lymph node assay for identification of contact allergens: a preliminary evaluation of in situ measurement of lymphocyte proliferation. *Contact Dermatitis* 1989;21:215–220.
61. Learn DB, Beard J, Moloney SJ. The ultraviolet C energy emitted from FS lamps contributes significantly to the induction of human erythema and murine ear edema. *Photodermatol Photoimmunol Photomed* 1993;9:147–153.
62. Vinson LJ, Borselli VF. A guinea pig assay of the photosensitizing potential of topical germicides. *J Soc Cosmet Chem* 1966;17:123–130.
63. Morikawa F, Nakayama Y, Fukuda M, et al. Techniques for evaluation of phototoxicity and photoallergy in laboratory animals and man. In: Fitzpatrick TB, ed. *Sunlight and man*. Tokyo: Tokyo Press; 1974:529–557.

Immunotoxicology and Immunopharmacology, Second Edition, edited by J. H. Dean, M. I. Luster, A. E. Munson, and I. Kimber.
Raven Press, Ltd., New York © 1994.

40

Guinea Pig Predictive Tests for Contact Hypersensitivity

David A. Basketter

Department of Biology, Unilever Environmental Safety Laboratory, Sharnbrook, MK44 1LQ, United Kingdom

Allergic contact dermatitis (contact hypersensitivity, skin sensitization) is a relatively common eczematous skin condition. The clinical aspects of this disorder form the subject of an excellent recent textbook (1). The mechanism(s) of contact hypersensitivity (reviewed in refs. 2 and 3) involves the immune recognition of chemical (hapten)-modified protein. However, it is the purpose of this chapter to provide a critical assessment of guinea pig predictive tests whose aim is to give a clear indication of the potential of a new chemical to cause contact hypersensitivity. Detailed descriptions of guinea pig tests and their relative merits are already available (4–7), so this chapter does not attempt to present an account of protocols or other aspects of test conduct except where it is of particular relevance. Instead, the main focus is on factors affecting the quality of test conduct, the further use of sensitized animals by rechallenge, the value of positive control studies, and the interpretation of test results for regulatory and risk assessment purposes.

Before proceeding, it is appropriate to provide definitions of some terms that will be used. *Hazard* is an intrinsic property of a substance, in this case the potential to cause contact hypersensitivity. The primary purpose of the guinea pig methods to be discussed is the identification of this specific hazard. The term *risk* is used *only* in relation to subsequent evaluation of an identified hazard in the context of exposure.

METHODS

Without exception, guinea pig predictive tests for contact hypersensitivity incorporate two essential phases. In the first, induction procedures are carried out in an attempt to stimulate a state of immune hypersensitivity. In the second phase, the guinea pigs are challenged to measure the extent to which contact hypersensitivity has developed. Control guinea pigs are sham treated at induction and then treated exactly as test animals at challenge. Within these minimal constraints, a substantial number of protocols have been developed (reviewed in refs. 4–7). However, from this wide range of options, just two assays have emerged as those most commonly performed (5) and as preferred by international agencies (8,9). The methods are the guinea pig maximization test of Magnusson and Kligman (10) and the occlusive patch test of Buehler (11). In this section, basic aspects of test conduct and key factors affecting test performance are considered. The comments are made in the context of a specific method but usually are generally applicable.

Guinea Pig Maximization Test (GPMT)

A great number of factors affecting the evaluation of sensitization potential in the GPMT were thoroughly investigated by Magnusson and Kligman (10). Their monograph concludes with the details of the optimum protocol. Some aspects may be of particular importance, however, and are highlighted in what follows.

The first stage of the GPMT induction phase involves intradermal injections of the test substance in various combinations with Freund's complete adjuvant. The concentration and vehicle selected from preliminary experiments should be irritating but not locally, or of course systemically, toxic. Since the assay is designed to maximize the chance of inducing hypersensitivity, the concentration should be the highest level producing an overt local irritation without other adverse effects. Ultimately, this is a matter of judgment, but it should be borne in mind that very high concentrations may lead to a lowering of the level of response (12,13) while the choice of a very low concentration (e.g., $<0.1\%$) might indicate the need to consider alternative vehicles.

The second component of the GPMT induction phase involves 48 hr occlusive topical application to the site where the intradermal injections were made. Again, based on the evidence of preliminary experiments, a concentration and vehicle should be selected that will be the maximum producing a moderately irritant response under these patch conditions. If a suitable irritant concentration cannot be achieved, the application site should be pretreated 24 hr earlier with 10% sodium lauryl sulfate (SLS) in petrolatum. At induction, the importance of concomitant irritation should not be underestimated. This is illustrated in the GPMT monograph (10), but to exemplify the point further, Table 1 contains results of testing isoeugenol at optimal concentrations and at suboptimal concentrations either with or without the use of SLS to restore the correct degree of irritancy at induction. The results demonstrate that irritancy is a major requirement for an optimal response. (See also the results noted by superscript *d* in Table 2). While it can be argued that SLS may promote skin penetration of an allergen, this was not the case in a recent study of a similar phenomenon in the mouse (14). There is evidence, although not in the guinea pig, that SLS causes keratinocytes to release cytokines, which may play an important role in the sensitization as well as the inflammatory process (15,16). In particular, SLS causes production of tumor necrosis factor-α (TNF-α), which promotes the migration of Langerhans' cells (LCs) to the draining lymph node (17).

TABLE 1. *Effect of irritation on the induction of contact hypersensitivity to isoeugenol*

Test protocol	Induction		Challenge result[a]
	II[b]	IP[c]	
Standard GPMT	0.15%	25%	30% (0.8)
Low concentration	0.03%	5.0%	0% (0.0)
Low concentration plus SLS	0.03% + 0.05% SLS	5.0% + 0.2% SLS	30% (0.8)

[a]Challenge was carried out at 0.05% isoeugenol, below the maximum nonirritant concentration. The results are expressed as the percentage of the test guinea pigs judged positive, followed in parentheses by the mean erythema score on those animals (scale 0–3).

[b]Induction injection concentration.

[c]Induction patch concentration.

The movement of antigen-bearing LCs to the draining lymph node is critical to the induction of sensitization and a direct quantitative relationship between these events has been reported (18).

In the second phase of the GPMT, an assessment is made of the extent to which contact hypersensitivity has been induced. This is done with a 24 hr occluded patch of the test substance applied at the maximum nonirritant concentration. The vehicle is likely to be the same as that used for the topical induction patch. The concentration is normally a little lower than that for the induction patch but is usually 1.0% or greater. However, the most important point is that the concentration is the highest that does not give rise to primary irritation, the appearance of which cannot be differentiated from that of an allergic response. The importance of this is demonstrated by the data in Table 2. In guinea pigs sensitized to isoeugenol, the substantially reduced response elicited by a suboptimal isoeugenol concentration can be restored by introduction of SLS in just sufficient concentration to provide a subthreshold level of irritation.

TABLE 2. *Effect of irritation on the elicitation of contact hypersensitivity to isoeugenol*

Test protocol[a]	Challenge result[b]				
	5.0%	1.0%	1.0% + SLS[c]	0.05%	0.05% + SLS[c]
Standard GPMT	100% (1.9)[d]	ND[e]	ND	30% (0.8)	90% (1.6)
Low concentration	ND	80% (1.2)[d]	ND	0% (0)	90% (0.9)
Low concentration plus SLS	ND	ND	100% (1.8)[d]	39% (0.8)	60% (1.0)

[a]Induction concentrations as in Table 1.

[b]The results are expressed as the percentage of the test guinea pigs judged positive, followed in parentheses by the mean erythema score on those animals (scale 0–3).

[c]SLS at 0.05%.

[d]These three tests give the results at optimal induction and elicitation concentration compared with fivefold reduced concentrations in the presence and absence of restoration of the irritancy component with SLS.

[e]ND, not done.

TABLE 3. *Comparison of the effect of clipping versus clipping and shaving fur prior to challenge*

Test protocol	Challenge result[a]	
	Clipped only	Clipped and shaved
GPMT of citral	10	90
GPMT of formaldehyde	0	100

[a]Results expressed as the percentage of test guinea pigs judged positive.

Another factor that can have an impact on both topical application stages of the GPMT, and indeed any other contact hypersensitivity test that incorporates epicutaneous treatment, is the nature of skin preparation. Magnusson and Kligman (10) concluded that it was necessary to remove guinea pig fur by clipping, followed by shaving. This ensures proper skin contact with the test substance, obviously a prerequisite for detection of contact hypersensitivity at the challenge phase. Data from this laboratory strongly support this conclusion (Table 3), and it has been observed that hairless guinea pigs have an enhanced contact hypersensitivity response (19). In addition, use of more than two patches on one flank at challenge can impair their occlusion, leading to a suboptimal response.

Buehler Occluded Patch Test

The Buehler test protocol employs only 6 hr occluded patch treatments at induction and elicitation phases (11,20). Neither intradermal injection of test substance nor Freund's complete adjuvant is used. However, though these differences may render the method a less sensitive indicator of contact hypersensitivity potential, when properly performed it identifies most important contact allergens (21,22).

Except in relation to intradermal injection, those comments made about the GPMT also apply to the Buehler test. For the induction phase, it is important to apply a definitely irritant concentration, but one that can be applied repeatedly to the same site. For the elicitation phase, challenge must be carried out with the maximum nonirritant concentration. At all stages, it is imperative that there is thorough contact between the patch loaded with test material and the skin. Experience in this laboratory shows that this may be achieved without the restraint recommended by Buehler (11), but it does demand tight occlusion of the patch to clipped and razored skin.

Many types of patch may be used for challenge. Relatively large fabric or filter paper patches, such as that recommended by Buehler (11,20), will hold a larger volume of test substance, but being not well delineated these can give rise to rather diffuse skin reactions with no well-defined limit. For this reason Finn chambers, Hill Top patches, or any other proprietary system with a lipped edge may be preferable. The key question is whether suitable results with positive controls can be obtained (see later discussion).

Assessment of Elicitation Reactions

The degree to which contact hypersensitivity has been induced is assessed by subjective scoring of challenge-induced skin responses. Control animals provide reassurance that skin irritation reactions are not present. The major component of the response is erythema, which is scored on an arbitrary scale, usually with five grades. Typically, the lowest grade is "no reaction" and the second is an indication for the investigator of an equivocal skin reaction not to be regarded as evidence of contact hypersensitivity without further support. The remaining three grades are weak, moderate, and strong erythema, all identifying a positive reaction.

Scoring of responses should be carried out on two occasions, 24 and 48 hr after patch removal. Experience shows that allergic reactions may only be positive at one or other time point, most commonly the later time. What should be done if reactions occur in the control guinea pigs? The extent of any response in sham-treated controls shows, under experimental conditions, the irritation potential of the test substance. Because of the preliminary experiments, it is very unlikely that the degree of response will be large. One approach then for a reaction in a test animal to be regarded as positive evidence of contact hypersensitivity is to raise the threshold which a test animal score must achieve by the maximum amount of irritation seen in the controls. Simple subtraction of the frequency of irritant responses in the controls from the frequency of response in the test animals is to be avoided. In addition, serious consideration should be given to rechallenge 2 weeks later on the unused flank with a reduced test concentration (see later discussion).

Rechallenge Procedures

There are several reasons why consideration should be given to the use of a rechallenge. Not the least is the ethical use of animals, since one ought to derive the maximum amount of information from the least number of animals: a rechallenge now may obviate the need for a completely new experiment in the future. Scientific reasons for rechallenge center on two aspects: the clarification of equivocal responses and further investigation, usually to aid risk assessment. Before discussing these in more detail, it is worth noting that it is easier to carry out a timely rechallenge if only one flank has been used for the first challenge, leaving the other in a naive state. Equivocal reactions may occur if either the first challenges are very weak or their significance is cast into doubt by the presence of irritation responses in controls. In the former case, a simple repeat challenge 2 weeks later on the opposite flank may suffice. In the latter situation, a similar repeat challenge but using a slightly lower (e.g., half) concentration of test substance is probably most appropriate. Changes to vehicles/patch type are not indicated unless the investigator has special knowledge clearly identifying this as the correct course of action. In either case, the challenge and rechallenge results should be looked at both individually and taken together. Although not a firm rule, it is reasonable to expect that a well-sensitized guinea pig will react to some degree at both challenges. In contrast, a weak reaction occurring at a single time point in only one challenge should cast strong doubt as to whether that guinea pig is really sensitized. The experience in my laboratory is that, except where animals are strongly sensitized, the results of rechallenge are often unpredictable. Rechallenges may be carried out for purposes related to risk assessment or to investigation of, for example, structure–activity relationships. Simple processes that may aid risk assessment could be to carry out an elicitation dose–response, to challenge with the test substance at its likely human skin contact level, perhaps in the relevant vehicle, or to evaluate potential cross-reactivities (e.g., with formaldehyde, if the test substance could be a formaldehyde releaser). The more investigative use of rechallenge procedures may include a consideration of chemical cross-reactivities (21,22) or an evaluation of the extent to which the allergic responses are due to impurities (23).

Positive Controls

It has become increasingly recognized that the existence of well-described and largely standardized protocols for contact hypersensitivity tests is not a guarantee that laboratories will achieve similar results for a single test substance in a particular protocol such as the GPMT or Buehler test. Indeed, wide discrepancies have been reported (5,24,25). The reasons lie most probably in differences in the detail of the technique, with some of the more critical aspects, such as skin preparation, having been described earlier. However, whatever the reasons for the differences may be, the simplest first step to achieve greater harmonization is in the setting of positive control standards.

Regulatory guidelines have suggested for many years that assays for contact hypersensitivity should be able to detect certain common contact allergens (26). Unfortunately, the substances listed were always those regarded as potent allergens. Thus they would not permit identification of all except the most poorly performed assays. For the same reason, Buehler's (27) recommendation for validation of his assay is flawed. He suggested the use of specific concentrations of 2,4-dinitrochlorobenzene (DNCB) and the resultant degree of sensitization this should give. However, since the quality of skin preparation and patch occlusion are critical aspects of his assay (11,20,25,27), it is unfortunate to have selected dilute solutions of DNCB in acetone, which contact and penetrate skin so easily. Unpublished experience in this laboratory demonstrated complete achievement of the Buehler targets with DNCB, but a complete failure of the same protocol to detect several common and strong human contact allergens such as formaldehyde and cinnamaldehyde.

Recently, Organisation for Economic Cooperation and Development (OECD) guidelines for guinea pig predictive tests for contact hypersensitivity have been updated (9). These new guidelines recommend the use twice a year of at least one moderately sensitizing contact allergen as a means of judging the quality of performance of a specific assay. The substances suggested were benzocaine, mercaptobenzothiazole, and hexyl cinnamic aldehyde, although this was not intended either as an exclusive or exhaustive list. Recent experience and typical results with these moderately sensitizing positive controls in two laboratories have been published (28). This laboratory has used one of these substances (hexyl cinnamic aldehyde) as a positive control for some years, obtaining very consistent results. The incidence of positives has rarely varied outside the range of 50% to 70%.

DATA INTERPRETATION

Regulatory Toxicology

In terms of regulatory toxicology, classification as a contact sensitizer is based on arbitrary thresholds of ≥30% for the GPMT and ≥15% for the Buehler test (29). For example, a chemical that results in a positive grading of ≥3 out of 20 test animals in the Buehler test is classified as a skin sensitizer and must be labeled in the EEC with the R43 phrase "may cause sensitization by skin contact." With the new positive control standards recommended by the OECD (9), negative test results on a new chemical will be unacceptable if the positive control data fail to meet the minimum standard of sensitivity (30% positive in the GPMT; 15% in the Buehler test).

Nevertheless, anomalies between laboratories will still arise. Under current regulations, data on a new chemical will be judged in an identical manner irrespective of whether the testing laboratory obtains a 30% or a 100% response with the positive control substance. Furthermore, the intensity of the contact hypersensitivity response to the new chemical is not taken into account, only whether it has attained the arbitrary classification threshold. This can have serious implications in the context of regulations such as the Dangerous Preparations Directive (29). Here the application of a warning label to a product only applies if the sensitizer is present at ≥1%. There is a failure to take into account the relative potency of the skin sensitizer in the context of the quality of the test performed in the particular laboratory.

Safety Evaluation

The results of a guinea pig test provide a good indication of the potential of a chemical to cause contact hypersensitivity, but this can only be assessed in the light of the test parameters and the experience with the particular method at the testing institution. Aspects to be considered are the test concentrations and vehicles, the magnitude of any responses (both frequency and degree), and the results of any rechallenges, including dose–response data and cross-challenges. If the safety evaluator knows the quality of assay conduct (hence the value of recent positive control data), then data on the new substance may be put into context.

The second part of the process must be to consider the nature and extent of human exposure to the chemical. Key factors in assessing risk include exposure concentration, duration, and frequency, the presence or absence of occlusion, the skin site exposed, the number of individuals exposed, and the existence of particularly susceptible subpopulations. If the chemical is to be incorporated into a product, it will be essential to appreciate the wide range of consumer habits and to consider foreseeable misuse of the product. The outcome of such safety evaluations demonstrates the value of a case-by-case analysis. Relatively strong contact sensitizers may be used quite safely under appropriate conditions, while weak sensitizers, including those that fail to cause any response in well-conducted guinea pig assays, can give rise to allergic contact dermatitis in humans if the exposure is sufficiently exaggerated.

Finally, it should be borne in mind that a very sensitive assay such as the GPMT does not provide an absolute standard. Not only may it fail to give positive results with recognized weaker human contact allergens (10,30,31), it may also appear to exaggerate the potential of some substances to cause contact hypersensitivity in humans (32).

SUMMARY

Guinea pig tests for contact hypersensitivity have been used successfully over many years to identify chemicals possessing the potential to cause skin sensitization (5,33). Procedures such as the GPMT (10) and the Buehler test (11) have been employed widely by toxicologists for this purpose (5,25). However, the sensitivity of these assays can vary quite widely between laboratories (5,9,24). Recognition of this fact, subsequent publication of validation criteria (27), and detailed explanations of test protocols (20,34,35) have not demonstrably improved the situation. Sources of variation are many, but those of prime importance and which probably explain the commonest causes of differences between laboratories have been described. They include proper selection of test concentrations, particularly in the context of achieving suitable levels of irritation, and thorough skin preparation prior to patch application.

The revision of Guideline 406 of the OECD (9) recommend positive control substances with moderate sensitization potential to set a minimum standard for test conduct. However, variation between laboratories will continue to exist. In addition, chemicals causing contact hypersensitivity do so in different ways (in terms of reaction chemistry and the requirement, or not, for skin metabolism) and with widely varying efficiency. Consequently, a proper assessment of this hazard can be made only on a case-by-case basis. This essentially follows the processes employed by toxicologists in safety evaluation of the use of chemicals shown to have the potential to cause contact hypersensitivity.

At present, it is difficult to see how *in vitro* methods could replace *in vivo* methodology. However, an alternative assay in the mouse, the local lymph node assay, offers the prospect of refinement and reduction of animal use while at the same time providing a robust and objective method that will be less susceptible to the sources of variation mentioned earlier (36–39). Furthermore, data on the OECD positive control substances compare favorably, in a regulatory sense, with that from the GPMT and Buehler test (28). Thus in the near future, this represents a promising route for further interlaboratory validation at an international level.

REFERENCES

1. Rycroft RJG, Menné T, Frosch PJ, Benezra C, eds. *Textbook of contact dermatitis*. Berlin: Springer-Verlag; 1992.
2. Kimber I. Contact sensitivity. In: Miller K, Turk J, Nicklin S, eds. *Principles and practice of immunotoxicology*. London: Blackwell Scientific Publications; 1992:104–124.
3. Scheper RJ, Von Blomberg BME. Cellular mechanisms in allergic contact dermatitis. In: Rycroft RJG, Menné T, Frosch PJ, Benezra C, eds. *Textbook of contact dermatitis*. Berlin: Springer-Verlag; 1992:11–27.
4. Andersen KE, Maibach HI, eds. *Current problems in dermatology, vol 14. Contact allergy predictive tests in guinea pigs*. Basel: Karger; 1985.
5. Botham PA, Basketter DA, Maurer T, Mueller D, Potokar M, Bontinck W. Skin sensitization—a critical review of predictive tests in methods in animals and man. *Food Chem Toxicol* 1991;29:275–286.
6. Maurer T. *Contact and photocontact allergens. A manual of predictive test methods*. New York: Marcel Dekker; 1983.
7. Andersen KE. Testing for contact allergy in experimental animals. *Pharmacol Toxicol* 1987;61:1–8.
8. EEC Council directive of 7 June 1988 on the approximation of laws, regulations and administrative provisions of the member states relating to the classification, packaging and labelling of dangerous preparations. *Off J Eur Comm* 1988;L187:14.
9. Organisation for Economic Cooperation and Development. *OECD guidelines for testing of chemicals*, No. 406. Skin sensitization. Adopted 12 June 1992.
10. Magnusson B, Kligman AM. *Allergic contact dermatitis in the guinea pig*. Springfield, IL: CC Thomas; 1970.
11. Buehler EV. Delayed contact hypersensitivity in the guinea pig. *Arch Dermatol* 1965;91:171–175.
12. Roberts DW, Basketter DA. A quantitative structure activity/dose response relationship for contact allergenic potential of alkyl group transfer agents. *Contact Dermatitis* 1990;23:331–335.
13. Basketter DA, Roberts DW. Structure/activity relationships in contact allergy. *Int J Cosmet Sci* 1990;12:81–90.
14. Cumberbatch M, Scott RC, Basketter DA, Scholes EW, Hilton J, Dearman RJ, Kimber I. Influence of sodium lauryl sulphate on 2,4-dinitrochlorobenzene induced lymph node acitivation. *Toxicology* 1993;77:181–191.
15. Brand CU, Hunziker T, Braathen LR. Isolation of human skin-derived lymph: flow and output of cells following sodium lauryl sulphate induced contact dermatitis. *Arch Dermatol Res* 1992;284: 123–126.
16. Enk AH, Katz SI. Early molecular events in the induction phase of contact sensitivity. *Proc Natl Acad Sci USA* 1992;80:1398–1402.
17. Cumberbatch M, Kimber I. Dermal tumour necrosis factor-α induces dendritic cell migration to draining lymph nodes and possibly provides one stimulus for Langerhans cell migration. *Immunology* 1992;75:257–263.
18. Kimber I, Dearman RJ. Investigation of lymph node cell proliferation as a possible immunological correlate of contact sensitizing potential. *Food Chem Toxicol* 1991;29:125–129.
19. Buehler EV, Krenzmann JJ, Sakr A, Xiao HG. Comparable sensitivity of hairless and Hartley strain guinea pigs to a primary irritant as a sensitizer. *J Toxicol Cutan Ocular Toxicol* 1990;9:163–168.
20. Ritz H, Buehler EV. Planning, conduct and interpretation of guinea pig sensitization patch tests. In: Drill VA, Lazar P, eds. *Current concepts in cutaneous toxicity*. New York: Academic Press; 1980:25–40.
21. Basketter DA, Goodwin BFJ. Investigation of the prohapten concept. *Contact Dermatitis* 1988; 19:248–253.
22. Barratt MD, Basketter DA. Possible origin of the skin sensitization potential of isoeugenol and related compounds. *Contact Dermatitis* 1992;27:98–104.

23. Lindup WE, Nowell PT. Role of sultone contaminants in an outbreak of allergic contact dermatitis caused by alkyl ethoxysulphates: a review. *Food Chem Toxicol* 1978;16:59–62.
24. Andersen KE, Boman A, Hamann K, Wahlberg KE. Guinea pig maximisation tests with formaldehyde releases: results from two laboratories. *Contact Dermatitis* 1984;10:257–266.
25. Robinson MK, Nusair TL, Fletcher ER, Ritz HL. A review of the Buehler guinea pig skin sensitization test and its use in a risk assessment process for human skin sensitization. *Toxicology* 1990; 61:91–107.
26. EEC Commission Directive of 25 April 1984 amending for the sixth time Directive 67/548/EEC on the approximation of the laws, regulations and administrative provisions relating to the classification, packaging and labelling of dangerous substances (Annex V). *Off J Eur Comm* 1984;L257:27:1.
27. Buehler EV. Comment on guinea pig test methods. *Food Chem Toxicol* 1982;20:494.
28. Basketter DA, Selbie E, Scholes EW, Lees D, Kimber I, Botham PA. Results with OECD recommended positive control sensitizers in the maximisation, Buehler and local lymph node assays. *Food Chem Toxicol* 1993;31:63–67.
29. EEC Commission Directive of 29 July 1983 adapting to technical progress for the fifth time Directive 67/548/EEC on the approximation of the laws, regulations and administrative provisions relating to the classification, packaging and labelling of dangerous substances (Annex V). *Off J Eur Comm* 1983;L257:1.
30. Goodwin BFJ, Crevel RWR, Johnson AW. A comparison of 3 guinea pig sensitization procedures for the detection of 19 reported human contact sensitizers. *Contact Dermatitis* 1981;7:248–258.
31. Holdiness MR. A review of contact dermatitis associated with transdermal therapeutic systems. *Contact Dermatitis* 1989;20:3–9.
32. Basketter DA, Scholes EW, Cumberbatch M, Evans CD, Kimber I. Sulphanilic acid: divergent results in the guinea pig maximization test and the local lymph node assay. *Contact Dermatitis* 1992;27:209–213.
33. Magnusson B. The relevance of results obtained with the guinea pig maximisation test. In: Maibach HI, ed. *Animal models in dermatology*. Edinburgh: Churchill Livingstone; 1975:76–83.
34. Buehler EV. A rationale for the selection of occlusion to induce and elicit delayed contact hypersensitivity in the guinea pig. In: Andersen KE, Maibach HI, eds. *Current problems in dermatology, vol 14. Contact allergy predictive tests in guinea pigs*. Basel: Karger; 1985:39–58.
35. Wahlberg JE, Fregert S. Guinea pig maximization test. In: Maibach HI, NJ Lowe, eds. *Models in dermatology*, vol 2. Basel: Karger; 1985:225–233.
36. Kimber I, Mitchell JA, Griffin AC. Development of a murine local lymph node assay for the determination of sensitization potential. *Food Chem Toxicol* 1986;24:585–586.
37. Kimber I, Hilton J, Botham PA. Identification of contact allergens using the murine local lymph node assay: comparisons with the Buehler occluded patch test in guinea pigs. *J Appl Toxicol* 1990;10:173–180.
38. Basketter DA, Scholes EW. A comparison of the local lymph node assay with the guinea pig maximisation test for the detection of a range of contact allergens. *Food Chem Toxicol* 1992;30:63–67.
39. Kimber I, Basketter DA. The murine local lymph node assay: a commentary on collaborative studies and new directions. *Food Chem Toxicol* 1992;30:165–169.

Immunotoxicology and Immunopharmacology, Second Edition, edited by J. H. Dean, M. I. Luster, A. E. Munson, and I. Kimber.
Raven Press, Ltd., New York © 1994.

41

Guinea Pig Predictive Tests for Respiratory Allergy

Katherine Sarlo and *Meryl H. Karol

*Procter & Gamble, Cincinnati Ohio 45239; and *Department of Environmental and Occupational Health, University of Pittsburgh, Pittsburgh, Pennsylvania 15238*

Allergic responses are adverse physiologic events that can be mediated by a variety of immunologic mechanisms. Respiratory allergic responses can also be rooted in several immunologic mechanisms although the immunoglobulin E (IgE) allergic antibody-mediated reactions are common responses to a variety of inhaled materials. Respiratory allergic responses can be associated with upper respiratory reactions (i.e., rhinitis and conjunctivitis) or more serious, potentially life-threatening asthmatic or anaphylactic responses. In the workplace, the prevalence of occupational asthma has been reported to range from 2% to 15% of the adult workforce and this condition has become one of the major causes of work-induced respiratory disability (these prevalence rates include immunologic and nonimmunologic causes of occupational asthma) (1).

Allergic respiratory responses can be classified as either *early* or *late onset*, depending on the time of onset after exposure to specific allergen. Clinically, these responses are identified by a decrease in forced expiratory volume in 1 sec (FEV_1). The early onset or immediate onset reactions occur within minutes to 1 hr after exposure to allergen. The late onset reactions occur hours after the initial exposure to allergen. Those individuals that experience both immediate and late onset reactions are said to have a *dual* response. The late onset reactions are most frequently observed in response to low molecular weight (LMW) chemical allergens as opposed to high molecular weight (HMW) allergens.

Immunologically mediated occupational asthmatic responses have been shown to be induced by a variety of agents. These agents can be HMW compounds (i.e., proteins) or LMW chemicals. LMW chemicals have broadly been classified as chemicals with MW<1000 daltons. Some of the HMW compounds associated with occupational allergic asthma (and other respiratory symptoms) include proteins derived from animal saliva and fur (e.g., laboratory animals), insect exoskeletons (e.g., cockroach and grain mite), proteins derived from plant materials (e.g., coffee bean and wheat), and enzymes derived from bacterial organisms (e.g., subtilisin and papain) (1). Some of the LMW compounds that have been associated with allergic respiratory reactions include isocyanates (e.g., toluene diisocyanate), anhydrides (e.g., trimellitic anhydride), transition metals (e.g., platinum salt), and certain pharmaceutical agents (e.g., cephalosporin) (1). LMW chemicals are generally too small to be recognized independently as foreign by the immune system. Rather, when these chemicals bind (haptenate) to a larger molecule (i.e., carrier protein), the chemical–carrier conjugate can be immunogenic and stimulate an antibody response. In addition, other as yet undefined mechanisms may be involved in asthmatic responses to inhaled chemicals since some individuals with clinical symptoms do not exhibit an allergic antibody response to the chemical. Therefore it can be difficult to diagnose immune-mediated respiratory allergic responses caused by LMW chemicals.

A variety of animal models have been developed to study immune-mediated respiratory reactions to foreign antigens. However, very few models have been developed as predictive tests for use in hazard identification and risk assessment in the area of respiratory allergy. This chapter focuses on those few guinea pig models that can be used by the toxicologist as predictive tests for respiratory allergy. In this chapter, we review the models, provide a critical assessment of the advantages and disadvantages of the models, as well as describe approaches for using these models in hazard identification and risk assessment.

CLINICAL DATABASE

To evaluate the validity of an animal model, it must be compared with the data obtained from clinical studies. Ideally, the clinical database would contain the following information:

A detailed history of individual exposure to the allergen including dates and lengths of exposure, as well as quantities involved.

The health status of the patient including indication and verification of atopy and smoking status.

Assessment of pulmonary function (FEV_1 and peak flow values) at the workplace, as well as away from work.

Evaluation of airway hyperreactivity.

Results of inhalation provocation challenge.

Determination of total and allergen-specific IgE and IgG.

Bronchial biopsy or bronchoalveolar lavage (BAL).

Whereas the above is the ideal situation, typically much less information is available for individual patients. Nevertheless, clinical studies have provided some information related to potencies and dose–response relationships of allergens, effects of chronic low-dose exposures, identification of populations susceptible to sensitization, and risk associated with continued exposure of skin test positive and radioallergosorbent test (RAST) positive individuals.

Clinical studies of sensitization have addressed the issue of dose dependency of sensitization to both HMW and LMW allergens. Using skin prick test results as an indication of sensitization, Juniper et al. (2) found the incidence of sensitization to detergent enzymes diminished as workplace atmospheric levels of the dust decreased. A similar finding was reported by Flood et al. (3). Regarding LMW allergens, Karol (4) detected IgE antibodies to toluene diisocyanate (TDI) only in workers who had reported accidental exposures or spills. Butcher et al. (5) found a correlation of skin test and RAST positivity with increasing exposure to TDI.

The influence of chronic low-dose exposure on development of sensitization has also been investigated for both classes of allergens. Juniper et al. (2) found that the conversions to skin test positivity typically occurred by 20 months of employment for both high- and low-exposure groups. Flood et al. (3) observed that reduction in dust levels coincided with a decreased conversioin rate and the time to conversion depended on the dust level. Regarding LMW allergens, Butcher et al. (5) found that sensitization to TDI, as evidenced by pulmonary responsiveness, usually became apparent during the first year of exposure; Venables et al. (6) noted that symptoms of TDI sensitization usually appeared in less than 3 years.

The epidemiologic studies have provided information related to characteristics of susceptible populations. Smoking may play a role in susceptibility to sensitization by pulmonary allergens. There appears to be increased susceptibility of atopic individuals to sensitization by HMW allergens, but not by those with LMW (2–5). Evidence supporting this conclusion has been obtained for numerous HMW and LMW allergens (1) and suggests a difference in mechanism of sensitization between the two types of allergens.

In spite of valuable information related to sensitization provided by epidemiologic studies, two questions vital to risk assessment remain unanswered: (a) What is the contribution of low-dose exposures and peak exposures to sensitization? (b) Which is the most relevant route of exposure to induce sensitization to LMW allergens? Validated (and calibrated) animal models may be ideal for addressing such issues.

GUINEA PIG AS AN ANIMAL MODEL

The guinea pig has been used for 90 years for study of anaphylactic shock (7) and for more than 70 years as a model for pulmonary hypersensitivity (8). It has been used for investigation of the pulmonary physiologic response as well as the immunologic response. Through passive immunization procedures, it has provided mechanistic information proving the ability of sensitizing antibodies to initiate immediate onset responses and, very recently, to induce pulmonary eosinophilic inflammation (9).

There are major benefits to the use of the guinea pig for study of hypersensitivity. The guinea pig is similar to humans in that the lung is the major shock organ for anaphylactic response to antigens; also, the animal responds to histamine, demonstrates both immediate and late onset types of allergic reactions, demonstrates neutrophil influx in late phase reactions and demonstrates eosinophilic inflammation and airway hyperactivity as a result of the allergic reaction (9–11). In addition, the animal is docile, relatively small, and comparatively inexpensive.

As with all models, there are disadvantages to its use. A disadvantage that severely limits the use of guinea pigs in mechanistic studies is the existence of only a few inbred strains. This shortcoming has resulted in a sparsity of reagents available to identify inflammatory cells through surface markers and is a major hindrance to mechanistic studies of asthma in this species. In addition, IgG1 is the major hypersensitivity antibody in the guinea pig; whereas in humans and several other rodent species, IgE is the prominent class of cytophilic antibody. Due to the lack of specific reagents for IgG1, it is difficult to use *in vitro* serologic assays to measure this antibody. Rather, the *in vivo* passive cutaneous anaphylaxis test is used to detect guinea pig allergic antibody.

In spite of these shortcomings, guinea pigs have been found to respond reproducibly to chemicals found to be allergenic in humans with appropriate histopathalogic changes and allergic manifestations. Its use in studies with TDI has led to recognition of the dose dependency of sensitization, when exposure occurs via inhalation of a chemical (12), and it appears suitable for investigations of mechanisms and treatments of asthma.

GUINEA PIG MODELS USED TO EVALUATE CHEMICALS AND PROTEINS AS RESPIRATORY ALLERGENS

In current guinea pig models for respiratory allergy, there are two major parameters that are measured as indicators of immunologic and pulmonary sensitivity to inhaled allergen: the presence of specific allergic antibody as a measure of immunologic sensitization to the allergen and the presence of pulmonary reactivity. Pulmonary reactivity or sensitivity can be detected by relatively simply methods (i.e., visual scoring of labored breathing) (13) to more complicated methods (i.e., whole-body plethysmography, which detects changes in respiratory rate, tidal volume, and plethysmograph pressure) (11,14). Pulmonary sensitivity can be manifested as immediate onset reactions and/or late onset reactions. In guinea pigs, elevation of body core temperature has been used as an additional measure to detect late onset pulmonary responses (15). For chemicals, detection of pulmonary sensitivity can be very important to the risk assessment process since mechanisms other than antibody-dependent reactions (i.e., lymphocyte directed) may play a role in allergic responses to inhaled chemicals. Therefore the development of an animal model that will display the late onset reaction is essential to the identification and assessment of risk associated with exposure to chemical allergens.

Proteins

Several routes can be used to sensitize guinea pigs to allergenic proteins. Two methods are currently available that utilize the respiratory tract as the route of exposure: inhalation and intratracheal instillation (13). No standard protocol exists for evaluating proteins as allergens via inhalation exposure although investigators have used variations of a protocol developed by Karol et al. (16) to sensitize guinea pigs. In this model, guinea pigs are exposed to protein aerosol for 10 min/d for 5 consecutive days. The animals receive no exposure on days 6 to 10 but are exposed to the same protein aerosol for 10 min/d on day 11 and onward. The first 5 days of exposure serve as the sensitization phase; whereas days 11 onward serve as the elicitation phase. Serum from each animal is collected at selected time intervals and analyzed for protein-specific antibody. If the animal is immunologically sensitized, allergic antibody to the protein will be present. If the animal possesses pulmonary sensitivity, immediate onset respiratory reactions can be elicited upon respiratory challenge with the protein aerosol. In some instances, late onset pulmonary reactions can also be elicited upon challenge with protein aerosol.

A modification of this protocol was successfully used by Thorne et al. (17) and Hillibrand, et al. (18) to sensitize guinea pigs to the occupational allergen subtilisin. Pulmonary sensitivity was detected in animals initially exposed to 150 μg subtilisin protein/m^3 for 15 min/d for 5 consecutive days. Both immediate and late onset reactions were reported. Animals initially exposed to 8 or 41 μg/m^3 subtilisin aerosol did not exhibit pulmonary sensitivity. However, specific antibody was detected in sera from animals exposed to these lower levels of subtilisin aerosol. Therefore immunologic sensitization to an occupational allergen can occur at exposure levels lower than those required for pulmonary sensitivity. As will be discussed later, such information is important to the risk assessment process since measures to prevent immunologic sensitization may be different from those measures needed to prevent pulmonary sensitivity.

In the guinea pig intratracheal model developed by Ritz et al. (13), animals are intratracheally dosed once per week for 10 consecutive weeks with protein allergen. After each weekly dose, they are observed for signs of immediate onset pulmonary sensitivity. The severity of the pulmonary response is scored by counting the number of normal respirations between diaphramatic contractions or spasms; the more severe the response, the fewer the number of normal respirations. Figure 1 shows tracings of normal respirations and diaphramatic spasms associated with immediate onset pulmonary responses. At selected times, sera are collected for measurement of allergic antibody titers to the protein. The model was developed using subtilisin as the model protein allergen since a threshold limit value (TLV) had been established for this material (19). In addition, a wealth of human data regarding the allergic response to this allergen in the exposed workforce provided a basis for comparing the responses of humans to the responses of the animal model.

The dose-dependent antibody response to subtilisin was found to be comparable in animals exposed via intratracheal instillation versus those exposed via inhalation (13). Such data suggest that instillation is an acceptable alternative for delivering antigen to the respiratory tract. The sensitivity of this model was suggested by observation of immunologic sensitization in animals after receipt of three doses of 100 ng of subtilisin protein. The intratracheal model has been used to compare new enzyme allergens with subtilisin for allergenic potency (20). Using antibody titer to

A

B

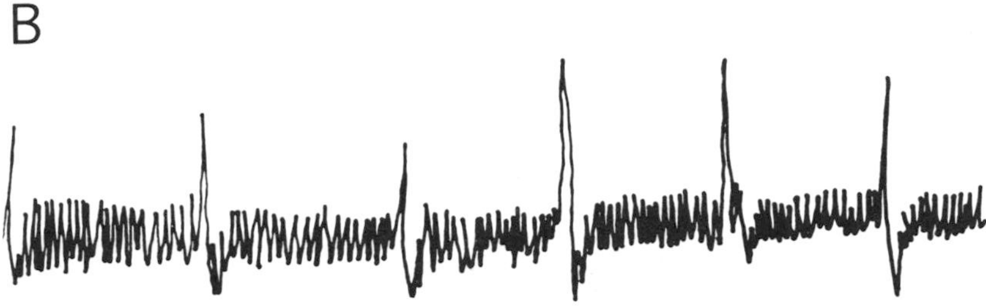

FIG. 1. Tracings of the respiratory pattern of guinea pigs with normal respirations (**A**) or with diaphramatic contractions associated with antigen-induced immediate onset pulmonary symptoms (**B**).

indicate sensitization, enzymes were found to differ in allergenic potency. Information of this type can be used for risk assessment, since these potency factors, together with the TLV for subtilisin, can be used to establish exposure guidelines for the new enzyme.

Low Molecular Weight Chemicals

Sensitization of guinea pigs to LMW chemicals is more difficult to detect compared with proteins since chemical–carrier conjugates are generally needed to measure immunologic sensitivity. It is the authors' experience that use of a homologous protein (i.e., guinea pig serum albumin) as the carrier molecule improves the serologic assays for detecting specific antibody to the chemical. A guinea pig inhalation model developed by Karol (12) has been used to examine the immunologic and pulmonary responses to TDI. This models has been adapted to evaluate responses to other chemical sensitizers. In this model, guinea pigs are housed in whole-body plethysmographs and exposed to chemical atmosphere for 3 hr/d for 5 consecutive days. The animals receive no exposure from days 6 to 21 but are exposed to chemical or chemical–carrier conjugate aerosols on day 22 onward to determine pulmonary sensitivity. Serum is collected from each animal at selected time points to measure antibody to the chemical. Investigators have used this model to examine immunologic and pulmonary sensitivity to chemicals such as TDI (12,14,22,23),

TABLE 1. *Sensitization following inhalation of low molecular weight allergenic chemicals*

Chemical (reference)	Exposure concentration	Antibody PCA	Antibody ELISA	Pulmonary sensitivity
TDI (12)	0.36 ppm	+	ND	+
	0.96 ppm	+	ND	+
	4.7 ppm	+	ND	−
TDI (22)	1.0 ppm	+	+	+
Des-N (14)	2.7 mg/m^3	ND	−	−
	9.5 mg/m^3	ND	−	−
TMA (22)	2.1 mg/m^3	−	+	−
	14.2 mg/m^3	+	+	−
	108.9 mg/m^3	+	+	−
TMA (14)	2.6 mg/m^3	ND	+	+
	62.4 mg/m^3	ND	+	+
PA (24)	0.5 mg/m^3	+	+	+
PA (23)	0.05–0.2 mg/m^3	−	−	−
	0.6–6.0 mg/m^3	+	+	+
Black B dye (23)	5.0 mg/m^3	−	−	−
	10.0 mg/m^3	+	+	−
	100 mg/m^3	+	+	−
Yellow mx4r (22)	1.47 mg/m^3	−	+	−
	94.0 mg/m^3	+	+	−

PCA, passive cutaneous anaphylaxis; ELISA, enzyme-linked immunoadsorbent assay; ND, not determined.

diphenylmethane diisocyanate (MDI) (21), trimeric hexamethylene diisocyanate (Des-N) (14), trimellitic anhydride (TMA) (14,22), phthalic anhydride (PA) (23), reactive black B dye (23), and procion yellow mx4r (22).

Pulmonary sensitivity, displayed as immediate onset and/or delayed onset responses, was detected in animals exposed to the isocyanates and the anhydrides and challenged with the appropriate chemical–protein conjugate. No pulmonary sensitivity was evident in the animals exposed to the dyes. Pulmonary sensitivity, elicited by challenge with the chemical alone, could only be demonstrated with TDI, MDI, and TMA. Immunologic sensitivity was detected to all the chemicals.

Table 1 summarizes data generated in four laboraties regarding initial exposure concentrations required to induce immunologic or pulmonary sensitivity to six different chemicals (12,14,21–24). In this summary, pulmonary sensitivity is defined as immediate onset responses elicited by chemical–carrier conjugate challenge. Although not indicated in the table, as the exposure concentration to the chemicals increased, the amount of detectable antibody also increased. For each of the chemicals tested by the different investigators, the presence of antibody and the antibody titer was not sufficient to predict pulmonary sensitivity. Animals with pulmonary sensitivity had antibody to the chemical but not every animal with antibody experienced pulmonary sensitivity when challenged either with the chemical alone or the chemical–protein conjugate. This relationship between antibody and pulmonary sensitivity is similar to that observed in the workplace with subtilisin exposure. In

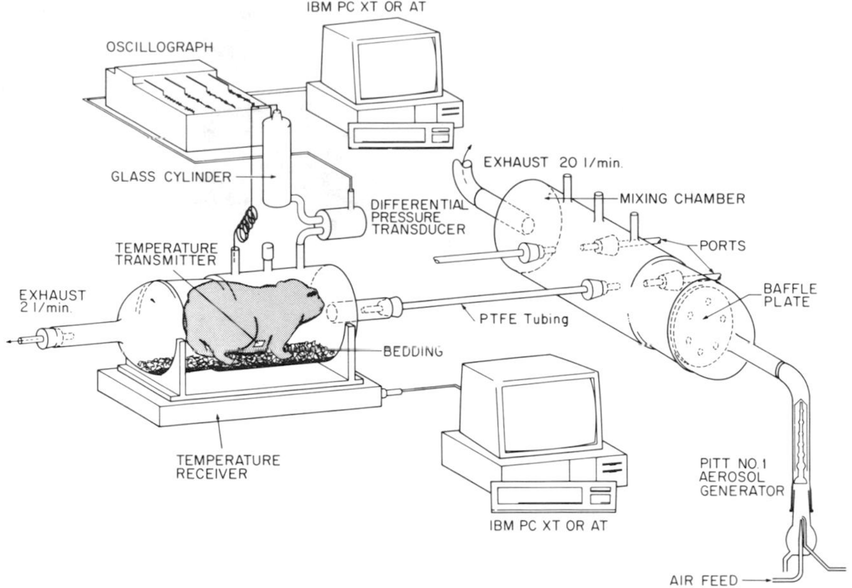

FIG. 2. Whole-body plethysmograph used for long-term passive monitoring of guinea pig respiratory rate and body temperature during and after inhalation exposure to antigen aerosol.

addition, like the subtilisin experience, immunologic sensitization to LMW chemical sensitizers as defined by hypersensitivity antibody can occur at exposure levels lower than those required to establish pulmonary sensitivity. In addition, certain chemicals (i.e., dyes) induced an antibody response in guinea pigs with no manifestation of pulmonary sensitivity to inhalation challenge with conjugate or free chemical. Therefore the role of antibody in pulmonary sensitivity is not fully understood.

Occupational asthma to LMW chemicals can be manifested as isolated late onset pulmonary reactions. The late onset reaction is believed to be rooted in an inflammatory response in the airways (25,26). It is not clear if this inflammatory response is dependent on antibody or other, as yet undefined, immunologic responses to the inhaled chemical. It is known that neurogenic mediators and viruses can trigger airway inflammation and asthma. Therefore the recognition of late onset and immediate onset pulmonary reactions in the guinea pig can be important to the assessment process since non-antibody-mediated mechanisms may be involved.

The characteristic feature of the late onset reaction is the gradual onset and recovery from symptoms. This characteristic, coupled with a variable time of onset of the response following exposure to the allergen, necessitates use of a passive monitoring system such as whole-body plethysmographs with dynamic airflow (Fig. 2) (27). Animals can be housed and continuously monitored for up to 20 hr after allergen exposure. Changes in breathing pattern, notably an increase in breathing frequency and a decrease in volume, are indicative of a late onset reaction. More detailed measures of changes in pulmonary function (i.e., changes in resistance) can be made during this time period by placing animals in head-only chambers with pneumotachographs for measurement of airflow. In addition, a febrile response (detected by monitoring radio transmitters implanted into the peritoneal cavity) is associated with the change in breathing pattern.

This model has been used successfully to detect late onset reactions in guinea pigs sensitized to ovalbumin (27) as well as MDI (21). For the ovalbumin-sensitized animals, 100% experienced immediate onset reactions, and half of these animals displayed late onset reactions. The occurrence of late onset reactions could not be predicted by the severity or kinetics of the immediate onset reaction. For the MDI sensitized animals, the late onset reaction was the typical pulmonary response upon challenge with the chemical. This is consistent with human pulmonary responses to MDI.

Several investigators have developed guinea pig injection models to examine the immunologic and respiratory responses to injected chemical. In two of these models, guinea pigs received either one or three intradermal injections of the highest tolerated dose of chemical (TMA or Des-N) (14,28). This was followed by serology approximately 2 weeks after the injection and inhalation challenge with free chemical or chemical conjugate a few days after serum collection. This regimen was successful in inducing allergic antibody to TMA and Des-N. Moderate to severe bronchoconstriction was elicited by inhalation challenge with high concentrations of free TMA (about 45 mg/m^3). Both of these injection models were successful in establishing conditions for elicitation of respiratory reactions upon challenge with free TMA. In a third injection model, guinea pigs were subcutaneously injected with several low doses of free chemical over a period of 4 weeks (induction doses), received a boost injection at week 6, and were evaluated for circulating antibody, tissue-fixed antibody, and respiratory reactivity to the chemical at week 8 (23). Table 2 summarizes the data generated for six chemicals: TDI, PA, reactive black B dye, MDI, and hexachloroplatinic acid (Pt). Dose–response relationships were observed between the induction doses of chemical and antibody titers or respiratory reactivity; the relationship was not the same for all the chemicals. For example, the greatest number of animals experiencing respiratory reactions upon challenge with chemical–conjugate was not always associated with the highest induction dose. In addition, for TDI, the greatest number of animals responding with immediate onset respiratory reactions did not correlate with the dose of chemical that induced the highest titers of IgG and IgG1 antibody. However, for PA, groups of animals with the highest allergic antibody titers were those that contained the greatest number of respiratory reactors. Therefore examination of dose–response relationships in injection models is as important as examination of these relationships in inhalation models.

TABLE 2. *Sensitization following subcutaneous injection of low molecular weight allergenic chemicals*

Chemical	Respiratory reactivity	Skin test reactivity[a]	Mean ELISA titer (SE)	Mean PCA titer (SE)
TDI[b]				
6.7×10^{-3} M	20%	100%	8960 (2200)	645 (106)
6.7×10^{-4} M	60%	90%	7800 (2050)	900 (350)
6.7×10^{-5} M	80%	100%	980 (150)	30 (10)
MDI				
6.7×10^{-3} M	80%	100%	220 (80)	79 (51)
6.7×10^{-4} M	40%	100%	170 (70)	5 (2)
6.7×10^{-5} M	60%	75%	40 (19)	5 (2)
PA[b]				
6.7×10^{-3} M	60%	80%	15360 (955)	220 (80)
6.7×10^{-4} M	90%	100%	4480 (1016)	1972 (522)
6.7×10^{-5} M	80%	100%	1040 (96)	313 (75)
TMA				
6.7×10^{-3} M	ND[c]	100%	10400 (3481)	1304 (480)
6.7×10^{-4} M	ND	100%	2400 (599)	336 (107)
6.7×10^{-5} M	ND	76%	287 (87)	64 (19)
Dye[b]				
6.7×10^{-3} M	0%	100%	170 (25)	0
6.7×10^{-4} M	0%	90%	500 (102)	0
6.7×10^{-5} M	0%	100%	460 (150)	30 (12)
Pt salt				
6.7×10^{-3} M	0%	63%	63%[d]	0
6.7×10^{-4} M	0%	88%	38%	0
6.7×10^{-5} M	0%	38%	25%	0
Controls	0%	0%	Negative	Negative

[a]Active cutaneous anaphylaxis for tissue-fixed allergic antibody.
[b]Data published in ref. 23.
[c]ND, not determined.
[d]Percentage of animals with IgG antibody in one-half dilution of serum.

ADVANTAGES AND DISADVANTAGES OF CURRENT GUINEA PIG MODELS

Table 3 summarizes the major advantages and disadvantages of the guinea pig models described previously. The guinea pig inhalation and intratracheal models for protein sensitization deliver the antigen to the relevant target organ, the respiratory tract. This is advantageous, since, for humans, the major route of exposure to occupational allergenic proteins, and likely for chemicals, is via the respiratory tract. This allows extrapolation of exposure data from the guinea pig models to the human situation. Both models allow the investigator to determine dose–response relationships between exposure and antibody response as well as pulmonary reactivity. The inhalation model has the added advantage of being able to detect late onset pulmonary responses. A disadvantage of the inhalation model is the need for specialized and expensive equipment for generation and monitoring of exposure atmospheres and detecting pulmonary reactivity. This can limit the number of doses that can be

TABLE 3. *Major advantages and disadvantages of guinea pig predictive models of allergy*

Model	Advantage	Disadvantage
Proteins		
Inhalation	Deliver antigen to respiratory tract Evaluate dose–response relationships Detect immediate and late onset pulmonary reactions	Expensive, time intensive Limited group sizes Need for specialized facilities and/or equipment
Intratracheal	Deliver antigen to respiratory tract Evaluate dose–response relationships Inexpensive, fast, no need for specialized facilities or equipment Can evaluate more than one compound at several doses	Bolus dose of antigen Cannot detect late onset pulmonary reactions
Chemicals		
Inhalation	Deliver chemical to respiratory tract; also skin exposure Evaluate dose–response relationships Detect immediate and late onset pulmonary reactions	Expensive, time and labor intensive Need for specialized facilities and/or equipment Need conjugate for serology Limited success of elicitation with free chemical Limited doses and group size
Intradermal injection	Induce antibody after one to three injections of free chemical Elicit pulmonary reactions via inhalation of free chemical	Cannot evaluate dose–response relationships Need specialized equipment and/or facilities Need conjugate for serology Only two chemicals tested; no standard doses for comparative purposes
Subcutaneous injection	Induce antibody after injection of free chemical Evaluate dose–response relationships Inexpensive, fast Six chemicals tested at equal molar doses for comparative purposes	Need conjugate for serology, pulmonary reactivity No elicitation of pulmonary reactions with free chemical

evaluated as well as increase the costs and time involved to conduct a study. The intratracheal model bypasses the need for sophisticated equipment, requiring only a restraining device and a lighted dosing needle. This allows for evaluation of both a greater number of animals and doses over the same period of time. The disadvantage to the intratracheal model is that the antigen is delivered at the tracheal bifurcation, bypassing the upper respiratory tract (i.e., nares). Also, the intratracheal model only detects immediate onset pulmonary responses. It has been suggested that intratracheal deposition of challenge antigen may cause some irritation that may interfere with the recognition of the pulmonary response. However, the moderate-to-strong allergic pulmonary reactions are clearly recognizable. The technique may only interfere with the detection of mild allergic pulmonary reactions. These disadvantages may not be significant since studies have indicated comparative antibody responses and pulmonary reactivity in animals exposed to subtilisin via the intratracheal and the inhalation route. A limitation of both models is the small number of proteins that have been evaluated as occupational allergens; mostly these are the detergent enzymes.

In the case of LMW chemicals, a major disadvantage common to all the models is the need for a chemical–carrier conjugate for serologic evaluation and, in some instances, evaluation of pulmonary sensitivity. Although serum albumin appears to be an adequate carrier protein for most of the chemicals evaluated in the animal models, other carrier proteins may be more relevant. For example, the very low antibody titers and lack of pulmonary reactivity in animals injected with the potent human allergen hexachloroplatinate may have been due to the inadequacy of serum albumin as the carrier protein for platinum. Chemical–carrier conjugates used in animal models must be characterized for hapten content, thereby requiring analytic techniques. The degree of haptenation of the protein by the chemical can alter the results of serologic assays. In addition, conjugates of the same chemical and protein (i.e., TDI and guinea pig albumin) prepared in the same manner by different laboratories have detected different titers of antibody in the same serum samples (22). Therefore preparation and standardization of chemical–protein conjugates can be viewed as a disadvantage for models of sensitization to LMW chemicals.

The advantages and disadvantages of the guinea pig inhalation model of evaluating LMW chemicals are similar to those described for proteins. In the inhalation model, the chemical antigen is delivered to the relevant target organ, the respiratory tract. In addition, since exposure of animals to the chemical is via whole-body exposure, there is skin contact with the chemical. It has been proposed that, for LMW chemical antigens, skin contact may play a role in respiratory sensitization (29; I Kimber, *personal communication*). A disadvantage to the inhalation model is the need for specialized equipment and facilities (e.g., negative-pressure rooms and modified fume hoods). Again, this limits the number of animals and doses that can be evaluated in a study as well as increases the cost and time involved to conduct a study. It has been estimated that the cost for conducting an inhalation study for one chemical at three concentrations at a not-for-profit laboratory is approximately $250,000.

The major advantage of the guinea pig inhalation model is the ability to evaluate late onset reactions. Similar to the human experience, isolated immediate onset reactions, isolated late onset reactions, and dual reactions can be elicited in this model. However, the model is still under development. Therefore its use as a predictive test is not clear. Currently, numerous endpoints are used to confirm the late onset reaction (i.e., breathing pattern, fever, pulmonary histopathology, BAL, and assessment of airway hyperreactivity). It is not clear which one of these endpoints will be most useful in a predictive test. In addition, only a limited number of materials have been evaluated in the model. A significant problem with the model results from the irritant properties of most chemical allergens. Since late onset reactions must be elicited via inhalation challenge with the chemical, the irritant properties of the material can cause a dose-dependent late onset alteration in breathing pattern that can be confused with a true late onset reaction. Therefore subirritant concentrations of chemical allergens must be identified by performing preliminary studies in naive animals with extended periods of monitoring for a response. These concentrations are then used for challenge.

The injection models developed for evaluating chemicals as allergens have the advantage of being technically simple to execute and less costly and time consuming than the inhalation model and lend themselves to standardization in several laboratories. In these models, one can quickly evaluate whether a chemical has the potential to form immunogenic and allergenic conjugates *in vivo* and stimulate a measurable antibody response. However, since delivery of the antigen is not via the respiratory tract, extrapolation of results obtained from injection models to respiratory exposure and development of allergic responses is limited. This can be remedied by conducting a limited number of comparative experiments using the inhalation and injection models to determine whether or not such extrapolations can be made (23). In the subcutaneous injection model, the dose–response (antibody titer) relationships can be evaluated for a particular chemical as well as for a series of chemicals since the doses can be standardized for comparative purposes. In the intradermal injection models, dose–response relationships cannot be evaluated since the animals receive one to three injections of the highest tolerated dose of chemical. However, in these models, elicitation of pulmonary sensitivity can be achieved by inhalation exposure with free chemical.

The exposure concentration of free chemical to elicit pulmonary responses in the guinea pig is much higher than that recognized to elicit responses in humans. No proposal has been made to extrapolate eliciting doses in the guinea pig to those required in the human. In addition, the data generated from the subcutaneous model indicate that elicitation (i.e., number of responding animals) cannot be predicted from the induction dose. For example, the highest injected dose of TDI yielded animals with the fewest pulmonary responses upon challenge with conjugate. Since the intradermal model uses the highest tolerated dose for induction, dose–response relationships for elicitation may also be missed in this model. Only two chemicals have been evaluated in the intradermal model. Other types of chemical allergens have not been tested in this model and whether the induction regimen is adequate for detecting sensitivity to a variety of chemicals has yet to be determined. Six chemicals, representing four different classes of chemical sensitizers (isocyanates, anhydrides, dye, and transition metal) have been evaluated in the subcutaneous injection model. Further testing of both models is needed using a variety of known human chemical allergens to determine the sensitivity and applicability of these models as predictive tests for respiratory allergy.

USING GUINEA PIG MODELS IN HAZARD IDENTIFICATION AND RISK ASSESSMENT

The guinea pig models described earlier have been used in both hazard identification and in risk assessment. For respiratory allergens, whether of HMW materials, such as proteins, or of LMW materials (i.e., chemicals), the induction of specific allergic antibody identifies the material as a hazard, that is, an allergen. Dose–response relationships between antibody and exposure and/or respiratory symptoms and exposure can be obtained from the guinea pig models and used for risk assessment. A considerable amount of information is available in the literature on human respiratory responses to occupational allergens. This information includes antibody responses, symptomatology and some exposure data. Incidence rates and prevalence rates can be determined from cross-sectional and longitudinal surveys. Exposure levels needed to elicit respiratory reactions can be determined by air monitoring at work or by controlled bronchial provocation tests. For certain known occupational respiratory allergens (e.g., subtilisin and TMA), TLVs have been established to protect a naive workforce from sensitization and an already exposed workforce from elicitation (19,30). Therefore evaluating the guinea pig models using allergens that have a supporting database in humans as well as recommended TLVs renders these models valuable for risk identification and assessment of new, potentially allergenic, materials.

For hazard identification, it is important to have methods that allow rapid identification of the potential allergenicity of a protein or LMW chemical. Models for hazard identification of protein allergens have not been described nor have structure–activity studies been reported. Until then, one assumes that respiratory exposure to amounts of a foreign protein can allergically sensitize some proportion of the exposed population. Therefore it is advisable to evaluate proteins as possible allergens in models developed for risk assessment (i.e., guinea pig intratracheal test). For LMW chemicals, hazard identification can involve structure–activity evaluation, protein or peptide binding, and the *in vivo* guinea pig injection models (14,23,28,31–33). The ability of injected free chemical to induce the formation of specific antibody indicates that the chemical has the ability to be immunogenic; the formation of allergic antibody suggests potential allergenicity. The ability to elicit pulmonary symptoms in the injection models may not be essential to hazard identification, since antibodies can be used to identify a chemical as a potential allergen. For example, reactive black B dye is a documented LMW chemical allergen and asthmagen in humans (34). Specific allergic antibody responses were obtained in the subcutaneous injection model and the inhalation model, yet pulmonary symptoms could not be elicited upon challenge with free chemical or chemical–protein conjugate. Therefore reliance on symptomatology to identify a chemical as a potential allergenic hazard can be misleading.

Four components are involved in risk assessment for respiratory allergens: (a) source assessment (what activity generates the exposure to the respiratory allergen), (b) exposure assessment (estimate or quantitate the concentration of allergen to which individuals can be exposed), (c) dose–response assessment (examine the relationship between allergen exposure and antibody production or pulmonary sensitivity), and (d) risk characterization (estimate the relative risk of sensitization to an allergen in a population or subpopulation of exposed individuals) (35). Information generated from the guinea pig models can be used in the dose–response assessment and, in some cases, the exposure assessment process. Identification of standard benchmark allergens for which there is epidemiologic data (i.e., exposure, sensitization rates, and pulmonary sensitivity) is critical for calibration of data from the guinea pig models to the human response. For example, subtilisin is a known human occupational allergen. A reasonable amount of information exists on human allergic responses to this allergen (2,3,36). In addition, the American Conference of Industrial and Government Hygienists (ACGIH) have set a TLV for subtilisin as 60 ng protein/m^3 to minimize sensitization of naive workers and elicitation of symptoms in the sensitized workforce. By comparing dose responses (antibody titers, pulmonary reactivity data) of guinea pigs exposed to a new protein to those responses generated to subtilisin, one can estimate the relative allergenic potency of the new protein for humans. The guinea pig intratracheal test has been used to compare antibody titers generated to a new enzyme with those produced to subtilisin to estimate the allergenic potency of the new enzyme (20). By using analogous information on human responses to known exposure levels of subtilisin, one can determine the potency factors for the new enzyme from the guinea pig model to establish exposure guidelines for the new enzyme. This process can be visualized by the diagram in Fig. 3. Confirmation of the adequacy of the exposure guideline for the new enzyme must be in humans. Confirmation in humans further supports the guinea pig model and builds confidence in the risk assessment process.

The value of antibody data when performing a risk assessment for chemical allergenicity must be stressed. For example, in the guinea pig inhalation study conducted by Thorne et al. (17) and Hillebrand et al. (18), guinea pigs exposed to 8 or 41 μg subtilisin protein/m^3 produced specific antibody but did not experience pulmonary reactivity upon challenge. Similarly, it has been noted that humans exposed to low levels of subtilisin can generate allergic antibody without expressing allergic symptoms (37). Therefore immunologic sensitization to an occupational allergen appears to occur at exposure levels lower than those required to initially elicit pulmonary sensitivity responses. This information is important in the assessment process since measures to prevent immunologic sensitization of an exposed workforce may be different from those needed to prevent pulmonary sensitivity.

A comparable approach can be used in the risk assessment process for LMW chemicals. Once a chemical has been identified as an allergen via the hazard identification process, further evaluation can be performed in the guinea pig inhalation model. A benchmark chemical allergen, such as TMA or TDI, can be used in the guinea pig inhalation model for comparative purposes. The ACGIH has established TLVs for both chemicals, which appear to protect humans from sensitization. Cross-sectional and longitudinal human epidemiologic data exist for both chemicals. Therefore, by comparing dose–response data for a new chemical to that gener-

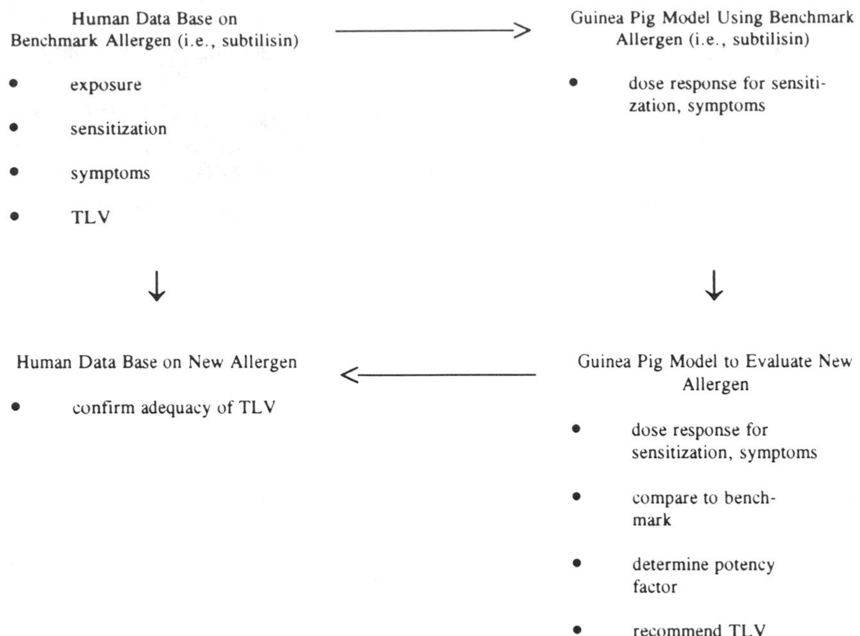

FIG. 3. Representation of how human and animal model data can be used to establish exposure guidelines for new occupational allergens.

ated by TMA or TDI, one can estimate the allergenic potency of the new chemical relative to the standard chemical allergen. In this manner, exposure guidelines and controls can be recommended to protect the workforce from sensitization to new allergenic chemicals.

REFERENCES

1. Chan-Yeung, M. Occupational asthma. *Chest* 1990;98:148s–161s.
2. Juniper CP, How MJ, Goodwin BFJ, Kinshott AK. *Bacillus subtilis* enzymes: a seven year clinical, epidemiological and immunological study of an industrial allergen. *J Soc Occup Med* 1977;27:3–12.
3. Flood DFS, Blofeld RE, Bruce CF, Hewitt JI, Juniper CP, Roberts DM. Lung function, atopy, specific hypersensitivity and smoking of workers in the enzyme detergent industry over 11 years. *Br J Ind Med* 1985;42:43–50.
4. Karol MH. Survey of industrial workers for antibodies to toluene diisocyanate. *J Occup Med* 1981; 23:741–747.
5. Butcher BT, Jones RN, O'Neil CE, et al. Longitudinal study of workers employed in the manufacture of toluene diisocyanate. *Am Rev Respir Dis* 1977;116:411–421.
6. Venables KM, Dally MB, Burge PS, Pickering CAC, Newman-Taylor AJ. Occupational asthma in a steel coating plant. *Br J Ind Med* 1985;42:517–524.
7. Paupe J. *L'allergie*. Paris: Presses Universitaire de France; 1984.
8. Ratner B, Jackson HC, Gruehl HL. Respiratory anaphylaxis: sensitization, shock, bronchial asthma

and death induced in the guinea pig by nasal inhalation of dry horse dander. *Am J Dis Child* 1927; 34:23–52.

9. Griffith-Johnson DA, Jin R, Karol MH. The role of purified IgG_1 in pulmonary hypersensitivity responses of the guinea pig. *J Toxicol Environ Health* 1993;40:117–127.
10. Griffith-Johnson DA, Karol MH. Validation of a non-invasive technique to assess development of airway hyperreactivity in animal model of immunologic pulmonary hypersensitivity. *Toxicology* 1991;65:283–294.
11. Karol MH, Stadler J, Underhill D, Alarie Y. Monitoring delayed onset pulmonary hypersensitivity in guinea pigs. *Toxical Appl Pharmacol* 1981;61:277–285.
12. Karol MH. Concentration-dependent immunologic response to toluene diisocyanate following inhalation exposure. *Toxicol Appl Pharmacol* 1983;68:229–241.
13. Ritz HL, Evans BLB, Bruce RD, Fletcher ER, Fisher GL, Sarlo K. Respiratory and immunological responses of guinea pigs to enzyme containing detergents: a comparison of intratracheal and inhalation modes of exposure. *Fund Appl Toxicol* 1993;21:31–37.
14. Pauluhn J, Eben A. Validation of a non-invasive technique to assess immediate or delayed onset airway hypersensitivity in guinea pigs. *J Appl Toxicol* 1991;11:423–431.
15. Thorne PS, Karol MH. Association of fever with late onset pulmonary hypersensitivity responses in the guinea pig. *Toxicol Appl Pharmacol* 1989;100:247–258.
16. Karol MH, Stadler J, Magreni C. Immunotoxicologic evaluation of the respiratory system: animal models for immediate and delayed onset pulmonary hypersensitivity. *Fundam Appl Toxicol* 1985; 5:459–472.
17. Thorne PT, Hillebrand J, Magreni C, Riley EJ, Karol MH. Experimental sensitization to subtilisin. I. Production of immediate and late onset pulmonary reactions. *Toxicol Appl Pharmacol* 1986; 86:112–123.
18. Hillebrand J, Thorne PT, Karol MH. Experimental sensitization to subtilisin. II. Production of specific antibodies following inhalation exposure of guinea pigs. *Toxicol Appl Pharmacol* 1987; 89:449–456.
19. Threshold limit values and biological exposure indices. *Am Conf Govt Ind Hyg Inc* 1990;38.
20. Sarlo K, Polk JE, Ritz HL. Guinea pig intratracheal test to assess respiratory allergenicity of detergent enzymes; comparison with the human data base. *J Allergy Clin Immunol* 1991;87:816a.
21. Karol MH, Thorne PS. Pulmonary hypersensitivity and hyperreactivity: implications for assessing allergic responses. In: Gardner DE, Crapo JD, Massaro EJ, eds. *Toxicology of the lung*. New York: Raven Press; 1988:427–448.
22. Botham PA, Hext PM, Rattray NJ, Walsh ST, Woodcock DR. Sensitization of guinea pigs by inhalation exposure to low molecular weight chemicals. *Toxicol Lett* 1988;41:159–173.
23. Sarlo K, Clark ED. A tier approach for evaluating the respiratory allergenicity of low molecular weight chemicals. *Fundam Appl Toxicol* 1992;18:107–114.
24. Sarlo K, Clark ED, Ferguson J, Zeiss CR, Hatoum N. Industion of type I hypersensitivity in guinea pigs following inhalation to phthalic anhydride. *J All Clin Immunol (in press)*.
25. Beasley R, Roche WR, Roberts JA, Holgate ST. Cellular events in the bronchi in mild asthma and after bronchial provocation. *Am Rev Respir Dis* 1989;139:806–817.
26. Saetta M, DiStefano A, Maestrelli P, et al. Airway mucosal inflammation in occupational asthma induced by toluene diisocyanate. *Am Rev Respir Dis* 1992;145:160–168.
27. Karol MH, Hillebrand JA, Thorne PS. Characteristics of weekly pulmonary responses elicited in the guinea pig by inhalation of ovalbumin aerosols. *Toxicol Appl Pharmacol* 1989;100:234–246.
28. Botham PA, Rattray NJ, Woodcock DR, Walsh ST, Hext PM. The induction of respiratory allergy in guinea pigs following intradermal injection of TMA: a comparison with the response to DNCB. *Toxicol Lett* 1989;47:25–39.
29. Karol MH, Hauth BA, Riley EJ, Magreni CM. Dermal contact with TDI produces respiratory tract hypersensitivity in guinea pigs. *Toxicol Appl Pharmacol* 1981;58:221–230.
30. Threshold limit values and biological exposure indices. *Am Conf Govt Ind Hyg Inc* 1990;41.
31. Agius RM, Nee J, McGovern B, Robertson A. Structure activity hypothesis in occupational asthma caused by low molecular weight substances. *Ann Occup Hyg* 1991;35:129–137.
32. Wass U, Belin L. An in vitro method for predicting sensitizing properties of inhaled chemicals. *Scand J Work Environ Health* 1990;16:208–214.
33. Gauggel DL, Sarlo K, Asquith TN. A proposed screen for evaluating low molecular weight chemicals as respiratory allergens. *J Appl Toxicol* 1993;13:307–313.

34. Docker A, Wattie JM, Topping MD, et al. Clinical and immunological investigations of respiratory disease in workers using reactive dyes. *Br J Ind Med* 1987;44:534–541.
35. Cohrssen JJ, Covello VT. *Risk analysis: a guide to principles and methods for analyzing health and environmental risks*. Springfield, IL: US Council for Environmental Quality; 1989.
36. British Medical Association. Biological effects of proteolytic enzyme detergents. *Thorax* 1976; 31:621–634.
37. Sarlo K, Clark ED, Ryan CA, Bernstein DI. ELISA for human IgE antibody to subtilisin A (Alcalase): correlation with RAST and skin test results with occupationally exposed individuals. *J Allergy Clin Immunol* 1990;86:393–399.

Immunotoxicology and Immunopharmacology, Second Edition, edited by J. H. Dean, M. I. Luster, A. E. Munson, and I. Kimber.
Raven Press, Ltd., New York © 1994.

42

Assessment of Contact and Respiratory Sensitivity in Mice

Ian Kimber and Rebecca J. Dearman

Immunology Group, Research Toxicology Section, ZENECA Central Toxicology Laboratory, Alderley Park, Macclesfield, Cheshire SK10 4TJ, United Kingdom

Allergy may take a variety of forms, those of greatest significance with respect to predictive toxicology and on which this chapter focuses being contact sensitivity (allergic contact dermatitis) and respiratory hypersensitivity. Allergy may be defined operationally as the adverse health effects that result from specific immune responses and, in the context of this chapter, immune responses to chemicals. The induction and expression of chemical allergy are clearly dependent on a variety of host factors, including genetic predisposition, environmental conditions, and health status, which together determine individual susceptibility. In practice, only a proportion, and frequently only a small proportion, of the exposed population will exhibit the symptoms of allergic disease.

Consideration of predisposing factors and the relative susceptibility of individuals is of course central to the accurate assessment of risk. The other key element in the risk assessment equation is identification of hazard and evaluation of the intrinsic ability of chemicals to provoke allergic responses. It is upon hazard identification that this chapter concentrates. As described elsewhere in this volume, the measurement of chemical sensitization potential has historically relied on the use of guinea pig predictive test methods. For a variety of reasons, however, there has in recent years been a growing interest in the use of the mouse for sensitization testing. Methods for the assessment of contact and respiratory sensitivity in this species are described in what follows.

CONTACT HYPERSENSITIVITY

The phenomenon of contact sensitization to low molecular weight (LMW) chemicals was first investigated rigorously using guinea pigs (1–3) and the first method designed specifically for sensitization testing was described in this species (4). Since then, a variety of tests have been described, all of which share certain common features (5,6). Guinea pigs are exposed by various routes and under various conditions to chemical. Subsequently, test and control animals are challenged with a subirritant concentration of the same material. Activity is measured usually by visual assessment of erythematous reactions, which develop at the challenge site over a period of 24 to 48 hr. Such methods, the most widely applied of which are the guinea pig maximization test described by Magnusson and Kligman (7,8) and the occluded patch test of Buehler (9,10), have served and will continue to serve toxicologists well. However, there is no doubt that guinea pig tests have certain limitations, not least of which is the fact that assessment of challenge-induced inflammatory reactions is commonly subjective and may pose interpretative difficulties when colored or irritant chemicals are evaluated (5,6,11). The desire and ability to consider alternative approaches to the measurement of skin sensitization potential have paralleled an increased understanding of the immunobiologic mechanisms that initiate and regulate the development of contact sensitivity. Much of this progress has derived from studies in the mouse and during recent years a number of novel methods have been described in this species (11,12).

The use of the mouse for studies of contact sensitization was facilitated by an increasingly sophisticated ability to dissect and characterize immune responses in this species and was heralded by the description of a method for the quantitative evaluation of contact hypersensitivity reactions following challenge of previously sensitized mice. Asherson and Ptak (13) demonstrated that contact reactions in mice could be measured as a function of challenge-induced increases in ear thickness. A number of novel predictive test methods based on this and related phenomena have now been proposed (11,12,14–17).

Mouse Ear Swelling Test and Related Assays

In 1986, Gad and colleagues (18,19) described the development and validation of a mouse ear swelling test (MEST). The method used a rigorous sensitization protocol requiring an intradermal injection of Freund's complete adjuvant followed by the daily topical application of the test chemical, for 4 consecutive days, to tape-stripped abdominal skin. Ten days following the initiation of sensitization, test and control (vehicle-treated) mice were challenged on one ear with the test compound and on the contralateral ear with the relevant vehicle alone. Ear thickness was measured 24 and 48 hr later and reactivity was recorded as a function of both the degree of specific ear swelling and the percentage of test animals displaying a positive response (18). On the basis of studies performed with 72 materials, it was argued that the MEST was of equivalent sensitivity to the guinea pig maximization test (GPMT) (18). However, despite the stringent sensitization regime employed, responses recorded with some chemical allergens were relatively weak and subsequent investigations have questioned the sensitivity of the MEST (20,21). A similar method, the mouse ear sensitization assay, which likewise requires the use of Freund's complete adjuvant, has been proposed by Descotes (22).

More recently, a modified procedure, the noninvasive mouse ear swelling assay (MESA), has been described by Thorne et al. (23,24). An important feature of this method is that animals are fed on diets supplemented with vitamin A acetate (VAA). The ability of mice maintained on diets enriched with VAA to exhibit enhanced contact hypersensitivity responses and the value of such animals in the identification of skin sensitizers as a function of challenged-induced increases in ear thickness have been reported previously by Miller and colleagues (25–28). The influence of VAA on delayed-type hypersensitivity is undoubtedly a consequence of augmented cell-mediated immune function (29,30). It has been claimed that the MESA provides a level of sensitivity comparable with many standard guinea pig tests (23,24) and the assay offers the added attraction of not requiring the use of adjuvant.

Challenge-induced reactions in the ears of previously sensitized mice can be measured also by analysis of the arrival into inflammatory sites of serum proteins or mononuclear cells. Cell localization has been measured both by the systemic injection of radiolabeled nucleic acid precursors (20,31,32) and by the injection of lymphoid cells labeled previously with ^{51}Cr (33). Alternatively, the quantitative evaluation of contact hypersensitivity reactions has been performed by measurement of [^{125}I]fibrin deposition (34). An alternative approach to measurement of elicitation reactions in mice is the flow cytometric analysis of cells infiltrating the challenge site. It has been found that local challenge of previously sensitized mice is associated with increased numbers of both CD4+ and CD8+ T lymphocytes in the inflamed tissue (35,36).

Operationally, it is possible to define contact sensitization as being the immunologic status required for a specific chemical to provoke a cutaneous inflammatory reaction at concentrations below those necessary to elicit a clinically similar reaction in a nonsensitized host. Consequently, the systemic changes resulting from local elicitation reactions can be exploited to measure contact hypersensitivity responses.

Systemic Responses

It has been found that local challenge of previously sensitized mice with subinflammatory concentrations of the inducing allergen causes an increase in serum levels of the acute-phase proteins haptoglobin and serum amyloid A (SAA). Challenge of sensitized animals with vehicle alone or challenge of nonsensitized animals with concentrations of the chemical allergen capable of eliciting responses in contact sensitized mice failed to provoke similar acute-phase responses (37). A correlation between serum concentrations of acute-phase proteins and challenge-induced increases in ear thickness was reported, the implication being that the serologic evaluation of acute-phase responses might provide an alternative or adjunct to conventional methods for measuring contact hypersensitivity reactions (37). It is now appreciated that an important molecular signal for the induction of acute-phase protein synthesis by hepatocytes during inflammatory responses is interleukin-6 (IL-6) (38). Perhaps not unexpectedly, plasma concentrations of this cytokine have been found to increase, in tempo with ear swelling responses, following challenge of sensitized mice (39).

Associated also with contact hypersensitivity reactions is an increase in the concentration of histamine found in serum. It has been suggested that the local release of vasoactive amines constitutes a mandatory first step in the development of contact allergic reactions (40). Although this issue remains unresolved, there is no doubt that the local inflammation induced following challenge of sensitized animals will be accompanied by the release of mediators such as histamine derived from mast cells. Studies in mice have revealed a dose- and time-dependent increase in serum histamine levels following challenge (41).

Taken together, the evidence summarized above suggests that serologic markers of acute inflammatory reactions may be used to measure quantitatively elicitation reactions in mice and presumably in other species.

All the approaches discussed thus far rely on analysis of the elicitation phase of contact allergy. An alternative strategy, the murine local lymph node assay, exploits instead events that characterize the induction phase of sensitization following first exposure to the chemical.

Local Lymph Node Assay

The induction of skin sensitization is associated with, and dependent on, immune activation of the lymph nodes draining the site of exposure (42–44). The theoretical basis of the local lymph node assay is that contact sensitization potential is measured as a function of the degree of activation provoked in the regional lymph nodes following topical application of the test chemical. Antigen-induced lymph node activation is characterized by an increase in node weight, the appearance of activated lymphocytes (pyroninophilic cells), and the stimulation of replicative deoxyribonucleic acid (DNA) synthesis by lymph node cells (LNCs). In preliminary investigations, each of these parameters was measured in draining (auricular) lymph nodes following repeated application of the test chemical to the ears of mice. Lymphocyte proliferative responses were evaluated *in vitro* following culture of LNCs in the presence or absence of an exogenous source of the T cell growth factor IL-2 (45–46). These analyses revealed that, of the measurements made, LNC hyperplasia represented the most sensitive and reliable correlate of lymph node activation. In subsequent studies, in an attempt to obviate the requirement for tissue culture and to simplify the procedure in the context of routine toxicity testing, LNC proliferative responses were measured *in situ* following the intravenous injection of [^{3}H]thymidine (47,48). Reactivity is measured as an index of isotope incorporation into the draining nodes of test animals relative to values obtained with vehicle-treated controls. The local lymph node assay has now been compared extensively with guinea pig predictive test methods (49–54) and has been the subject of interlaboratory validation studies (53–56). Currently, the recommended protocol requires the use of CBA/Ca strain mice, which receive three consecutive daily applications of various concentrations of the test chemical to the dorsum of both ears. Five days following the initiation of treatment, test and control (vehicle-treated) mice receive an intravenous injection of [^{3}H]thymidine. Animals are sacrificed 5 hr later, the draining auricular lymph nodes are excised and pooled, and a single cell suspension of LNCs is prepared and processed for β-scintillation counting. Chemicals are classified as "sensitizers" or "not strong sensitizers"; the criterion for a positive response being a threefold or greater increase in isotope incorporation compared with vehicle control values (56). Experience to date indicates that the local lymph node assay provides a rapid, cost-effective, and accurate method for the identification of chemicals considered to possess moderate or greater skin-sensitizing potential. The assay is able to detect also many materials that, on the basis of guinea pig test procedures, possess only weak sensitizing activity. Compared with guinea pig methods, the local lymph node assay offers a number of significant advantages, not least of which is the fact that the endpoint of the test is objective and quantitative. Moreover, activity in the local lymph node assay is unaffected by the color of the test material and skin irritants cause either no, or only comparatively modest, effects and do not compromise interpretation (56). Many of these advantages are, of course, shared by the more sensitive ear swelling tests, particularly the MESA and MEST, described earlier.

A particular attraction of the local lymph node assay is that LNC proliferative responses not only provide an indicator of sensitizing activity but also correlate with the extent to which sensitization will occur. There is evidence available that indicates that the efficiency of sensitization and the severity of contact allergic reactions induced following challenge are determined by the vigor of lymphocyte proliferative responses in lymph nodes draining the site of first exposure (57,58). These data confirm that LNC proliferation is a relevant marker of sensitizing activity and suggest that measurement of proliferative activity may permit direct comparative evaluation of contact sensitizing potential. For such comparative studies it may be appropriate to measure sensitization not as proliferative activity at a defined period following exposure, as is the current practice, but rather as the concentration of test material required to provoke a positive local lymph node assay response. This approach has already been used to some effect in assessing the relative potential of a variety of biocides to cause contact sensitization (59).

In recent years modifications to, and new applications of, the local lymph node assay have been proposed, including a potentially important contribution to the analysis of structure–activity relationships in contact sensitivity (60–65).

Progress with the local lymph node assay and the MEST has begun to impact on the regulatory environment. A new Organisation for Economic Cooperation and Development (OECD) test guideline published in 1992 (66) recognized as a significant advance on both ethical and scientific fronts the development and validation of these methods. This new guideline states that either the local lymph node assay or the MEST can now be employed as a first stage in the assessment of contact sensitization potential. "If a positive result is seen in either assay, a test substance may be designated a potential sensitizer, and it may not be necessary to conduct a further guinea pig test. However, if a negative result is seen, a guinea pig test must be conducted" (66).

Other Sensitization Phenomena

The activation of T lymphocytes during the induction phase of contact sensitization and the resultant clonal expansion of allergen-reactive cells can be exploited to investigate responses to skin-sensitizing chemicals *in vitro*. Lymphocyte blastogenesis assays have been described in which cells isolated from the lymph nodes of previously sensitized mice are cultured in the presence of the inducing allergen and an appropriate source of antigen-presenting cells (67–70). Under suitable conditions, LNCs from sensitized mice, but not from control animals, will mount a secondary proliferative response *in vitro*. Such assays provide a method of confirming immunologic sensitization and of investigating cross-reactivity between chemical allergens.

The initiation of lymph node activation during the induction phase of contact sensitization is dependent on the arrival in the nodes of sufficient allergen in an appropriate form. There is compelling evidence that epidermal Langerhans' cells play a pivotal role in this process. Following exposure to sensitizing chemicals, Langerhans' cells, a significant proportion of which bear antigen, are induced to migrate from the skin, via the afferent lymphatics, to the draining nodes. While in transit to the lymph nodes, Langerhans' cells are subject to phenotypic and functional maturation and assume the characteristics of immunostimulatory dendritic cells (reviewed in ref. 71). It has been proposed previously that the arrival of dendritic cells in the draining lymph nodes may provide a potentially useful biologic marker of skin-sensitizing activity (11). While the number of dendritic cells that arrive in draining lymph nodes does appear to correlate with the vigor of the induced LNC proliferative response (72), the complexity of techniques required for the accurate enumeration of lymph node dendritic cells prohibits the use of such measurements in the context of routine toxicity testing. Furthermore, it is apparent that cutaneous trauma, other than that resulting from local exposure to chemical allergens, can induce Langerhans' cell migration from the epidermis and the accumulation of dendritic cells in draining lymph nodes. Both irradiation with ultraviolet B (UVB) light and topical application of skin irritants have been shown to provoke the arrival in draining nodes of dendritic cells (73,74).

Finally, as a consequence of the arrival in draining lymph nodes of antigen-bearing dendritic cells and the subsequent stimulation of T lymphocyte activation, cytokines will be produced and released. It has been shown that activated draining lymph node cells elaborate a variety of cytokines including IL-1, IL-2, IL-3, and IL-6, granulocyte–macrophage colony-stimulating factor (GM-CSF), and interferon-γ (IFN-γ) (70,75–77). Recently, we have been interested particularly in the production by activated LNCs of IL-6 and have explored whether measurement of this cytokine in the supernatants of draining LNCs might provide an alternative endpoint for the local lymph node assay. Studies to date indicate that chemicals with a moderate or greater potential to induce contact sensitization stimulate the production of detectable levels of IL-6, while nonsensitizing chemicals, including nonsensitizing skin irritants, do not (78). A molecular, rather than cellular, read-out for the local lymph node assay would provide several potential benefits including the possibility of batch analysis and more exacting interlaboratory studies. Investigation of IL-6 production by draining LNCs is continuing.

RESPIRATORY HYPERSENSITIVITY

A variety of chemicals has been implicated as causing occupational respiratory hypersensitivity, frequently, but not invariably, associated with the presence of specific immunoglobulin E (IgE) antibody (79–81). Unlike the situation that pertains to contact hypersensitivity, there are no widely accepted methods available for the prospective identification of chemical respiratory allergens. Progress toward the development of appropriate model systems has derived almost entirely from studies in the guinea pig and, in particular, from the analysis of inhalation or intratracheal challenge-induced changes in respiratory function of previously sensitized animals (82–85). There has been only a single systematic attempt to measure respiratory sensitization potential in mice. This method, the mouse IgE test (86,87), is based on the assumption that chemicals capable of causing respiratory hypersensitivity will induce the quality of immune response necessary for the stimulation of IgE antibody production. In comparative experiments, the nature of immune responses provoked in mice by a series of chemical allergens was investigated. It was found that topical exposure of mice to known chemical respiratory allergens induced responses characteristic of the selective activation of T helper (T_H2) cells (87–91). Such cells represent a discrete functional subpopulation of T_H lymphocytes, which, when activated, produce IL-4, a cytokine necessary for the synthesis of IgE antibody (92,93). Conversely, contact allergens known or suspected not to cause respiratory hypersensitivity induced instead responses consistent with T_H1 cell activation (87–91). A product of T_H1 cells, IFN-γ, inhibits IgE antibody responses (92,93). A key observation was that, presumably as a consequence of the preferential stimulation of T_H2 cell-type responses and IL-4 production, topical exposure only to chemical respiratory allergens caused in mice an increase in the serum concentration of IgE. No such changes in IgE concentration were observed as a result of exposure to chemical allergens considered not to cause respiratory hypersensitivity (86). The mouse IgE test therefore seeks to identify chemicals with the potential to cause respiratory hypersensitivity as a function of induced increases in the serum concentration of this immunoglobulin. The practice currently is to measure changes in serum IgE levels 14 days following the initiation of exposure. The exposure regime is straightforward and noninvasive. Mice receive two topical applications of the test material, the second exposure being 1 week following the first (86).

Clearly, there is some way to go in defining the sensitivity, selectivity, and potential utility of this method and presently both internal and interlaboratory validation studies are planned or in progress.

CONCLUDING COMMENTS

Significant advances have been made in characterizing the nature of immune responses induced in mice by chemical allergens. In parallel, new approaches to the identification and classification of chemical sensitizers have emerged. It is arguable that all chemical allergens have some potential to cause contact hypersensitivity, at least in animal models. The implication is that accurate predictive tests for contact sensitization will necessarily identify also chemical respiratory allergens. If such is true, then it is reasonable to begin to consider a structured approach to allergy testing in which the first step is evaluation of skin-sensitizing activity. Chemicals that prove positive in such assays could then be classified as being allergenic and as having the potential to cause contact hypersensitivity. Further definition, and evaluation of respiratory sensitizing activity, would require additional analysis, including possibly use of the mouse IgE test. The judicious use of such an approach would permit not only the identification of chemical allergens but also prediction of the type or types of allergic reaction they are likely to elicit.

A more thorough understanding of the important immunobiologic events that occur during the development of sensitization and that influence the severity of allergic reactions has already permitted progress toward hazard assessment. Definition of relative potency based on relevant dose–response relationships should provide a sound basis for accurate risk assessment.

REFERENCES

1. Polak L. *Immunological aspects of contact sensitivity. An experimental study. Monographs in allergy*, vol 15. Basel: Karger;1980.
2. Landsteiner K, Jacobs JL. Studies on the sensitization of animals with chemical compounds. *J Exp Med* 1935;61:643–646.
3. Landsteiner K, Chase MW. Experiments on transfer of cutaneous sensitivity to simple compounds. *Proc Soc Exp Biol Med* 1942;49:688–690.
4. Draize JH, Woodward G, Calvery HO. Methods for the study of irritation and toxicity of substances applied topically to the skin and mucous membranes. *J Pharmacol Exp Ther* 1944;82:377–390.
5. Andersen KE, Maibach HI. Guinea pig sensitization assays. An overview. In: Andersen KE, Maibach HI, eds. *Contact allergy predictive tests in guinea pigs. Current problems in dermatology*, vol 14. Basel: Karger; 1985:263–290.
6. Oliver GJA, Botham PA, Kimber I. Models for contact sensitization—novel approaches and future developments. *Br J Dermatol* 1986;115:53–62.
7. Magnusson B, Kligman AM. The identification of contact allergens by animal assay, the guinea pig maximization test method. *J Invest Dermatol* 1969;52:268–276.
8. Magnusson B, Klingman AM. *Allergic contact dermatitis in the guinea pig*. Springfield, IL: CC Thomas; 1970.
9. Buehler EV. Delayed contact hypersensitivity in the guinea pig. *Arch Dermatol* 1965;91:171–177.

10. Ritz HL, Buehler EV. Planning, conduct and interpretation of guinea pig sensitization patch tests. In: Drill VA, Lazar P, eds. *Current concepts in cutaneous toxicity*. New York: Academic Press; 1980:25–40.
11. Kimber I. Aspects of the immune response to contact allergens: opportunities for the development and modification of predictive test methods. *Food Chem Toxicol* 1989;27:755–762.
12. Kimber I. Contact sensitivity. In: Miller K, Turk J, Nicklin S, eds. *Principles and practice of immunotoxicology*. Oxford: Blackwell Scientific Publications; 1992:104–124.
13. Asherson GL, Ptak W. Contact and delayed hypersensitivity in the mouse. I. Active sensitization and passive transfer. *Immunology* 1968;15:405–416.
14. Botham PA, Basketter DA, Maurer T, Mueller D, Potokar M, Bontinck WJ. Skin sensitization—a critical review of predictive test methods in animals and man. *Food Chem Toxicol* 1991;29:275–286.
15. Botham PA. Classification of chemicals as sensitizers based on new test methods. *Toxicol Lett* 1992;64/65:165–171.
16. Botham PA. Animal models for predicting hypersensitivity reactions to small molecules. In: Dayan AD, Hertel RF, Heseltine E, Kazantzis G, Smith EM, Van der Venne MT, eds. *Immunotoxicity of metals and immunotoxicology*. New York: Plenum Press; 1990:75–82.
17. Kimber I, Dearman RJ. Approaches to the identification and classification of chemical allergens in mice. *J Pharmacol Toxicol Methods* 1993;29:11–16.
18. Gad SC, Dunn BJ, Dobbs DW, Reilly C, Walsh RD. Development and validation of an alternative dermal sensitization test: the mouse ear swelling test (MEST). *Toxicol Appl Pharmacol* 1986;84:93–114.
19. Gad SC. A scheme for the prediction and ranking of relative potencies of dermal sensitizers based on data from several systems. *J Appl Toxicol* 1988;8:361–368.
20. Cornacoff JB, House RV, Dean JH. Comparison of a radioisotopic method and the mouse ear swelling test (MEST) for contact sensitivity to weak sensitizers. *Fundam Appl Toxicol* 1988;10:40–44.
21. Dunn BJ, Rusch GM, Siglin JC, Blaszcak DL. Variability of a mouse ear swelling test (MEST) in predicting weak and moderate contact sensitization. *Fundam Appl Toxicol* 1990;15:242–248.
22. Descotes J. Identification of contact allergens: the mouse ear sensitization assay. *J Toxicol Cutan Ocular Toxicol* 1988;74:263–272.
23. Thorne PS, Hawk C, Kaliszewski SD, Guiney PD. The noninvasive mouse ear swelling assay. I. Refinements for detecting weak contact sensitizers. *Fundam Appl Toxicol* 1991;17:790–806.
24. Thorne PS, Hawk C, Kaliszewski SD, Guiney PD. The noninvasive mouse ear swelling assay. II. Testing the contact sensitizing potency of fragrances. *Fundam Appl Toxicol* 1991;17:807–820.
25. Miller K, Maisey J, Malkovsky M. Enhancement of contact sensitization in mice fed a diet enriched in vitamin A acetate. *Int Arch Allergy Appl Immunol* 1984;75:120–125.
26. Katz DR, Mukherjee S, Maisey J, Miller K. Vitamin A acetate as a regulator of accessory cell function in delayed-type hypersensitivity responses. *Int Arch Allergy Appl Immunol* 1987;82:53–56.
27. Maisey J, Miller K. Assessment of the ability of mice fed on vitamin A supplemented diet to respond to a variety of contact sensitizers. *Contact Dermatitis* 1986;15:17–23.
28. Maisey J, Purchase R, Robbins MC, Miller K. Evaluation of the sensitizing potential of 4 polyamines present in technical triethylenetetramine using 2 animal species. *Contact Dermatitis* 1988; 18:133–137.
29. Malkovsky M, Dore C, Hunt R, Palmer L, Chandler P, Medawar PB. Enhancement of specific antitumor immunity in mice fed a diet enriched in vitamin A acetate. *Proc Natl Acad Sci USA* 1983; 80:6322–6326.
30. Malkovsky M, Edwards AJ, Hunt R, Palmer L, Medawar PB. T cell-mediated enhancement of host-versus-graft reactivity in mice fed a diet enriched in vitamin A acetate. *Nature* 1983;302:338–340.
31. Eipert EF, Miller HC. Contact sensitivity in mice measured with thymidine labelled lymphocytes. *Immunol Comm* 1975;4:361–372.
32. Vadas MA, Miller JFAP, Gamble J, Whitelaw A. A radioisotopic method to measure delayed type hypersensitivity in the mouse. I. Studies in sensitized and normal mice. *Int Arch Allergy Appl Immunol* 1975;49:670–692.
33. Sabbadini E, Neri A, Sehon AH. Localization of non-immune radioactively labelled cells in the lesions of contact sensitivity in mice. *J Immunol Methods* 1974;5:9–19.
34. Mekori YA, Dvorak HF, Galli S.J. ^{125}I-Fibrin deposition in contact sensitivity reactions in the mouse. Sensitivity of the assay for quantitating reactions after active or passive sensitization. *J Immunol* 1986;136:2018–2025.

35. Stern ML, Munson AE. L3T4$^+$ and Lyt-2$^+$ cell surface antigens as indicators of an allergic contact hypersensitivity response. *Arch Dermatol Res* 1990;281:1–5.
36. Stern ML, Brown TA, Munson AE. Lymphocyte cell surface markers as indicators of an allergic contact hypersensitivity response. *Toxicologist* 1990;222:886(abst).
37. Kimber I, Ward RK, Shepherd CJ, Smith MN, McAdam KPWJ, Raynes JG. Acute-phase proteins and the serological evaluation of experimental contact sensitivity in the mouse. *Int Arch Allergy Appl Immunol* 1989;89:149–155.
38. Castell JV, Gomez-Lechon MJ, David M, et al. Interleukin 6 is the major regulator of acute phase protein synthesis in adult human hepatocytes. *FEBS Lett* 1989;242:237–239.
39. Kimber I, Cumberbatch M, Humphreys M, Hopkins SJ. Contact hypersensitivity induces plasma interleukin 6. *Int Arch Allergy Appl Immunol* 1990;92:97–99.
40. Van Loveren H, Meade R, Askenase PW. An early component of delayed-type hypersensitivity mediated by T-cells and mast cells. *J Exp Med* 1983;157:1604–1617.
41. Kimber I, Cumberbatch M, Coleman JW. Serum histamine and the elicitation of murine contact sensitivity. *J Appl Toxicol* 1991;11:339–342.
42. Oort J, Turk JL. A histological and autoradiographic study of lymph nodes during the development of contact sensitivity in guinea pigs. *Br J Exp Pathol* 1965;46:147–154.
43. Turk JL. Cytology of the induction of hypersensitivity. *Br Med Bull* 1967;23:3–8.
44. Parrott DMV, de Sousa MAB. Changes in the thymus-dependent areas of lymph nodes after immunological stimulation. *Nature* 1966;212:1316–1317.
45. Kimber I, Mitchell JA, Griffin AC. Development of a murine local lymph node assay for the determination of sensitizing potential. *Food Chem Toxicol* 1986;24:585–586.
46. Kimber I, Weisenberger C. A murine local lymph node assay for the identification of contact allergens. Assay development and results of an initial validation study. *Arch Toxicol* 1989;63:274–282.
47. Kimber I, Hilton J, Weisenberger C. The murine local lymph node assay for identification of contact allergens: a preliminary evaluation of in situ measurement of lymphocyte proliferation. *Contact Dermatitis* 1989;21:215–220.
48. Kimber I, Weisenberger C. A modified local lymph node assay for identification of contact allergens. In: Frosch PJ, Dooms-Goossens A, Lachapelle J-M, Rycroft RJG, Scheper RJ, eds. *Current topics in contact dermatitis*. Heidelberg: Springer-Verlag; 1989:592–595.
49. Kimber I, Hilton J, Botham PA. Identification of contact allergens using the murine local lymph node assay: comparisons with the Buehler occluded patch test in guinea pigs. *J Appl Toxicol* 1990; 10:173–180.
50. Basketter DA, Scholes EW. Comparison of the local lymph node assay with the guinea-pig maximization test for the detection of a range of contact allergens. *Food Chem Toxicol* 1992;30:65–69.
51. Basketter DA, Scholes EW, Cumberbatch M, Evans CD, Kimber I. Sulphanilic acid: divergent results in the guinea pig maximization test and the local lymph node assay. *Contact Dermatitis* 1992;27:209–213.
52. Basketter DA, Selbie E, Scholes EW, Lees D, Kimber I, Botham PA. Results with OECD recommended positive control sensitizers in the maximization, Buehler and local lymph node assays. *Food Chem Toxicol* 1993;31:63–67.
53. Kimber I, Hilton J, Botham PA, et al. The murine local lymph node assay: results of an interlaboratory trial. *Toxicol Lett* 1991;55:203–213.
54. Basketter DA, Scholes EW, Kimber I, et al. Interlaboratory evaluation of the local lymph node assay with 25 chemicals and comparison with guinea pig test data. *Toxicol Methods* 1991;1:30–43.
55. Scholes EW, Basketter DA, Sarll AE, et al. The local lymph node assay: results of a final interlaboratory validation under field conditions. *J Appl Toxicol* 1992;12:217–222.
56. Kimber I, Basketter DA. The murine local lymph node assay: a commentary on collaborative studies and new directions. *Food Chem Toxicol* 1992;30:165–169.
57. Kimber I, Shepherd CJ, Mitchell JA, Turk JL, Baker D. Regulation of lymphocyte proliferation in contact sensitivity: homeostatic mechanisms and a possible explanation of antigenic competition. *Immunology* 1989;66:577–582.
58. Kimber I, Dearman RJ. Investigation of lymph node cell proliferation as a possible immunological correlate of contact sensitizing potential. *Food Chem Toxicol* 1991;29:125–129.
59. Botham PA, Hilton J, Evans CD, Lees D, Hall TJ. Assessment of the relative skin sensitizing potency of three biocides using the murine local lymph node assay. *Contact Dermatitis* 1991;25: 172–177.

60. Kimber I, Weisenberger C. Anamnestic responses to contact allergens: application in the murine local lymph node assay. *J Appl Toxicol* 1991;11:129–133.
61. Pfennig K, Ziegler V. Detection of allergens by lymph node assay. *Z Haut Kr* 1991;66:959–963.
62. Basketter DA, Roberts DW, Cronin M, Scholes EW. The value of the local lymph node assay in quantitative structure–activity investigations. *Contact Dermatitis* 1992;27:137–142.
63. Scholes EW, Basketter DA, Lovell WW, Sarll AE, Pendlington RU. The identification of photoallergic potential in the local lymph node assay. *Photodermatol Photoimmunol Photomed* 1992;8:249–254.
64. Gerberick GF, House RV, Fletcher ER, Ryan CA. Examination of the local lymph node assay for use in contact sensitization risk assessment. *Fundam Appl Toxicol* 1992;19:438–445.
65. Ikarashi Y, Tsuchiya TA, Nakamura A. Detection of contact sensitivity of metal salts using the murine local lymph node assay. *Toxicol Lett* 1992;62:53–61.
66. OECD guidelines for testing of chemicals, No 406. Adopted 12 June 1992.
67. Robinson MK. Optimization of an in vitro lymphocyte blastogenesis assay for predictive assessment of immunologic responsiveness to contact sensitizers. *J Invest Dermatol* 1989;92:860–867.
68. Robinson MK, Sneller DL. Use of an optimized lymphocyte blastogenesis assay to detect contact sensitivity to nickel sulfate in mice. *Toxicol Appl Pharmacol* 1990;104:106–116.
69. Gerberick GF, Ryan CA, Fletcher ER, Sneller DL, Robinson MK. An optimized lymphocyte blastogenesis assay for detecting the response of contact sensitized or photosensitized lymphocytes to hapten or prohapten modified antigen presenting cells. *Toxicol in Vitro* 1990;4:289–292.
70. Kimber I, Gerberick GF, Van Loveren H, House RV. Chemical allergy: molecular mechanisms and practical applications. *Fundam Appl Toxicol* 1992;19:479–483.
71. Kimber I, Cumberbatch M. Dendritic cells and cutaneous immune responses to chemical allergens. *Toxicol Appl Pharmacol* 1992;117:137–146.
72. Kimber I, Kinnaird A, Peters SW, Mitchell JA. Correlation between lymphocyte proliferative responses and dendritic cell migration to regional lymph nodes following skin painting with contact-sensitizing agents. *Int Arch Allergy Appl Immunol* 1990;93:47–53.
73. Moodycliffe AM, Kimber I, Norval M. The effect of ultraviolet B irradiation and urocanic acid isomers on dendritic cell migration. *Immunology* 1992;77:394–399.
74. Cumberbatch M, Scott RC, Basketter DA, Scholes EW, Hilton J, Dearman RJ, Kimber I. Influence of sodium lauryl sulphate on 2,4-dinitrochlorobenzene-induced lymph node activation. *Toxicology* 1993;77:181–191.
75. Marcinkiewicz J, Chain BM. Antigen-specific inhibition of IL-2 and IL-3 production in contact sensitivity to TNP. *Immunology* 1989;68:185–192.
76. Hopkins SJ, Humphreys M, Kinnaird A, Jones DA, Kimber I. Production of interleukin-1 by draining lymph node cells during the induction phase of contact sensitization in mice. *Immunology* 1990;71:493–496.
77. Marcinkiewicz J, Chain BM. Further studies on the regulation of lymphokine biosynthesis in contact sensitivity. *Cytokine* 1990;2:344–352.
78. Dearman RJ, Hope JC, Hopkins SJ, Debicki RJ, Kimber I. Interleukin 6 (IL-6) production by lymph node cells: an alternative endpoint for the murine local lymph node assay. *Toxicol Methods* 1993;3:268–278.
79. Chan-Yeung M, Lam S. Occupational asthma—state of the art. *Am Rev Respir Dis* 1986;133:686–703.
80. Salvaggio JE, Butcher BT, O'Neil CE. Occupational asthma due to chemical agents. *J Allergy Clin Immunol* 1986;78:1053–1057.
81. Karol MH. Occupational asthma and allergic reactions to inhaled compounds. In: Miller K, Turk J, Nicklin S, eds. *Principles and practice of immunotoxicology*. Oxford: Blackwell Scientific Publications; 1992:228–241.
82. Karol MH, Stadler J, Magreni C. Immunotoxicologic evaluation of the respiratory system: animal models for immediate- and delayed-onset pulmonary hypersensitivity. *Fundam Appl Toxicol* 1985;5:459–472.
83. Botham PA, Rattray NJ, Woodcock DR, Walsh ST, Hext PM. The induction of respiratory allergy in guinea-pigs following intradermal injection of trimellitic anhydride. A comparison with the response to 2,4-dinitrochlorobenzene. *Toxicol Lett* 1989;47:25–39.
84. Pauluhn J, Eben A. Validation of a non-invasive technique to assess immediate or delayed onset of airway hypersensitivity in guinea pigs. *J Appl Toxicol* 1991;11:423–431.
85. Sarlo K, Clark ED. A tier approach for evaluating the respiratory allergenicity of low molecular weight chemicals. *Fundam Appl Toxicol* 1992;18:107–114.

86. Dearman RJ, Basketter DA, Kimber I. Variable effects of chemical allergens on serum IgE concentration in mice. Preliminary evaluation of a novel approach to the identification of respiratory sensitizers. *J Appl Toxicol* 1992;12:317–323.
87. Kimber I, Dearman RJ. The mechanisms and evaluation of chemically-induced allergy. *Toxicol Lett* 1992;64/65:79–84.
88. Dearman RJ, Kimber I. Differential stimulation of immune function by respiratory and contact chemical allergens. *Immunology* 1991;72:563–570.
89. Dearman RJ, Kimber I. Divergent immune responses to respiratory and contact chemical allergens: antibody elicited by phthalic anhydride and oxazolone. *Clin Exp Allergy* 1992;22:241–250.
90. Dearman RJ, Spence LM, Kimber I. Characterization of murine immune responses to allergenic diisocyanates. *Toxicol Appl Pharmacol* 1992;112:190–197.
91. Dearman RJ, Basketter DA, Coleman JW, Kimber I. The cellular and molecular basis for divergent allergic responses to chemicals. *Chem Biol Interact* 1992;84:1–10.
92. Mosmann TR, Coffman RL. Heterogeneity of cytokine secretion patterns and functions of helper T cells. *Adv Immunol* 1989;46:111–147.
93. Mosmann TR, Schumacher JH, Street NF, et al. Diversity of cytokine synthesis and function of mouse $CD4^+$ T cells. *Immunol Rev* 1991;123:209–229.

Subject Index

Note: Page numbers in italic indicate figures; those followed by *t* indicate tables.

D

G

H

Q

R